1 MONTH OF
FREE
READING

at
www.ForgottenBooks.com

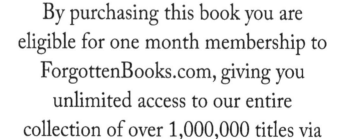

By purchasing this book you are eligible for one month membership to ForgottenBooks.com, giving you unlimited access to our entire collection of over 1,000,000 titles via our web site and mobile apps.

To claim your free month visit:

www.forgottenbooks.com/free899950

ISBN 978-0-265-85599-7
PIBN 10899950

Nothnagel's Practice

DISEASES OF THE LIVER
PANCREAS

AND

SUPRARENAL CAPSULES

BY

LEOPOLD OSER, M.D.
Professor of Internal Medicine,
University of Vienna

EDMUND NEUSSER, M.D.
Professor of Internal Medicine,
University of Vienna

HEINRICH QUINCKE, M.D.
Professor of the Practice of Medicine,
University of Kiel

G. HOPPE-SEYLER, M.D.
Professor of Internal Medicine,
University of Kiel

EDITED, WITH ADDITIONS

BY

REGINALD H. FITZ, M.D.
Hersey Professor of the Theory and Practice of Physic, Harvard University

AND

FREDERICK A. PACKARD, M.D.
Late Physician to the Pennsylvania Hospital and to the Children's Hospital, Philadelphia

AUTHORIZED TRANSLATION FROM THE GERMAN, UNDER THE
EDITORIAL SUPERVISION OF

ALFRED STENGEL, M.D.
Professor of Clinical Medicine in the University of Pennsylvania

PHILADELPHIA, NEW YORK, LONDON
W. B. SAUNDERS & COMPANY
1903

PREFACE.

THE excellence of the series of monographs issued under the editorship of Professor Nothnagel has been recognized by all who are sufficiently familiar with German to read these works, and the series has found a not inconsiderable proportion of its distribution in this and other English-speaking countries. I have so often heard regret expressed by those whose lack of familiarity with German kept these works beyond their reach, that I was glad of the opportunity to assist in the bringing out of an English edition. It was especially gratifying to find that the prominent specialists who were invited to co-operate by editing separate volumes were as interested as myself in the matter of publication of an English edition. These editors have been requested to make such additions to the original articles as seem necessary to them to bring the articles fully up to date and at the same time to adapt them thoroughly to the American or English reader. The names of the editors alone suffice to assure the profession that in the additions there will be preserved the same high standard of excellence that has been so conspicuous a feature in the original German articles.

In all cases the German author has been consulted with regard to the publication of this edition of his work, and has given specific consent. In one case only it was unfortunately necessary to substitute for the translation of the German article an entirely new one by an American author, on account of a previous arrangement of the German author to issue a translation of his article separately from this series. With this exception the Nothnagel series will be presented intact.

ALFRED STENGEL.

EDITOR'S PREFACE

TO SECTIONS ON DISEASES OF THE PANCREAS AND OF THE SUPRARENAL CAPSULES.

SINCE the publication of the original edition of this volume, the surgical importance of the consideration of diseases of the pancreas has been made especially manifest by the comprehensive treatises of Körte and of Mayo Robson.

It has been the privilege of the editor to avail himself of the writings of these authors, and especially to refer to the important contribution of Mayo Robson with regard to the etiology and treatment of chronic pancreatitis. His observations are a most significant addition to those of Opie concerning the influence of gall-stones in the etiology of acute pancreatitis.

Reference to Opie's work on this subject, and to the investigations by him, Flexner, and others on fat necrosis, will be found among the additions made by the editor.

It will be noted that the possible significance of the islands of Langerhans in the structure, function, and disease of the pancreas, made so prominent by Opie and others, did not appear till after the publication of the German edition.

It is especially agreeable to observe the familiarity of Professor Oser with the writings of English and American investigators, and to acknowledge his courtesy in recognizing their influence in renewing interest in the diseases of the pancreas.

The additions made to the section on Diseases of the Suprarenal Capsules which seem especially noteworthy are the investigations on the active principles of suprarenal extract by Abel and Crawford, v. Fürth, Takamine, and others, and the discoveries concerning the therapeutic properties of suprarenal extract.

The editor wishes to acknowledge his obligation to Dr. Elliot P. Joslin for his assistance in revising the translation, and especially for his aid in collaborating the results of the chemical, physiologic, and therapeutic researches which have been made within the past few years.

REGINALD H. FITZ.

EDITOR'S PREFACE

TO SECTION ON DISEASES OF THE LIVER.

It is my sad duty to write this preface to the section on Diseases of the Liver in place of the editor, Dr. Frederick A. Packard, whose untimely death occurred while the volume was going through the press. Those who knew him mourn the loss of a man of singularly pure and lovable character, of intense earnestness of purpose, and yet of entire simplicity; and the profession has lost in him a distinguished member, of great accomplishment and great promise. Dr. Packard's careful clinical work and his interest in the diseases of the liver marked him as the most suitable person to edit the excellent monograph of Quincke and Hoppe-Seyler, and a survey of the pages of this work will show the numerous critical additions, some of which embody contributions that appeared after the German edition, and others expressions of his own views regarding subjects under discussion. It is unnecessary to refer to the many topics which seemed to him to require amplification, but in general his practical and clinical interest will be seen to have led him to devote especial care to diagnosis and treatment, including the surgical procedures that have recently found their place in this field. With these additions the articles on diseases of the liver are brought fully up to date, and have no equal in our language.

ALFRED STENGEL.

CONTENTS.

DISEASES OF THE PANCREAS.

BY DR. L. OSER, OF VIENNA.

DISEASES OF THE SUPRARENAL CAPSULES.

BY DR. E. NEUSSER, OF VIENNA.

DISEASES OF THE LIVER.

BY DR. H. QUINCKE AND DR. G. HOPPE-SEYLER.

DISEASES OF THE PANCREAS.

BY

L. OSER, M.D.

PREFATORY NOTE.

THE pancreas, perhaps, presents a greater contrast between its physiologic importance and the lack of clinical knowledge concerning its affections than any other organ of the human body.

It is known that this is one of the most important glands concerned in metabolism, and, thanks to exact physiologic investigations, it is also known that its functions are manifold; the conclusion, therefore, is justified that pathologic disturbances of its structure are followed by grave injury to the vital functions of the body; yet the positive knowledge of the pathology of the pancreas is very slight when compared with that of the pathology of the neighboring organs, the liver, the intestines, etc.

Despite the energetic initiative of Friedreich, further investigation has progressed but slowly, although his classic treatise on diseases of the pancreas presented at the time, in the most suggestive form, the sum total of clinical knowledge on the subject, small as it was. A decided impulse, however, was given to investigators in this field by the persistent advance in surgery after Lister's imperishable work. Surgery influenced the question from two sides. It now for the first time became possible to take into consideration the solution of certain questions by means of experiments upon animals. Only on the soil prepared by Lister could v. Mering and Minkowski establish the important fact of experimental pancreatic diabetes. On the other hand, the clinicians learned no less through therapeutic surgery. Certain processes, as cysts, abscesses, necroses, tumors, and chronic inflammations, which had generally been brought to view only by anatomists, were now placed within the realm of diagnostic knowledge.

Within the past ten years interest in the pancreas has increased. A great impulse was given by American physicians, especially through the brilliant work of Fitz and Senn. The valuable and comprehensive treatises of Seitz and Nimier concerning several important subjects appeared in the same period. The surgeons Gussenbauer (1883), Senn, Ruggi, Krönlein, Biondi, Sendler, Riedel, and others, and in more recent times and in an especially prominent manner, Korte, published communications, and the noted operators of all lands made known the brilliant results of the newly created pancreatic surgery. The pioneer experiments of v. Mering and Minkowski aroused eager investigation on all sides, and pathologic anatomy was greatly enriched by the valuable work of Orth, Balser, Langerhans, Ponfick, Chiari, Tilger, Olivier, E. Fraenkel, and others, and especially by the important treatises of Dieckhoff and Hansemann. A careful table of statistics and numerous monographs on different themes appeared during this same period.

Notwithstanding this impulse, it must be admitted that we unfortunately stand at the very entrance of clinical knowledge. A correct diagnosis of a disease of the pancreas is an event almost worthy of publication. This open acknowledgment should not alarm us, but should incite to renewed investigations.

When I undertook to describe the present state of our knowledge of the disease of the pancreas, I was well aware of the great difficulties to be encountered. The reports of cases are entirely too few to enable us to use them as a basis of clinical classification. I could only combine these reports, and, therefore, was obliged to give more space to statistics than was their due as almost the only foundation of our present knowledge.

I was aware from the first that, on account of the many-sided character of the subject to be treated, nothing noteworthy could be accomplished without efficient aid. The expression of this desire brought a rich response. Prof. Zuckerkandl has had the kindness to sketch the descriptive and topographic anatomy with especial reference to the clinical point of view. Some facts have thus been brought to light which should interest the clinician as well as the surgeon.

Prof. Weichselbaum had the goodness to place at my disposal the results of the postmortem investigations at the Vienna Pathologic Institute for the last ten years. Dr. Zemann, the prosector, undertook to examine, with his usual thoroughness, the autopsies in my hospital which were appropriate for the purpose, and also contributed an interesting report on the results secured by him elsewhere. He examined also most of the microscopic preparations obtained from experiments on animals. To all these gentlemen I express my most heartfelt thanks.

Pathologic material is only sparingly at the disposal of the clinician. A substitute, although not entirely satisfactory, can be gained from experiments upon animals. Thanks to the advances of surgery, it is possible to produce different pathologic processes in the pancreas of animals, to study their course during life and the anatomic conditions after death, and to examine these at a much earlier stage than is possible in the human body.

The accomplishment of this plan was rendered possible by the co-operation of my assistant, Dr. Katz, and the support of several younger colleagues. Several important morbid processes, as abscess, hemorrhage, induration, necrosis, and fat necrosis, were produced in animals. The course during life could be watched and immediately after death anatomic preparations could be secured.

The experiments upon animals permitted the testing of the various alterations of the functions of the pancreas when partially or wholly destroyed. They were undertaken in a laboratory of the polyclinic. During 1893 and 1894 Dr. Theodore Zerner, Jr., conducted the operations, and later, with the aid of my assistant physicians in the hospital and in the polyclinic, the operations were performed by Dr. Katz, who has also carried on many laborious chemical investigations. To all these gentlemen I owe a debt of gratitude, but especially to my assistant, Dr. Katz, for his help in many different ways.

The further I advanced in my work, the more was it impressed upon me that innumerable questions were to be solved, and that it would need many energetic workers from the most varied branches of theoretic and practical medicine to raise our knowledge of the diseased pancreas approximately to the level which would correspond to its physiologic importance.

I have made it especially my task to describe the present condition of our knowledge on the subject, to point out where it was deficient, and to stimulate to new work.

Because of the variety and amount of the material to be mastered, and on account of the relatively short time which was at our command, the question could in most cases be only suggested; the answer was impossible. The conviction is forced upon me that it needs only appropriate effort to bring many of these dark questions into the brightest light. The experiments upon animals in particular make it possible for the pathologist, the clinician, and the pathologic anatomist to gain an insight into the more deep-seated processes, to test the disturbances of function produced by morbid conditions induced at will, to study the minute histologic changes in their various stages, and to compare them with the observations made at the sick-bed and in the autopsy-room.

The pessimistic view that clinical studies are and will remain without practical value is certainly not justified. Already surgeons have shown us that by correct knowledge of certain pathologic processes in the pancreas, and by interference at the right time, many cases can be cured. We have learned also from the surgeons to speak of the hopeful prevention of certain diseases. Is it not conceivable that the medical treatment of pancreatic disease may be broadened by rational methods, as already has happened for the neighboring organs, for instance, the intestines and biliary passages, with which the pancreas is so intimately associated?

It is to be hoped that the time will come and is not far distant when it will be possible to present that clinical representation of the diseases of the pancreas which so vitally important an organ deserves.

PROFESSOR OSER.

DISEASES OF THE PANCREAS.

GENERAL CONSIDERATIONS.

I. ANATOMIC INTRODUCTION.

BY PROF. EMIL ZUCKERKANDL.

THE pancreas lies behind the stomach, crosses the spinal column at a point corresponding to the first lumbar vertebra, and extends from the concavity of the loop of the duodenum to the mesial surface of the spleen on the left. The length of the gland varies from 15–21 cm. (6–8 inches).

The form of the organ is not regular, but can for the greater part be compared with an elongated triangular prism. The right end represents the thickest part, and is called the head; the middle portion with the three surfaces clearly pronounced is the body, while the left pointed end is called the tail; these three portions of the pancreas show no distinct lines of demarcation. Such a line may be thought of only where the head and body are joined, as this is the thinnest portion of the gland.

The head of the pancreas, distinguished by its breadth, lies attached to the concavity of the duodenum. When the head of the pancreas is especially thick, it may, by overlapping the sides of the intestinal loop, inclose nearly a third of the tube. From the middle of the head a process (lobe) extends upward as well as downward; the upper smaller lobe, if well developed, extends to the superior horizontal part of the duodenum. The lower larger lobe (*pancreas parvum*) follows the distal portion of the duodenum, and when well developed extends to the point at which the duodenum merges into the jejunum.

Between the head and body of the pancreas there is a groove for the superior mesenteric vessels. If the portion of the pancreas in front of this groove is cut through, the superior mesenteric artery is to be seen; also the union of the two mesenteric veins and the splenic vein, forming the portal vein.

This groove may be imagined to have been developed in the following way: the narrow body of the gland failed to attach itself to the left end of the much broader head, but passed from the ventral surface of the head of the pancreas into the axis of the gland close to the duodenal wall. Thus only is to be explained the development of a broad groove between the ventral surface of the head and the dorsal surface of the body. The body of the gland is thinnest in the region of this groove, a condition probably dependent upon the disposition of the large intestinal vessels.

The ductus choledochus is embedded in a furrow which is, as a rule, soon transformed into a canal at the back of the head and at the side of the gland toward the duodenum. Hence a part of the common bile-duct varying in length from 0.5 to 3 cm. is buried in the gland. The side of the glandular canal turned toward the duodenal wall is thin, as it usually consists of only a few lobes. This view is in direct opposition to that of O. Wyss,* according to whom the ductus choledochus traversed the pancreas only five times in 22 autopsies. From the location of the duct it is easy to see how readily enlargement and tumors of the pancreas may lead to compression and obstruction of the ductus choledochus.

The body of the gland has three surfaces: a ventral, in front, a dorsal, behind, and a caudal, below. One might also speak of a rectilinear surface, because the gland lies attached to the duodenal wall by a broad terminal surface. The ventral surface of the pancreas is free and has a delicate peritoneal covering. The dorsal surface lies upon the posterior wall of the trunk, while the caudal surface is attached closely to the transverse mesocolon. This last-mentioned surface is wide only at the left of the duodeno-jejunal flexure; at the right of this loop, however, and in the region of the superior mesenteric vessels, where the body of the pancreas is thinnest, it has a blunt edge.

Opposite the caudal surface the gland is bordered by the so-called (anterior) edge. In this there are two long grooves for the splenic vessels. The anterior shorter groove contains the artery, the posterior longer one carries the vein; but it sometimes happens that there is only a single furrow present for both vessels.

The tail of the gland, which really represents only the left end of the organ lying next to the spleen, is the least firmly attached portion of the pancreas. Occasionally a portion of the mesentery containing a lymph node lies between the tail and the mesial surface of the spleen, thus permitting a certain mobility to the tail of the pancreas.

Regarded as a whole, the pancreas shows, in addition to the form already described, a distinct **S**-shaped bend (Fig. 1), which is plainly seen in preparations hardened *in situ*. The gland is thus bent by the neighboring organs, including the spinal column and the stomach. Since the posterior abdominal wall is uneven and the pancreas lies over the marked prominence of the spinal column, the corresponding portion of the body of the gland must be bent convexly forward.

This convexity appears all the more sharply defined because on each side there are depressions produced by the stomach. The depression on the left, extending from the prominence to the tail (*impressio gastrica*), is large and is caused by the posterior wall of the stomach, which crosses the gland. The depression found at the right of the prominence (*impressio gastroduodenalis*) is considerably smaller and is determined by the position of the pylorus and the first part of the duodenum (Fig. 1).

Consistency.—The pancreas has the firm texture which characterizes the other salivary glands. This organ, however, consists of large lobes, and the individual lobules are easily separated from each other in couse-quence of the loose texture of the interacinous connective tissue.

Excretory Ducts.—Under normal conditions the pancreas has two excretory ducts: the pancreatic duct (*ductus Wirsungianus*) and the

* "Zur Aetiologie des Stauungsicterus," *Virchow's Archiv*, Bd. xxxvi, 1866.

accessory pancreatic duct (*ductus Santorini*). The former (Fig. 2) traverses the entire length of the gland, closely following the axis. In its course from left to right, the duct increases in diameter through the reception of numerous side branches. When it reaches the head, the

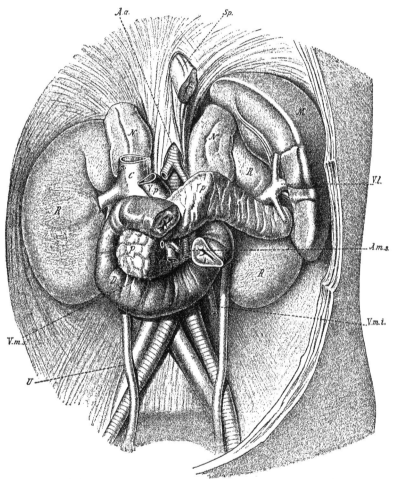

FIG. 1.—Relation of the pancreas to the duodenum and to the organs of the posterior abdominal wall: *P*, Pancreas; *D*, duodenum; *R*, kidney; *N*, suprarenal gland; *M*, spleen; *Sp*, esophagus; *U*, ureter; *A.a*, aorta and celiac axis; *C*, vena cava inferior; *V.p*, vena portæ; *V.m.s*, vena mesenterica superior; *V.m.i*, vena mesenterica inferior; *A.m.s*, arteria mesenterica superior; *V.l*, vena lienalis.

pancreatic duct turns backward and downward and unites at the end with the common bile-duct, both passing obliquely through the wall of the intestine and entering a little pouch lined with mucous membrane known as the *diverticulum Vateri*. The entrance to this pouch is indicated by a longitudinal fold of mucous membrane (*plica longitudinalis*), which contains the mouth of the diverticulum, in which is a papilliform projection (*papilla major*, Fig. 2). This papilla lies in the projection of the pancreas parvum, near the place where the left wall of the duodenum becomes the dorsal wall; hence it is more posterior than anterior. When this portion of the duodenal diverticulum is incised, the upper part shows two openings, that of the ductus choledochus, and, further in, the opening of the pancreatic duct; the two are separated from each other by a narrow band.

The caudal portion of the diverticulum is covered with delicate valve-like projections considered by Ch. Sappey to prevent the entrance of the intestinal contents into the two ducts.

The *ductus pancreaticus accessorius* (Fig. 2) is limited to the head of the gland. It runs above the duct of Wirsung, with which its left end communicates by means of a wide opening. Near its entrance into the intestine the accessory duct is reduced in size. The opening of the ductus Santorini in the mucous membrane of the duodenum is marked by a small, wart-like prominence 2 to 3 cm. above and rather behind the diverticulum Vateri (*papilla minor*, Fig. 2).

For a long time the accessory duct was regarded as inconstant, but Cl. Bernard,[*] Verneuil,[†] Sappey,[‡] and very recently Hamburger,[§] have shown that it is constantly present. Hamburger found the duct always present in the 50 cases examined by him; Sappey, in 17 preparations, never found it wanting; in one case, however, he found the right part of it obliterated. There are no reports of the frequency of this obliteration.

As the pancreas lies immediately in contact with the wall of the intestine, its excretory duct passes directly from the gland into the latter.

The presence of two ducts in the pancreas is explained by the fact that the gland develops from prohypoblastic projections. A single gland results from their fusion, and their excretory ducts thus communicate with each other. It needs no detailed description to show the importance of the two ducts; it is sufficient to mention the fact that in the case of the obliteration of the main duct the accessory duct can carry off the secretion.

Blood-vessels.—The pancreas is supplied with blood-vessels which communicate with the celiac artery, the superior mesenteric artery, and the portal vein. The arteries arise as follows: .

(a) From the splenic, which sends a number of branches into the gland.

(b) From the undivided trunk of the hepatic artery, which at times sends a large branch downward on the posterior side of the pancreas; this branch anastomoses with the arteria colica media and gives off smaller arteries for the head of the pancreas.

(c) From the gastro-duodenal artery, which by means of the upper pancreatico-duodenal branch nourishes the head of the pancreas. The arteria pancreatico-duodenalis superior, in its course toward the duodenum, lies in a groove on the ventral surface of the head of the pancreas.

(d) From the arteria pancreatico-duodenalis inferior, which also supplies the head of the gland, and likewise sends a lateral branch into the body of the gland· on the concave border of the duodenum it forms an

*Ph. C. Sappey, " Traitè d'anatomie descriptive," T. 4, Paris, 1873.
†Ibid., *loc. cit.*   ‡Ibid., *loc. cit.*
§ "Zur Entwicklung der Bauchspeicheldrüse des Menschen," *Anat. Anz.*, 1892.

arch with the arteria pancreatico-duodenalis superior. The arteria pancreatico-duodenalis inferior rises from the trunk of the superior mesenteric artery or from the arteria colica media, which also sends some branches to the pancreas.

The splenic artery provides chiefly for the body and tail of the pancreas, while the other arteries supply more especially the head.

The veins follow in general the course of the arteries. The vena pancreatico-duodenalis superior empties into the gastro-duodenal vein. The vena pancreatico-duodenalis inferior empties into the superior

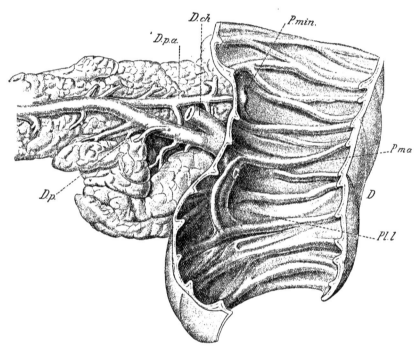

FIG. 2.—Pancreas and duodenum. In the former the ducts are shown. The duodenum is so opened as to show the papillæ. *D*, Duodenum; *P.maj.*, papilla major; *P.min.*, papilla minor; *P l.*, plica longitudinalis; *D.p.*, ductus pancreaticus; *D.p.a.*, ductus pancreaticus accessorius; *D.ch.*, ductus choledochus.

mesenteric vein and the superior mesenteric vein into a lateral branch of the vena colica media. The vena lienalis collects the blood from the veins which accompany the pancreatic branches of the splenic artery.

The blood-vessels which are to be considered in operations on the pancreas are the glandular branches arising from the splenic, superior mesenteric, hepatic, and gastro-duodenal arteries, as well as the corresponding veins. But, in addition to these, sometimes one and sometimes another of the larger blood-vessels lying in the depressions on the gland may fall into the field of operation. In larger tumors of the gland even more distant vessels, as the cœliaca, hepatica, gastrica sinistra, and,

according to Krönlein,* even the colica media, may be of importance.†
According to K. Franz,‡ the origin of the arteria mesenterica superior
and colica media may be found in a space the upper border of which lies
behind the pancreas, while the lower limit is 5 cm. below this gland.

Of anomalous vessels which might be involved in operations on the
pancreas, the following are to be mentioned:

(*a*) The hepatic artery, when its branches (the right and left) arise
separately, as not rarely happens; the left branch from the celiac artery
and the right branch arising from the portion of the superior mesenteric
artery covered by the gland. In the latter case the arteria gastroduodenalis is usually given off from the right branch.

(*b*) The two hepatic branches which arise separately from the celiac.

(*c*) The hepatica communis, which arises, not from the celiac, but from
the superior mesenteric.

(*d*) The arteria suprarenalis sinistra, which is given off from the celiac
and therefore passes through the bursa omentalis.

Lymph-vessels are present in large numbers; these are divided,
according to the situation of the lymph-nodes into which they enter,
into the upper (accompanying the splenic artery), lower (with the superior mesenteric artery), on the right (along the head of the pancreas),
and on the left (in the mesentery of the tail of the pancreas).

Nerves.—The nerves of the gland arise from the solar plexus.

Structure of the Gland.—The pancreas is a branched alveolar gland
with terminal alveoli as the essential constituents of the organ. The
secretory cells of the alveoli present a different appearance according to
the state of activity of the gland. The protoplasm at the bottom of the
cell is homogeneous, while that next to the free surface is granular.
This different condition of the two zones depends upon the physiologic
condition of the gland. In hunger the lower zone of the cells is wide
and well provided with granules; after an abundant secretion has taken
place the cells, on the whole, are somewhat smaller and the granules are
fewer. The protoplasmic upper zone increases in corresponding ratio.
If the gland has secreted for some time, then there is a complete lack of
granules and the whole cell consists of homogeneous protoplasm.

It must be assumed, therefore, that during the resting period of the
gland peculiar granules are formed at the expense of the protoplasm,
and that they are the predecessors of the secretion (zymogen granules).
During secretion these gradually disappear, while at the same time the
fluid secretion appears in the lumen. The zymogen granules, however,
have not as yet been seen in the secretion.

After secretion the cells enlarge, attain their original volume, and
again begin to form zymogen granules. The excretory ducts are lined
by a cylindric, simple epithelium; goblet cells occur, but isolated, in the
pancreatic duct (A. A. Böhm and M. v. Davidoff).

[The islands of Langerhans were first described by Paul Langerhans,§

---

* "Klinische und top. Beitrage zur Chirurgie des Pankreas," *Beiträge zur klin.
Chirurgie*, Bd. xiv, Tübingen, 1895.

† It has happened that the arteria colica media had to be ligated, and gangrene
of the transverse colon resulted. In such a case it would be advisable, in conjunction
with the operation on the gland, to undertake resection of this part of the intestine.

‡ "Ueber die Configuration der Arterien in der Umgebung des Pankreas," *Anat.
Anz.*, Nr. 19, 20, 1896.

§ "Beiträge zur mikroskopischen Anatomie der Bauchspeicheldrüse," Inang.
Diss., Berlin, 1869.

in 1869. He called attention to the presence in the lobules of the pancreas of groups of small, spherical or polygonal cells differing in appearance from the ordinary cells of the gland. Laguesse * designated them "ilots" of Langerhans, and they have been the subject of repeated investigation, especially of late years, as the possible source of the supposed internal secretion of the gland. They have been regarded as lymph-follicles or pseudo-lymph-follicles, as blood-glands, and as resembling the hypophysis and the carotid and coccygeal glands. It is generally admitted, however, that, in the adult at least, they are not, as a rule, in continuous relation with the efferent duct of the gland. It was found by Kühne and Lea † that they corresponded to groups of dilated and tortuous capillaries resembling renal glomeruli. Opie ‡ has recently studied these structures, and finds them more numerous in the tail than elsewhere in the gland.—ED.]

Anomalies of the pancreas are relatively rare; they concern the gland itself, or the presence of pancreatic tissue in atypical places in the intestinal tract, or, still more rarely, the inclosure of atypical tissue in the stroma of the pancreas. The following may be mentioned among the peculiar anomalies of the pancreas:

(*a*) Cases in which—as described, for instance, by J. Hyrtl §—a portion of the head of the gland becomes separated and lies behind the mesenteric artery and superior vein, or an accessory pancreas as large as a dollar, with an excretory duct opening into the pancreatic duct, lies under the head of the gland at the inner side of the descending part of the duodenum (J. Engel ‖).

(*b*) Separation of the head or tail of the pancreas, as described by J. Hyrtl.** In the one case the tail of the pancreas was detached and was connected with the gland only by a duct which communicated with the duct of Wirsung. In a second preparation made from the body of a newborn child, Hyrtl saw the head of the gland separated from the body. In the space between the two parts were the superior mesenteric artery and vein. A pedicle ½ inch long, and formed simply of the pancreatic duct, united the two.

(*c*) The case of A. Ecker,†† in which the descending portion of the duodenum was surrounded by a ring of pancreatic tissue. Across the above-mentioned portion of the intestine was found a strip of gland which arose from the head of the pancreas and surrounded the duodenum by a continuous ring. The excretory duct of the abnormal piece of gland proceeded from the pancreatic duct, ran forward, and ended in the neighborhood of the main duct in fine branches. Finally:

(*d*) A case observed by me, in which the groove for the superior mesenteric artery and vein formed a canal in consequence of the union of the descending lobe with the body of the gland.

The second group of anomalies concerns, as already mentioned, the occurrence of pancreatic tissue in atypical places, and such accessory

---

* *Journ. de l'Anat. et Phys.*, 1896, xxxii, 208.

† "Untersuch. a. d. Phys. Inst. d. Univ. Heidelberg," 1882, ii, 488.

‡ *Johns Hopkins Hosp. Bull.*, 1900, xi, 205.

§ "Topograph. Anatomie."

‖ "Ueber Krankheiten des Pankreas und seines Ausführungsganges," "Medicin. Jahrb.," Wien, 1840.

** "Ein Pancreas accessorium und Pancreas divisum," *Sitzungsber. d. kaiserl. Akademie*, Bd. lii, Wien, 1866.

†† "Bildungsfehler des Pankreas," etc., *Zeitschr. f. rationelle Medicin*, 1862.

pancreatic glands have been observed (a) in the stomach, (b) in the duodenum, (c) in the jejunum, and (d) in the ileum.

Accessory Pancreas in the Stomach.—J. Klob[*] found such a formation in the middle of the greater curvature, inclosed between the serous and muscular coats. According to Klob, the gland had no excretory duct, but, as Zenker justly remarks, Klob may have overlooked the duct.

E. Wagner [†] observed an accessory pancreas in the anterior wall of the stomach near the lesser curvature, midway between the cardia and the pylorus. The gland, which was situated in the submucosa, was 2 inches long, 2½ inches thick, and 3½ inches broad.

C. Gegenbaur [‡] found in the lesser curvature, 2 cm. distant from the pylorus, in the submucosa, an accessory pancreas which was 14 mm. long and 6 mm. thick.

Finally, Weichselbaum [§] describes a case in which, at the bottom of a diverticulum near the pylorus, there was a nodule of the size of a hemp-seed which showed the structure of the pancreas. He found also in the anterior duodenal wall an accessory pancreas as large as a bean and covered by the serous coat.

Accessory Pancreas in the Wall of the Duodenum.—To this class belongs the above-cited case of Weichselbaum and also the observation of Zenker, of an accessory pancreas on the convex border of the duodenum opposite the head of the pancreas.

Accessory Pancreas in the Wall of the Jejunum.—Klob [||] found an accessory pancreas in the dorsal wall of the first loop of the jejunum.

F. A. Zenker [**] adds several similar cases. Twice he found the accessory pancreas quite near the duodenum; in a third preparation it lay 16 cm., and in a fourth 48 cm., below the duodenum.

Accessory Pancreas in the Wall of the Ileum.—The first description of such an anomaly is that by Zenker.[††] Fifty-four centimeters above the cecal valve this investigator observed an intestinal diverticulum, with a mesentery containing a large amount of fat, and in which was the accessory pancreas.

E. Neumann [‡‡] also saw an accessory pancreas in connection with an intestinal diverticulum in a child. The diverticulum was 2 feet above the cecal valve and its tip was connected by a pedicle with an accessory pancreas as large as a pea. The excretory duct of the gland entered the diverticulum.

The last case in this category is described by C. Nauwerck.[§§] This author found hanging free in the abdominal cavity, 2.3 m. above the cecal valve, a pancreas 9 cm. long, provided with a serous covering. The excretory duct opened into a deeper portion of the intestine. As a Meckel's diverticulum was present 80 cm. above the cecal valve, it is probable that in this case, as in those of Zenker and Neumann, the diverticulum, to which the accessory pancreas was related, was not a Meckel's

---

[*] "Kleinere Mittheilungen," *Zeitschr. d. Gesellsch. d. Aerzte*, Wien, 1859.
[†] *Archiv f. Heilkunde*, 1862.
[‡] "Nebenpankreas in der Magenwand," *Reichert's Archiv*, 1863.
[§] "Nebenpankreas in der Wand des Magens und Duodenums," *Bericht d. Rudolf-stiftung*, 1884.
[||] *Loc. cit.*
[**] "Nebenpankreas in der Darmwand," *Virchow's Archiv*, Bd. xxi.
[††] *Loc. cit.*
[‡‡] *Archiv f. Heilkunde*, Bd. xi, 1870.
[§§] "Ein Nebenpankreas," *Ziegler's Beiträge*, Bd. xii, 1893.

diverticulum, but a malformation of some kind—a conclusion which seems well justified.

[On the contrary, the observation of J. H. Wright * suggests that the development of an accessory pancreas may be connected with the persistent remains of the vitelline duct. He found a nodule of pancreatic tissue about 3½ mm. in diameter in the vicinity of an umbilical fistula which had existed since birth in a child of twelve years. An efferent duct leading to the surface was not found. The peritoneal cavity was opened and explored, but the finger found no connection between the fistula and the intestine.—ED.]

Finally, it is to be noted that in all forms of accessory pancreas except that described by Klob [and Wright] an excretory duct of the gland could be found.

The third kind of anomaly was described by Klob.† This anatomist dissected a body the pancreas of which showed a spherical enlargement of the tail. Further investigation disclosed that the enlargement was due to the inclusion of an accessory spleen.

Abnormalities of Excretory Ducts.—The following have been observed:

(a) Lack of an accessory duct.

(b) Three openings on the *plica longitudinalis,* of which two belonged to the pancreas and one to the bile-duct (Fr. Tiedemann ‡).

(c) Four openings in papilliform prominences of the mucous membrane of the duodenum. Of these, the uppermost corresponds to the accessory pancreatic duct, the second, which is situated about 1.5 cm. lower and flanked by an obstructing valve, corresponds to the ductus choledochus. About 0.5 cm. below the latter opening was a third eminence with the opening of the ductus Wirsungianus; finally, about 1 cm. deeper is the opening of a duct also at the top of a fold of mucous membrane originating in the head of the pancreas (original observation).

(d) A solitary duct; this passes through the whole length of the gland and opens on the papilla minor. The end of the duct accordingly corresponds to the ductus Santorini. The ductus choledochus alone opens into the diverticulum Vateri (original observation).

(e) The typical two ducts are present; the ductus Santorini runs to the papilla minor, which is normally situated, while the ductus Wirsungianus, on the other hand, opens into the terminal portion of the ductus choledochus. The papilla major is lacking. In place of it is found a groove limited by wide folds of mucous membrane. The upper ends of the two folds are united, and at this point is found a larger opening, the mouth of the ductus choledochus. The other portion of the groove is crossed by transverse bands; it is clear, therefore, that in this case there is a cleft of the diverticulum Vateri (original observation).

Topography.—In contradistinction to the liver and spleen, the pancreas does not lie in the greater peritoneal sac, but in the bursa omentalis, which represents an accessory space of the peritoneal cavity. In this bursa we distinguish an anterior and a posterior wall; the former is composed of the posterior wall of the stomach, the gastro-splenic ligament, and the anterior layer of the great omentum; the posterior wall is formed by the posterior layer of the great omentum. A passage leads from the right into this bursa, and is bounded anteriorly by the lesser

---

* *Jour. Boston Soc. Med. Sci.,* 1901, v, 497. † *Loc. cit.*
‡ "Ueber die Verschiedenheiten der Ausführungsgänge der Bauchspeicheldrüse," etc., *Meckel's Archiv,* Bd. IV.

omentum, posteriorly by the parietal peritoneum of the abdominal wall, and above and below by the fusion of the liver and duodenum with the parietal peritoneum. The entrance of the passage into the bursa is marked by a fold (plica gastro-pancreatica) running from the celiac end to the lesser curvature of the stomach and concealing the vasa gastrica sinistra, while toward the right the passage opens into the peritoneal sac through the foramen of Winslow. The lobus Spigelii is situated in the passage.

To expose the hidden position of the pancreas, even after the abdominal cavity is opened, the anterior layer of the greater omentum must be separated from the greater curvature of the stomach. The omental bursa can also be opened by cutting through the lesser omentum, but this method is advisable only in the case of small tumors of the head of the pancreas.

The peculiar position of the pancreas is readily understood when the development of the mesogastrium is considered. The anlage of the gland is carried into the mesogastrium, which, stretched between the vertebral column and the greater curvature of the stomach, lies free, like the mesentery of the small intestine. This condition of the mesogastrium persists in most mammals, and explains the great motility of the gland in these animals. In man, a mesogastrium free on both sides is found only as a temporary stage of development. Later the pancreas becomes fixed because the portion of the mesogastrium corresponding to this organ is fused with the parietal peritoneum of the posterior abdominal wall.

When the fusion is complete, three layers are to be recognized in the posterior fold of the great omentum; the upper is united to the pancreas, the middle to the upper surface of the transverse mesocolon, and the lower portion hangs free over the coils of the intestine. It seems noteworthy that the caudal surface of the pancreas reaches the line of attachment of the transverse mesocolon, whence it results that the gland is visible when the transverse mesocolon is raised, especially when there is a lack of fat.

The anterior layer of the great omentum is more simple; it extends from the greater curvature of the stomach to the free lower edge of the omentum, where it becomes the posterior layer of this structure.

From the description given it may be assumed that the pancreas is neither retroperitoneal nor free in the bursa, but, as a formation of the mesogastrium, projects into the cavity named and is drawn over to its ventral surface by the free dorsal plate of the mesogastrium.

Of the topical relations of the gland to neighboring structures, that to the stomach is especially important. In a circumscribed spot just below the cardia a typical adhesion is found between the posterior wall of the stomach and the posterior abdominal wall. That large portion of the posterior wall of the stomach which lies adjacent to the impressio gastrica pancreatis, on the other hand, usually remains free. Not rarely, however, the above-mentioned fusion of the stomach extends further downward. The stomach and the pancreas may be united by bands, or the union may be formed by broad adhesions.

Similar alterations occur also in the region of the pylorus. The upper horizontal part of the duodenum is fused with the head of the pancreas and the gastro-duodenal artery runs in the connective tissue forming the line of union. The stomach and the duodenum, therefore, cover the greater part of the pancreas, but one portion of it lies in the projection of the lesser omentum, especially in that of the upper horizontal part of the duodenum.

The upper portion of the omental bursa lying behind the stomach is divided by adhesions into small recesses, and sometimes is wholly obliterated.

The attachments described, leaving out of consideration the pathologic cases, which may simulate them, belong to the category of physiologic processes of fusion, which lower down establish connections between the two layers of the great omentum.

That the fixation of the posterior wall of the stomach interferes with the mobility of the stomach can easily be understood. Under ordinary conditions the stomach, excepting at its attached portion, is freely movable. The ligaments and mesogastrium oppose no obstacle to its distention, free motion being allowed by the considerable length and purse-like structure of the great omentum, which has the sole purpose of securing extensive displacement and distention of the stomach.

Extensive adhesions diminish, however, the distensibility at least of the posterior wall of the stomach. They are of importance especially in connection with tumors of the pancreas and with adjoining ulcers of the stomach, since the latter give rise to adhesions resembling those produced by other pathologic processes.

The length of the pancreas, as well as its sharply limited surfaces, will explain the fact that small tumors of that organ show different topical relations according to the place or the surface from which they arise. A tumor of the head of the pancreas will show a different position and different topical relations to the neighboring organs from those exhibited by a tumor of the tail of the gland. Of the neighboring organs,

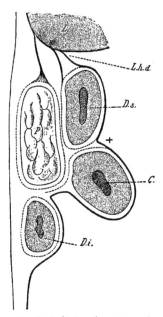

FIG. 3.—Sagittal section of the region of the pancreas corresponding to the curve of the duodenum (schematic): *P*, Pancreas; *L*, liver; *D.s*, pars horizontalis duodeni; *C*, colon transversum; *L.h.d*, ligamentum hepatoduodenale.

the stomach, the transverse colon, and the liver are of first importance. Tumors of the anterior surface of the gland will project into the bursa and approach the stomach, the ligamentum gastro-colicum, or both, but will not affect the transverse colon (see Figs. 4 and 5). If, moreover, the tumor is not so large as to hinder the movement of the stomach downward, then the relation to the gastro-colic ligament will be dependent on the fulness of the stomach; for the empty and therefore contracted stomach approaches the diaphragm, causing a marked widening of the ligament, while the full stomach extends down to the transverse colon, producing a marked narrowing of this band. When the tumor develops at a place where the anterior surface of the gland is covered by the lesser omentum, the growth, by pushing the omentum before it, may adhere to the abdominal wall between the lesser curvature of the stomach and the liver.   If the tumor grows from that portion of the head of the pancreas to the anterior side of which the upper horizontal portion of the

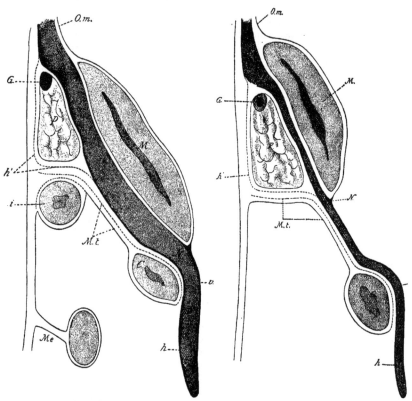

FIG. 4.—Sagittal section of the region of the pancreas immediately to the right of the flexura duodenojejunalis (schematic) : *P*, Pancreas; *G*, artery on its upper edge; *M*, stomach; *D.i*, pars horizontalis inferior duodeni; *C*, colon transversum; *M.t*, the two layers of the transverse mesocolon; *M.e*, mesentery of the small intestine; *v*, anterior, *h*, posterior layer of the great omentum; *N*, omental bursa; *O.m*, lesser omentum.

FIG. 5.*—Sagittal section of the region of the pancreas to the left of the flexura duodenojejunalis (schematic) : *P*, Pancreas; *G*, artery at the upper edge of the gland; *M*, stomach; *v*, anterior, *h*, posterior layer of the great omentum; *N*, omental bursa; *O.m*, lesser omentum; *M.t*, the two plates of the transverse mesocolon.

duodenum is attached, it may easily cause compression of this portion of the intestine, especially as in this region the lower surface and right end of the gland are flanked also by the duodenum (see Fig. 3 †).

* The heavy line (Figs. 3–5) represents the layers of the great omentum; the dotted line represents the place where either the great omentum is united with the transverse mesocolon, or·(as in *h'*) the pancreas is united with the parietal peritoneum.

† This diagram was prepared from a sagittal section through the abdominal cavity of a human embryo. In the adult the part designated by a cross (+) is

Tumors on the left of the duodeno-jejunal flexure, where the lower surface of the gland lies directly on the transverse mesocolon, will have a tendency to crowd between the above-mentioned mesenteric plate and the posterior layer of the great omentum. If the enlargement of the growth is uniform on all sides, it will grow upward into the omental bursa and downward toward the central region of the abdominal cavity, arching the transverse mesocolon. The transverse colon lies in this case on a level with the tumor, while the stomach lies above it. If the growth of the tumor is more lateral, it will crowd either into the bursa or into the central region of the abdomen; in the former case the transverse colon lies at the lower border of the tumor, and in the latter case at the upper border.

Relation to Blood-vessels and Organs of the Posterior Abdominal Wall.—It has been shown that the pancreas is very closely related to the large blood-vessels. These are the superior mesenteric vessels, the portal veins, the splenic and gastro-duodenal vessels, all of which lie in grooves of the gland. It may be remarked concerning the splenic vessels that they lie free and project considerably above the tail of the pancreas.

A less intimate relation exists between the gland and the organs of the posterior abdominal wall, the crura of the diaphragm, the vena cava inferior, the aorta, the left adrenal gland, and the left kidney. There is direct contact between the pancreas, the vena cava inferior, the left adrenal gland, the left kidney, and the spleen. The lower lobe of the pancreas lies directly on the vena cava inferior, the body lies on the left adrenal, and the tail on the left kidney and on the mesial surface of the spleen. A space lies between the gland, the crura of the diaphragm, and the aorta because other structures intervene. Between the right crus of the diaphragm and the pancreas lie the vena cava inferior and some lymph-nodes; lymph-nodes are likewise found between the body of the pancreas, on the one hand, and the aorta and left crus of the diaphragm on the other. The left adrenal also intervenes between the gland and the crus of the diaphragm on the corresponding side.

II. REMARKS ON THE PHYSIOLOGIC CHEMISTRY OF THE PANCREATIC JUICE AND ON PANCREATIC DIGESTION.*

AMONG all the glands of the digestive system, the pancreas has the most varied activity, since by means of its secretion all three groups of food-stuffs are changed into soluble, absorbable substances.

PHYSICAL CHARACTERISTICS OF THE PANCREATIC JUICE.

The knowledge of the physiologico-chemical activity of the pancreatic secretion has been acquired by the study of the secretion secured from temporary and permanent fistulæ. The appearance of the secre-

lengthened. In consequence of which the space between the duodenum and transverse colon is enlarged.

* From a collection of the most important facts, made by Dr. A. Katz.

tion varies according as it is obtained from a temporary or permanent fistula.

1. The **secretion from a temporary fistula** probably best corresponds with the condition in the organism. It represents a clear, colorless, tough, viscous fluid of strongly alkaline reaction. On cooling to 0° C. (32° F.), a gelatinous substance separates, soluble in sodium chlorid and in weak acids, and consisting of a myosin-like body, which is never wholly free from ferment. Pre-formed peptone, leucin, or tyrosin is never present in the fresh secretion. By the action of alcohol a precipitate is formed, which is for the greater part soluble in water and contains a crude ferment, which, at 40° C. (104° F.), changes albuminous bodies into the well-known products of digestion.

2. The **secretion obtained from a permanent fistula** is, as a rule, a thin fluid, which foams on shaking and has a low specific gravity. On cooling, no gelatinous substance separates.

The pancreatic juice is a material which readily putrefies. On standing in the air, a fecaloid odor quickly arises, and on the addition of chlorin water a red coloring-matter is rapidly formed, and later indol also is produced.

Relatively normal pancreatic secretion has been investigated by Herter and Zawadzki. The fluid examined by Herter came from an enlarged duct of Wirsung, which had been compressed at the place of exit by a carcinoma. It was clear yellow in color and strongly alkaline in reaction. Albumin, peptone, and sugar were not present. The ash was very rich in alkaline phosphates. The three ferment actions of the pancreas could be shown. Besides this, Herter investigated the contents of two pancreatic cysts. In these three analyses the following results were found:

	I.	II.	III.
Total solids	24.1%	24.1%	23.8%
Organic constitutents	17.9%	14.9%	18.5%
Ash	6.2%	9.2%	8.7%

Zawadzki analyzed the secretion of a pancreatic fistula which remained in a young woman after extirpation of a cystic pancreatic tumor. The analysis of the juice, which was a very effective digestive, resulted as follows:

Dry constituents	13.59%; of which
Proteids	9.20%
Mineral constituents	0.34%

The rest of the dry constituents were soluble in alcohol.

3. **Ferments.**—The ferments are contained in the gland in the form of zymogens. They become effective only after long exposure to the air or through the influence of weak acids. The isolation of the pure ferments is attended with great difficulty, and, in spite of the many attempts which have been made, no one has yet wholly succeeded.

(a) *Trypsin.*—The power of the pancreatic juice to digest albumin was first observed by Bernard, and more closely studied and demonstrated by Corvisart. This action is due to a ferment, which is called trypsin by Kühne, who made a most careful study of it, and obtained it in the purest possible form.

The secretion of trypsin in carnivora is not continuous, but is closely related to the taking of food. The secretion is most abundant from four to seven hours after eating. In the glands of animals which had not eaten for some time, no ferment could be found by Lewaschew, Heidenhain, and others, while the later investigations of Cavallo and Pachon, as well as Dastre, showed that the trypsin ferment could be obtained from the pancreas of dogs after five to twelve days of starvation.

When precipitated with alcohol, trypsin forms an amorphous, colorless powder which easily dissolves in water, forming a clear straw-yellow fluid, which even when alkaline is relatively stable. It dissolves fibrin almost instantly at incubator temperature. Trypsin is much more energetic in its action than pepsin. The presence of water is quite sufficient for the beginning of the hydrolytic action; no definite reaction is required as with pepsin, although differences in reactions of the digestive fluids are not without influence on the intensity of the action of the ferment. This is entirely checked by the presence of free hydrochloric acid. If there is sufficient albumin present so that the hydrochloric acid exists only in the combined form, the deleterious influence is not noticeable.

Trypsin, moreover, is not destroyed by hydrochloric acid. According to Lindberger, if in a digestive mixture in which there is too much hydrochloric acid the quantity is lessened by dialysis, or removed entirely, the trypsin becomes again effective.

The influence of the organic acids found in the intestinal canal was investigated by Lindberger with the following results: Acetic acid in a strength of 0.01%, especially if bile and sodium chlorid were also present at the same time, had a favorable influence, in many cases even hastening the action of the trypsin. In no instance were the small amounts used injurious. Lactic acid also had a favorable influence on the processes of digestion. In the presence of 0.02% of lactic acid and 1% to 2% of bile and of sodium chlorid, the solution of the fibrin took place more quickly than in an alkaline fluid.

The acid reaction of the intestinal contents of the dog was estimated by Lindberger as equal to 0.005 to 0.01 to 0.02% of HCl. The last amount is very rarely observed.

The organic acids formed in the intestine cannot, therefore, be considered as having any injurious influence on trypsin digestion.

The *influence of bile* on trypsin digestion was very carefully investigated by Chittenden and Cummings, with the following results: If bile be added to a neutral solution of trypsin, the influence of the ferment is not essentially altered; if the ferment solution is alkaline, its action is somewhat checked. Sodium taurocholate and glycocholate exert but slight influence on the proteolytic action. Taurocholic acid, however, added to a neutral solution, hinders the process decidedly. In a pancreatic juice which contains 0.1% of combined salicylic acid, the ferment action is greatly strengthened by the addition of 10% of bile. In the presence of combined hydrochloric acid, this addition has no influence.

[Rachford * has called attention to the fact that the nearer an animal is to the carnivorous type, the more surely are the bile and pancreatic juice to be pressed into the intestine through one duct and the more closely to the pylorus is this duct situated. He used freshly secreted pancreatic juice and bile for the study of the action of bile on proteolytic digestion. Thus he showed that the presence of bile increased the proteolytic action of the pancreas about one-fourth.

Fibrin half saturated with hydrochloric acid was digested by pan-

* *Jour. of Physiol.*, xxv, 2, p. 165.

creatic juice more slowly than neutral fibrin, while fibrin nine-tenths saturated showed marked retardation of digestion. The proteolytic action of pancreatic juice was not wholly lost even if free hydrochloric acid was present. Similar results were obtained when bile was also present with the acid.—ED.]

The *effect of temperature* on fresh pancreatic secretion and on solutions of Kühne's trypsin was investigated by Biernacki. Pure pancreatic secretion remains effective at 55° C. (133° F.). A trypsin solution in 0.2% sodium carbonate loses its efficiency after warming for five minutes at 50° C. (122° F.), while a temperature of 45° C. (113° F.) causes a marked weakening of the action, and at 40° C. (104° F.) its action is most effective. The addition of salts in concentration of 0.05 to 4% protects the ferment from the influence of higher temperature. Each salt has a certain concentration in which its influence is most energetic. The addition of a mixture of two salts is especially favorable. Such mixtures may be heated to 60° C. (140° F.) without injuring the ferment. Amphopeptone which is free from salt and antipeptone in concentrations of 0.5 to 5% have a similar protective influence. Starch and sugar had no influence. In neutral and acid solutions, the bodies named have no effect whatever and the ferment is destroyed at 45° C. (113° F.). In a dry condition the ferment may be heated for hours to 100° C. (212° F.) without losing its power (Salkowski).

Changes of the albuminous bodies by trypsin: The hydrolytic decomposition of albuminous bodies is carried further through the action of trypsin than by any other ferment. A number of amido-acids arise as ultimate products of the decomposition: leucin, asparagin, lysatin, lysin, and also tyrosin and ammonia. The whole albuminous molecule, however, is not divided in this general manner. According to the careful investigations of Kühne and his students, the albuminous molecule is made up of two groups of substances in about equal parts, which behave differently toward trypsin and are known as the hemi- and the anti-group. Antipeptone and hemipeptone are the result of the action of trypsin on the ampho-deutero-proteoses and the amphopeptones which are formed in the stomach. The antipeptone energetically opposes any further action of the digestive ferments. The hemipeptone is broken up into the above-mentioned products. According to the recent investigations of Siegfried, antipeptone is identical with sarcolactic acid obtained by him from muscle.

The production of crystalline products of the decomposition of the albuminous bodies was formerly ascribed to the influence of bacterial action. Even very recently Duclaux attributes it to bacteria, which he asserts are never absent in the experiments with pancreatic juice. The majority of authors, among them Kühne and Chittenden, regard these bodies as the direct products of trypsin digestion.

Leucin and tyrosin may be regarded as the main representatives of these substances. Kühne, and later Chittenden, also found them in the digestive fluids in no inconsiderable amounts. Thus the former, in one experiment, found 9.1% leucin and 3.8% tyrosin.

Asparagic acid was found by Salkowski and Radziejewski in the digestion of blood-fibrin, and is to be regarded as amido-succinic acid.

Glutamic acid, or amidopyrrhotartaric acid, has been shown by Knieriem in the digestion of wheat-gluten.

Lysin and *lysatinin* were obtained by Hedin in the digestion of blood-fibrin with trypsin. Drechsel was able to obtain urea directly from lysatinin, by boiling with baryta water. His experiments are therefore of great interest, because they show that urea could be produced directly from albumins by simple hydrolytic decomposition. Drechsel asserts that normally about one-ninth of the urea excreted originates in this way. In the breaking up of the albumin molecule, hypoxanthin (xanthin?) is produced, and also a body, tryptophan, which gives a beautiful violet color by the action of chlorin and bromin water. The latter, in its elementary composition, shows a close relationship to the animal coloring-matters, bilirubin, melanin, etc. Nencki, to whom we owe this knowledge, expresses the view that tryptophan will eventually be brought into relation with the development of certain animal coloring-matters.

Products resembling ptomains result from putrefaction of the pancreas when mixed with albuminous bodies, but this is to be ascribed to bacterial influence and not to the action of the ferment. Werigo, however, asserts that in perfectly sterile pancreatic infusions pentamethylendiamin also is found, but in his experiment the quantity was very small: from 33 lbs. of pancreas he could secure only a few grams.

One of Chittenden's experiments shows that the decomposition of albumin into crystalline products takes place in the intestinal canal of an animal. He fed a dog with 400 gm. of meat and killed it six hours later; ¾ gm. of a mixture of leucin and tyrosin was obtained from the intestinal contents.

The utilization of the albumins is much less when the pancreatic juice is lacking in the intestine than when it is present. According to Abelmann, the total is much more deleterious than the partial extirpation of the gland. In the former case 44%, in the latter 54%, is absorbed. When pancreatic emulsion is given with meat, absorption reaches 74% to 78%. Renzi also has shown that the amount of nitrogen in the feces was greater after extirpation of the pancreas. The utilization of the albumins is still less if fat is fed at the same time. Abelmann was able to recognize macroscopically bits of muscle in the stools.

Influence of the spleen on the formation of trypsin: The assertion was made by Schiff that the spleen during digestion secreted a juice which had the function of converting pancreatic zymogen into trypsin. This view is supported by later investigations of Herzen, which show that in the extract of the spleen at the time of digestion a ferment must be present having the property of changing zymogen into an active trypsin. This view could not be confirmed by the experiments of Ewald, Buffallini, Cavallo, and Pachon. Herzen, however, tries to support it in a later work.

[Bellamy * confirms Herzen's work. He believes that the ferment which is formed in the spleen and changes the zymogen into trypsin reaches the pancreas through the blood; that if the spleen is removed the pancreas is in a state of permanent atrypsia, though the zymogen will continue to be secreted; that the zymogen will then be converted into trypsin, as Pawlow has shown, through the agency of the mucous membrane of the small intestine.—ED.]

(b) *Steapsin.*—The fat-digesting ferment has not hitherto been isolated and preserved in a permanent form. The experiments in this direction were either performed with extract of pancreas, or the changes in its behavior to fats were ascertained after operation upon the gland of an

* *Jour. of Physiol.,* xxvii, p. 323.

animal. The emulsifying influence of the pancreatic juice does not need the assumption of a peculiar ferment; sufficient explanation is to be found in the viscosity of the secretion and in the presence of alkalis and soaps. The fat emulsion formed by the pancreatic secretion is far more permanent and complete than that obtained in any other way.

The influence of the pancreatic secretion in decomposing fat into fatty acids and glycerin was known to Claude Bernard. If neutral butter was mixed with particles of the gland at an incubator temperature, an acid reaction soon set in. Berthelot showed the action of the ferment by the use of monobutyrin, which is synthetically prepared and easily decomposed; Nencki used tribenzoicin, the triglycerid of benzoic acid, combined in a manner analogous to that of the neutral fats. His investigations are the first which, by excluding the influence of the cleaving fungi, ascribed the decomposition of the esters to the unformed ferments of the pancreatic juice.

The formation in the intestinal canal of the fatty acids from the neutral fats has probably the purpose of facilitating the absorption of the fats, since it was shown by Brücke and Gad that fats containing fatty acids are more easily absorbed than those having a neutral reaction. The favorable influence of bile on the decomposition of fat was shown by Nencke, and later by Rachford, Hédon, and Ville.

Their investigations permit the assumption that the conditions for the decomposition of the fats are best in the duodenum, while in the small intestine the conditions appear to be most favorable for its emulsification. Bile and pancreatic secretion, working together, are necessary for the absorption of the fat into the circulation. Claude Bernard found in the rabbit, whose ductus choledochus and pancreaticus open separately into the intestine, that the chyle vessels contain milky chyle only below the place of opening of the bile-duct into the intestine. Dastre was able to establish the same facts experimentally in the dog. The most thorough investigations on the fate of the fat in the intestinal canal when the pancreatic juice is lacking have been made by Abelmann. After the total extirpation of the pancreas, unemulsified fat was not utilized, except when the animals were fed upon the minced pancreas of a hog. However, a cleavage took place in the intestine, probably through the action of bacteria. The results of the investigations will be referred to more in detail in a later section (p. 84).

In a dog which had survived for twenty-five days the extirpation of the pancreas and the resulting diabetes, Baldi was able to show large amounts of fat in the stools after feeding with fatty meats. In the stools there was an oleaginous, fatty mass which was not solid at the temperature of the room in spite of the fact that the fat at the time of its introduction had had a much greater consistency. If the small amount of fat in the stools of a dog having a biliary fistula is compared with the amount obtained from the stools in this case, it must be concluded that the pancreas plays a much more important rôle than the liver in the digestion of fat.

The fat-cleaving ferment seems to pass over into the blood-serum. According to Hanriot's experiments, this ferment, which he calls lipase, must have an important part in the circulation of the fat in the organism.

(c) *Pancreatic Diastase.*—The influence of the pancreatic secretion and of the infusion of the gland on starch is, in its introductory stages, identical with the diastatic influence of malt extract. The difference lies in the fact that if the temperature is maintained for a longer time at 40° C. (104° F.), a part of the maltose changes into grape-sugar, which is not possible in the case of malt diastase. On the other hand, no ferment inverting cane-sugar is present in the pancreas. The transition products are the same as in salivary digestion. The final product consists mostly of maltose with a small amount of dextrose. In salivary digestion the formation of grape-sugar does not usually take place. Glycogen as well as starch is changed by the pancreatic ferment; inulin and cane-sugar are not altered.

According to the investigations of Martin and Williams, the presence of bile hastens the diastatic influence of the pancreas; the same is true of sodium glycocholate. Glycocholic acid hinders the action because of its acidity. The organic acids, if they are present in any considerable amounts, have an injurious influence. According to Hofmeister's results, the presence of 0.01 to 0.03% of lactic acid, or of 0.008 to 0.04% of acetic acid, increases the diastatic fermentation; 0.04% or 0.05 to 0.06% decreases it; and it is suspended by 0.05% lactic acid or 0.08% acetic acid. It is a peculiar fact that in the presence of sodium chlorid the acetic acid shows its injurious influence much earlier than in the absence of that salt. The influence of the diastatic ferment is very quickly destroyed by mineral acids.

After removal of the pancreas, 60 to 80% of amylaceous substances are utilized. Recently Hess has performed some experiments in which the absorption of starch was reduced to the minimum only after subsequent removal of the salivary glands. Very recently, Rohmann found in the gland a second diastatic ferment forming isomaltose.

In the newborn, the diastatic ferment does not occur, but is produced in the first months of extra-uterine life.

(d) *The milk-coagulating ferment of the pancreas:* If milk is mixed with weak pancreatic secretion, the casein, after a transformation into metacasein, becomes coagulated. Cooked pancreas loses this power, so that this peculiarity must be referred to a ferment existing in the gland. This is not identical with trypsin, as pure trypsin produced by Kühne's method does not show this peculiarity; the influence of trypsin and of the milk-coagulating fluids of the pancreatic juice may be shown by external agents to be markedly different. If on mixing milk and pancreatic juice, no coagulation takes place, we can easily produce it by the addition of sodium chlorid or magnesium sulphate. Pure casein solutions also are coagulated by this ferment.

[Weinland * has shown that the pancreas in dogs produces a ferment, lactase, which breaks up milk-sugar into dextrose and galactose, and that this ferment is increased after feeding with milk-sugar. In a further communication † he shows that milk-sugar acts on the digestive tract in such a manner as to excite or increase the production of this ferment in the pancreas. The blood is not the medium through which the milk-sugar acts.—ED.]

4. **Fate of the Pancreatic Ferments in the Organism.**—The presence of trypsin in the urine was asserted by Grützner and v. Sahli. As the influence of putrefactive organisms seems not to have been sufficiently excluded in their experiments, Leo has undertaken a new series of investigations, and has come to the conclusion that trypsin is never found in the urine. In the feces, also, it was sought in vain. In order

* *Zeitsch. f. Biol.,* 1899, Bd. xxxviii, p. 607.   † *Ibid.,* 1900, Bd. xl, p. 386.

to ascertain more exactly its function in the intestine, Leo killed a dog in the process of digestion and by ligatures divided the intestine into five parts and investigated each part separately for the presence of trypsin. In the lower portions of the intestine no ferment was demonstrable. Tarulli, on the contrary, found in the normal urine a ferment having the same influence as trypsin. The amount varied according to the time of day. In cases of long inanition, an increase of the ferment was parallel with the decrease of the leucocytes of the blood. In order to ascertain the conditions of pancreatic secretion, the pancreatic duct of a dog was tied, when large amounts of enzymes appeared in the urine. In a second dog, after the extirpation of the pancreas, the ferment disappeared entirely from the urine. This also happened in a patient with diffuse malignant degeneration of the gland.

5. **Pancreatic Secretion.**—(*a*) *Innervation.*—The dependence of the pancreatic secretion on nervous influence is shown by the fact that it has been possible to cause the production of an efficient secretion by reflex excitation. Gottlieb was able to stimulate the gland to secretion by the introduction into the stomach or intestine of certain substances, as oil of mustard, dilute sulphuric acid, or concentrated solutions of sodium carbonate. Likewise it was possible, by a pretense of feeding, to cause activity of the gland. Evidently the secretion of the acid gastric juice acts as a stimulator of the function of the gland.

[Pawlow *: "The energetic action of acid upon the pancreatic gland is one of the most constant facts in all the physiology of the pancreas. Acid is so powerful an excitant of the pancreatic gland that it is the agent above all others which is capable of forcing the activity of the gland." Red pepper and mustard inserted into the stomach instead of hydrochloric acid have not the slightest exciting action on the pancreas. Pawlow explains the contrary results of Gottlieb † on the ground that the strength of the solutions of pepper and mustard which he employed destroyed the mucosa to such an extent that, the centripetal nerves themselves were excited and not their peripheral extremities. The reader is referred to Pawlow's lectures for the further discussion of this and other questions relating to the physiology of the pancreas.—ED.]

By direct stimulation of the nerve it has also been possible to establish the dependence of the secretion upon the vagus and splanchnic nerves. The frequent failure of the earlier experimenters is explained by the fact that the vasoconstrictor fibers of the abdominal cavity are easily stimulated with the other nerves, and the anemia of the pancreas resulting from this stimulation makes it impossible to cause the production of pancreatic juice. After excluding this source of error, Pawlow and his students, Mett and Kudrewetzky, were able to show that the main course of the stimulating nervous influence ran in the vagus; this could be shown with certainty by stimulation of the peripheral stump of the vagus in the abdomen, especially after a higher section of the cord. The splanchnic is to be regarded as the inhibitory nerve of the pancreas (Morat). The results of experiments in this line, however, are by no means so clear as those regarding vagus excitation. After consecutive stimulation of the sympathetic, the secretion caused by stimulation of the vagus is increased in amount and density, and the amount of ferment is also increased (Kudrewetzky). Section of the sympathetic

* " Le Travail des Glandes Digestives," Paris, 1901, p. 185.
† *Arch. f. exp. Pathol. u. Pharmakol.*, Bd. xxxiii.

plexus supplying the vessels of the gland leads to an abundant secretion (paralytic pancreatic juice—Bernstein). According to Popelski, a pupil of Pawlow, the nerves in the gland limiting its secretion run along the straight line parallel to the attachment of the pancreas to the duodenum. [E. Wertheimer and Lepage * severed the vagi and thoracic sympathetic, and having curarized the animal kept it alive by artificial respiration. In such an animal dilute solutions of hydrochloric acid (0.5%) markedly increased the secretion of pancreatic juice if they were inserted not only into the duodenum, but also into the jejunum and ileum for one-fourth to one-third of its length. Below the appendix the acid was without effect, and the same held true of injections into the blood. In other experiments the dorsal and lumbar cords were cut in addition, and the duodenum and jejunum divided. The abdominal organs were thus completely severed from the central nervous system, but the acid acted in quite the same way as before. Wertheimer therefore concludes that the centers are in the celiac and mesenteric ganglia.

Popielski † obtained similar results and by methods similar to those of Wertheimer, only he carried the investigation one step further by destroying the celiac ganglion in addition to the other structures above mentioned. He was therefore forced to the conclusion that the dilute hydrochloric acid acts on the gland itself or the nervous apparatus contained in it.—ED.]

(*b*) *Effect of Different Foods on Pancreatic Secretion.*—Wassilieff found that the amount of ferment was essentially different with various foods. Meat increased the amount of tryptic ferment and decreased its amylolytic power. A bread-and-milk diet had the opposite effect. After the formation of a permanent pancreatic fistula, only bread and milk should be given to the animals at first. Walter arrived at similar results. He asserted so marked an adaptability of the pancreas for the work of digestion that the existence of a very sensitive peripheral nerve apparatus in the mucosa of the digestive canal must be recognized.

(*c*) *Pancreatic Secretion in Fever.*—Stolnikow investigated the secretion of the gland in the beginning of fever, and found it increased; later it was diminished, and finally ceased. The amount of ferment in the gland is likewise at first increased; in fever of longer duration, however, there is a decided diminution. But the gland is never entirely free from the ferment, even when the secretion is entirely stopped. The addition of an ichorous fluid hinders the influence of the ferment only when it is present in large amounts.

III. GENERAL PATHOLOGY AND SYMPTOMATOLOGY.

THE physiologic significance of the pancreas is clear up to a certain point. It is known what function belongs to this gland in the collaboration and assimilation of food-stuffs, and what and how much it has to do; later another, the so-called internal function, which relates to the change of sugar, will be shown. One would think that in the event of a disturbance in the function of the pancreas from disease of this organ

* *Jour. de Physiol.*, III, 5, pp. 689–708.
† *Pflüger's Archiv*, LXXXVI, 5, 6, p. 215.

such distinct symptoms would result that the recognition of this disturbance both qualitatively and quantitatively would be very easy. The facts of the case, however, are quite different. Characteristic pathologic symptoms are rarely found in diseases of the pancreas. The explanation is as follows:

1. For each physiologic function of the pancreas which concerns digestion, a compensatory organ is present, which is qualified to do the work left by the failure of the pancreatic function. The stomach* takes care of the digestion of the proteids, the bile and to a certain extent the intestinal juice provide for the emulsification of the fats, while amylolysis is the work of the salivary glands and certain intestinal glands. Even the decomposition of fat is not the exclusive function of the pancreas. In the lower part of the intestine there are micro-organisms which participate in this work and even carry further the decomposition of the free fatty acids into lower carbon compounds (Hédon and Ville).

2. The anatomic structure is of importance. As a rule, in man the pancreas has two excretory ducts, and whenever one of these is obstructed or the portion of the gland corresponding to this duct is incapable of function, the other duct assumes its duties vicariously. The fact that the liver has only one duct explains the constancy of the pathologic symptoms in case of obstruction of this duct.

3. A large portion of the gland may be destroyed or become incapable of function and the rest will be entirely sufficient for the work required. A considerable portion of the gland may be destroyed by acute or chronic inflammation, by hemorrhage, necrosis, new-formations, or cysts, and the remainder of the gland may perform the function sufficiently, especially with regard to the internal function. But this is also conceivable for the digestive action, if at least one excretory duct is available. These facts will be found illustrated in a great number of cases.

4. Diseases of the pancreas are frequently combined with diseases of neighboring organs. They may occur as a part of the symptom-complex of diseases of the stomach, of the intestine, of the bile-passages, and of the liver. Ulcerations or tumors of the stomach may extend to the pancreas and there excite inflammation, ulceration, or tumor formation. An extension from the intestine is the most frequent occurrence. Different processes, which are common in the small intestine, simple catarrhs, bacterial processes, deep-seated inflammations, and new-formations may be transferred from the intestine to the pancreas. They may lead to inflammations of the pancreatic duct or of the parenchyma of the gland, to obstruction of the pancreatic duct, or to cyst formation. From the neighboring lymph-glands, also, different pathologic processes may extend to the pancreas.

From the bile-passages inflammations or new-formations may extend to the pancreatic ducts and cause acute or chronic inflammations or new-formations in the parenchyma of the gland. Concretions in the bile-

---

* [Volhard (Zeit. f. klin. Med., 1901, XLII, p. 414) has again called attention to the digestion of fat in the stomach which was first suggested by Marcet (The Med. Times and Gazette, New Series, 1858, vol. XVII, p. 210) and confirmed by Cash, Ogata, and others. His conclusions are as follows: The gastric juice contains a fat-splitting ferment which is produced chiefly in the mucous membrane of the fundus. It can be extracted with glycerin and will pass through a Clay filter. Its action is hindered and finally destroyed by pepsin-hydrochloric acid.—ED.]

passages may lead to closure of the pancreatic duct, with the usual consequences.

On the other hand, it happens in many cases of diseases of the pancreas that the neighboring organs are likewise affected. Many pathologic processes have their seat in the head of the pancreas and may in consequence lead to compression of the ductus choledochus, to icterus and its consequences.

Inflammations, especially acute purulent processes, may extend to neighboring organs and new formations of the pancreas may be continued to the latter. Compression of the intestine with symptoms of obstruction may result from ulceration, hemorrhage, abscesses, neoplasms, and cysts. Severe pain may be produced by pressure upon the neighboring ganglia of the inflamed, hemorrhagic, neoplastic, or cystic gland.

Very confusing pictures may arise through these manifold combinations, because the symptoms which depend upon the diseases of the neighboring organs may be much sharper and more definite than the disturbances arising from the diseased pancreas itself.

The facts mentioned explain sufficiently why the really characteristic symptoms, so far as they are known, are only rarely recognized, and why during life in most cases only such symptoms come to light as are common to diseases of the pancreas and a large number of diseases of the organs adjacent to the pancreas.

The symptoms, according to their pathologic importance, form three groups:

A. Characteristic symptoms.

B. Symptoms which, according to the views of older or more recent authors, are to be referred to disease of the pancreas, although no very satisfactory proof has been brought forward.

C. Symptoms which, although important and significant, show no features peculiar to a diseased pancreas.

A. FIRST GROUP.

The characteristic symptoms which point to disturbances of the manifold functions of the pancreas are, naturally, in spite of their relatively rare occurrence, the important and determining ones; they accordingly demand a detailed and comprehensive representation in the general consideration, because they do not occur in any special diseases of the pancreas, but are symptoms of different processes, manifestations of a disturbance of function, which may be produced by various causes.

1. DIABETES AND GLYCOSURIA AS SYMPTOMS OF DISEASES OF THE PANCREAS.

The title indicates precisely the limits of my treatment of this subject. It is not purposed to discuss here the whole question of diabetes, which is reserved in this handbook for the pen of a more distinguished writer. It is only suggested why and how glycosuria or diabetes may be a symptom of disease of the pancreas. The facts which relate to the occurrence of diabetes in diseases of the pancreas will be noted only, the prevalent views and hypotheses which are advanced to explain these facts will be mentioned, and the many loop-holes in our knowledge which must remain to be filled by later investigators will be indicated.

In the search for an organ which should be responsible for the mysterious pathogenesis of diabetes, the pancreas was long since thought of. The earliest noteworthy communication in this direction was published in 1788 by Cowley, who found diabetes in an alcoholic patient thirty-four years old who was also very fleshy. At the autopsy the pancreas was found to be filled with small calculi, some as large as peas, firmly embedded in the substance of the gland; they were white and raspberry shaped. In 1821 Chopart mentioned a case of diabetes with calculi in the pancreas. Bright reported in 1833 the case of a diabetic, nineteen years old, who had also jaundice and fatty stools and died of marasmus. At the autopsy he found the head of the pancreas changed into a hard, nodular tumor which was firmly united to the duodenum; the ductus choledochus was closed at its entrance into the duodenum and the gland was atrophied. Elliotson described the case of a diabetic, forty-five years old, who had fatty stools. At the autopsy the pancreatic duct, including the large lateral branches, was found filled with concretions. Other similar communications were published by Fles, Hartsen, v. Recklinghausen, Munk, and Silver.

Since then the pathogenesis of diabetes has often been ascribed to the pancreas. Frerichs, Seegen, and Friedreich mention the not infrequent concurrence of diabetes and pancreatic disease, without, however, expressing any decided views on the question. Friedreich says regarding it: "According to my opinion, the combination of pancreatic disease with diabetes has to be regarded in different ways. We must distinguish between preceding affections of the pancreas, as cancer, chronic indurative inflammation, stone formation, etc., in the course of which secondary mellituria occurs, and primary diabetes, in which a secondary disturbance of nutrition of the pancreas (simple atrophy, fatty degeneration) takes place." Among 30 cases of diabetes mellitus in the postmortem records of the Vienna General Hospital atrophy of the pancreas, sometimes of high degree or combined with fatty change, was found by Seegen 13 times; once numerous calculi were found in the Wirsungian duct and once the pancreas was changed into a gray indurated band.

According to Frerichs, atrophy, fatty degeneration, and induration of the pancreas are frequently found in diabetes. He laid especial weight on two cases in which diabetes was directly associated with an acute disease of the pancreas which ended in suppuration.

A very pronounced stand on this question is taken by French authors. Bouchardat was the first, in 1875, to suggest the dependence of diabetes on disease of the pancreas, resting his conclusions on his own observations and those of older writers. Soon afterward Lancereaux developed his theory of *diabètes maigre*, in which he claimed to have found always changes in the pancreas. His pupils, Lapierre and Baumel, brought forward new clinical facts to support the theory of pancreatic diabetes. In Germany an attitude of reserve was maintained toward the new doctrine.

The pancreatic theory first received a firm support through the fundamental experiments of v. Mering and Minkowski, and since their investigations this subject has remained not simply in the foreground of discussion, but the diseased pancreas has been accepted as a cause of diabetes by a large number of investigators, physiologists, clinicians, and pathologists; many of these even claiming that it is possible that the pancreas alone is responsible for the occurrence of diabetes.

In order to explain with the greatest possible objectivity the present stand on this important question, it seems best to state the results of experimental and clinical investigations up to the present time and to examine into their value.

(a) EXPERIMENTAL PANCREATIC DIABETES.

For the purpose of ascertaining the function of the pancreas and the symptoms after elimination of the organ, attempts long ago were made to extirpate the pancreas in animals. The first of these experiments were made by L. Brunner, who removed a portion of the gland from young dogs. The animals lived and showed no changes. Later Bernard attempted the extirpation of the pancreas. He was unsuccessful with dogs, and declared it impracticable. In birds death occurred from marasmus eight to ten days after extirpation. Berard and Colin found no disturbances of digestion after extirpation of the pancreas. After death only small bits of intact pancreas were found in the animals. Schiff also had negative results. He was able to keep alive only birds, ravens and pigeons, for some time after extirpation of the entire organ. In 1881 Martinotti declared the extirpation of the pancreas in dogs to be possible. These animals were said to show no abnormality afterward. After the removal of the pancreas, nuclear division was found in the glands of Lieberkühn as an indication that these glands were acting vicariously for the extirpated organ. In none of the communications above mentioned was it stated whether sugar was found in the urine in these animals after extirpation of the gland.

Of most decided importance in this connection were the experiments described in 1889 by v. Mering and Minkowski, who succeeded in a perfectly unquestionable manner in producing genuine diabetes with all the manifestations of this well-studied disease of man. At about the same time de Dominicis reached nearly the same result, which, however, was published somewhat later.

Through the epoch-making discovery of v. Mering and Minkowski, a solid foundation for the first time was laid for further investigation in the hitherto rather barren discussion concerning pancreatic diabetes; further advance was next made by Minkowski alone. A large number of investigators of all countries then studied this subject: de Dominicis, Lépine, de Renzi and Reale, Hédon, Gley, Thiroloix, Gaglio, Capparelli, Harley, Schabad, Sandmeyer, Seelig, Rumbold, etc.

With few exceptions all these investigators confirmed the views of v. Mering and Minkowski, but a number of very interesting and important details were also brought to light. Although at present a satisfactory solution of the diabetes mystery is still in doubt, yet a path has no doubt been opened which may lead to the desired end.

The attempt to produce diabetes by extirpation of the pancreas has not succeeded in all animals. Minkowski was able to produce it in dogs, in a cat, and in a pig. Harley also had positive results in cats. In rabbits, Minkowski had no positive results, while Hédon produced diabetes in several instances by the injection of olive oil into the ductus Wirsungianus of rabbits and by this means caused certain changes of tissue. The glycosuria, however, occurred first three to five weeks after the operation and lasted but a short time. The experiments on rabbits of Weintraud, who resected portions of the intestine in order to remove the pancreas as thoroughly as possible, and found sugar temporarily on the day after the operation in two cases, were not convincing, as glycosuria may easily occur after similar severe operations.

In pigeons and ducks, Minkowski found no glycosuria after extirpation of the pancreas. After 15 out of 19 operations performed on ducks, Weintraud found no sugar in the urine, but in four of the series the excretion of the sugar was demonstrated. Kausch, who very recently again experimented on ducks, always removed at the same time the adjacent piece of the duodenum, as a complete separation of the pancreas was not possible in any other way. In nearly all cases (76 out of 83) the amount of sugar in the blood was increased. The same result occurred in 17 geese, but in these animals the amount of sugar in the blood increased much more slowly after the operation than in ducks. Occurrence of sugar in the urine was noted in relatively few of the ducks operated upon. Kausch concluded from his experiments that in ducks the extirpation of the pancreas caused essentially the same changes as in mammalia. The difference consists only in the fact that ducks use up the increased sugar in the blood, which is not the case in dogs. In birds of prey Langendorf and Weintraud found a glycosuria until the death of the animals, while in ravens the result was inconstant. In frogs and turtles, Aldehoff had positive results. In the former the glycosuria appeared slowly and developed only four to five days after the operation. In turtles it occurred in the first twenty-four to forty-eight hours. In every case the animals died after the operation. Minkowski was not able to show the presence of sugar in the urine of frogs. Marcus generally had positive results in his experiments on frogs. Velich's experiments showed that in nine out of fifteen frogs from which the pancreas was removed glycosuria developed after the operation. Capparelli operated on eels; glycosuria occurred twice in eleven cases.

By far the most constant results are obtained in the operations on dogs, on which the most numerous experiments have been performed. The results of these experiments form the foundation for the following statements.

An essential difference exists between the results of a total and a partial extirpation of the pancreas.

According to Minkowski, the total removal of the gland regularly results in diabetes. This view is supported by Hédon, Gley, Gaglio, Capparelli, Harley, Schabad, Sandmeyer, Seelig, Rumbold, and Dutto. Lépine and Thiroloix noted the absence of diabetes only in those cases in which the animals had been starved for some time before the operation. Other authors, as de Dominicis, de Renzi and Reale, Rémond, and Cavazzani deny the constancy of diabetes after the extirpation of the pancreas.

De Dominicis is to be regarded as the main supporter of the theory of the inconstancy of the glycosuria. He assumes, however, that the removal of the gland or its elimination according to his method is always followed by the other symptoms of diabetes, as emaciation, phosphaturia, etc.

Reale noted the occurrence of glycosuria in only 75% of the cases. In experiments undertaken by himself in company with de Renzi, diabetes resulted in 18 out of the 22 dogs on which they operated. Rémond is likewise convinced·that glycosuria does not always occur after total extirpation of the pancreas. Of three dogs which survived the operation for some time, only two were affected with diabetes. Also, in two dogs the gland which had become indurated by ligation of the excretory duct was removed without causing diabetes. In a third, fatal cachexia was observed, without glycosuria. The brothers Cavazzani also were not always able to show the occurrence of glycosuria after extirpation of the pancreas. In opposition to all these objections, Minkowski strongly maintains that the absence of the glycosuria can only be explained by the assumption that in the experiments mentioned the gland was not totally extirpated.

After complete removal of the pancreas the excretion of sugar, according to Minkowski, is as follows: The time of the first appearance of sugar after the operation varies in different cases. Frequently it occurs after the first hour following the operation. Often it does not occur until later, and its first appearance has been observed on the third day.

These differences are in part based on the condition of the gland at the time of the operation. In those cases in which diabetes did not appear until the third day, the gland at the time of its removal appeared very hyperemic and its function was evidently active. On the other hand, the kind and amount of nourishment given the animal before the operation are of great importance in determining the occurrence of glycosuria.

As a rule, the excretion of sugar increases in intensity, and, even when no nourishment is given, it generally reaches its maximum of 8% to 10% on the third day.

That the amount of carbohydrate present in the organism is related to the amount of the gradually increasing excretion of sugar is shown by the experiment of Minkowski, from which it appears that in the dog which had been abundantly fed beforehand on meat and bread the ratio between the sugar and the total nitrogen (D : N) increased most rapidly.

The further course of the sugar elimination is essentially dependent on the nourishment. With abundant nourishment, an amount of 10% to 12% in the day's excretion of 1 to 1½ liters is not at all rare. Even after complete withdrawal of nourishment as long as seven days the sugar does not entirely disappear from the urine. With a pure meat diet or in starvation, a constant relation generally exists between the sugar and the total nitrogen (D : N). This ratio is usually about 2.8 : 1. All the grape-sugar introduced with the food may be found in the urine.

When the affection has lasted for some time and the physical strength of the animal begins to diminish, the intensity of the excretion of sugar also diminishes, especially with the occurrence of complicating diseases.

The views are widely different with regard to the cause of this diminution of intensity of the diabetes after the long continuance of the disease. Lépine, de Renzi and Reale, and Hédon assume that it is due to a vicarious assumption of the duties of the pancreas by other organs. Minkowski, on the other hand, believes that the cause is to be sought in a disturbance of sugar production, "perhaps also in a decomposition of the sugar under the influence of pathologic processes; for instance, under that of pathogenic bacteria." He bases his view on an experiment which shows that even the dextrose introduced into the body leaves it without being utilized. If it were really a question of a better function of the powers regulating the digestion of sugar, then it would be impossible to explain this continual impossibility of utilizing the sugar added to the organism. It perhaps may be a question of toxicogenic influences. Capparelli was able to show that injections of emulsified pancreas into the peritoneum of marasmic animals with diminished excretion of sugar caused the apparent weakness to disappear and at the same time produced an increase of the glycosuria, thus forming additional proof that the lessening of the output of sugar did not indicate any improvement in the diabetes.

Our own experiments correspond in the main with the results communicated by other experimenters.

EXPERIMENT OF NOVEMBER 14, 1893.—The pancreas of a dog was entirely extirpated. November 15th: Dog quite well. Bile pigment in the urine but no sugar. November 16th: No sugar in the urine. November 17th: The dog takes some milk. In the urine was found 4.8% of sugar. November 18th: Amount of sugar, 4.8%. November 20th: The dog ate some meat the day before; very much debilitated. No sugar. November 21st: Killed by bleeding. Amount of sugar in the blood 0.16%. After the meat was eaten, the stools were rich in undigested meat; tuft-like arrangement of the fat-acid needles; few bacteria. After autopsy, adhesive peritonitis.

Result: (a) Appearance of the excretion of sugar on the third day after the operation; (b) disappearance of the excretion of sugar before death, normal amount of sugar in the blood; (c) in the stools, much undigested meat.

EXPERIMENT OF FEBRUARY 24, 1894.—Total extirpation of the pancreas under morphin narcosis. The operation lasted two and one-half hours. February 25th: Traces of sugar in the afternoon urine. February 26th: Amount of sugar, 1%. An intense diabetes developed without polyuria or azoturia. The maximum amount of sugar in the urine reached 13.6%. On the sixth of April the animal died of exhaustion, and 6.8% of sugar was observed in the urine two days before death.

Result: (a) Excretion of sugar on the day after the operation (traces), 1% on the second day, and 7.5% on the next day. (b) The maximum excretion of sugar reached 13.6%. Two days before death 6.8% was present in the urine. (c) The amount of indican in the urine was increased, but the excretion of sulphuric acid showed no marked variation from the normal. The animal lived forty-one days after the operation.

EXPERIMENT OF JUNE 19, 1894.—Total extirpation of the pancreas. June 20th: The urine contained traces of sugar. Indican was present in moderate amount. June 21st: Urine icteric and contained 0.8% of sugar. June 22d: In the urine 3.1% of sugar and the indican increased. June 23d: In the urine 2.4% of sugar, no acetone. June 24th: Dog found dead. Hemorrhagic exudate in the abdominal cavity.

Result: The glycosuria occurred on the day after the operation, but did not reach a high degree.

After partial extirpation, v. Mering and Minkowski found no glycosuria when the greater part (one-fourth to one-fifth) of the gland was left behind. On the basis of later experiments, Minkowski asserts that after partial extirpation of the pancreas the occurrence of glycosuria is determined not so much by the size of the piece of the pancreas that is left as by the condition of the gland after the operation. In two cases diabetes of the severest form followed this operation, once after five days and the second time after three days; in both cases the autopsy showed that the portion of the gland remaining was entirely destroyed.

At times the occurrence of the diabetes can be prevented by the presence of very small and morbid bits of gland. For instance, Thiroloix reports an experiment on a dog weighing 33 lbs., in which no diabetes occurred for twenty-seven days. At the autopsy a piece of sclerotic pancreas weighing 1½ gm. was found. In other cases glycosuria occurred, even although pieces of pancreas weighing 3 or 4 gm. had been left behind.

Minkowski was able to show the most varied degrees of diabetes after partial extirpation of the pancreas. In 15 of 32 cases transient glycosuria was found; in three cases, where one-eighth to one-twelfth of the gland was left, a diabetes of the lightest form developed as an alimentary glycosuria. In one case where the largest part of the gland was removed and only a small portion remained, after having been transplanted beneath the skin of the abdomen a diabetes of moderate severity developed.

These observations therefore appear of the greatest importance, because they show that even mild cases of diabetes are referable to pancreatic disturbances.

In order to show that the diabetes was not caused by some unavoidable injury to nerves during the operation, Minkowski performed the following experiment: In one case he removed all attachments of the pancreas to the mesentery, so that it remained in connection only with the duodenum; in two other cases, after ligating the ductus Wirsungianus, he severed all connections with the duodenum. In none of these cases did diabetes occur. The same result was shown by other experiments of Minkowski. If the partial extirpation was so managed that the portions of the gland which were left behind in the one experiment were removed in the other, then the influence of accidental injuries or nerve lesions would be shown. As in all these cases no diabetes occurred, it proves that the cause of the diabetes is not to be sought in the accidental injuries.

Sandmeyer, after partial extirpation of the pancreas with progressive atrophy of the portions of the gland remaining, observed a progressive diabetes, which, after some months, ended fatally. In a dog in which the vessels of the portion of the gland remaining had been ligated, diabetes of a light form soon appeared, three months later increased in intensity, and lasted until death. In a second case, in which the blood-vessels had remained intact, the first traces of sugar appeared seven weeks after the operation; only after twelve months was there an increase in the excretion of sugar, and only after thirteen and a half months did permanent diabetes develop, which eight months later caused the death of the animal experimented upon. At the autopsy the remains of the piece of gland which had been left behind were found adherent to the posterior wall of the stomach, midway between the pylorus and cardia. This remnant was 2.5 cm. long, 0.5 to 1.0 cm. wide, and 0.36 gm. in weight, of firm consistency, and showed no trace of glandular tissue. Moreover, in the lowest portion of the duodenum a particle of about the size of a pea was found, which felt soft and had a distinctly lobular character. On microscopic examination the piece attached to the stomach showed no trace of gland structure. The piece found on the duodenum consisted for the most part of very slightly changed gland tissue.

We may mention the following of our own experiments upon partial extirpation of the pancreas:

EXPERIMENT OF JANUARY 4, 1894.—*A* dog of medium size, weighing about 8 kilos, was operated upon under morphin narcosis. The large excretory duct of the pancreas was tied. Isolation from the intestine of a portion of the middle. Extirpation of the two lateral portions.

January 5th: Urine amber yellow. Specific gravity 1054, alkaline, 145 c.c. Total nitrogen 3.13%, 4.54 gm. in 145 c.c. Amount of sugar 3.0%, 4.35 gm. in 145 c.c. $N : D = 1 : 1.04$. Indican moderate in amount.

January 6th: Urine brownish-yellow, clear, acid. Total nitrogen 5.42%. Indican increased. Bile pigments present. Sugar not present.

January 7th: The dog received in the forenoon $\frac{1}{2}$ liter milk. No sugar in the urine. Traces of albumin and bile pigments are present. The total nitrogen reached 2.2%.

In the next days sugar was never demonstrable in the urine. With pure meat diet the dog excreted no sugar. The amount of the combined sulphuric acid was lessened. It reached: January 11th: Total SO_3, 0.606; combined SO_3, 0.032; ratio, 1 : 19.2. January 12th: Total SO_3, 0.662; combined SO_3, 0.022; ratio, 1 : 22.3. January 13th: Total SO_3, 0.394; combined SO_3, 0.069; ratio, 1 : 20.2.

On administration of grape-sugar, glycosuria occurred; after 10 gm. had been administered, traces of sugar appeared in the urine. For five days the animal received 220 gm. of horse meat and 50 gm. of sugar. During this time the amounts introduced and the amounts excreted were as follows:

January 26th:	N in the food,	13.32 gm.;	in the urine,	9.69 gm.;	sugar,	1.90 gm.
January 27th:	" " "	11.22	" " " "	10.68 "	"	3.04 "
January 28th:	" " "	11.75	" " " "	10.84 "	"	2.10 "
January 29th:	" " "	17.88	" " " "	10.25 "	"	1.80 "
January 30th:	" " "	13.00	" " " "	11.13 "	"	2.40 "

The total nitrogen in the stools during the time of the experiments reached 1.96 gm. In all, the amount of nitrogen introduced was 67.17 gm.; sugar, 250 gm. The total amount of nitrogen excreted was 52.55 gm.; sugar, 11.24 gm.

The estimation of fat in the stools yielded in 10 gm. of air-dried stool:

Ethereal extract	1.407 gm.	
Neutral fat	0.544 gm.	51.63%
Free fatty acids	0.494 gm.	46.04%
Soaps	0.025 gm.	2.33%

After introduction of cane-sugar glycosuria occurred. The cane-sugar was in part excreted as such.

On the 15th of May another operation was undertaken on the same dog, and the remaining piece of the pancreas, as far as possible, was removed. In this operation only a piece as large as a walnut remained behind. On May 16th the urine contained 2.2% of sugar. On the next day no sugar was present. The same was true later. The dog was sick, feverish, and vomited several times.

After the dog recovered he received on the 25th of May 50 gm. of grape-sugar. The urine secreted later was levorotatory. Subsequent additions of grape-sugar, 5 to 10 gm., gave a negative result as concerned the production of glycosuria.

June 27th: Subsequent laparotomy, from which the dog died.

From this experiment the following conclusions may be drawn:

1. Every operation on the pancreas was followed by transient glycosuria.

2. With exclusive meat diet, after 10 gm. of grape-sugar, a slight glycosuria occurred, and after 50 gm. it was more intense. Cane-sugar also caused alimentary glycosuria.

3. The food was well assimilated and the glycogen content was increased.

4. In the stools the free fatty acids and soaps appeared less than in the normal.

EXPERIMENT OF OCTOBER 3, 1894.—In this operation, all of the pancreas was removed except the descending portion. The spleen appeared remarkably large. In the intestine occasional transparent areas.

October 4th: Urine amber yellow; specific gravity 1024. Sugar not present. Phenylhydrazin test negative. Reduction test positive. Albumin not present. Acetone not present. Indican in small amounts.

October 5th: Urine brownish-yellow; specific gravity 1037. No albumin, no sugar. Urobilin, small amount. No bile pigments.

October 6th: Some vomiting after taking milk. Distinct urobilin reaction in the urine. Indican somewhat increased.

October 7th: The dog was very ill. Urine as on the preceding day. Indican in large amounts.

The stools were pultaceous and contained very numerous desquamated epithelial cells, mostly degenerated, but partly recognizable by their structure; they also contained a few bacteria, but no fat drops,

October 8th: Dog found dead. On section, a peritonitis was found.

EXPERIMENT OF JULY 10, 1894.—In a dog the lateral portions of the gland, with the exception of the duodenal piece, were extirpated.

The first day after the operation the urine was contaminated by vomited matter. Sugar could not be shown in it. The stools evacuated after the feeding of milk contained on microscopic examination numerous fat droplets.

July 16th: The dog was found dead. Cause of death, peritonitis suppurativa.

Results: In the experiments on partial extirpation of the pancreas we never succeeded in causing severe diabetes, but only transient glycosuria. In some cases sugar was never found in the urine.

If from the results hitherto communicated the conclusions are justifiable that the diabetes is not caused by nerve lesions or nerve injuries inflicted during the extirpation of the pancreas, the experiment performed by Minkowski of transplanting portions of the gland under the skin of the abdomen proves this conclusion even more conclusively and incontrovertibly.

He was able in dogs to separate the extreme end of the descending portion of the gland and to implant it under the skin of the abdomen, without injuring the arteries leading to that part. Under favorable conditions the implanted piece healed under the skin of the abdomen. Then the intra-abdominal portion of the gland was removed and no glycosuria occurred, not even the alimentary variety. The subsequent removal of the piece embedded under the skin produced the symptoms of a severe diabetes. The piece of pancreas embedded under the skin continued to secrete. Minkowski was able in five cases to form fistulæ, through which flowed a secretion which digested starch, and to a less degree fibrin. If the transplanted piece of gland is insufficiently nourished, then a slight degree of diabetes may develop.

It is not necessary that the secretion should be entirely intact. In one case Minkowski ligated a vein which passed upward from the transplanted piece, and yet no diabetes was observed. This experiment showed that a direct relation existed between the secretory function of the pancreas and that function which has to do with the production of sugar. Almost simultaneously with Minkowski, but independently of him, Hédon experimented, with like results. After extirpation of the intra-abdominal portion of the gland he observed emaciation of the animal experimented upon and increased secretion of nitrogen. At times Hédon also saw transient glycosuria after extirpation of the intra-abdominal portion of the gland. The removal of the implanted part of the gland was always followed by severe diabetes. The excretion of sugar was even greater than that following total extirpation of the pancreas, perhaps because the operation was less severe and the nutrition of the animals was unaffected, since they continued to feed as usual.   According to Hédon, the extirpation of the transplanted portions of the gland must be undertaken while the strength of the animal is good.   If the reverse is the case, the result is not direct.   This operation was followed only by a slight elimination of sugar in a dog whose common duct was tied at the same time, since the animal was in a wretched condition.

Thiroloix later obtained the same result.   He concluded from his experiments that the pancreas possessed an internal and an external secretion, the former controlling the sugar transformation, and that both were wholly independent of each other.   This view satisfactorily explains the instance where severe diabetes results despite the unaffected secretion from the implanted portions of the pancreas.   Evidently the internal secretion must have suffered.   Thiroloix found in the implanted portions cystic degeneration as well as intact pancreatic tissue.

Another view regarding the subject of implantation is held by de Dominicis.   He implanted from one-third to one-fourth of the gland beneath the skin of three dogs and found that the extirpation of the intra-abdominal portion of the pancreas was immediately followed by glycosuria to the extent of 100, 90, 80% respectively.   In two of the dogs, after the abdominal portion of the gland was extirpated, there was neither glycosuria nor any other evidence of the absence of pancreatic juice from the intestine.   At the autopsy it appeared that the implanted portion of the gland was not wholly freed from the duodenum, but was attached at one point.   In another case, after the removal of the intra-abdominal portion of the gland, all the disturbances arose which are due to the absence of pancreatic juice from the intestine.   Even after the removal of the transplanted piece there was no glycosuria.

These results have not been confirmed by other observers, but de Dominicis explains their experiments in the light of his theory by assuming, on the one hand, that the absence of pancreatic juice from the intestine is of essential importance in the production of glycosuria, while, on the other hand, after the extirpation of the intra-abdominal and transplanted portion of the pancreas the manifestations of diabetes with and without glycosuria develop.

The experiments with transplantation show with great certainty that the local extirpation of the pancreas is the cause of the diabetes and that the latter is the manifestation of the loss of a definite function of the pancreas.

Whether this attribute belongs to the pancreas alone or exists in other organs is not at present determined.   Minkowski considers it "more probable" that it is a special function of the pancreas.   De Renzi and Reale characterized the salivary glands as those organs the removal of which may result in diabetes.   Minkowski showed that in this event the glycosuria never reached a high degree and never lasted long.   This conclusion was reached also by Hédon, who tied the ductus Wirsungianus in a dog, extirpated the vertical branch of the pancreas, and in one operation removed all the eight salivary glands.   As a result of this operation only a slight glycosuria, lasting one day, occurred.

In like manner the glycosuria developing after resection of the intestine is not a true diabetes.   Weintraud, under the direction of Minkowski, resected different portions of the intestine, the pieces being of different size.   At times a glycosuria occurred, which, however, quickly passed away without further consequences. Lépine claims for the duodenal glands the characteristic of being able to take in part the place of the pancreas in its sugar-destroying (glycolytic) function. Falkenburg saw glycosuria develop after removal of the thyroid gland. All these experiments, as well as those especially of Hédon, Thiroloix, and Seelig, prove by no means conclusively that there are indeed other organs which may act vicariously for the pancreas in its influence on sugar metabolism.

Through the experiments which led to the production of pancreatic diabetes in animals a number of important and interesting results have been brought to light, which cannot here be referred to more in detail.

The relation to pancreatic diabetes of phloridzin diabetes, piqûre, and many other forms of diabetes variously brought about have been studied, and it has been shown that there are indeed various ways which lead to the excretion of sugar in the urine.

The loss of the digestive function of the pancreas which naturally results from the extirpation of this organ leads to severe disturbances of nutrition, to emaciation, and to rapid diminution of strength, and causes changes which become evident in the stools and in the urine. These important factors will again be referred to.

A thorough investigation of sugar metabolism requires studies into the fate of the glycogen stored in the liver, in the muscles, and in the leucocytes after the extirpation of the pancreas. On the one hand, hyperglycemia, and, on the other, disappearance of the glycogen from the liver, the muscles, and the leucocytes, are facts which are stated by all authors to occur after removal of the pancreas.

Nearly all authors who have made this theme a subject of experimental research have concerned themselves with the theory of the causation of diabetes after extirpation of the pancreas. This is the more intelligible since if a satisfactory explanation of experimental pancreatic diabetes is found, an essential factor is certainly discovered which may lead to the clearing up of the mystery of diabetes. Unfortunately, in spite of much labor, experiment, and speculation, and although much enthusiasm has entered into the work, no hypothesis has yet been found which can be regarded as wholly satisfactory.

Before the convincing experiments of Minkowski and v. Mering, there were certain clinical observations which indicated a relation between the pancreas and diabetes, and explanations were sought for such a relation.

Bouchardat assumed that in the absence of pancreatic secretion the stomach undertook the task of digesting the starches. In consequence, a perverted function of the stomach resulted. The blood was over-filled with sugar and the liver was no longer in condition to store this excess.

Popper believed that the liver formed the bile acids from the fatty acids resulting from the splitting-up of fat and from glycogen. If the cleavage of the fat was not accomplished by the pancreas, then the glycogen alone was changed into sugar, and when in excess was excreted with the urine.

Zimmer ascribed to the pancreas the duty of changing glucose into lactic acid. If the function of the pancreas be lessened, then the sugar must pass over into the blood unchanged.

All these hypotheses are pure speculations, and have been devised to explain the connection of the pancreas with diabetes, a connection which had been only assumed, but not demonstrated.

After the experimental proof of this connection presented by v. Mering and Minkowski, these experimenters, on the basis of their observations, could suggest only the choice of two hypotheses: (1) Either something abnormal is accumulated in the organism after the extirpation of the pancreas,—that is, the pancreas has normally the power of destroying an injurious substance as it is formed,—or (2) a normal function is lacking —that is, the pancreas normally has the power of regulating the consumption of sugar.

The former hypothesis was withdrawn by Minkowski on the basis of later experiments and only the second was considered plausible. Von Mering and Minkowski attempted to bring forward experimental proof of the existence of an injurious substance. They transfused a healthy animal with the blood of one at the acme of sugar excretion. A positive result of this experiment would have had great significance. From the negative results which actually were obtained nothing could be decided, for the healthy dog has all the conditions in his normal pancreas necessary for destroying this injurious substance when it is present. Of just as little value was the experiment of Hédon, who injected the blood of a diabetic dog into an animal which, after extirpation of the pancreas and when fed on meat, excreted only traces of sugar in the urine. After the transfusion there was no increase of sugar excretion in the urine.

Although the assumption of Minkowski that the diabetes after extirpation of the pancreas is to be ascribed to the retention of some substance —that is, to a kind of auto-intoxication—cannot wholly be disregarded, still his deductions regarding glycogen metabolism, sugar consumption, and blood diastasis in diabetic dogs offer weighty reasons against it. Most authors incline to the view of Minkowski that the pancreas produces something which influences the consumption of sugar in the organism, and that the diabetes occurring after the extirpation of the pancreas is due to the cessation of this production. This function is characterized as the internal secretion or, as Hansemann asserts, the positive function. According to the experiments of Thiroloix and Minkowski, this internal secretion is independent of the secretion of the pancreatic juice. Transplanted pieces of the pancreas may continue to secrete pancreatic juice and yet glycosuria occur, and, on the other hand, the secretion of the juice may cease in such transferred portions of the gland without the development of diabetes.

Although authors so generally agree that the digestion of sugar is regulated by such an internal secretion, yet there is quite a difference in the views regarding the nature and kind of influence of the internal secretion. The hypotheses regarding this point advanced by French writers deserve a somewhat more extended mention.

1. *Lépine's hypothesis:* On the basis of numerous experiments and studies, Lépine reached the conclusion that glycolytic ferment was produced in the pancreas, passed from the pancreas into the lymph, and thence into the blood, where it was contained in the white blood-corpuscles. The consumption of the sugar in the tissues takes place through the influence of this ferment. If, through failure of the corresponding function of the pancreas, this ferment is wanting, hyperglycemia and diabetes result.

Claude Bernard knew that the quantity of sugar in the blood diminished after venesection. Lépine gave the term glycolysis to this process and attributed it to the presence of a ferment chiefly produced in the pancreas. The extirpation of the gland, therefore, would result in the disappearance of the ferment or its considerable diminution, in case small quantities of it are produced in other organs and there give rise to the accumulation of sugar in the blood, hyperglycemia, and glycosuria.

The glycolytic power of the blood was ascertained by Lépine and Barral in the following way: They determined the amount of sugar in two portions of blood, one of which was examined immediately after it was drawn, the other after it had remained for one hour in the incubator at 37° C. (98.6° F.); in the second portion the experiment showed a diminution in the amount of sugar. In order to meet the objection that perhaps the glycogen which was present was transformed into sugar, a third portion was then heated to 54° C. (129.2° F.) in order to destroy the glycolytic ferment and then allowed to stand for one hour in the incubator. The amount of sugar was not changed. Thereby the absence of glycogen could be excluded.

On the basis of these experiments, no doubt could be admitted as to the fact that glycolysis occurs in the blood. It was only necessary to prove that this destruction of sugar was brought about through the action of a ferment and was not a postmortem phenomenon. Lépine next advanced an indirect proof of the ferment character of the substance which caused the glycolysis. He had shown, on the one hand, that heating the blood to 54° C. (129.2° F.) was sufficient to hinder the glycolysis, and that, analogous to the conduct of other ferments, lower temperatures delayed its occurrence, while it was most intense at 50° to 52° C. (122° to 125.6° F.). The production of fluids with powerful action by centrifuging the blood with sodium chlorid solution presented a direct proof of the existence of a soluble body in the blood; Lépine undertook to prove that it was of the nature of a ferment by changing the diastase of the saliva and pancreatic juice into a glycolytic ferment. By treating these fluids with 1% sulphuric acid, he claims to have transformed the amylolytic into a glycolytic enzyme.

That this ferment is not of postmortem origin is shown by the fact that the injection of a few drops of sterilized oil into the ductus Wirsungianus and stimulation of the nerves of the pancreas are sufficient to cause an increase of the glycolytic action of the blood. These experiments at the same time show the close relationship between the glycolytic ferment and the pancreas; they were confirmed by a further experiment of Lépine, in which he showed that electric stimulation of the peripheral stump of the vagus nerve increased the glycolytic power of the blood, while this influence was absent in animals in which the pancreas had been extirpated. On the basis of all these experiments and observations it could be assumed that the glycolytic ferment was formed in the pancreas, taken up by the white blood-corpuscles, and carried into the circulation; but as the sugar is found only in the blood plasma, it will in reality appear first when the white blood-corpuscles are destroyed. The glycolytic action of the blood observed outside of the organism is accordingly dependent on two factors: the richness of the blood in ferment and the rapidity with which the leucocytes are destroyed. According to Lépine, this is influenced not only by the pancreas, but also by other organs, especially the duodenal glands, which appear to take part in the production of the ferment.

The experiments on 150 dogs carried on by Lépine likewise showed that a diminution of the glycolysis in the blood went hand in hand with the extirpation of the pancreas. In man also he found a greater or less diminution, but did not venture to generalize on these facts. Very recently Lépine claims to have caused a diminution of the glycosuria in some diabetics by the use of the glycolytic ferments produced from diastase.

Signorini also found that the pancreas had a marked glycolytic power. He believed that glycolytic characteristics could also be ascribed to the urine; this agrees very well with the assumption of a ferment, so much the more as, after heating, the power of destroying sugar is lost.

Mansel Sympson also found that pancreatic extract had a glycolytic function, and that if sugar solutions were treated with it, the amount of sugar was much diminished after ten hours' stay in the incubator. On boiling, this extract lost its power.

Although this theory was apparently so well founded, yet a number of weighty objections removed its firm basis. The consideration of the process as a vital one, the ferment nature of the glycolytic agent, the constancy of its presence, and especially its diminution after extirpation of the pancreas as well as in human diabetes, were all questioned.

Shortly after Lépine's first publication, Arnaud took the ground that it was not a fermentative action, but a peculiarity inherent in the blood. Lépine and Barral could easily contradict this view by the proof that it was not easy to procure a fluid of glycolytic action by washing out the blood-corpuscles in the centrifuge with sodium chlorid solution.

In Lépine's experiment of changing diastase into glycolytic ferment in order to establish the ferment character of the glycolytic agent, Nasse was not able to confirm Lépine's results. Although Lépine has lately taken the opposite stand, yet it appears from more recent experiments that the transformation of the one ferment into the other is scarcely probable.

The most weighty objection against Lépine's theory was, however, raised by Seegen, who showed that the process of glycolysis could hardly be regarded as vital. It can be shown that chloroform, which destroys the life of the cell, does not affect the glycolytic action; that the passage of air through contaminated blood at a high temperature causes considerable destruction of sugar; and especially that in the second and third hours after the removal of the blood the glycolysis is greater than in the first, increasing, therefore, at the time when the vital conditions in the blood are becoming poorer.

Physiologic experiments also were made to show that glycolysis was not a vital process. Arthus examined the fluid blood drawn from the jugular vein of a horse and was unable to show any destruction of sugar, in spite of the fact that the blood was apparently alive. On the other hand, he added sodium fluorid to the blood taken from the vein, and in this way checked glycolysis, which was not stopped if a certain time intervened between the removal of the blood and the addition of the sodium fluorid. The value of this experiment was denied by Lépine; but it has recently been shown by the experiments of Colenbrander that glycolysis stands in close relation with the postmortem destruction of the white blood-cells, since the injection of leech extract, which preserves the leucocytes, in contrast to other substances which restrict coagulation, hinders the destruction of sugar.

By these facts, confirmed by other investigators, a specific glycolytic power of the blood is rendered very doubtful. It seems as if we are concerned in the consumption of sugar in the blood, with a property of one or more of the various tissues to act as oxygen-carriers (Spitzer).

From this preliminary statement we can readily understand the contradictions found by various authors (Sansoni, Kraus, Minkowski) in their investigations of the glycolytic ferment of normal and pathologic, especially of diabetic blood. Lépine also, in his investigations on diabetics, found no constancy in the diminution of the glycolytic ferment, while his experiments on 150 dogs gave a constant diminution in the amount of ferment, although it varied in degree. From his standpoint, he reached the very justifiable conclusion that diabetes was not a nosologic unit, and was not produced exclusively by changes in the pancreas.

Experiments performed by A. Katz gave results corresponding perfectly with the data mentioned, and showed that the doctrine of the glycolytic ferment rested on a very insufficient foundation.

(a) In spite of numerous attempts, he was unable by the action of 1% sulphuric acid on the ordinary diastase of trade, as well as on the extremely active taka-diastase, to transform them into the glycolytic ferment.

(b) An increase of the glycolysis could be caused by the addition of blood poisons, as sodium taurocholate. So, for instance, in one experiment, the percentage of the loss of sugar in the unchanged blood was 17.41%, and after the addition of the sodium taurocholate it reached 30.84%; in a second experiment before the addition it reached 20.34%, and afterward 51.97%.

(c) Glycolysis could also be increased by preventing the coagulation of the blood by the addition of leech extract immediately after the blood was removed from the vein.

(d) A diminution of the glycolytic action also takes place in blood prevented from coagulation by the injection of peptone. In one experiment the peptone did not have the desired effect and the blood taken after the injection was clotted. The loss of sugar before the injection was 65%, and afterward 63%. In another experiment, in which the blood did not coagulate after the injection of peptone, the loss of sugar before the injection was 71.85%, and afterward 52.10%. From these experiments the conclusion is permissible that there is a parallelism between glycolysis and the postmortem process of coagulation of the blood, and that, accordingly, the glycolysis runs parallel with postmortem changes.

(e) In order to diminish the percentage of loss of sugar it is sufficient to increase the amount of sugar in the blood by the injection of sugar. In one case the amount of sugar in the blood before the injection was 0.226%, but fell to 0.146% after the blood had remained for two hours in the incubator; after the injection of 30 gm. of grape-sugar the percentage was increased to 1.019, but after two hours in the incubator it was lowered to 1.017. Glycolysis therefore had not taken place. In another case the sugar-content was 0.221%, and after three hours' stay in the warm oven it reached 0.191%; after the injection of the sugar the amount of sugar-content was increased to 1.706%, but after three hours it had fallen to 1.604%. The percentage of loss was at first 14%, and later only 5.4%, although an absolutely larger amount of sugar had been decomposed.

A diminution in the percentage of destruction of sugar can, therefore, be brought about by simply increasing the absolute amount of sugar, without causing any lesion of the pancreas. Even with the assumption of a glycolytic ferment, therefore, the diminution of the percentage of loss of sugar in a given time by no means warrants the conclusion that an injury of the pancreas is involved.

Very recently Lépine transferred the stage of activity of the glycolytic ferment from the blood to the tissues. By so doing, as Minkowski mentions in a critical review, he has eliminated a great portion of the above-mentioned objections, and the "assumption of such a ferment no longer appears impossible," although the conclusive proof of it still is lacking.

2. *Hypothesis of Chauveau and Kaufmann:* In opposition to those theories which explain the diabetes after extirpation of the pancreas as due to a diminution in the destruction of sugar, Chauveau and Kaufmann assume an increase of the production of sugar in the liver. Regarding the sugar-producing function, the liver and pancreas appear to them to be closely related and dependent upon each other. The pancreas, through the mechanism of the nervous system, regulates the production of sugar in the liver. An inhibitory center for this function is situated in the medulla oblongata and a stimulating center in the upper part of the cervical cord. The former is in relationship with the sympathetic system through the rami communicantes of the upper cervical nerves, the latter through the rami communicantes of the upper portion of the dorsal cord. The pancreas exerts a reversed action on these two centers.

If the spinal cord is cut below the fourth pair of cervical nerves and above the sixth dorsal nerves, then only the inhibitory center acts, as above the point of section fibers run from it to the sympathetic. The center for stimulation of glucose formation in the liver is, however, thrown out of service, and therefore extirpation of the pancreas can no longer lead to diabetes.

If the medulla oblongata between the atlas and occiput is cut across, then the influence of the inhibitory center is lost and that of the stimulation center prevails, so that hyperglycemia and glycosuria occur. They are, however, not so severe as after extirpation of the pancreas, as in this case only the loss of one inhibition is concerned, while in the extirpation of the pancreas, which stimulates the inhibitory center and inhibits the stimulation center of the liver, there is a twofold restriction of sugar production, and therefore the hyperglycemia and glycosuria must be considerably increased.

This theory, which considered it necessary to appeal to nervous influences in explaining the condition of pancreatic diabetes, was not, however, supported. In a later work Kaufmann showed that, even when all nerves leading to the liver were divided, diabetes developed after extirpation of the pancreas. The influence of the pancreas on the liver, therefore, can be exerted directly without the intervention of the nerves. Under this assumption, the transplantation experiments are explained in a perfectly natural way, since the products of internal secretion of the pancreas have a direct influence on the liver.

The close relation found by Chauveau and Kaufmann between the pancreas, the liver, and the nervous system would teach, further, that disturbances of the internal secretion of the pancreas with all their consequences may be caused by changes outside of the gland, and so appear to justify those attempts to refer all cases of diabetes to one and the same type, which is represented by that form produced by extirpation of the pancreas.

The soundness of the theory of Chauveau and Kaufmann was attacked especially by Minkowski, who contested its very foundation. Chauveau and Kaufmann hold that the consumption of sugar is not diminished in pancreatic diabetes, and support their opinion by an experiment which showed that the blood of the femoral vein in comparison to that of the femoral artery is poorer in sugar in the same ratio after extirpation of the pancreas as in normal animals. Seegen had already raised well-founded objections regarding the exactness of this method.

Minkowski, on the basis of his experiments, considers it absolutely certain that in experimental pancreatic diabetes there is no increase in the production of sugar, but that a disturbance takes place in the consumption of sugar. He has recently in a critical review called attention to the following experiment: A diabetic dog, after going without food for several days, received gradually 100 gm. of grape-sugar, after which it excreted in the urine 107.5 gm. of sugar besides 4.55 gm. of nitrogen. Before the sugar was given the animal excreted 115 c.c. of urine, in which were 7.8% sugar and 2.33% nitrogen. This excess in the elimination of sugar can be explained only by the fact that the sugar introduced passed off unconsumed.

The same objections may be raised against—

3. *The hypothesis of the brothers Cavazzani:* They declare that the occurrence of diabetes after extirpation of the pancreas is due to changes in the liver. It could be established experimentally that the amount of sugar in the blood of the liver is considerably increased by stimulation of the celiac plexus. An analogous irritation may be caused by extirpation of the pancreas. In consequence of this there is an overproduction of sugar in the liver, an increased metabolism in the same, and a degeneration of the parenchyma of the organ. The exclusion of the pancreatic digestion leads to a diminished consumption of the albuminous bodies and to emaciation. The combination of the two results may explain fully the pathogenesis of diabetes. The results of transplantation of the pancreas also contradict this theory.

None of the hypotheses mentioned can hold their ground as against the justified objections. The most persistent of all, that of Lépine, is not sufficiently established. It still remains for future investigators to advance the solution which shall perhaps satisfactorily settle the whole diabetes question.

If the results of the experiments upon animals, so far as they interest us here, are collected, the following conclusions are reached:

1. In a number of species of animals the total extirpation of the pancreas produces genuine diabetes.

2. In partial extirpation, glycosuria and diabetes may be entirely absent. Frequently there is a transient or alimentary glycosuria. In a number of cases diabetes of moderate or considerable severity developed. This occurred when the portion of the gland remaining gradually atrophies and becomes unfitted for its internal function.

3. It is established that diabetes occurs through the failure of a special —the internal—function of the pancreas, and neither through a nerve lesion nor through the loss of the external—that is, the digestive—function of the pancreatic juice.

4. We are still entirely in the dark concerning the nature of this internal function.

(b) CLINICAL AND PATHOLOGIC-ANATOMIC EXPERIENCE.

Although for some time, as before mentioned, attempts have been made at the sick-bed and by postmortem examinations to discover the relation between the pancreas and diabetes, an evident advance of the investigations in these directions was made soon after the important and luminous discovery of v. Mering and Minkowski. Investigations have been made more frequently, and, therefore, more has been discovered. In the light of animal experimentation, the older results gained increased significance and an extensive material has gradually been collected, since not only clinicians, but especially pathologic anatomists, who for a long time were skeptical, gave important and well-founded contributions.

Notwithstanding, a final solution of the question is still remote. There are yet enough unsettled points and gaps in our knowledge, and there is still necessity for hard study, abundant statistics, and fundamental investigation of individual cases, before a full understanding of the relation between diabetes and the diseased pancreas can be reached.

In order to judge as objectively as possible, it is recommended:

1. To review, in brief, the existing clinical and anatomic material, and especially the clinical cases of diabetes in which changes of the pancreas have definitely been established.

2. To investigate in these cases whether the disease of the pancreas is to be regarded as the cause or the effect of the diabetes, or whether both are co-ordinate, being accidentally associated.

The older material collected before the positive experiments on animals succeeded has already been considered. There are still some statistical communications to be mentioned, and these will be tabulated. Mention should be made also of the following evidence:

Frerichs (1884), in diabetes, found the pancreas normal 28 times and atrophied 12 times. The weight varied from 1 to 5 ounces. Once almost the whole pancreas had undergone complete fatty degeneration and the ductus Wirsungianus was filled with a large concretion 3 cm. thick and 4 cm. long, in addition to numerous mortar-like fragments. In another case in the head of the gland there was a carcinoma with cyst-like dilatation of the duct and closure of the ductus choledochus. Once the pancreas was changed into an abscess as large as an apple, and in one case peripancreatitis and pancreatitis hæmorrhagica purulenta were present.

Windle (1881), among 139 cases, found the pancreas normal in 65, 38 times there was simple atrophy, 11 times atrophy with fatty degeneration, 3 times atrophy with concretions in the Wirsungian duct, 5 times induration, and 3 times carcinoma; hyperemia, coffee-colored pigmentation, and small hemorrhages were present each in one case. Among four of his own patients he found two with atrophy and cloudy swelling of the cells, one with atrophy and increase of connective tissue, and one with marked shrinkage. Since the first communications of v. Mering and Minkowski, the increased interest of authors in diabetes in its relations to the pancreas has expressed itself in abundant and more detailed statistics as well as by a number of concise pathologic works.

Dieckhoff examined 19 cases of diseases of the pancreas. In 7 of them diabetes had been present, once in case of hemorrhage in the neighborhood of the pancreas with destruction of the gland, twice in chronic pancreatitis, once in subchronic pancreatitis, twice in simple atrophy, and once in chronic indurative pancreatitis with lipomatosis and fat necrosis.

Hansemann investigated the protocols of the Berlin Pathologic Institute in the last ten years and found the following statistics:

Diabetes without disease of the pancreas .... 8 cases.
Diabetes without any statement concerning the pancreas .... 6 "
Diabetes with disease of the pancreas .... 40 "
Diseases of the pancreas without diabetes .... 19 "

Among the 40 cases of disease of the pancreas in which diabetes occurred there were 36 cases of simple atrophy, 3 cases of fibrous induration, 1 complicated case.

Hale White found among 6000 autopsies at Guy's Hospital between 1883 and 1894 the pancreas diseased in 99 cases, among which 16 were cases of atrophy; in 13 of these diabetes had occurred.

One of my assistants, Dr. Sigmund Bloch, has, with the kind consent of Prof. Weichselbaum, examined the protocols of the General Hospital at Vienna for the years 1885 to 1895, and in 18,509 autopsies he found the following data:

Diabetes with disease of the pancreas .... 12 cases.
Diabetes without disease of the pancreas * .... 10 "
Diabetes without any statement concerning the pancreas ...64 "
Disease of the pancreas without diabetes .... 89 "

In cases of diabetes atrophy was found 8 times, fat necrosis twice, pancreatitis suppurativa once, necrosis circumscripta once. In 86 cases of diabetes, therefore, diseases of the pancreas occurred 12 times. In 89 cases of diseases of the pancreas there was no diabetes. If we take simply the years 1894 and 1895, in which the "normal" pancreas was also expressly noted, the following data are given:

Diabetes with diseases of the pancreas .... 8 cases.
Diabetes with normal pancreas .... 10 "
Diabetes without any statement concerning the pancreas .... 9 "
Pancreatic disease without diabetes .... 31 "

Seegen has collected the results from the autopsy records at the General Hospital from 1838 to November, 1892. He found among 122 cases of diabetes, changes in the pancreas 34 times. If we supplement these figures by the results of the estimate made by Dr. Bloch up to the end of 1895, it results that among 161 cases of diabetes examined in the General Hospital, changes of the pancreas were observed 42 times.[†]

* These cases come from the years 1894 and 1895, in which it was expressly mentioned in the protocols that the pancreas was normal. In the earlier protocols, if no disease of the pancreas in diabetes is mentioned no statement is made about the pancreas, so that we cannot say with certainty that the pancreas was normal, although this can probably be assumed.

† In the statistics given by Seegen diseases of the pancreas in diabetes seem more frequent than in the protocols examined by Dr. Bloch. These differences are due to the subjective comprehension of the pathologist. At one time pigmentations, soft consistency, etc., are explained as postmortem phenomena and are not mentioned, while at another time they are stated as existing.

The statistics, so far as they were accessible to me,* arranged according to the kind of disease,† give the following tables:

I. ATROPHY.

AUTHOR.	AGE.	SEX.	CONDITION OF THE PANCREAS.	REMARKS.
Bouchardat: cited by Lapierre.	?	?	Atrophy of the pancreas.	
Caplick: Diss. Kiel, 1882.	12½	M.	Small, very pale.	Died in coma.
Cruppi: Diss. Göttingen, 1879.	27	M.	Marked atrophy with induration.	Died with symptoms of fever.
Dieckhoff: "Beitr. z. path. Anat. d. Pankr.," 1896.	57	M.	Pancreas very thin, smooth, weighing 39 gm.	Diabetes for years.
	27	F.	Pancreas weighs 30 gm. Macroscopically and microscopically, no essential change, only smaller than normal.	Diabetes for 2½ years.
Frerichs: "Ueber don Diabetes," 1884.	37	F.	Small, flabby, tough, weighs 45 gm. Fibrillar connective tissue, with small remains of acini.	Diabetes for 2 years.
	25	F.	Very flabby and tough. Fibrous connective tissue with remains of acini. Gland cells small and transparent.	Thin, had disease of the lung and died in coma.
Griesinger: "Arch. f. Heilk.," 1859, p. 44.	?	?	Atrophy of pancreas.	
Hartsen: "Donders' Archiv," III.	?	?	High degree of atrophy. Gland not recognizable.	Liver filled with small abscesses.
	?	?	Similar findings.	Liver hypertrophied and contains colloid.
Jaksch: "Prager med. Woch.," 1883, p. 193.	13	M.	Marked atrophy. Duct narrowed. Details of the gland indistinct. The groove for vena lienalis is very wide.	Acute course in 22 days after first symptoms. Death in coma.
Klebs: "Handb. d. path. Anat.," 1868, p. 536.	?	F.	Narrow and smooth.	
	?	F.	Weighs 25 gm.	
Lancereaux: "Bull. acad. méd.," 1877.	61	F.	But little of pancreas left. Connective-tissue bridge. Head and tail atrophied. Plexus normal. Duct. Wirsung. obliterated. Fatty degeneration of epithelium.	

* It is easily understood that in the following tables not all the published cases of diabetes with diseases of the pancreas are given. In the numerous reports of hospitals, of pathologic institutes, in collections of references, and in the clinical reports which have been published, of course numerous cases are found which belong to this list.

† A strict division according to the kind of disease is impossible, because manifold combinations occur. There is a combination of new-formations, cysts, calculus, inflammation with atrophy and calculi with cysts and fibrous degeneration, carcinoma with chronic pancreatitis, lipomatosis with indurative pancreatitis, etc. In the table "Atrophy" the corresponding cases of atrophy without any combination are given so far as possible.

I. Atrophy.—(*Continued.*)

Author.	Age.	Sex.	Condition of the Pancreas.	Remarks.
Lancereaux: "Bull. acad. méd.," 1877.	29	M.	Small, weighs 10 gm., soft. Cells of acini, atrophied, fatty, degenerated.	Diabète maigre, duration 1¼ years. Tuberc. pulmon.
	40	M.	Atrophied. Duct obliterated. Tuberculosis pulmon.	Diabète maigre for two years. 6% sugar.
	51	M.	Atrophy of pancreas. Head and neck quite thin.	Diabète maigre for 1¼ years. Four hundred gm. of sugar per day. Suppurative pleurisy.
Lecorché: "Arch. gén. Méd.," 1861.	45	M.	Atrophy.	
Leroux: Cited by Wegeli.	14	—	Atrophy of gland cells of pancreas with normal arrangement of connective tissue.	6.1% to 7.1% sugar in the urine.
Leva: Cited by Wegeli.	12	—	Atrophy.	3.3% to 6.5% of sugar in urine.
Le Nobel: Maly J. B. 1886, p. 449.	61	M.	Atrophy of pancreas and disease of liver.	2.27% sugar in urine after food rich in carbohydrates, maltose. Neither indol nor skatol in feces.
Noltenius: Diss., 1889.	20	F.	Small, pale, brownish-red.	Died in coma.
	12	M.	Small, reddish-gray, weighs 50 gm.	
	50	F.	Highly atrophied. Small concretions in duct.	
Schabad: "Zeitschr. f. klin. Med.," 1894, p. 108.	22	M.	Size much diminished. Pigmented atrophy of gland cells. Spots of connective-tissue growth.	
Schaper: Diss., 1873.	20	M.	Atrophied. Lobules shrunken. Fatty degeneration of epithelium.	Diabetes after injury to the skull.
Scheube: "Arch. f. Heilk.," 18. Bd., p. 389.	27	M.	Pancreas atrophied.	Marked emaciation.
Seegen: "Diab. mell.," 1893.	35	M.	Flabby, small, dark-red, acinous structure unrecognizable in many places. Epithelial cells fatty degenerated.	
Silver and Irving: "Trans. of the path. Soc.," 1878.	19	M.	Pancreas hard, atrophied, granulated.	Emaciation. Phthisis.
Thiroloix: "Diabète panc.," 1892.	45	M.	Pancreas changed into a fibrous band. Duct. Wirsung. much narrowed. Small cyst in head. Gland tissue still visible.	Acute beginning. Duration about 2 years. Disappearance of the glycosuria about 24 days before death.
Williamson: "Med. Chron.," 1892, 3.	?	?	Pancreas atrophied.	

Hansemann's table contains 36 cases of simple atrophy:

Sex.	Age.	Condition of Pancreas.	State of Nutrition.
F.	24	50 gm., pale red, flabby.	Marasmic.
M.	22	50 gm., thin, atrophied.	Marasmic.
M.	62	Small and thin.	Emaciated.
M.	30	Atrophied.	Fat.
F.	66	Very thin, 14 cm. long, head 3.5, tail 1.5, duct widened. Pars Wirsung. wholly lacking.	Emaciated.
F.	55	Body quite atrophied, toward the tail somewhat more substance, but also marked atrophy. Cicatricial retraction	Well nourished.
M.	60	Very small and atrophied.	Well nourished.
M.	14	Small and flabby.	Poorly nourished.
M.	42	Atrophied.	Marasmic.
M.	?	Small and atrophied.	Emaciated.
F.	55	Atrophied.	Emaciated.
F.	53	Atrophied.	Much emaciated.
M.	40	Atrophied.	Emaciated.
F.	17	Atrophied, 50 gm.	Very well nourished.
M.	26	Atrophied, very flabby.	Emaciated.
M.	25	Atrophied, 50 gm.	Emaciated.
M.	25	Atrophied.	Emaciated.
M.	30	Atrophy with induration.	Emaciated.
M.	48	Small, atrophied.	Emaciated.
M.	29	Small, atrophied.	Emaciated.
M.	33	Atrophied.	Marasmic.
M.	39	Atrophied.	
F.	18	Atrophied.	Marasmic.
F.	25	Half as large as normal.	Marasmic.
M.	50	Atrophied.	
M.	32	Much atrophied, 24 gm.	Emaciated.
F.	15	Small, flabby.	Emaciated.
M.	?	Atrophied.	Emaciated.
F.	66	Atrophied.	Well nourished.
M.	31	Flabby, pale, 65 gm.	Emaciated.
F.	67	Much atrophied.	
M.	22	Atrophied.	Marasmic.
M.	32	Fibrous degeneration with atrophy.	Emaciated.
F.	36	Atrophied, 35 gm.	Moderate.
M.	30	Atrophied, 50 gm.	Emaciated.
M.	42	Beginning atrophy and interstitial inflammation, 97 gm.	

To these hitherto published cases I wish to add three recent original observations, in which microscopic investigations of the pancreas were made.

1. A. R., clerk, twenty-one years, entered hospital March 31, 1896. Emaciation for several months, almost unquenchable thirst, great hunger. Body-weight 45 kg. Amount of urine 5000. 7.7% sugar. Specific gravity 1040. No albumin, no acetone. In spite of diabetic diet, 6.7% sugar increased to 8.1%. Goes to Carlsbad. On returning, 3%. Reentered hospital January 2, 1897. Evident phthisis,

great weakness, much acetone, 45 kg. Sugar 3.3%. February 1st, coma, death. The anatomic diagnosis (prosector, Dr. Zemann) was marasmus eximius from diabetes mellitus. Phthisis tuberc. lobi super. pulm. dextr. Infilt. lobular. tuberculosa pulmonis sinistri. The pancreas was quite firm, pale yellow, the lobules large. Microscopic examination showed atrophy of the pancreas. Weight 66 gm.

2. S. B., merchant, thirty-seven years. Admitted December 31, 1896. For two years marked hunger and thirst. At the time of admittance passed 10 liters of urine per diem. 6.4% sugar. Body-weight 44 kg.; before he was sick usually 80 kg. Increasing emaciation, 40 kg. 6% sugar. January 30, 1897, coma, death. Anatomic diagnosis (prosector, Dr. Zemann): Diabetes mellitus, tuberculosis pulmonum, catarrhus ventriculi chronicus, marasmus. Pancreas macroscopically flabby, reddish-yellow on section, the acini quite small, soft, separated from each other by very loose connective tissue and some edematous fat tissue. Weight 70 gm. Microscopically: Size of gland lobules diminished and these are separated by quite abundant fat tissue, which, however, is undergoing serous degeneration. The gland cells small, markedly granular, and filled with fat drops.

3. A. L., workman, thirty-five years. Admitted September 30, 1895. Since February, 1893, has had great hunger and thirst; has been in Carlsbad twice on account of diabetes. At the time of admission the amount of urine was 4 liters, specific gravity 1026, 4.5% sugar, acetone 0.026. Body-weight 47 kg. Sugar decreased to 3.1% and even to 2.3%. The patient left the hospital March 27, 1896, and reentered April 20, 1896. At the time of admission he voided 5 liters of urine per day, specific gravity 1035, sugar 3.7%, much acetone, and great weakness. Could take but little nourishment. Coma, April 30th, death. Anatomic diagnosis (prosector, Dr. Zemann): Diabetes mellitus, tuberculosis circumscripta chronic. apic. pulmonum, catarrhus ventriculi chronicus, marasmus eximius. Macroscopic examination: Pancreas quite narrow and very thin, flabby, poor in blood, the lobules small. Microscopic examination: The lobules of the pancreas somewhat small, the epithelium in a high degree of fatty degeneration and partly transformed into fat detritus. All the changes evidently related to the marasmus.

From the results of the autopsies at the General Hospital, the following cases may be added:

1. 1892: Man aged fifty-five. Results of autopsy: Acetonemia, tuberculosis subacuta et chronica pulmon., atrophia pancreatis.

2. 1894: Woman aged fifty-four. Encephalomalacia multipl. cerebr. ex endarteriitide luetica, pneumonia hypostatica, atrophia pancreatis.

3. 1894: Man aged sixty. Cirrhosis hepat. alcohol., tumor lienis chronicus, atrophia pancreatis pigmentosa.

4. 1894: Man aged sixty. Cirrhosis hepat., ascites, atrophia pancreatis.

5. 1895: Woman aged (?). Edem. acut. pulm. et cerebri, atrophia pancreatis.

6. 1895: Woman aged twenty-two. Tuberculosis chronica glandul. bronch. ad hil. sin. subsequente tuberculosi hujus pulm., atrophia pancreatis, degenerat. ren., struma levis gradus, exophthalmos.

7. 1895: Man aged sixty-one. Acetonæmia c. degeneratione parenchym. hepat., ren. et cordis adipositate affect., encephalomalacia multipl. hemisph. sin. cerebri region. gyr. central. et in corpore striat. ex embolia, endarteriitis chronic. deformans cum ulceribus ad arcum aortæ, atrophia pancreatis eximia, hyperost. tibiæ ex lue.

8. 1895: Man aged forty. Atrophia pancreatis, induratio callosa cand. pancreatis, tuberculosis pulm. The pancreas was surrounded by abundant fat tissue, the tail transformed into a callus, elsewhere indurated, considerably narrowed, in its calloused portion embedded in indurated fibrous tissue; was indurated; the lobules project from the cut surface as white granules.

II. FATTY DEGENERATION.

AUTHOR.	AGE.	SEX.	CONDITION OF THE PANCREAS.	REMARKS.
Baumel: "Montpell. méd."	50	M.	Fatty degeneration of acini. Slight increase of interstitial tissue.	Abundant fat tissue. Death from pneumonia. Large amount of sugar.

II. Fatty Degeneration.—(*Continued.*)

Author.	Age.	Sex.	Condition of the Pancreas.	Remarks.
Caplick: Diss., 1882.	38	M.	Pancreas changed into mass of fat. Small, dense tumors in pancreas. Duct ending blindly. Normal pancreas substance seen near the ductus choledochus.	Duration of diabetes 6 years. Death from erysipelas.
Chiari: "Zeitschr. f. Heilk.," 1896.	74	M.	Infiltrated with abundant fat tissue. Microscopically marked lipomatosis. Increase of interlobular and interacinous tissue.	Death from meningitis suppur.
	51	M.	Pancreas thin, soft. Micros.: Fatty degeneration of cells.	Death from gangræna pulmon.
	44	M.	Pancreas small. Fatty degeneration of cells.	Death from tuberculosis.
Dieckhoff: "Beitrag z. path. Anat. d. Pank.," 1895.	60	M.	Lipomatosis of pancreas. Old chronic interstitial pancreatitis. Areas of fat-necrosis.	Diabetes for 11 years. Sugar between 6.4% and 1.5%. An inebriate. Hemorrhage of stomach before death. Numerous erosions in stomach.
Friedreich: "Krankbeiten d. Pankr.," 1878.	?	?	Pancreas dimin. in size. Substitution of fat tissue. Here and there, remains of acini undergoing fatty degeneration.	Diabetes for 5 years. Death in coma.
Guelliot: "Gaz. méd.," 1881.	67	M.	Pancreas enlarged, substitution of fat, a cyst in head. A few remains of glands surrounding the normal duct.	Disease lasted 1 year and 9 months. Death in collapse.
Hoppe-Seyler: "Deut. Arch. f. klin. Med.," 1894.	57	F.	Pancreas entirely changed to fat. No remains of fat tissue. Calcification of blood-vessels.	Diabetes insipidus with transient glycosuria.
Thiroloix: "Diabète pancreat.," 1892.	32	M.	Pancreas has undergone fatty degeneration, small, of 50 gm. weight. Duct. Wirsung. permeable.	Sudden onset. Death from pneumonia. Disease lasted 5 years.

III. INDURATIVE PANCREATITIS.

Author.	Age.	Sex.	Condition of the Pancreas.	Remarks.
Buss: Diss., 1894.	?	?	Induration of pancreas.	Brown pigmentation of some organs, especially of liver. Hemachromatosis (v. Recklinghausen).

III. INDURATIVE PANCREATITIS.—(*Continued.*)

AUTHOR.	AGE.	SEX.	CONDITION OF THE PANCREAS.	REMARKS.
Cantani u. Ferraro: "Il Morgagni,"1883, p. 1.	38	M.	Pancreas small, thin, fibrous for the greater part, but in some places penetrated by fat. Only in the tail are there areas of gland tissue.	Marasmus, acetonemia.
	47	M.	Small, flabby, body fibrous, remaining portions better preserved.	Emaciation. Death from pneumonia.
	50	M.	Small, granular connective tissue between the lobules.	Emaciation. Death from pneumonia.
Dieckhoff: "Beitr. z. path. Anat. d. Pankr.," 1896.	67	M.	Chronic indurative pancreatitis. In head, a walnut-sized cavity with cream-like contents. Marked development of fat tissue.	Diabetes for about 1 year. Between 5.0% and 1.3% sugar. Large, hard liver. Resistance in left hypochondrium.
	4	M.	Pancreas small, flabby, and light, 60 gm. weight. Microscop. exam.: subacute interstitial inflammation, with recent small-celled infiltration, partly diffuse and partly in areas.	Eight months before death, sugar in the urine after taking cold; after trauma 6 months later, repetition of the glycosuria. Death in coma.
Fles: "Donders' Arch.," III	?	?	Pancreas entirely changed to connective tissue. No gland tissue recognizable even microscopically.	Liver small. Liver cells decreased in size.
Hadden: "Path. Soc. of London," 1887, 1891.	65	F.	Marked increase of connective tissue in pancreas.	
	38	M.	Marked connective-tissue sclerosis.	
Hansemann: "Zeitschr. f. klin. Med.," 1895.	45	M.	Pancreas large, very hard. On the cut surface and on the free surface are acini separated from each other by bands of connective tissue; some acini red, others white. Pancreatitis interstitialis.	Death in coma. 4% sugar. Corpulent man.
	58	M.	Fibrous induration of pancreas. Arteria lienalis tortuous.	Syphilis. Bronchitis. Dilatio et hypertrophia cordis. Endarteritis obliterans. Encephalomalacia.

III. INDURATIVE PANCREATITIS.—(*Continued.*)

AUTHOR.	AGE.	SEX.	CONDITION OF THE PANCREAS.	REMARKS.
Hansemann: "Zeitschr. f. klin. Med.," 1895.	49	M.	Pancreas entirely degenerated. None of the substance present, except a thin layer of connective tissue, which surrounds the enlarged duct. Around the head, more marked connective-tissue growth. Mouth of canal in duodenum obliterated. Artery not tortuous. Wall thickened.	Marasmus. Death in coma.
Noltenius: Diss., 1888.	46	M.	Marked induration of the pancreas.	
Obici: "Soc. di Bologna," 1893.	?	?	Interstitial pancreatitis in the neighborhood of the blood-vessels and lymph-vessels.	Disappearance of glycosuria for a short time under a pure meat diet.
Rowland: "Brit. Med. Jour.," 1893.	57	F.	Fibrous degeneration of the pancreas. Lime concretions in the connective tissue.	Death in coma.
Roque, Devic and Hugounenq: "Rev. de méd.," 1892, p. 995.	39	M.	Pancreas small, connective tissue increased. Cells small and do not stain (postmortem phenomenon).	Duration of diabetes, 2 years. Death in coma.
Rühle: Cited by Dieckhoff.	20	M.	Cirrhosis of the pancreas. Enlargement of duct. In the head, cysts the size of an apple with blood-clot.	Diabetes mellitus for one year. Sugar at last alternating. At the end ascites. Edema of lower extremities and anuria at times.
Seegen: "Diabet. Mellit.," 1893.	?	?	Pancreas changed to a gray calloused band. In the region of the head, remains of granular structure.	
Williamson: "Brit. Med. Jour.," 1894.	52	M.	Pancreas dense and heavy. On microscopic examination, cirrhosis. Changes in spinal cord.	Diabetes and paresis of right arm muscles.

A case of connective-tissue growth in the pancreas of a diabetic, mentioned by Tylden and Miller, is also to be added. Indurative changes were found also in the cases recorded by Frerichs, Lancereaux, Dieckhoff, Goodmann, and Lépine, and listed in Tables I, II, VI, and X.

The case of Baumel may also be added to this table, in which pancreas, spleen, and stomach were found closely grown together.

An interesting anatomic condition has kindly been communicated by Dr. Zemann:

K. W., maid-servant, forty-five years of age, died December 20, 1896. Clinical diagnosis: Diabetes mellitus.

Result of postmortem examination: Extensive ichorous carcinoma of the left large and small labia of the vulva with phlegmonous inflammation in the region of the mons veneris and of the groins. Beginning gangrene of the skin on both sides, especially on the right. Chronic tuberculosis of the apices of the lungs with induration. Acute, lobular, tuberculous infiltration of the lungs. Nearly complete cicatricial shrinkage of the pancreas, which is replaced by a small cavity, also a duodenal fistula just at the pylorus, the results of chronic ulcerative pancreatitis. Diabetes mellitus.

On raising the liver, there appears in place of the lesser omentum a dense, white, radiating mass of cicatricial tissue, by which the lesser curvature of the stomach is much shortened and closely approximated to the liver; the contiguous portion of the capsule of the left lobe of the liver is white, thickened, and opaque, the fibrous tissue in the portal fissure is only slightly thickened. After cutting through the transverse mesocolon, there is seen in place of the pancreas a nodule about the size of a hazelnut, which is inclosed in very dense, white, fibrous tissue, radiating from the former, and by which the upper transverse piece of the duodenum and the pylorus are drawn and firmly attached to the nodule. On cutting the nodule open a transverse, egg-shaped cavity, about 12 mm. in the greatest diameter, is exposed; this occupies the right portion of the whole nodule, while the remaining left portion consists of connective tissue, which incloses a group, larger than a pea, of pale-yellow, soft lobules of pancreatic structure. In the cavity is found a turbid, thick, slimy, dirty reddish-gray fluid, in which are fine sand-like particles and a hard concretion about 4 to 5 mm. long, 1 mm. thick, and of irregular shape. The inner surface of the cavity is lined with smooth, delicate, grayish-red tissue. The wall, with the exception of the left portion, is formed of a layer of somewhat dense white tissue, 2 or 3 mm. thick, and calcified in places. On the right, the wall contains an opening, scarcely as large as a millet-seed, through which the closely approximated upper portion of the duodenum is entered. The orifice of the duodenum, about 1 cm. from the pylorus, lies in a funnel-shaped pocket which is bounded by a thick projection of mucous membrane. The remains of the head of the pancreas, forming a mass 3 to 5 mm. thick, are found close to the duodenum. The lobules of this remnant of the pancreas are very small, and are separated by considerable intervening tissue. The pancreatic duct is not permeable.

IV. CALCULI.

AUTHOR.	AGE.	SEX.	CONDITION OF THE PANCREAS.	REMARKS.
Baumel: "Montpell. méd.," 1882.	50	M.	Pancreas incrusted with fine concretions. About the atrophic acini, abundant connective tissue. Stones weigh together 1.2 gm. and consist of $CaCO_3$.	Cause of death tuberculosis.
Capparelli: "Il Morgagni," 1883.	?	F.	Pancreatic fistula for years. Discharge of calculi. No autopsy.	After closure of the fistula, diabetes developed.
Chopart: cited by Klebs.	?	M.	Fatty stools, calculi in pancreatic duct.	
Cowley: "London Med. Journal," 1788.	35	M.	Calculi as large as a pea wedged in gland substance. Pancreas atrophied.	Inebriate, very corpulent.
Elliotson: "Med.-chir. Transact.," 1833.	35	M.	Duct as far as the lateral branches obstructed by calculi.	Fat in stools.

5

IV. CALCULI.—*(Continued.)*

AUTHOR.	AGE.	SEX.	CONDITION OF THE PANCREAS.	REMARKS.
Fleiner: "Berl. klin. Wochenschr.," 1894, p. 38.	40	M.	Calculus in duct. Gland almost wholly sclerotic, in the tail only was there some gland tissue.	Inebriate. Much emaciated.
Frerichs: "Diabetes," 1884.	?	?	In the duct, together with numerous fragments of calculi, were two spindle-shaped concretions. Gland, with the exception of a few acini, wholly degenerated.	
Freyhan: "Berl. klin. Wochenschr.," 1893.	35	M.	In the duct, calculi consisting of calcium carbonate. Duct enlarged with lateral pockets. Pancreas atrophied, no gland structure. Fatty degeneration.	Insidious beginning of diabetes. Up to 3.1% sugar in urine. Pulmonary tuberculosis.
	?	F.	Duct dilated. In the tail, firmly fixed in the canal, was a hard calculus as large as a plum-stone, consisting mostly of calcium carbonate. Gland entirely changed into fat and connective tissue.	1.8% sugar in the urine. Pulmonary tuberculosis. Disappearance of glycosuria before death.
Gille: "Soc. d'anat.," 1878.	?	M.	Calculus wedged in duct. Gland atrophied.	
Holzmann: "München. med. Wochenschr.," 1894.	68	M.	Concretions found in the feces.	Traces of sugar after the attacks of colic.
Lancereaux: 1877, "Bull. de l'acad. méd."	42	M.	Syphilis. Dilatation of both ducts. Calculi of various size.	
	?	?	Cited by Giudiceandrea without further details.	
Lancereaux: "Bull. acad. méd.," 1888.	45	F.	Mouth of ductus Wirsung closed by calculi. Growth of connective and fatty tissue. Gland tissue atrophied.	Colic and fatty stools before the beginning of diabetes. Diabète maigre. Duration 5 months.
Lancereaux: 1888. "Bull. de l'acad de méd. de Paris," Seance 8ᵉ, mai, 1888, cited by Giudiceandrea.	25	F.	Body of gland atrophied. Hard calculi of the size of peas.	
Lichtheim: "Berlin. klin. Wochenschr.," 1894.	36	M.	Calculi in duct. Fibrous degeneration with almost total disappearance of gland tissue.	
Lusk: Cited by Giudiceandrea	?	M.	Pancreas showed almost complete calcification of the gland.	

IV. CALCULI.—(*Continued.*)

AUTHOR.	AGE.	SEX.	CONDITION OF THE PANCREAS.	REMARKS.
Moore: "Path. Soc. London," 1884.	40	M.	In the pancreatic duct, numerous irregularly contoured calculi consisting of CaCO₃. Marked enlargement, especially in the head. No obstruction.	
Müller: "Ueber Icterus," "Zeitschr. f. klin. Medicin," Bd. XII, S. 84.	21	M.	Dense, nodular. Duct much enlarged. Containing several yellowish-white concretions of the size of a cherry-stone, with cylindric dilatation behind them. Gland substance atrophied. Concretions in the lateral branches.	Diabetes for two years. 3% to 6% sugar. Death from phthisis pulmonalis. Caries of the petrous bone. Stools always abundant, yellow, foamy, and of the consistency of thin porridge.
Munk u. Klebs: "Naturforscherversammlung," 1869.	?	?	Calculus formation. No remains of gland visible macroscopically. Behind the omental bursa in the connective tissue surrounding the blood-vessels single groups of cells were to be found with the microscope.	
Nicolas u. Mollière: "Bull. méd.," 1897.	47	M.	Ductus Wirsung. obstructed by calculi, opens into a cavity filled with pus which comprises the central portion of the pancreas. Sclerosis of the gland. Fistula from the pus-cavity into the duodenum near the pylorus.	Occasional attacks of colic. Melena. Symptoms of diabetes 2½ months after the beginning of the disease: sugar reached 179 gm. a day. Caseous pneumonia. Duration of disease, six months. Stools normal.
v. Recklinghausen: "Virch. Arch.," 1864.	26	M.	Large and small concretions in the much widened duct. Pancreas changed to a tumor consisting of fat.	Gangrene of lungs. Diabetes for some time.
Rörig: Cited by Wegeli.	10½	?	In an accessory pancreatic duct a calculus which entirely filled the lumen. Behind it, a cyst filled with pancreatic juice.	Diabetes.
Seegen: "Diab. mell.," 1893.	?	?	Duct dilated by concretions to the size of a raven's quill. Concretions also in finest branches.	

V. CARCINOMA.

Author.	Age.	Sex.	Condition of the Pancreas.	Remarks.
v. Ackeren: "Berl. klin. Wochenschr.," 1889.	49	M.	Carcinoma in head and tail of pancreas. Carcinoma of pylorus.	Maltose in urine. Many muscle-fibers in stools.
Bouchard: "Malad. par rallent. de la nutr."	?	M.	Carcinoma in the head of the pancreas.	
Bouchardat: Cited by Lapierre.	?	?	Carcinoma pancreat.	
Bright: "Med. Chir. Trans.," 1833.	49	M.	Carcinoma of the pancreas, of cartilaginous density.	Rapid cachexia. Severe icterus.
Courmont u. Bret: Clinique, 1894.	64	M.	Carcinoma of the head of the pancreas, with sclerosis of the whole gland. Parenchyma of liver changed.	Diabetes after trauma. Fracture of rib. Icterus. Disappearance of sugar.
Dieckhoff: "Beitr. z. path. Anat. d. Pank.," 1896.	75	F.	Cylindric-celled carcinoma of head of pancreas. Chronic interstitial and purulent pancreatitis.	In the urine taken after death there was a positive phenylhydrazin test.
Dreschfeld: "Med. Chron.," Apr., 1895.	?	?	Pancreas firm, dense, and infiltrated with cancer. Almost no normal tissue. Portal vein compressed by the new growth.	Duration of disease three months. Stabbing pains in epigastrium. Vomiting. Ascites. Hematemesis. Death in collapse.
Duffey: "Dublin Journal," 1884.	24	M.	Carcinoma pancreat. Gland substance entirely disappeared.	Duration of disease 2 months. Dysenteric diarrhea. Death in collapse.
Fothergill: "Brit. Med. Jour.," 1896.	53	F.	Pancreas entirely destroyed. Carcinoma of peritoneum, mesentery, and omentum.	Repeated cramps. Icterus. Tumor distinctly felt in abdomen. Operation. Hematemesis. Death.
Frerichs: "Ueber d. Diabet.," 1884.	?	?	Head of pancreas changed into medullary carcinoma and fused with the duodenum. Dilatation of duct of Wirsung. Atrophy of gland.	
Galvagni: "Rif. med.," 1896.	63	M.	Diagnosis of cancer of the pancreas.	Duration of disease, 6 months. Marked glycosuria.

V. CARCINOMA.—(*Continued.*)

AUTHOR.	AGE.	SEX.	CONDITION OF THE PANCREAS.	REMARKS.
Kesteren: "Path. Trans.," 1890.	60	M.	Primary carcinoma of pancreas.	Transient glycosuria, disappears after appropriate diet. Icterus. Pustule formation on skin.
Macaigni: Cited by Thiroloix.	69	F.	A large, very hard cancer of the head of the pancreas, replacing one-half of the gland, the rest of which was apparently normal. Compression of bile-ducts.	Transient glycosuria for 7 months, then 11 months cachexia without glycosuria. Disease lasted 23 months.
Martsen: Thèse, 1890.	?	?	Scirrhus of head of pancreas. Complete obliteration of ductus Wirsung.	Fatty diarrhea. Diabetes.
Masing: "Petersburg. med. Wochenschr.," 1879.	46	M.	Scirrhus in head of pancreas as large as child's fist. Duct. choled. compressed, dilated.	Sick 7 months. Neuralgia cœliaca. Icterus. Nothing objectively demonstrable.
Mirallié: "Gaz. des hôpit.," 1893.	?	?	Carcinoma of pancreas.	Fifty-eight gm. sugar a day.
Servaes: "Berl. klin. Wochenschr.," 1878.	?	?	Carcinoma of pancreas.	Severe celiac neuralgia for years. The last three years, bronzed skin.
Suckling: "Lancet," 1889.	33	M.	Carcinoma of pancreas.	Rapid emaciation. Jaundice. Stools ash-colored.
Thiroloix u. Lancereaux: "Diàbete pancreat.," 1892.	60	F.	Epithelioma in head of pancreas. Obliteration of duct of Wirsung. Sclerosis and atrophy of the remaining portions of gland.	Duration about 7 months. No polyphagia. Azoturia. Sudden death.

Besides these are the cases of Collier, Marston, Santi, Musmeci, Choupin, and Moll, concerning which I have no further information.

VI. CYSTS.

AUTHOR.	AGE.	SEX.	CONDITION OF THE PANCREAS.	REMARKS.
Bull: "New York Med. Jour.," 1887.	?	?	No autopsy. Pancreatic cyst containing 3½ liters.	Tumor for 10 months. Fatty stools, 5% sugar. Death 3½ months after operation.

VI. Cysts.—(*Continued.*)

AUTHOR.	AGE.	SEX.	CONDITION OF THE PANCREAS.	REMARKS.
Churton: "Brit. Med. Jour.," 1894.	35	M.	Pancreas changed into fibrous mass. Remains of a cyst in duodenal portion. Duct partially obliterated.	Exploratory puncture. After it, circumscribed peritonitis. Laparotomy, drainage. After 5 months, collection of pus behind stomach. Second laparotomy. Death. Diabetes.
Goodmann: "Philadel. Times," 1878.	55	M.	Large cysts, in tail. Gland tissue atrophied. Fibrous tissue in head.	Diabetes. Steatorrhea.
Horrocks and Morton: "Lancet," 1897.	56	M.	Large cyst with thick fibrous wall. Inner surface smooth, with small projections. No normal pancreatic tissue. Duct of Wirsung impermeable.	In urine, some albumin and much sugar. Patient died on the next day after aspiration of the cyst.
Malcolm Mackintosh: "Lancet," 1896.	?	M.	Large cyst under and behind the spleen, with some pancreatic tissue on posterior and lower part of cyst-wall.	Marked polyuria. Death in coma 11 days after discovery of sugar in urine. Disease lasted ½ year.
Mulert-Zweifel: Dissert., 1894.	64	F.	Pancreatic cyst removed by operation.	Transient glycosuria.
Nichols: "New York Med. Jour.," 1888.	49	M.	Large serous cyst of pancreas. No trace of gland tissue.	Diabetes.
v. Recklinghausen: "Virchow's Archiv," 1864.	40	M.	Large cystic tumor, probably caused by partial ectasia of the obliterated duct.	Diabetes for 4 years. 4% to 5% sugar.
Riegner: "Berlin. klin. Wochenschr.,"1890.	23	M.	Pancreatic cyst. Operated upon.	Traces of sugar. Many muscle-fibers in stools.

VII. ABSCESS.

AUTHOR.	AGE.	SEX.	CONDITION OF THE PANCREAS.	REMARKS.
Atkinson: "Med. News," 1895.	45	F.	Pancreatitis suppurativa, abscess breaking through into the intestine.	Acute beginning of disease, vomiting, pain. Tumor in epigastrium. Pus in stools one day before death. Slight glycosuria.

VII. Abscess.—(*Continued.*)

AUTHOR.	AGE.	SEX.	CONDITION OF THE PANCREAS.	REMARKS.
Frerichs: "Ueber den Diabetes," 1884.	27	F.	Head of pancreas normal, rest of the gland surrounded by a cyst. On posterior wall the atrophied pancreas.	Acute disease of the pancreas, ending in suppuration. 6% to 7% sugar. Tuberculosis.
Frerichs: "Diabetes," 1884.	31	F.	Pancreas, with the exception of the head, changed into an abscess the size of an apple. The pus-sac completely closed off, not communicating with the surrounding tissues.	Cardialgia. Icterus. Sudden onset of diabetes. As high as 600 gm. of sugar daily; on animal food 40 to 50 gm. Pulmonary tuberculosis. Duration of disease, 6 months.
Frison: "Recueil méd. mil.," 1876.	28	M.	Pancreas enlarged to three times its natural size, infiltrated with pus, a large abscess in the tail. Small abscess in liver. Gallbladder dilated.	Afebrile uterus. Anorexia, adynamia. Two months later, edema, polyphagia, polydipsia. Sugar in urine.
Harley: "Trans. path. Soc.," 1862.	58	M.	Head of pancreas contains a quantity of pus. Enlargement. Duct dilated. Gall-stones present.	Glycosuria developed three weeks before death.

In the reports of the autopsies of the General Hospital the following case is found: Acetonemia. Pancreatitis suppurativa et necrosis tel. adipos pancreat. Tumor hypophyseos. Acromegalia.

VIII. HEMORRHAGE.

Sarfert, in 1895, reported a case of pancreatic apoplexy in a man aged thirty-nine on whom laparotomy was performed on account of symptoms of intestinal obstruction. Death soon afterward. In the urine removed after death 1% sugar was found. At the autopsy, the pancreas, infiltrated with blood, was transformed into a mass resembling spleen tissue. Cutler's communication is dated the same year. Diabetes developed in a woman of fifty-two years. At the autopsy the pancreas was found, enlarged to twice its size, firm, dry, dark. Disseminated fat necrosis in the surrounding tissue.

Among the cases reported by Dieckhoff, there is one of hemorrhage into the pancreas, which, however, was certainly not the cause of the diabetes:

A woman of middle age suffered for years from diabetes. During the last year, in repeated examinations, no sugar was found in her urine. About four weeks before death she was attacked with severe pains in the abdomen, which lasted until death. At the autopsy a large effusion of blood was found surrounding the left kidney, the suprarenal capsule, and in part the pancreas; the blood formed a compact mass. A portion of the gland was quite well preserved, no alteration being recognizable. The fat tissue within and around the pancreas showed several isolated patches of necrosis.

IX. NECROSIS AND FAT NECROSIS.

Silver observed alterations of the pancreas, regarded by Hansemann as necrotic, in a diabetic aged twenty-three. Israel found gangrene of the pancreas with diabetes in a work-woman aged twenty-seven.

In the reports of autopsies at the General Hospital, the following pertinent cases are found:

1. Woman aged fifty-one. Glomerulonephritis, necrosis circumscripta in cauda pancreatis.
2. Man aged forty-nine: Hyperæmia cerebri, alcoholism. chron. (inebriate). Necrosis incip. tel. adipos. pancreatis.
Woman aged nineteen. Necrosis text. adipos. in regione pancreatis.

In the following table the cases are given in which no macroscopic alterations were found, but in which microscopic changes were seen:

X. MICROSCOPIC CHANGES.

Author.	Age.	Sex.	Condition of the Pancreas.	Remarks.
Bond and Windle: "Brit. Med. Jour.," 1883.	17	M.	Pancreas macroscopically normal. Microscopically, epithelium swollen and granular.	Death in coma after 4 days.
Caplick: Diss., 1882.	19	M.	Pancreas normal. Hyperemic.	
Fleiner: "Berl. klin. Wochenschr.," 1894.	57	F.	Tissue preserved only in the head. Nuclei poorly stained. (According to Hansemann, a postmortem change.)	
Harnack: "Arch. f. klin. Med.," 13, 1874.	33	M.	Pancreas macroscopically normal, microscopically shows fatty degeneration.	Diabetes for over one year; 600 to 800 gm. sugar. Intestinal catarrh. Slight glycosuria at the end.
Lépine: "Rev. méd.," 1892.	40	M.	Pancreas macroscopically normal, microscopically shows periacinous sclerosis.	
	54	M.	The same condition.	Death in coma.
Notta: "Union méd.," 1881.	25	M.	Pancreas somewhat enlarged, macroscopically normal, microscopically shows marked fatty degeneration of the glandular epithelium.	Marked emaciation, fatty stools, death in extreme marasmus.

Changes in the pancreas have been found, as appears from the above data, in 188 cases of diabetes; and of these, 78 cases showed atrophy, 10 cases fatty degeneration, 22 induration, 24 calculi, 24 cancer, 9 cysts, 6 abscess, 3 hemorrhage, 3 necrosis, 2 fat necrosis, and 7 showed only microscopic changes.

Can the conclusion be drawn from these facts that disease of the pancreas is the cause of diabetes? Certainly not. Although doubtless these figures * could actually be multiplied many times, and from the frequency of diabetes the number of cases in which disease of the pancreas could certainly be found at the autopsy would be very much greater, yet nothing would be proved.

To solve the question with certainty in a statistical way would be a matter of great difficulty. It would be necessary to know in large numbers of cases how often diabetes occurred in pancreatic diseases and how frequently pancreatic diseases occurred in diabetes, and only from constant or nearly constant relations could conclusions be drawn which would be available under certain conditions which will later be explained.

The figures at hand for this purpose are too few and too dissimilar to admit comparisons and conclusions.

A few data, as already mentioned, exist with regard to the question of the frequency of pancreatic diseases in diabetes. Windle found the pancreas changed 74 times in 139 cases of diabetes. Hansemann found in the protocols of the Berlin Pathologic Institute 54 autopsies of diabetics, among which changes were recorded in the pancreas 40 times.

The reports of autopsies at the General Hospital in Vienna give changes in the pancreas 42 times in 151 cases of diabetes.

Concerning the frequency of pancreatic diseases in general there are no available statistics, for the reason that in autopsies the pancreas is not always sufficiently studied, and where the diagnosis of the presence of some acute or chronic disease is evident, as tuberculosis, pneumonia, typhoid, etc., the pancreas is rarely examined in detail.

With regard to the frequency of diabetes in diseases of the pancreas, some significant figures are given.

Dieckhoff investigated 19 cases of diseases of the pancreas, in 7 of which there was diabetes; no other cases of diabetes at this time were examined after death.

Hansemann found 59 cases of diseases of the pancreas, among which diabetes was present in 40. In 54 cases of diabetes postmortem examinations were made.

Among 18,509 autopsies in the Vienna General Hospital between 1885 and 1895, pancreatic diseases were noted 96 times, and in 12 of them there was diabetes. There were 86 autopsies of diabetics.

These data are, of course, striking, but still not convincing, because it can be stated with certainty that the number of changes in the pancreas in general, aside from those in diabetes, is much greater than the number given in the report of the autopsies. Atrophy especially, which is the condition so frequently found in diabetes, and which certainly is often found as marantic atrophy in old age and in cachexia, is regarded as irrelevant and is rarely noted. Tuberculosis of the pancreas, according to Kudrewetzky, is a frequent disease, and yet it is seldom mentioned in reports of autopsies.

It will be shown in a special portion that diabetes occurs in diseases of the pancreas by no means so frequently as would be supposed from the reports of autopsies quoted. It will be seen that in acute and chronic inflammations, abscess, cysts, carcinoma, etc., diabetes is a relatively rare symptom.

There is, then, a contradiction between the anatomic and clinical facts,

* The numbers given in abstract, for instance, those from Seegen's statistics from the Vienna General Hospital, are not included

which can be decided only by frequent investigation on the part of clinicians and anatomists.

But even taking it for granted that the relations between pancreatic disease and diabetes, which, according to the autopsy reports given up to the present time, are shown in relatively few cases, were expressed constantly and in large numbers, it would still not always be proved that the disease of the pancreas found was the cause of the diabetes. If one should express in figures from the reports of autopsies the frequency of tuberculosis and diabetes and the frequency of the coincidence of the two diseases, he would find a large and probably constant number, and yet there is no doubt that tuberculosis is not the cause of the diabetes.

A similar relation would be found also between diabetes and diseases of the kidney, and yet it is established for most cases that there is no renal diabetes.

When clinical diabetes and anatomic affection of the pancreas are asserted, there are three possibilities: (1) That the diabetes is the result of the change of the pancreas; (2) that the diabetes is the cause of the change of the pancreas; (3) that the diabetes and the disease of the pancreas are co-ordinated but are independent of each other. Only when the two last possibilities can positively be excluded could even the existing few instances be regarded as of positive value.

But this proof is not to be furnished without an exhaustive study of the individual cases. On the contrary, it is known definitely that there are cases of secondary diseases of the pancreas in diabetes. It is an undeniable fact that cachectic atrophy of the pancreas is found in diabetes. The only difference of opinion relates to the recognition as examples · of cachectic atrophy of a greater or less number of the cases of pancreatic atrophy frequently found in diabetes, and not a few clinicians and pathologists until most recently have inclined to the view that all the atrophies are secondary.

The rare cases of necrosis also can be considered as secondary processes. The latter doubtless may exist side by side. When in the course of a diabetes which has existed for years, a cyst, carcinoma, an acute or chronic inflammation, a hemorrhage, or a fat necrosis develops, we certainly have not the right to bring these lesions into etiologic relation with the diabetes.

The fact which has long been known, that diseases of the pancreas certainly occur as conditions resulting from diabetes, and also quite independently of it, has caused such distinguished investigators as Seegen and Frerichs to take so reserved a point of view. The frequent coincidence of affections of the pancreas with diabetes was known to them, and from it they came to the conclusion that in a number of cases the disease of the pancreas was possibly the cause of the diabetes.

Only through animal experimentation did the familiar facts receive new light, and since in the mean time the number of reported cases was essentially increased, there was a greater certainty in the significance of the concurrence of diabetes and diseases of the pancreas. In order to use the results of animal experimentation in the solution of the questions under consideration, it is necessary to investigate whether the data obtained from animals can be applied to man. It is evident that not all species of animals act alike, and that many are refractory. The most constant results are obtained in dogs.

A positive proof that in man an experimental pancreatic diabetes may arise cannot, of course, be produced. There are, however, some suggestions which may be regarded in the light of such an experiment.

Diabetes developed after a pancreatic cyst had been operated upon by Zweifel. In a woman sixty-four years old there was under the left ribs a tumor which finally grew rapidly. At the operation the tumor was found to be a pancreatic cyst. It was extirpated. A piece of the pancreas 3 cm. long remained. Before the operation the urine was free from sugar. On the ninth day after the operation sugar appeared at times in the urine. It was independent of the food taken. After four weeks there was still sugar in the urine, and three weeks later it was no longer present. In a case of suppuration and necrosis of the pancreas operated upon by Körte there was no sugar in the urine during the stay in the hospital, but later permanent diabetes developed.

Although these cases cannot be regarded as absolute proof that the results in animals can without reservation be applied to man, and that the former are essentially an analogue of the partial extirpation of the pancreas with consequent diabetes in the dog, nevertheless such a conclusion, I think, should be given careful consideration.

This assumption would gain essential support if the facts hitherto known concerning diseases of the pancreas in diabetes could be so utilized that they would harmonize with the experiments on animals.

There are two recent communications, each published by a representative pathologic anatomist, Hansemann and Dieckhoff, who have tried to establish this harmony.

Hansemann propounds the following question: Is there any objection to transferring to man the results of the experiments on dogs? He divides the existing material into three groups.

1. Diabetes without diseases of the pancreas. There is no doubt that there are cases in which, even with the most careful investigation, neither macroscopic nor microscopic changes can be recognized. Hansemann has distinctly found them. This fact obviously does not deny that there is a diabetes in man, attributable to alterations of the pancreas, analogous to the experimental diabetes in animals.

2. Diseases of the pancreas without diabetes. Those cases in which the pancreas is only partly diseased are separated from those in which a total destruction has taken place. In experiments on animals diabetes after partial extirpation is very inconstant, and generally is lacking. This observation corresponds with the fact that in man also diabetes is frequently lacking if the pancreas is only partially diseased.

Hansemann examined 19 of his own cases of disease of the pancreas without diabetes, and found in most of them, even when the organ macroscopically seemed to be totally diseased, that there was enough normal gland tissue to explain the lack of diabetes. Among them, to be sure, were some cases of total destruction of the organ by diffuse carcinoma, and Hansemann explained these by the hypothesis that even cancerous cells may be able to carry on the internal function of the pancreas although they are of no value as regards the secretory function. In like manner, Lubarsch explains the absence of Addison's disease in primary tumors of both adrenals. However ingenious this hypothesis, it cannot be regarded as proof. It takes for granted that which is to be proved.

The cases of total destruction of the pancreas by hemorrhage, suppuration, or necrosis without diabetes, Hansemann explains by reference to the animal experiment, in which the time between the extirpation and the appearance of the glycosuria varied, although the interval was usually short. When the above pathologic processes ran a rapid course, it is clear that there was not time for the occurrence of diabetes. Since in man the glycosuria disappears not infrequently a short time before death, so in the rapidly fatal course of pancreatic necrosis "the disappearance of sugar from the urine may immediately follow the period of incubation." Hansemann admits that this inference is not conclusive.   .

3. Diseases of the pancreas with diabetes. The following varieties are distinguished:

(*a*) Cases in which the disease of the pancreas is a result of the diabetes (cachectic atrophy).

(*b*) Cases in which the diabetes is explained by the total or very widespread destruction of the pancreas.

(*c*) Cases in which the disease of the pancreas assumes the character of an accidental affection with which the diabetes stands in no definite causal relation.

(*d*) A typical variety of disease constantly accompanied by diabetes—namely, the genuine granular atrophy of the pancreas. This discovery of Hansemann in partial disease of the pancreas is of especial interest.

The most frequent lesion in diabetes is atrophy. Hansemann distinguishes two forms: The cachectic, which is rare, and the diabetic, which is more frequent. According to Hansemann, the two varieties are distinguished macroscopically and microscopically.

"In cachectic atrophy the pancreas is sharply defined from the surrounding tissues; the adjacent fat tissue has disappeared corresponding to the general emaciation. The organ is cylindric; that is, its thickness and its height are about equal. It is also of firm or moderate consistency, according to the condition of digestion (even when it has not undergone self-digestion). On microscopic examination the lobules appear small, the individual cells are small, and the stroma is scanty. Gland cells and stroma are atrophied. There is no especial pigmentation of the cells.

"In diabetic atrophy the pancreas is usually flabby and somewhat dark colored. The color is due to the condition of the connective tissue and to the small veins within it. The gland is especially diminished in its transverse diameter and is transformed into a flat structure. The gland lobules are small. The surrounding connective or fat tissue extends into the organ, so that the latter often is removed with difficulty. At times large adhesions and new-formed bands unite the pancreas with the surrounding tissues. Under the microscope the secreting cells show no especial change aside from the atrophy; there are particularly no opacity, fatty degeneration, nor extensive pigmentation. The stroma, however, has not become scanty, as in the cachectic atrophy, but the gaps caused by the diminution in size of the gland lobules are more or less obliterated. It is largely fibrous, but here and there are recent patches of cellular infiltration. Thus an active process is added belonging to the group of interstitial inflammations, and presenting a decided similarity to certain forms of granular atrophy of the kidney."

Hansemann describes cases showing an early stage of this process with signs of an acute interstitial inflammation, and includes in this series the initial stage of the cases described by Lépine as *sclérose périacineuse.*

According to Hansemann, the genuine granular atrophy of the pancreas inevitably leads to diabetes, as the geniune atrophied kidney presents from the beginning characteristic symptoms, while the other affections cause diabetes only when they have continued long enough.

This observation of Hansemann is especially noteworthy; it requires confirmation, however, in two ways:

1. Does this condition actually occur only in diabetes? It may be possible that this process occurs also without diabetes, since at autopsies the pancreas often is not carefully examined and is rarely examined microscopically, especially in certain groups of diseases of other organs. In such instances another explanation might be given.

2. It might well be wished that the genuine, granular atrophy of the pancreas suggested and described anatomically by Hansemann, and maintained always to be associated with diabetes, should find general acceptance and be recognized with the same certainty as granular atrophy of the kidney. This question cannot be decided from reports of autopsies. The few cases investigated by us disclosed, as before mentioned, only cachectic atrophy. The material necessary to prove or disprove Hansemann's view can be collected only very slowly. There is no doubt that a solid foundation for the existence of a pancreatic diabetes would be laid were Hansemann's view correct, but the assumption urgently needs proof.

The communications of Lépine on *sclérose périacineuse* of the pancreas in diabetes alone give evidence in its favor. Hansemann concludes that "there is no case in man which opposes the transference of the results of the experiments on dogs to men."

Dieckhoff proceeds from the certainly surprising fact that in 19 cases of pancreatic disease most carefully examined by him diabetes existed in 7, no examination was made for sugar during life in one, and diabetes was absent only in 11 of the patients. During the same period no other cases of diabetes were examined postmortem in the Pathologic Institute. Dieckhoff asks three questions:

1. Is every case of diabetes referable to changes in the pancreas? Dieckhoff asserts that this question will hardly be answered in the affirmative in the light of the sugar-puncture and the presence of such changes in the fourth ventricle in diabetes as tumors, cysticerci, and sclerosis.

2. What diseases of the pancreas cause diabetes? Experiments and anatomic observations have shown that diffuse diseases attacking the whole organ are more liable to cause diabetes than diseases which attack certain areas. Slight changes in the pancreas, according to Dieckhoff, can be assumed to be related to the diabetes, only when changes in the fourth ventricle are excluded by the postmortem examination, and especially by the most careful microscopic investigation.

The pathologic changes which are found in the pancreas are various, but they have this in common, that they affect to a greater or less extent the whole organ and cause its destruction.

Dieckhoff collects from the literature and from his own experience 53 cases of severe diseases of the pancreas with diabetes, as follows:

Acute pancreatitis....................................... 5
Chronic pancreatitis ....15 + (4?)
Carcinoma 4
Degenerative atrophy, lipomatosis 21
Cysts 4

[The theory of Lépine that one of the functions of the normal pancreas was to produce a glycolytic ferment influencing the consumption of sugar in the organism, and the loss of which was regarded as the cause of diabetes, appears to have been materially strengthened by recent investigations. It was suggested by Laguesse,[*] Schäfer,[†] and Diamare [‡] that the islands of Langerhans probably furnished this internal secretion, and Ssabolew [§] endeavored to solve this question experimentally. He found that the cells of these islands were more granular in fasting dogs than in those fed chiefly with carbohydrates and in whose blood sugar had been introduced. He found also that twenty days after ligation of the excretory duct the islands persisted, although the gland became atrophied. Furthermore, in two cases of diabetes he was unable to find islands of Langerhans in the pancreas. He therefore came to the conclusion that the islands were blood-glands and bore some relation to the utilization of sugar in the organism.

W. Schulze[‖] tied a ligature around portions of the pancreas and found the islands unchanged after eighty days, although the actual tissue of the gland was extensively replaced by fibrous tissue. He inferred that the portions of the gland which persist after ligation influence sugar metamorphosis, since diabetes results from total extirpation of the gland, but does not take place when the excretory ducts are tied and a successful transplantation has been made.

E. L. Opie [**] directed his attention especially to the conditions of the islands of Langerhans in diabetes. He recognized two varieties, an interlobular and an interacinar, of chronic pancreatitis. The islands of Langerhans are affected in the former only when the sclerosis is extreme, and in 11 cases of interlobular pancreatitis diabetes was present in but one, and was of a mild type. The pancreas, however, showed a very advanced degree of inflammation and the islands were altered. In two out of three cases of interacinar pancreatitis, on the other hand, the islands of Langerhans were invaded by the new-growth of fibrous tissue, were atrophied, and diabetes was present. In two other cases of diabetes, in one of which the pancreas was soft and of a gray-yellow color, there was hyaline degeneration of the islands, and to such an extent in one case as to prevent their recognition.

Opie showed that when diabetes is caused by a lesion of the pancreas the islands of Langerhans are injured or destroyed, and when the pancreas is diseased and there is no diabetes the islands are relatively unaffected. In chronic interacinar pancreatitis with diabetes the sclerosis may be so slight as to be definitely recognized only with the microscope, and where there is extreme sclerosis or atrophy without involvement of the islands of Langerhans there is no diabetes.

Weichselbaum and Stangl [††] examined the pancreas in 18 cases of diabetes, and found more or less striking alterations of the islands of Langerhans in all of them. They were diminished in number, absolutely and relatively, to a remarkable degree, and those which were seen were

* *Compt. Rendu Soc. de Biol.*, 1893. v, 819, *Journal de l'Anat. et Phys.*, 1896, xxxii, 208.
† *Lancet*, 1895, ii, 321.
‡ *Intern. Monatsschr. für Anat. u. Phys.*, 1899, xv, 177
§ *Centralbl. f. allg. Path. u. path. Anat.*, 1900, xi, 207.
‖ *Arch. f. mikr. Anat. u. Entwickelungsgesche*, 1900, lvi, 491.
** *Jour. Boston Soc. Med. Sci.*, 1900, iv, 251; *Jour. Exp. Med.*, 1901, v, 397, 528.
†† *Wiener klin Woch.*, 1901, xiv, 968.

more or less altered. In two cases they were hemorrhagic; many islands were atrophied and irregular in shape, as if compressed. Others were so homogeneous as to suggest obliterated renal glomeruli. Although in all cases the pancreas was atrophied, the atrophy differed from other varieties in the predominant affection of the islands of Langerhans.

Further confirmation of Opie's statements has been made by Wright and Joslin.* Portions of the pancreas from nine cases of diabetes were examined, and in two hyaline change in the islands of Langerhans were found. In the remaining seven cases there were no lesions of the pancreas except in one in which there was a fibrinous cellular exudation in the fibrous septa of the gland. Herzog† examined the pancreas in five cases of diabetes with results well in accord with those above mentioned. As Opie justly remarks: "What has been learned concerning the relation of the pancreas to diabetes is the relation of the islands of Langerhans to the disease."—ED.]

3. How are the changes in the pancreas without diabetes to be explained? In slight or circumscribed affections, as in the experiments on animals, sugar is not likely to occur in the urine. In extensive, diffused alterations a remnant of the gland sufficient for the function concerned always may be present. Even the microscopic examination does not positively settle this question.

It is most difficult to explain these cases without diabetes in which the anatomic changes are often much more severe and extensive than in the cases with diabetes. Dieckhoff collects nine such cases, in which the pancreas was almost entirely destroyed and yet there was no diabetes. He explains this by the rapid course of the disease or by complications, as abscess or peritonitis, under which circumstances there was also no diabetes in the animals experimented upon. But this assumption does not explain all the cases. When disease of the pancreas exists a long time without diabetes, it is possible that the severe complicating disease is also to be regarded as a cause; "it is then necessary to conclude that the relation between the changes of the pancreas and the excretion of sugar in man are not so simple as in the dog."

If the results of animal experimentation, the tabulated collections of clinical and anatomic facts, the critical remarks concerning the previously mentioned statistics, and the attempts of Hansemann and Dieckhoff to reconcile the clinical and anatomic facts with the results of animal experimentation are borne in mind, it must be agreed that there is no difficulty in explaining the conditions found in man in the light of the experiments on animals.

The cases of total or very extensive destruction of the pancreas with diabetes are analogous to the total extirpation of the pancreas and explain the occurrence of diabetes.

The cases of atrophy not due to cachexia and affecting nearly the whole gland, of fatty degeneration, induration, calculus formation, with extensive atrophy or fatty change, of new formations or cysts replacing the whole organ, belong in the category of total extirpation.

Limited diseases of the pancreas, abscess formation, and carcinoma, like partial extirpation, may cause a severe diabetes. The latter occurs in the experiments on animals when the rest of the gland gradually dies. All the instances of focal and partial diseases of the pancreas do not be-

* *Jour. of Med. Research*, 1901, VI, 360.
† *Trans. Chicago Path. Soc.*, 1901, V, 15.

long in this series. In such cases the assumption is plausible that the pancreatic disease and diabetes occur simultaneously. This view is not in opposition to the experiments on animals.

There are two objections to the transference to man of the results of the experiments on animals:

1. There are cases of diabetes without any demonstrable changes in the pancreas. Neither the most careful macroscopic nor the most searching microscopic examination shows any noteworthy changes. A list of such cases is included in the following table:

XI. NORMAL PANCREAS IN DIABETES.

AUTHOR.	AGE.	SEX.	CONDITION OF THE PANCREAS.	REMARKS.
De Bary: Wegeli, 1895	9	F.	Pancreas smooth, flabby, pale, microscopically normal.	
Cantani and Ferraro: "Il Morgagni," 1883.	53	F.	Pancreas normal. Microscopically no staining of nuclei (a postmortem phenomenon).	
	30	M.	The same condition.	
Heubner: Wegeli, 1895.	?	?	Pancreas not atrophied. Twelve cm. long.	
Hirschfeld: "Zeitschr. f. klin. Med.," 1896.	61	F.	Pancreas narrow, 76 gm. No anomaly, either macroscopic or microscopic.	
	55	M.	Pancreas normal, 93 gm.	
	56	F.	Pancreas normal, 93 gm.	
Lépine: "Lyon med.," 1891.	40	M.	Normal microscopic appearances in liver and pancreas.	
Obici: "Boll. Scienze med.," 1893.	?	?	No changes in pancreas.	Severe diabetes of rapid course.
Sandmeyer: "Deut. Arch f. klin. Med.," 1892.	9	F.	Pancreas normal.	Death in coma.
Thiroloix: "Diabète pancreat.," 1892.	28	M.	Macroscopically and microscopically normal.	Sudden onset. Very marked polyuria.
	69	F.	Pancreas and solar plexus normal.	Emphysema. Dilatation of heart.
	58	M.	Pancreas normal.	Death with symptoms of uremia.
	60	F.	Pancreas normal.	Death from pneumonia of right side.
Williamson: "Brit. Med. Jour.," 1894.	21	F.	Pancreas small, weight light. Microscopically no changes.	Rapid course of disease.

The pancreas in diabetes is elsewhere very frequently mentioned as normal; Hansemann mentions 8 such cases. Among the reports of autopsies at the General Hospital, the pancreas is characterized as normal in ten instances, but it is not stated that a microscopic examination was made.

Closely allied are the conditions like cachectic atrophy, in which the alterations of the pancreas are distinctly to be regarded as results of the diabetes, or the cases in which the pancreatic disease followed the diabetes, or those in which the alterations probably were not present in life, but are to be regarded as evidence of an autodigestion. Table X doubtless contains such cases. Also to be included are those cases in which, as mentioned before, partial disease of the pancreas and the diabetes are concurrent as accidental conditions without causal relations.

There is no difficulty in explaining this list, if it is assumed that diabetes is no isolated disease, but may result from various causes.

This is not the place to further investigate this subject, but there is no doubt from the present state of our knowledge, that transient and permanent glycosuria may occur from causes other than those which are referred to the pancreas. It is not denied that the time may come when it shall be discovered that the pancreas alone plays the leading part in the pathogenesis of diabetes.

At present it is not justifiable to decide that the pancreas is the sole cause of diabetes. By assuming that there are various causes of diabetes, all the cases may be explained; for example, those in which the pancreas is perfectly normal both macroscopically and microscopically, those in which there are secondary changes in the gland which with certainty are not to be regarded as the cause of the diabetes, those in which there are slight changes, to be considered as postmortem processes of digestion, and also the instances of localized affections in which the greater portion of the gland is normal. The cause of the diabetes which may accompany all of these conditions, according to our present knowledge, is to be sought elsewhere than in the pancreas.

2. The real difficulty lies in the fact that extensive diseases of the pancreas, which have led to a destruction of the whole organ, are not infrequently without diabetes. In the following table a list of such cases is given:

XII. TOTAL DESTRUCTION OF THE PANCREAS WITHOUT DIABETES.

AUTHOR.	AGE.	SEX.	CONDITION OF THE PANCREAS.	REMARKS.
Dieckhoff: "Beitr. z. path. Anat. d. Pankr.," 1896.	?	M.	Tail of pancreas sequestrated, the rest partly destroyed by suppuration and partly beset with areas of fat necrosis. Purulent peritonitis.	
	60	M.	Pancreas contains numerous greenish-yellow masses of pus; in some places firm, indurated substance. Gelatinous cancer of duodenum. Hepatic abscess. Circumscribed abscess between stomach and omentum.	
Hansemann: "Zeitschr. f. klin. Med.," 1895.	52	F.	Pancreas cancerous throughout. Numerous metastases.	
	41	M.	Diffuse carcinoma of pancreas.	
	56	M.	Large primary carcinoma involving the whole gland.	
	33	M.	Whole pancreas transformed into a tumor of size of man's head. Cancer of pylorus.	

6

XII. Total Destruction of the Pancreas without Diabetes.—(*Continued.*)

AUTHOR.	AGE.	SEX.	CONDITION OF THE PANCREAS.	REMARKS.
Litten: "Charité-Annalen," 1877.	45	M.	Pancreas and solar plexus entirely concealed in a glandular mass infiltrated with carcinoma. Medullary carcinoma of stomach, omentum, left kidney, and left ureter. Both adrenals and abdominal glands infiltrated. Cancerous metastasis in duodenum.	Duration of disease one year. Gradual, then very marked decline. Pain in left lumbar region. Urine: albumin, blood, no sugar. Stools normal.
	28	M.	Pancreas changed into a callus, without trace of gland structure, embedded in degenerated lymph-glands. Primary carcinoma ventr. Carcinoma of diaphragm, liver, and lymph-glands. Peritonitis carcin.	Pains in right hypochondrium. Ascites. Urine normal. Appetite good. About three months in duration.
	43	F.	Pressure atrophy of pancreas, replaced by edematous connective tissue. Single small remnants of glands, with nuclei which do not stain. General dropsy. Medullary swelling of epigastric and mesenteric lymph-glands, fused with neighboring organs (pancreas).	Always healthy. Duration of disease 2½ months. High degree of dropsy, hydrothorax and ascites. Otherwise no symptoms. Urine normal.
	59	F.	Primary carcinoma of pancreas with entire destruction of the organ. Cancerous embolism of portal vein. Diffuse infiltration of liver. Gastric ulcer. Swelling of abdominal lymph-glands.	Ascites for 3 months. Pains in right hypochondrium during the last weeks. No disturbances of digestion. Urine normal.
Ziehl: "Deutsche med. Wochenschr.," 1883.	34	F.	Primary carcinoma of pancreas, growing around the aorta and both adrenals.	Once intermittent fever. Acute beginning with chill, fever, and pains in epigastrium. After one month, repeated hematemesis. Emaciation. After 4 weeks, ascites, icterus, attacks of pain in epigastrium daily; collapse. Duration of disease, 9½ weeks.

Hansemann describes also some cases in which, however, the microscopic examination showed that gland substance was present.

The cases in which the pancreas is apparently entirely destroyed, while on microscopic examination normal gland substance can be shown, have their analogue in the experiments on animals. The whole gland apparently has been extirpated, permanent diabetes did not follow, and after death, a portion of the normal gland has been found. Those cases, on the other hand, in which, in spite of entire destruction of the pancreas, diabetes has not developed, do not correspond to the results of experiments on animals. Hansemann, in speaking of a case in which the whole pancreas was transformed into a tumor (carcinoma) of the size of a man's head, but which, on account of defective data, he did not consider sufficiently conclusive, says: "If a new similar observation were made with especial inquiry on this point, then I admit we should have to confess that there are exceptions, and with this admission, however rare the exceptions might be, the whole theory would lose much of its force."

In spite of the attractive hypotheses which have been advanced, we have at present no satisfactory explanation of the lack of diabetes in many cases of total destruction of the pancreas. For instance, in the chronic cases of totally destroyed gland in which no carcinoma was found, even Hansemann's hypothesis is not sufficient for explanation, and a gap exists which still is to be filled.

Notwithstanding the important experiments on animals, there still remains much that is unexplained in the question of pancreatic diabetes in man, and further investigation is required to solve satisfactorily the whole question.

The following conclusions only are to be drawn at present:

1. The undoubted presence of diabetes when the pancreas is microscopically and macroscopically perfectly normal indicates, in connection with other experimental and clinical facts (sugar-puncture, disease of the fourth ventricle, etc.), that there are various causes of diabetes.

2. Diseases of the pancreas may be regarded as one of these causes, as is shown by a number of clinical and anatomic facts, which fully correspond with the results of experiments on animals.

3. The absence of diabetes in man in the not infrequent cases of total destruction of the pancreas cannot at present be definitely explained. It is, however, possible that on further investigation a satisfactory explanation in harmony with the results of experiments on animals may be found. Facts, however, may be brought to light which in various directions will indicate that there is a difference in man and animals in the method of origin of pancreatic diabetes.   ·

2. FATTY STOOLS (STEATORRHEA) AS A SYMPTOM OF DISEASES OF THE PANCREAS.

In the physiologic considerations the influence of the pancreatic juice on the digestion of fat has been stated, especially its emulsifying property and its influence on the cleavage of fat, and the question now is whether in the diminution or total destruction of this pancreatic function, through disease or entire destruction of the gland, symptoms of disturbed fat digestion would be demonstrable in the stools.

As the emulsification and cleavage of the fat are functions not belonging exclusively to the pancreas, but are carried on also by the bile and through the agency of intestinal bacteria, it can readily be understood that these symptoms will not occur regularly.

In order to decide this question, it is desirable to examine the results of experiments on animals, and also to learn the clinical facts.

(a) EXPERIMENTAL RESULTS.

From experiments which caused the degeneration of the pancreas by means of the injection of fat, ether, and other substances into the main excretory duct, Claude Bernard came to the conclusion that the pancreatic juice had the following functions: (1) The cleavage of neutral fats; (2) the emulsification of these fats; (3) the promotion of the absorption of the fats through the presence of the pancreatic juice in the intestine.

Soon after Bernard's communication appeared, the experiments were repeated in France and Germany with various methods, and other results were obtained.

Frerichs tried to destroy the pancreas by numerous ligatures and fed the animals with fat; at the postmortem examination the lacteals were found more or less filled with white chyle. Herbst had the same result. Weinmann caused pancreatic fistula in dogs, fed the animals on food rich in fat, and found no fat in the feces. It must certainly be stated that these experiments show absolutely nothing, because, according to Weinmann's statement, a portion of the pancreatic juice might have reached the intestine through a second pancreatic duct.

Bernard's teachings were opposed by Bidder and Schmidt in Germany, and by Bérard and Colin in France. The latter investigators extirpated the pancreas in five dogs and left only that portion lying next the portal fissure. The animals lived for eight months and showed absolutely no changes of the digestive functions and the feces contained no undigested fat.

Schiff injected paraffin into the main excretory duct in dogs; he claims that the digestion of fats went on normally.

Hartsen extirpated the pancreas in pigeons; the digestion of the fats is said to have been disturbed by this proceeding. The feces of the birds operated upon contained three times as much ether extract as the feces of healthy birds on the same food. Langendorff tied the pancreatic duct in pigeons, but was unable to confirm Hartsen's results.

Pawlow, by tying the Wirsungian duct of rabbits, caused atrophy of the gland. The absorption of fats was not disturbed, at least the feces appeared normal. The same result was obtained by Cash, Arnozan, and Vaillard. On the other hand, Senn, after extirpation of the pancreas in dogs and cats which lived several days after the operation, found in the feces much undigested fat. Martinotti (1888) extirpated the pancreas in dogs, but not thoroughly, and probably not with the view of studying the influence of the pancreatic juice on the digestion of fat; he made no estimate of the amount of fat in the feces; but decided, because the animals did not diminish in weight, that the absorption of the fat had not suffered.

The most thorough experiments were carried on by Abelmann, who, under the guidance of Minkowski, made metabolism experiments in the most careful manner on dogs from which the pancreas had been partially or wholly extirpated. He tried to ascertain the quantity of fat in the stools after the administration of certain definite amounts of fat, and also to estimate in the feces the amount of unchanged neutral fat, fatty acids, and soaps. From his experiments it appeared that when the pancreas was entirely lacking, non-emulsified fat was not at all absorbed, and emulsified fat only in small amount (18.5%). The absorption of fat in the form of milk resulted much more favorably: on the administration of large amounts, 30%, and with smaller amounts, 53%. In case of partial extirpation, small amounts of emulsified fat were about half used up; after the administration of larger amounts of 70 to 150 gm. the consumption was not so good (lowest value 31.5%). Milk was very well used up to 80%. Administration of pig's pancreas as food facilitated the absorption of fat after the extirpation of the pancreas. Abelmann concludes that all fat with the exception of milk needs unquestionably the influence of the pancreas for its absorption.

Sandmeyer, in his experiments, found variable results: Non-emulsified fats were not utilized or slightly absorbed or from 30 to 78% was taken up; 42% of emulsified fat was absorbed. Like Abelmann, he was able to obtain a better utilization of the fat by the addition of pancreas to the food.

The brothers Cavazzani, after extirpation of the pancreas, found that the fat was not used up. A dog the pancreas of which was extirpated a few weeks before, rejected fat but ate soap with great eagerness. After a while there was a better absorption of the fat, since the bile assumed a portion of the function and acted energetically on the fats.

Baldi, as previously mentioned, fed dogs from which the pancreas had been extirpated with meat from which the fat had not been removed, and was able to observe in the stools large amounts of oily fat, which was not solid at temperature of the room, in spite of the fact that the fat of the meat was solid. So high a degree of steatorrhea was never observed after tying the bile-duct.

Rosenberg, by cutting the pancreatic duct and tying the arteries and veins, produced atrophy of the gland; the feces evacuated in large amounts were clayey and showed a large amount of fat.

In one of our experiments on animals Katz found a surprising diminution in the cleavage of fat after partial extirpation of the pancreas and tying of the main excretory duct. The analysis of the feces, the absolute amount of which was not abnormally large, gave the following result:

Neutral fats...51.63%
Fatty acids..46.04%
Soaps..2.33%

(b) CLINICAL EXPERIENCES.

There are three groups of clinical experiences with fatty stools: (1) Fatty stools in diseases of the pancreas; (2) diseases of the pancreas without fatty stools; (3) fatty stools without diseases of the pancreas.

1. The statistics of the **concurrence of fatty stools and diseases of the pancreas** are quite numerous.

Kuntzmann (1820) was probably the first who associated fatty stools with diseases of the pancreas. He described the abundant evacuation of fat in the stools of a man who died from induration of the pancreas with obliteration of the Wirsungian duct, chronic jaundice, and dropsy.

R. Bright, in 1833, reported 7 cases of pancreatic disease, in 3 of which fatty stools were found. As Lloyd states, "icterus was the only symptom common to all of Bright's observations."

Since then the interest of authors has been directed to the concurrence of fatty stools and diseases of the pancreas. At first Lloyd and Elliotson published similar communications. Gould, in 1847, reported a case of calculus and cyst of the pancreas with a large amount of fat in the stools.

Reeves in 16 cases of fatty stools found diseases of the pancreas 11 times: fatty degeneration, cancer, induration of the head with closure of the Wirsungian duct, cysts in the head of the pancreas with obliteration of the pancreatic duct and ductus choledochus, concretions in the ductus pancreaticus, and 6 times there was simultaneous disease of the liver; in only 5 cases was the pancreas intact. Griscom reported 24 cases (14 fatal) in which fatty stools occurred; 8 times an affection of the pancreas was shown at the autopsy; there was no postmortem examination of four of the patients. Moyse gives a similar report.

The communication of Fles, 1864, is of especial interest. A diabetic who had eaten much bacon and fat meat evacuated with the stools such a quantity of fat that it could be skimmed from the surface of the feces by the ounce. The fat disappeared from the stools when an emulsion prepared from the pancreas of a calf was given to the patient. As soon as the emulsion was omitted, the fatty stools again occurred. This experiment was repeated several times with like results. At the autopsy there was so complete a disappearance of the pancreas that only connective tissue with scarcely any recognizable traces of gland substance remained. At the same time, however, there was also atrophy of the liver.

Ancelet collected from the literature 16 cases of steatorrhea in diseases of the pancreas, in 5 of which the pancreatic duct, as well as the ductus choledochus, was closed. In three cases the former alone was closed and in one there was also a pancreatitis.

Silver's case was one of diabetes with fatty stools in a man thirty-two years old. The entire pancreas had undergone fatty degeneration; it was partly calcified and no gland substance was present.

Friedreich reported 2 cases of steatorrhea. In both, jaundice was present.

Bowditch (1852) reported diarrhea with a large amount of fat in the feces in a case of carcinoma of the pancreas. Carcinoma of the liver and jaundice also were present.

Molander and Blix described a case of steatorrhea in carcinoma of the pancreas. Icterus was present. There was a similar condition in Ziehl's case; a large amount of fat in the stools, about 50% of the dry feces; there were also closure of the ductus choledochus and jaundice. Demme found an abnormal amount of fat (64% to 73.3%) in the asbestos-like feces of a case of congenital syphilis and atrophy of the pancreas. There were also jaundice of the skin, perihepatitis, and gummata of the liver.

There were fatty stools in the cases of pancreatic cyst reported by Goodmann, Bull, and Gould; also in the cases of cancer which were published by Clark, Besson, Marston, Martsen, Rocques, Luithlen, Labadie-Lagrave, Pott, Maragliano, and Mirallié. Jaundice was noted by Gould, Clark, Pott, Maragliano, and Mirallié.

Harley reported a case of pancreatic abscess with fatty stools and jaundice.

In a case of fibro-adenoma of the pancreas successfully operated upon and recently reported by Biondi, fatty stools were found, also traces of sugar and jaundice.

Steatorrhea has been observed also in calculi of the pancreas; in addition to the cases already mentioned by Clark, Gould, Reeves, are those of Capparelli, Copart, Cowley, and Lancereaux. In the case described by Lichtheim, numerous fat crystals were found.

A communication of Le Nobel is of interest. A diabetic sixty-one years old observed that his stools contained much fat. Although there was no jaundice, the stools were colorless and contained an abundance of fat. There was an entire absence of all biliary constituents, as well as of hydrogen sulphid, indol, skatol, leucin, and tyrosin. The feces had a sour odor like rancid butter, but no fecal smell. Microscopically no micro-organisms were present, but there was an abundance of fatty acid crystals without soaps. Bile pigments and bile acids were absent. No autopsy was held.

Le Nobel thought that the lack of fat-acid salts, the absence of all products of putrefaction in the stools, and the occurrence of maltose in the urine were positive evidence of an affection of the pancreas.

Clay-colored stools abounding in nitrogen and fat were found by Hirschfeld in 6 cases of diabetes. According to him, this sign, in connection with the colic frequently observed in this patient, might be used to place cases of this kind in a special category and to indicate that a disease of the pancreas was of pathogenic importance.

The following observation is from my own experience, and further details will be given in the section on cancer:

In a woman thirty-nine years old there had been diarrhea since the summer of 1892. The patient became emaciated, yet the appetite remained good. Fecal evacuations appeared regularly at night, were unusually copious, of the consistency of thick porridge and of cadaverous odor, chocolate-colored, and always abundantly covered with fat rings. On the 11th of January, 1893, I saw the patient for the first time, and found steatorrhea. The investigation of the stools gave the following result: Large in amount and of the consistency of thick porridge; in the sediment were scattered white particles. Microscopic examination: (1) Very numerous fragments of striated muscle, in the main with well-preserved structure; (2) numerous fat-acid needles and fat-drops; (3) bacteria and detritus.

After drying the stools for several days on the water-bath in order to determine the amount of fat, there were obtained 4.6325 gm. of solid substance, in which 2.1265 was fat, representing 45.9% of the dried residue. The ether extract consisted almost entirely of neutral fat. On the 18th of January I found in the epigastrium a distinct hard, round tumor, which was diagnosticated as carcinoma of the head of the pancreas. In March, jaundice developed. At the beginning of April an exploratory laparotomy was undertaken and the diagnosis was confirmed.

2. The literature of **diseases of the pancreas without** fatty stools is abundant. In the special portion of this section but few statements are made regarding the presence of fatty stools in diseases of the pancreas. In many cases nothing is said about the condition of the stools, and only in the rarest instances are exact chemical investigations under-

taken, so that the lack of a positive statement can in no case be regarded as evidence to the contrary. From the earlier collections of cases, it may be mentioned that Ancelet in 330 instances of disease of the pancreas found fatty stools 28 times.

Statements also appear concerning the lack of fatty stools when the pancreas is totally destroyed; thus, Litten reports four cases of total degeneration of the pancreas with normal stools and without diabetes.

Hartsen, in two diabetics, in whom the autopsy showed atrophy of the pancreas amounting almost to total disappearance of the gland, in spite of the daily administration of 8 to 10 teaspoonfuls of cod-liver oil, was unable to show the presence of any unusual amount of fat in the stools.

The most important work in this connection is that of Friedrich Müller. In two cases investigated by him, one of total obliteration and the other of cystic degeneration of the pancreas, he was unable to find any increase over the normal amount of fat in the feces, although sufficient fat was given in the food. The feces, examined with the naked eye, microscopically, and chemically, were similar to the dejections of a normal individual.

Müller attributes the occurrence of fatty stools in diseases of the pancreas to disturbances in the secretion of bile, which in a very large number of observations take place at the same time; this conclusion is due to the fact that the withdrawal of bile always leads to the poor absorption of fat. From his investigations carried on with jaundiced patients, Müller comes to the following conclusions:

(a) If the bile is excluded from the intestine, the absorption of fat suffers very considerably. In his experiments, when there was a total lack of bile, 55.2% to 78.5% of the fat in the food was evacuated with the feces, while in the normal individual only 6.9% to 10.5% is found.

(b) If the pancreatic juice is excluded from the intestine, there is no increase of fat in the stools, and it is doubtful whether steatorrhea is a symptom of purely pancreatic diseases.

(c) The absence of pancreatic juice causes no quantitative change in the condition of the fat of the feces. The cleavage of the neutral fats is a function of the pancreatic juice. In three cases in which there was an obstruction of the Wirsungian duct and a degeneration of the gland, a much smaller cleavage of the fat than normal was demonstrable (39.8% as compared with 84.3%). Müller concludes that when there is a lack of pancreatic juice, the cleavage of the fats goes on less energetically than normally.

3. Fatty stools without alteration of the pancreas.

(a) An abnormally large quantity of fat may occur in the stools of a healthy man when so large an amount of fat is taken with the food that all cannot be absorbed by the intestine.

(b) Steatorrhea occurs when bile is absent from the intestine, as is shown especially by the investigations of Nothnagel, Gerhardt, and Müller.

(c) The fat is increased in the stools, although the amount of fat in the food remains the same, when there is disease of the mucous membrane of the intestine and of its lymphatics, especially of the mesenteric glands, rendering the absorption of the fat difficult or impossible. The abundant fat in the stools is thus explained in extensive atrophy of the mucous membrane of the small intestine, in amyloid disease and tuberculosis of the same, in caseation of the mesenteric glands, in chronic tuberculous peritonitis, and perhaps in some catarrhal processes (Nothnagel).

It is evident from the clinical facts reported that the presence of fatty stools alone is not of value in the recognition of diseases of the pancreas, because steatorrhea may arise from different causes. The formerly well-accredited doctrine of the importance of steatorrhea in the recognition of diseases of the pancreas has recently been discredited especially on account of the thorough work of Friedrich Müller, whose results we have learned.

Müller's proof is twofold. He shows the presence of fatty stools in the absence of any affection of the pancreas, especially when bile is excluded from the intestine, and he finds a normal amount of fat in the stools in undoubted disease of the pancreas. Müller says that it is difficult to believe that there are no fatty stools when the pancreatic juice alone is excluded from the intestine, especially as there have been no accurate metabolism experiments either on animals or man.

At present, however, there are very suggestive and convincing experiments in this direction. Metabolism experiments on animals have been carried on by Minkowski, Abelmann, Sandmeyer, Cavazzani, Baldi, and Rosenberg, and on man by Hirschberg. The experiments on animals show with some variations that after extirpation, as well as after destruction of the gland tissue, there is a poorer consumption of the fats, with the exception of that of milk. That the increased or diminished fat absorption is to be ascribed to the lack of the pancreatic juice in the intestine is shown by the fact that in several experiments there was a better absorption of fats when the animals were at the same time fed with the minced pancreas of a pig.

There is still much that is not clear in the experiments on animals; for instance, there is at present no answer to the question why in the absence of the pancreatic juice bile does not supply its place.

Do the results of the experiments on animals harmonize with the clinical facts, especially with the somewhat diverging results of Müller's series of experiments? Müller was certainly correct in assuming that it is not justified, in the relatively frequent cases of disease of the pancreas and fat stools occurring at the same time with jaundice, to refer the steatorrhea with certainty to the disease of the pancreas, because the exclusion of bile from the intestine is alone sufficient to explain the poor fat absorption; but, on the other hand, the possibility must be admitted, because of the results of experiments on animals, that in these cases the consumption of the fat was poor even without jaundice.

Müller says also that it is difficult to believe that there are no fat stools when the pancreatic secretion alone is excluded.

Abelmann explains the two cases of pancreatic disease without fatty stools investigated by Müller, as well as all similar negative cases, by the assumption that a portion of the pancreas, even if very small, still acts normally. For the case of pancreatic cyst which Müller investigated, this idea is plausible. For the other case, however, in which there was a closure of the Wirsungian duct by concretions, as a result of which the gland atrophied, this explanation is applicable only on the assumption that there was a second pancreatic duct through which some pancreatic juice reached the intestine.

It must be admitted on the basis of experiments on animals that steatorrhea may occur in total or very severe disease of the pancreas. The relative infrequency of its occurrence undoubtedly depends on the fact that the bile assumes a vicarious function, and that the presence of a second excretory duct furnishes the pancreas a means of furthering the digestion of fat even in case only a small bit of the gland is connected with the open duct.

The infrequency of the statements regarding the presence of fatty stools in diseases of the pancreas may also be explained by the fact that examinations of the stools, and particularly metabolism experiments, are rarely made and especially are recognized only in striking instances. The most of the diagnoses of diseases of the pancreas are made either by an operation or by a postmortem examination, and careful examinations of the stools are rarely made before the operation or autopsy. One therefore can say nothing of most of the cases, and only a few data appear concerning Müller's important observation regarding the deficient cleavage of fat in diseases of the pancreas.

It cannot, therefore, be positively stated at present what the conditions really are, as the literature gives no standard of judgment. Investigations are lacking on animals as well as on man. The knowledge regarding the absorption of fat has still many unsettled points. It is probably to be explained by the experiments on animals why, in total extirpation of the pancreas, the bile does not perform its function, and. why the experiment with the simple ligation of the excretory duct, even where there was only one, caused no essential disturbance in the absorption of the fat. There is a contradiction also between the experiments on animals and the observations in man in regard to the cleavage of fat. After total extirpation of the pancreas, Abelmann found normal fat-cleavage, while Müller showed a disturbed cleavage of the fats but no steatorrhea. It is mysterious and entirely unexplained why, after partial extirpation of the pancreas, although so conducted that no pancreatic juice could reach the intestine, up to one-half of small amounts of non-emulsified fat and up to 80% of milk were used up, while after total extirpation no emulsified fat was absorbed. In both cases there was an entire lack of pancreatic juice in the intestine, and yet there was this difference. Exact metabolism experiments in man are needed also, in order to ascertain whether, in case of simple obstruction of the ductus choledochus, the digestion of fat does not show essential qualitative and quantitative differences according to the open or closed condition of the pancreatic ducts and whether the disturbance in fat-cleavage observed by Müller really occurs only in affections of the pancreas, and how these facts are to be brought into harmony with the diametrically opposite results in the experiments on animals.

In spite of the many gaps and obscurities, it must be asserted, on the basis of experiments on animals and of a small series of clinical and anatomic facts, that there are cases of fatty stools which under certain conditions indicate directly a disease of the pancreas.

What is known at the present time can be stated as follows:

1. Steatorrhea alone gives no evidence which points to disease of the pancreas.

2. It is possible that disturbed fat digestion is caused by a disease of the pancreas when there are neither jaundice nor disease of the intestine.

3. The probability that a disease of the pancreas exists increases and

may become certain when, jaundice being absent, symptoms still occur which point to the pancreas, as, for instance, defective consumption of nitrogen (azotorrhea), diabetes, or a tumor in the region of the pancreas, as in the case observed by me.

4. There may be diabetes and at the same time poor absorption of fat without disease of the pancreas.

5. It cannot, at present, be stated positively to what extent the disturbed cleavage of fats, which is certainly an essential function of the pancreas, may be used as a pathognomonic symptom of an affection of the pancreas. Müller's cases give a positive indication.

3. FAULTY DIGESTION OF ALBUMIN (AZOTORRHEA).

Experiments on animals give some evidence concerning the defective digestion of albumins. Abelmann found that when the pancreatic juice was lacking, the albuminous substances were partly absorbed, to the extent of about 44% in dogs which were without pancreas and 54% in dogs which still possessed a small piece of the gland. The variations in absorption were ascribed by Abelmann in part to the poorer consumption of the fat introduced at the same time, since steatorrhea certainly exerts an influence on the absorption of the other food-stuffs. When pig's pancreas was given with the meat, in the one series 74% and in the other 78% of the nitrogen administered was absorbed. After the administration of pure pancreatin only 47% in the one case and 55% in the other was absorbed. The feces had a penetrating odor and visibly contained undigested muscle-fibers when meat was given.

De Renzi also found increased nitrogen in the feces after total extirpation of the pancreas in animals. A similar observation was made by the brothers Cavazzani.

Sandmeyer found large amounts of well-preserved, striped muscle-fibers in the feces of animals fed with meat and bread after total extirpation of the pancreas. After partial extirpation 62% to 70% of the albuminous bodies were used up.

Undigested bits of meat in the feces were found also by Rosenberg. The disturbed digestion of albumins was shown in a very marked way in one of our experiments after total extirpation, which was followed also by diabetes. Large pieces of undigested meat were found mingled with the stools after the first meat was taken. On microscopic examination, numerous muscle-fibers with unchanged structure were distinctly recognized. On the other hand, no change in the appearance and composition of the stool could be shown in an animal which lived with severe diabetes for forty-one days after the operation.

After partial extirpation no increase in excretion of nitrogen could be noted. The dog fed with meat was able to use no inconsiderable amounts of nitrogen from the food given.

The oldest and most remarkable clinical statement is that of Fles, previously mentioned. He found in the stools of a diabetic very numerous unchanged and perfectly well-marked bundles of striated muscle-fibers. The muscle-fibers disappeared from the stools when a calf's pancreas was daily fed to the patient, and were found when the calf's pancreas was omitted from the diet.

Harley mentions the occurrence of large amounts of undigested muscle-fiber in the stools of a patient with pancreatic abscess. Le Nobel also observed large amounts of undigested muscle-fiber in a patient's stools. A similar observation was made by v. Ackeren in a case of carcinoma of the pancreas. In a case of pancreatic cyst, Küster saw large amounts of undigested muscle-fiber in the feces even when the amount of meat in the food was very limited. In a case of calculus of the pancreas in a diabetic patient reported by Lichtheim the stools were found very rich in striated muscle-fibers.

In the case of cancer of the head of the pancreas previously communicated by me, very numerous bits of striated muscle-fibers were found, in the main with the structure distinctly preserved.

The diminished consumption of nitrogen was found in several diabetics by Hirschfeld. Upon an average, the feces contained, of the food introduced: 35.2% of the dry substance; 31.8% of the nitrogenous substance; 34.8% of the fat. The normal quantity is from 6% to 7%. In these cases there was no postmortem proof of disease of the pancreas.

The presence in the stools of numerous undigested muscle-fibers is certainly an important feature and deserves especial attention.

The azotorrhea alone does not permit the diagnosis of an affection of the pancreas, since the digestion of albuminous bodies is not exclusively the function of the pancreatic juice. When this sign is combined with the absence of jaundice and faulty digestion of fat or disturbance of the cleavage of the fat, and if neither gastric nor intestinal disease is demonstrable, the suspicion is wholly justified that a disease of the pancreas is present. The probability is materially increased when diabetes also exists, and becomes a certainty if a tumor in the region of the pancreas is demonstrable, as in the case observed by me.

B. SECOND GROUP.

1. CHANGES IN THE URINE.

It would be of decided importance if evidence of a disease of the pancreas could be found in the urine.

The statements on this point already made unfortunately are not conclusive.

Acting on my advice, and from the beginning of our investigations, A. Katz has paid special attention to this subject, but has been unable to obtain results in favor of the pathognomonic value of changes in the urine in disease of the pancreas.

Especial weight was laid on the excretion of indican. Since this is derived from indol, which arises in pancreatic digestion under the influence of bacteria, an important diagnostic value for the recognition of disease of the pancreas has been assigned to the quantitative estimation of indican in the urine.

Gerhardi was the first who, in the year 1886, made the diagnosis of disease of the pancreas as the cause of the mechanical disturbance of the intestine on account of lack of increase of indican in a case of obstruction of the small intestine. Jaffe found, after ligating the small intestine, an enormous increase in the excretion of indican, although ligation of the large intestine had little or no effect on this excretion. In obstruction of the large intestine the indican is increased only when inflammatory changes occur and the small intestine participates in the disturbance.

In Gerhardi's patient there were several symptoms which indicated an obstruction in the uppermost portion of the intestine, but as there was no abnormal increase of the indican in the urine, and especially no peritonitic symptoms, a loss of function of the pancreas or a disease of that gland was suspected. The autopsy confirmed this assumption of Gerhardi.

This view appeared to be supported by experiments on animals. Pisenti has estimated the amount of indican in the urine of dogs before and after tying of the pancreatic duct. He found in one case, before the operation, 11.70 to 19.90 mg. of indican *pro die;* after the operation, 4.30 to 4.20 mg. *pro die.* In a second case, before the operation, 15.0 to 21.0 mg. of indican *pro die;* after the operation, 6.0 to 9.0 mg. of indican *pro die.* The estimation of the indican was made according to the method given by Salkowski. After the administration of pancreas peptone to dogs, the pancreatic duct of which had been tied, there was an increase of the indicanuria.

Some of the very few clinical observations which have been made support the assumption of Gerhardi, while others refute it. Stefanini, in a case of purulent pancreatitis, and Biondi, in a case of adenoma of the gland, observed lack of indicanuria. On the other hand, Schlagenhaufer asserts directly the increase of the indican in a case of syphilitic interstitial pancreatitis.

The results obtained by Katz are in diametrical opposition to the statements of Pisenti. The former examined the amount of indican in the urine in the majority of our experiments on animals and showed very positively that there was absolutely no diminution in the amount of indican after lesions of the pancreas. In many cases a marked indicanuria could be proved. The amount of indican was greater and its increase could be shown distinctly in the days following the attack, especially in those cases in which the animals took no nourishment after the operation, and even when they died quickly from duodenal necrosis. There was no diminution in the excretion of indican also in the animals which long survived the operation. On a pure meat and milk diet, abundant amounts of indican were found in the urine. De Renzi also could show no change in the amount of indican in the urine in his experiments on animals, even after total extirpation of the pancreas.

From these observations it is evident that the presence or absence of a disease of the pancreas is not to be concluded from the amount of indican in the urine.

The variations in the excretion of the indican may be founded on factors which have no direct relation to the activities of the pancreas. The conditions of absorption of the intestinal mucous membrane which are independent of the secretion of pancreatic juice, or processes in the organism which have their scat outside of the intestine, may have an influence on the excretion of indican.

The latter assumption is favored by the fact·that during inanition, in sulphuric-acid poisoning, in progressive anemia, in cholera nostras and Asiatica, in spite of the rapid passage of the intestinal contents, an increase of indican in the urine is to be shown. It is interesting that Hennige refers the increase of indican in cholera and lead-colic to an alteration in the pancreatic juice caused by nervous influences.

The excretion in the urine of certain carbohydrates may be added to the symptoms which are regarded as characteristic of diseases of the pancreas. Maltose in rare instances, as well as glucose, has been found in the urine. Le Nobel observed, in a man sixty-one years old, who suffered from fatty stools and glycosuria, a reducing substance in the urine, corresponding, as he thought, to maltose. Von Ackeren, in a case of pancreatic carcinoma, found a like substance, and regarded its presence as pathognomonic of diseases of the pancreas. Later investigators were not able, however, to find maltose in the urine of diabetics. At any rate, the occurrence of maltose is very rare.

The presence of pentose in the urine is of greater diagnostic importance, according to Salkowski. Only a few cases heretofore have been known in which this pentatomic sugar has been found in the urine. It was shown first by Jastrowitz and Salkowski in the urine of a morphin-eater, who for a time suffered from glycosuria.

Ferdinand Blumenthal reported the cases of two individuals in whose urine the presence of pentose was observed for some time, both independently of the diet and without further disturbance of the general condition. There was also a diminution in the amount of indican in the urine in both cases. Hammarsten found in the pancreas a nucleo-proteid containing mucin, which on cleavage gave rise to a pentose.

Salkowski found that the pentosazon extracted from the urine was identical with the pentosazon obtained from the pancreas. The melting-point, the form of crystallization, the external appearance, the reaction to heat, and the solubility corresponded so perfectly in the two preparations that the identity of the two substances was to be assumed "with a degree of probability bordering on certainty." On the basis of this observation, Salkowski believes "that the pentosuria depended on an abnormally increased formation and destruction of the nucleo-proteid which forms the pentose, and as this nucleo-proteid predominates in the pancreas, the pentosuria is presumably to be regarded as an affection of this organ."

This conclusion was supported apparently by the statements of Külz and Vogel, who found pentose in the urine of starving dogs which had become diabetic after extirpation of the pancreas. The presence of pentose was frequently shown also in diabetes in man. They examined the urine of 80 diabetics; in only 4 cases was there no pentose, in 12 cases the pentose test was weak or doubtful, in 64 cases it showed distinctly the red coloration from the use of the Tollen reagent (phloroglucin and fuming hydrochloric acid). As foods of plant origin very frequently contain pentose, the pentosuria may doubtless be of purely alimentary origin in many cases.

The statements of Salkowski and Blumenthal are opposed to this positive evidence. The former never found pentose with the glucose in 9 diabetics. Blumenthal investigated 10 severe cases of diabetes, among which were the 9 cases examined by Salkowski, and was unable to find pentose with the grape-sugar. A diabetic who in seven weeks, under strict diet, showed a diminution in the amount of sugar from 6.5% of glucose in 3500 c.c. of urine to none at all, never had pentosuria, although the morning and evening urines were daily examined for pentose.

The cleavage of the nucleo-proteid of the pancreas, although the most prominent, is certainly not the sole source of pentosuria. In the cell-nucleus are found still other bodies belonging to the group of nucleo-albumins, the cleavage of which with dilute sulphuric acid also gives rise to pentose. In consequence, the pentose may arise from the nucleinic acid distributed throughout the animal body (Blumenthal).

Pentosuria was constantly found by Capparelli after the injection of morphin. The assumption is probable that in this case the pancreas is not specially involved.

The occurrence of fat in the urine, lipuria, is mentioned by the older authors as a result of disease of the pancreas. Tulpius describes a case in which fat was excreted with the feces and in the urine. Elliotson reports a like condition. In neither case was there an autopsy to confirm the diagnosis of disease of the pancreas.

Fat was found by Clark in the urine of a woman for a long time, and later fatty stools also occurred. At the autopsy carcinoma of the pancreas and nutmeg liver, with a very small amount of bile in the gall-bladder, were found.

Bowditch reported the case of a man on the surface of whose urine numerous fat-drops were found. At the autopsy cancer of the liver and of a large portion of the pancreas were observed.

Lipuria certainly cannot be utilized in the diagnosis of disease of the pancreas, since it results from most diverse causes. (See Lipuria, by Senator, "Diseases of the Kidneys.")

The changes hitherto described have been regarded by many as characteristic of diseases of the pancreas, but unfortunately their claim is not justified. In brief, the condition of the urine in diseases of the pancreas has no especial peculiarities.

The appearance of the urine is, as a rule, not altered. The dark pigmentations noticed in bronzed diabetes are not to be ascribed directly to the disease of the pancreas, but probably originate in the disturbance of general metabolism and in the alteration of the liver. The jaundice often present in pancreatic diseases of course changes the color of the urine. Turbidity of the urine is found in cases of lipuria. The specific gravity of the urine is altered only when it is increased by the diabetes resulting from disease of the pancreas.

The reaction of the urine is more strongly acid than normal, according to the observations of Jablonski on dogs with pancreatic fistulæ and external discharge of pancreatic juice. Before the operation there was 0.013% of oxalic acid, but after the establishment of the fistula the oxalic acid was 0.156%. Jablonski attributes this increase of acidity to diminished alkalinity of the blood, from the loss of alkalis contained in the pancreatic juice, and he succeeded in producing a normal acidity of the urine by injecting a weak soda solution. There are no observations upon man relating to this point.

The amount of urine is affected by disease of the pancreas only when diabetes occurs. In bronzed diabetes, in spite of the excretion of sugar, the polyuria seems not so strongly marked as in the other forms of glycosuria. De Dominicis, in his experiments, observed an increase of the amount of urine independently of the excretion of sugar. In our experiments, however, no abnormal increase of the amount of urine could be shown either as the result of pancreatic lesions or of extirpation of the pancreas.

The amount of urea in the urine was, as a rule, greatly increased. The azoturia generally was in proportion to the glycosuria. In some of the cases observed by de Dominicis, Hédon, and Thiroloix, azoturia without glycosuria occurred after extirpation of the pancreas. Azoturia, however, does not occur constantly in the experiments on animals. After partial extirpation, it could not be shown.

There are no statements regarding the excretion of the urea-containing constituents of the urine—urea, uric acid, and ammonia. The excretion of the chlorids appears to be unaltered by disease of the gland. The excretion of the phosphates is increased. De Dominicis assumes that an increase of phosphoric acid is a characteristic of pancreatic lesion even in those cases in which there is no glycosuria. The excretion of sulphuric acid obviously is increased in cases of azoturia.

Katz has devoted especial attention to the relation between the total sulphuric acid and the ether-sulphuric acids as a measure of the processes of decomposition going on in the intestine. According to his investigations, the amount of combined sulphuric acids showed no essential variation from the normal after total as well as after partial extirpation of the pancreas. Considerable variations were shown, as have been observed in dogs under other conditions, and were dependent upon the variation in the absorption of the food. When a dog was fed with easily and rapidly absorbed fish, Katz found small amounts of ether-sulphuric acid,—0.032, 0.022, 0.069 gm. daily,—the relation to the excretion of the total sulphuric acid being 19.2, 22.3, 20.2.

When the dog made diabetic by extirpation of the pancreas was fed with pure meat, Katz found the amounts to vary very considerably; relatively they were very high—0.076, 0.089; but also as low as those above mentioned—0.024, 0.025, 0.033, 0.039. The variations in the relative amounts were, of course, correspondingly great according to the differences in the absolute amounts of ether-sulphuric acid and were between 21.0 and 4.5. These investigations of Katz do not permit the recognition of any constancy in the excretion of the ether-sulphuric acid after complete exclusion of the pancreatic juice from the intestine, as in the case mentioned, and the reason for the differences must be found in the varying conditions of intestinal resorption.

Acetone and acteo-acetic acid are not regularly found after extirpation of the pancreas. Minkowski observed them especially when there was marked emaciation of the animals experimented upon. After extirpation of the pancreas Baldi found a considerable increase of acetone. In the normal animal the daily amount varied between 0.0 and 0.105 gm., while the amount of acetone excreted on the second day after the operation reached 1.043 gm., on the third day 0.652 gm., and fell later to 0.385 to 0.282 to 0.049 gm.

According to Minkowski, oxybutyric acid did not occur constantly in the urine and was excreted in small amounts. The diabetic organism is able to oxidize the oxybutyric acid introduced even after extirpation of the pancreas. The amount eliminated may, therefore, be smaller than the amount originating in the organism. Its occurrence might perhaps be regarded always as a complication of diabetes; it was present, especially in the larger amounts, at a time when the amount of sugar was diminished (Minkowski).

BRONZED DIABETES.

This peculiar disease, which has been associated with affections of the pancreas, deserves mention at the close of the consideration of the changes in the urine occurring in disease of the pancreas.

Trousseau was the first to report a case which may be regarded as *diabète bronzé.* Servaes described a patient with pancreatic carcinoma, bronzed skin, and diabetes.

The clinical picture and the anatomic lesions were stated most carefully and thoroughly by Hanot and Chauffard. They reported two cases. Letulle, in the same year (1882), published two new observations. In 1886, Hanot and Schachmann reported another case.

In 1888, Brault and Galliard published a new observation. Barth demonstrated a striking specimen in the Société d'anatomie. In 1892, Gonzales Hernandez mentioned another case in his thesis. In 1893, Palma reported two cases of diabetes with cirrhosis of the liver and bronze coloring of the skin. In 1895, Mossè and Daunic, in a man thirty-nine years old, who had suffered from diabetes for about a year, observed a dark brown color of the skin, moderate polyuria, 4 to 5 liters daily, marked glycosuria, and azoturia. At the autopsy the liver showed the picture of Hanot's pigmentary cirrhosis. The pancreas was somewhat yellower than normal, firm, slightly sclerosed, and showed also on microscopic examination the picture of pigmentary sclerosis. The adrenals were normal.

Buss described, in his dissertation in 1894, a case of diabetes mellitus with cirrhosis of the liver, atrophy of the pancreas, and general hematochromatosis. In 1895, de Massary and Potier reported another case at the Société d'anatomie. In the same year Marie published a striking case in a man fifty-one years old who, about four months before, had been attacked with the symptoms of diabetes mellitus and with edema of the lower extremities. The average daily amount of urine was 2.5 to 3.5 liters, and that of the excretion of sugar 40 to 50 gm. The liver was distinctly enlarged. There was difficulty in breathing, sleeplessness, and distention of the abdomen. Six days before death there was no sugar in the urine.

Aucher reported another observation in the Société d'anatomie. In their theses appearing in 1895, Achard and Dutournier took up the subject of bronzed diabetes. Rendu and Massary reported at the Société des hôpitaux the case of a strong man affected with diabetes and subsequent brown coloration of the surface of the body. The disease lasted about half a year. Jeanselme at the same meeting referred to two cases observed by him. One was the case of a man who had worked for ten days with litharge and red oxid of lead and then sickened with symptoms of a severe diabetes accompanied by discoloration of the skin, with a daily excretion of 5 to 7 liters of urine containing from 150 to 337 gm. of sugar. In the second case the disease developed as the result of an injury in the region of the umbilicus. The disease lasted five and a half months. Hitherto only 22 cases of the disease have been reported.

Marie gave the following picture of the disease based on these observations: Bronzed diabetes occurs especially in men between forty and sixty years of age. The youngest patient was thirty-seven, the oldest sixty-one years old. Among the etiologic factors are alcoholism, malaria in the case of Hernandez, and in one of Jeanselme's lead-poisoning and in the other injury. The diabetes generally begins suddenly. Gastrointestinal disturbances early occur, also diarrhea or affections of the respiratory apparatus. The characteristic symptoms of diabetes, polydipsia and polyuria, are, as a rule, not so strongly marked as in the other varieties of this affection. The urine is generally dark, beer-colored, and free from bile pigments. The abdomen is swollen and its veins

7

distended, the liver is greatly enlarged, and the spleen is somewhat increased in size. At first there is little or no ascites; later, accumulations of 6 to 8 liters of fluid have been observed in the abdomen.

Hanot and Chauffard, in one patient, noted a lymphangitis of the abdominal wall. Digestion is frequently delayed. Toward the end of life diarrhea often is observed. The patients become rapidly and extremely emaciated. In Brault's case 55 pounds were lost in six months. Finally, edema of the lower extremities and cachexia develop.

The discoloration of the skin is general and uniform. Spotted pigmentation is not seen. In contrast to Addison's disease, there is no pigmentation of the mucous membranes. The color is not always bronze-like; in many cases the skin is blackish-gray, with a metallic luster, like the broken surface of cast-iron. Under certain circumstances, despite the characteristic change in the liver and internal organs, the pigmentation of the skin is much less distinctly marked. The course of the disease is, as a rule, very rapid. The longest duration—two years— was in the case reported by Letulle; the shortest was five and a half months, in a patient of Jeanselme and five months in Marie's case. In the last few days of life fever occurs, as a rule, and sugar disappears from the urine.

The most striking of the anatomic changes takes place in the liver. This organ is large and hard; only very exceptionally, as in two questionable cases of Palma and Lucas-Champonnière, is there noted a diminution in the size of the liver. Its color is brownish-red, "like old red leather," its surface is generally uneven, rarely smooth. The gall-bladder appears filled at times with colorless bile. Slate-gray coloring is seen also in the intestine, mesentery, omentum, and in the lymph-glands, especially in those of the abdomen. The spleen is rust-colored and sclerosed.

The pancreas in most cases is sclerosed, rust-colored, and its excretory duct is patent. The heart, as a rule, is normal, flabby, reddish-yellow. In the lungs, tuberculosis is frequently demonstrable. On microscopic examination there are found in the liver granular degeneration of its cells, increase of the connective tissue, and deposition of pigment, especially in the interstitial tissue, less frequently in the liver-cells.

In the pancreas the spaces in the connective tissue are much enlarged and much pigment is deposited both in them and in the cells. This pigment is of yellow-ochre color, rich in iron, and evidently to be regarded as a derivative of the blood coloring-matter. The development of the pigment is located in the liver by Hanot and Chauffard, and is regarded by them as an increase of its chromatogenic function. It is supposed that this pigment is transferred through the lymphatics from the liver to other organs.

Letulle opposes this view by calling attention to the fact that the deeply pigmented cells are dead, and believes that the hemoglobin is locally reduced. Brault and Galliard consider the cirrhosis as the primary, and the degeneration of the blood as the secondary, condition.

Marie thinks that the hemoglobin is decomposed through some unknown cause and is transformed into the pigment. The latter is eliminated in part by the lymphatic system and thus causes degeneration, irritation, and connective-tissue growth in the various organs.

Achard states that the changes in the liver have nothing to do with the diabetes, and that the latter is to be regarded solely as the result of the changes in the pancreas. This view regarding the chronologic course of events Buss considers improbable.

Jeanselme explains the mechanism of the development of bronzed diabetes in the following way: First there is the degeneration of the red blood-cells in the capillaries of the gland parenchyma; the yellow ochre pigment originating in this way reaches the secretory epithelium and a sclerosis develops in all the organs overladen with pigment. If a sclerosis of the pancreas is added to the sclerosis of the liver, diabetes develops, and then is to be regarded as a purely secondary phenomenon.

Rendu and Massary think the formation of the yellow ochre pigment takes place in the cells as a consequence of the normal metabolism. After the destruction of the cells the pigment reaches the connective-tissue spaces and is carried from them to the several organs by the lymph-cells.

The diabetes cannot be made answerable for the disturbance of cell activity, as Hanot and Chauffard originally claimed, since a like change in the skin is repeatedly seen without diabetes; thus, it was observed in malaria in 1889 by Kelsch and Kiener, in 1895 by Brault in two cases without diabetes, and most recently by Letulle, Gilbert, and Grenet in hypertrophic cirrhosis of the liver.

Reference may here be made to the cases in which affections of the pancreas occur without mellituria, but with bronzed coloration of the skin. Aran found the condition in a woman twenty-five years old in whose pancreas caseous foci were found containing cavities from softening. Jenni has mentioned an ashen-gray color of the face in a case of cancer of the pancreas. Kappeller and Moritz observed two cases of this affection, in which there was a bronzed color of the skin.

2. EMACIATION.

The earlier authors regarded an especially marked degree of emaciation as a characteristic symptom of diseases of the pancreas. It is not surprising that this occurs in cases of diabetes or carcinoma, but it may be found also without these; for instance, when there are cysts. In Küster's case the patient lost 33 lbs. in four months. Küster and Riegner ascribed the emaciation to the poor digestion of proteids. The weight not infrequently has increased rapidly after a successful operation.

The cachexia in carcinoma of the pancreas at times presents certain peculiarities, which, however, are not to be regarded as pathognomonic, as has been claimed by many, especially French, authors. It indeed often develops much more quickly and intensely than in other carcinomata of the upper abdomen. There is much weakness and prostration, which cannot be explained by the inanition alone. The subject will again be considered in the section on carcinoma.

The occurrence of diseases of the pancreas in fat persons will repeatedly be noted in the special part of this article. Very acute processes, especially, as hemorrhages, the so-called hemorrhagic pancreatitis, necrosis, and fat necrosis, are found quite often in corpulent people.

3. SALIVATION OR SIALORRHOEA PANCREATICA, AND DIARRHOEA PANCREATICA.

The spitting or vomiting of large quantities of fluid resembling saliva has been regarded as characteristic of diseases of the pancreas.

The cause was assumed to be an increased secretion of saliva or of pancreatic juice due to reflex excitation.   In two cases of cysts, reported by Battersby and Ludolf, a flow of saliva is noted.   Holzmann also reports salivation during the colic produced by pancreatic calculi.   A similar observation was made by Capparelli and Giudiceandrea in lithiasis. From the rarity of its occurrence, it is evident that there is no causal relation between this symptom and diseases of the pancreas.

It may be, as Friedreich justly suggests, that the flow of saliva is referable to concurrent disease of the stomach.   The thin viscid stools supposed to be composed of pancreatic juice and regarded as characteristic are of no greater importance.   From the older literature Friedreich mentions the following experience reported by Levier.   In the cholera epidemic at Bern from 1861 to 1864, a large amount of leucin was found in the evacuations.   "The idea can by no means be excluded," writes Friedreich, "that there may have been an actual hypersecretion of the pancreas, an accompaniment of a peculiar form of acute epidemic intestinal catarrh."

Senn has recently suggested a causal relation between the profuse diarrheas occurring at times with cysts and a degeneration of the parenchyma of the gland.   Lichtheim also, in a case of pancreatic calculus with diabetes, suggests the obstinate diarrhea as an important sign.

Peculiar diarrheas may occur in consequence of the rupture of a pancreatic cyst into the intestine.   Such was observed in Nothnagel's clinic in Vienna.   A tumor was demonstrable in the region of the pancreas, but it disappeared after the evacuation of diarrheic stools and the vomiting of a bowl full of alkaline fluid containing grayish-red and reddish-brown shreds.   This result is obviously not identical with pancreatic salivation.   There is no further proof of this condition in recent communications.

C. THIRD GROUP.

This includes the symptoms which frequently occur in diseases of the pancreas.   They present no peculiarities which point to the pancreas, with the exception of a distinctly palpable or visible tumor in the region of the pancreas.   They are mostly morbid signs which may occur in the most diverse diseases of the digestive organs and are often the expression of a combination of diseases of various organs, as has already been stated in the introduction to the general part (p. 17).

1. **Tumor or resistance.** A circumscribed or diffuse tumor, or an elevated, distinctly palpable, abnormal resistance, corresponding to the position of the pancreas, may be found in acute or chronic inflammation (abscess or induration), in cysts or new formations of the pancreas. A more or less sharply defined tumor or an indefinite resistance in the upper portion of the abdomen may be found in some cases of abscess, as in the cases reported by Kilgour and Percival.   In Graeve's case, also, an increased resistance was found.   Thayer observed in the middle line above the umbilicus, a deep-seated resistance, which could not be separated from the liver.

If a pancreatic abscess has ruptured, and a bursal abscess or a retroperitoneal collection of pus has developed, then a fluctuating tumor may be found in the epigastrium (Körte, Rosenbach, Werth-König, Casper-sohn-Hansen).

As will be stated in the special part, a palpable tumor may be recognized also in chronic induration. Riedel once felt beneath the abdominal wall a tumor of the size of a fist consisting of the head of the pancreas, which proved to be caused by chronic inflammation. The presence of a tumor in cases of cysts and neoplasms will be sufficiently treated in the special part.

2. **Jaundice** is a frequent symptom of diseases of the pancreas. The anatomic position of the bile-duct, as has been shown in the preceding communication of Zuckerkandl, gives a satisfactory reason for this condition. According to his investigations, it is easily understood that when the ductus choledochus extends at least a half centimeter into the head of the pancreas, it may be compressed, even to entire closure, if the head is swollen or atrophied. Such swellings eventually may subside if the cause is temporary, as an inflammatory enlargement which may resolve. Many cases of so-called catarrhal jaundice may perhaps depend on such resolving swellings of the head of the pancreas.

Jaundice may develop in like manner in chronic induration of the pancreas, as in Hjelt's patient. Jaundice not infrequently develops from the pressure of cysts on the ductus choledochus. It may arise, however, in other ways.

In a case described by Gould, the jaundice was transient, and, probably, was produced by duodenal catarrh. Cruveilhier refers to a scirrhus at the mouth of the ductus choledochus which caused both jaundice and, by closure of the pancreatic duct, also a pancreatic cyst. In a case described by Phulpin, a gall-stone in the ductus choledochus caused jaundice, and, by compression of the ductus Wirsungianus, also a pancreatic cyst. In Friedreich's case an annular cancer of the duodenum produced jaundice and dilatation of the Wirsungian duct with numerous sac-like diverticula by compression of this duct.

Jaundice is found most frequently in cancer of the pancreas. As a rule, it develops slowly and insidiously, but steadily. The jaundice may diminish toward the end of life. As the skin becomes pale and anemic, the yellowish color becomes less intense.

Mirallié noted 82 instances of jaundice in 113 cases of primary cancer of the pancreas. Among 36 additional cases collected by me, jaundice is noted 21 times; thus, in 149 cases jaundice is present in 103. The jaundice may be due also to disease of some neighboring organ which accompanies the affection of the pancreas. Diseases of the liver and of the biliary tract, especially gall-stones, extension of pancreatic diseases, particularly new-formations, to the liver and biliary tract, metastases in the liver, and, lastly, catarrhal processes may also cause the jaundice.

3. **Different kinds and degrees of pain and painful sensations** play an important part in diseases of the pancreas. Without doubt, diseases even which extensively invade the pancreas may run their course without pain. In cancer, for example, pain may be absent throughout the whole course of the disease, as in the case described by Friedreich, in which there was neither spontaneous pain nor tenderness. Also, in the case reported by Stiller no severe pain occurred. It may be absent even in abscess of the pancreas (Nathan). The pains may be occasional or continuous, and in the latter case temporary exacerbations may occur.

The occasional pains may have the character of colic or of cardialgia. They occur in acute as well as in chronic affections of the pancreas.

The colicky pains are oftenest caused by stagnation of secretion due to closure of the excretory duct or of the ducts in the interior of the organ by concretions or by some other mechanical factor hindering the free evacuation of the secretion. The colic therefore occurs most frequently in calculus formation, compression of the excretory and secretory ducts by new-formations, scars, indurative inflammation, or hemorrhage. It is to be assumed also that catarrhal processes which lead to swelling of the mucous membrane at the outlet of the pancreatic duct may cause colicky pains. Not infrequently so-called nervous gastralgias may be referred to such stagnation of secretion.

The pains in hemorrhage have mostly a colicky character; that is, they diminish or entirely disappear at times, and then return with increased violence. In tumor-formation, also, the pains may be only occasional. In pancreatic cysts the pains may occur in paroxysms and have the character of cardialgias or biliary colic, when the cyst develops in the head of the pancreas. The colic at times occurs with great violence, fainting, and symptoms of collapse. In cancer, also, pains may at times occur, and present the characteristics of colic and cardialgia. They may represent the exacerbation of neuralgic pains produced by pressure on neighboring ganglia, or be due to stagnation of secretion from compression of the excretory duct, or, lastly, there may be a real biliary colic, when the ductus choledochus is embedded in the carcinomatous mass.

The continuous pains are of various kind and intensity, often remittent and occasionally with paroxysmal exacerbations, but frequently increasing gradually; they are present in acute and chronic processes in the pancreas, as pancreatic abscess, hemorrhage, gangrene, indurative pancreatitis, and tumor-formation. The pains may come on suddenly with great severity, as is usually the case in abscess of the pancreas, in hemorrhage, and in the so-called hemorrhagic pancreatitis and in gangrene. In tumor-formation—cyst or carcinoma—the pains, as a rule, come on gradually and increase in severity with the growth of the tumor.

The pains in cancer may be of especial violence and of peculiar character. In the section on this subject their characteristics will be considered in detail. To what extent the celiac ganglion or nerve-trunks arising from it are concerned in the production of these pains it is impossible to state at present. The designation "celiac neuralgia" was long since chosen for these pains. Although there is no proof that the pain is related to the celiac ganglion, it is very probable that pressure or traction on this ganglion actually causes severe pains.

Pains of different kinds may of course be produced by the combination of disease of the pancreas with diseases of neighboring organs. When the stomach or intestine overlaps it or becomes adherent to it, constant or remitting pains may be produced by the peristaltic movement dependent upon the function of these organs. Intense continuous pain may arise also from participation of the peritoneum. Concurrent affection of other neighboring organs, as the liver, bile-passages, and lymph-glands, will give rise also to different kinds of pain.

More or less extreme sensitiveness to pressure in the epigastrium, in the region corresponding to the pancreas, is found in connection with the most diverse processes in this gland. It must be mentioned, however, that in many acute and chronic processes, even when diffused, it is especially noted that there is no sensitiveness to pressure.

In a number of cases merely vague, troublesome sensations, not to be regarded exactly as pain, occur in the region of the pancreas. These are the discomfort, sense of distress, feeling of pressure, fulness, and tension, which are especially unpleasant in certain positions of the body.

4. **Pressure on adjacent organs** may produce severe results in the course of the disease. Compression of the intestine first deserves consideration. The stomach, especially the pyloric portion, may also be compressed under certain conditions, and stenosis with dilatation of the stomach thus may be caused. This occurred in a case operated upon by Bardeleben; the diagnosis before the operation was closure of the pylorus by a compressing tumor. At the operation multiple carcinosis of the liver and peritoneum were recognized and no relief could be afforded. After death cancer of the head of the pancreas, compressing the pylorus, was found.

The compression of the intestine may give rise to stenoses, and symptoms of obstruction may arise. Not infrequently symptoms of intestinal obstruction are the first marked evidence of disease of the pancreas, and in a number of cases laparotomy has been undertaken because intestinal occlusion was diagnosticated. At the operation the obstruction was sought in vain.

Such instances of real or apparent obstruction of the intestine occur in various diseases of the pancreas. They are recorded in acute processes, as in the cases of Nathan, Fitz, Hirschberg, Sarfert, McPhedran, Parry Dunn and Pitt, Gerhardi, Balser, Rosenbach, Caspersohn, v. Bonsdorff, Hovenden, Simon and Stanley, Allina.

The intestine may be narrowed or entirely closed by growing tumors. Intestinal occlusion may be due to cysts, as was found in the cases of Brown and Hagenbach, and transient obstruction was noted in the case of Lardy.

Intestinal occlusion is reported in carcinoma by Kerckring, de Haen, Mondière (2 cases), Holscher, Teissier, Tanner, Salomon, Wrany, Stansfield.

Hindrance of intestinal function, meteorism, and constipation are frequent symptoms of disease of the pancreas. In pancreatic carcinoma Kellermann found constipation 60 times, diarrhea 12 times, and in 9 cases alternate constipation and diarrhea. By pressure on the portal vein, ascites, enlargement of the spleen, and dilatation of the hemorrhoidal veins may develop and edema of the lower extremities may result from pressure on the vena cava. One or the other ureter may be compressed by tumors, and thus hydronephrosis develop (Recamier, Reeve).

5. **Vomiting and nausea** are remarkably frequent, and are nearly constant signs of disease. They may appear at the beginning and persist throughout the disease. The various combined affections—the colic, the peritoneal disturbance, the intestinal obstruction, etc.—likewise lead to vomiting.

Nausea and vomiting are usually present at the beginning of abscess-formation, and vomiting is likewise found frequently in chronic interstitial pancreatitis; there is vomiting also in hemorrhage, although in exceptional cases there is only nausea, or gastric disturbance may be entirely lacking. There may be vomiting of blood (Hooper) or vomiting of a dark brown fluid (Fearnside). Vomiting is a very frequent symptom of cancer. Blood may be mingled with the vomitus, or pure blood may be vomited, especially when there has been perforation into the cavity of the stomach or into the duodenum.

Vomiting frequently occurs in cysts also; at first only at intervals, during the attacks of colic, but later with greater frequency—perhaps after each administration of food.

6. **Abnormalities of the** stools have already been discussed in different places in this section. The frequency of constipation and the occasional occurrence of diarrhea have repeatedly been mentioned. Certain characteristic peculiarities of the stools, steatorrhea and azotorrhea, have been reported in detail.

Bloody stools occur at times in cancer. Such cases have been reported by Bohn, Friedreich, Kobler, Mariani, Molander and Blix, and Wesener. The hemorrhages were generally caused by ulceration of the intestine. Pancreatic cysts by rupture into the intestinal cavity also may cause bloody stools. In Pepper's case a cyst of the head of the pancreas broke into the duodenum and caused hematemesis and bloody stools. A pancreatic abscess may break into the intestine, and blood and foul pus pass off with the stools (Percival, Atkinson).

A sequestrated pancreas also may be evacuated with the stools (Rokitansky-Trafoyer, Chiari-Schossberger). Sometimes pancreatic calculi are found in the stools, as in the cases cited by Leichtenstern and Minnich.

7. **Dyspeptic disturbances** are very frequently recorded: altered appetite and sense of hunger, especially anorexia, distaste for meat, discomfort after meals, sensations of pressure, fulness, epigastric tension, especially after meal-time, heart-burn, eructation, nausea, etc.

It is clear that it cannot be considered that all these difficulties are to be ascribed to the pancreatic affection. They are mostly to be regarded as resulting from a simultaneous disease of the stomach and intestine.

8. **Fever** is found at times in acute as well as in chronic affections of the pancreas. In pancreatic abscess and in bursal abscess there is generally an irregular fever with intercurrent chill. Pancreatic abscess also may run its course without fever. The combination with peritonitis naturally becomes a source of fever.

In cancer the fever generally depends upon complications, as cholangitis with abscess-formation in the liver, subsequent pancreatitis, and metastases in the lungs and pleura. The fever also may be related to the development of the tumor (Kobler).

Fever may arise in cases of cysts also, in consequence of the occurrence of pancreatitis or of the suppuration of the cyst. In gangrene and necrosis the fever may develop from the metastatic pleuritis, pericarditis, leptomeningitis, etc. In cases of pancreatic calculi fever is at times noted. In the patients of Bonet and Galeati the type was tertian; but it could not be assumed with certainty that the fever had any relation to the lithiasis.

In the case reported by Minnich and Holzmann fever (37.7° to 38.3° C.—99.9° to 101° F.) was shown during the colic. Subnormal temperature has been found especially in the last stage of cancer (Bard and Pic). It is found not infrequently as a manifestation of collapse in various acute processes in the pancreas.

IV. GENERAL STATISTICS AND ETIOLOGY.

TRUSTWORTHY statistics can be obtained under only two conditions: When the diagnosis can be made with certainty during life, and when there is a postmortem examination. These two conditions are not fulfilled in diseases of the pancreas. These affections are rarely to be recognized with certainty during life, and the anatomic statistics are not sufficiently complete, because the pancreas is not examined frequently enough at autopsies, certainly not with the same thoroughness as are the liver and kidney.

In the diseases which are the most frequent causes of death, as tuberculosis, cardiac and renal diseases, infections, cachexias of different kinds, and senile marasmus, it is probable that the pancreas is seldom examined thoroughly, and yet there is no doubt that tuberculosis causes frequent changes in this gland, and that in cachexias and marasmus atrophy of the pancreas is by no means rare. Statements about the pancreas are rarely found in postmortem records of the above-mentioned diseases.

It is probable that another, even large series of diseased processes in the pancreas escapes observation, because not being recognized during life, healing takes place and no obvious trace is found at a subsequent postmortem examination.

Catarrhal inflammations of the pancreatic duct, continued from the intestine or from the gall-bladder, circumscribed acute or chronic inflammations, slight hemorrhages, disturbances of pancreatic secretion, formations of concretions, are certainly recovered from, as will later be shown. All of these processes are rarely recognized during life. After death, traces might exceptionally be found, but even if traces were present, search for them is rarely made.

Pancreatic diseases, consequently, are by no means so rare as is repeatedly assumed. It is not at all clear why of the entire series of digestive organs—stomach, intestine, liver, pancreas—the latter alone should especially be protected from disease; why diseases of the blood-vessels, gland parenchyma, secretory canals of the blood, should spare only the pancreas whose vital functions are so important and manifold, while under quite similar conditions the neighboring organs are so frequently attacked. If the attention were given to the pancreas which it certainly deserves on account of its physiologic importance, the limited experience now at hand would certainly be enlarged.

Although it is very probable, from the above statements, that diseases of the pancreas occur much more frequently than is known, yet it must be recognized that the number of fatal diseases of the pancreas is certainly much less than that of the neighboring organs. Tumors and general acute and chronic inflammatory processes occur without doubt more rarely in the pancreas than in the other organs of digestion. Statistics are continually being published, and even cases following a regular course are considered worthy of communication. This speaks decidedly for the relative rarity of severe diseases of the pancreas which, if marked, certainly would not be overlooked at autopsies.

The figures which hitherto have been given are insufficient as a basis for the determination of the absolute frequency of diseases of this organ. Claessen has collected all previous to 1842, and there are 322° cases, 193 in men and 129 in women. It will be seen in the special part that the data which have become known in the last few years are relatively much more numerous.

Recent statistics have been published by Hansemann. In ten years there were found in the postmortem records of the Berlin Pathological Institute (Charité and Augusta-hospital) 59 cases of disease of the pancreas, 40 with diabetes and 19 without this condition. Among the 19 cases, necrosis of the gland and fat necrosis were not included.

In the postmortem records of the Vienna General Hospital from 1885 to 1895 the following statistics were found:

Diseases of the pancreas with diabetes ....12 cases.
Diseases of the pancreas without diabetes ....84 "
                                                            96 "

The figures recorded in the years 1893 to 1895 show that there has been increased attention directed to this matter of late years. In these three years 49 cases have been reported, as against 47 in the seven preceding years. Claessen states that more men than women suffer, 193 of the former and 129 of the latter. In Hansemann's statistics a similar relation was noted, there being 42 men and 17 women. In the postmortem records of the Vienna General Hospital, among 94 cases, 42 were men and 52 were women.

Diseases of the pancreas may occur at any age. In late fetal life and in the newborn indurative pancreatitis, depending on inherited syphilis, is by no means rare. When there is a syphilitic affection of the liver in such children, syphilitic pancreatitis is frequently found. In early childhood and youth cancers have been noted. Bohn found cancer of the pancreas in a child seven months old, Kühn in a girl two years old, and Dutil in a boy of fourteen. Cysts occur even in infancy. Railton found a cyst in a girl six months old, Lynn in a boy two years old, v. Petrykowski in a girl three and a half years old, and Fenger in a girl eight years old. The last three cases were operated upon successfully. MacPhedran describes a case of acute pancreatitis in a boy nine months old. In the special part the age is tabulated in a number of the diseases.

Claessen gives the following statistics with regard to the relative frequency at different ages. Among 262 cases there were found:

In the newborn.. 5 cases.
In the first year .... 2 "
From the first to the tenth year .... 20 "
From the tenth to the twenty-fifth year 41
From the twenty-fifth to the sixtieth year 156
Beyond the sixtieth year............................. 38 "

The postmortem records of the Berlin and Vienna Pathologic Institutes for a term of ten years show the following relative frequency of these diseases at the different periods of life:

BERLIN PATHOLOGIC INSTITUTE.

Age.	Number of Cases.
From 10 to 20 years	4
" 21 to 30 "	12
" 31 to 40 "	12
" 41 to 50 "	11
" 51 to 60 "	9
" 61 to 70 "	5
" 71 to 80 "	4
	57

In two cases there is no statement regarding the age.

VIENNA PATHOLOGIC INSTITUTE.

AGE.	NUMBER OF CASES.
From 10 to 20 years	3
" 21 to 30 "	5
" 31 to 40 "	11
" 41 to 50 "	21
" 51 to 60 "	24
" 61 to 70 "	23
" 71 to 80 "	7
" 81 to 90 "	1
	.95

In one case no statement was made concerning the age.

The etiology of pancreatic diseases is usually obscure. The heretofore mentioned causes—as, prolonged use of mercury, misuse of tobacco and drastic cathartics, pregnancy (Mondière), suppression of the menses (Schönlein)—are scarcely deserving of mention. The influence of syphilis and alcohol is undoubted. These certainly are a cause of chronic inflammations of the gland.

Acute purulent processes are of bacterial origin and are to be attributed to the admission of organisms from the intestine or from the bile-passages. This subject will be treated more in detail in the special part.

Chronic pancreatitis is, no doubt, due to a similar etiologic factor. Various processes which promote the entrance of micro-organisms, cholelithiasis, for instance, may give rise to chronic pancreatitis.

Catarrhal processes in the pancreatic ducts resulting from the continuation of catarrh from the intestine and biliary tract produce stagnation of secretion and its results. The secretion may become stagnant from other causes: for example, the formation of calculi in the pancreas, compression of the excretory duct by indurations, scars, tumors, calculi in the ductus choledochus, etc. Chronic pancreatitis and cyst formation may result.

The influence of injury in the production of cysts and hemorrhages is well established. Atrophy of the pancreas certainly may be a manifestation of general cachexia and marasmus. Autodigestion of the pancreas is also to be mentioned as a cause of pathologic changes. In the section on Necrosis and Fat Necrosis this question is more thoroughly treated.

Venous hyperemia and stasis may result from disease of the heart, lungs, and liver. The continuance of processes which have their seat in the neighborhood (neoplasms of the stomach, duodenum, and liver, and ulcers of the stomach) may include the pancreas. Metastases of inflammatory or neoplastic character may attack the pancreas.

In acute and chronic infectious diseases there are various alterations of the pancreas: parenchymatous degeneration in acute infectious diseases, and gumma and tuberculosis as a part of general syphilitic and tuberculous infection.

V. GENERAL THERAPY.

FROM the rarity with which a correct diagnosis * of pancreatic disease can be made specialized treatment is 'not often possible. The patients with pancreatic disease recover or die generally without the disease being recognized; therefore, apart from surgical treatment, a specific treatment affecting the diseased organ is usually not attempted. Therapeutic suggestions are sufficiently numerous, the older physicians having recommended a long list of medicaments and methods of treatment.

Claessen enumerates the remedies suggested: Eyting saw a chronic pancreatitis wholly cured by chlorin and iron; Landsberg states that scirrhus was cured by "nitro-muriatic acid, foot-baths, tamarind whey, and laxative pills." Calomel has been recommended as a specific by various writers (Brera, de Haën, Harder, Berlioz, Claessen). Nasse claimed to have seen a very strikingly favorable effect from the use of corrosive sublimate in a severe case of chronic inflammation with induration of the pancreas. In all these cases of so-called cure there is no proof of a correct diagnosis; therefore the value of these observations is very problematical.

When we can recognize the etiologic factors, a rational therapy is possible. Syphilis doubtless plays an important part in the production of pancreatic diseases, and the antiluetic treatment of chronic inflammation or of gumma of the pancreas in a syphilitic patient might have favorable results.

Diseases of the intestine may have a decided influence on the occurrence of affections of the pancreas, and the rational treatment of catarrh and bacillary affections of the intestine may have a protective and healing influence on the pancreas.

The connection between chronic inflammations of the pancreas and cholelithiasis has definitely been established by recent experience. There is no doubt that the timely removal of calculi from the gall-bladder or bile-ducts can save the pancreas from inflammation and is influential in promoting the resolution of existing inflammation.

Other affections of the liver and biliary tract also are of influence in the production of diseases of the pancreas, and if the former can be directly treated, disease of the pancreas may be prevented and existing disturbances of the pancreas perhaps may be relieved.

If alcoholism, arteriosclerosis, acute and chronic infectious diseases, affections of the heart, lungs, kidneys, and those causing disturbances of general nutrition, as diabetes (from extra-pancreatic causes), obesity, etc., which are of importance in the etiology of diseases of the pancreas, are checked, the dangers of impending diseases of the pancreas are lessened, or if actually existing, their course may indirectly be alleviated.

For years much has been hoped from organotherapy in pancreatic diseases, but unfortunately no material advance has been made in this direction. Pepsin, and later pancreatin, were the first used, long before the present era of modern organotherapy. Some of the results obtained in patients gave much promise. Under this head belongs the case already mentioned of Fles, who gave to a diabetic, who passed in the stools much

---

* The diagnosis of pancreatic diseases in general has been thoroughly considered in the section on General Pathology and Symptomatology, and the diagnostic value of the individual symptoms has been given at length.

fat and undigested meat, calf's pancreas with the food, and in consequence caused an improvement in the digestion of fat and meat. The pancreas was finely minced in a mortar, rubbed with 6 ounces of water, and strained. The resulting milk-like fluid was taken after meals. Each day an entire calf's pancreas was used. The case described by Langdon-Down also could here be mentioned: A man fifty-two years old, suffering from diabetes, fatty stools, and great emaciation, was greatly improved after the administration of pancreatin (Friedreich).

Organotherapy in the treatment of diseases of the pancreas has been strongly supported by the results of experiments on animals, as shown in a previous section. Abelmann, experimenting on animals from which the pancreas had been removed, found a marked improvement in the digestion of fats and proteids after pig's pancreas was added to the food. Sandmeyer also saw an improvement of fat-digestion after adding pancreas to the food. De Renzi, Cavazzani, and others had similar results.

It is evident that when diabetes was supposed to be related to changes in the pancreas, the attempt was made to treat the diabetes by the administration of pancreas or pancreatic preparations, and numerous reports have been made. The question has not yet reached a satisfactory conclusion. Some authors report favorable results, while with others the reverse is the case.

Since it is possible only in rare instances to make a diagnosis of pancreatic diabetes with certainty during life, because other characteristic features are usually lacking, organotherapy was often used when the pancreas certainly was not the cause of the diabetes. The negative results in these cases are of course not convincing, either for or against the value of this treatment. But even in the cases with positive results, strict proof is generally lacking that a disease of the pancreas is the necessary cause of the diabetes, and the objection certainly is justified that any improvement is to be referred to other factors than the administration of pancreas or preparations of pancreas.

Among the positive results, the following may be mentioned:

Battistini obtained pancreatic juice from the fresh gland of a calf or sheep by maceration with physiologic salt solution or with glycerin. After filtration of the extract through sterilized paper and dilution of the glycerin extract with water, 5 c.c. at first, and afterward 15 to 20 c.c. were injected. In a man thirty-seven years old, the amount of urine before treatment was 4200 c.c., in which were 110 gm. of sugar; after three injections the amount of urine was 4110 c.c. containing 89 gm. of sugar. Later there were fever and a further diminution of the glycosuria. The amount of urea remained unchanged.

In a woman thirty-nine years old the amount of urine fell from 3800 c.c. to 2000 c.c., the amount of sugar from 111 gm. to 43.04 gm. After the injection of 15 c.c. the result was still more significant and continuous; the amount of sugar reached only 3 to 5 gm. and the patient felt stronger, although her weight did not increase.

In two diabetics, Hale White either gave internally 2 ounces of fresh pancreas or injected two drops of extract each morning and evening. The amount and specific gravity of the urine did not change, the urea in one case remained unaltered and in the other increased. The excretion of sugar was unaffected in one case but diminished in the other. The subjective condition of each patient was improved.

In two cases Wood found improvement of the general condition, and in one there was a diminution in the amount of sugar. Rémond and Rispal saw decrease in the excretion of sugar in one case of *diabète maigre* after injection of pancreatic extract.

Sibley Knowsley used the freshly expressed juice or the slightly cooked gland. The result in one severe case of diabetes was very favorable; the weight increased about 700 gm. and the subjective troubles and glycosuria diminished.

Lisser used pancreatic enemata. The ox or sheep pancreas was minced finely, allowed to stand for twenty-four hours with an equal amount of physiologic salt solution, and 2 gm. of sodium bicarbonate were added to it after being slightly warmed. From 50 to 120 gm. were given daily in the form of an enema to a man seventeen years old who for three months had suffered from a severe diabetes with daily amounts of urine equal to 10 to 14 liters and an amount of sugar equal to 6.25%. After 34 enemata, the daily amount of sugar fell from 875 gm. to 425 gm.; but when the remedy was omitted, the excreted sugar became 916 gm. and then fell to 256 gm. The body-weight increased about $4\frac{1}{2}$ pounds. In a second case also the result was very favorable. The weight increased $8\frac{1}{2}$ pounds. In the latter case diarrhea occurred after the enemata had been used two or three weeks.

Bormann used the gland in a diabetic thirty years old. With a strict diet of meat the patient excreted 1500 to 2300 c.c. of urine with 30 to 60 gm. of sugar, and with a diet of milk and meat 30 to 110 gm. After he had eaten on each of three days a slightly broiled pancreas, the amount of sugar was 17 gm., and four days later 40.5 gm. As the patient refused to take the gland, the juice was given in an enema. After four days the amount of sugar was 14.6 gm. and then increased to 30.3 gm. The sugar remained quite constant at this level, in spite of the fact that the patient received a daily subcutaneous injection of $1\frac{1}{2}$ c.c. of pancreatic extract. His subjective condition and his strength improved. The weight increased, the thirst and amount of urine had diminished.

Ausset gave the pancreas of a calf internally to a man who daily excreted 38 gm. of sugar. After two days the excretion of sugar had fallen to 4.0 gm. On the ninth day the glycosuria had entirely disappeared. The urine remained free from sugar for a month.

Among the negative results, the following may be mentioned:

Comby tried injections of the pancreatic juice of a guinea-pig, prepared after Brown-Séquard's method, in a diabetic twenty-five years old. One-half c.c. was injected at first every second day, and later every day. The daily amount of urine reached 7 to 10 liters, the excretion of sugar varied between 800 gm. and 1000 gm., and the amount of urea had increased to 75 gm. The injections were well-borne, but were without influence on the course of the disease.

In two severe cases of diabetes Mackenzie used the juice expressed from the fresh pancreas in daily doses of 15 gm. The amount of urine diminished during the treatment. The subjective symptoms, especially the thirst, became less. The glycosuria was not influenced.

Fürbringer, and also Renvers, used glycerin extract of pancreas in two diabetic patients without result.

Goldscheider used pancreatic extract in six cases of diabetes without any result. Senator had negative results with pancreatin.

In a diabetic fifteen years old Williams tried the injection of extract of pancreas, and later undertook the implantation of the gland of a sheep which had just been killed. The patient, however, died comatose. In two cases he gave the gland in part internally and in part subcutaneously; in the first case no result was to be noted, and in the second the result was probably to be ascribed to the diet and the administration of codeïn.

The most recent communications concerning the treatment of pancreatic diabetes with preparations of pancreas are those of Hugounenq and Doyon. They found that the excretion of sugar was not diminished.

In conclusion, mention may be made of an observation by Mairet and Bosc, who found that in healthy men the injection of an emulsion of pancreas caused fever, acceleration of the pulse, weakness, increase of the amount of urine and of the excretion of urea. After injection of the glycerin extract of pancreas in 21 epileptics, an increase in the paroxysms was observed.

In a number of diabetic cases which were admitted to the Rothschild Hospital, I also have tried organotherapy. The preparations chiefly used were such as had earlier been tried with reference to their physiologic activity. The "zymine" tabloids and pancreaticum siccum of Merck, introduced by Burroughs, Wellcome and Co., had the desired activity. In addition, pancreatic enemata prepared according to Lisser's direction were tried. The pancreatic preparations recommended by Knoll were not used.

The experiments were made with eight diabetic patients, and the following results are briefly sketched:

1. H. R., man sixty-one years old, admitted on the 24th of December, 1895. Amount of urine 2 liters, specific gravity 1031, sugar 1.2%, no acetone. January 19, 1896, sugar 2.7%. From the 20th of January daily administration of 2 zymine tabloids. February 5th, sugar 3.3%.

2. R. W., woman thirty-eight years old, admitted January 20, 1896. At the time of admission, amount of urine 4½ liters, specific gravity 1030, sugar 6%, much acetone, body-weight 45.5 kg. March 27th, amount of urine 5 liters, 3.5% of sugar, much acetone, body-weight 44 kg. From the 7th of April, 0.5 gm. of pancreatin of Merck was given three times a day. April 19th, 5 liters of urine, 5% of sugar.

3. A. L., man thirty-five years old, admitted September 30, 1895. At the time of admission, 4.5% sugar, 0.026% acetone, acetic acid, specific gravity 1026, day's amount 4 liters, body-weight 47 kg. December 5th, 2.3% sugar, 45.6 kg. body-weight. December 22d, 2 zymine tabloids, from January 3d 3 tabloids daily. January 20th, 3.1% sugar, 46.5 kg. body-weight. March 16th, 43.5 kg. body-weight. March 27th, 1896, discharged. Admitted again April 20th, the patient very miserable, 3.7% sugar, 5 liters urine, large amount of acetone. Coma. Death. At the autopsy, marantic atrophy of the pancreas was found.

4. J. R., man forty-five years old, admitted February 6, 1896. At entrance, 3½ liters of urine, specific gravity 1032, sugar 3.8%, 60 kg. body-weight. From the 16th of February three zymine tabloids daily, sugar 1.4%, 3 liters. March 10th, 4.2% sugar, 3½ liters urine in one day, tabloids omitted. March 21st, 3 tabloids again. March 26th, 4 liters urine, 6.4% sugar. April 4th, 0.5 gm. daily pancreatin. April 15th, 4.2% sugar, 3½ liters urine.

5. M. M., man sixty-two years old, admitted March 27, 1896. At entrance, body-weight 50 kg., 5 liters urine, 3.2% sugar, no acetone. After diabetic diet, 5 liters urine and 1.4% sugar. From April 4th, 0.5 gm. pancreatin daily. April 17th, 3 liters urine and 1.9% sugar. May 19th, 3 liters urine, 1.9% sugar, and 49.5 kg. body-weight.

6. A. R., man twenty-one years old, admitted March 31, 1896. At entrance, sugar 7.7%, specific gravity 1040, daily amount 5 liters, no acetone, body-weight 45 kg. April 15th, after diabetic diet, sugar 6.7%, body-weight 46 kg., urine 5 liters. Three times a day, 0.5 gm. pancreatin. May 4th, body-weight 48 kg., 6.3% sugar. May 7th, pancreatin omitted on account of severe abdominal pains. The patient left the hospital May 31st, and reentered January 2, 1897, in a miserable condition. Phthisis, 8 liters urine, specific gravity 1032, sugar 3.3%, much acetone, body-

weight 45 kg. Death February 1st, coma. At the autopsy, marantic atrophy of the pancreas was found.

7. J. J., woman fifty-four years old, admitted March 2, 1897. Diabetes for ten years. In the year 1891, 8% sugar. At entrance, body-weight 56 kg., urine 3½ liters, specific gravity 1030, traces of albumin, 4.4% sugar, large amount of acetone. The following table shows the data noted by Dr. Katz. From March 7th to March 24th the patient received 15 pancreatic enemata made according to Lisser. March 24th, the patient complained of severe colicky pains in the region of the stomach, combined with oppression. The patient had previously often suffered from anginoid

Date.	Amount.	Sp. Gr.	Nitrogen.	Ammonia.	Sugar.	Acetone.	P_2O_5.	Remarks.
March 4.	—	1.030	0.447%	0.060%	4.4%	0.022%	—	
" 6.	—	—	0.746%	0.054%	4.5%	—	—	
" 7.	2000	—	0.794% 15.90 gm.	0.062% 1.25 gm.	5.6% 112 gm.	—	—	First pancreatic enema.
" 8.	—	1.032	0.654%	0.057%	5.4%	0.022%	—	
" 9.	2750	1.034	0.660% 18.16 gm.	0.063% 1.724 gm.	5.2% 165.2 gm. 3.0 g	0.020% 0.550 gm.		
" 10.	4000	1.030	0.587% 23.49 gm.	0.041% 1.649 gm.	4.8% 192 gm.	0.022% 0.863 gm.		
" 11.	3750	1.031	0.587% 22.02 gm.	0.044% 1.660 gm.	4.9% 183.8 gm.	0.0167% 0.628 gm.		
" 12.	4250	1.030	0.514% 22.09 gm.	0.025% 1.041 gm.	4.6% 195.5 gm.	0.018% 0.750 gm.		
" 13.	3250	1.030	0.660% 21.43 gm.	0.046% 1.419 gm.	4.6% 150.2 gm.	—		
" 14.	3500	1.031	0.573% 20.04 gm.	0.052% 1.833 gm.	4.6% 161.7 gm.	—	—	
" 15.	3500	1.031	0.743% 26.03 gm.	0.067% 2.331 gm.	4.5% 159.9 gm.	0.025% 0.877 gm.	—	
" 16.	3250	1.030	0.735% 23.89 gm.	0.045% 1.463 gm.	4.8% 157.3 gm.	—		
" 17.	3500	1.031	0.521% 18.25 gm.	0.054% 1.881 gm.	5.3% 175.8 gm.	—		
" 18.	3000	1.030	0.654% 19.62 gm.	0.049% 1.484 gm.	4.6% 138.6 gm.	—		
" 19.	3500	1.027	0.668% 23.37 gm.	0.041% 1.443 gm.	4.51% 157.9 gm.	0.015% 0.527 gm.	0.0539% 1.887 gm.	
" 20.	3500	1.028	0.721% 25.24 gm.	0.045% 1.584 gm.	4.29% 140.2 gm.	—	—	
" 21.	3750	1.022	0.579% 21.71 gm.	0.044% 1.665 gm.	4.62% 173.3 gm.	—	—	
" 22.	4250	1.026	0.865% 36.78 gm.	0.058% 2.476 gm.	4.18% 177.6 gm.	—	—	
" 23.	3500	1.035	0.545% 18.08 gm.	0.041% 1.419 gm.	4.95% 173.3 gm.	0.022% 0.770 gm.	0.0775% 2.713 gm.	
" 24.	3000	1.024	0.491% 14.73 gm.	0.037% 1.135 gm.	4.51% 135.3 gm.	—	—	Last pancreatic enema.
" 25.	4250	1.025	0.731% 31.08 gm.	0.042% 1.794 gm.	4.62% 196.4 gm.	0.032% 1.360 gm.	1.0358% 5.772 gm.	
" 26.	2500	1.025	—	0.061% 1.53 gm.	4.51% 112.8 gm.	0.031% 0.775 gm.	0.0768% 5.370 gm.	
" 27.	2750	1.031	—	—	3.52% 96.7 gm.	—	—	

attacks. March 25th, vomiting after indigestion, repeated several times during the day. Tongue dry, pulse 120, temperature normal. March 27th, collapse, coma. March 28th, death. At the autopsy were found: Degeneratio myocardii adiposa ex endarteriitide chron. arter. coron. Cirrhosis hepatis in potatrice. Tumor lienis chronicus. Catarrhus ventric. et intest. chronicus. Diabetes mellit. The pancreas large, dense, infiltrated with much fat tissue, which also lies between the lobules of the pancreas. The lobules, on section, appear sharply defined, separated from each other by loose connective tissue; reddish-gray. Weight 97 gm. Microscopic examination showed nothing pathologic. (Prosector, Dr. Žemann.)

8. Ch. Sch., woman twenty-four years old, admitted March 9, 1897. The examinations of the urine during the whole stay at the hospital were made by Dr. Katz in the same thorough manner as in the preceding case. At entrance, amount of urine 3000 c.c.; specific gravity 1038; sugar 5.9%, 177 gm. a day; acetone 0.015%, 0.458 gm. a day. March 19th, 3500 c.c. urine, specific gravity 1033, sugar 4.73%, 165.5 gm. in the day's amount, 0.021% acetone, 0.752 gm. of acetone in the day's amount of urine. Pancreatic enemata for nine days. March 28th, 2500 c.c. urine, specific gravity 1036, sugar 5.17%, 128.3 gm. in the day's amount of urine. On leaving the hospital, April 8th, the amount of urine was 2000 c.c., specific gravity 1035, sugar 5.6%, 112.2 gm. per day.

The experiments showed, therefore, that the administration of pancreatic preparations was without influence on the course of the diabetes. The variations observed, now an increase and now a diminution in the excretion of sugar, certainly had no connection with the treatment, and much more probably were due to the diet or other factors. In several of these cases, on account of the large amount of acetone or on account of advanced phthisis, a strict diabetic diet could not be ordered, and many patients avoided the diet prescribed despite the most careful watching. It is, therefore, not strange if figures appear which are to be explained only by the increased ingestion of sugar.

Among all these cases there was not one which could be shown positively to be one of pancreatic diabetes. Many of the patients presented during life the perfect picture of *diabète maigre*. They were relatively young, thin, and the diabetes pursued a rapid course. It was certain that some adhered strictly to the prescribed diet, and yet a great deal of sugar always was excreted. The complication with tuberculosis, mentioned by Lancereaux, was likewise present. Peculiar pancreatic symptoms, as changes in the digestion of fat and proteids, etc., did not appear. In two fatal cases changes were found in the pancreas, but they were by no means such as could be claimed with certainty to be the cause of the diabetes. On the contrary, the assumption was justified that these were conditions of general marasmus produced by the diabetes. The experiments made by us, therefore, are not conclusive. It may still be possible that in cases of genuine pancreatic diabetes organotherapy would have a favorable influence.

There is but little experience in the effect of pancreatic preparations on diseases of the pancreas. In one of my cases I believe I can justly assume a favorable influence of such preparations on the digestion of fats. Although the diagnosis of disease of the pancreas was not established by an autopsy, yet such marked symptoms were present that there seems to be scarcely any doubt.

The case was as follows: J. N., forty-nine years old, many years before had an attack of pneumonia and malaria; for several years had frequent attacks of disturbance of digestion after errors of diet; seven months before our observations began had noticed pains in the epigastrium gradually increasing in severity; the patient felt these pains running across the upper portion of the abdomen. They were generally independent of eating, were sometimes slighter and sometimes more severe after a meal. The patient lost flesh. As there was at the same time migraine, ringing in the ears, general weakness, and no abnormal objective signs, the diagnosis had been neuralgia or neurosis.

When I saw him for the first time, there were circumscribed tenderness in the epigastrium and slight yellow color of the sclerotic in the urine; there was a faint reaction of bile-pigment, but no sugar. Under observation the jaundice became daily more intense, the stools were wholly free from bile, and the quantity was remarkably large in comparison to the relatively small amount of nourishment.

The examination of the stools gave the following results: Stools formed, white, perfectly free from bile, of salve-like consistency. Microscopic examination: (1) A few remains of distinct muscle-fibers, with the structure well preserved *; (2) few vegetable cells; (3) fat-drops; (4) very numerous fat-acid needles; (5) bacteria, detritus. The examination of the urine resulted as follows: Specific gravity, 1018; acid; indican in large amounts; no abnormal constituents.

The sensitiveness to pressure in the epigastrium increased and a resistance to the right of the median line and extending along the same could be recognized. The resistance became more and more marked and on certain days, especially when the stomach was empty, a hard mass very sensitive to pressure was very distinctly to be felt extending from the right across the median line of the abdomen; it moved somewhat downward at each inspiration. The stomach was not dilated. The liver increased gradually in size, the gall-bladder could be more and more distinctly palpated as a pear-shaped tumor, and the poor digestion of fat and proteids became more and more pronounced.

The coincidence of all these symptoms made the diagnosis of carcinoma of the head and body of the pancreas seem very probable. The pains across the epigastrium for months, the emaciation, the gradually increasing jaundice, even to perfect closure of the ductus choledochus, the poor digestion of fats and proteids, the appearance of a tumor corresponding in position to that of the pancreas, the growth of this tumor, the lack of symptoms which would point to a pyloric or duodenal cancer or to cholelithiasis, all justified the diagnosis of cancer of the pancreas.

Merck's pancreatin, 1 gm. daily, was given to this patient, and the stools examined some days later showed a decided improvement in the digestion of fats. Repetition of the examination gave the same result. The patient also expressed himself as feeling better, and did not feel so weak as formerly. From news which I received some weeks later from the patient, I was able to decide that no essential change had occurred in his condition. This is the only case in which I could persuade myself that there was a real improvement in the digestion of fats and proteids from the administration of preparations of pancreas.

[Salomon † increased the digestion of fat in a mild case of diabetes with fatty stools by the administration of fresh pancreas in capsules or spread on bread. In the periods before and after medication 51% and 85% respectively of the fat ingested were unabsorbed, during the intervening period when the pancreas was given but 19% of the fat was unassimilated. In another experiment upon the same individual pankreon was used instead of the fresh pancreas. In the preliminary period 38.4% of the ingested fat escaped absorption; in the next period 1 gm. pankreon was given five times daily and the percentage of undigested fat fell to 21.3.

Joslin ‡ increased the digestion of fat 50% by the use of ox-bile given in pill-form.—Ed.]

The recommendation may well be made that further experiments in

---

* The patient in the last few days had eaten only a very small amount of scraped beef.

† *Berl. klin. Wochen.*, 1902, p. 45.

‡ *Jour. of Experimental Med.*, 1901, p. 513.

this direction should be undertaken. It is to be assumed that in disturbances of digestion which are caused by lack of the pancreatic juice a better utilization of the food would be brought about by the use of active pancreatic preparations. For this purpose the pure gland, as in the earlier cases, or pancreatic preparations should be used.

It is doubtful from experience thus far whether an efficient organotherapy for the diseased pancreas can be found like that for diseases of the thyroid.

Surgery, in the last few years, has been successful in the treatment of diseases of the pancreas. Cysts, abscesses, necroses, even tumors of the pancreas have been operated upon with brilliant results. To be sure, some operations were performed even before the time of Lister, as by A. Petit, Caldwell, Kleberg and Wagner, Wandesleben, but it was Gussenbauer who, by successfully operating on a cyst, opened the way for pancreatic surgery.

Under Special Considerations the details of this important achievement will be given, and it is to be expected that, with the advance of our knowledge of diseases of the pancreas, a rational surgical therapy will be placed on a firmer foundation. Symptomatic treatment alone is all that is left for the clinician, in the present state of our knowledge, when the etiologic treatment earlier described fails or is without hope. The narrow field of the physician's activity is limited. Its object is to lessen pain, to provide sufficient nourishment, the eventual introduction of artificial feeding, the increasing of strength, in order to gain time, that a process capable of recovery may end favorably, and the alleviation of distressing symptoms caused by such complications as jaundice.

SPECIAL CONSIDERATIONS.

I. INFLAMMATIONS OF THE PANCREAS.

So far as present anatomic and clinical data show, the inflammations of the pancreas are, on the whole, rare diseases. Among the 18,509 autopsies which were conducted in the Vienna General Hospital during the years 1885 to 1895, only 15 cases are found noted—1 of hemorrhagic pancreatitis, 9 abscesses (primary and secondary), and 5 cases of chronic indurative pancreatitis.

Inflammations of the pancreas undoubtedly occur more frequently than is thought, because there are curable forms leaving no traces, as will appear later.

In general we can distinguish the following varieties *:

(1) Acute hemorrhagic pancreatitis; (2) suppurative pancreatitis; (3) necrotic pancreatitis; (4) chronic indurative pancreatitis.

The variety of disease characterized by Friedreich and others as acute parenchymatous pancreatitis, and which is found especially in severe infectious diseases, ought not, as Dieckhoff states, to be included among the inflammations, but rather among the retrograde disturbances of nutrition.

Mixed forms also may occur; thus, purulent inflammations with hemorrhages, purulent inflammations with indurative pancreatitis, purulent and chronic indurative inflammations with necroses.

1. ACUTE HEMORRHAGIC PANCREATITIS.

There is no doubt that slight degrees of hemorrhage occur in the course of both acute and chronic varieties of inflammation. Hemorrhages into the pancreatic tissue occur easily, as it appears, under certain conditions. This may be based on the anatomic structure (Fitz). Hemorrhages easily arose, in our experiments upon animals, in the attempt at extirpation of a portion of the gland or of the whole gland and in the artificial inflammations.

The term hemorrhagic pancreatitis is used by many authors to repre-

---

* A catarrhal pancreatitis is also mentioned by many authors. The inflammatory processes in the parenchyma of the gland which take their origin from catarrhs of the excretory duct will be referred to in the following description. Doubtless there is a catarrhal inflammation of the excretory duct, which runs its course without inflammatory changes in the gland itself. A clinical presentation of this process appears impossible in the present condition of our knowledge, as neither the anatomic data nor the clinical symptoms are clear enough to enable a distinct picture of the disease to be formed. Further investigation must be made in order to permit clinical recognition of these processes, probably of not infrequent occurrence and also curable.

116

sent a process with characteristic symptoms in which more or less extensive hemorrhage, affecting a large part of the entire gland, stands in the foreground.

It is a mooted point whether in these cases the hemorrhage is only the consequence of the inflammation, or whether the hemorrhage is primary and the inflammation secondary, or whether there is simply a hemorrhage in which, because of the rapid course or for some other reason, no inflammatory processes at all develop.

Neither the pathologists nor the clinicians are agreed in their understanding of the process. Orth says regarding it: "Parenchymatous pancreatitis is generally connected with hemorrhages, which were in many cases so considerable that the extravasated blood escaped through the pancreatic duct into the intestine. It is possible that some of the fatal hemorrhages are to be regarded as symptoms of a pancreatitis." Birch-Hirschfeld mentions two cases which indicate the existence of a hemorrhagic pancreatitis leading quickly to death. According to Ziegler, hemorrhages may occur in the region of the pancreas as the consequence of inflammations, and may be so severe that the intrapancreatic connective tissue and the fat tissue are filled with blood, hematomata thus being formed. An opposite view is advanced by Dieckhoff. He states that in an exact investigation of the cases known it has been shown that a great part of the cases characterized as hemorrhagic pancreatitis had another cause for the hemorrhage, and the inflammatory phenomena were due to the hemorrhage. Dieckhoff considers it not improbable "that in an acute inflammation, through injuries of the vessel-wall, minute hemorrhages can occur in the pancreas as in other inflamed organs. This variety does not, however, receive the designation hemorrhagic pancreatitis, which term is rather applied to those cases where hemorrhage predominates and where frequently the proof is absent."

The same divergency of views exists among the authors who consider the subject from the clinical point of view. Fitz takes the most decided position; he describes hemorrhagic pancreatitis as an independent affection from the clinical point of view, separates it from the hemorrhages, and collects from the literature 17 illustrative cases.

Fitz assumes, to be sure, that the anatomic signs are not clear enough, but considers himself justified in assuming the presence of an inflammation if the symptoms indicate it. When the general symptoms of inflammation are present, says Fitz, and when the pancreas is described as infiltrated with blood, then such a combination of symptoms and lesions is to be reckoned rather among the inflammations than among the hemorrhages.

Seitz, in a thorough and comprehensive study, investigated all the known cases pertaining to this subject, and came to the conclusion that inflammation as cause of considerable hemorrhage into the pancreas is, up to the present time, "not so clearly and positively shown as we might wish." He does not deny the possibility of its occurrence, but inclines to the view that, so long as the opposite is not shown, the inflammatory symptoms are to be regarded as consequences of the hemorrhages. These inflammations, which may reach the highest degree, become much more probable through the communication of the pancreas with the intestine, through the great tendency of the gland to decomposition, and through the proximity of the peritoneum and through the chemical peculiarities of the pancreatic secretion.

In spite of the observation of Seitz, so apt in many respects, the idea of a hemorrhagic pancreatitis is maintained in recent publications, as those of Körte, Jung, Dettmer, Cutler, Parry, Dunn and Pitt, etc.

The divergence of views just described is easily explained. In the clinical form of the process, which some term pancreatic apoplexy and others term hemorrhagic pancreatitis, there is absolutely no means by which it can be decided whether the hemorrhage is the result of an inflammation or the inflammation is a result of the hemorrhage, or whether there is simply a severe hemorrhage without any inflammation at all.

In all cases the pathologic picture is about as follows: Usually there is the sudden onset of the symptoms, violent pains in the region of the stomach and umbilicus, nausea, vomiting, frequently the appearance of intestinal obstruction, immediate occurrence of collapse with feeling of anxiety, great rapidity of pulse, dyspnea, rapid loss of strength, death from exhaustion in a few hours or at longest in a few days.

This distinction between inflammation with hemorrhage and hemorrhage with inflammation cannot in most cases be seen in the body after death, and so it happens that one author regards as a pure hemorrhage the same case which another considers as inflammation. Of the 17 cases which Fitz regards as examples of hemorrhagic pancreatitis, Seitz recognizes no one of them as proved with certainty, and he considers it also more probable in all the cases that the inflammation is a secondary process. Even the cases which are generally regarded as hemorrhagic pancreatitis—those of Löschner, Oppolzer, Osler and Hughes, Hirschberg, Birch-Hirschfeld—do not, according to Seitz, present the proof that the inflammation was the cause of the hemorrhage.

Loschner's case: An inebriate, twenty-six years old, dyspeptic for five years, mostly in consequence of faults of diet. About three weeks before the last sickness there were repeated attacks of colic. Suddenly continuous torturing pain in the upper abdominal region with great restlessness, vomiting of stomach-contents, constipation, slight fever, on the fourth day of the disease collapse, epigastrium distended, very sensitive to pressure; burning, often stabbing pains, which extend to the right toward the duodenum and to the left toward the spleen and also radiate backward and toward the right shoulder; the constipation persistent, death from collapse. At the autopsy the pancreas was found dense, more than twice as thick as normally, of a violet color externally. On cutting into the gland, a large amount of dark blood gushed forth, the individual acini were greatly enlarged, dark-colored, and traversed with vessels distended with blood; the intervening cellular connective tissue was infiltrated with blood, the mucous membrane of the excretory duct appeared dark red. In the head of the pancreas a finely granular, yellow exudation was seen here and there between the acini.

Seitz rightly suggests that in this case it was not thoroughly shown that a primary inflammation existed. Just as little is it shown in the case described by Oppolzer.

A strong, previously healthy man had severe cardialgic attacks, which constantly increased. On entrance, there were great restlessness, vomiting of abundant bilious masses, very frequent pulse, cold extremities, drawn face, severe pain in the region of the stomach, increasing on pressure, constipation, high fever; death three days after admission into the hospital. At the autopsy the pancreas was found enlarged to three times its normal size, and on section a bloody exudation was seen between the dark-red acini; the surrounding tissues were infiltrated with blood.

In this case, also, there is no proof that an inflammation was the primary process. In the case of Hirschberg there were symptoms of intestinal obstruction in a very fleshy woman fifty-six years old, on whom laparotomy was performed on the fourth day after the beginning of the disease. Death at the end of five hours. At the autopsy the pancreas was found greatly enlarged, black from hemorrhages, there was fatty degeneration and general peritonitis. Signs of fat necrosis were seen at the operation as well as in the corpse.

It is not shown positively in the cases of Birch-Hirschfeld also that the inflammation preceded the hemorrhage.

Hawkins also came to the same conclusion as Seitz and Dieckhoff. It is questionable, says Hawkins, whether the cases of acute hemorrhagic pancreatitis in general are not to be regarded as primary hemorrhages with secondary inflammatory processes. "If the patient survives the first attack, it is certainly clear that secondary changes must occur, analogous to the conditions in renal infarction." Although we must grant that Seitz, Dieckhoff, and Hawkins are right in the assumption that the hemorrhage is in most cases to be regarded as the primary factor, yet some facts are to be mentioned which do not easily dispose of the idea that inflammatory processes may be the cause of the disease which runs so rapid a course. These facts are as follows:

1. Seitz has suggested the following question as one of the most important supports of his reasoning: Why are there no cases of immediately fatal inflammation reported without hemorrhage? The most recent literature reports two such observations. Cayley describes a case of acute pancreatitis in a man thirty years old who had previously been healthy; probably alcoholic. Three days before admission to the hospital, without definite cause, pains began in the stomach, constipation, but no severe feeling of sickness. Ol. ricini and laudanum were ordered. On the next day, continuous pain; in spite of this, the patient continued to work. Then there was vomiting. On the third day the condition became more threatening and the patient was brought to the hospital.

Status præsens: Deep collapse, extremities cold, skin moist, pulse about 150, scarcely perceptible, slight cyanosis, irregular respiration, temperature 37.0° C. (98.6° F.), falling to 35.2° C. (94.4° F.), violent vomiting of milk, no symptoms of regurgitation of intestinal contents, severe pain, sensitiveness to pressure in the epigastrium, abdomen not distended, everywhere tympanitic, liver dulness normal, anuria, small evacuation of stools after enema, collapse despite stimulants; a fluid stool before death, which occurred on the fourth day of the illness.

Autopsy: Body very rich in fat, great omentum and retroperitoneal tissue overladen with fat, liver shows marked fatty degeneration, heart enveloped with fat, about ¼ liter of bloody serum in the peritoneal cavity, the peritoneum over the pancreas and intestine dull, injected, and reddened, but showed no fibrinous exudation. Tissue about the pancreas infiltrated with bloody serum, the fat tissue here and in the adjacent mesentery shows distinct fat necrosis. On lying in the water, a milky fluid exuded, which was regarded by Völcker as saponified fat. The pancreas was enlarged, reddened, somewhat brittle, the lobules pale red, transparent, resembling salmon, doubtless in a condition of coagulation necrosis, organ edematous with bloody serum. Pancreatic duct normal, containing no calculi. Although there was a general infiltration of bloody colored serum in and around the pancreas, yet neither hemorrhage nor suppuration was to be shown in the gland. Other organs normal.

On the basis of his observations, Cayley comes to the conclusion that hemorrhages are not an essential factor in the pathologic picture of acute pancreatitis.

The absolute proof is not brought forward that there was really an inflammation, as an exact microscopic examination of the case was not made, although it is certain that the clinical picture of the preceding case corresponds to an acute hemorrhagic pancreatitis, on account of the epigastric pain for one or two days, the sensitiveness to pressure, vomiting, the sudden occurrence of collapse, which lasted until death on the fourth or fifth day of the illness, and although there was certainly no hemorrhage in the gland. Certainly fat necrosis was present, and it may be that the same factor which led to this lesion caused the changes in the pancreas, either directly or in the way of the fat necrosis (see section on Fat Necrosis). Likewise an analogous case reported by Kennan does not give absolute proof.

A woman thirty-eight years old was attacked with vomiting and pains in the upper abdomen. The discomforts persisted, the abdomen became distended, on the day afterward some urine was evacuated, but after that the anuria was complete. On the day of admission to the hospital there was collapse, subnormal temperature, pulse scarcely to be felt, cold sweat, no vomiting, pain slight, sensorium perfectly free, no jaundice, obstipation. On the next morning, death. Duration of the disease, forty-two hours.

At the autopsy the woman was very well nourished; the great omentum very rich in fat, adherent in places to the peritoneum of the pelvis; slight peritonitis; adhesions between the intestinal coils; large intestine, especially the descending colon, injected in places, of a very dark color in the region of the splenic flexure, with numerous dark-colored extravasations of blood on its surface; the main mass of inflammation in the neighborhood of the head of the pancreas. The pancreas itself was markedly infected and enlarged, "evidently by inflammatory changes." The ductus choledochus and gall-bladder contained numerous, whitish, faceted calculi. One of these was found in the duodenum; they were about the size of a pea and possessed a dark nucleus.

The passage of a gall-stone into the duodenum, Kennan thinks, may have been sufficient to produce lesions which rendered possible the entrance of infectious organisms through the duct into the pancreas. In this case also there was no careful microscopic examination, and it is not shown whether an inflammation really existed, although the possibility cannot be denied that in this, as well as in the case just described, primary inflammatory processes were present.

2. Some cases are reported in the literature in which an inflammatory process certainly existed with the hemorrhage, and in which it must be granted that the inflammation was possibly the primary factor.

1. Zahn's case: Waiter twenty-one years old, previously always healthy; fourteen days before he suffered from a pain in the neck, which had disappeared completely for eight days, when on the 19th of February he suddenly on awakening felt pain in the region of the umbilicus. The pains were so severe that he had to return to his bed, and they lasted until the following day. On entering the hospital, there was cyanosis of the hands and feet, small, scarcely perceptible radial pulse. The patient complained of fulness and weight at the pit of the stomach, the abdomen was distended and sensitive to pressure, especially in the region of the cecum, with occasional eructation and nausea. On the next day there was at first slight, but later constantly increasing delirium. There was diarrhea, urine normal. On the fourth day there was slight jaundice; the temperature varied between 36.0° C. (96.8° F.) and 37.6° C. (99.7° F.). Death February 27th. The clinical diagnosis was pyosepticemia arising from the intestine.

At the autopsy there was found, besides cloudy swelling of the kidney and liver, a fibrinopurulent inflammation of the peritoneum. The mesocolon in its whole extent, even to the rectum, thickened by a large amount of blood, extravasated between its layers. The root of the mesentery was also suffused with blood. On more careful investigation for the origin of the hemorrhage, the walls of the portal vein near its beginning were found thickened by inflammatory exudation and in the interior there was a firmly adherent white thrombus. The vein was also compressed by the enlarged pancreas in which inflammatory changes were to be distinctly recognized on cross-section. It was opaque where not discolored with blood. The pancreatic duct contained a thick brown fluid; its wall, as well as the pancreatic tissue lying next to it, were colored brown. It opened by a very narrow mouth somewhat below the ampulla of Vater into the intestinal lumen.

PLATE I.

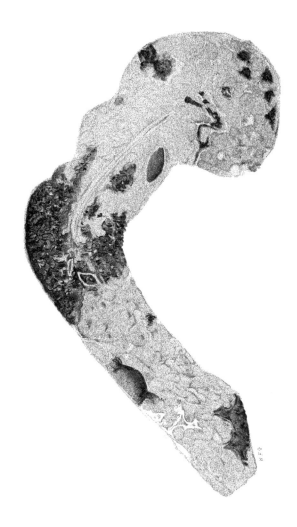

ACUTE HEMORRHAGIC PANCREATITIS OF FOUR DAYS' DURATION.
(From the Warren Anatomical Museum of Harvard Medical School, Boston.)

The great majority of the pancreatic cells showed cloudy swelling, part of them had undergone fatty degeneration and part hyaline degeneration. The pancreatic duct contained altered red blood-corpuscles, brown pigment, distinct round cells and epithelial debris, fat drops, and finely granular detritus. Epithelial cells were no longer found on the wall of the duct. This was abundantly filled with small round cells and red blood-corpuscles. The interacinous connective tissue had a similar appearance. It was everywhere filled with round cells, which were most abundant in the neighborhood of the veins, especially those obstructed by white thrombi. The arterial wall appeared normal, the lumen of the vessels empty.

The bacteriologic examination of very thin sections showed numerous and quite large colonies of very small bacteria in the pancreatic duct. Colonies were found in considerable numbers in the connective tissue surrounding the canal, also in the inter-acinous connective tissue and in the wall of the portal vein.

Doubtless this was a case of parasitic (acute) pancreatitis, but it does not follow that this was the primary process. It might easily be imagined that the passage of microbes from the intestine was rendered possible by the occurrence of a preceding hemorrhage in the pancreas, and that, therefore, the inflammation was a secondary process.

The conditions in a case described by Kraft were still less conclusive:

The patient had sudden severe pain in the region of the stomach, vomiting, and obstinate obstruction of stools, so that laparotomy was undertaken on account of a supposed intestinal obstruction. At the operation, after the evacuation of a brownish, turbid fluid, there was no sign of a peritonitis nor of an intestinal obstruction. The death of the patient soon followed, and the pancreas was found embedded in clotted blood, double in size, and beset with yellow and dark red foci. The connective tissue of the great omentum and ascending mesocolon and the retroperitoneal tissue appeared infiltrated. The microscopic examination of the pancreas showed bloody infiltration and numerous leucocytes between the acini. The latter appeared degenerated in spots, which were composed of granular detritus, with few poorly preserved nuclei.

The fact that the liver was fatty, that evidences of inflammation previously not recognized were found at the autopsy, prevents the origin of the hemorrhage from being regarded as simply inflammatory. On the one hand, it may be assumed that the fatty degeneration might have been the cause of the hemorrhage, for yellowish foci were present in the pancreas; on the other, the evidence of a recent peritonitis shows that it might have been possible that the small-celled infiltration did not precede the hemorrhage, but rather developed in consequence of it.

The conclusion is just as difficult whether the hemorrhage or the small-celled infiltration was the primary condition in the case observed by Haidlen of acute pancreatitis after delivery.

The patient, a woman thirty-three years old, during the seventh, ninth, and tenth months of pregnancy had suffered from severe pains of such intensity that perforative peritonitis was suspected. In the sixth week after delivery attacks of violent pain in the region of the pylorus occurred quite suddenly. Vomiting, sensitiveness to pressure in the pit of the stomach, finally collapse. The skin was very pale, the pulse was from 110 to 120, and signs of intestinal obstruction appeared. On the second day of her sickness the pains diminished somewhat, the collapse, the coldness of the extremities increased more and more, meteorism became more marked, pulse was 130 to 140. Death after ninety-six hours. At the autopsy no marked peritonitis; the pancreas was enlarged and changed into a brownish-red mass suffused with blood. The peritoneum also was slightly hemorrhagic. Under the microscope a small-celled infiltration of the pancreatic tissue was seen in addition to the extravasation of blood.

The case which Dittrich describes as genuine inflammation of the pancreas also suggests that the inflammation was secondary.

A prisoner twenty-one years old made an attempt to hang himself in his cell, was rescued, and became conscious.   From that time he had severe colicky pains in the lower abdomen, which continued uninterruptedly until death the day after in collapse.   Four weeks before death he was said to have had an attack of colic which lasted eight hours.

At the autopsy, the pancreas was found 16 cm. long, and 3.5 cm. thick through the middle; its tissue was very loose, easily torn, and to a great extent infiltrated with extensive hemorrhages.   In the head of the pancreas the normal structure and color of the organ could be distinctly recognized with the naked eye.   But the tissue here also was loose.   The middle portion and the tail were changed into a dark-brown mass, almost confluent from the slightest pressure.   If the head of the pancreas were compressed with a knife, large quantities of a reddish-gray, thick, puriform fluid could be scraped from the cut surface; on microscopic examination it appeared that the whole organ was invaded by an inflammatory process characterized anatomically by a dense small-celled infiltration, observable in many places."

Although it was shown in this case that there was a wide-spread inflammation, yet there was no positive proof that the inflammation preceded the hemorrhage.

There can be no doubt, according to the above communications, that the hemorrhage and inflammation existed at the same time, but it is well enough apparent also how difficult it is even at the autopsy to decide whether an idiopathic hemorrhagic pancreatitis exists.   This decision can be made much less easily at the bedside.

Although, as mentioned earlier, the possibility cannot be denied that there is an acute idiopathic pancreatitis, which runs its course generally with severe hemorrhage, very rarely without hemorrhage and without suppuration, yet in the present condition of our knowledge a clinical separation of these processes from the severe hemorrhages with or without inflammation is impossible.   It therefore will be most appropriate to postpone clinical presentation of this subject to the section on Hemorrhages.

It was impossible to decide these questions by experiments on animals. It will be shown later that hemorrhages, abscesses, chronic inflammations, necroses, and fat necroses could be successfully produced in animals in different ways, but it was not possible to produce a hemorrhagic pancreatitis—that is, a primary pancreatitis without suppuration, which gives rise to hemorrhages—in order to prove the correctness of the view maintained by many authors that inflammation of pancreatic tissue is to be regarded as the primary feature in hemorrhagic pancreatitis.

It was possible, as will be shown later, by means of parenchymatous injections of 5% chlorid of zinc solution, or by injection of $\frac{1}{40}$ normal sulphuric acid into the Wirsungian duct, to cause hemorrhages into the pancreas resulting in death within twenty-four hours.   At the autopsy, however, only more or less extensive hemorrhages with destruction of the tissue of the pancreas were found, but no signs of inflammation.

2. SUPPURATIVE PANCREATITIS, PANCREATIC ABSCESS.

Historical.—Among the earlier writers are found solitary instances concerning the occurrence of suppuration in the pancreas.

Lieutaud mentions that in the last century cases of pancreatic abscess were observed.   The cases of Riolanus, Bonz, and Gaultier are referred to by Ancelet.   Claessen calls attention to a preparation in the Anatomical Museum at Strassburg which, according to Bécourt's description, showed several foci of pus in inflamed tissue. He cites especially the communication of Blancard, 1688, in which a child who had died of smallpox showed small masses of pus on the surface of the pancreas; in addition, Tonnellé reports two cases of suppurative pancreatitis in puerperal fever.

Döring found an abscess between the pancreas, transverse colon, and mesentery, containing about 4 ounces of a yellowish, offensive pus, originating apparently from the pancreas.

Baillie saw a pancreas notably enlarged, in which a large quantity of thin pus was found. Tulpius (1652) gives a somewhat more detailed description of a patient from whom a caseous tumor of the testicles had been removed some years earlier. The disease developed with symptoms of fever, pain in the abdomen, and very great dyspnea. At the autopsy the pancreas was found filled with smeary pus which oozed from the cut surface. The aorta and vena cava were compressed by the gland and made impermeable. Portal (1803) describes the case of a man who had earlier suffered from gout. After two or three spells of vomiting, collapse and rapid failure occurred. The whole pancreas was involved in the process of suppuration and embedded in pus. Claessen mentions also a case of suppuration of the pancreas with calculus formation, described by Fournier.

In the literature accessible to me up to the end of 1896 there were 46 cases. The number of cases which have been made known may be essentially larger, as only a part of those which have been examined after death have been published in detail, and many may have been overlooked. In reports from hospitals and autopsies pancreatic abscesses are not infrequently mentioned without further details, and pancreatic abscesses occur still more frequently, which run their course during life under wrong diagnoses and are not examined after death. Primary and secondary suppurative pancreatitis may be distinguished according as the process originates in the pancreas, or proceeds from a neighboring organ, or occurs through metastases.

A. PRIMARY SUPPURATIVE PANCREATITIS.

Pathologic Anatomy.—Small, multiple foci are found distributed throughout the entire gland or are limited to individual portions of the same, or purulent foci varying in size from that of a walnut to that of an egg or even larger are to be found as the result of the confluence of small abscesses.

Multiple abscesses are described by Drasche, Friedreich, Moore, Fraenkel, Musser, Dallemagne, Greve, Dieckhoff (3 cases), Leichtenstern. Extensive collections of pus in the pancreas were found in the cases of Salmade, Portal, Gendrin, Baillie, Perle, Fletcher, Kilgour, Riboli, Habershon, Frison (2 cases), Moore, Hansemann, Körte (2 cases), Macaigne, Dieckhoff. Isolated abscesses in the pancreatic tissue have been described by Fournier, Percival, Harley, Roddick, Nathan, Smith, Shea, Moore, Bamberger, Fitz, Thayer, and in the reports of St. George's Hospital. No especial reference to other cases is possible.

Necrosis of small or large parts of the gland may develop from the suppuration, or the whole gland may degenerate and lie as a sequestrum in the large pus-cavity. The pus assumes at times an ichorous character, and then gangrene of a part or the whole of the gland all the more easily occurs. Such abscesses and putrid cavities, which contain gangrenous portions of the pancreas, may be cured by operative interference (Körte, Thayer). They may also be evacuated through the intestine during life (Chiari), and thus be cured. In such cases it can by no means always be decided whether the inflammation or the necrosis is primary.

Peripancreatic abscesses (foci of pus in the omental bursa) may be brought about by various causes; thus, for instance, by suppurating lymph-glands, by peritonitis, or by continued inflammation (Orth), and necrosis and sequestration of a larger or smaller portion of the pancreas may thus result.

A reactive inflammation, a circumscribed peritonitis (Dieckhoff), at times is found in the neighborhood of the pancreas infiltrated with pus. The pancreatic abscess sometimes becomes encapsulated, as in the cases of Frison, Musser, Moore, Roddick, Smith, Dieckhoff.

Abscesses of the pancreas may break into the omental bursa, and then the large pus-cavity above mentioned may develop as the result of the closure of the foramen of Winslow and appear encapsulated. The pus may burrow into the retroperitoneal tissue, extending in different directions on the right as far as the right kidney, but far more frequently on the left to the spleen, following the course of the descending colon, even to the pelvis (Körte). This extension to the left is typical, as has been established by Körte with injections in the dead body.

Pancreatic abscesses and peripancreatic foci of pus may perforate into the stomach and intestine. Hoggarth and also Atkinson mention a case of rupture into the intestine. In Fletcher's case, the abscess of the head of the pancreas broke into the duodenum. In Drasche's case two abscesses perforated into the stomach and into the duodenum. Abscesses of the omental bursa also may rupture into a portion of the intestine (Langerhans, Hansemann, Chiari, Rosenbach). In most of these cases gangrene of the pancreas was the cause of the inflammation.

Rupture of a pancreatic abscess may lead to a general peritonitis (Friedreich, Moore, Perle, Dieckhoff). In one of Moore's cases a pancreatic abscess had ruptured into the abdominal cavity and had perforated the pancreatico-duodenal artery. Not infrequently in such cases there is thrombosis of the vena portæ, vena lienalis, or the vena mesenterica superior or inferior (Drasche, Bamberger, Musser). Thrombosis of the femoral vein is also mentioned in the case described in the reports of St. George's Hospital. Körte found a parietal thrombus in the splenic artery. Through the mediation of such thromboses, abscesses may easily develop in other organs. Drasche found an hepatic abscess as large as an egg; there were several abscesses in the liver in the second of Frison's cases; Smith found an abscess in the diaphragm above the spleen and abscesses in several small lymph-glands in the neighborhood. Klob saw the posterior wall of the stomach, in which there was an abscess beneath the mucous membrane, firmly adherent to the pancreas. Körte found several splenic abscesses, the largest of which communicated with a subphrenic abscess. In one of Dieckhoff's cases, and in a patient of Greve there was suppuration of a lymph-gland. Whatever may be the changes observed in the body, it is noteworthy that the spleen is not, as a rule, enlarged; not even when there is thrombosis of the splenic vein or portal vein (Dieckhoff). Kilgour, Stefanini, and Greve mention a slight enlargement of the spleen. A mild degree of jaundice was found in the cases of Shea, Moore, Riboli, Roddick; Frison and Greve reported marked jaundice. In the first of the last-mentioned cases several abscesses were found in the liver; in the last there were swollen lymph-glands in the portal fissure and along the celiac artery.

Etiology.—The following have been mentioned as causes of primary suppurative pancreatitis, although without any proof whatever: alcoholism, misuse of tobacco, pregnancy (Mondière), suppression of menstruation (Schönlein), use of mercury. Whether suppurative pancreatitis may arise from an injury, a push or blow on the epigastrium, is also doubtful.

The entrance of pyogenic micro-organisms is necessary for the production of an acute suppurative pancreatitis. As Dieckhoff states, there are the three following possibilities:

1. A hematogenous origin, in which the pyogenic irritant enters into the pancreas through the blood. Only metastatic processes are brought about in this way.

2. Suppuration penetrates from the neighborhood; for instance, from an ulcer of the stomach extended to the pancreas.

3. The pyogenic irritant enters from the intestine through the excretory duct.

The last form alone is to be considered in primary pancreatic abscess. Orth has already presented this as the cause of primary suppurative pancreatitis. "A catarrh of the duct—*sialodochitis pancreatica*—is caused by concretions in the excretory duct and becomes transformed into a suppurative inflammation by the entrance of inflammatory excitants from the intestine."

Virchow has already shown that in the salivary glands the inflammation proceeds from the gland-ducts and thence extends to the gland lobules. Hanau also showed that a like course was pursued in the infectious diseases in the so-called metastatic inflammations of the salivary glands. According to Hanau, the process originates from a suppurative inflammation of the larger salivary ducts, then attacks the smaller branches, and, continuing from the central intra-acinous ducts, it causes a purulent liquefaction of the gland lobules.

According to Dieckhoff's investigation, suppurative pancreatitis runs a similar course. He showed the advance of the process from the larger to the smaller excretory ducts. A purulent liquefaction of the tissue proceeded from the minutest excretory ducts of the gland and resulted in the formation of the actual abscess. In a case of gelatinous cancer of the duodenum described by him, he says: "The pyogenic organisms have certainly wandered from the intestine, perhaps from ulcerated portions of cancer, into the excretory duct of the pancreas and have produced there a desquamative catarrh. The liquefactive process has begun in the central intra-acinous ducts." In a second case in which a gall-stone was found in the ductus Wirsungianus, the suppuration certainly originated from the excretory duct. The enlargement of this by the gall-stone gave opportunity for the entrance from the intestine of pyogenic agents. A similar condition was observed in two other cases reported by Dieckhoff.

Different investigations have been made into the nature of the microorganisms. In a case of suppurative pancreatitis reported by Fitz, four different kinds of bacteria were isolated in the bacteriologic examination carried on by Jackson and Ernst: (1) A fluorescent bacillus which liquefied gelatin and was half as large as the bacillus of tuberculosis; (2) a bacterium similar to Staphylococcus pyogenes citreus; (3) short, thin, non-liquefying rods, which formed gray, wrinkled membranes on the surface of agar and gelatin cultures; (4) very large numbers of a small, plump bacillus, which did not liquefy gelatin and formed superficial colonies 2 or 3 mm. in size in the vicinity of the point of inoculation.

Dallemagne in 1892 makes an additional bacteriologic report. He isolated from the contents of an abscess pure cultures of a bacterium which is easily stained with methylene-blue, does not take the Gram stain, and forms on gelatin round, grayish-yellow colonies with irregular borders and dark center. Good development in meat-broth at 37° C. (98.6° F.); coagulates milk and gives no indol reaction. After intraperitoneal injection of 1 c.c. of the culture into a rabbit death followed in twenty-four hours with the symptoms of infectious peritonitis. The bacterium belongs probably to the proteus group (Hauser). Macaigne saw pneumococci in the abscesses.

Körte twice saw rod-like bacteria resembling intestinal bacilli, and once streptococci. In the cases investigated bacteriologically by Dieckhoff and Lubarsch, they were twice able to show with certainty microorganisms from the group Diplococcus pneumoniæ of Fraenkel. Twice these were shown only microscopically. Once Bacterium coli commune occurred alone. "It appears, therefore," says Dieckhoff, "as if the primary suppurative inflammations of the pancreas were only exceptionally caused by the invasion of organisms from the intestinal canal." It is always difficult to explain why pancreatic inflammations are relatively so rare in view of the frequency of the occurrence of microorganisms in the intestine and in the vicinity of the opening of the Wirsungian duct. The same factor which explains the relative infrequency of abscesses of the liver probably prevails here, although space and opportunity enough are given for entrance of pus organisms through the bile-ducts. Doubtless there must be also, as is suggested by Dieckhoff, a special disposition, a pathologic change or a lack of secretion, in order to produce the soil that is peculiarly fitted for the development of the pus organisms.

In purulent parotitis Hanau assumes a suppression of the secretion as the condition of the entrance into the gland of the pus organisms. Dieckhoff proposes a similar postulate for the development of suppurative pancreatitis. As a rule, however, such pathologic changes are shown in but few instances. Among the pathologic processes which are seen in some cases, and possibly explain the disposition to suppuration, the following may be mentioned:

1. Fat necrosis: This was shown by Fitz, Körte, Thayer, etc. Also in a case of diabetes which was examined after death in the Vienna General Hospital in 1895, in addition to a suppurative pancreatitis, there was found a fat necrosis between the lobules of the pancreas. In 1887 there were observed an abscess with necrosis of the pancreas and a necrosis of the subserous fat tissue. In Körte's third case the fat necrosis was "very marked." The patient was a man twenty-two years old, not corpulent. Thayer saw a wide-spread disseminated fat necrosis in the omentum.

It might be possible that the necrotic fat tissue facilitates the entrance of pus organisms (Dieckhoff). But this is not proved, for fat necrosis occurs quite frequently. On the other hand, it might be possible that the fat necrosis is a consequence of the inflammation, as

Dieckhoff considers very probable from the evidence furnished by two of his cases.

2. Circumscribed chronic indurative pancreatitis occurs after long-continued suppuration (Klob, Perle, Shea, Musser). The induration is to be regarded as the consequence and not as the cause of the inflammation.

3. The retention of secretion, the obstruction of the excretory duct by concretions, or compression of the duct by tumors or scars may be assumed with great probability as causes of the development of pancreatic abscess.

Alterations in the secretion or its stagnation and the development of catarrhal processes occur in this way (*sialodochitis pancreatica*, Orth), and the immigration of pus organisms from the intestine may arise as in analogous processes in the liver. In the case of Roddick several stones were found in the enlarged duct. Orth states that "the stones are generally present." In one of Dieckhoff's cases there was a gallstone in the ductus Wirsungianus. Shea found an ascaris 17 cm. long partly in the pancreatic duct and partly in the duodenum; Drasche also found one in a pancreatic abscess. It is possible, however, that in these cases the ascarides entered after the development of the abscess.

Dilatation of the pancreatic duct in consequence of compression by tumors has been reported a number of times. Dieckhoff found an ulcerating cancer at the mouth of the duct. At the Vienna General Hospital in 1892 an autopsy was held of a case of lymphosarcoma of the duodenum with abscess in the head of the pancreas.

Nevertheless the etiology of suppurative pancreatitis is not clear, and there is no satisfactory reason for the rarity of this affection when contrasted with the great frequency of micro-organisms in the intestine.

Dieckhoff rightly suggests that the cause of suppuration is to be sought, not in the gross anatomic changes of the pancreas, but in other factors, among which are the following:

1. The micro-organisms which have been found as the cause of suppuration of the pancreas (Diplococcus Fraenkel, Streptococcus) are not constantly present in the intestine.

2. It is possible for certain pathogenic organisms to become active in consequence of an alteration of the pancreatic and intestinal juices, such as occurs, for instance, in cholelithiasis with stagnation of the bile in the biliary tract.

3. The variable virulence of the fission fungi may be of consequence.

[The recognized importance of cholelithiasis in the etiology of acute pancreatitis has especially been emphasized by Opie.* He suggests that in certain cases the common bile-duct and the pancreatic duct may be converted into a continuous closed channel by an impacted gall-stone at the outlet of the two ducts in the duodenal papilla. The entrance of bile into the pancreatic duct thus may be permitted by retrojection. Halsted † and Opie showed that the injection of bile into the pancreatic duct of dogs caused an acute hemorrhagic pancreatitis accompanied by fat necrosis.—ED.]

Pancreatic abscesses may be produced experimentally in different ways. Claude Bernard found suppuration of the pancreas to occur after the injection of mercury. Körte produced pancreatic suppuration in

---

* *Am. Jour. Med. Sci.*, 1901, cxxi, 27. *Johns Hopkins Hosp. Bull.*, 1901, xii, 182.
† *Johns Hopkins Hosp. Bull.*, 1901, xii, 179.

animals by the injection of fresh perityphlitic pus into the tissue of the pancreas, also by the injection of bacteria (taken from a pure culture from fresh perityphlitic pus), and by cutting into the substance of the gland with the production of an extravasation of blood.

The injection of fresh cultures of staphylococci into the excretory duct, with subsequent tying of the duct near the head, led to the formation of an extensive abscess in the part isolated by the ligature, and caused death on the fifth day. Injection of oil of turpentine combined with the implantation of an excised piece of gland into the abdominal cavity likewise caused an abscess. In 16 experiments with the injection of pyogenic organisms or of substances irritating chemically there was the formation of an abscess in four.

By the injection of oil of turpentine to which soot was added we produced an abscess, as the following record shows:

October 26, 1896: The pancreas is drawn forward. From 0.1 to 0.2 c.c. Ol. terebinth. to which some soot was added were injected in three places in the body, in one place in the head, and in one in the tail of the gland. At the time of injection the black fluid was extensively diffused within the parenchyma of the gland. Several subperitoneal hemorrhages between the lobules.

October 27th: The animal vomited somewhat in the night. The vomitus and a little feces were mixed with the urine. Fever. Urine and vomitus, 340 c.c., brownish-yellow. Specific gravity 1025. Acid reaction. Traces of sugar. Indican in small amounts.

October 28th: No vomiting, fever, the animal drank some milk. Urine brownish-yellow, 220 c.c., albumin in small amounts. Nucleo-albumin is present. No sugar, no acetone. Indican somewhat increased. Bile pigments present.

October 29th: The dog was found dead in the morning.

The autopsy showed: Abdominal wound closed. Spleen small. Liver jaundiced. Kidneys not enlarged, capsule strips off easily. Pancreas swollen and markedly injected. The most striking changes at the point of injection on the posterior surface of the organ. In the decidedly swollen head was an area about the size of a hazelnut sharply separated from the normal portion, black, and surrounded by suppurating tissue. The tissue around the suppurated part is strongly injected. At a greater distance from the place which is so changed there is normal tissue, appearing somewhat swollen, but showing a normal structure.

The place of injection in the body of the gland shows analogous changes. On the anterior surface is an abscess about the size of a hazelnut, stained black in the middle by the injected soot. In its vicinity the pancreas is swollen, the peritoneal covering smooth and shining. A bridge of normal tissue about 3 cm. long connects this portion of the gland to the tail.

In the latter was a spot the size of a hazelnut, stained black and surrounded by purulent and hemorrhagic infiltration.

Figure 6 * illustrates a cross-section through a part of the abscess.

As can be seen in figure 6, the suppuration extends between the lobules, and can be seen in places between the acini.

Statistics.—According to the data known at present, primary pancreatic abscess occurs in men more frequently than in women. Among the 46 cases upon which these statistics are based, there are found, so far as is specified, 28 men and 11 women; in the autopsy reports of the Vienna General Hospital from 1885 to 1895 there were 3 men and 2 women.

The following statements regarding the age are noted in 30 cases:

1 to 10 years	.... 1 (10 days)	51 to 60 years	 3
21 to 30 "	11	61 to 70 "	 2
31 to 40 "	 6	71 to 80 "	 1
41 to 50 "	 6		——
			30

* Figures 6, 7, 13–16 are drawn by Mr. Wenzl from sections by Dr. Katz.

Most of the cases, therefore, are between the ages of twenty and thirty years. Fitz's table gives a similar result. Among 21 cases which Fitz mentions, there are 17 men and 4 women. According to age, they are distributed as follows:

```
20 to 25 years  ............................................3
25 to 30   "    ............................................4
30 to 35   "    ............................................2
35 to 40        ............................................2
40 to 45        ............................................3
50 to 55   ::   ............................................1
55 to 60        ............................................1
60 to 65        ............................................1
65 to 74        ............................................1
```

Symptoms.—The disease generally begins suddenly or after the occurrence of some disturbance of digestion or attacks of biliary colic (Körte) with severe pains in the epigastrium, which not infrequently radiate over the whole abdomen. Cases are described, however, in which there are no pains (Nathan). In some cases the pains are in the region

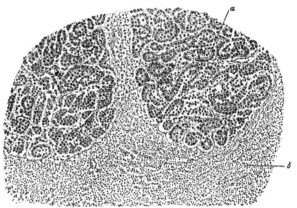

FIG. 6.—*a*, Normal gland tissue; *b*, abscess.

of the spleen or gall-bladder, the latter being sensitive to pressure. There is almost constantly epigastric tenderness. Vomiting, or at least severe retching, nausea, and eructation are usually present even at the beginning. The vomitus is stained with bile or is described as a fibrillated brown fluid. These symptoms of course are not characteristic, and correspond to an acute gastro-enteritis, if the prostration, which is at times very pronounced at an early stage, does not point to a more severe disease.

The process is generally accompanied by fever, which takes an irregular course with chills occurring at irregular intervals. At times there is no fever. As a rule there is constipation, although diarrhea has been observed either in the first twenty-four hours or as profuse, colliquative stools at a later stage of the disease. At times the constipation alternates with the diarrhea (Riboli). Blood and foul pus are often found in the stools in consequence of the rupture of an abscess into the intestine (Percival and Atkinson). In one case (Harley) the stools contained much fat and albumin.

9

The liver is at times enlarged, the spleen slightly enlarged (Greve), but at times is surprisingly small, even in those cases in which, at the autopsy, the splenic or portal vein is found thrombosed. The intestines are distended and tympanitic. In some cases free fluid or other signs of peritonitis could be shown in the abdominal cavity.

The epigastrium shows the most important changes. It appears distended and tympanitic, and in some cases a more or less distinctly limited tumor or an indefinite resistance is found in the upper part of the abdomen. Such a swelling was present in the cases reported by Kilgour, Percival, Musser, and Fournier. In Greve's case an increased resistance was found. Thayer found in the middle line above the umbilicus a deep-seated resistance, which could not be defined from the liver; percussion over this area gave a tympanitic sound and the tumor was quite sensitive on palpation. If the pancreatic abscess has ruptured and a bursal abscess has developed or a retroperitoneal collection of pus has formed, a fluctuating tumor may be recognized, as a rule extending to the left, but more rarely to the right. Such a condition was reported by Körte in his cases, in two of which certainly there were pancreatic abscesses.

In his other cases, as well as in those cited by him (Rosenbach, Werth and König, Caspersohn-Hansen), large quantities of pus were found in which either necrosis of the pancreas was the primary factor, or it was at least doubtful whether the suppuration was the result of the gangrene or the latter was the result of the suppuration. The place in which the tumor is felt, as Körte states, differs somewhat according to the point of exit of the pus and according to its development within the peritoneum, in the omental bursa, or behind the peritoneum in the posterior wall of the abdomen.

Collections of pus originating in the head or body of the pancreas will cause a swelling in the middle line or to the right or the left of that line. If the suppuration begins in the tail of the pancreas, the swelling is to be felt in the upper left portion of the abdomen. The percussion note of the resistance or of the tumor is dull (Kilgour). Large bursal abscesses or retroperitoneal collections of pus likewise are dull on percussion (Körte, Rosenbach, Werth-König, Caspersohn-Hansen). In Thayer's case there was a tympanitic sound on percussion over the resistance. The pus presents, as Körte found, certain peculiarities. He found twice in the omental bursa yellow contents like thick broth, mixed with many yellow, tallow-like fragments and brownish, discolored shreds. Microscopic examination showed fat-crystals, yellow pigment, and either no pus cells or a few which were undergoing fatty degeneration. There was found in the pus a bright brownish fluid mixed with yellow necrotic fragments, which on microscopic examination were seen to consist of fat.

Körte leaves it undecided whether the clumps of fat contained in the pus and in the discharge from the wound are to be attributed to existing, disseminated fat necrosis or to the influence of the pancreatic juice.

The following statements relate to the condition of the urine: In one case normal urine was found, except that the specific gravity was 1002; in Stefanini's case 1005. Bamberger showed the presence of peptone; Musser and Körte, albumin. Harley, Frison, Atkinson, and Frerichs found sugar, and Stefanini notes the absence of indican.

Jaundice is quite frequently found; according to Fitz, in nearly one-fourth of the cases. This may be caused by obstruction of the ductus choledochus by the swelling of the head of the pancreas, or by compression of the bile-duct by the abscess. In one case there was an abscess in the liver with dilatation of the bile-duct.

Fitz mentions bronzed skin in one case. Körte found in four of his patients (abscesses and necrosis) a grayish-brown color of the skin with very dry, desquamating epidermis. The autopsy in one of the cases showed necrosis of the fat tissue in the left adrenal. In the more chronic cases there were marked emaciation, edema, and petechiæ; and death occurred in consequence of exhaustion or sudden collapse.

Diagnosis.—The initial symptoms, the violent pain in the epigastrium, generally extending over the whole abdomen, vomiting, nausea, eructation, atypical fever, constipation or diarrhea, sensitiveness to pressure in the epigastrium, feeling of severe sickness, and prostration are such universal symptoms, and may belong to so many processes, that it cannot even be suspected that a disease of the pancreas is in question.

When, however, a more or less painful tumor appears in the epigastrium, the pancreas may be thought of, and the diagnosis of the nature of the diseased process first becomes possible when with fever a large collection of pus has formed in or behind the omental bursa and is associated with fever. It is impossible to diagnosticate small or multiple abscesses within the substance of the pancreas. It is probable that there is a collection of pus in or behind the omental bursa, when, associated with the above-mentioned symptoms so strongly characteristic of inflammation, there is an epigastric tumor disconnected with the liver, spleen, and stomach, dull or with a muffled tympany on percussion and situated behind or between the stomach and colon, as can be shown by inflating these organs.* Distinct fluctuation is rarely to be felt. Körte found indistinct fluctuation in two cases of abscess in the omental bursa, and Thayer, though unable to demonstrate fluctuation in the case in which he made the diagnosis of acute pancreatitis, nevertheless had the impression that the tumor contained fluid.

Examination under narcosis and the preliminary emptying of the stomach and intestine (Körte) are to be recommended for the purpose of deciding upon the location and nature of the tumor. Körte considers that exploratory puncture in the lumbar region should be performed without hesitation when there is retroperitoneal extension of the inflammation; it establishes the diagnosis more certainly, especially when turbid fluid mixed with fragments of fat escapes. Körte considers exploratory puncture not wholly advisable when the pus lies in or behind the bursa, and this procedure then should be employed only where it is to be followed immediately by the evacuation of the pus.

Although the diagnosis of a collection of pus in or behind the omental bursa under favorable circumstances can now be made with some degree of probability, yet this condition does not always prove that there is a suppurative process in the pancreas as the cause of the abscess, for abscesses so situated may originate from various causes. Hemorrhage of the pancreas, necrosis, or the rupture or suppuration of a cyst may be the primary factor. The collection of pus in the bursa may also originate

* For seat of pancreatic tumors see section on Cysts.

from an ulcer or cancer of the stomach or duodenum or from lymph-glands. The history may then give some indication.

The view of the pancreatic source of the disturbance would be justified when there were no symptoms of ulcer or cancer of the stomach or of duodenal disease, when the process was of sudden onset without precursory symptoms but with the rapid development of the maximum symptoms of inflammation, and when, as in the cases of Frison and Harley, and others, there was diabetes. The diagnosis of pancreatic abscess cannot be made beyond a certain degree of probability, and mistakes in diagnosis are unavoidable even with the most careful observation.

It often happens that the disease is first correctly recognized during an operation. The condition of the pus, the large amount of fat, the presence of necrotic fragments, give valuable evidence for diagnosis.

The correct diagnosis at times is made only during the treatment of the wound, when a pancreatic fistula develops, from which characteristic pancreatic juice is evacuated. In the present condition of our knowledge it is absolutely impossible to make a correct diagnosis in the great majority of pancreatic abscesses, especially in those in which general peritonitis is combined with the local process.

Prognosis and Course.—Suppuration of the pancreas is certainly a fatal disease if the abscess does not rupture into the intestine (Chiari), which is very rare, or if the surgeon's knife does not open it at the right time.

The course may be acute, subacute, or chronic. There have been cases which ended in death in a few days, and, on the other hand, patients with pancreatic abscess are known to have lived eleven months and more.

Treatment.—Radical relief is not to be expected from medical treatment. The evacuation of the abscess by surgical methods offers the only means of permanent relief.

Senn, in 1887, first proposed this method of treatment, and Fitz, Seitz, and Nimier, from the theoretic point of view, assigned the treatment of pancreatic abscess to the surgeon. The cases of Körte and Thayer were first successfully operated upon, with the exception of that of Wandesleben, operated on before the days of antisepsis.

Körte makes the following statement concerning the method of operating: "If the presence of pus in the omental bursa is shown on investigation, the operation should take place from the front, as in the treatment of pancreatic cysts. The incision is best made in the middle line. If the tumor lies distinctly on one side, the incision may be carried to that side. When the gastro-colic ligament is exposed, an exploratory puncture is made if this has not been done earlier, the abdominal cavity being protected by gauze. A piece of the gastro-colic ligament large enough for incision and drainage is then sewed to the abdominal wall and the upper and lower parts of the abdominal incision are united by a row of sutures.

"When the abdominal cavity is thus perfectly protected, the gastro-colic ligament is divided with a dull instrument, as a hollow sound or blunt forceps, and the abscess is opened. The opening is enlarged with dressing forceps. After the purulent contents have escaped, a drainage-tube is inserted and the cavity is washed out with sterile water or a very weak solution of lysol. Fragments of dead tissue are removed with the pus or drawn out with the dressing forceps. The subsequent treatment consists in washing out the cavity and in introducing gauze around the drainage-tube. If the seat of the pus is largely retroperitoneal with burrowing toward the left lumbar region, it is desirable to make an oblique incision through the abdominal wall similar to that for extirpation of the kidney. The peritoneum should then be detached with a blunt instrument toward the tail of the pancreas and the abscess opened. The pus frequently has burrowed downward as far as the brim of the pelvis.

"The skin surrounding the incision of either operation should be well anointed with zinc paste, in order to prevent corrosion."

B. SECONDARY ACUTE SUPPURATIVE PANCREATITIS.

The secondary variety may arise in various ways:

1. By extension of an inflammatory process from a neighboring organ, and especially from ulcer of the stomach. Observations on this point have been made by Thierfelder and Chiari. The former found, in a case of ulcer of the stomach at the base of which lay the pancreas, small abscesses in the connective tissue around the duct of Wirsung and penetrating the gland. Chiari also reports a similar case. Dieckhoff describes secondary suppuration of the pancreas in a gelatinous cancer of the duodenum.

Several cases of secondary suppuration of the pancreas are found among the autopsies of the Vienna General Hospital in the last ten years. In 1887 a woman twenty-one years old was examined after death, and the anatomic diagnosis of abscess of the head of the pancreas from suppuration of the inferior vena cava was made. In 1888 an abscess of the liver and of the pancreas were found, the result of pylephlebitis, in a man twenty years old. In 1889, in the case of a man seventy-nine years old, the following diagnosis was made: Carcinoma duodeni et diverticuli huius, dilatatio ductuum pancreaticorum, abscessus multiplex pancreatis cum perforatione in duodenum. The following anatomic diagnosis was made in 1892 in a man thirty years old: Lymphosarcoma duodeni valde exulceratum cum abscessibus capitis pancreatis et phlegmone textus cellulosæ retroperitonealis.

2. Metastatic abscesses may occur in the pancreas in the course of pyemia and puerperal fever; such cases, however, are rare (Orth). In the reports of autopsies at the Vienna General Hospital for the last ten years no such case is found.

3. The possibility of the occurrence of a metastatic pancreatitis in the course of a parotitis has repeatedly been considered. It is well known that in this affection metastases take place in the testes, ovaries, mammary glands, and labia majora. Mondière has mentioned parotitis also among the causes of metastatic pancreatitis.

Friedreich refers to the following cases which have been interpreted by many authors to signify that the pancreatic disease was the result of a metastasis from the parotitis. Canstatt, in the chapter on epidemic parotitis, mentions the occurrence of metastases to the pancreas. Battersby relates that the symptoms of a pancreatic disease became more evident after the disappearance of saliva from the mouth. Andral and Mondière state that either of the parotid glands may swell in the course of diseases of the pancreas. Roboica observed a case of severe parotitis in a man who suffered from a severe, deep-seated pain in the epigastrium after the parotitis suddenly disappeared. This pain also disappeared quickly, whereupon swelling of the testes occurred, after which parotitis returned. Schmackpfeffer relates the following case: In a syphilitic girl who was pregnant, the sublimate cure was begun after delivery. After the disappearance of the syphilitic symptoms, severe salivation set in. When this diminished there was abundant diarrhea with marked thirst, fever, nausea, anxiety, and a deep-seated pain in the region of the stomach radiating toward the right hypochondrium. The diarrhea was profuse, the stools watery, resembling saliva, and yellow; suddenly the diarrhea ceased and there occurred a painful swelling of both parotids, but without salivation. The pulse became small and intermittent. The patient died in collapse the following night. At the autopsy the pancreas was found swollen, reddened, very rich in blood, and of considerable consistency. Both parotids were inflamed.

"However little the symptoms just mentioned," says Friedreich, "seem sufficient to indicate the existence of a metastatic pancreatitis, yet the possibility of its presence ought not to be overlooked, in view of the last observation."

In the examination of the more recent literature there appears no report which could be interpreted to mean that pancreatitis occurs as a metastatic process after parotitis. Among reports of autopsies at the Vienna General Hospital in the last ten years there is one which suggests the occurrence of parotitis after a secondary pancreatic abscess. In a man seventy-nine years old the following conditions were present: Carcinoma cap. pancreatis cum infiltr. partiali choledochi et stenosi ejus subsequente dilatatione viarum biliferarum. Icterus univers. Carcinoma secundarium hepatis. Suppuratio partis centralis tumoris capitis pancreatis et cholangitis subsequente parotitide bilaterali et phlegmone colli cum pharyngitide et laryngitide phlegmonosa.

It is impossible to produce at present a clinical picture of secondary suppurative pancreatitis.

3. NECROTIC PANCREATITIS.

The consideration of this variety is most appropriate in the section on Necrosis.

4. CHRONIC INDURATIVE PANCREATITIS.

PATHOLOGIC ANATOMY.

The characteristic feature of this form of inflammation is the thickening and fibrous transformation of the interstitial tissue, with destruction of the substance of the gland. The changes in the gland may be primary, as in those varieties of inflammation which arise from the acute form, or from certain inflammatory processes to be further considered later, and which originate in the gland or in the ducts and lead secondarily to an increase of the connective tissue. It more frequently happens that the increase of interstitial connective tissue is primary and leads to degenerative changes and destruction of the gland.

The inflammatory process may be diffused over the entire gland or may affect only certain portions. In the former instance even the alteration need not be spread uniformly throughout the entire gland, but may be conspicuously limited to certain portions, especially the head.

A. Inflammations of the Entire Gland.

Two groups can be distinguished, in general, according to the origin of the inflammatory process from the blood-vessels or from the excretory ducts and gland cells.

The first group includes the indurative processes which occur in consequence of disease of the blood-vessels, arteriosclerosis, and endarteritis obliterans, especially when resulting from syphilis and alcoholism. The second group includes the chronic indurative processes which develop in consequence of closure, narrowing, obturation, and inflammation of the excretory ducts. In many cases it is impossible to separate these two groups sharply from each other, because there are many transitional and mixed forms.

1. **Chronic Indurative Pancreatitis Originating from the Blood-vessels (Hematogenous Variety, Dieckhoff).**—(*a*) *Indurative Pancreatitis, due to Endarteritis Obliterans.*—The blood-vessels of the pancreas are very frequently affected in the arteriosclerotic and endarteritic processes taking place throughout the body in general. They cause in this organ as in others a hyperplasia of connective tissue, and, in addition, produce throughout the entire gland or in individual portions of the same such secondary changes as fatty degeneration, atrophy, hemorrhage, and necrosis of the gland.

The characteristic changes of a typical obliterating endarteritis are given in the case described by Hoppe-Seyler of a diabetic woman fifty-seven years old.

The process was far advanced and the pancreas represented merely "a clump of fat tissue." Yet the histologic investigation showed the close relation between a previous chronic interstitial inflammation and the existing fatty degeneration. The celiac, gastroduodenal, and splenic arteries, especially the last, were markedly calcified, and the smaller branches, which penetrated into the substance of the gland, were thickened.

Hoppe-Seyler describes the development of the disease in the following manner: "The blood-vessels first become diseased, their walls thickened, their lumen narrowed or obstructed. In consequence there are disturbances of nutrition in the parts supplied by them, notably thickening of the connective tissue around the gland acini and degeneration and disappearance of the gland-cells. The interacinous fat tissue increases in proportion to the disappearance of gland tissue; indeed, it becomes so excessive that the pancreas is reduced almost to a mass of fat which may be larger than the normal pancreas." The process is regarded by Hoppe-Seyler as analogous to that found in the atrophied kidney.

Fleiner reports a similar case, also in a diabetic. This observer was able to distinguish the following pathologic processes in the pancreas: (1) Chronic obliterating endarteritis with hyaline degeneration of the vessel-wall, leading to a general narrowing of the arterial current and consequently to a greater or less degree of disturbance of nutrition, tending especially to hyperplasia of the connective tissue and atrophy of the parenchyma; (2) acute arterial thrombosis and subsequent tissue necrosis; (3) septic infection of the necrotic parts of the tissue and beginning suppuration.

Bacterium coli commune and another unidentified bacterium were isolated from the parenchymatous juice of the pancreas. It is worthy of mention that Hansemann regarded the poor staining of the nuclei in both of the cases as the result of postmortem changes.

The above processes are a transition to those which have of late been frequently recognized as chronic, indurative pancreatitis in diabetes, since the changes in the pancreas in this disease have oftener been sought for than formerly in consequence of the results of the experimental extirpation of the pancreas. Although atrophy of the pancreas and fatty degeneration of the gland are most frequently found, yet there are not a few cases in which a chronic interstitial pancreatitis, in consequence of changes in the blood-vessels of the gland or in their vicinity, is found at the autopsies of diabetics.

Lépine assumes theoretically that the primary alterations of the pancreas, at first without change in the macroscopic appearance of the gland, must be found in the neighborhood of the veins. In the course of the last few years he has been able to make some observations in support of his view, and similar contributions have since appeared, especially in French literature.

Lépine, for instance, has observed *"sclérose periacineuse"* once in a man forty years old and again in one fifty-four years old. In both patients the macroscopic appearance of the gland was altered. Especially careful investigations were made by Lemoine and Lannois in three diabetic cases, in each of which the pancreas showed the like sclerotic induration of its connective tissue. The microscopic examination of the apparently normal organ showed that the hyperplasia of the connective tissue was especially connected with its veins and the lymph-vessels, and that there was both a considerable periacinous sclerosis, which separated the lobules by strong trabeculæ of connective tissue, and an intercellular sclerosis, which had given rise to a hyperproduction of the connective tissue lying between the individual cells.

It is to be especially mentioned that, in spite of these marked microscopic changes of the gland-substance, nothing abnormal was to be discovered on macroscopic examination, a point which strongly indicates the need of more exact microscopic observations, if chronic interstitial inflammation of quite marked degree is not to be overlooked. Similar conditions in diabetes visible to the naked eye, as induration and atrophy of the gland, had been mentioned by a number of authors.

In the table headed "Indurative Pancreatitis" (page 62), and also in Tables I, II, and VI, pages 58, 61, and 69, similar cases are described, and among them that form of atrophy which Hansemann regards as the consequence of interstitial inflammations analogous to the granular atrophy of the kidney. It is, however, in most cases difficult to decide whether the process takes its origin from the blood-vessels or from the excretory ducts. Pancreatic sclerosis and excretion of sugar in the urine do not, however, by any means necessarily concur, as numerous cases show.

Obici mentions two cases of interstitial pancreatitis, one of which showed the picture described by Lépine of *"sclérose periacineuse"* in its most perfect development, without any glycosuria. Hansemann also saw two cases of induration of the pancreas, in which there was no diabetes during the life of the patient. In one of these cirrhosis of the liver was found, indicating that this case is to be regarded rather as one of pancreatic induration depending on chronic alcoholism.

The following case described by Rosenthal (1892) is on the borderline of the forms of chronic interstitial pancreatitis due to syphilis:

A girl sixteen and a half years old a year previously had chlorosis, in the course of which there were frequent attacks of fainting. Previously she had always been healthy; nothing was learned regarding any hereditary conditions (tuberculosis, syphilis). Her appearance became worse and worse, and finally rapid emaciation set in. For some weeks before her admission to the hospital she complained of backache, difficulty in urinating, and stabbing pain in the chest. Finally there was increased frequency of respiration and marked distention of the abdomen.

On entrance, the physical examination resulted as follows: Skin pale, temperature 37.8° C. (100.04° F.), pulse 120, respiration 60. In the lungs there was diffuse catarrh, the heart normal. The abdomen was markedly distended and contained free fluid. The liver projected somewhat beyond the edges of the ribs, was smooth and hard; the spleen was not enlarged.

During the seven weeks' stay at the hospital puncture of the abdomen had to be undertaken repeatedly; there was edema of the lower extremities with progressive failure of strength, and the patient died after the occurrence of symptoms of collapse. During the whole course of the disease there was no fever at any time, the urine was always normal, the stools now loose, now constipated, and again of normal consistency. The rapid failure of strength and the high degree of emaciation were especially noteworthy, the latter being such as is observed only in malignant neoplasms or in advanced tuberculosis.

The autopsy revealed as follows: Pylephlebitis chronica cum induratione pancreatis, stenosis levis et thrombosis parietalis venæ portæ. Ascites. Bronchopneumonia multiplex. Œdema leve glottidis. Degeneratio amyloides lienis.

The pancreas was of normal size, the head appeared especially thick, but the structure could be distinctly recognized in places. Microscopically the alteration of the pancreas appeared as chronic interstitial pancreatitis and proliferating lymphangitis. The connective tissue appeared especially increased between the single acini. In the head and the extreme end of the tail, masses of round cells were found lying in the much dilated lymph-vessels.

This result led Rosenthal, in spite of the previous history, to regard the case as one of latent congenital syphilis.

(b) *Chronic Indurative Pancreatitis from Syphilis.*—An increased growth of connective tissue occurs very frequently in syphilis. Chronic pancreatitis is frequently observed, especially in the congenital variety. Rokitansky has suggested that induration of the pancreas, with similar but much more frequent alteration of the liver with or without gummata, occurs in syphilis. In 23 cases of hereditary syphilis more or less pronounced changes in the pancreas were found by Birch-Hirschfeld in 10 children. In the severest cases the entire gland appeared swollen, doubled in size, very firm, white and shining, the structure entirely obliterated. On microscopic examination the interstitial tissue was found so greatly increased that the acini appeared to have entirely disappeared, and the organ seemed rather an actual fibroid than a gland. In some places the growth of connective tissue extended into the individual acini and caused the disappearance of the epithelium. Round, oval, and spindle-shaped cells were embedded in places in the connective tissue. Blood-vessels with thickened walls were only sparingly found. In cases in which the changes were not so extreme, there were found only a moderate growth and widening of the interacinous connective tissue, with slight compression of the lobules of the gland, but without disappearance of the epithelium, changes which previously were described by Oedmansson. The entire organ then appears enlarged and of a pale gray color. According to Birch-Hirschfeld, this change develops in the last months of fetal life. The most marked and most advanced alterations of the gland were found in a fetus which died in the fifth month but was delivered at the normal end of pregnancy.

In the communication in Gerhardt's "Handbook of Children's Diseases," Birch-Hirschfeld states that he has found induration of the pancreas 27 times in 124 cases of congenital syphilis. Hecker, in 1869, showed similar changes in the pancreas in 22% of the cases. Wegner, in his article on hereditary bone-syphilis, mentions three cases of induration of the pancreas. In the body of a girl who died shortly after birth, Huber found a long and wide pancreas, which was not very hard and showed interacinous increase of connective tissue, in addition to pronounced syphilitic changes in the liver and in the bones.

In 18 cases of hereditary syphilis Müller observed marked changes in the pancreas in two. In a fetus which was delivered dead at the fifth month there was found a considerable periacinous growth of granulation cells, which compressed the gland lobules and apparently led to the formation of numerous miliary syphilomata. The second case described by him, of a child born dead at the normal end of pregnancy, belongs rather to the type of interstitial pancreatitis. The bands of connective tissue were widened and infiltrated with cells. Large accumulations of lymphoid cells were found in place of the gland acini, the normal structure of the gland was retained only in single portions of the pancreas. Cases of syphilitic interstitial pancreatitis have been described by Friedreich, Demme, and Chiari. In the autopsy of an eight-months' fetus, Beck found a pancreas which was much enlarged, very thick, and nearly as hard as cartilage. Huebner has recently reported the case of a boy three and a half years old in whom he found, in addition to a high degree of syphilis of the liver, an enormous syphilitic infiltration of the pancreas, causing an increase in the size of the organ from fourfold to sixfold. Analogous conditions have been mentioned by earlier authors, although they were not always attributed to syphilis. Thus, von Osterloh and Cruveilhier described such anatomic changes without expressing any opinion as to their actual etiology. In chronic pancreatitis developed in constitutional syphilis the increased connective tissue shows generally rather a succulent character, and its inflammatory origin is indicated by the abundant infiltration of round cells, while in the cases observed in adults the connective tissue is firmer, denser, and more like scar tissue.

Thus, Drozda found a distinctly marked chronic pancreatitis in a man thirty-four years old who for years had suffered from syphilis. The patient four years before had jaundice; for three years there were periodical disturbances of digestion with vomiting and defined pain in the epigastrium, repeated distress, and attacks of fainting. The swelling of the cubital and inguinal glands showed the presence of a syphilitic dyscrasia. There was at first scarcely anything demonstrable objectively except a constant sensitiveness in the region of the stomach. Ascites occurred subsequently, followed by general edema. Bilious, and later also bloody, vomiting were often observed. Nothing abnormal could be discovered in the urine and stools. The temporary swelling of the parotid during the course of the disease was of interest; it was followed by purulent otorrhea of the right ear. Death occurred in collapse after about two and a half months of the above severe symptoms. At the autopsy the pancreas was found transformed into a hard callus. The original structure was still to be recognized in places only in the head of the gland. In some parts caseous masses were found embedded within the dense tissue. In the liver also were seen several indurated spots and an indurated scar was in the stomach. The spleen was increased to twice its size. In addition, there were chronic Bright's disease, general anemia, ascites, and dropsy.

In a case of visceral syphilis in an officer forty-six years old, Chvostek found in the tail of the pancreas several cicatricial retractions, which gave a lobulated appearance to the affected portion. Of the three cases of induration in diabetes found by Hansemann and mentioned in Table III (page 63), two had a syphilitic history. Dieckhoff reports the histologic findings in a case of interstitial pancreatitis also to be referred probably to a syphilitic condition. Cranial syphilis, pulmonary tuberculosis, and cancer of the stomach were found at the autopsy. Induration of the pancreas was quite distinct under a low power of the microscope. The connective tissue was largely arranged in circular bands surrounding the blood-vessels, excretory ducts, and gland-lobules; the intralobular tissue was increased in many of the last.

(c) *Chronic Indurative Pancreatitis from Alcoholism.*—Chronic alcoholism may cause a hyperplasia of the stroma of the pancreas, as it may produce serious changes in the connective tissue of the liver. Hence, such a pancreas may be spoken of as cirrhotic, although it does not appear yellow. Hansemann also protests against this use of the term, which may give rise to mistakes. Friedreich, in a most instructive case, already has described the occurrence of such changes in the pancreas associated with cirrhosis of the liver.

Chvostek (1876), in an inebriate twenty-nine years old, found the pancreas of cartilaginous density, tough, of the color of gray fat with a tinge of red, and with large lobes. Communicating cavities as large as beans, with smooth, firm, fibrous walls and soft, dark-gray contents, were found in the parenchyma. The liver appeared tenacious, tearing with difficulty, brownish-gray in color, finely granular, and brittle. Yellowish-brown, sharply circumscribed friable portions about the size of a walnut were found in different places in the parenchyma. There was also thrombosis of the portal vein. The case is to be regarded probably as one of interstitial pancreatitis dependent upon chronic alcoholism and complicated with pylephlebitis, to which latter lesion the further changes in the pancreas were attributable.

The patient for about ten months had suffered from repeated cardialgic attacks lasting two or three hours; later there were stabbing pains in the upper abdomen, and, finally, tension in the lower portion, with increasing ascites, temporarily disappearing, but then reappearing, and not to be prevented despite puncture. There were sensitiveness to pressure in the hepatic region, and, in the left hypochondrium, dulness extending downward to the lower border of the tenth rib and in front to three finger-breadths below the level of the costal cartilages. The appetite at first was normal, but later there were anorexia, nausea, retching, and toward the end of life, vomiting. Diarrhea alternated with constipation. Nothing abnormal could be shown in the urine. The temperature of the body remained normal throughout the disease. At the end of about fourteen months there were sudden dyspnea, severe pain in the lower part of the abdomen, marked meteorism and vomiting, death finally coming in collapse.

Hansemann (1894) also, as previously mentioned, found the pancreas very thick, markedly indurated, and the lobules not easily displaced in a man thirty-seven years old with cirrhosis of the liver.

Dieckhoff describes a very instructive case. A man sixty years old, alcoholic, had diabetes for eleven years. The amount of sugar in the first ten years varied between 6.4% and 1.5%; in the last year, between 2% and 4%. The patient, who in general felt well, after some physical exertion had a sudden hemorrhage from the stomach and died. The anatomic diagnosis was as follows: Cirrhosis of the liver, lipomatosis of the pancreas, and old, chronic interstitial pancreatitis. Dieckhoff dates the beginning of the pancreatic disease and the cirrhosis of the liver from the time when the diabetes first developed.

Among the five cases of chronic interstitial pancreatitis which are recorded in the autopsy reports of the Vienna General Hospital in the last

ten years, there is found also one case of hepatic cirrhosis in an inebriate.

The cases of chronic interstitial pancreatitis associated with chronic
interstitial nephritis should be considered after those due to alcoholism.
Tylden and Miller (1891) showed that the simultaneous occurrence of these
two processes must be very frequent, since among 15 patients with chronic
nephritis a like alteration of the pancreas was found in eight.

The previously described alterations of the pancreas designated simple
diabetic atrophy by Hansemann bears a close resemblance to certain
forms of granular kidney. The case observed by him proves that this is
to be regarded as due to an interstitial pancreatitis. In a man forty-two
years old who died with symptoms of acute phthisis after transient glycosuria and acetonuria had been shown, the lobules of the pancreas were
found widely separated by connective and fat tissue. On section, abundant, somewhat reddened gland substance was seen. Microscopically the
parenchymatous cells were not perceptibly changed. Wide capillaries
and small vessels abounded in the stroma. There was no thickening of
the vessel-walls. Inflammatory foci of small cells were numerous. The
case is important because, according to Hansemann, it shows the early
changes in the pancreas after disease of short duration: chronic fibrous
and recent small-celled inflammation of the stroma.

2. **Chronic Indurative Pancreatitis Originating from the Excretory Ducts.**—(*a*) *From Inflammation of the Excretory Ducts (Sialangitis
pancreatica).*—This variety may perhaps be the more frequent and has the
same etiology as the acute (suppurative) inflammation. It may develop
in connection with any process which favors the immigration of micro-
organisms, especially with cholelithiasis and cancer (Dieckhoff).

Among the cases described by this author, there are two in which
cholelithiasis is to be regarded as the starting-point of the pancreatitis.
In one of these the ductus choledochus was found much enlarged as far as
the entrance of the hepatic duct, and this as well as its larger branches
also were enlarged. In the fundus of the gall-bladder was a concretion
consisting of several stones closely packed together. The tissue of the
pancreas apparently was densely fibrous, permeated by very large veins
and widely dilated arteries. Occasional islands of parenchyma of a dirty
gray color and of moderately firm consistency projected slightly above
the cut surface.

Chronic interstitial pancreatitis was found also in a second case of
cholecystitis, hepatitis, and jaundice, and in one of cylindric-celled cancer
of the pancreas. In two of the cases mentioned there was diabetes.

According to Dieckhoff, the process develops as follows: "The connective tissue increases around the blood-vessels, excretory ducts, gland-
lobules, and nerve-trunks. In the further course of the disease the intralobular tissue, which separates the acini from each other, is increased. The
fat tissue also is increased; at the same time, fatty degeneration and disappearance of the parenchyma occur. The sclerosis may become so extreme
that, finally, the entire organ is changed to a fibrous band and remains of
gland-tissue can hardly be found even with the microscope."

The cases of indurative pancreatitis in cholelithiasis are of great practical interest, and Riedel has made very interesting and important communications on this subject. "In connection with gall-stones," says
Riedel, "there is a severe inflammatory process in the head of the pancreas, which leads to the formation of a large tumor; an enlargement of

iron-like density develops in a suspicious spot—namely, at the exit of the pancreatic and common bile-duct; starting originally from continued inflammation, it assumes a certain independent character, lasts for months and eventually years, until, after the removal of the cause of the disease, resolution takes place. This inflammation results not merely from a calculus in the common duct, but also may be caused by a concretion in the gall-bladder."

Riedel found induration of the head of the pancreas three times in 122 cases of gall-stones. One of the cases will serve as an example:

A man sixty-two years old was suddenly attacked in June, 1892, with biliary colic followed by jaundice. In the summer of 1893 there were repeated attacks of jaundice which became permanent and very severe. Cachexia. Liver enlarged. No ascites. Operation, August 8th, showed the liver without nodular tumors, gall-bladder large, filled with bile, containing a single large calculi. Cystic and common ducts extraordinarily wide, containing dark bile without calculi. In the head of the pancreas a tumor of iron-like density of the size of a small apple which was believed to be certainly cancerous. Cholecystenterostomy. The wound ran its course without reaction. Jaundice became gradually less, and after four weeks entirely disappeared. Stools colored. Patient recovered quickly, soon regained his former weight, and two and a half years after the operation was perfectly healthy. No tumor of the pancreas was perceptible either before or after the operation.

An autopsy showed that a pancreatitis exists in such cases. The microscopic examination of the tumor revealed interstitial pancreatitis. A new-formation could be excluded with certainty.

[Robson * lays especial stress upon the production of chronic pancreatitis by existing or probably pre-existing gall-stones, and publishes a number of cases in support of this view.—Ed.]

(b) *From Closure of the Excretory Duct.*—If the excretory duct is obstructed,—by concretions, for instance,—or is impassable for any other reason, there gradually arises an enlargement of the ducts in the gland, combined with a destruction of the gland-cells and an induration of the interstitial tissue. Experiments on animals have shown this conclusion to be correct. Pawlow tied the ductus Wirsungianus in rabbits and found the following very striking histologic changes: The cells of the tubules are diminished in size, an interstitial increase of connective tissue occurs, beginning in the greatly dilated ducts and extending between the tubules, gradually assuming extreme proportions and causing the destruction of a portion of the secreting parenchyma. Langendorff obtained similar results in pigeons after tying the pancreatic duct. The interstitial growth of connective tissue and atrophy of the pancreas were greater in them than in rabbits.

A similar process occurs in man after closure of the ductus Wirsungianus. Concretions in particular are the cause of such an interstitial inflammation of the pancreas. The following cases are mentioned as typical:

Fleiner had under observation a man forty years old who for some years had suffered from marked cardialgia. For several days he complained of great hunger and thirst. There was sugar in the urine. Four months after admission into the hospital he died of pneumonia, after severe diarrhea. Calculi were found in the excretory duct of the pancreas. The histologic changes were especially marked in the tail of this gland. In stained sections it could be seen with the unaided eye that only a few dark stained portions of gland tissue remained preserved. The main mass of the section of the gland was composed of thick connective tissue, poor in cells and rich in fibers, in which were scattered large and small masses of round cells, rather in connection with the excretory ducts than with the blood-vessels. Acini, alone or in

* *Lancet*, 1900, ii, 235; *Trans. Am. Surg. Assoc.*, 1901, xix, 144.

small groups or irregularly formed masses of epithelial cells scattered through the tissue, were separated by broad bands of fibrous tissue. The gland-cells were small, the protoplasm scanty, the nuclei well preserved and stained. The interacinous tissue was infiltrated in many places with small cells. The small excretory ducts of individual acini showed in many places a considerable, often quite irregular, bulging and widening of the lumen. In many places the lining epithelium was well preserved; in others it was desquamated and the lumen was filled with degenerated epithelium, round cells, and a finely granular, opaque mass. Small-celled infiltration of the wall and of the surrounding connective tissue was often to be seen.

Baumel describes the following case:

In a negro fifty years old, addicted to alcohol and much emaciated, diabetes was found. Death was due to tuberculosis. The apparently normal pancreas was full of calculi, which were found both in the head and in the tail of the pancreas, in the ductus Wirsungianus, and in the terminal pouches of the ducts. The shape of the stone was fitted to the space in which it was embedded and the concretions apparently interfered both with the removal of the juice and the activity of the gland. Nevertheless the pancreas was normal in appearance and size. On microscopic examination the blood-vessels were found increased, their walls thickened, and the lumen widened. Thick fibrous trabeculæ proceeded from their walls and so divided as to enlace the gland-tubules. The lobules were separated from each other by the marked growth of connective tissue and many of them were destroyed. The walls of the excretory ducts were the seat of an active growth and transformation of connective tissue, which were perhaps more marked than in the blood-vessels. The ends of the excretory ducts were surrounded by fibrous trabeculæ and filled with small cells, which at times completely occluded the lumen (Nimier).

Von Recklinghausen describes a case similar in many respects. There was a chronic inflammation of the ducts of the pancreas, probably caused by the formation of calculi, which led to fatty degeneration of the gland. In a case reported by Harley the closure of the Wirsungian duct was caused by a growth of connective tissue at the duodenal opening. In addition to an abscess in the gland, there was found hypertrophy of the pancreatic tissue caused by chronic inflammatory swelling.

B. Chronic Circumscribed Indurative Pancreatitis.

Localized affections of the pancreas, mostly secondary and due to the advance of inflammatory processes from the neighborhood, are much more frequent than general inflammation of the gland. As an illustration may be mentioned the inflammation of the pancreas extending to the gland from an ulcer of the stomach or duodenum. When an ulcer has penetrated to the pancreas and has exposed this to a large extent, according to Orth's description, the base is uneven and coarsely granular. The elevations are reddish-yellow or slightly brownish-yellow, and correspond to separate portions of the parenchyma. Dense, white, streaked bands of callous fibrous tissue are found between the divisions of the gland. On cross-section the bands, gradually narrowing, extend from the interstitial tissue in which they originated for some distance into the parenchyma. The ulcerative process often attacks the pancreatic tissue itself, parts of which may even be destroyed, and thus small branches of the excretory ducts may be opened and their secretion be poured on the base of the ulcer, thus preventing its healing. This process is generally found in the head of the pancreas and in that portion lying adjacent to the lesser curvature of the stomach.

Similar secondary processes of inflammation may be caused by aneurysm of the abdominal aorta or celiac artery, by ulcerating cancer, by preverterbal chronic inflammatory processes (Orth), and lastly by concretions which become fixed in the common duct, as it passes through the head of the pancreas. Riedel's cases also belong to this series.

Circumscribed inflammation also may be caused by such limited inflammatory processes in the gland itself as may be due to a defined obliterating endarteritis caused by syphilis or by the obstruction of a lateral duct by concretions.

Senn has produced indurative pancreatitis in animals by injury of the gland tissue and by ligation of the excretory duct.

Indurative processes have frequently been seen after partial extirpation in the study of experimental pancreatic diabetes, by Sandmeyer, for instance. The most extensive recent experiments have been made by Körte. After various injuries the gland was found denser in the injured portion. Here the interstitial connective tissue was markedly increased to such an extent that the gland-tissue became atrophied and in many places entirely disappeared. The portions beyond the ligature were atrophic and sclerosed. Injections of the pure culture of the colon bacillus led to a more or less extensive interstitial inflammation. Injections of oil of turpentine caused a very intense sclerotic inflammation. Where chronic inflammation was caused by oil of turpentine and the gland was injured four or five weeks later (by crushing, tearing, or cutting), a still more considerable growth of connective tissue occurred.

In our experiments also a demonstrable indurative pancreatitis developed, at times after the injection into the parenchyma of alcohol and zymine.

EXPERIMENT OF FEBRUARY 2, 1895.—Small dog. Pancreas drawn forward. In each of four different places 0.3 c.c. of spirit. vini rectificati was injected. In the middle portion of the pancreas a circumscribed hematoma appeared immediately after the injection, while in the other places only a slight elevation of the peritoneum resulted.

February 3d: Temperature 39.1° C. (102.4° F.). Animal takes very little milk. No urine passed.

February 4th: Temperature 37.4° C. (99.3° F.). Takes some milk. Urine reddish-yellow, turbid. Amount 190 c.c. Specific gravity 1046. Sugar 0.6%. Indican in large amount. Albumin not present. Turbidity on addition of acetic acid.

February 5th: Animal received some milk. Cutaneous wound gaping, stitches cut through. No suppuration. Iodoform bandage. Dog quite lively. Temperature 37.9° C. (100.2° F.). Urine reddish-yellow and turbid, 185 c.c. Sugar not present. Indican in large amount.

February 6th: Urine mixed with stools. The latter contain numerous desquamated intestinal epithelium, detritus, bacteria, and fat-drops.

February 7th: Urine 1050, brownish-yellow. No sugar. Indican in abundant amount.

February 9th: Urine brownish-yellow. Indican in small amount (moderate reaction). Sugar, marked reaction with Fehling's test, phenyl-hydrazin test doubtful. Stools formed. Large in amount, few flakes turning blue with iodin-potassium iodid (starch?).

February 13th: Urine shows a very strong reaction with Fehling's test.

February 16th: Condition the same. Wound quite closed.

March 15th: In addition to bread, the dog received 20 gm. of cane-sugar. Urine 75 c.c. After inversion with sulphuric acid, reduction very marked, although previously only slight.

March 20th. The pancreas appears harder after total extirpation, the fibrous tissue thickened.

March 21st: Dog found dead.

EXPERIMENT OF FEBRUARY 12, 1896.—In each of five different places in the pancreas injections were made of 0.2 c.c. of a 5% zymine solution. In some of the places there were small hemorrhages, which were checked by compression.

February 14th: No sugar in the urine.

February 20th: Animal dead.

On section the pancreas appears somewhat thicker, in the two spots there were hemorrhages of the size of a pinhead, the interstitial tissue was somewhat denser, the lobules everywhere distinctly visible. On microscopic examination the fibrous trabeculæ between the lobules appeared enlarged.

Similar macroscopic and microscopic appearances were seen by Katz and Winkler in their experiments, more complete reports of which will be given in the section on Fat Necrosis.

EXPERIMENT OF JUNE 22, 1897.—Medium-sized, long-haired dog. After opening the abdominal cavity, the pancreas was drawn forward and ligatures were tied around the gland in nine different places. The pancreas became red during the operation; the lacteals were injected.

June 23d: 0.25% of sugar was present in the urine.

June 24th: Traces of sugar in the urine.

June 26th: Urine free from sugar. The dog frequently vomited the milk taken.

June 29th: Dog quite cheerful, appearance normal. On account of great restlessness could not be kept in the cage. The urine was examined at times and always found free from sugar.

September 4th: Recent laparotomy. In this operation several peritoneal adhesions were found. The pancreas appears considerably smaller, very hard and firm. This is extirpated. Operation very difficult on account of numerous adhesions.

September 6th: Dog found dead.

The pancreas taken at the time of operation appeared distinctly smaller than normal, white, glistening, hard, and firm. On cutting into the organs, the normal gland structure is indistinct and white bands appear between the lobules.

Examined with the microscope, as is shown in figure 7, these bands are composed of fibrillated tissue, which appears to penetrate also into the gland-lobules.

Symptoms.—Most of the cases of indurative pancreatitis have first been recognized at the autopsy, and only exceptionally was the diagnosis made during life, and even then only when the abdominal cavity was opened at an operation. This fact indicates clearly that there are no known pathognomonic symptoms which point with certainty to chronic inflammation of the pancreas.

In the histories of the cases collected the symptoms mentioned are mostly general and indefinite—sensations of pressure in the region of the stomach and umbilicus, disturbances of digestion, vomiting, heartburn, epigastric tenderness, cardialgia, colicky pains, constipation or diarrhea, jaundice, meteorism, hiccough, emaciation, general weakness, at times splenic tumor, wholly afebrile or slightly febrile condition. These symptoms have such a varied significance that they may occur in every possible alteration of the digestive apparatus. This is the more easily understood, since in chronic pancreatitis other parts of this apparatus are likewise affected, for gastro-enteric processes and diseases of the biliary tract and of the liver are not infrequently the causes of the chronic pancreatitis, and in other cases the same factor which causes the pancreatitis produces also pathologic changes in other portions of the digestive system.

Arteriosclerosis, endarteritis, syphilis, alcoholism, cholelithiasis, are recognized as causes of indurative pancreatitis, and it is easily understood that the anatomic changes produced by these processes in organs near the pancreas cause symptoms which often appear much more prominent in the clinical picture than the much rarer characteristic symptoms of pancreatic affection. Arteriosclerosis, syphilis, and alcoholism certainly do not affect only the pancreas, but, in the stomach, intestine, and liver, cause changes which give rise to disturbances of function; these may be noticed earlier than the manifold signs of disturbed nutrition, which have so little that is characteristic. The general poor nutrition, increasing at times even to cachexia, the high degree of emaciation, and the progressive anemia are by no means factors diagnostic of affections of the pancreas, since they occur in the course of chronic and deep-seated diseases. When disease of the bile-passages or of the intestine gives rise to chronic inflammation of the pancreas, there are objective and subjective symptoms which generally obscure or, more accurately, do not allow to be recognized the symptoms produced by the disease of the pancreas. The jaundice observed at times may be caused by pressure of the enlarged head of the pancreas on the common duct. It may, however, be caused by gall-stones, which have given rise to the pancreatitis, or by a catarrh

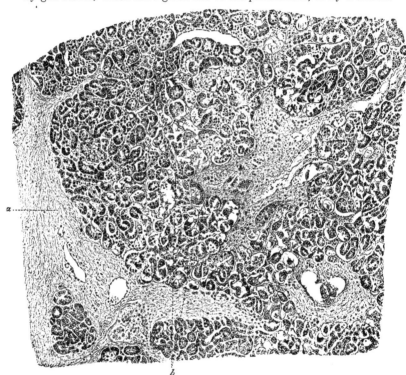

FIG. 7.—*a*, Increased fibrous tissue; *b*, fat necrosis of parenchyma.

of the duodenum and of the bile-passages. If other symptoms, which will be mentioned later, do not point to the pancreas, the jaundice offers nothing especially characteristic, even when it develops gradually and is persistent. When chronic pancreatitis is due to closure of the excretory ducts, then the colic and disturbances of digestion which eventually occur may be regarded only as symptoms of retention or suppression of secretion, without indicating an indurative inflammation.

Signs due to the inflamed pancreas may become prominent in a small number of cases of chronic pancreatitis. These are as follows:

1. The occurrence of a tumor in the region of the pancreas: There is
10

no positive evidence that the entire enlarged, calloused pancreas can be felt during life through the abdominal wall, as can the hard band at times found in the corpse after the abdomen has been opened. Some esteemed writers have stated that they have been able at times in especially thin individuals to palpate the normal pancreas. I have never succeeded in so doing, although for several years I have frequently tried.

When the head of the pancreas is the seat of the induration, and is considerably thickened, enlarged, and hard, it may be felt through the anterior abdominal wall. There is certainly one such instance. Riedel, in his three cases of chronic pancreatitis in cholelithiasis, was twice able to feel a tumor of iron-like density in the head of the pancreas during the operation, but only once did he feel through the abdominal walls a tumor as large as the fist in the head of the pancreas. He thought it the gall-bladder filled with calculi on account of its mobility, change of position with respiration, and superficial position. In another case a tumor of the head of the pancreas as large as a small apple could not be felt by Riedel either before or after the operation.

It is easily understood from this experience of Riedel that such a pancreatic tumor might compress neighboring organs and thus occasion severe symptoms, the cause of which might not be recognized during life. In Hjelt's case, for instance, of indurative inflammation of the head of the pancreas, in addition to small cysts, there was severe jaundice from compression of the common bile-duct. Jaundice also was present in the cases of Dejerine, Demme, Dieckhoff, etc. Ascites may occur from pressure on the portal vein, and dropsy by pressure on the inferior vena cava (Rigal), according to Friedreich. There was ascites also in the cases reported by Chvostek, Drozda, and Rosenthal, although probably attributable to other causes.

2. Diabetes: In the general part and in various places in this section a number of cases are given in which diabetes existed during life and chronic pancreatitis was demonstrated after death. Diabetes certainly may occur in the course of this lesion. It must be mentioned, however, that in none of the cases was the diagnosis of interstitial pancreatitis made, although the presence of the diabetes was recognized. In the cases reported by Riedel no sugar was present in the urine.

3. Fatty stools: This sign is very rare. In a newborn child Demme observed a papular rash which almost disappeared after 10 sublimate baths. On the twelfth day of life slight jaundice occurred with painful distention of the abdomen and the stools became paler, grayish-white, and fatty. Fat content 64.0% to 73.3%. In the urine were traces of bile-pigment, small amount of albumin, no formed elements. Death from scleroderma. At the autopsy the pancreas was found atrophied from chronic pancreatitis. Fibrous degeneration of the head. Acini not recognizable.

Friedreich mentions that fatty stools have been found at times, but does not describe the cases. In a patient whose diagnosis varied between chronic pancreatitis and catarrhal closure of the ductus Wirsungianus, he found "in the thin, grayish-yellow stools large and small clumps, greasy, tallow-like, and consisting of solid fat in considerable quantity."

Individual observers—Rosenthal, for instance—state expressly that the stools were perfectly normal. It is certain, however, that the quality of the stool has been only rarely observed, and that in many cases at least, it would always be possible on more careful observation to discover characteristic changes.

Diagnosis.—The obscurity of the symptoms indicates that the diagnosis of chronic pancreatitis is very rarely possible, and even then is probable only to a certain degree. The distinction between cancer and induration, especially in the early stage of the former, is difficult even when all the cardinal symptoms are present, as palpable tumor either of the entire pancreas or of the head, diabetes, fatty stools, and jaundice. Even if chronic inflammation of the pancreas were suggested from the existence of syphilis, alcoholism, or arteriosclerosis, the possibility of a new-formation in the pancreas could not be excluded.

Riedel's cases show that even large tumors are not felt through the intact abdominal walls, that even when the abdominal cavity is open inflammation cannot be distinguished from new-formation, and that one must wait a half-year or more before the true condition is known. If the tumor disappears, it was inflammation; if it grows and the patient dies, it was carcinoma.

Chronic pancreatitis may be confounded not merely with cancer of the pancreas, but also with cancer of the duodenum, portal fissure, common bile-duct, and lymph-glands, and with tumors of the vertebræ.

It is hardly possible to more than suspect indurative pancreatitis even when diabetes occurs in an alcoholic patient with cirrhosis of the liver or in a syphilitic patient, since enlargement of the pancreas is rarely observed and the thickened and indurated gland is seldom felt. Riedel's observations show that secondary pancreatitis is not so very rare in the course of cholelithiasis. If surgeons in operating for relief from gall-stones pay more attention to this matter, as is to be anticipated, indurative pancreatitis will be more often diagnosticated, at least at operations, and data will be obtained for the recognition of the disease in its earlier stages.

If such affections of the pancreas can resolve and heal perfectly after existing for years, it may positively be assumed that inflammations of the pancreas capable of undergoing resolution are much more frequent in disease of the bile-passages and duodenum than has been supposed, and have hitherto escaped recognition because they present no characteristic symptoms. It is a well-known fact that many patients suffering from gall-stones, even without permanent jaundice, become so very weak and rapidly emaciated that the development of a cancer is suspected, and yet, after a long time, the patients wholly recover. It is always possible that in such cases the pancreatitis may be recovered from without operation; that the stone in the gall-bladder, which kept up the inflammation of the pancreas, has passed out by the natural passages, and that the pancreas then has returned gradually to the normal condition, as happened in Riedel's patient after a successful operation. At present the diagnosis of such a pancreatitis cannot be made, but it may be approximated if pancreatic symptoms are sought for in analogous cases.

Since in Riedel's cases a correct diagnosis was eventually established only a long time after successful surgical treatment, so medical treatment may succeed in many cases in healing processes whose nature first becomes clear after they are recovered from.

Prognosis, Duration, and Course.—Since it is almost impossible to make a diagnosis, it is almost as difficult to give a prognosis; that is, it will be a rare exception when it can be foretold what is to be the course of the disease.

Although most of the cases, especially those due to arteriosclerosis, are to be regarded as incurable, yet there is no doubt, according to the most recent experience, that there are curable varieties, and it is impossible at present to state whether these or the incurable kinds predominate. Recovery certainly is to be thought of. When the cause which leads to chronic pancreatitis can be eliminated, as gall-stones or calculi in the pancreatic ducts, or curable intestinal processes, or perhaps syphilis in many instances, recovery is possible, but only in the earlier stages when atrophic processes have not already led to destruction of the gland, obstruction of the circulation, or cyst formation. Riedel's observations show that a cure is possible even when there is a considerable tumor.

The disease runs a slow course and the process may extend over years in favorable as well as in unfavorable cases.

Treatment.—The rational treatment of chronic pancreatitis has been rendered possible by the information obtained from surgery of late years. Surgical experience has taught that if the cause which has led to the pancreatitis can timely be removed, an integral restitution is possible up to a certain point. In this respect cholelithiasis holds the first rank. Inflammation of the pancreas is one of the many dangers which may arise in the course of cholelithiasis and may pursue an independent course, even after removal of the gall-stones, and prove dangerous to life if the process is not arrested at the right time. There is consequently a further indication for the operative treatment of cholelithiasis, which is demanded to prevent in time the further development of a secondary pancreatitis not amenable to medical treatment.

Preventive treatment should be considered for other processes also which may lead to pancreatitis, such as syphilis, alcoholism, and catarrhal inflammations of the intestine, which may be continued to the pancreatic ducts and cause them to be inflamed.

Surgical experience also offers a guide to the rational treatment of other varieties of chronic pancreatitis, although there are no facts in support of this view.

II. NEOPLASMS.

1. CARCINOMA.

Carcinoma is the most important and frequent of the new-formations in the pancreas; in the light of our present knowledge it is perhaps to be considered the most common disease of the pancreas. The view is undoubtedly correct, though at present not capable of proof, that certain affections of the pancreas—as diseases of the blood-vessels, circulatory disturbances, inflammations, catarrhal processes in the excretory ducts, atrophy, fatty degeneration, tuberculosis, etc.—occur much more frequently than has been recognized on account of defective investigations. The relative frequency of cancer to other diseases of the pancreas is probably about the same as in other organs, in which cancer certainly does not assume the highest statistical importance. Carcinomata are much more rarely overlooked than other affections which perhaps are recognizable only on microscopic examination, which is generally omitted.

The earlier literature and the contained statistics are of but little value in consequence of the frequency with which chronic inflammations of the pancreas were confused with scirrhus. There is some evidence with regard to the frequency of cancer of the pancreas, although the primary are not separated from the secondary varieties. Remo Segré collected the cases of pancreatic tumor observed in the Ospedale maggiore in Milan during nineteen years, and found 132 cases in 11,500 autospies—127 carcinomata, 2 sarcomata, 1 syphiloma, and 2 cysts.

Biach found the following results among 18,069 autopsies in the Vienna General Hospital: 1270 carcinomata, 22 pancreatic carcinomata; 5065 autopsies in Wiedener Hospital, 514 carcinomata, 6 pancreatic carcinomata; 477 autopsies in Rudolf's Hospital, 221 carcinomata, 1 pancreatic carcinomata. Therefore among 23,611 autopsies there were 2005 cancers, of which 29 were in the pancreas. Thus he finds 8.5% of cancers, of which 1.5% were pancreatic cancers.

From Biach's collection of the carcinomata observed in the Wiedener Hospital for the years 1860 to 1866, the following results show the relative frequency of the occurrence of this neoplasm in the stomach, liver, and pancreas:

	1860.	1863.	1864.	1865.	1866.
Stomach	29.54%	28.80%	21.15%	25.53%	34.42%
Liver	27.27%	23.07%	21.15%	21.28%	18.03%
Pancreas	2.27%	3.85%	1.92%	2.13%	1.64%

In this statement also the primary and secondary tumors are not distinguished.

Eppinger's statistics are based upon 1314 autopsies. Among these there were 308 cancerous neoplasms in the different organs. The pancreas was involved in 19 cases (5.5%). Only two cases (0.6%) were certainly primary in the pancreas.

Among 3950 autopsies, Soyka found 313 carcinomata, of which 3 (1%) were primary in the pancreas. Among 313 cases of cancer, Wrany found the pancreas involved 6 times. Among 639 autopsies in individuals dying of different diseases, Forster found pancreatic cancer 6 times, and it was always secondary. Among 467 autopsies of cancerous patients, Willigk found pancreatic cancer 29 times.

The primary cancer of the pancreas is certainly much rarer than the secondary variety, but primary carcinoma of the pancreas is by no means a very rare disease. Friedreich collected only 15 cases. In statistics published in the year 1893 by Mirallié, 113 cases of primary carcinoma of the pancreas are reported. He eliminated all cases from consideration in which a cancer was found at the same time in any other organ, since it would render doubtful the primary origin of the tumor; he excluded also those cases in which he was unable to get any detailed account. It may certainly be assumed that among the cases excluded by Mirallié there were some which were primary, for metastases after primary carcinomata of the pancreas are by no means infrequent.

To the above mentioned I have been able to add, up to 1896, 36 additional cases of primary cancer. There are recorded in the reports of the Vienna General Hospital, from 1885 to 1895, 32 cases of primary cancer of the pancreas.* The number of actual cases is, of course, much greater. If the report of a large hospital or the autopsy reports of an anatomic institute are examined, there will always be found individual cases of primary cancer which are not published elsewhere. Since it is well known that

* In the literature from the beginning of 1896 to July, 1897, the following cases are found: Abbe, Aigner (4 cases), Bandelier (5) cases, Fothergill, Gade, Gorbatowski, Hale White (2 cases), Lütkemuller, Maxson (2 cases) Russel.

primary cancer of the pancreas is by no means rare, only such cases
usually are published in which the diagnosis can be established or in which
special features appeared during life or after death.

It cannot be decided with certainty whether all cases described as
primary pancreatic cancer really originate in the pancreas, since there
are many cases, as Dieckhoff states, in which it is not possible, even at the
autopsy, to answer exactly this question. "It not infrequently happens
that a cancer which to the unaided eye gives at first the impression of a
primary carcinoma of the pancreas shows on microscopic examination
that it originates from the glands of the duodenum, an occurrence which is
especially emphasized in a careful study made by Olivier." This writer
concludes that it may happen that a neoplasm which, on macroscopic
examination, appears as a primary tumor of the pancreas, originates in
the duodenum and actually presents, after it has secondarily affected the
pancreas, all the characteristics of an interstinal cancer.

It may be at times, as Orth suggests, that even a microscopic examination does not insure a positive conclusion, "since cylindric-celled cancers
may proceed even from the pancreas,—that is, from its excretory ducts,—
and the transition of the atypical growth of gland acini into cancerous
alveoli, observed by some investigators, is by no means always so easily
established in primary tumors."

Secondary carcinoma of the pancreas is far more frequent. This can
be determined from the earliest statistics of Gussenbauer and Winiwarter.
These observers examined the autopsy reports of the Vienna Pathologic
Institute from 1817 to 1873 with reference to the relation of cancer of the
stomach to its metastases. Among 61,287 autopsies there were 903 cases
of cancer of the stomach. In these, there were 100 metastases in the
pancreas, the liver was the seat of secondary cancer 259 times, the mesentery and intestine 173 times, the lymph-glands and pancreas 94 times.
Among 542 cases of primary cancer of the stomach limited to the pylorus,
there were metastases in the pancreas in 34.

The frequency of gastric cancer permits a conclusion to be drawn as to
the frequency of secondary pancreatic cancer, since more than 10% of
the metastases after cancer of the stomach affect the pancreas, which
organ is not infrequently also the seat of metastases from cancers elsewhere.

PATHOLOGIC ANATOMY.

Seat of the Neoplasm.—The head of the gland is the most frequent
seat of the neoplasm according to the earlier statistics of Ancelet, who
collected 200 cases without discriminating between the primary and secondary forms. The tumor was found in the head 33 times, in the body
5 times, twice in the tail, and 88 times it affected the entire pancreas.
Among 73 cases of primary and secondary cancer of the pancreas collected by Biach the head was affected 19 times, the body 13 times, and
the whole gland 31 times. The seat of the cancer was not stated in 19
cases. In one case the upper edge of the gland alone was diseased. Remo
Segré found the seat of the tumor 35 times in the head, 19 times in the entire
gland, twice in the middle, and once in the tail. Mirallié writes: "In
general, the head of the pancreas is the seat of the disease." Among
78 cases in which sufficient details were given for classification, the head
was found the seat of the new-growth 39 times, the whole organ 19 times,

the tail 4 times, head and body 3 times, middle portion and tail once, middle portion once, head and tail once; in 10 cases no exact statement was made.

In the autopsy reports of the Vienna General Hospital from 1885 to 1895, the following data were found: Among 32 cases of primary carcinoma it was found in the head in 20 cases, twice in the body, 3 times in the tail, and once throughout the entire gland. In 6 cases no exact statements were given regarding the location. Among 53 cases Boldt found the head diseased 25 times and the entire gland more rarely.

Variety of Cancer.—The most frequent form is fibrous cancer with hard, dense nodules. Soft medullary cancer and cylindric-celled and gelatinous cancers are rare. Medullary cancers are reported by Allen, Harrison, O'Hara, v. Hauff, Kernig, Lubarsch, Mariani, Molander and Blix, and Wrany. Cylindric-celled cancers have been described by Wagner, Pott, Strümpell, Wesener, and Dieckhoff (two cases and a mixture of medullary and cylindric-celled cancer). Gelatinous cancer is reported by Lücke-Klebs and Mosler; alveolar cancer by Bruzelius and Key and by Seebohm (hard scar-like tissue with alveolar structure and epithelioid cells). Adenocarcinoma by Seebohm and by Ruggi.

Segré found among his cases 29 of fibrous cancer, 19 of medullary, 2 of combined, and 1 of melanotic cancer. Of the 32 cases of cancer which were examined postmortem in the Vienna General Hospital from 1885 to 1895, 19 are noted as scirrhus, 1 as medullary, 1 as adenocarcinoma, and 3 as gelatinous (one of which was a gelatiniform fibrous cancer). In 8 cases the exact characterization was not given.

Cancer of the pancreas may proceed from the glandular epithelium or from the cells of the excretory ducts. "In general," says Dieckhoff, "the conclusion may be justified that, in the pancreas, as in other organs, cancer with ill-defined forms of epithelium originates from the glandular epithelium, while cancer with typical and conspicuously cylindric cells originates from the epithelium of the excretory ducts, and a number of small alveolar cancers even with less typical cylindrical epithelium also originate from the epithelium of the excretory ducts."

He coincides with the view of Olivier, who, on the basis of a careful investigation of three cases of cancer, comes to the following conclusion: "Primary cancer of the pancreas may proceed from the epithelium of the small ducts even when 'la faible proportion des formations neoplastiques canaliculaires'—as Dieckhoff designates the small alveolar cancer—does not give the appearance of a cylindric-celled cancer." Dieckhoff somewhat modifies this view in a foot-note in which he refers to a case of medullary cancer observed by Lubarsch, where, "in spite of the large alveolar character of the new-growth, the origin from the excretory ducts was known by the fact that the cancerous strands penetrated as large bands into the normal pancreatic tissue, in which, however, there were no excretory ducts; Thierfelder has described a similar condition in his case of pancreatic cancer."

Size of the Tumor.—The pancreas in the great majority of cases is enlarged. The nodes are described as being as large as a pigeon's egg, a hen's egg, a goose-egg, or as large as a child's fist. Exceptionally, larger tumors are found. Terrier extirpated a neoplasm of the size of the head of an adult and weighing $5\frac{1}{2}$ pounds. In Sauter's case the tumor was of the size of a man's fist. Bard and Pic found a tumor of the size of the head of a fetus. Isch-Wall found a tumor as large as a mandarin orange.

At times the pancreas appears smaller than normal, shrunken (Kühn, Mosler), or of normal dimensions (Bard and Pic).

The portion of the pancreas not affected by the cancer is either normal or hardened or atrophied by the new-formation of connective tissue.

Extension to neighboring organs frequently takes place, and all tissues in the neighborhood of the cancerous pancreas may be involved in the neoplasm. In many cases it is certainly difficult to say positively what is the origin of the carcinoma.

Most frequently the liver, stomach, duodenum, gall-bladder, the larger bile-passages, and the neighboring lymph-glands are involved. The cancer may extend also to the omentum, the mesentery, the large intestine, the kidney, the spleen, to the aorta and the portal vein, the vertebral column, to the diaphragm and through this to the pleuræ and lungs.

Metastatic nodules are found most frequently in the liver, but they are also observed in the skin, heart, lungs, and pleura, in the cardia, in the dura, in portions of the large intestine (cecum, rectum), in the plexus hepaticus and spermaticus, and in the ovary. Not infrequently a general carcinosis develops. The primary seat of the cancer, however, is doubtful in many cases.

The growing tumor compresses the neighboring organs and obstructs the cavity of adjacent hollow organs and canals. The frequent seat of the neoplasm in the head of the pancreas and the relation of the latter to the ductus communis choledochus explain the frequent compression of this duct.

It is easy to understand that when the head is degenerated, a mechanical hindrance to the flow of bile must frequently result from pressure on the common duct, since, according to the investigations of Zuckerkandl, this duct for about $\frac{1}{2}$ to 3 cm. traverses the gland tissue in the head of the pancreas.

Courvoisier found cancer as the cause of obliteration of the ductus choledochus from disease of the pancreas in 55 out of 66 cases. It is evident that the ductus Wirsungianus may be compressed or even involved in the neoplasm. Dilatation of the duct, and at times even a cyst-formation in the pancreas (according to Boldt, in about one-third of the cases), are necessarily present beyond the obstruction of the ductus choledochus and ductus Wirsungianus. The intimate relation between the head of the pancreas and the duodenum easily leads, when cancer develops in the head of the pancreas, to compression and obturation of the duodenum (de Haën, Mondière 2 cases, Teissier, Holscher, Wrany, Stansfield, Tanner, Salomon). In the case reported by Wesener the cancer was fused with the duodenum, and in Mariani's case it had become attached to the concavity of the duodenum.

Pyloric stenosis also may result from the compression, as in the cases of Bardeleben-Klemperer and Pilliet. Rahn reports compression of the cardia, and Petit states that the entire stomach was compressed and crowded toward the anterior wall of the abdomen. The colon was compressed, Battersby; the ureters, Recamier, Soyke, Bard and Pic; the vena portæ, Faendrich, Molander and Blix, Wrany; the aorta, Teissier, Andral, Choupin and Molle, Battersby; the splenic artery and vein, Sandwith; superior mesenteric artery and vein, Williams. Compression of the inferior vena cava occurs not infrequently. According to Boldt, the aorta and vena cava inferior were compressed in about 10 cases, the aorta alone in 5 cases. The compression of the thoracic duct also is noted. Thrombosis of the portal vein was found in the case of Wesener.

Ulcers, which may perforate, result from degeneration of the cancer. Such cases are described by v. Hauff, perforation through the abdominal wall at the navel; Campbell, through the posterior wall of the stomach. Ulceration of the tumor after its growth into the stomach or into the duodenum is reported by Muhry, Albers, and Kopp; perforation into the portal vein, noted by Bowditch, Molander and Blix, Litten; ulceration of the celiac artery by Cash.

ETIOLOGY AND STATISTICS.

The causes of the development of cancer of the pancreas are entirely unknown. The influence of heredity, predisposition, poor nourishment, and abuse of alcohol as etiologic factors is entirely hypothetic. Traumatic factors are noted only in the rarest cases. In Clurg's case the patient attributed his disease to the pressure of a quantity of coal in the region of the stomach. Schupmann's patient blamed the lifting of a heavy body.

Cancer of the pancreas is found more frequently in men than in women; both earlier and later statistics are agreed on this point. Da Costa found among 37 cases, 24 men and 13 women; Ancelet among 161 cases, 102 men and 59 women; Bigsby among 28 cases, 16 men and 12 women; Boldt among 56 cases, 35 men and 21 women; and Mirallié noted 69 men and 37 women in his 106 cases. In addition to the above, I have found, up to the beginning of 1896, statements regarding 21 men and 20 women. Including Mirallié's cases, there are 90 men and 57 women, hence 61.2% of the cases are men. This proportion is changed somewhat by the autopsy reports of the Vienna General Hospital from 1885 to 1895. Among 32 cases, 12 were men and 20 women.

The age most frequently concerned is between forty and seventy years. According to Boldt, the greatest number of cases, 18, were found between fifty and sixty years; between forty and fifty there were 11 cases, and between sixty and seventy there were 10 cases. The following table is based upon 73 cases:

YEARS.	CASES.
0 to 1	1 (Bohn, 7 months)
1 to 10	1 (Kühn, 2 years)
11 to 20	1 (Dutil, 14 years).*
21 to 30	3
31 to 40	14
41 to 50	19
51 to 60	20
61 to 70	10
71 to 80	4
	73

SYMPTOMS.

The symptoms of primary pancreatic cancer, according to the time of their occurrence, can be divided into three groups:

1. The disturbances of function of the pancreas and of its nerves and

* Bandelier has recently reported the occurrence of cancer in a boy thirteen years of age.

canals resulting from alteration of the pancreatic tissue during the beginning and development of the neoplasm.

2. The arrest of function of neighboring organs invaded by or involved in the extension of the growth from the pancreas.

3. The result of metastases and of general carcinosis.

This grouping cannot be strictly adhered to because many of the symptoms differing in intensity and quality are present in all three groups, and, therefore, should be considered in the description of each. Besides, our knowledge of the pathology of the pancreas is still so defective in many respects that the symptoms of the first group, which are caused by the partial failure of pancreatic function, generally disappear entirely and show nothing characteristic. Striking symptoms generally occur first when the cancer of the pancreas affects the function of neighboring organs, when, as one might say, it becomes cultivated. The following attempt to represent the frequency and importance of the symptoms is based upon published experiences, since a single observer has but little opportunity to discuss them from his own observation on account of the rarity of recognizable diseases of the pancreas.

Disturbances of digestion are generally given as the first symptoms, diminished appetite and hunger, distress after eating, sense of pressure, fulness in the epigastrium, especially after meals, heartburn, eructation, nausea, retching. It cannot be decided that these symptoms are attributable to the development of the cancer.

It is possible that catarrhal processes of the stomach or of the small intestine precede or accompany the disease of the pancreas, and that the dyspeptic disturbances are due to them. In the course of the disease these symptoms appear much more pronounced. Complete anorexia frequently develops, also a loathing for food, especially for meat, and the aversion may become so extreme that all nourishment is refused. Numerous observations show that this distaste for food does not take place simply in case of the extension of the disease to the stomach. In certain cases the appetite suffers little or none. The patients eat well and with satisfaction, but become continually more and more emaciated, as was the fact in a case which I shall later describe. The disturbance of the appetite does not depend upon the carcinoma itself, as may be seen in a number of the cases, in which, on account of closure of the ductus choledochus by a pancreatic cancer, cholecystenterostomy was performed. After the anastomosis had been established and the jaundice had disappeared, the appetite became good at times, although temporarily, and the patient's weight increased (Reclus, Regnier, Terrier, Kappeller-Socin, Ruggi).

Severe disturbances of digestion develop when there is a dilatation of the stomach with all the consequences of stagnation of the gastric contents from compression of the duodenum or pylorus. The frequent vomiting of an earlier stage becomes the rule (Mirallié, Strümpell, Ziehl, Drozda). Blood may be mixed with the vomitus, or the latter may consist of pure blood, when the tumor has perforated into the cavity of the stomach or into the duodenum.

The examination of the gastric contents, which only rarely has been made after a test-breakfast, repeatedly shows an entire lack of free hydrochloric acid, although the stomach was entirely free from disease (Bottelheim). In the case of Klemperer-Bardeleben, in which the pylorus was compressed by a tumor of the pancreas and the contents of the stomach could not pass through the pylorus, the examination showed 2.6% hydrochloric acid. On strong suction, there escaped from the stomach about 50 to 80 c.c. of a greenish fluid, which distinctly contained mucin and bile pigment.

The signs of disturbed digestion indicative of a loss of the function of the pancreas are rarely found in the stools. Fatty stools are noted several times. Mirallié mentions nine cases: Besson, Garnier, Marston, Musmeci, Rocques, Luithlen, Labadie-Lagrave, Pott, Mirallié. In addition, fatty stools were noted by Bowditch, Clark, Friedreich, Maragliano, Marsten, Molander, and Blix and Ziehl. The last found silver-gray stools, three-fourths of which consisted of acicular fat-acid crystals. The chemical examination showed that one-fourth of the weight was due to fat, half to water, and the remaining fourth to other substances.

The case observed by me in which this symptom was especially striking was as follows *:

M. M., born in 1854, manufacturer's wife, family healthy. Father and mother still living. Has borne three children and had one abortion. After the abortion, in 1889, she had a posterior parametritis. At this time there was also an intramural uterine fibromyoma as large as a fist in the posterior wall. In 1890 and 1891 she felt relatively well, but on account of anemia and the persistence of the parametritis exudation she took a course of treatment at Franzensbad. In the summer of 1892 she was taken ill with diarrhea and became emaciated. Her appetite, however, was good. The stools were regularly evacuated at night, were uncommonly copious, of the consistency of thick broth, of offensive, extremely bad odor, chocolate in color, and always plentifully covered with fat-drops, in spite of the fact that she ate as little fat as possible. At the end of December, 1892, the rather large woman weighed only 100 pounds.

On physical examination, the lungs and heart were normal; abdomen flat, not painful on pressure. In the uterus was a myoma the size of a fist; in the urine no albumin and no sugar.

January 11, 1893, I saw the patient for the first time and the stools were thoroughly examined, with the following result: Stools moderate and like thick broth; white particles were scattered in the sediment.

Microscopic examination: (1) Very numerous fragments of striated muscle-fibers, in the main with well-preserved structure; (2) numerous fat-acid needles and fat-drops; (3) bacteria, detritus.

Chemical examination: After several days' drying on the water-bath in order to estimate the amount of fat, 4.6325 gm. of dry residue were obtained, in which there were 2.1265 gm. of fat; that is, 45.9%. The ether extract consisted predominantly of neutral fat.

At a subsequent examination, on January 28th, I found in the epigastrium a hard, round tumor, the size of a nut, the seat of which I located in the head of the pancreas. My diagnosis was carcinoma capitis pancreatis. In March the patient stayed for two weeks in Hungary, and there menstruated profusely and developed jaundice.

April 6, 1893, an exploratory laparotomy was undertaken in Eder's Sanitarium by Professor Albert in the presence of Professors Schauta, Hochenegg, and Director Schopf. After cutting through the great omentum, especially the gastrocolic ligament, an attempt was made to isolate the tumor, which was found connected with the head of the pancreas. It appeared firmly attached to the surrounding structures, especially to the vena cava, so that it was necessary to give up the extirpation. The much reduced patient became steadily weaker after the operation and died on the 13th of April. No autopsy was performed.

A similar condition was reported by me (see page 113) in a case in which the diagnosis of cancer of the pancreas could be made only with great probability.

The disturbance of the digestion of proteids deserves especial attention. Besides the above observations in pancreatic cancer, there is only

* The history was kindly supplied to me by Director Schopf.

one other on this subject—that of v. Ackeren. The latter quotes also a very similar case reported by Le Nobel.*

In another case, to be mentioned later, and which may be regarded as cancer of the pancreas, there was a similar condition in the stools. It may probably often occur that many undigested muscle-fibers could be found in the feces on microscopic examination; Küster, for instance, having found them in a case of probable pancreatic cyst.

Bulky stools are a striking symptom, as has already been mentioned. They were present in one of the cases described by me, and were due to the fact that a large part of the food passed out undigested. It might be claimed that this disturbance of digestion was due to the diseased pancreas, since there was no jaundice at first. The patient generally recognizes that he is evacuating a surprisingly large amount of feces in relation to the food he is taking. This symptom should certainly attract the attention of the physician. I have a number of cases in mind in which from this symptom I concluded that the pancreas was diseased. In a man over seventy years old there was diabetes. Later jaundice developed, which slowly increased and became very intense. There was found in the epigastrium to the right of the spinal column a resistance, which gradually increased in size. Aside from the rapid emaciation and persistently advancing cachexia, the most surprising symptom was the daily evacuation of very abundant, firm masses of fecal matter. On microscopic examination of the stools, many muscle-fibers and undigested vegetable cells were seen; fat in abnormal amounts was not present. Unfortunately no autopsy was allowed, but the assumption of a cancer of the pancreas seems fully justified in this case.

Such changes in the stools are certainly rare. Although in most of the publications no statement is made concerning the feces, yet in a number of cases it is expressly stated "stools normal."

Acholic stools and disturbances of digestion dependent on the want of bile often occur on account of the frequency with which the outflow of bile into the intestine is hindered by a growing cancer in the head of the pancreas.

Bloody stools occur frequently, and have been reported by Bohn, Freidreich, Kobler, Mariani, Molander and Blix, Wesener. Hemorrhage occurs in ulceration of the duodenum or some other portion of the intestine, after the cancer has spread to these parts. Constipation or diarrhea often occur as manifestations of disturbed intestinal function. Constipation is the more frequent. Kellermann found it 60 times in the reports of cases investigated by him, while diarrhea was observed only 12 times; in 9 cases diarrhea alternated with constipation, and in the others the consistency of the stools was either noted as normal or no statement was made concerning them. In case of extension of the growth to the intestine or of compression of the latter by the tumor, there may be stenosis leading even to complete closure. Hagenbach mentions eight such cases (Kerckring, de Haën, Mondière 2 cases, Holscher, Teissier, Tanner, Salomon), and describes Kerckring's case as follows: A man forty years old suffered for six days from irremediable obstipation, and died after having vomited fecal matter for three days. The pancreas, enlarged to three or four times its natural size, had completely compressed the ileum.

Pain is one of the symptoms which generally accompany the process

* In Maly's "Jahresbericht" regarded as atrophy (see General Considerations, pp. 59 and 92).

from beginning to end. It is rarely wholly absent. In one of the cases reported by Friedreich the absence of pain, either spontaneous or on pressure, in the upper abdomen was very surprising; in Stiller's patient also severe pains and cramps were lacking during the whole course of the disease. In a number of patients there were moderate pains, a feeling of pressure and tension in the epigastrium, a feeling of distress behind the stomach, sensitiveness to pressure, which increased during and from peristalsis. As a rule, however, the pains are very severe, either continuous or paroxysmal, and assume the form of cardialgia and colic. The continuous pains are seated in the epigastrium and radiate in all directions, especially into the right hypochondrium, when the cancer is in the head of the gland. They may radiate toward the chest, shoulder, abdomen, and back, and are of great intensity, being further increased by movement and by taking food. The patients may be unable to define exactly the kind of pain. They call it burning, boring, tearing, drawing, stabbing; but when it is most severe, they say only that they suffer beyond endurance.

The nature and intensity of the pain, which is rarely so severe in other tumors of the upper abdomen, have led to the assumption that it was due to pressure upon or stretching of the celiac ganglion or the nerve-trunks proceeding from it, and, therefore, it has been designated celiac neuralgia. Similar suffering is seen only in the severe crises of tabes or other diseases of the central nervous system, but these disappear after a few days or one or two weeks, while the pains arising from pancreatic cancer, perhaps with ever-increasing intensity, last to the end of life.

Constant or paroxysmal pains of another kind may arise, due to the adhesion of the pancreas to movable neighboring organs in consequence of the extension of the cancer to the adjacent peritoneum, every movement of which leads to stretching and pain.

The paroxysmal pains come next, and are regarded as cardialgia, colic, perhaps biliary colic. They are of various duration and intensity and may originate from different causes. They are either paroxysms of the neuralgia previously mentioned as attributed to the participation of the celiac ganglion, or attacks of genuine pancreatic colic caused by stagnant secretion in the ductus Wirsungianus or in other secretory ducts of the pancreas, when they are compressed, stretched, or entirely closed by the cancerous growth within them. The pain may be actual biliary colic if the outflow of the bile is so disturbed by pressure on the ductus choledochus or by its involvement in the growth of the cancer, or by a bend of the common bile-duct, that concretions form, or if, as is not rarely the case, a cholelithiasis is actually present. True gastralgias also may be present, when the growth extends into the stomach and ulcerates or constricts the pyloric orifice. Intestinal colic arises when the action of the intestine is disturbed by the pressure on it of the cancer or cancerous glands, or when the coils become adherent in consequence of cancerous peritonitis. The continuous pains not infrequently are combined with the paroxysmal variety; the continuous, more or less intense pain is intensified at times, and, thus increased, may last for several days. Sensitiveness to pressure occurs in addition to spontaneous pains. This is present almost without exception, but there is, at times, pain produced by pressure so intense that the patients cannot bear the slightest touch.

Jaundice is one of the most frequent symptoms of cancer of the pancreas. In most cases it does not first occur when the cancer extends beyond the pancreas, but arises from alterations in the pancreatic tissue and from pressure of the neoplasm on the common bile-duct in consequence of the usual passage of this duct through the head of the pancreas. Jaundice not infrequently is the first indication of the disease. It may occur suddenly after an attack of colic, and then is attributable to cholelithiasis. As a rule, it develops gradually, insidiously, and when it has once appeared it increases, slowly but unceasingly advancing until it has all those peculiarities which are presented by jaundice from complete closure of the ductus choledochus. It always increases progressively although with differing rapidity. The skin, especially that of the face, becomes dark brown, and finally is almost black. The jaundice may apparently diminish toward the end of life, as sometimes happens in other varieties of permanent closure of the excretory bile-ducts. The color due to the bile-pigment seems to be less pronounced than before because the skin becomes anemic and pale. In many cases jaundice is slight at the onset, and first appears distinctly or increases in intensity toward the end. In a number of cases there is no jaundice. Mirallié found it 82 times in 113 cases; in addition, it was noted 21 times in the 36 cases above referred to; hence, it has been reported 103 times in 149 cases. Jaundice was entirely lacking at first, and only appeared later in the patient reported by me as having marked fatty stools. In the cases of Ramey and Kellermann, in which the head of the pancreas was considerably enlarged and hardened, no trace of yellow color was found in the skin. The retention of the bile is associated with all its consequences, as acholic, silver-colored stools, itching, slow pulse, weariness, bile pigment in the urine, and xanthopsia.

In a later stage of the process the jaundice may be due to compression of the bile-ducts by the development of metastatic nodules in the liver, and thus jaundice may occur, even when the primary seat of the cancer is not in the head, but in the tail of the pancreas.

The liver and gall-bladder are altered in connection with the stagnation of bile. These alterations, according to many writers, have especial peculiarities by which pancreatic carcinoma is said to be characterized.

Bard and Pic state their experiences as follows: "The liver, as a rule, is hard, the edges are frequently sharp, but the organ is always small or at least but slightly enlarged. It is generally only slightly painful on pressure, except in the neighborhood of the tumor caused by the enlarged gall-bladder. The pain and tenderness associated with the condition are commonly most intense in the epigastrium. The liver has never been found hypertrophied, hard, and mammillated, as is so frequently the case in cancer of the digestive tract. These negative qualities form the most important characteristics of the disease, and do not depend on the absence of metastases in the liver; on the contrary, generalization of the cancer in the liver is almost an absolute rule. Although the liver is not enlarged in consequence, it is because metastatic cancer of the liver secondary to cancer of the pancreas is quite different from primary cancer of the liver secondary to cancer of the digestive tract. In the former case the secondary nodules are small, not elevated above the surface, and do not increase essentially the size of the liver."

These conclusions were reached by Bard and Pic on the basis of seven cases, but surely cannot be regarded as the general rule. It is first to be mentioned that in the cases communicated by Bard and Pic there are some in which there is considerable enlargement of the liver. In Case 1 the liver overlapped the false ribs about 8 cm. To be sure, two months later, at the autopsy, it was not found enlarged. In Case 3 the liver overlapped the false ribs about four finger-breadths. At the autopsy, performed one and a half months later, the liver was not enlarged. In Case 5 the liver was enlarged even after death. Enlargement of the liver with and without metastases in it is not infrequent. Mirallié found enlargement of the liver in 17 cases. Besides these, hepatic enlargement with metastases is mentioned in the cases of Friedreich, Biach, Bohn, Maragliano, Kellermann, Munkenbeck, Reinhardt, Aigner, and Bandelier; and without metastases in those of Rankin and of Dieckhoff (two cases). Enlargement of the liver without any statement of the presence or absence of metastases is mentioned by Miller, Rufus Hall, and Reclus. Before the Société anatomique, 1887, Moutard-Martin demonstrated a liver the lower edge of which extended beyond the umbilicus; Chopin and Molle also refer to hypertrophic liver. In the two cases of Cochez the liver was enlarged and hypertrophic without secondary nodules. The liver was enlarged in two of my patients with jaundice. In a number of cases an enlargement first exists, but later the volume becomes diminished even below the normal size. In the case of Mirallié the liver was at first markedly hypertrophic, the lower border was smooth and sharp and extended to the level of the umbilicus; two and a half months later the lower border could be felt three finger-breadths below the false ribs, and two months afterward, hence five months after the first examination, the liver extended scarcely below the false ribs and it was difficult to feel the lower edge. According to Mirallié and Cochez, therefore, there are two stages to be discriminated: the first that of enlargement of the liver, the second that of diminution in size, atrophy, analogous to the course of biliary cirrhosis. The size of the liver, therefore, will depend on the duration of the changes in it. If they have lasted but a short time, the liver will be enlarged; if hepatic cirrhosis has had time to develop, a more or less pronounced atrophy will be present.

Even this wholly plausible explanation will not fit all cases. When metastases form, the liver may be enlarged even at the terminal stage, and even when the process has lasted a long time, especially since the small nodules regarded by Bard and Pic as characteristic are not always present. Nodules as large as those in metastatic cancer of the liver may occur when the primary tumor is not seated in the pancreas.

Several medullary nodules of secondary cancer as large as a walnut were found within the liver in Friedreich's second case. In the case reported by Kellermann the liver contained nodules of various size, one as large as an apple being found on the anterior surface of the right lobe. It certainly must be granted that small nodules only are found much more frequently. This may be due to the generally rapid course of pancreatic cancer.

It is true that in a number of cases, in spite of the presence of jaundice, the liver was not only not enlarged, but was stated to have been normal or even diminished in size. Suckling and Wescner, for instance, found it small in spite of intense jaundice. In the cases of Drozda, Klemperer, and Stiller, the liver did not exceed the normal limits. Such statements are often made.

It is therefore to be stated that there is no characteristic outline of the liver in all cases of cancer of the pancreas, but the liver frequently shows such changes as are caused by the gradually advancing closure of the bile-duct and the resulting biliary cirrhosis, as well as those resulting from the development in it of secondary nodules. In a large number of cases a scanty secretion of bile and early atrophy are caused by the rapid occurrence of cachexia and extreme anemia, and the liver assumes such a shape as rarely takes place in chronic jaundice produced by gradual closure of the common duct from other causes. The diagnostic importance of this factor will be considered later more in detail.

The gall-bladder is almost always distended, and under favorable conditions is to be felt as a sensitive pear-shaped tumor, smooth, soft, or tense and at times fluctuating, usually displaceable with the respiratory movements, situated on the outer edge of the right rectus, either toward the middle or more toward the side, often reaching to or below the level of the navel. The gall-bladder may be grasped, at times drawn forward and pushed laterally, and its relation to the liver above can rarely be determined. The reason why no mention is made of an enlarged gall-bladder in many of the cases reported is probably due to the fact that the examination was not sufficiently exact or that the enlargement could not be determined during life. In the case of Reclus the gall-bladder could not be palpated; but at the time of the operation it was found to be twice the size of the fist.

A special diagnostic value in distinguishing between pancreatic cancer and calculus in the common duct was ascribed by Courvoisier and later Terrier to this enlargement of the gall-bladder, to which Battersby, and especially Bard and Pic, had previously called attention. The calculus in the duct usually causes atrophy and shrinkage of the gall-bladder. Hanot explains this relation by the infection of the bile-passages so often present in the formation of calculi. The micro-organisms cause an inflammation of the wall of the gall-bladder with formation of fibrous tissue, the retraction of which diminishes the size of the gall-bladder. In pancreatic cancer, on the other hand, such an infection rarely occurs, and therefore the mechanical distention of the gall-bladder is not prevented.

It should further be mentioned that the gall-bladder may also be normal or contracted in pancreatic cancer, and that a distended gall-bladder may be found when there is an impacted calculus in the common duct in case of obturation of the ductus choledochus by stone. The gall-bladder was not enlarged in the cases of Choupin and Molle, Moncorge and Kellermann. Cochez found a shrunken gall-bladder in two cases, and thinks that its condition depends upon the seat of the obstruction. The frequent atrophic condition resulting from obstruction by impacted calculi is due to the injuries, producing stenosis of the canal, following the passage of the calculus from the hepatic and cystic ducts into the common duct. On the other hand, the obstruction in pancreatic carcinoma is situated in the head of the pancreas, and the reservoir can distend at pleasure. If, on the contrary, the cystic or hepatic duct is compressed by the cancer or degenerated glands, an atrophy of the gall-bladder will result.

Distention of the gall-bladder is not infrequently found in cases with calculi in the common duct, even when there is not a combination with cancer of the pancreas. In the course of a year I had two such cases in the hospital. Cholecystotomy was performed on both; in one concretions were found in the distended gall-bladder; in the other there was empyema of the gall-bladder. The concretions in the ductus choledochus were found at the autopsy.

It can be stated merely that when chronic jaundice is due to cancer of the pancreas, as a rule, the gall-bladder is distended, but it may also be shrunken.

[R. C. Cabot * recently reports the data derived from 30 autopsies and 56 operations. Of the 86 cases, 57 were of obstructing gall-stone in the common duct and 29 were of obstruction from other causes, almost invariably from cancer of the pancreas. In but two of the 57 cases of calculus was the gall-bladder distended; while in the 29 cases, the gall-bladder was distended in all but two.—ED.]

A tumor may be felt when the alterations of the pancreas have reached a certain degree. This possibility is relatively rare because the pancreas lies concealed behind the left lobe of the liver and the stomach. In about one-fourth or one-fifth of the cases it is said to be possible to feel the tumor or at least a distinct resistance. It is then a question whether the distended gall-bladder has not ₍been₎ confounded with the tumor. The difficulty is appreciable if the relations are recalled which at times are to be observed in operations for calculi. Even when the abdomen is opened, an impacted stone in the common duct is found with difficulty by the palpating finger, and sometimes is first discovered at the autopsy.

The tumor must have reached a certain size to be surely felt, not only on account of its deep situation, but also on account of the frequent extreme tenderness. In a later stage, when ascites is present, the palpation is still more difficult or impossible.

The tumor is smooth or rough, nodulated, spherical, rarely sharply limited, and is situated, when the head of the pancreas is involved, to the right of the spine at or somewhat below the region of the pylorus. In the case observed by me the tumor was the size of a nut, nearly round, and was prominent. As a rule, there is no mobility, but there are cases in which the tumor can be displaced (Stein, v. Hauff, Klemperer). In the last case there was movement on respiration, while in mine the tumor was fixed and did not move with respiration.

The tumor does not, as a rule, appear to the palpating finger as large as it actually is. Every surgeon knows how easily one is deceived in estimating the size of an abdominal tumor. An extensive tumor will often be felt only as an ill-defined resistance. The possible differences in size were earlier mentioned. The tumor may show pulsation, transmitted from the aorta (Andral, Battersby, Teissier, Labadie-Lagrave, Charlton-Bastian). This pulsation at times causes the growth to be confounded with aortic aneurysm.

In a number of cases it may be possible to feel two tumors, the distended gall-bladder and the pancreatic cancer. Frerichs describes a case with closure of the ductus choledochus and intense jaundice, in which during life he made the correct diagnosis of pancreatic cancer. He found a hard, uneven, immovable, deep-seated tumor to the left of and somewhat higher than the distended gall-bladder, which also was palpable.

Symptoms may arise in consequence of the modification of function of the neighboring organs due to the pressure of the tumor on them. Pressure on the pylorus and on the common duct causes symptoms of gastric dilatation and jaundice. Through pressure on the intestine, meteorism may develop in the portions situated in the upper part of the abdomen; obstruction and fecal vomiting may develop.

Ascites may result from pressure on the portal vein, and progresses continuously and reappears quickly after puncture. It has nothing char-

* *Medical News*, 1901.

acteristic and runs its course like the ascites of cirrhosis of the liver. The ascitic fluid is serous and only rarely contains chyle. Flavio Santi has reported two such cases.

The ascites may originate from the development of metastatic nodules in the peritoneum. The swelling of the spleen which sometimes occurs, and the hemorrhoids also, may be referred to compression of the portal vein. Pressure on the vena cava leads to edema of the lower extremities. Pressure on a ureter may lead to hydronephrosis (Recamier). Cachexia is one of the most essential and constant features, and is dependent upon the rapid and continuously diminishing nutrition, emaciation, and associated feeling of great fatigue and debility.

In rare cases the nutrition remains good for a long time, as happened in the cases of Frerichs, Caron, Macaigne, and Mirallié, in which emaciation occurred late, but then rapidly led to exhaustion. As a rule, the cachexia is prominent and occasionally appears more intense than would be expected from the other symptoms. Indeed, it may at times be the only abnormality pointing to severe disease of the pancreas, aside from ill-defined disturbances of digestion and more or less pronounced epigastric pain. Many authors consider the cachexia caused by pancreatic cancer as especially characteristic of that disease, particularly because of its rapid course and great intensity, which exceeds that caused by cancer elsewhere. They assume that the peculiarity of the severe cachexia is due, not simply to the cancer, but also to the absorption of pancreatic juice.

Whatever one thinks of the cause of the cachexia in pancreatic cancer it may be regarded as fairly established by the testimony of many esteemed authors that the cachexia in this disease as a rule develops much more quickly and with greater intensity than in other cancerous affections in the upper abdomen. One peculiarity especially is frequently pronounced and manifest in the cachexia caused by pancreatic cancer— namely, the great weakness and prostration, which cannot be explained by the inanition alone. There are conditions of debility with attacks of fainting, or at least tendency to fainting. The sensation of weakness may be too great for words, and in consequence the patient avoids expressions of suffering, because it is worse to bear than the violent pains. The patients lie quiet and apathetic, and consequently present such a picture of disease as is much more rarely met in other degenerative processes in the abdomen.

The above group of symptoms is absent in many cases and cachexia, emaciation, and debility are dependent upon faulty nutrition or disturbed digestion.

The examination of the urine may give weighty and important evidence. The amount of urine may be decidedly increased, and some authors mention polyuria, without the presence of sugar (Kappeller, Moutard-Martin).

Albumin occurs very frequently. (Bard and Pic, 4 cases; Bruzelius, Choupin and Molle, Dreyfus, Drozda, Kellermann, Kühn, Krieger, Klemperer, Musmeci, Rankin, etc.) Kobler mentions peptonuria. The presence of sugar in the urine is very important. Mirallié showed that in 50 cases sugar was found 13 times (v. Ackeren, Bouchard, Choupin and Molle, Collier, Frerichs, Lancereaux, Macaigne, Marston, Mirallié, Musmeci, Santi, Servaes, Suckling). Besides these cases, sugar was demonstrated in the urine by Bright, Courmont and Bret, Dieckhoff, Dreschfeld, Duffey, Fothergill, Galvagni, Kesteren and Massing.* Alimentary glycosuria was found by Parisot and Dutil.

Mirallié thinks that sugar would be more frequently found if the examination were earlier made. He supports this view by the fact that in a number of cases (those of Marston, Frerichs, Collier, Macaigne, Mirallié) sugar was certainly found, but disappeared a longer or shorter time before death. In the case of Courmont and Bret also the sugar disappeared with the progress of jaundice. In Kesteren's case it occurred only temporarily, and disappeared on a diabetic diet. Mirallié found that in the 35 cases in which there was no sugar, the examination was made just before death, and if the examination had been made earlier, sugar possibly might have been found, as in the above mentioned five cases. This assumption of Mirallié can be proved only by further observations. It is probable that mention would have been made by the patient of other symptoms of diabetes, as polyuria or polydipsia, and would have led the physician to make earlier an examination of the urine or would have been referred to in the history of the case.

Many cases of cancer of the pancreas doubtless run their course without sugar in the urine, and even when the pancreas is completely destroyed no sugar has been found, as in the cases of Ewald, Hansemann, Litten, Ziehl.

The separation of the course of pancreatic cancer into two stages, one with and one without sugar in the urine, as attempted by Mirallié, is not justified by the facts known at present.

Fat, in rare cases, has been found in the urine. To the best of my knowledge, the earlier observations of Clark and Bowditch are the only ones reported. As a rule, the urine presents no other deviation from the normal than that due to the small amount of food and the poor nutrition in general. The amount of urea is diminished. According to the statement of Mirallié, we have the following data: Arnozan found 12 gm. daily; Lancereaux, 12 to 20 gm.; Dreyfus, 13 gm.; Bard and Pic, 17 and 6 gm.; Moutard and Martin, 7 to 15 gm.; Terrier, 14 to 18 gm.; Saguet-Lucron, 7, 15, and 14 gm.; Le Gendre, 6 to 8 gm.; Bret, 14 gm.; Musmeci, 2 to 15 gm.; Klemperer, 9 to 10 gm.; Caron, 2 to 20 gm.; Mirallié, 4 gm.

According to Sahli, the urine in pancreatic cancer shows the loss of another function of the pancreas. As is well known, salol is broken up in the intestine into salicylic acid and phenol. This cleavage is said to be brought about by the pancreatic juice, and is therefore absent in cancer of the pancreas. According to Mirallié, two examinations have been made with reference to this point. Lucron found the cleavage of salol normal and De Hue found none.

Fever is one of the rarest symptoms. The temperature usually is normal or subnormal, corresponding to the cachexia. If fever is present, it depends, in the first instance, on complications, as infectious cholangitis with pus in the liver as observed in a case in the Rothschild Hospital, or peritonitis or the development of metastases in the lungs, pleuræ, etc. It may also occur that fever is associated with the development of the tumor. In Kobler's case the fever is directly attributed to the tumor.

Bard and Pic lay especial stress upon subnormal temperature. The hypothermia at the end may, they say, be worse in certain cases on ac-

* Two such observations are said to have been reported by Bouchardat and Martsen in the theses of Lapierre and Giorgi; these theses were not accessible.

count of abundant, numerous hemorrhages; but in the majority of cases
it cannot be explained by any complication. The deep collapse with
considerable fall of temperature below the normal is frequently found
in the terminal stage of pancreatic cancer; it follows a long period of low
temperature and seems to depend directly upon the lesion of the pancreas.
In the cases observed by me the temperature was normal except in one in
which there was elevation of temperature combined with chill in consequence of suppurative hepatitis.

Certain alterations of the skin may occur rarely; bronzed color, as in
Addison's disease, is now and then mentioned (Jaccoud), also the hemorrhages, as in purpura and metastatic nodules in the skin. Various symptoms may occur as a result of metastatic processes in various organs, but
their consideration is not now fitting. Mention should be made of glandular swellings, especially of the occasional occurrence of such in the
supraclavicular glands, because this has led to a diagnosis in many cases.

DIAGNOSIS.

The cardinal symptoms, which may lead to the correct diagnosis, are
the following: jaundice with its consequences in the liver and gall-bladder,
tumor, pain, cachexia, emaciation, and the chemical disturbances which
are caused by the loss or alteration of the pancreatic function, and which
are manifest in the urine or feces.

Jaundice and tumor are the most prominent of the above symptoms.
When both of these are absent, it is probably impossible to make a correct
diagnosis. However pronounced are pain and cachexia, no inference can
be drawn from them. Diabetes and fatty stools are such rare symptoms
in cancer of the pancreas that when present, some other disease of the
pancreas is first to be thought of, unless there is also jaundice or a palpable tumor in the region of the pancreas.

Jaundice and tumor, therefore, are the most important signs in
diagnosis, and it will be considered under what conditions these two factors may become so characteristic that the diagnosis can be established
with certainty or probability. Jaundice in pancreatic cancer usually has
definite characteristics. It is chronic, as a rule develops gradually,
rarely abruptly, commonly advances steadily, never diminishes or disappears, but may appear to fade shortly before death.

It is clear that jaundice, with these characteristics, must always be
present when the retention is one which develops gradually and when the
stenosis increases gradually to complete closure. This type of jaundice,
therefore, must always be found in all cases of gradually increasing compression of the common duct, as from tumors of the duodenum or pylorus,
tumors or swollen lymph-glands in the portal fissure, or the head of the
pancreas, either inflamed or containing a gumma. A similar form of
jaundice may be caused by flexure of the common duct or by slowly contracting adhesions. Jaundice may slowly develop without appreciable
remission in consequence of concretions which at first merely narrow
the common bile-duct, but later, from further additions, completely obstruct it.

It may be very difficult or even impossible to distinguish between
these different causes. The question most frequently arises whether the
persistent jaundice is caused by a stone in the common duct or by a cancer
in the pancreas. As a rule, in cancer it develops gradually; suddenly in

calculus. The exceptions already have been mentioned that a gradual development is possible with impacted calculi and a sudden development in cancer of the head of the pancreas. When a stone is in the common duct, the liver is more frequently large and the gall-bladder small; in pancreatic cancer the liver is more frequently of normal size or only slightly enlarged, while the gall-bladder is much distended. We have seen, however, a large liver in a considerable number of cases of cancer of the pancreas, and not simply from metastases; on the other hand, we know that in closure of the common duct by concretions there may be a stage in which the liver is atrophied and small, and that often in an early period of cholelithiasis there is only a moderate enlargement of the liver. It is probably true that the gall-bladder is enlarged in most cases of cancer of the pancreas, but there are frequent exceptions, and one finds at times a shriveled gall-bladder. It may happen also that on the most careful examination the enlarged gall-bladder cannot be felt. On the other hand, it is not so rare that the gall-bladder is enlarged from a calculus in the common duct. In such cases a decision is reached by the evidence of a preceding colic or pronounced cachexia. The diagnosis is frequently first established at the operation. The most difficult question, and often impossible to answer, is whether the cancer of the head of the pancreas or of a neighboring organ causes the jaundice. According to Bard and Pic, a large liver and a slowly developing cachexia indicate degeneration of the neighboring organs; a normal or only slightly enlarged liver and a rapid cachexia indicate cancer of the pancreas. It has been stated, however, that a large liver and not infrequently a slowly developing cachexia occur in cancer of the pancreas. On the other hand, it is to be assumed that even in an early stage of the degeneration of the organs near the pancreas only small metastatic nodules are to be found in the liver.

The second cardinal symptom, the tumor, is demonstrable in only a small number of cases, about one-fifth to one-fourth, and in most cases it will be doubtful whether the object felt is really the degenerated pancreas. Surgical experience shows clearest what difficulties may be encountered. Inflammatory swellings of the pancreas, as Riedel has recently stated and illustrated by some very instructive cases, may appear to the palpating finger of "iron-like density," even when the abdominal cavity is open, and only the subsequent course of the disease shows that there was no cancer. The differential diagnosis between inflammatory and cancerous tumors of the head of the pancreas, says Riedel, "is almost impossible at the operation, if there is no ascites." The inflammatory pancreatic tumor is just as hard as cancer, and the jaundice in the two cases may be equally severe. In a long duration of the affection experience teaches that "the cancer will always lead to ascites, while the inflammatory affection will not."

Cancer of the duodenum, common duct, or portal fissure, lymph-gland tumors, aneurysms of the hepatic artery, products of chronic inflammation of a tuberculous nature, even cancers of the colon and pylorus, may here give rise to confusion.

By palpation alone, without reference to the other clinical symptoms, it is generally impossible to form a correct opinion. In the case repeatedly mentioned by me, in which there was a deep circumscribed resistance in the region of the head of the pancreas and the stomach was apparently normal, I should not have ventured to make a diagnosis of carcinoma of the pancreas if fatty stools had not been present.

The distinction between tumors of the pancreas and cancer of the pylorus or colon is usually based upon the fixation of the first and mobility of the last. In doubtful cases the diagnosis can be made positive by distending the stomach and colon, by the chemical and microscopic examination of the contents of the stomach and intestine, the demonstration of symptoms characteristic of stenosis attributable to constriction of the pylorus or colon, as well as by other clinical signs which indicate either a disease of the stomach or intestine or an affection of the pancreas. These methods of investigation also fail when, as is not rarely the case, the cancer of the pancreas extends to the neighboring organs or compresses them.

It is much more difficult and often impossible to discriminate tumors of the pancreas from tumors arising in the duodenum or extra-hepatic biliary passages. The tumors which narrow the canal of the duodenum above the papilla of Vater, and which, as a rule, pursue the course of the cancer of the pylorus, as also those producing constriction below the papilla, may under favorable circumstances be distinguished from tumors of the pancreas, provided the latter do not narrow the duodenal canal, by certain characteristic signs. These have clearly been presented by Nothnagel in the volumes on "Diseases of the Intestines and Peritoneum" and "Diseases of the Stomach."

The diagnosis of tumors of the duodenum which do not cause stenosis and cancers of the ampulla, on the contrary, frequently cannot be made. It has already been shown that the microscopic examination may leave it doubtful whether the cancer is of the pancreas or duodenum. How, then, can clinical methods make the diagnosis clear?

The suggestions made by Bard and Pic for differential diagnosis will again be mentioned. The cachexia may show peculiarities which are of diagnostic value. Its development is not infrequently as rapid as it is intense, a cachexia præcox, such as rarely occurs in other cancers. It is known how slowly the cachexia usually develops in mammary, uterine, and even in rectal carcinomata. On the contrary, in cancer of the pancreas it is early pronounced. The great weakness with tendency to fainting, the uncomfortable sensations, the extreme prostration, are essential symptoms, often striking and of importance in diagnosis because they are rarely seen in such severity in cancers proceeding from other parts of the digestive apparatus. There are, however, cases in which the cachexia develops but slowly, and depends only on the poor absorption of food. This is best shown by the cases in which after cholecystenterostomy a prolonged improvement takes place with increased appetite, weight, and ability to work, as in the cases of Kappeler, Reclus, and others.

It has already been mentioned that the pains in pancreatic cancer are, as a rule, more intense than in other tumors of the upper abdomen; that they may be peculiar not merely on account of their intensity, but also on account of their characteristics and the feeling of distress which accompanies them, perhaps the result of a combination of intense pain and a high degree of prostration. These characteristics are less frequent in cancers of the duodenum, pylorus, liver, gall-bladder, and common duct than in cancers of the pancreas, and the cause may lie in pressure on the solar plexus or its involvement in the pathologic conditions. This celiac neuralgia differs in quality and quantity from the other varieties of pain in the upper abdomen, and although pain cannot be measured or weighed, and the individual sensitiveness of the patient of course plays the first part, yet the objective impression which this pain at times makes on the observer is so pregnant that it may, in connection with the other cardinal symptoms, establish the diagnosis. It is never safe to make a definite diagnosis from the character of the pain alone, because pancreatic pains, however caused, appear alike, and because, in spite of all that has been said, it is impossible to give a sharply defined, readily understood presentation of so-called "celiac neuralgia."

It has already been mentioned that cancer of the pancreas may run its course with little or no pain, and that the suffering described and attributable to the special involvement of the celiac ganglion not infrequently is entirely absent.

The disturbances of digestion among the remaining symptoms are usually not characteristic. Even if a part of the pancreas is degenerated, and the whole or a large part of it is diseased, the loss of pancreatic function is not striking, because other organs may vicariously assume its work. The results of the examination of the stools and urine are of diagnostic value, especially in connection with all, or at least a number of, the cardinal symptoms, only when fatty stools occur, particularly in the absence of jaundice, and when the digestion of proteids is notably poor or when diabetes is present. Unfortunately, the loss of function of the pancreas causes no symptoms in far the greater number of cases of pancreatic cancer, and, therefore, is only exceptionally to be considered of value in connection with the diagnosis.

In the absence of jaundice the diagnosis will rarely be correctly made. If there is no tumor to be demonstrated, and no definite indications, as fatty stools or diabetes, call attention to the pancreas, no conclusions are to be drawn from the cachexia, however rapidly it may develop, "even with such pancreatic characteristics" as the severe prostration and extreme degree of debility mentioned by French authors, or from the pains, although so peculiar as to lie within the obscure boundaries of celiac neuralgia.

The concurrence of jaundice slowly proceeding but always advancing, generally associated with a large gall-bladder and frequently with a liver of normal size or only slightly enlarged, the distinct, slowly growing tumor in the region of the head of the pancreas, the rapidly developing cachexia, the peculiar severe pains, combined with marked feelings of weakness, and, in addition, such alterations of the feces and urine as the occurrence of fatty stools, of moderate passages of undigested muscle-fibers, or distinct diabetes, give so striking a picture that they justify a positive diagnosis of cancer of the pancreas. All these symptoms, however, rarely occur together. The tumor is lacking in about one-fourth of the cases; fatty stools, disturbed proteid digestion, and diabetes are relatively rare; and, accordingly, the certainty of the diagnosis is essentially narrowed.

The deep, chronic, progressive jaundice with extreme dilatation of the gall-bladder, the rapidly developing emaciation and cachexia with usually subnormal temperature, and the lack of any marked enlargement of the liver, form a group of symptoms which, according to Bard and Pic, if rightly understood and at the right time, make the diagnosis of cancer of the pancreas as easy and certain as, for instance, the diagnosis of cancer of the stomach. These writers assert that cancer of the pancreas can only be confounded with certain manifestations of cholelithiasis or with cancer of the neighboring organs—namely, primary cancer of the liver and bile-passages, and of the stomach and duodenum with generalization in the liver. In rare instances cholelithiasis presents the above-mentioned group of symptoms. If there is a stone in the common duct, the jaundice has not the gradually increasing and progressive character, the dilatation of the gall-bladder is neither so frequent nor so marked, and the general condition never shows that rapid change which is peculiar to "pancreatic cachexia." In addition, the temperature is low, as Bard and Pic found 6 times in 7 cases, while in cholelithiasis there was usually fever. In cancer of the liver the jaundice is frequently lacking or not so intense, the liver is always enlarged and painful, and ascites almost constantly develops. Cancer of the bile-passages is much rarer and the course not so rapid, and it is always combined with enlargement of the liver. When metastases occur in the liver in consequence of primary cancer of the digestive tract, jaundice does not develop until late, and secondary nodules form in the liver and rapidly increase in size. In cancer of the ampulla the course is much slower, the secondary nodules in the liver much larger, and therefore this organ is always enlarged.

Although these statements contain much that is true, there are many objections that may be raised. In the first place, it is very questionable whether the group of symptoms is of such frequency as believed by Bard and Pic, and permit in the "immense majority" of cases the diagnosis of cancer of the pancreas to be easily and safely made. There is no jaundice in about a fourth of the cases, and it is difficult to show from the statistics at hand whether it is present in the majority of the remaining three-fourths.

It is obvious that the liver is frequently enlarged, that the gall-bladder is at times not distended, and that the cachexia may develop slowly even in pronounced cases of cancer of the pancreas. This group of symptoms occurred in none of the three absolutely demonstrated cases of cancer of the head of the pancreas under my observation. There was no jaundice in the first case, it appeared late in the second, and in the third the condition seemed to be one of infectious cholangitis with abscess of the liver. The pathologic picture of the disease presented by Bard and Pic did not occur in the patient referred to by me (page 113), in whom the diagnosis of cancer of the pancreas was established only with great probability. In another case in which I suspected cancer of the pancreas on account of the marked jaundice, rapidly developing cachexia, and intense, peculiar pains, a cancer of the common duct extending to the duodenum was found at the autopsy. The liver scarcely reached beyond the border of the ribs and the gall-bladder was about the size of a goose-egg. A chronic, slowly developing jaundice without being preceded by colic may certainly, even if only exceptionally, occur in the case of calculi which are incarcerated in the common duct and gradually increase in size; the gall-bladder may appear distended, the liver, on account of the cirrhosis, be not especially enlarged, and a certain degree of cachexia may develop, which is difficult to separate from the "*cachexie pancreatique*."

On the other hand, a cancer of the pancreas doubtless may assume the characteristics of cholelithiasis; that is, after the sudden occurrence of jaundice it may pursue a slow course with gradually occurring cachexia and violent paroxysmal pains which resemble biliary cramps, especially when pancreatic colic arises from closure of the duct of Wirsung. Cholecystenterostomy undertaken repeatedly with the idea that stones are present offers a proof. In such cases after a successful operation there has often taken place a more or less persistent improvement in the condition and in the nutrition, only to be explained by the assumption that the cachexia has become relieved for the time being, and to a certain extent by the removal of the harmful effects of the jaundice.

The discrimination between cancer of the pancreas and that of the adjacent organs, especially of the duodenum and bile-passages, will always be difficult, since the size of the metastases in the liver and the nature of the progress, regarded by Bard and Pic as of diagnostic value, are very irregular. There is certainly a period in each process when there are no metastases, and, therefore, no means of differentiation.

Relative frequency alone can be utilized in differential diagnosis. Cancer of the small intestine, on the whole, is rarer than cancer of the pancreas, more frequently and earlier causes duodenal stenosis, but less often a rapidly advancing cachexia. The grouping of symptoms presented by Bard and Pic occurs without doubt in a number of cases of cancer of the pancreas, and it, therefore, will be possible, although by no means certain, to make the diagnosis of pancreatic cancer with some degree of probability because a similar grouping of symptoms rarely occurs in other diseases which might be confounded, and because many of them, as cancer of the duodenum and portal fissure, are, on the whole, more infrequent.

If there is a tumor in the region of the pancreas and the stools and urine present the alterations previously mentioned, and if there is also some ascites, there can be no doubt about the diagnosis.

Primary cancer of the pancreas gives a complicated picture of disease. Various combinations of the cardinal symptoms occur, some of which are attributable to severe diseases of the neighboring organs and depend upon the location, kind, size, stage of development, disturbances of function, whether local or produced in neighboring organs, the complications, and other circumstances, perhaps unknown, which cause either a rapid or a slowly progressing disturbance of nutrition. The possibility or impossibility of the diagnosis depends on the various combinations, some of which make the diagnosis easy and safe. Such cases, however, are rare, and a positive diagnosis is hardly possible without a demonstrable tumor and pancreatic symptoms.

In a second series of cases the diagnosis is only more or less probable. Most of the diagnoses hitherto correctly made belong to this class, including those based on the "Bard-Pic group of symptoms." Even in this series of cases the proof of a tumor will essentially raise the degree of probability. The differentiation between cancer of the pancreas, duodenum, and bile-duct must always be made only with a certain degree of probability.

A tumor near the head of the pancreas, intense jaundice, slightly enlarged liver, large gall-bladder, a certain degree of cachexia, and even pancreatic symptoms may occur without cancer and be due to a stone in the common duct with induration of the head of the pancreas. Even laparotomy in such cases as observed by Riedel may not enable the decision to be made between cancer and induration.

In the majority of cases the diagnosis is impossible, unless suspecting and guessing are confounded with knowledge. It may be stated as probably certain that a positive diagnosis, as a rule, is only made very late in the course of the disease. Even if the views of Bard and Pic are accepted, the small secondary nodules in the liver which form an essential feature do not appear until late. If cancer of the pancreas can be successfully operated upon,—and a few successful attempts have already been reported,—the surgeons certainly will not be satisfied with a diagnosis made only after the occurrence of secondary nodules in the liver.

DURATION, COURSE, AND PROGNOSIS.

Since the nature of the early symptoms is wholly uncertain, the duration of the disease is also indefinite. In some cases only two or three months elapsed from the appearance of the first symptoms to the time of death (Litten, Laborde). In other cases the disease is said to have lasted over two years (Molander and Blix, Crampton), and even, as Dieckhoff mentions, three or four years (Canfield, Bowditch, Battersby). According to a collection of cases published by Da Costa, the duration of the disease varied from two months to two years. A case under my observation (1880), in which purulent hepatitis caused death, lasted from the first symptoms to death, somewhat over fifty days; in two other cases rather more than a half year intervened.

It is evident that the great variations in the duration of the disease depend on individual conditions, the quick or slow growth of the tumor, its histologic characteristics, the interference with the function of neighboring organs, complications, hemorrhages, etc. The average duration of the disease stated by many authors is given as six months, and coincides with the facts.

In most cases death is at the end of a high degree of marasmus, but it may be sudden, as in the cases of Campbell, Huber, and Litten. The prognosis is unfavorable while surgery accomplishes so little. There have been but a few cases of neoplasm in the pancreas cured by operation. The hope of the physician unfortunately depends wholly upon a wrong diagnosis. Recovery is possible only when the symptoms suggestive of a pancreatic cancer are due to a chronic interstitial pancreatitis, a gumma, or an impacted calculus in the common duct.

TREATMENT.

The medical treatment of cancer of the pancreas is merely symptomatic. The chief indications are the relief of pain by narcotics and the best possible nourishment, at first by the mouth, and, when this is no longer possible, by means of nutrient enemata. The possible value of organotherapy has previously been stated. It will always be desirable to try some pancreatic preparation, which may improve the digestion of the food. The formula used by Boas is especially to be recommended for this purpose:

R. Pancreatin.
  Natr. carbon.. .... āā 0.5
M. f. pulv. comprim.
Sig.—Two to four tablets to be used a quarter of an hour after meals.

The jaundice and associated itching are to be treated merely as symptoms. If the obstruction is absolute, nothing, of course, can be accomplished by cholagogues. In an early stage it might, perhaps, be possible by increasing the pressure from behind or by diluting the bile to cause a temporary improvement. The most effective cholagogue— namely, the administration of mixed diet, largely of meat—is generally counterindicated by the marked anorexia, especially for meat. Sodium salicylate, 0.5 to 1.0 gm. several times a day, by the mouth or rectum, can be taken only for a short time, as the appetite lessens still more under its use. Of the other cholagogues which are recommended, the salts of the bile-acids in the form of the Fel tauri depuratum siccum (Naunyn) are to be mentioned. Little is to be expected of salol, euonymin, or podophyllin. Diuretics and the treatment of the skin are especially desirable to relieve the jaundice and the annoying sequels connected with it. Some of the unpleasant features may be lessened by the use of mineral water, especially that containing an abundance of carbonic acid, and in large amounts, when there is no vomiting, for the flushing of the vascular system, or the administration of fluids by the rectum, when there is no diarrhea.

Active sweating is contraindicated by the decided weakness. Diuretics also, as diuretin or caffein, are probably of doubtful value.

Itching of the skin, at times very troublesome, claims especial attention, and must be treated as in other cases of chronic jaundice. The most effectual treatment consists in warm baths, especially when soda has been added in the proportion of $\frac{1}{4}$ pound to the full bath, or in the form of bran baths. Unfortunately the application of the baths is often very difficult or impossible on account of the extreme weakness and severe pain, which cause the patient to shun anxiously every movement. Washing the skin with dilute vinegar, a teaspoonful, according to Leichtenstern, to a liter of the decoction of bran of almonds, or weak carbolic acid solution 1% to 2% (to be avoided if there are excoriated spots), or rubbing with fresh lemon-peel, or spraying with 1% to 2% of salicyl-alcohol or 1% to 2% of menthol-alcohol is beneficial.

Where the itching of the skin was very severe, Leichtenstern has used menthol (Menthol 5 to 10 gm., Spir. vini, Æther. āā 50.0 gm.) by means of the atomizer with temporary benefit. Spraying the skin with menthol gave decided relief.

R. Menthol 5.0
   Zinci oxydati
   Amyli
   Talci................................. āā
   ad pulv. quantitatem 100.0

Washing with hot water, often as hot as the patient can bear it, is frequently beneficial. The severe pain, when present, often requires the subcutaneous injection of morphin, and this remedy will give the most effectual relief to the itching.

Radical treatment is to be hoped for only from an operation, and immediate prospect of such relief is very slight. Gussenbauer was the first to suggest this, at the time when he reported his operation upon a pancreatic cyst, in the following words: "I consider it possible that we shall be able in this way to operate upon other tumors of the pancreas, when by larger experience and accurate study the suspected disease can be diagnosticated with certainty." Senn, in 1888, expressed the opinion that partial extirpation was possible under certain circumstances. The most favorable condition would be present when the tail of the gland is first affected, and the disease does not perforate the capsule. In such cases the excision of the splenic end of the pancreas would present a prospect of permanent cure without endangering the digestive processes, "as still enough of the gland would remain in connection with the intestine to maintain pancreatic digestion."

Billroth in two cases partially resected the pancreas. In the one he

removed a portion of the head of the pancreas with cancer of the pylorus,
in the other the tail was removed with a sarcoma of the spleen. Krönlein, who recently has carefully studied this question, believes "that
primary carcinoma of the head of the pancreas can be extirpated only exceptionally and under the most favorable circumstances, especially when
the tumor is a dense, circumscribed scirrhus, which is suspected by the
demonstration of a palpable tumor in the region of the pancreas, but
which causes the fewest possible symptoms referable to the bile-passages,
the intestine, and the stomach. A positive diagnosis will, of course, be
possible only after laparotomy has been performed and the tumor exposed. Primary cancer of the body and tail of the gland, especially of
the latter, in general presents favorable conditions for extirpation, provided the tumor is circumscribed and limited to the pancreas and is not
adherent to the surrounding tissues."

The first successful operation on a pancreatic cancer was performed by
Professor Ruggi in Bologna in 1889. The description of the case in
brief is as follows:

Woman fifty years old, frequent menstrual disturbances for the last fifteen years.
Of late the distress more marked, tumor observed in the abdomen, use of baths of the
salts of iodin ineffectual.

Present condition: Abundant panniculus adiposus of the abdominal walls, some
free fluid in the peritoneal cavity, two tumors in the abdomen, the lower a fibromyoma uteri, and between them a distinct line of demarcation; the upper tumor is on
the left side and extends from the left hypochondrium toward the umbilicus. The
posterior limit corresponded to the extended mid-axillary line, the anterior to the
extension of the parasternal line. The longer diameter was oblique and measured
about 25 cm. Surface smooth, hard, sensitive to pressure, tumor displaceable downward and forward, still more upward and backward, and disappears completely
under the border of the ribs. In a half-sitting posture it reappears. Spleen, liver,
kidney normal; in the urine nothing abnormal. Anorexia, nausea, poorly nourished.
Profound melancholy. Retroperitoneal adenosarcoma arising from the kidney or
pancreas suspected.

Operation: Incision in the region of the left loin, across and somewhat obliquely
downward and forward close under the border of the ribs; after the escape of the
ascitic fluid the tumor drawn forward, small intestine clinging to it, great omentum
adherent to the anterior surface. The tumor, which belongs to the pancreas, is quite
diffuse and is as soft as brain. The intestine detached with blunt instruments, the
omentum tied and separated, drainage, sutures in layers, healing in seven weeks.
During convalescence good appetite, disappearance of melancholy. Patient wholly
recovered. Tumor weighs 1 pound 7 ounces. The microscopic examination
showed adenocarcinoma of the pancreas.

Gade reports a second case of successful recovery. In a woman
forty-nine years old a cancer as large as a child's head in the tail of the
pancreas was extirpated. There were no metastases. The anatomic
examination showed giant-celled cancer. According to Nimier, Terrier
performed a still bolder operation, but with fatal result.

Woman, fifty-one years old; for five years a gradual enlargement of the abdomen, menopause one year ago, emaciation, loss of strength, disturbances of digestion.

Present condition: Skin of abdomen traversed by subcutaneous network of
veins, abdomen not symmetric, left side more prominent. In the umbilical region
an irregular, three-lobed tumor, lying to the left; one lobe lost in the depths of the
abdomen, the two upper tumors lie to the left and right. The tumor at the right is
rounded below; that on the left is irregular below, shows a marked depression by
which it can be grasped, and the consistency found to be greater than in other portions. The tumor on the right side fluctuates and is not movable from above downward, although slightly movable transversely. The whole tumor dull on percussion
and is surrounded by a tympanitic zone. In the urine no albumin and no sugar;
urea 26.50 gm. Specific gravity 1024.

December 3, 1892, operation: Incision in the median line. Tumor covered by omentum. This was cut through and a violet surface appeared, and fluctuation was apparent. Exploratory puncture negative. After enlargement of the incision the tumor was drawn forward, found to be three-lobed and without connection to the organs of the pelvis. Terrier believed the tumor to be mesenteric. Markedly distended veins, especially in the right portion. After raising it from the peritoneal cavity, needles were inserted, elastic ligatures applied, the upper part cut off, thermocautery, marked hemorrhage, ligation of numerous veins. The separated mass weighed 5½ pounds; pancreatic tissue on the surface of the pedicle, which was left outside; incision closed in two layers. Some hours after the operation, small pulse, rapid respiration, subnormal temperature, death in the evening. Autopsy: Pancreas is represented by a thin layer of gland tissue in the loop of the duodenum, which surrounds the pedicle of the tumor. The tumor was as large as the head of a powerful man. Histologic investigation resulted in the diagnosis: Epithelioma cysticum pancreatis.

As palliative operations, cholecystotomy to carry off the bile or cholecystenterostomy to cause the bile to flow into the intestine are performed much more frequently than extirpation of pancreatic cancer. These operations certainly are performed much more frequently than is mentioned in the literature and here noted.

According to the publications of Nimier (up to 1893), cholecystotomy in two operations was first performed by Socin in 1887 (the patient died of inanition); cholecystotomy at one operation was performed by Mackay, Chandelux, Jordan Lloyd, Krieger, Frey, Gersuny-Bettelheim, Reynier (2 cases), Herringham, Mayo Robson, Bennet, Duncan and Parry, Boeckel, Rufus B. Hall, and Terrier. An operation performed by Russel (1895) may be added. In all cases death occurred a short time after the operation, although in many there was temporary improvement. It is peculiar that in the case described by Gennett the feces regained their normal color after the laparotomy. Krönlein also reports a cholecystotomy performed by him in a case of pancreatic cancer. Death ten days after the operation. There is certainly no justification for cholecystotomy, as the loss of the bile only hastens inanition.

Cholecystenterostomy has been performed as follows:

1. Monastyrski: Death three months after the operation; in the mean time stools of normal color.

2. Kappeller: The patient, fifty-five years old, after the operation (June, 1887) at first regained normal appetite, increased 14 lbs. in bodyweight, was able to resume work, and felt well up to the end of January, 1888. Then pain returned, although the patient was able to continue his duties up to July; December 22d, death occurred in consequence of cachexia, one and a half years after the operation.

3. Socin: Woman, fifty-one years old; the patient left the hospital after her weight had increased 11 pounds.

4. Terrier performed cholecystenterostomy, July 13, 1889; improvement of appetite after the operation, general condition not bad until the end of 1889; died at the end of March, 1890, more than eight months after the operation.

5. Reclus: Man, thirty-six years old; cholecystenterostomy performed August 13, 1892; three and a half months after the operation the color of the stools normal, appetite good, liver did not project beyond the false ribs, increase in weight 24 lbs., and patient felt well. Death occurred the first of June, 1893, and cancer of the pancreas was found.

6. Paul Reynier: Cholecystenterostomy, January, 1893; after the operation increase of strength and weight, but patient died in June, 1893.

7 and 8. Terrier: Two rapidly fatal cases after the performance of cholecystenterostomy.

Tillaux attempted cholecystenterostomy in two operations on a man thirty-eight years old; death from exhaustion some days after the operation. A recent communication is from Abbe, who, in a case of cancer of the head of the pancreas, made an anastomosis between the gall-bladder and duodenum with the Murphy button; good result.

The method of cholecystenterostomy introduced by Winiwarter is better justified than simple cholecystotomy. It may possibly prolong life, and for some time make the condition endurable.

2. SARCOMA.

Primary sarcoma of the pancreas is certainly very rare. Secondary sarcoma, especially the melanotic variety, has been observed a number of times in the pancreas. Chiari describes an extensive melanotic sarcoma of the pancreas. Isham found at an autopsy a spindle-celled sarcoma weighing 25 pounds. The primary seat of the neoplasm could not be stated positively. As the pancreas was not found, Isham assumed that the tumor arose from this organ. Neve describes a secondary lymphosarcoma. In the autopsy reports of the Vienna General Hospital from 1885 to 1895, a metastatic lymphosarcoma of the head of the pancreas and a lymphosarcoma of the duodenum with infiltration of the pancreas were noted. According to Orth's conclusion, all tumors formerly described as melanotic cancers probably belong under this head.

The rarity of primary sarcoma of the pancreas is apparent from the fact that in most of the works on pathologic anatomy (for instance, Orth, Birch-Hirschfeld, Ziegler) it is stated only briefly that primary sarcoma of the pancreas occurs very rarely. Klebs does not speak at all of sarcoma. Friedreich knew only one positively proved case, which was found by Paulicki in the body of a young man who died of pulmonary and intestinal phthisis and presented no symptoms during life. On microscopic examination a small-celled sarcoma was found. Litten considers it difficult to decide whether this was really a case of sarcoma or of tuberculous disease.

Two other cases are cited by Senn:

1. Mayo: Man, thirty-five years old; duration of disease eight months, digestive disturbances, variable appetite, extreme anemia. The autopsy showed the pancreas much enlarged, of cartilaginous density, individual nodules were recognized as medullary sarcoma.

2. Lépine and Cornil: Man, sixty-two years old; sick for eleven months, obstinate vomiting for seven months. Head of the pancreas much enlarged, pylorus thickened, its lumen narrowed, metastases in both kidneys. Microscopic examination showed sarcoma. There are recent observations from Litten, Machado, Chvostek, Briggs, Schueler, Krönlein, Neve and Aldor.

Litten's case was that of a boy four years old, who was very well nourished until a few weeks before death; but had abdominal pain both spontaneous and on pressure. On palpating the abdomen, large tumors could be felt. Rapid emaciation and diarrhea occurred. Urine normal. The abdomen was greatly distended, the tumor very painful, both spontaneously and on movement, and of enormous size. At the autopsy the whole abdomen was found filled with the neoplasm. It was hard to determine the place of origin. The entire pancreas was transformed into an enormous tumor. There was not merely an involvement of the head of the pancreas, but the tumor was formed by disease of the entire gland and its surroundings, and the fact that it was an abnormally large pancreas was distinctly to be recognized from the conformation of the tumor and its acinous structure. The microscopic examination made by Virchow showed a small-celled sarcoma, which bore a marked resemblance to a lymphosarcoma.

Nimier's report gives information regarding a successful operation by Briggs on sarcoma of the pancreas. A woman, forty-five years old, had in the upper abdomen a hard, smooth, globular, easily movable tumor. Puncture caused the escape of a coffee-colored fluid, which contained a large number of small bodies resembling degenerated hydatids. On opening the abdomen the tumor was found adherent to the omentum, transverse colon, and stomach. A ligature was applied above the adhesions and the tumor was removed with the tail of the pancreas. Recovery without accident. The microscopic examination showed the tumor to be sarcomatous with old hydatids. Hooklets were found in the fluid obtained by puncture. It was, therefore, a case of an echinococcus which had undergone sarcomatous degeneration.

Schueler's case concerned an alcoholic thirty-eight years old, who had a sudden attack of vomiting a year before; later ravenous appetite, then again vomiting after eating, constipation, stools yellowish-brown. Pains in the stomach and back.

Present condition: Emaciated, pale, without fever, pain in the cardiac region and below the border of the ribs, radiating to the left to the vertebral column. Pain especially after eating, eructation, obstipation, abdomen below the xiphoid process very sensitive to pressure, abdominal wall very tense, palpation difficult, edge of liver somewhat higher than normal, spleen not enlarged, no free hydrochloric acid in the gastric contents. The liver was constantly smaller than normal. In the left hypochondrium in the region of the left lobe of the liver there was found a tense, elastic, somewhat fluctuating tumor, of the size of a hen's egg and sensitive to pressure. The exploratory puncture gave brownish-red fluid; stools loose; otherwise nothing abnormal. The tumor increased in size, vomiting finally became fecaloid, death in collapse in three months.

At the autopsy there was found below the stomach a large cystic tumor reaching down to the pelvis, distinctly fluctuating, cyst-wall very thin; cyst contained 2 liters of a fluid colored like chocolate or coffee; pancreatic artery eroded in one place; there remained only a piece of the pancreas as large as a walnut, in which was a tumor as large as a hazelnut. There was beneath the spleen a tumor the size of a goose-egg; the rest of the pancreas was changed into a hemorrhagic cyst.

Microscopic examination: Numerous large spindle cells; sarcomatous metastases in the right and left pleuræ, in the third and fifth thoracic vertebræ, and in the ribs.

Krönlein extirpated a primary sarcoma:

Woman sixty-three years old. Three years before admission there was at the level of the umbilicus a tumor of the size of a walnut, which gradually increased and became somewhat painful on pressure. In 1894 the tumor was as large as the fist, movable vertically and laterally, descending on inspiration. Liver dulness extended 10.5 cm. above the border of the ribs. On admission, in 1894, the skin and sclera were yellow; in the filtered gastric contents there was no free hydrochloric acid. At the operation it was seen, after the omental bursa had been sufficiently opened, that the tumor lay behind the pylorus, the pyloric part of the stomach, and the adjacent duodenum, and without doubt belonged to the head of the pancreas. The posterior portion of the stomach, pylorus, and the upper part of the pars verticalis duodeni were fused with the tumor. After the ligation of many vessels (the pancreatico-duodenal artery and the middle celiac artery and vein were tied in two places and cut through), the tumor could be set free. About 40 ligatures were necessary to tie the vessels exposed during the operation. Death seven days later. At the autopsy there was found a circumscribed gangrene of the transverse colon for about 16 cm. Microscopic examination by Ribbert showed an angiosarcoma.

Neve found a sarcoma of the pancreas in a man forty-four years old, and Aldor in a man forty-five years old. That latter patient dated his first symptoms five months previous, complained of severe pain in the left hypochondrium, and had fever at times. At the autopsy the pancreas was transformed into an irregular, uneven tumor of the size of a man's fist, adherent to the spleen and transverse portion of the duodenum, and still more strongly to the stomach. The middle of the fundus showed a perforation of the size of an apple, with ragged edge. The further macroscopic and microscopic examination resulted in the diagnosis of medullary sarcoma.

In conclusion might be mentioned the typical angiosarcoma of the pancreas observed by Lubarsch and referred to by Dieckhoff. The same statements concerning diagnosis and treatment apply as in cancer.

Adenoma also is mentioned in the recent literature, and one case was especially interesting because recovery followed successful operation. Biondi describes this case as fibroadenoma of the head of the pancreas. Two years after its extirpation the patient was well.

A communication is made by Cesaris-Demel of a case of "adenoma acinoso del pancreas." The structure of the growth was similar to that of the pancreas. Its interstitial tissue, as well as that of the pancreas, was thickened. The author concludes that cirrhosis of the pancreas developed upon a syphilitic basis incited the formation of the tumor.

Neve described a case of adenoma in a woman fifty years old. There was a glandular tumor in the region of the pancreas, adherent to the duodenum; the latter was somewhat narrowed. Common duct narrowed and included in the tumor.

III. TUBERCULOSIS.

TUBERCULOSIS of the pancreas was considered until very recently to be a very rare disease. Claessen wrote as follows in his monograph of 1842: "Recent observations have shown without doubt that tubercles occur in the pancreas. Clermont Lombard believes that he is able to determine their relative frequency in it as compared with other organs; according to his investigations, among 100 cases in children tubercles were found in the pancreas 5 times. Similar observations appear in the works of Varnier, Glatigny, Nasse, Bouillaud, Mitivié, A. Petit, Venables, Harless, and Schmidt, to which may be added the observation of Reynaud, who found them in apes, and of Emmert, who noted their presence in cats. The tubercles were limited to the pancreas only in the rarest cases; in most of these they were present at the same time in several other organs, especially in the lungs and the liver."

This view of Claessen's is not, however, accepted in the text-books of pathologic anatomy which have later appeared. On the contrary, pancreatic tuberculosis is everywhere regarded as an uncommonly rare disease; thus, by Rokitansky, Förster, and Klebs. Cruveilhier mentions only tuberculous disease of the lymph-glands on the surface of the pancreas. Louis and Lebert doubt its occurrence. According to Friedreich, "tubercles are found very rarely in the pancreas as a large or small collection of miliary granulations in the form of a more or less cheesy nodule, associated with chronic tuberculosis and phthisis of the lungs and intestine. What is usually regarded as tubercle of the pancreas belongs rather to the group of chronic cheesy inflammations."

Tuberculosis of the pancreas is regarded in the recent text-books also as a rare disease. According to Birch-Hirschfeld, in addition to caseous processes in other organs large cheesy nodules are found in the pancreas, and miliary tubercles are present in the neighboring interstitial tissue. Orth states that a disseminated, general miliary tuberculosis may be seen exceptionally, whereas a partial miliary tuberculosis around large cheesy foci is somewhat more common. Such appearances are not so rare in the pancreas, especially near its surface; but, as a rule, they do not lie chiefly within the gland, but usually in the lymph-glands, which are embedded entirely or in part in interstitial tissue. Ziegler in his latest ·edition briefly states that tuberculosis, on the whole, rarely leads to pancreatic disease.

There are but few collections of cases besides those recorded by Claessen; in the earlier literature there are also the communications of Martland, Sandras, Berlyn. Aran found in 1846, in addition to tuberculosis of the abdominal lymph-glands and spleen, a tuberculous abscess in the tail of the pancreas of the size of a hen's egg, the walls of which were about 2 cm. thick and contained numerous softened tubercles as large as hemp-seed. The patient had suffered from violent epigastric pains, was deeply bronzed, and had frequent vomiting. Roser and Barlow reported cases of miliary tuberculosis in children, in which miliary tubercles were found also in the pancreas. Chvostek describes a case of chronic tuberculosis of the pancreas in which the gland was considerably enlarged and entirely changed into a firm, fibrous mass, inclosed in which were several foci as large as walnuts; there was no trace left of actual gland tissue. The pancreas, thus altered, produced marked obstruction of the descending part of the duodenum.

Mayo describes a case of which Senn's opinion of a primary disease of the pancreas may be accepted.

The patient, thirty-eight years old, was sick for sixteen weeks, bedridden for seven weeks. The first symptoms consisted of pain in the abdomen, radiating from the right hypochondrium toward the spinal column. Twenty-eight days before death jaundice developed; later, dyspnea. A large tumor was felt above the umbilicus, a short time before death; the right arm and right side of the neck were edematous. At the autopsy an effusion into the right pleura was found and the gallbladder was distended; the head of the pancreas was enlarged, forming an irregular spherical mass, 10 cm. in diameter, which compressed the bile-duct. The rest of the gland was enlarged. In places there was a normal gland tissue; elsewhere it was infiltrated with tubercular masses which at two or three points were softened and transformed into thick pus. There was a secondary affection of some lymph-glands, the thymus, and the kidneys.

Bruen recently reported a case of tubercular disease of the pancreas the details of which I was unable to obtain. The most thorough investigation on this subject was made by Kudrewetzky in Chiari's Pathologic-Anatomic Institute. He found that "the percentage of tuberculosis of the pancreas to tuberculosis elsewhere in the human body appears so high that this disease can by no means be regarded as so great a rarity as has previously been the case. Of 128 cases of tuberculosis examined successively, and in which tuberculosis of the pancreas was sought for, there were 12 positive cases—namely, 9.37%. Among 18 cases of general

12

miliary tuberculosis, Kudrewetzky found pancreatic tuberculosis **6** times; thus, 33.33%. Children furnished the greatest number. Kudrewetzky found 44.44% of pancreatic tuberculosis in tuberculous children. He emphasizes the fact that tuberculosis of the pancreas occurs only in connection with tuberculosis of other organs; that is, as a secondary condition.

"In the majority of the cases the blood-vessels furnish the channel for the distribution of the bacilli of tuberculosis. Under favorable circumstances an infection with the tubercular virus may arise from mere contact. It cannot be denied that some of the bacilli may enter the pancreas through the excretory duct, although there is no proof of this view. When the bacilli have entered the tissue of the pancreas, they cause either a miliary or a chronic tuberculosis. The former variety occurs as well in the chronic as in the miliary tuberculosis of other diseased organs. The chronic variety, on the contrary, is found only in chronic tuberculosis of other organs. The tubercles are situated usually in the actual gland tissue, in consequence of which whole groups of acini are destroyed by them and very soon suffer degenerative changes, hence such a tubercle always has a more or less cheesy center and only a narrow peripheral zone free from necrosis and frequently containing giant cells. The bacilli of tuberculosis are always present and are scattered throughout the entire tuberculous mass, often in enormous numbers. In the chronic form of tuberculosis of the pancreas large tuberculous masses may form, which, since they spread over the whole gland, may sometimes produce disease of the entire gland. In such cases there is, on the one hand, destruction of a large portion or even of the entire gland and a corresponding loss of the function of the organ; on the other hand, cavities form which may open, for instance, into the stomach."

Paul Sendler has very recently made a very interesting communication of practical importance on tuberculous disease of the lymph-glands of the pancreas as follows: A woman fifty-four years old, from a healthy family, was well until the beginning of the present illness, about nine months previously. Since then she has suffered from loss of appetite, feeling of pressure in the stomach, vomiting at times, discomfort independent of food, and emaciation.   •

Present condition: Delicate, pale, thin woman; palpation shows above the umbilicus, almost exactly in the middle line, a slightly nodular movable tumor. When the stomach is inflated, the tumor is no longer to be felt distinctly. In the urine, neither albumin nor sugar.

Laparotomy: Behind the stomach a nodular hard tumor is felt. In the head of the pancreas is a grayish-yellow tumor, nearly of the size of a walnut, which is sharply defined from the surrounding tissues. The tumor was extirpated, hemorrhage stopped by ligatures; convalescence only interrupted by an abscess in the abdominal wall and a periphlebitic abscess in the lower part of the thigh. The patient has since been perfectly well (nine months after the operation). On microscopic examination the tumor was found to be a tuberculous lymph-gland of the pancreas.

The symptomatology of pancreatic tuberculosis is not at present perfectly clear. The cases of Mayo and Sendler show that a tumor in the region of the pancreas may be due also to tuberculosis. Other signs pointing to the pancreas have been absent in all the reported cases, unless the bronzed skin in Aran's case is excepted.

Under existing conditions it is impossible to make a correct diagnosis.

In Sendler's case the explanation was clear only on microscopic examination after the operation.

Senn has already suggested the surgical treatment of this affection, especially in consequence of the cases of Aran and Mayo. The only successful result, as above stated, was that obtained by Sendler.

IV. SYPHILIS.

SYPHILIS of the pancreas produces two lesions: chronic indurative pancreatitis and gumma. The two may occur together. Rokitansky has already mentioned two kinds of syphilitic disease of the pancreas.

Indurative pancreatitis due to syphilis has already been described in the section on Chronic Indurative Pancreatitis, page 137. It occurs principally as a manifestation of congenital syphilis, and is quite frequent. The few known cases of indurative pancreatitis in acquired syphilis are mentioned in the same section.

The gumma is much rarer. Rokitansky mentions the occurrence of gummous inflammations, without entering into further details. Lancereaux found, in many patients who died of visceral syphilis, that the pancreas was indurated either diffusely or in circumscribed areas, and in one case there was a circumscribed gumma.

Rostan describes, in addition to multiple gummata, two tumors of the pancreas, whose gummous character was established by microscopic examination, in a man who, fourteen years before, had had a primary lesion. Klebs observed several gummous nodules in the pancreas of a fetus six months old. Among 124 cases of congenital syphilis Birch-Hirschfeld found gumma of the pancreas twice. In the case of indurative pancreatitis described by Beck, miliary gummata were found.

Schlagenhaufer has carefully studied the following case of indurative and gummous pancreatitis.

A much emaciated married man, thirty-four years old, died after a short illness of bilateral lobular pneumonia. In the urine a reducing substance was found; acetone and indican were increased. The autopsy showed lobular pneumonia and purulent bronchitis in both lungs, subacute splenic tumor, fibrous pleuritis on both sides and chronic interstitial pneumonia with bronchiectasis, syphilitic scars in the liver, gumma in the pancreas, together with indurative syphilitic pancreatitis, syphilitic induration of both testes and adrenals with gummata in those on the right side, syphilitic scars in the prepuce, chronic catarrh of the stomach and duodenum.

The pancreas was 15 cm. long, the head unusually dense and hard; on section the glandular lobules were to be seen, but appear small and atrophied (separated from each other by broad stripes of connective tissue). The portion adjoining the head of the pancreas was strongly curved for 4 cm.; on cutting into this portion a round, yellow, not sharply limited nodule was found, as large as a hazelnut, and softened in the center, surrounded by a broad zone of connective tissue; in which here and there, especially in the posterior portions of the pancreas, were solitary, well-preserved gland-lobules. The tail of the pancreas seemed macroscopically to be normal. The ductus Wirsungianus was permeable. The larger blood-vessels, both in the pancreas and its vicinity and in the rest of the body, were normal.

Microscopic examination resulted as follows: The head of the pancreas, which, as above mentioned, was very dense and hard, showed a great increase of intra-acinous connective tissue; the lobules were separated from each other by a wavy fibrous tissue, poor in cells, which extended into them as more or less broad bands, somewhat richer in cells, which so separated the acini that in places they formed small islands, in part necrotic, in part almost wholly destroyed.

The larger blood-vessels, as well as the excretory ducts, were intact. Various appearances were found in the part evident to the naked eye as gummous. The nodule with central softening was a typical gumma: the cheesy necrotic center, containing isolated nuclei, was surrounded by a broad zone of round cells. Adjoining this was connective tissue, quite rich in cells, completely replacing the gland parenchyma—the excretory ducts alone remained—and in which were scattered numerous miliary gummata in various stages of development; the smallest with cheesy center and radiating spindle cells, the larger with markedly cheesy center and spindle cells radiating about a circle of round cells, and large confluent gummata, with one or several giant cells. Toward the surface of the pancreas the connective tissue became poor in cells, surrounded the gland lobules, and caused them to atrophy to a greater or less extent.

The blood-vessels in this part were also abnormal from alterations indicative of syphilis. The adventitia, for instance, was studded with numerous small accumulations of round cells, the intima was hyperplastic, so that the lumen of the vessel appeared here and there much narrowed. There were no pathologic changes in the tail of the pancreas on microscopic examination.

In conclusion, mention may be made of a case reported by Chvostek and Weichselbaum of probably syphilitic disease of the pancreatic vessels. In a soldier twenty-three years old they found patches of endarteritis with the consequent formation of aneurysm in numerous arteries, especially in the pancreatico-duodenal artery, probably due to syphilis. A clinical description of syphilis of the pancreas is impossible in the present stage of our knowledge.

What is to be said regarding the symptoms, course, diagnosis, and treatment of indurative pancreatitis has already been discussed. If diabetes, fatty stools, azotorrhea, and resistance in the region of the pancreas appear in a syphilitic person, one would be justified in thinking of the pancreas. The diagnosis of syphilitic disease of the pancreas has never been made, so far as I am aware.

V. CYSTS.

CYSTS without doubt belong to the few diseases of the pancreas which can rightly claim clinical and practical importance. Since surgery has taken possession of this subject, and since recovery has been brought about in a relatively large number of cases by operative treatment, clinical interest in this question has been increased and some advance has been made in the knowledge of this condition with respect to the method of origin, diagnosis, and course.

The domain of cysts is the most fruitful portion of the territory of pancreatic diseases, clinically so sterile; it is therefore justifiable to give considerable attention to this subject. Cysts of the pancreas are rare. The literature available to me contains but 134. No doubt its occurrence is more frequent.*

Since animal experimentation teaches very little with regard to the nature of this affection, our knowledge of cysts of the pancreas is based almost entirely upon reports of cases; and since our knowledge of the subject is only to be advanced by study of these cases, it is justified on account of the practical importance of cysts to enter more closely into details.

NATURE AND DEVELOPMENT OF CYSTS OF THE PANCREAS.

There are many gaps in our knowledge of the nature and method of origin of pancreatic cysts. There are relatively few reports of autopsies and exact pathologic investigations, and insight into the more exact relations is rarely obtained at an operation.

Three varieties of cysts are to be distinguished:

A. RETENTION CYSTS.

Dieckhoff, Tilger, and other authors agree with the earlier view, which was formerly generally accepted, that most of the pancreatic cysts

* The cases considered were as follows: Agnew, Albert (2 cases), Anandale, Anger, Ashhurst, Bamberger, Barnett, Baudach, Bécourt, Bozemann, Brown, Bull, Challand-Rabow, Chew and Cathcart, Churton, Cibert, Clare, Clutton, Cornil, Cruveilhier, Curnow, Dieckhoff, Dixon, Dreyzehner, Durante, Eve, Fenger, Filipow, Finotti (2 cases), Fisher (2 cases), Flaischlen, Giffen, Goiffey, Goodmann, Gould (4 cases), Gross, Gussenbauer (3 cases), Hagenbach, Hartmann, Heinricius (2 cases), Herczel, Hersche, Hinrichs, Hjelt, Horrocks and Morton, Holmes, Hoppe, Hulke, Karewski (2 cases), Klob, Kootz, Kramer, Kühnast, Küster, Kulenkampf, Lardy, Ledentu, Lindner, Littlewood, Lloyd Jordan (2 cases), Lobstein, Ludolph (2 cases), Lynn, Malcolm Mackintosh, Martin, Martin and Morison, Mayo, Michailow (2 cases), Mumford, Newton-Pitt-Jacobson, Nichols, Ochsner, Osler, Parsons, Pepper, v. Petrykowski, McPhedran, Phulpin, Railton, v. Recklinghausen, Reddingius, Reeve, Richardson (2 cases), Riedel (2 cases), Riegner, Rotgans, Salzer (2 cases), Savill, Schnitzler (2 cases), Schröder (2 cases), Schwarz (2 cases), Senn, Stapper, Steele, Stieda, Stiller, Störk, Subotic, Swain, Thiersch, Thiroloix-Pasquier, Thorén, Tilger, Tobin, Tremaine, Treves, Tricomi, Trombetta, de Wildt, Witzel, Wölfler, Wyss, Zawadzki, Zukowski, Zweifel.

It is certain that all cases have not been published, and that others exist in hospital reports, lectures, etc., and are found with difficulty. Certain cases could not be considered, because exact data were lacking; thus, for instance, Bas in his dissertation asserts that Heinricius has successfully made four incisions and two extirpations; Malthe also reports incision twice with recovery. Körte, in his "Beitrag zur chirurgischen Behandlung der Pancreas-Entzündungen," mentions two operations conducted by him. A number of cases also may have been overlooked. In a large number the diagnosis is not made during life, and hence the cyst escapes recognition if no autopsy is made. Some, perhaps many, of the cases are not cysts of the pancreas. If there is no autopsy, it is often difficult, even after operation, to decide whether the cystic tumor really originated from the pancreas.

were caused by retention of the gland secretion, the outflow of which is hindered in some way. Senn suggests a modification of the retention theory. He considers as the result of his experiments on animals "that the closure of the pancreatic duct is not the only or the most important cause of the development of the pancreatic cyst." Among all the cases of ligation of the pancreatic duct which he performed on different animals, he never saw the development of a pancreatic cyst, or any tendency to such formation, although without doubt the portion of the pancreas which was cut off continued to secrete, as was shown by the experiments in which external pancreatic fistulæ were established. The single visible result of the closure was always a moderate dilatation of the duct beyond the ligature. "The most important etiologic factor in the development of pancreatic cysts," says Senn, "must be sought in the hindrance to the absorption of the pancreatic juice, which must depend either on a change of the pancreatic juice by the admixture of pathologic non-absorbable substances, or on a lessened activity of the absorbing vessels. The closure of the pancreatic duct probably may cause stagnation and accumulation of pathologic products, but can never be the sole cause of retention of the pancreatic juice in an otherwise normal gland."

These remarks of Senn's, which are chiefly based on experiments on animals, merely express the thought that retention is neither the only nor the most important factor in the pathogenesis of cysts, but they cannot be intended to mean also that the stagnation of secretion plays no part at all.

The assumption is justified that the retention of secretion represents an essential, even if not the most important, factor in the occurrence of the cyst. The results of experiments on animals cannot straightway be transferred to the pathogenesis of pancreatic cysts in men. Senn caused a sudden closure of the excretory duct, while in far the greater number of cases of closure observed in men, the condition develops gradually. In the cases of sudden closure, as by concretions, the formation of cysts rarely occurs.

The development of cysts from retention is seen in other organs, especially in the salivary glands, physiologically so closely allied to the pancreas, and the occurrence of retention cysts in them is placed entirely beyond question. Senn's remarks certainly deserve consideration in so far as they demonstrate that cyst formation does not follow all cases of retention, that simple dilatation frequently results, and that in the occurrence of true cysts other factors are of usually great influence, especially the activity of the retained secretion and the condition of the absorbent vessels. In many cases of closure of the excretory duct there may not be cyst formation because the function of the accessory duct is still preserved.

An experiment recently performed on an animal by Thiroloix succeeded in producing a cyst.

He tied the accessory duct in a dog and injected into the Wirsungian duct 7 c.c. of a mixture of soot and carbolized liquid vaselin. The vertical branch of the gland was resected. Two months later a second laparotomy. The pancreas was black and very hard. A piece 2 cm. large of the sclerosed and a portion of the normal tissue apparently as large as a hazelnut were resected. Three weeks later the dog was killed. In the splenic portion of the pancreas a large cystic cavity was found, which contained a fluid as clear as water and a considerable number of hard, irregularly shaped calculi, of the size of a pinhead. The wall was several millimeters thick and was formed of very dense connective tissue; the Wirsungian canal was much dilated and filled with small calculi. The parenchyma of the gland was as hard as wood and difficult to cut.

In this case the formation of the cyst was the result of indurative pancreatitis. The occurrence of a chronic pancreatitis has repeatedly been observed, as will be seen also in pancreatic cysts in men.

Some authors object to the retention theory of the origin of large pancreatic cysts, because the hindrance to the outflow of the secretion often could not be shown, and therefore look for the etiologic factor in the inflammation of the gland itself. Doubtless such chronic inflammations frequently exist; but the explanation given by Tilger and Dieckhoff, for instance, for the pathogenesis of such cysts—namely, that the stagnation of secretion is produced by the induration—certainly seems very plausible.

The common factor in all such cases is the retention of secretion, and this justifies including them all under the term retention cysts.

The outflow of the secretion may be hindered in different ways: By compression or obturation of the secretory duct or by a combination of both factors.

(a) The most frequent cause is chronic indurative pancreatitis, in which compression and constriction of the ducts result from a new-formation of connective tissue, and consequently a stagnation of the secretion can take place. By such interstitial growths the duct may be bent, and by the contracting force of the newly formed connective tissue the excretory duct may become widened in places, and in the widened ducts the secretion can easily undergo such a chemical change that it assumes a firmer, more tenacious character, still further preventing its outflow. Dieckhoff thus explained the origin of the cyst in his case:

In a merchant thirty-six years old, who rapidly became emaciated, there was found in the left mesogastrium an oblong tumor with the long diameter running from above downward. On puncture, a dark-red fluid was evacuated. At the laparotomy a cyst was found in connection with the pancreas. The cyst was sewed to the abdominal wound and drained. Recovery good. Patient was able later to resume his former occupation. Two years later jaundice developed. One year later, frequent attacks of colic, regarded as due to gall-stones. Then rapidly increasing ascites. Great loss of strength, death. At the autopsy the pancreas was found changed into a dense, firm mass which compressed the vena portæ. In the head of the pancreas were the remains of a cyst-wall. The rest of the gland consisted of an extremely firm mass, with pancreatic structure in only a few places, in which were numerous large and small cavities, corresponding to the excretory ducts. From some of the spaces purulent fluid escaped, in others were yellowish and brownish concretions, some as large as beans.

According to Dieckhoff, the development was as follows: First, from some unknown cause, a chronic indurative pancreatitis developed, beginning in the head of the pancreas and advancing insidiously; in consequence, enlargements of the excretory ducts, caused partly by the traction of the growing connective tissue and partly by the stagnation of secretion. The increasing dilatation of several cysts and disappearance of the intervening walls resulted in the formation of one large cyst, that operated upon. As the inflammation of the pancreas later advanced it led to the pathologic condition last described.

The like occurrence of a chronic interstitial pancreatitis has been regarded in many other cases as the cause of the cyst formation.

In a man fifty-five years old who had steatorrhea and diabetes, Goodmann found, in addition to tuberculosis of the pancreas, a voluminous tumor in the tail, containing yellowish-green fluid. The cavity of the cyst was surrounded on all sides by thick, firm walls, and was nowhere connected with the ductus Wirsungianus, which ended near the tumor. At the place of transition from the head to the body of the gland, the duct showed a pocket-like enlargement, which contained masses resembling concretions. The gland tissue was atrophied. The head was changed into fibrous tissue, which sent out into the neighborhood fibrous bands compressing the excretory ducts and surrounding the blood-vessels.

A similar condition is mentioned in the case of Hagenbach, Hjelt, Martin, Tilger, and others.

(b) The ductus Wirsungianus may be closed from without. At the autopsy of a man who had suffered for months from jaundice, Cruveilhier found, in addition to marked dilatation of the gall-bladder, a tumor on the surface of the pancreas filled with watery fluid, following the long axis of the gland, and frequently showing transverse projecting folds from the interior. The tumor proved to be the much dilated ductus Wirsungianus, and as the cause of the dilatation was found a small scirrhous tumor closing the duodenal orifice of the duct and the ductus choledochus, which opened just at this point.

In the cases reported by Virchow and Friedreich the compression was due also to duodenal tumors. Such a closure may be caused likewise by peripancreatic scars or swollen lymph-glands and adhesions, especially in the neighborhood of the head of the gland (Hoppe). In Phulpin's case a gall-stone wedged in the ductus choledochus was the cause of compression of the lumen of the pancreatic duct from without.

In a woman seventy-four years old, who for a year had suffered from jaundice and was greatly emaciated, several stones were found in the greatly dilated gall-bladder, and, in addition, there was a concretion impacted in the ductus choledochus, at a distance of about 2 cm. from the diverticulum Vateri. The ductus choledochus above this place was enormously dilated and showed a lumen almost equal to that of the small intestine. The pancreatic duct was compressed and enlarged at the place where it crossed the stone impacted in the excretory duct of the gall-bladder; on the distal side it was as large as the index-finger; on the other side it was normal. The pancreas appeared to have undergone cystic degeneration. About twenty cysts as large as hazelnuts were visible on the surface and collapsed on cutting into the gland, with the evacuation of contents resembling normal pancreatic juice. The development of the numerous cysts was probably due to the fact that the accessory duct of the gland was congenitally obliterated, and, therefore, there was no outlet for the pancreatic secretion.

An impacted gall-stone in the ductus choledochus compressing the Wirsungian duct was present also in the earlier case reported by Engel, and more recently in those of Horrocks and Morton.

(c) Obturation of the Wirsungian duct by concretions. The pressure of the enlarged sac filled with fluid on the surrounding tissue leads to the formation of large cysts, whose contents at times show similar concretions. In a case reported by v. Recklinghausen, a cyst was formed of the size of a child's head. In Gould's case the retention cyst was so large that it could be felt through the abdominal walls.

The following communication with reference to this variety has recently been made by Tricomi:

In a woman twenty-two years old a fluctuating tumor in the epigastric region developed with cramps. On exploratory puncture, a fluid was found containing albumin and diastase. Laparotomy was performed and 800 c.c. of a turbid yellow fluid were evacuated in which were necrotic pancreatic tissue, and small, very friable concretions. The ductus Wirsungianus was obstructed by a stone which lay some distance from its mouth.

The obturation of the ductus Wirsungianus may result from other factors.

Durante operated on a girl who came to the hospital suffering from a tumor of the right hypochondrium. In spite of the evacuation of the contents of the cyst, the patient died two days after the laparotomy. At the autopsy an *Ascaris* lumbricoides was found wedged in the ductus Wirsungianus. The lumen of the duct was almost entirely closed in consequence, and the portion lying beyond appeared markedly dilated. A further result was softening of the gland, the remains of which were found as soft bodies in the interior of the fibrous wall of the cyst.

(*d*) It is probable, but not certain, that a catarrhal affection may close the ductus Wirsungianus, as in the case of the ductus choledochus. In a case reported by Curnow, in which there was an enlargement of the duct and concretions, it appeared as if the duodenal orifice was closed by catarrhal inflammation and the pancreatic secretion was inspissated.

(*e*) Neoplasm in the pancreas, especially in the head, may compress or obliterate the excretory duct and thus dilate the secretory duct beyond the stenosis. There are no known cases of the occurrence of cysts in this manner.

B. CYSTIC NEOPLASMS (PROLIFERATION CYSTS).

Proliferation cysts (Dieckhoff) belong to a second, much more rare series of cases of cyst formations, and are to be regarded as the expression of the formation of cysts in tumors or as a primary cystic degeneration of the pancreas, analogous to that of the kidneys, testes, or mammary gland (Nimier), since there is no proof that there is a stagnation of the pancreatic secretion.

The following are instances: .

The case of Baudach (cited from Dieckhoff): A man forty-one years old died of phthisis pulmonum. During life, with the exception of a slight sensitiveness to pressure in the epigastrium, there had been no symptom present which could have indicated any disease of the pancreas. At the autopsy a globular cyst as large as an orange was found in the middle of the pancreas. The contents were brownish-red, turbid, somewhat viscid, in which were numerous disintegrated white and red blood-corpuscles, granular detritus, granular corpuscles, and epithelial cells for the most part altered and disintegrated, but a few were well preserved, some with one very large, not excentric nucleus, and others with several nuclei. The cyst was distinctly multilocular; between the walls were projecting beams and villous excrescences. In some places the wall was 3 cm. thick and showed also a lobulated sinuous structure with numerous depressions and pockets. In this part were the remains of the primary adenomatous neoplasms with increased blood-vessels and secondary myxomatous degeneration. The neoplasm, according to Baudach, was an angioma myxomatosum intercaniculare or an adenoma.

The case of Hartmann (cited from Nimier): A woman fifty-three years old for some time had suffered from disturbances of digestion. For three months she felt ill. She complained of loss of appetite, great weakness, emaciation, vague pains in the left side at the level of the umbilicus, where was a rapidly growing tumor.

For several months the patient could not endure fatty foods. In the morning there was frequent nausea, but never any vomiting. There was always constipation, but the stools were of normal appearance. On palpation a tumor was found to the left of the umbilicus, as large as two fists, dense, hard and smooth on the surface, extending on the right to the umbilical line, and on the left to the loin. It was easily distinguishable from the liver. The stomach appeared dilated. The urine was normal. Laparotomy was performed and the tumor proved to be a cyst, from which, on puncture, 7 ounces of chocolate-colored fluid were evacuated. Well for some weeks after the operation, then persistent vomiting set in and the patient died of general inanition. At the autopsy nodules of secondary cancer were found in the liver. The duodenum was compressed. Between the transverse colon and the greater curvature of the stomach there was a fistula which entered an empty cyst.

In addition, the pancreas was filled with cysts. Their formation began where the arteria mesenterica crossed the pancreas. The cysts, from the size of a pea to that of the fist, surrounded the vena portæ and were connected above with the left lobe of the liver, and one was connected with the wall of the stomach. They contained viscous or reddish fluid. The head of the gland only appeared normal. The intact ductus Wirsungianus passed through this agglomeration of cysts. The histologic examination showed that it was a case of cystic epithelioma of the pancreas.

In a case operated upon by Lücke, Klebs found, in addition to the large cyst, a section of macerated tissue, which showed all the characteristics of a colloid cancer.

At the autopsy of one case, Menetrier saw a large cyst in the pancreas as large around as the head of a fetus at full term, also numerous smaller cysts. In the liver also similar changes were to be found. According to Gilbert's microscopic examination, this was a case of a cylindroma of the pancreas.

Zukowski's case: In a woman thirty-six years old a tumor had gradually been forming in the abdomen for two and three-fourths years. It was considered a cystic ovary. The abdomen was unequally distended. Tumor extended two hand's-breadths above the umbilicus and showed distinct fluctuation. At the laparotomy a brownish-red fluid, containing much albumin and cholesterin, was evacuated. The inner wall of the cyst was quite smooth, only in places thickened by projections. A mass of papillary excrescences as large as a pigeon's egg projected from the posterior surface.

Thiroloix and Pasquier report a case which showed a great resemblance to congenital cystic degeneration of the kidneys. In a woman ninety-three years old, who died of bronchitis, the pancreas was found changed into a tumor consisting of 5 or 6 cysts, of the size of hen's eggs. The cysts did not communicate with each other. Between them was found fatty tissue in which were numerous small cystic spaces. The head of the pancreas was also beset with miliary cysts and infiltrated with fat. The parenchyma of the gland in all portions except a part of the tail resembled a sponge. The ductus Wirsungianus was normal and entirely permeable. The fluid filling the spaces was alkaline, light-colored, and clear and contained epithelial detritus and lymphoid cells in addition to much albumin. On microscopic examination the wall of the larger cyst appeared formed of fibrous, non-vascular connective tissue. The spongy portions of the gland were penetrated by walls formed of connective tissue and cellular trabeculæ. The cells were embryonal in character: small, round, crowded together, and having a nucleus which stained poorly. In places they appeared to have an alveolar arrangement.

The case reported by Garrigues, in which small daughter cysts were found, might belong to this series (Orth).

The case reported by v. Petrykowski is to be placed here; in this a cystic tumor of the pancreas of an adenomatous character was removed from a boy three and a half years old.

According to a communication from Cibert, Poncet removed from a woman twenty-six years old a tumor of the size of the head, which contained three liters of brown fluid and, according to the histologic examination conducted by Dor, was regarded as a teratoma or fetal adenoma.

The cases of Riedel, Martin, and the second case of Salzer from the Rothschild Hospital (Zemann-Oser) probably belong in this series of cystic neoplasms.

[The border-line between proliferating cysts and cystomatous cancer is not always to be sharply drawn, as is illustrated by the case of multilocular cystoma of the pancreas reported by Fitz * and that of Ransohoff.†—Ed.]

C. APOPLECTIC CYSTS.

The question whether hemorrhages can give rise to the formation of cysts in the pancreatic tissue is still undecided, and most recent authors either dispute it or consider it uncertain.

It is well known that cysts frequently have bloody contents, and

* *Trans. Assoc. Am. Phys.*, 1900, xv, 254.   † *Am. Med.*, 1901, ii, 138.

it is almost the rule, as will appear subsequently, that the cystic contents are tinged with blood or contain more or less of this fluid. The presence of bloody or blood-stained contents is so frequent that, as Kütser thinks, it is almost pathognomonic of pancreatic cysts.

Most of the cysts containing blood are retention cysts, and there can be no doubt regarding their origin and that of the hemorrhage into the cyst. That the cyst is preformed and that the hemorrhage into it is secondary is shown without doubt by the situation of the cyst, its relation to the secretory ducts, the demonstrable hindrance to the outflow of the secretion through closure of the main excretory duct or of the secretory ducts by obturation or compression, mostly caused by chronic inflammation, leading to sclerosis of the gland and obstruction to the discharge.

In many of the cases fresh hemorrhage could be shown. It occurred between the exploratory puncture and the evacuation of the cyst at the operation; hence the contents of the cyst removed at the operation contained much more blood that that evacuated by puncture. In one of Küster's cases there was a hemorrhage during the operation.

Apart from these cysts, which have the same etiology, there are others mentioned in literature, of a different nature and which present at least the possible interpretation that hemorrhage was the primary and cyst formation the secondary factor. Such cysts are mostly large, solitary, develop in the tail of the pancreas, and the contents are markedly hemorrhagic; they show no relation to the excretory ducts and there are also no changes which point to a preceding chronic indurative inflammatory process. Ledentu was the first to suggest that cysts might develop from hemorrhages into the pancreatic tissue in two cases referred to by him. The first of these cases was reported by Anger.

A man seventy-two years of age suffered in his youth from a severe injury with fracture of several of the left ribs. At the autopsy Anger found a tumor of the size of a child's head at the level of the left kidney; the stomach lay in front of the tumor and below it the transverse colon. The tumor contained blood and fresh clot. The inner surface was irregular and resembled in structure the left ventricle or the "Vessie à colonnes." The wall was very thick in many places and was calcified. The microscopic examination showed the presence of glandular elements of the pancreas, and this aided in the diagnosis of a cyst of the tail.

Anger was in doubt whether there was a hemorrhage into the pancreatic tissue with a resulting cyst, or whether the hemorrhage was the result of the rupture of a vessel in a preformed cyst. Ledentu assumes the hemorrhage to be the primary factor, especially with reference to a second case, which he reported as follows:

A man twenty-six years old received a blow on the abdomen two and a half months before death. A tumor of the size of a child's head developed in the head of the pancreas. The Wirsungian duct was not involved.

Ledentu refers to the literature up to that time, and cites the observations reported by Bécourt, Gould, and Parsons concerning cysts with hemorrhagic contents. In Gould's cases there was certainly a dilatation of the excretory duct, while in the two other cases there was no satisfactory interpretation.

Following Ledentu, Friedreich has accepted this view, and distinguishes between hemorrhagic cysts—that is, retention cysts with bloody contents—and apoplectic cysts. Under certain circumstances "large hemorrhagic foci develop in the pancreas, often, perhaps, in connection with pre-existing alterations of the blood-vessels. The so-called apoplectic cysts, arising secondarily from such hemorrhages, are of course to be distinguished in their nature and genesis form those hemorrhagic cysts which are caused by hemorrhages into the contents of pre-existing cysts. Perhaps Stork's case from the earlier literature belongs to the same category."

A woman twenty-eight years old, otherwise well, was attacked with severe vomiting during her menses, and the menstrual flow consequently ceased; there were fainting, palpitation of the heart, coldness of the extremities, and great feeling of anxiety. A pulsating tumor appeared in the epigastrium. After the latter symptoms had lasted for three and a half months, bilious vomiting suddenly reappeared, accompanied with diarrhea, and death occurred after general emaciation and weakness. At the autopsy the pancreas was changed to a large sac, weighing 13 pounds, and was filled with bloody, in part lamellated contents. Its development could be referred to a laceration of the blood-vessels in the center of the pancreas.

On examination of the abundant literature of pancreatic cysts published since Friedreich's treatise, it must be admitted that Tilger and Dieckhoff are correct in asserting that there are no cases of apoplectic cysts positively established. Among the more recent authors, however, many are found who support Friedreich's point of view; Orth says: "Large circumscribed hemorrhages into the pancreas may be absorbed, and, like the small ones, leave a pigmentation or cause the formation of cysts the inner surface of which appears rust-colored from pigment." Senn, Schroeder, Kühnast, and Nimier also assume that cysts may develop in consequence of pancreatic hemorrhages. At the autopsy of an inebriate seventy-five years old, with marked cirrhosis of the liver, Kühnast found, in addition to a cyst in the body of the pancreas filled with blood and as large as an apple, that "the pancreatic duct, very much dilated, could be followed for 6 cm., then continued into the cystic portion, in which, by careful search, it could be here and there discovered. It could not be determined that it communicated with the large cyst." In the absence of an accurate microscopic examination, Tilger could not support Kühnast's view.

Tilger, the most decided opponent of Friedreich's theory, supports his view by the thorough study of his own case. There can be no doubt that in this case there was not an apoplectic cyst in Friedreich's sense. There certainly was a high degree of chronic interstitial inflammation and increase of connective tissue in the tail of the pancreas, especially noticeable around the lobules, and the hemorrhage was of the secondary kind, largely due to erosion of the blood-vessels by the pancreatic secretion.

Although there is some justification for Tilger's view that in the cases hitherto presented no convincing proof has been given of the existence of apoplectic cysts, yet, on the other hand, the possibility cannot be put aside that cysts may develop from hemorrhages, as suggested by Nimier. Hemorrhages very easily occur in the soft, vascular pancreatic tissue, as can frequently be observed in experiments on animals, and it would not be impossible at the outset that such hemorrhagic cysts might occur.

Some traumatic cases are mentioned in the literature, which allow the interpretation that hemorrhage was the primary factor. Littlewood's case is in point:

A man thirty years old fell from his horse and received a kick in the abdomen. Thirteen days later a tumor was found in the epigastrium and in the left upper portion of the umbilical region. On exploratory puncture dark blood was evacuated. For seven days the swelling increased slowly, but afterward it advanced rapidly with severe pain. At a second puncture, 10½ oz. of an alkaline, sage-green fluid were evacuated. Laparotomy was then performed, the cyst was opened, and its walls were stitched to the abdominal wall. The cyst-fluid contained serum-albumin and trypsin, and possessed diastatic and fat-emulsifying properties and coagulated milk (Nimier).

It must certainly be admitted that in this case it is possible that hemorrhage into the pancreatic tissue took place as a result of the injury (the first puncture brought pure blood); that in consequence of the hemorrhage and tearing of the pancreatic tissue the secretion from the latter became mixed with the blood; that the cavity became enlarged by the digestive power of this secretion, consequently when laparotomy was performed the cyst was found to contain fluid possessing the digestive properties of pancreatic juice. At all events, it would be difficult to explain by any other assumption the appearance of pure blood at the first puncture, and the characteristic contents of a pancreatic cyst only at a later puncture.

Paltauf supports Nimier's assumption that pancreatic cysts may develop from hematomata with simultaneous laceration of the duct. Paltauf believes that the possibility of such a method of origin must be granted for various reasons (anatomic and histologic). In one preparation he was able to "convince himself positively that such a hematoma was a pancreatic cyst."

From what has been stated it is evident that it by no means has been positively shown that the so-called apoplectic cysts arise from hemorrhage into the pancreatic tissue; but, on the other hand, it is impossible to exclude the possibility that under certain circumstances after injury, cysts may arise in consequence of the hemorrhage.

[In this connection especial attention should be called to the communication of Lloyd * concerning a method of origin of hemorrhagic cysts. This writer makes it very probable that many so-called pancreatic cysts of traumatic origin are collections of fluid in the omental bursa, the result of a localized inflammation of this portion of the peritoneum. It is readily apparent that blood and even pancreatic secretion might be present in the contents of the "cyst" from laceration of a portion of the pancreas at the time of the injury.—ED.]

PATHOLOGIC ANATOMY.

SHAPE OF THE CYSTS.

The shape of the cyst varies as it originates from the ductus Wirsungianus or from the smaller canals within the gland. If the constriction of the duct is near the entrance into the intestine, either the main duct alone is distended or its branches also may be enlarged. In the former case there is a rosary-like dilatation of the whole excretory duct. Virchow reports such a case, and designates it *ranula pancreatica* from its analogy with the formation of cysts in the salivary glands. The dilatation was caused by a soft, villous duodenal tumor, which obstructed the common opening of the ductus choledochus and Wirsungianus.

Many small cysts are formed (*acne pancreatica*, Klebs) when numer-

* *Brit. Med. Jour.*, 1892, II, 1051.

ous small ducts are constricted by pathologic processes, most frequently fibrous tissue formation in consequence of indurative pancreatitis, perhaps also by accumulation of catarrhal secretion. When there is partial cystic dilatation of the ductus Wirsungianus, very capacious sacs form, sometimes spherical, sometimes oblong (Klebs); the former being more frequently seen.

The size may vary. It is worthy of note that pancreatic cysts are described as much smaller by the anatomist than by the surgeons. Virchow has seen sacs as large as a fist; v. Recklinghausen, likewise Birch-Hirschfeld, describe one as large as a child's head; Klebs and Orth mention cysts of a size greater that that of a child's head. The majority are from the size of an orange to that of a child's head, but surgeons have reported much larger cysts; thus, Bozemann reports one containing 11 liters; Salzer, Richardson, as large as a man's head; Wölfler, twice the size of a man's head; Stapper, containing 20 liters; Hersche, almost as large as a man's head, etc. The wall of the cyst consists chiefly of dense, firm, fibrous connective tissue, poor in cells. Its thickness varies, but it is usually 2, 3, or 4 mm., and may even reach 3 cm. Portions of unaltered pancreatic tissue are found not infrequently in the cyst-wall. Salzer found in the case operated upon by him that the posterior external surface of the cyst was formed of pancreatic tissue. The rest of the wall consisted of connective tissue poor in cells but calcified and containing pigment cells.

In Dieckhoff's case there were in the wall pancreatic lobules with distinctly dilated excretory ducts. The interacinous connective tissue was increased in various degrees. Most of the gland cells were quite small, yet provided with nuclei which stained well, and lobules which merely diffusely stained were found only in places.

The lining of the cyst is generally smooth, shining, and free from epithelium. In some cases, however, cylindric epithelium is found here and there, probably the remains of the epithelial lining of the former excretory ducts. A similar condition was found in the cases of Martin and Zukowski. In Salzer's case the inner surface of the cyst was bare of epithelium and showed comb-like projections and septa, the remains of the original cysts, now transformed into a large single cavity.

The clotted remains of previous hemorrhages are often seen in the form of a gray, sandy coating on the inner wall (Martin). Large or small deposits of fat are not infrequently seen in places. Under certain circumstances there may be circumscribed necroses of the wall or of the remains of pancreatic tissue attached to it (Tricomi).

The large blood-vessels run along the outer wall of the cyst and often form a most unpleasant complication at the operation. The large arteries and veins visible on the surface do not always belong to the vascular supply of the cyst itself. For instance, Salzer saw the splenic vessels on the surface of a cyst and their mistaken ligation led to serious consequences.

The cyst is more frequently seated in the tail than in the head of the gland.

Among 134 cases examined with reference to this point, in 90 there was no statement regarding the location; in 14 the whole pancreas was involved; in 15 the tail was affected; in 11 the head and in 4 the middle portion of the gland was involved.

The amount of fluid contained in the cyst varies considerably and corresponds to the size of the cyst, which is often enormous. In Stapper's case, as already mentioned, there were 20 liters; in Osler's 18 liters were evacuated and in Bozemann's 11 liters; Riedel and Lardy each report 10 liters; in the cases of Wölfler, Salzer, and Zukowski there were 5 liters. The contents in general vary from 1 liter to 3 liters.

It is seldom that the contents of the cyst resemble water, light colored and transparent (Kramer, Schroeder, Cruveilhier, Thiroloix and Pasquier, Kulenkampf). They are usually more or less turbid, slimy (Dixon, Gussenbauer, Salzer, Gross, v. Recklinghausen, Railton, Malcolm Mackintosh, Richardson, and others), syrup-like and gelatinous (Gould), colloid (Ludolph), purulent (Herczel, Ashhurst).

The color is rarely bright yellow (Hjelt, Tricomi, Küster), sometimes yellowish-green (Goodmann, Stapper), green (Flaischlen, Newton-Pitt-Jacobson, Littlewood). In most cases it is light brown, coffee-brown, or reddish-brown in color. When the quantity of blood in the contents is large, and if a long time has elapsed after the hemorrhage, the color is chocolate-brown, an appearance which has repeatedly been reported by different observers. In the majority of cases there is such an admixture of blood. Küster, indeed, thinks, as already mentioned, that the presence of a small amount of blood in a cyst of the upper abdomen punctured for the sake of diagnosis is characteristic of a pancreatic cyst.

The contents of the cyst at times are exclusively or chiefly liquid or partly clotted blood in consequence of the marked tendency for hemorrhage to take place within the cavity, and Friedreich classifies such as hematoma of the pancreas, in contradistinction to the so-called apoplectic cyst originating from hemorrhage into the tissue of the pancreas. Such cysts containing much blood are reported by Störk, Parsons, Pepper, Anger, Gussenbauer, Thiersch, Baudach, Challand and Rabow.

The extravasated blood generally shows marked changes. Gussenbauer found altered red and white blood-corpuscles and clumps of pigment. A deposit of blackish-brown masses is found at times in the wall (Parsons, Gussenbauer). Recent hemorrhages into cysts also were sometimes noted (Parsons, Küster).

The reaction of the fluid, as a rule, is alkaline; only once is it noted as acid (Bozemann); in the cases of Kramer, Hersche, and Wölfler the reaction was neutral.

The specific gravity was ascertained in but few cases: Tremaine, 1007; Richardson, 1008; Horrocks and Morton, 1009; Hinrichs, 1015; Tilger, 1015; Stappe, 1019; Bozemann, 1020; Hersche, 1028. Complete analyses are given by Hinrichs, Kulenkampf, and Hoppe.

In 100 parts of the fluid the following percentages were found:

	HINRICHS.	KULENKAMPF (SECRE-TION FROM THE FISTULA).
Dry substance	3.25%	1.222%
Organic material	2.55%	0.809%
Ash	0.80%	

HOPPE.	
Alcoholic extract	0.87%
Aqueous extract	0.49%
Inorganic salts	0.57%
Fat	0.02%
Urea	0.12%
Residue	2.60%
Water	97.40%

The organic substances in Kulenkampf's case consisted of albumin precipitated by alcohol, 0.365%; other organic materials, 0.807%.

There are some statements regarding the amount of albuminous substances. In one of Küster's cases the amount of albumin reached 3%; in Wölfler's case, 1.5%; in Tilger's, 0.56%; in Stapper's, 6.49%; and in Tremaine's, 10%.

Serum-albumin and serum-globulin of the proteid substances have been found. Littlewood noted in his case the presence of metacasein. In Tilger's case peptone was said to have been present in the contents of the cyst. Obviously, blood pigment is found in a more or less changed form in the cases where hemorrhages had taken place. A large amount of mucus is exceptional. Gussenbauer is authority for its occurrence in his case, which he designates a mucous cyst.

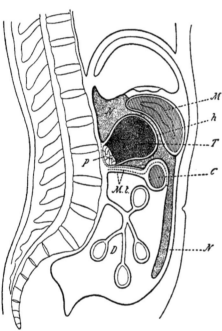

Of other organic substances, sugar has been found in rare cases: Bull, 2.7% (diabetes); Tremaine, traces of sugar, and Gussenbauer likewise. Cholesterin is more often found, and in well-formed crystals, by Zukowski, Wölfler, Lardy, Swain, v. Petrykowski, etc. The amount of urea is stated in Hoppe's case to have been 0.12%.

Leucin and tyrosin, which are rarely seen in the contents of cysts, were found in the cases of Tilger, Newton Pitt, and Jacobson. Ferments were not always present in the cystic contents. The cases of Witzel, Swain, Salzer (2), Brown, Stiller, Steele, Thiersch, and Richardson were especially investigated with

Fig. 8.—Tumor of the ventral surface of the pancreas projecting into the bursa. The stomach lies in front of, the colon below, the tumor. *M*, Stomach; *C*, transverse colon; *P*, pancreas; *D*, coils of intestine; *N*, omental bursa; *M.t*, the two layers of the transverse mesocolon; *h*, posterior layer of the great omentum; *T*, tumor.

reference to the presence of ferments, but none were found. The three ferments, however, were found in the cases of Hinrichs, Subotic, Flaischlen, Tricomi, Richardson, Littlewood and Phulpin; they were present also in the secretion from the fistula in the cases of Kulenkampf and Richardson.

Diastase was found in the cases of Lardy, Wölfler, Cathcart, Hersche, Fisher, de Wildt, Barnett, Schroeder, Martin and Morison, Schnitzler (2), Tilger, Küster, Lindner, Stapper, Cibert. Trypsin was noted by Gussenbauer and Stapper. Steapsin is reported in the cases of Küster, Lindner, Schroeder, Tilger, Cibert.

SITUATION OF THE CYST.

Professor Zuckerkandl has shown in the anatomic introduction that tumors of the pancreas, according to their location or the surface from which they arise, the direction of their growth, and their size, present fle e topical relations to the neighboring organs, especially to the stomach, transverse colon, and liver.

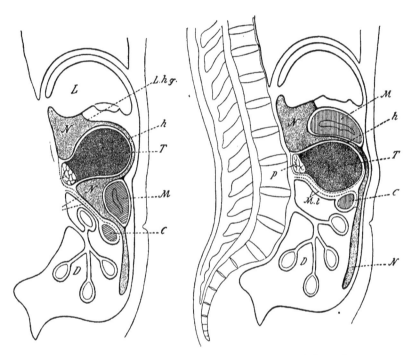

FIG. 9.—Tumor projecting into the omental ursa, pushing the lesser omentum forward. tomach and colon ·lie below the tumor. *L*, lver; *M*, stomach; *C*, transverse colon; *P*, ancreas; *D*, coils of intestine; *N*, omental ursa; *L.h. g*, ligamentum hepatico-gastricum lesser omentum); *M.t*, the two layers of the ransverse mesocolon; *h*, posterior layer of the reat omentum; *T*, tumor.

FIG. 10.—Tumor symmetrically developed in all directions, projecting between the posterior layer of the great omentum and transverse mesocolon. Stomach above, colon below the tumor. *M*, Stomach; *C*, transverse colon; *P*, pancreas; *D*, Coils of intestine; *N*, omental bursa; *M.t*, the two layers of the transverse mesocolon; *h*, posterior layer of the great omentum; *T*, tumor. The anterior layer of the great omentum, which is pushed forward between the stomach and colon, corresponds to the gastrocolic ligament.

To complete this consideration Professor Zuckerkandl has prepared the accompanying diagrams, which show the topographic relations of tumors of the pancreas to neighboring organs in five different ways. The situation of the cysts of the pancreas, which form the largest tumors developing in the pancreas, corresponds to the accompanying diagrams. The third variety (Fig. 10) is found most frequently. The cyst pushes the gastrocolic ligament forward, the stomach lies above and the colon below the cyst. Smaller cysts may be found directly behind the stomach and

13

show no palpable projection. In figure 8 a larger tumor of this region is represented, as was found in Swain's case. The cyst lay behind the stomach and contained a liter of dark brown fluid. Hersche's case corresponded to the fifth variety (Fig. 12). "The colon embraced the upper border of the spherical tumor, which projected toward the front."

Ochsner also may have seen a similar relation. "The cyst-wall first became apparent when the omentum and intestinal coils which projected into the wound were pushed back." The second variety (Fig. 9) was found in the cases of Riegner and Karewski. In the former the "gastro-

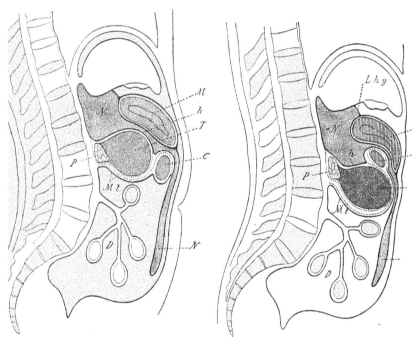

FIG. 11.—Tumor of the same region, developed on one side, growth largely toward the omental bursa. Stomach lies above the tumor, and colon in front of the lower portion. *M*, Stomach; *C*, transverse colon; *P*, pancreas; *D*, coils of intestine; *N*, Omental bursa; *M.t*, the two layers of the transverse mesocolon; *h*, posterior layer of the great omentum; *T*, tumor.

FIG. 12.—Tumor of the same region developed on one side, growth largely downward toward the mid-abdomen. Tumor lies below the colon and stomach. *M*, Stomach; *C*, transverse colon; *P*, pancreas; *D*, coils of intestine; *N*, omental bursa; *L.h.g.* gastrohepatic ligament; *M.t*, the two layers of the transverse mesocolon; *h*, posterior layer of the great omentum; *T*, tumor.

hepatic ligament was tightly stretched by the tumor." "After the cyst was evacuated, the sharp edge of the liver appeared in the upper and the stomach in the lower angle of the wound." After evacuation of the cyst, Karewski saw the stomach and colon ascend, and the left lobe of the liver appear in the wound. It is easily understood that there are many transitions between the several varieties, and that the position of the neighboring organs does not correspond to the diagrams in the case of very large tumors, which "almost fill the whole abdomen," as in Riedel's case.

Salzer's case also is atypical. The tumor began three finger-breadths below the xiphoid process and reached nearly to the symphysis. The upper end of the tumor extended behind the upper portion of the stomach. The transverse colon surrounded the lower surface of the tumor and lay behind the symphysis.

The place of origin and the direction of growth of the tumor explain the seat of cysts of the pancreas in the middle of the abdomen and again toward the side.

COMPLICATIONS.

Manifold complications are caused by the relation of cysts of the pancreas to their surroundings. Among these are concerned the adhesions already mentioned. Large pancreatic cysts may cause not simply pressure upon and displacement of other organs, as the liver, stomach, colon, small intestine, and kidney, but may compress also the hollow structures. Jaundice may arise from compression of the common duct, as in the cases of Gross, Bécourt, Hoppe, Hjelt, Wyss, Friedreich, Dixon, Salzer, Gould, Stapper, Phulpin, Newton Pitt and Jacobson, Cruveilhier, Horrocks, and Morton. There was compression of the duodenum in the cases of Hagenbach and Hartmann.

Compression of the right ureter was reported by Reeve. Dreyzehner observed an interesting case of axial twist of the right kidney. Ascites from compression was observed in the cases of Battersby, Anger, Küster, Tilger, and Dieckhoff. Cholelithiasis was reported by Phulpin and Curnow. Calculi in the pancreatic duct were seen by v. Recklinghausen, Goodmann, Tricomi, Dieckhoff, Clarc, Gould, Michailow, and Curnow. An ascaris was found by Durante in the Wirsungian duct. Cirrhosis of the liver was seen by Hjelt, Klob, Phulpin, and Clark.

Rupture of a cyst of the pancreas is rare. In Pepper's case a cyst of the head of the pancreas ruptured into the duodenum, and there were hematemesis and bloody stools. Reddingius also reports the rupture of a large cyst of the pancreas into the duodenum. Peabody mentions the rupture of a pancreatic cyst into the abdomen.

ETIOLOGY.

With the assumption that most pancreatic cysts are to be regarded as retention cysts, their etiology must be represented by the conditions which lead to the stagnation of secretion. It has already been stated that the most frequent cause of stagnation of secretion is chronic indurative pancreatitis, and mention should first be made of those causes which give rise to this inflammation. These are discussed in detail in the section on chronic indurative pancreatitis.

Cysts are much more rarely formed in consequence of calculi in the pancreas, catarrhal strictures, and compression or distortion of the excretory ducts by peripancreatic thickenings and adhesions, impacted gallstones wedged in the common duct compressing the Wirsungian duct, and neoplasms in the pancreas or its vicinity.

In the great majority of cases the cause of the formation of the cyst is obscure. Immoderate eating and drinking are frequently mentioned as a cause. It is possible in such cases that chronic pancreatitis leading to stagnation of secretion and to the formation of a cyst is caused by frequent attacks of gastritis and enteritis and by alcoholism.

Antecedent injury is quite often mentioned as a cause in the history of the cases reported. This is noted in 27 cases (Ledentu, Kulenkampf, Senn, Küster, Fenger, Steele, Lindner, Chew and Cathcart, Karewski (2 cases), Riegner, Richardson, Fisher (2 cases), Littlewood, Lloyd (2 cases), Barnett, Martin and Morison, Newton Pitt and Jacobson, Schnitzler, Brown, Lynn, Tilger, Michailow, Tobin, Eve).

Walter Henry Brown reports a striking case. A man seventeen years old was well until March, 1893. After a fall from a locomotive there was a swelling of the abdomen. Splashing sounds were audible on shaking. On puncture, the evacuation of bloody fluid. After six weeks the puncture was repeated, with the same result. Well until the end of June. Then he fell from a beam, and immediately afterward there was severe illness with fecal vomiting.

Present condition: Abdomen tense, markedly swollen, no passage of feces or gas. Urine: specific gravity 1039, small amount of albumin Laparotomy evacuation of large quantities of blood-stained fluid. Drainage. For a week quite well with escape of large amounts of fluid through the drain. Sudden exacerbation. Swelling, distention, great tenderness of the abdomen, swelling to the left of the median line near the navel. On the next day pains greater, vomiting, second laparotomy. A dense cyst behind the stomach, which was pushed upward, and the great omentum. On puncture of the cyst, a peculiarly offensive dark fluid was evacuated. Its wall was stitched to the abdominal wound. Drainage. No ferment was found in the evacuated fluid. From that time the condition was good, the fluid flowed out through the drain. At times great pain, normal temperature. A week after the operation, pancreatic ferments were found in the fluid. Seven weeks later all the fluid was evacuated, condition excellent. In his remarks Brown observes that the case is important, because two organs, the pancreas and peritoneum, were injured. The fluid which was first evacuated evidently came from the peritoneum. The cyst of the pancreas developed slowly.

Barnett reports a similar case:

A man twenty-four years old after falling from a wagon suffered from dyspepsia and debility. After eight weeks, symptoms of a pleuritic exudation. Evacuation of 8 ounces of a turbid, dark fluid. This came from the peritoneum and entered the thoracic cavity after rupture of the diaphragm. At the end of a week an elastic, round tumor was found in the epigastrium. Percussion over it gave dulness. On aspiration 300 c.c. of an alkaline, turbid, albuminous fluid were evacuated. Renewed swelling. The tumor was punctured a second time.

The fluid last obtained contained a ferment, saccharifying starch. At the laparotomy a cyst was found at the right of the stomach and near the stomach and liver and above the intestine. Cyst was sewed to the abdominal wall and drained. After five months the man was perfectly well and was able to resume heavy work.

It is not easy to understand how injury can lead to cyst formation in the protected position of the pancreas. The great vulnerability of the organ, shown also in experiments on animals, and the tendency to hemorrhages may here play important parts.

The injury may cause the tearing of small excretory ducts and the escape of secretion, or cause hemorrhage, resulting in inflammation ending in the formation of scars and the contraction and constriction of small excretory ducts. The origin of apoplectic cysts could be easily understood if, as was earlier considered, their existence could be established. The occurrence of hemorrhages into the pancreas from injury are easily explained, and if a cyst could result from hemorrhage, the traumatic origin of the former is readily understood.

It is possible that the trauma may act through the nervous system. Many authors advance this view. Thus, Fischer believes that, as in the Goltz experiment, a blow upon the abdomen may lead to severe nervous disturbances, and he explains the symmetric hemorrhages which sometimes occur in the adrenals as the effect of injury to the sympathetic nervous system. He regards the fat necrosis resulting from trauma as a trophoneurotic disturbance. Compression of the excretory ducts and stagnation of secretion and, therefore, cyst formation might always occur, according to Fischer, in consequence of such an occurrence of hemorrhage into the pancreatic tissue.

It is stated that the formation of cysts takes place after infectious diseases, typhoid fever, influenza; and in such cases the cause has been sought in the action of bacillary toxins upon the gland either directly or through the mediation of the nervous system.

It is obvious from the above that there is much which is hypothetic in the etiology of cysts, and much that is obscure still remains to be cleared up.

STATISTICS.

The following relation of age and sex is determined from the consideration of 134 cases:

Years.	Men.	Women.		
½ to 10	3	+ 1	=	4 (Railton ½ year)
11 to 20	5	+ 4	=	9
21 to 30	1	+ 2	=	31
31 to 40	2	+ 1	=	31
41 to 50		+	=	5
51 to 60		+	=	14
61 to 70		+	=	3
71 to 93		+	=	6
Age not given		+	=	8
	60	+ 61	=	121
Neither age nor sex was given in 13 cases				13
				134

The number of women suffering from pancreatic cysts is, according to this table, scarcely larger than that of the men. Those most frequently diseased are between twenty and forty years of age. In men the greatest number is reached during the fourth and in women during the third decade.

SYMPTOMS.

Various obscure disturbances of digestion, pains, and loss of weight often precede for a long time the development of the pancreatic cyst. This may be explained by the fact that the original disease which gradually leads to the formation of the cyst produces dyspeptic disturbances and pains, while the lowering of the general nutrition is due to the actual disturbance of digestion.

Chronic pancreatitis, as has already been shown, is the commonest cause of cyst formation, and the digestive function and the general nutrition must be variously influenced, according to the extent of the pancreatitis, the degree of the stagnation of secretion, and the resulting hindrance to the physiologic function of the gland.

When the cyst has once begun, and is growing, disturbances of function in other organs naturally arise, and the resulting symptoms are added to those dependent upon the affection of the pancreas. Pains are among the most frequent symptoms of cyst of the pancreas, but are inconstant. They may be paroxysmal or persistent, the latter especially when the cyst is large. They are felt either in the epigastrium, and then are designated cardialgias, or they may be referred to the right or left border of the ribs, according to the development of the cyst in the head or tail of the pancreas. When the pains are on the right, they are easily regarded as biliary colic.

The pains may radiate in all directions into all regions of the abdomen, sometimes along the loins toward the sacrum, or they are sometimes referred to the navel. Doubtless these wide-spread pains are caused by the size of the tumor, and especially by the rapidity of its growth. The pains may occur at longer or shorter intervals as colic, and may then be of great severity, sufficient to produce fainting and symptoms of collapse. It may be questioned in such cases whether pressure on the solar ganglion is the cause of pain.

It is not easily understood how such a constant, gradually increasing pressure should cause such severe pain only at times. As a matter of fact, attacks of colic very frequently occur in pancreatic cysts, and always represent a characteristic peculiarity of them (Leube), since a similar colic does not occur in other cystic tumors of the upper abdomen.

Colic frequently precedes the dilatation of the duct of Wirsung, and the gradual formation of a cyst occasioned by the formation of calculi or other causes which temporarily or permanently obstruct the outflow of secretion. However, there certainly are pancreatic cysts in which the pains are not so violent, although they are periodic, and it is expressly stated in a series of cases that there is no pain at all. Violent continued pains may be present after the cyst has once formed. There is at times considerable sensitiveness to pressure over the tumor. It is to be noted, however, that in many cases there is an actual lack of sensitiveness and of spontaneous pains especially in the region of the tumor. Conspicuous dyspeptic difficulties before and after the formation of the tumor often occur. Not infrequently mention is made of a preceding gastric catarrh, nausea, morning vomiting, and anorexia. It is assumed that the process causing pancreatitis and the simultaneous or preceding catarrhal condition of the stomach and intestine may be the cause of these symptoms. Large tumors must naturally interfere with function, especially with the mechanism of the stomach and intestine, and these disturbances may result in consequence of the size of the tumors. It is obvious that they are not characteristic, as similar symptoms occur in many diseases of the digestive tract.

Vomiting is frequently noted in the histories of patients. At the outset it occurs only at the time of the colic, as it is an accompaniment of biliary, intestinal, and renal colic; later it becomes more and more frequent, and under some circumstances may follow each meal, probably in consequence of the displacement of the stomach and intestine or by interference with their mechanical function. The vomitus consists either of the food taken, or is an alkaline fluid at times bile-stained, at times bloody.

Marked hematemesis also may occur, especially when a cyst filled with blood ruptures into the stomach or into the upper part of the intestine. Cysts so small as not to be palpable may perforate, as reported by Pepper. In a case observed in Nothnagel's clinic, a cyst ruptured into the intestine some days after a liquid stool had been evacuated, and a bowlful of a thin, grayish-red liquid, containing several reddish-brown shreds, was vomited. The reaction was alkaline. On microscopic examination there were mucin and bacteria, but no blood-corpuscles.

The action of the bowels is sometimes normal or there is constipation or diarrhea. The constipation is explicable when there are large tumors by the hindrance to intestinal peristalsis. The diarrhea was formerly regarded as characteristic. Authors have described as pancreatic diarrhea, celiac flux, or pancreatic flux, the passage of thin viscous material supposed to consist of pancreatic juice, and have regarded it as a form of diarrhea especially characteristic of diseases of the pancreas (see General Considerations, page 99). In Nothnagel's case above mentioned there were liquid stools after the disappearance of a tumor previously palpated, and which surely had ruptured into the intestine.

In some cases of cysts of the pancreas there were peculiar changes in the stools, which certainly must have had some relation to the disease of the pancreas. In those of Bull, Goodmann, and Gould, fatty stools were mentioned as a symptom. In the case last named, there was at the same time jaundice. In by far the greater number of cases of pancreatic cysts in which the stools have been examined—although this was relatively rare—it was expressly stated that there was no steatorrhea. It is noteworthy that there was an abnormal proteid digestion in some instances. Küster found large numbers of undigested muscle-fibers in his case even when the amount of meat in the food was very limited. Riegner also found many undigested muscle-fibers in the stools.

The displacement and compression of certain portions of the intestine by a large tumor may influence the condition of the stools. Slight degrees of pressure may slightly diminish evacuation of the bowels (Martin), or, as in the case reported by Lardy, may flatten the colorless stool. There was complete intestinal obstruction in the cases of Brown and Hagenbach and temporary obstruction in Lardy's case.

The jaundice appearing in cysts of the pancreas may be explained by · the compression of the ductus choledochus by the tumor. In a case reported by Gould the jaundice was transitory, and may have been caused by a duodenal catarrh. Jaundice is not always caused by the pressure of the pancreatic cyst on the common duct. In the case described by Cruveilhier, a scirrhus situated at the exit of the common duct caused both jaundice and, by closure of the Wirsungian duct, a cyst of the pancreas. In the case reported by Phulpin, a gall-stone lay in the ductus choledochus and caused, on the one hand, jaundice, and, on the other, a cyst of the pancreas, by compression of the duct of Wirsung. In the case reported by Friedreich, also, an annular cancer of the descending portion of the duodenum closed the common duct, produced jaundice, and at the same time compressed the duct of Wirsung, which entered the duodenum separately from the common duct and caused its dilatation, with the production of numerous saccular diverticula.

The ureter also may be compressed by a large tumor, and thus the outflow of urine from the kidney be prevented, as in Reeve's case, in which the right ureter was obstructed. Ascites and edema of the lower extremities may result from the interference with the circulation in the abdomen, as in the case of all large abdominal tumors.

Certain changes in the urine deserve especial mention, particularly the occurrence of sugar. Diabetes is mentioned in nine cases (Bull, Churton, Goodmann, Horrocks, and Morton, Malcolm Mackintosh, Nichols,

v. Recklinghausen, Riegner [traces of sugar], Zweifel-Mulert). In the case operated upon by Zweifel there was no sugar previous to the operation. Afterward the urine sometimes contained sugar and at times it was absent. There are reports from the autopsies of six of the cases. Nichols found that the pancreas was wholly destroyed by the formation of the cyst. Goodmann saw atrophy and Churton observed fibrous degeneration of the pancreas (see page 70). Küster reports polyuria. Albuminuria is mentioned several times.

Fever is often recorded, and may depend upon the accompanying diseases, peritonitis, hemorrhage into or suppuration of the cyst. Salivation is to be mentioned among the symptoms which have been attributed to diseases of the pancreas. It is obviously not characteristic, because it has been observed only twice (Battersby, Ludolph). The interference with the action of the stomach in these cases may have been of importance in producing this condition.

General emaciation is one of the most frequent symptoms. It occurs almost constantly, and is rarely noted as absent. It may be very great and rapidly occur. In Küster's case the patient lost 15 kg. in four months. When the formation of the cyst is complicated with a malignant neoplasm, as in the case of Hartmann, the emaciation is not striking, and is sufficiently explained by the cachexia associated with the development of the neoplasm. The cause of the disturbance of nutrition and the feeling of weakness is equally obvious when there is diabetes. The emaciation, however, occurs in very many cases in which there is neither a neoplasm nor diabetes. In such cases the cause cannot be satisfactorily explained. It may be that in many cases, as in those of Küster and Riegner, a faulty proteid digestion contributes to the poor nutrition, but it also may be, especially in large tumors, that the interference with the function of other vital organs is responsible for the emaciation, or, as Küster claims, the participation of the nervous system, especially of the celiac plexus, may exert an injurious influence on the general nutrition. All this, however, is at present mere hypothesis. It is certain that very frequently there is emaciation, and that after successful operation there is often a rapid increase of weight and of strength.

Among the objective symptoms, the physical conditions and the demonstrable tumor are especially important. The abdomen is flat or retracted (Hagenbach) but exceptionally, as in the case of small cysts. As a rule, it is more or less distended and swollen. The distention is limited to one or another region, and eventually the entire abdomen is involved, according to the seat and size of the tumor. In far the greatest number of cases the distention takes place in the epigastrium. The left epigastrium, the mesogastrium, and the left hypochondrium are more frequently the seat of the tumor than the right half of the body, because the tail and the body of the pancreas are more frequently the seat of the development of the cyst than is the head.

Large tumors may descend and occupy the meso- and hypogastrium, or may be found simply in the hypogastrium, as in Treves's case, where the tumor lay between the umbilicus and pubes. Very large tumors fill the whole abdomen, as in the cases reported by Riedel, Ludolph, and Hulke. The distention of the abdomen from large tumors is at times uniform. Its circumference, under such conditions, may increase enormously, as in Martin's case, in which it reached 61 inches.

As a rule, the distention is rather localized, and the tumor projects distinctly on inspection of the abdomen. The surface of the tumor is generally smooth and is tensely stretched. Fluctuation is common when the cyst is hyperdistended, but the sense of fluctuation is indistinct and may even be wholly absent. On percussion over the tumor there is either flatness or a dull tympanitic resonance, the latter depending upon the situation of the tumor behind the stomach and colon. The modified tympanitic zone may be at the upper or lower border of the tumor or in both places, or over the entire tumor, according to the relations of the stomach and colon to the cyst. The character of the resonance may change according to the distention of the stomach and intestine with air and solid contents. The relation of the tumor to its surroundings as determined by percussion will further be considered in the section on diagnosis. The tumor is sometimes movable with respiration, and in certain cases has been moved laterally.

DIAGNOSIS.

Cysts of the pancreas belong to the few diseases of that organ the recognition of which is possible during life. The knowledge and successful treatment of pancreatic cysts are due, above all, to surgery, which has reached the pancreas in its triumphal progress into the previously closed region of the viscera.

"The diagnosis of the formation of a cyst in the pancreas," says Friedreich, "will of course be possible only in those cases in which the tumor has reached a considerable size." In 1878 he could state nothing of a diagnosis actually having been made during life. In 1883 Gussenbauer came very near making the diagnosis of a pancreatic cyst, being in doubt only between a cyst of the pancreas and one of the adrenal gland.

Following Gussenbauer, Senn in 1885, and in 1886 and 1887 Küster, Bull, and Subotic, made correct diagnoses. Wölfler was the first to make this in a woman. According to the published reports of cases at hand, the diagnosis was correctly made before an operation in 27 instances. It must be stated, however, that it is by no means sure that pancreatic cysts were actually present in all these cases. In most of them the cyst was not extirpated, but merely drained after one or two incisions, and the diagnosis, as a rule, was based solely on the fact that the cysts lay in the upper abdomen, did not communicate with the liver or kidney, and the contents were diastasic or emulsified fat. As is explained later, these are not positive proofs. Absolute proof is furnished only when pancreatic secretion, with all its qualities, including that of proteid digestion, is found; or when undoubted pancreatic juice escapes from the fistula following the operation.

An examination of the literature shows that these cysts are confounded with the most diverse processes, oftenest with ovarian cysts and echinococci of the liver. Pancreatic cysts have been mistaken also for aortic aneurysms, for cysts of the peritoneum or of the retroperitoneal tissue, of the mesentery, of the adrenal, of the kidney, of the spleen, for abscesses of the abdominal wall, for echinococci of the omentum, for perinephritic abscess, for omental tumors, etc. The diagnosis of a pancreatic cyst, then, is first to be considered when there is a palpable or visible tumor. Months or years may elapse between the beginning of the disease and the development of the tumor, and during this time it is impossible to make the diagnosis. If in chronic pancreatitis dilatation of the gland ducts and consequent cyst formation has resulted from the gradual constriction of excretory ducts, then, as has been stated in the section on Pancreatitis, it will rarely be possible to more than suspect such a disease of the pancreas. An exact diagnosis beyond a certain degree of hypothesis, or at the most probability, will in such cases be wholly impossible.

The suspicion of a disease of the pancreas may certainly be aroused if there are occasional colic resembling celiac neuralgia, steatorrhea, many undigested muscle-fibers in the stools, or diabetes. The diagnosis of cyst first becomes possible when there is in the upper abdomen a visible or palpable tumor in which there is also fluctuation.

The results of physical examination are important, and first of all palpation, which through resistance fixes the position and size of the tumor, and makes fluctuation evident. Percussion establishes the presence of dulness, tympany, or modified tympany over the tumor.

It is important to establish the previously mentioned relation of the tumor to the stomach, colon, and small intestine. In order to determine this point, the distention of the stomach with carbonic acid is recommended, by means of the administration of tartaric acid and sodium bicarbonate, or with atmospheric air, and the filling of the colon with fluid or with air.

The distention of the stomach with air is the most effective, as has previously been stated. When it is inflated with carbonic acid, the quantity of gas set free from the carbonated mixture cannot be accurately determined, while if air is used it may be introduced gradually and the stomach is distended slowly, thus rendering the condition much clearer. The intestine may easily be distended with a tube having two bulbs attached.

The determination of the situation of the cyst with reference to the colon and stomach is one of the most important aids in diagnosis. The difficulty and not infrequent impossibility of a differential diagnosis is in many cases apparent from the numerous wrong diagnoses which have been made.

The situation and size of the cyst cause it to be confounded with various tumors arising from other organs than the pancreas, but showing similar physical conditions. The following tumors situated in the upper abdomen are especially to be considered: echinococcus of the liver, spleen, mesentery, or peritoneum; hydronephrosis; dropsy of the gall-bladder; abscess of the abdominal wall; aneurysm of the aorta and its branches; soft apparently fluctuating sarcoma of the liver; cysts of the omentum or mesentery; cysts or collections of fluid in the omental bursa; cysts of the kidney or adrenal bodies.

Many of these possibilities of error may be avoided by greater care in examination. Thus, aneurysm of the aorta or its branches, abscess of the abdominal wall, peritoneal tumor, or sarcoma of the liver may easily be excluded. The chief difficulty lies between echinococcus of the liver and cyst of the pancreas, since echinococci of the spleen, peritoneum, and omental bursa are very rare. In this case percussion may decide, but it must be tried both in the recumbent and upright positions of the patient. When the stomach is inflated, it will lie in front of the pancreatic cyst, while in echinococcus of the liver, especially of the left lobe, the stomach, as a rule, lies behind the tumor. In many but not in all cases it will be possible to find between the liver and the cyst a tympanitic area which becomes diminished on deep inspiration.

The mobility of the tumor is of uncertain value in the differentiation, as pancreatic cysts also may be movable with respiration. If the patient is examined in the upright position, it may happen, as Küster suggests, that the cyst will descend, and then it may be possible to recognize a distinct tympanitic area between the liver and the cyst, which could not be ascertained when the examination was made in the recumbent position.

Puncture, which, however, is certainly not entirely free from danger, permits more exact differentiation between echinococcus of the liver and pancreatic cyst. Other cystic tumors of the liver do not attain so large a size, for cystic enlargements of the bile-ducts are small; hence puncture with the Pravaz syringe, recommended especially by Küster, may clear up the diagnosis. Other surgeons also consider that puncture in these cases is not wholly free from danger, because echinococcus fluid or pus, even if there is suppuration of the echinococcus sac, may possibly flow into the peritoneal cavity.

Karewski considers exploratory puncture dangerous, because other organs may be injured. In one of his patients he penetrated the stomach in spite of the fact that he was able to prove the presence of the stomach above the cyst. The stomach was pressed flat between the cyst and the abdominal wall, and only a small portion of it lay above the cyst. A possible puncture of the colon would not be wholly free from risk. Küster, on the contrary, regards the danger of exploratory puncture as very slight, since the escape of echinococcus fluid and pancreatic secretion causes only temporary disturbances.

According to my humble opinion, an operation should be undertaken whether there is an echinococcus cyst or one arising in the pancreas, because the operation will first definitely decide the nature of the cyst.

The examination of the contents of the cyst in echinococcus of the liver shows clear watery fluid, free from albumin, in which on microscopic examination there are either hooklets or at least an absence of all morphologic elements, which likewise is to be regarded as characteristic. If, however, the echinococcus is sterile and the sac contains pus, the presence of hooklets indicates the existence of an echinococcus. Puncture may decide also between a cyst in the tail of the pancreas and echinococcus of the spleen. Other cystic tumors in the spleen are very rare, although Küster found in it a cavity larger than the fist.

The distinction between pancreatic cyst and hydronephrosis is difficult, and in many cases is first made evident by the examination of the liquid contents. The history at times may give a clue. Hydronephrosis should first be thought of if there are renal colic, lumbar pain in the vicinity of the tumor, and urinary difficulties, or the previous escape of renal concretions or a characteristic condition of the urine.

If the fluid at the operation is due to hydronephrosis, the sediment will contain epithelium from the calices or pelvis of the kidney. The fluid will also contain urea, which is rarely absent, and then only late in the disease; also uric acid and so-called mucin and metalbumin or paralbumin (Senator). Pancreatic cysts may be confounded also with chylous cysts or cysts of the mesentery. Chylous cysts, according to Küster, seldom, if ever, lie above the navel, since they correspond to the position of the receptaculum chyli just above or just below the umbilicus.

Mesenteric cysts are characterized by great mobility, which is lacking in cysts of the pancreas. As Hochenegg states, the mesenteric cyst which is seated somewhere in the vicinity of the navel may so be pushed upward as to disappear completely beneath the costal cartilages, and downward as far as the entrance to the pelvis. Pancreatic cysts never show such a degree of mobility. The large cysts which almost entirely fill the abdomen are echinococcus cysts of the liver and ovarian cysts. The means of differentiating the former have already been stated. The presence of a tympanitic area between the liver and tumor is in favor of a pancreatic cyst.

The confusion between pancreatic and ovarian cysts is most frequent and most easily understood. An ovarian tumor is usually first thought of in consequence of its greater frequency and the relative rarity of cysts of the pancreas. The history in such cases aids in the distinction, and women can often state where the tumor appeared first. The prominence of pancreatic cysts is above the navel, a position which contraindicates an ovarian tumor. Thorough, careful percussion in different positions of the body permits the recognition of even very large ovarian tumors, according to the experience of Küster. "Large ovarian tumors fill at least one iliac fossa so completely that there is no tympanitic resonance below the tumor. On the other hand, they rarely reach so near the liver and diaphragm that it is impossible to recognize a tympanitic area above them. Nevertheless, it would scarcely happen that a pancreatic cyst descending from the upper abdomen would so completely fill only one side of the pelvis that no tympanitic zone could be distinguished between the upper border of the pubic bone and the tumor. But when it is suspected that there may be a pancreatic cyst, the inflation of the stomach with carbonic acid offers an excellent means of discrimination; for the stomach must lie in front of the pancreatic cyst, while the ovarian cyst must crowd it backward."

The examination of the fluid from the cyst permits the distinction in many but not in all cases. The objections to exploratory puncture with the Pravaz syringe have already been stated. Disagreeable results may follow the escape of pancreatic fluid, or the contents of a suppurating cystoma of the ovary, or the epithelial contents of a dermoid cyst. The last-mentioned tumors rarely become so large as to be confounded with cysts of the pancreas.

The value of the examination of the cyst fluid has been overestimated by many. The contents of undoubted pancreatic cysts may, during their long continuance, undergo such changes after prolonged retention that they present none of the specific peculiarities of the pancreatic secretion. But even when certain characteristics are present, they prove nothing. Great weight has formerly been placed on the diastatic ferment, but this has proved erroneous. Von Jaksch found small quantities of a saccharifying ferment, at times transforming starch, in ascitic fluid and in the contents of abdominal cysts of other origin than the pancreas. It must be proved at least that the fluid after the addition of starch not only possesses reducing qualities, but maltose must be formed, for other diastatic fluids do not change starch to maltose (v. Jaksch).

The diagnostic value of the frequently mentioned emulsifying quality is not much more satisfactory. It is undoubtedly absent in many pancreatic cysts, but, as Frerichs has already stated, a slight emulsifying action on fats may be possessed by other cystic fluids of alkaline reaction and by transudates.

The presence of trypsin in the fluid is the real test and this is often absent in the contents of pancreatic cysts.

If a fistula results, the secretion may represent pure pancreatic fluid, even if the fluid escaping at the time of the operation has none of the physiologic qualities of the pancreatic secretion. The presence of blood in the contents of the pancreatic cyst is, as Küster states, an important diagnostic sign. Hemorrhagic contents occur only in an ovarian cystoma, with a twisted pedicle, but such tumors are relatively small, and do not extend to the upper abdomen (Küster). There are, however, enough pancreatic cysts in which there is no blood.

Küster regards the presence of fat granular corpuscles as characteristic of pancreatic cysts, but, as Karewski asserts, these may be absent. On the other hand, fat granular corpuscles may be found as the product of fatty degeneration of epithelium even in the contents of an ovarian cyst.

In spite of the above-mentioned numerous means of diagnosticating pancreatic cysts there is at times difficulty in making a diagnosis, which in many cases is first positively established after the operation or at a postmortem examination.

DURATION AND COURSE.

The statements widely differ regarding the time between the appearance of the first symptoms of a pancreatic cyst and the period when it is first seen, diagnosticated, and operated upon. Doubtless there are acute cases, while, on the other hand, the process very frequently extends over a period of years. The onset can rarely be stated with certainty, and is possible only when it follows injury. In all other cases no positive clue to the beginning of the process can be drawn from the vague statements of the occurrence of colic, disturbances of digestion, pain, etc. If, as in most cases, chronic pancreatitis must be regarded as the cause, the beginning of the disease is naturally obscure and only approximately to be determined.

Cysts may develop very rapidly after trauma. In Littlewood's case an epigastric swelling occurred thirteen days after the kick of a horse. Three weeks after a trauma, Kulenkampf found a painful tumor in the epigastrium. In Fisher's case fever, hematemesis, melena, and a small tumor developed a few days after a fall from a wagon; three weeks later an operation was performed. In a boy two years old whose case was reported by Lynn, there was collapse and vomiting after the child was run over; three weeks later a swelling of the abdomen was noted.

In contrast with this rapid development, there are certainly many cases in which the cysts have existed for years. In such, the growth is often periodical after being quiescent for a long period, or the enlargement is very slow. Pregnancy causes no increase in size (Mayo).

The assertions concerning the long duration are naturally to be accepted with considerable hesitation, because the physician can depend only on the statements of the patient, which cannot be further controlled. Thus, Hulke reports the existence of a tumor since childhood in a woman forty-seven years old. That a cyst may last sixteen years is definitely established by Martin. The first operation was performed in 1873 and an irremovable tumor was found behind the large intestine and mesocolon. In 1889 the abdomen increased rapidly in size and an operation was performed. In the case observed in my hospital and reported by Salzer, the cyst had certainly existed for twelve years. A woman thirty-five years old, operated upon by Clutton, is said to have had a tumor in the left side of the abdomen for twenty years. In most cases one to three years elapse between the first symptoms of the disease and the time when the cyst was observed.

PROGNOSIS.

Pancreatic cysts may come to a standstill, and are then sometimes found unexpectedly at a postmortem examination. In very rare cases the cyst may rupture into one of the neighboring hollow organs, as the stomach, with consequent hematemesis, or into the intestine with subsequent hemorrhagic stools or the evacuation of watery alkaline contents. If such a communication between the cyst and intestine exist for some time, there may be a thoroughly characteristic rise and fall in the size of the tumor, and the latter may wholly disappear at times, but at the next examination be again distinctly palpable. Operation exercises the most favorable influence upon the course.

TREATMENT.

Nothing is to be expected from the internal treatment of pancreatic cysts. The formation of the cyst cannot be avoided even when its most frequent cause, chronic interstitial pancreatitis, can positively be diagnosticated. The progress of the disease perhaps might be influenced by a timely treatment if there were positive indications that the condition was caused by gall-stones or syphilis.

The great advance of surgery has included the pancreatic cyst in its field of successful treatment. Fifteen years ago Gussenbauer first introduced an effective means of operating and was successful, and now the number of cases of recovery increases from year to year. One hundred and one operations with 81 recoveries are to be found in 134 cases. Although it is by no means sure that in all of these pancreatic cysts were present, yet the facts mentioned must be accepted, and there is no doubt that the percentage of recoveries will become far more favorable as the method of operation is now quite well established and it is unnecessary to make any new experiments in this direction.

The following methods of operating have been employed: (1) Simple puncture; (2) Récamier's procedure; (3) total extirpation; (4) partial extirpation with subsequent drainage; (5) incision in two operations with drainage; (6) single incision with drainage.

1. Puncture was undertaken 7 times with 5 fatal results.

Dixon, simple puncture; Hagenbach, laparotomy, puncture, death from "ileus"; Horrocks and Morton, puncture and aspiration; Lloyd, puncture; Railton, puncture twice, the first time with aspiration and the second time with drainage; Lynn, puncture with aspiration, recovery; Stiller, exploratory puncture, recovery(?).

2. Récamier's procedure was tried but once; then by Ledentu. At intervals of two to three days the cyst was cauterized five times with caustic potash; perforation then took place at the base of the eschar;

after two and a half days, death from peritonitis. The stomach was opened by the cauterization.

3. Total extirpation was performed 11 times, two being fatal.

Recovery in the cases of Bozemann, Cibert, Clutton, Eve, Heinricius (2 cases), Martin, Schroeder, Zweifel. Death in the cases of Riedel and Salzer.

4. Partial extirpation 12 times with 4 fatal results.

Recovery in the cases of Filipow, Emmet Giffin, Hersche, v. Petrykowski, Schroeder, Tobin, Trombetta, Zawadzki. Death in those of Hulke, Kootz, Ludolph, and Zukowski.

5. The incision in two operations was performed 12 times, one proving fatal (diabetes).

Recovery in the cases of Albert (2 cases), Annandale, Dreyzehner, Fenger, Finotti (2 cases), Kulenkampf, Steele, Subotic, Thiersch. Death from diabetes in Bull's case three and a half months after the first incision.

6. The single incision was performed 58 times with death in seven (but independent of the operation in four).

Recovery in the cases of Agnew, Ashhurst, Barnett, Brown, Chew and Cathcart, Dieckhoff, Flaischlen, Fisher (2 cases), Goiffey, Gould (2 cases), Gussenbauer (3 cases),* Herczel, Hinrichs, Holmes, Karewski (2 cases), Kramer, Küster, Lardy, Lindner, Littlewood, Lloyd, Ludolph, Martin, Mayo, Mumford, Newton, Ochsner, Osler, McPhedran, Richardson (2 cases), Riedel, Riegner, Schnitzler (2 cases), Senn, Swain, Schwarz, Stapper, Thoren, Tremaine, Treves, Tricomi, de Wildt, Witzel, Wölfler. Death in the cases of Churton: second laparotomy on account of collection of pus behind the stomach, Durante: two days after the operation uncontrollable vomiting, Gould; peritonitis, Hartmann; death from cancerous cachexia seven weeks after the operation, Reeve; death from "fever" three months after the operation, Savilli; spontaneous rupture of a pancreatic cyst, puriform infiltration behind the pancreas, laparotomy, suture of the sac, death in collapse; Schwarz, sepsis.

The method which is now chiefly used and the details of which are given by Gussenbauer is the completion of the operation at once, the wall of the cyst being stitched to the abdominal wound and the cavity drained.

Appendix.—There are but few observations regarding the occurrence of echinococcus in the pancreas. Claessen mentions several doubtful cases of Chambon de Montaux, Portal, and Engel. Heller states that echinococcus occurs rarely in the pancreas, and cites the case of Seidl. Tricomi asserts that seven cases are noted in the literature, but does not mention any of them. According to Nimier, Briggs extirpated an echinococcus sac which had undergone sarcomatous degeneration. Hooklets had been found in the fluid obtained by puncture.

VI. HEMORRHAGE.

HEMORRHAGE into the pancreatic tissue occurs relatively often. This statement, however, applies only to slight punctate hemorrhages, such as occur in diseases of the heart, lungs, and liver, as manifestations of stasis, in hemorrhagic diathesis (scorbutus, purpura, morbus maculosus Werlh.),

* A fourth case of successful operation by Gussenbauer was omitted by mistake.

eclampsia (Schmorl, Lubarsch), phosphorus-poisoning, acute exanthemata or other infectious diseases, and in various inflammatory processes in the pancreas itself.

In acute and chronic pancreatitis the hemorrhages are either fresh, often microscopically minute, or, if old, are evidenced by round or oblong, small, pigmented foci or spaces and gaps, which are filled with a more or less discolored serous fluid and are limited by dense, rust-colored walls which project toward the interior (Klob, Friedreich). The ready occurrence of hemorrhage into the pancreatic tissue may be due to the anatomic structure of the organ and its vessels. Klebs seeks for the cause of the hemorrhages in the corroding action of the pancreatic secretion, and Fitz calls to mind the fact known to anatomists that when the arteries are injected, the fluid used easily escapes from the pancreas—a result which may, to be sure, as Dieckhoff suggests, be due to postmortem changes.

Pancreatic hemorrhages easily occur, as already mentioned, in different experiments on animals, as total or partial extirpation, and artificially produced inflammations.

Large hemorrhages into the pancreas may, at times, in spite of their extent, be only incidental and without essential influence on the course of the disease and the final outcome. They are then generally connected with extravasations of blood in other organs, and are results of severe circulatory disturbances. Doubtless such a condition would be much more frequently discovered and would be better known if the reports of autopsies relative to this matter were published.

In the reports of postmortem examinations in 1894 at the General Hospital in Vienna, two cases of hemorrhage in the pancreas are noted —one from aortic insufficiency, the other in emphysema. To the cases of this kind mentioned in literature belongs that reported by Gerhardt-Kollmann, relating to a woman forty-seven years old, who died with emphysema, diffuse bronchial catarrh, anasarca, ascites with evidence of a high degree of stasis, and marked cyanosis.

At the autopsy the peritoneum over the convexity of the duodenum was found suffused with a considerable hemorrhage. Less extensive hemorrhages were found between the individual pancreatic lobules, while the retroperitoneal tissue behind the pancreas as far as the hilus of the spleen was infiltrated with blood. There was a group of smaller ecchymoses in the large intestine behind the cecum.

The emphysema in this case is doubtless to be regarded as the cause of death, and the pancreatic hemorrhage as a secondary result of stasis. Kollmann reports a similar case in which a patient with mitral stenosis and left-sided pleuritic exudation died suddenly.

At the autopsy the peritoneum was found suffused with blood in the region of the pylorus in consequence of a subperitoneal hemorrhage. The mucous membrane of. the stomach, markedly injected, showed small ecchymoses in two places, while the mucous membrane of the duodenum was suffused with blood along the convexity; the hemorrhagic infiltration extended from the curvature of the duodenum into the retroperitoneal tissue along the pancreas to the hilus of the spleen. The tail of the pancreas was hyperemic and showed a larger amount of hemorrhage than the head. The appearance of the pancreas gave no evidence of fatty degeneration. The semilunar ganglion was found entirely surrounded by the hemorrhagic infiltration.

It is probably impossible to decide whether in this case the sudden death is to be ascribed to the diseased heart or to the pancreatic hemorrhage so affecting the semilunar ganglion as to have caused an arrest of the function of the heart by reflex action.

The communication of Rehm probably belongs under this head: A female mill operative thirty-seven years old was choked by a man and died a short time afterward. At the autopsy extravasations of blood from the size of a bean to that of a hazelnut were found in the connective tissue around the head of the pancreas, in the peritoneal covering of the diaphragm, and over the left kidney. Rehm attributed the death to suffocation from throttling, while Zenker, who made a report on the same case, regarded the hemorrhage into the pancreas as the cause of death, by its reflex influence on the nerve plexus there situated. Reubold supported Rehm's view, regarding the death as due to the throttling, and reports an analogous case: A man fifty years old hanged himself in prison. At the autopsy the middle third of the pancreas was dark red; the gland-lobules of the same portion contained numerous punctate hemorrhages, and from 6 to 10 separate spots could be distinguished in each lobule; there were larger hemorrhagic infiltrations between the lobules.

Reubold also reports two cases in which there were hemorrhages into the pancreatic tissue, the one of morphin-poisoning and the other of bleeding to death. All the organs of the latter patient were found bloodless, but there was quite a large hemorrhagic infiltration of about one-third of the head of pancreas; there were a few ecchymoses also in the stomach. Large pancreatic hemorrhages have been observed also in other cases of extreme anemia; thus, in a puerpera observed by Lawrence, possibly a case of pernicious anemia, as held by Seitz, the pancreas was of a uniform, deep, dark red color, and from the outside felt dense. Large hemorrhages affecting the pancreas alone are of much greater interest, and, at times, involve the whole organ and the surrounding tissue, and are the actual cause of death. They are not very rare, Dieckhoff having collected 62 such cases.

ETIOLOGY.

The causes of the hemorrhage can be established in but a few cases. The following factors are to be considered, most of which are based upon the able publication of Seitz.

1. **Disease of the blood-vessels** (atheroma, fatty degeneration, alteration of the vessel-walls from alcoholism, syphilis, etc.) is to be regarded as the most frequent cause. The anatomic structure of the pancreas, already mentioned, favors the rupture of atheromatous vessels. Fitz includes among these anatomic factors the presence of numerous small vessels immediately influenced by the powerful aortic pressure, the great variation in their fulness in consequence of the action of the diaphragm and abdominal muscles, the stasis caused by the variations in the distention of the stomach and intestine,.and, finally, the slight counterpressure from the surrounding tissue, almost wholly composed of glandular cells.

The following cases serve to illustrate the course:

The second case of Prince: A woman sixty-five years old, much addicted to liquor; fell down-stairs while intoxicated, then went out and came home drunk. At daybreak she was found dead. The autopsy showed atheroma of the middle cerebral artery, also of the coronary arteries, and slight mitral stenosis. The subperitoneal tissue about the pancreas was moderately infiltrated with fresh blood. The tissue of the gland showed marked hemorrhagic infiltration throughout the whole organ, especially in the head.

Draper: Sudden death from pancreatic hemorrhage. A woman forty-four

14

years old was found dead in her bed. She drank alcoholic liquors, but was rarely intoxicated, and the evening before was perfectly well. In the morning she complained of headache, returned to her bed, and later was found dead. At the autopsy the pancreas was seen infiltrated with blood throughout its whole extent, there was a moderate amount of blood in the retroperitoneal tissue, and eight ounces of reddish fluid in the peritoneal cavity.

Draper: Duration of the illness three-quarters of an hour; death from pancreatic hemorrhage. A type-setter thirty-one years old, intemperate, was attacked while in perfect health with sudden pains in the epigastrium, nausea, collapse, and died forty-five minutes later. The autopsy showed the pancreas and surrounding tissue infiltrated with blood; the heart was friable, the intima of the aorta showed a pre-existing endarteritis, the splenic artery was tortuous, its intima rough and of a finely granular appearance. On microscopic examination of the pancreas the gland cells appeared granular, and there was blood in the interlobular tissue.

Seitz includes in this series the cases of Draper (three besides those mentioned), of Reynolds and Gannet (in a corpulent man sixty-six years old), of Williams (in a man seventy years old with peripheral arteriosclerosis), of Challand and Rabow, Whitney and Homans, Putnam and Whitney, Driver and Holt.

Driver and Holt: Slender man, fifty-eight years old, awakened with severe abdominal pains, vomiting, great exhaustion. Pale, pulse very weak. Death in thirty minutes. The duodenal half of the pancreas was bluish-red, in strong contrast to the yellowish-gray splenic end. The darker part was infiltrated with blood, which lay in the interlobular tissue and could be easily scraped from the cut section.

Seitz regards the observation of Fearnside as a case of pancreatic hemorrhage from uremic vascular sclerosis in atrophy of the kidney:

A farmer forty-nine years old, not especially large, had for a year frequent deeply seated pains in the region of the stomach with emaciation, and for three months numerous and violent attacks of pain. Three days before death he had a sudden attack of fearful pain with fainting and vomiting of dark-brown fluid, and the next day jaundice developed. Hiccough, abatement of the pain. On the day of death Fearnside noted collapse, distention of the abdomen, and a deep-seated tumor between the xiphoid process and the umbilicus. At the autopsy it was found that the tumor felt during life was formed by the pancreas. The enlargement involved the entire organ, especially the right end of the gland, which was brownish-black and almost completely changed into a pap-like, pulpy mass.

The case shows also how many interpretations may be placed upon such observations. Seitz thought it possible that the case was one of pancreatic hemorrhage in consequence of uremic vascular sclerosis, because the kidneys were small, indurated, and with an ill-defined cortex. Fearnside regarded chronic pancreatitis as the cause, and Fitz thought that a hemorrhage had taken place into a malignant tumor of the pancreas.

Seitz reports an original observation in which he attributed the suddenly fatal pancreatic hemorrhage to syphilitic changes in the vessels.

A muscular man twenty-eight years old was suddenly attacked with abdominal pain, and collapse soon followed. Vomiting, fainting; after six hours, death. At the autopsy a large collection—some 2 quarts—of blood was found in the peritoneum. Tissue between the stomach, duodenum, transverse colon, spleen, and pancreas was extensively infiltrated with blood. The bleeding point could not be located exactly, but probably one of the branches of the celiac axis had ruptured. The pancreas appeared perfectly normal, except for the hemorrhagic infiltration which had penetrated into the connective tissue between the lobules and only sparingly into the lobules. Seitz suspected that the case was one of syphilis, because the patient had undergone syphilitic treatment on account of chronic iritis and opacities of the vitreous body. On microscopic examination, Seitz found an endarteritis of the branches of the celiac, which extended into the surrounding glandular tissue and formed a small-celled tumor. Seitz regarded syphilis as the only explanation of this process. •

2. Fatty **degeneration of the gland-cells and excessive** fatty **infiltration of the pancreas** are to be considered as the cause of the hemorrhage in a number of cases. There may be also fatty degeneration of the vessel-walls and consequent ease of rupture. On account of the fatty degeneration of the gland parenchyma, the blood-vessels lose their support, can no longer sufficiently resist the blood-pressure, and rupture. The changes affect mostly the smaller vessels, but the larger ones also may be involved in the lesion.

Alcoholism, general adiposity, and marasmus lie at the bottom of the process. It is doubtful whether there is not probably a primary disease of the pancreas as a cause for the obesity. It is certainly conceivable that at a certain stage in disease of the pancreas before there is diabetes an excessive development of fat may take place in accordance with the recognized relations between diabetes and obesity so clearly established by von Noorden.

Bauer (Ziemssen's clinic) reports an appropriate communication:

Enormous fatty degeneration of the pancreas, old and recent hemorrhages. There was a spot resembling an ulcer in the head of the considerably enlarged pancreas, and which seemed to have broken through the peritoneum and caused hemorrhage in it. Peritonitis.

Fatty degeneration of the gland and compact capillary hemorrhages occurred also in the case reported by La Fleur of a man fifty years old who had suffered from digestive disturbances for several years and was suddenly attacked by violent pains in the stomach, vomiting, and died in collapse.

In the case of Hooper: Sudden violent pain, vomiting, and collapse after frequently recurring gastric disturbances—"biliary attacks." Sickness lasted two days. At the autopsy, small extravasations of blood were found in the gland-follicles throughout the pancreas. Fatty degeneration was regarded as the cause of the hemorrhage (Seitz).

Zenker reported three cases of pancreatic hemorrhage with sudden death. In all three there were fatty degeneration and extreme hemorrhagic infiltration of the pancreas. Zenker did not regard the loss of blood as the cause of death, but believed that the influence of nerves was to be thought of, as in Goltz's experiment, in which repeated blows on the abdomen of frogs gives rise to diastolic cardiac paralysis. Zenker supported this view by the fact that he had found in two cases very striking venous hyperemia of the solar plexus with perfect integrity of the ganglion cells and nerve-fibers. Friedreich opposed this hypothesis by the statement that no mention was made in Zenker's case of the hyperemia and dilatation of all the vessels in the abdomen constantly observed in Goltz's experiment, and therefore must have been absent. He offers "as a cause of the fatal apoplexy an irritation of the semilunar ganglion and the solar plexus from pressure due to the rapid hemorrhagic swelling of the pancreas," and "a consequent reflex disturbance of the heart (reflex paralysis?)."

Recent communications have been made by Sticker and Kotschau. The former observed in a woman seventy-eight years old the occurrence of sudden death with violent colic-like pains a short time after she had suffered from vomiting, diarrhea, and pain in the left hypochondrium. Although there was no autopsy Sticker explained the symptoms in accordance with a second case observed by him.

A very fat woman, twenty-four years old, suffered from attacks of dyspnea, palpitation, and cramps in the stomach, in one of which death occurred. At the autopsy the liver was found much enlarged and fatty, and there were fresh hemorrhages in the center of the pancreas and a large infarction in its vicinity. The pancreas appeared transformed into a large mass of fresh blood which had forced the tissue apart and to a certain extent had disintegrated it. The ductus Wirsungianus was indicated only by a red thrombus of the size of the little finger, which extended to the papilla Vateri.

Sticker did not regard the simple fatty condition of the pancreas and its surrounding tissues as the sole predisposing cause of the hemorrhage, since he had never seen anything similar in other organs. He thought rather that the pulling and tearing of the pancreas by the excessively fat mesentery, increased by the movements of the body, easily gave rise to interruptions of continuity in the pancreas and caused hemorrhage. The hemorrhage spread more and more in consequence of the advancing fatty change. The occurrence of the colic indicated a renewal of the hemorrhage.

Kotschau saw a woman twenty-four years old who was attacked by frequent cardialgic pains. On physical examination nothing abnormal was found. The pains ceased after an injection of morphin. The next night the patient complained of nausea, tension, and a feeling of fulness in the abdomen, collapsed quickly, and died the same night. The patient was accustomed to liquor. At the autopsy all the internal organs were extremely fatty, there were numerous fat necroses in the peritoneum of the intestine, and abundant ecchymoses in the mucous membrane of the stomach. The liver and kidneys showed extreme fatty changes. There were several calculi in the gall-bladder. The heart was fatty to a marked degree. The pancreas lay behind the stomach as a black, structureless mass, tensely filled with blood and as large round as a man's arm. Kotschau also regarded the traction on the pancreas of the root of the mesentery and the fatty intestines as the source of hemorrhage.

3. **Fat necro**sis in the gland or in its vicinity is mentioned by many authors as the cause of pancreatic hemorrhage. Balser first attracted attention to the importance of this after an analogous condition in the bone-marrow had been shown by Ponfick. According to Balser, such a hyperplasia of young fat cells may occur in certain places in very fat individuals. Even in the marantic a surrounding inflammation may occur through which the blood-vessels are affected. Various degrees of hemorrhage may be the consequence.

Balser reports three similar cases.

The first case was that of a very strong fat woman, thirty-two years old, who was attacked by violent vomiting and severe pain in the loins and back four weeks before her entrance into the hospital. Fever, pain in the head, extraordinary swelling of the body, dyspnea. Sudden death in five days. At the autopsy there were found areas of fat necrosis from the size of a pea to that of a bean. A cavity was formed similar to an abscess by the adhesion of the transverse mesocolon to the mesentery, and it contained a liter of fluid, in which were bits of necrotic fat tissue of different size. The dead portions of fat tissue were often surrounded by a hemorrhagic zone of rust-red to dark-brown color. The pancreas lay in the cavity.

The appearances in the other two observations of Balser were similar, but the hemorrhage in the pancreas was much more intense.

In a case reported by Gerhardi, the hemorrhage was so great that an enormous swelling of the pancreas resulted, and in consequence compression and obstruction of the duodenum developed. In this case also the microscopic examination showed that there was necrosis of the fat tissue with hemorrhage into the surrounding tissue. Similar communications regarding cases of fat necrosis with hemorrhage have been presented by König, Marchand, Pinkham and Whitney, Guillery, Hirschberg, and more recently by Simon and Stanley, Cutler (2 cases), Sarfert (3 cases), Parry, Dunn, and Pitt and Rachmaninow. It must be stated, however, that in these cases the causal relation between the fat necrosis and the hemorrhage is not established (see section on Fat Necrosis).

A case observed by Simon and Stanley, and regarded as hemorrhage of the pancreas, was that of a woman sixty-three years old. For five days there had been pain and distention of the abdomen, slight jaundice, and later the vomiting was fecaloid and dark-brown. Two years before there had been, it was claimed, a similar attack. Laparotomy was performed on account of symptoms of intestinal obstruction. No occlusion was found. Death occurred a short time afterward. Autopsy: Body very fat, fat necrosis of the peritoneum. Pancreas much enlarged, infiltrated with blood, and showing fat necrosis. There were hemorrhages also toward the pelvis. The adhesions found depended perhaps on the earlier attack.

In a case reported by Cutler as "hemorrhagic pancreatitis," the patient was a woman fifty-two years old, and had 6.1% sugar. Disease lasted six days.

Sarfert's first case ("apoplexy of the pancreas") was that of a man thirty-nine years old, who, after carrying a heavy load, was suddenly attacked by pain in the left side of the abdomen. Nausea and retching. In the night, repeated vomiting, gradual swelling of the abdomen, constipation. On admission: Collapse, dyspnea, pulse scarcely perceptible; temperature 37.8° C. (100.04° F.), palpation painful, especially in the region of the stomach, where was a dense resistance on deep pressure. Hiccough, vomiting. Diagnosis: Ileus, internal strangulation. Laparotomy: Intestine dark-blue, distended, no incarceration; death after the operation. Autopsy two hours after death. Pancreas double in size, infiltrated with blood, and transformed into a mass resembling the spleen. Numerous fat necroses in the mesentery, omentum, and peritoneal fat tissue. Urine obtained after death contained 1% sugar.

In the case of pancreatic hemorrhage reported by Parry, Dunn, and Pitt, there were symptoms of intestinal obstruction in a man sixty years old. Laparotomy. Death four hours later. At the autopsy numerous small white or orange-colored areas of fat necrosis were found not far from the pancreas. This organ large, indurated, and on section infiltrated with blood.

4. **Hemorrhages in pancreatic cysts** are not uncommon. In the section on Cysts this condition was thoroughly considered (pages 186 and 190).

5. Cases of **hemorrhages from the disintegration of neoplasms** have been reported by Cash and Huber.

The first case was that of a woman sixty-one years old who had been sick for a long time, with constipation, attacks of pain in the umbilical region, nausea, and emaciation. Twice hematemesis occurred, the last time two hours before death. At the autopsy the stomach was distended with blood; pancreas enlarged, nodular, infiltrated with cancer; in the center was a large ulcerating cavity connected with the stomach by a ragged opening. A branch of the celiac artery also was opened.

Huber's case was a muscular, corpulent brewer, thirty-five years old, who had several attacks of pain in the epigastrium, which were regarded as the result of cholelithiasis; about eight months after the first attack of colic he suffered again from a violent pain in the region of the stomach. Soon afterward the pulse became exceedingly small and death suddenly occurred. At the autopsy a tumor of the head of the pancreas was found which surrounded the common duct. The gross appearances of the tumor corresponded with those of Förster's carcinoma simplex, and in addition, there were numerous pigmented and hemorrhagic spots.

In Baudach's case, previously mentioned, the hemorrhages occurred in consequence of erosion of the vessels in an angioma myxomatosum.

6. **Hemorrhage from embolism of a pancreatic artery** is reported in a case observed by Mollière.

7. **Trauma** may give rise to extensive hemorrhage in various organs of the abdomen, among which the pancreas and the surrounding subperitoneal connective tissue are included, or the pancreas and the surrounding connective tissue alone may be the seat of the hemorrhage.

Nimier distinguishes three groups of traumatic pancreatic hemorrhages:

(*a*) The pancreatic hemorrhage is the direct and immediate consequence of the trauma. An extensive or pure hemorrhagic extravasation takes place suddenly in the spaces of the great omentum.

(*b*) The trauma may cause hemorrhage and a rupture of the ductus Wirsungianus, and, in consequence, an admixture of pancreatic secretion. A cyst, therefore, forms in addition to the various symptoms of reactive inflammation. The contents are due to the activity of the escaped fluids modified by the inflammatory products of the neighboring tissue.

(*c*) The trauma affects an already diseased pancreas, and in such cases even a slight injury may cause hemorrhage.

The cases of Prince and of Foster and Fitz belong to the traumatic hemorrhages.

Prince gives the history of a strong porter, twenty-two years old, who, being in prison for eight days before the beginning of the disease, complained of a severe pain in the lower part of the abdomen immediately after turning a handspring. Eight days later there was a sudden violent cramp in the stomach. Soon collapse occurred, and for about fourteen days a moderate fever, temperature varying between 36.0° C. and 39.0° C. (96.8° F and 102.2° F.). Diarrhea. Vomiting. Meteorism. Increasing collapse. Death. At the autopsy, the region of the pancreas was black, consisting of dead, gangrenous shreds.

It is probable that a pancreatic hemorrhage had occurred and gradually ended in gangrene. It is certainly remarkable, as Seitz declares, that so slight an injury as turning a handspring should have produced such a hemorrhage, and it certainly is questionable whether there was not some other predisposing cause of the hemorrhage. [The trauma in this case was not from "das drehen eine Handmühle," as in the original German, but from turning a handspring, a much more violent procedure. —Ed.]

It is at least doubtful, as Seitz maintains, whether in the case of Foster and Fitz the hemorrhage was not the effect of the trauma upon pre-existing fatty degeneration of the vessels or from the production of fat necrosis. The man, fifty-nine years old and weighing 200 pounds, was thrown from a wagon, apparently without having suffered any injury, and four days later was attacked with pains in the abdomen and vomiting, and died on the tenth day.

The second of the groups suggested by Nimier includes only the cases of hemorrhagic cysts due to trauma, and consequently has been sufficiently considered in the section on Cysts.

8. **Inflammations of the pancrea**s may give rise to more or less severe hemorrhages. The relation of extensive hemorrhage to inflammation has been thoroughly discussed in the section on Hemorrhagic Pancreatitis.

Hemorrhagic pancreatitis belongs to the unsolved questions concerning the pancreas. The same case will be called by one author "hemorrhagic pancreatitis," and by another "apoplexy."

It is certain that the hemorrhage often exists alone or with subsequent inflammation; it is possible that an idiopathic inflammation may give rise to an extensive hemorrhage. Further observations and investigations will solve these important questions. Without doubt different factors act together in the production of hemorrhage, as is evident from the previously reported cases; for example, disease of the blood-vessels, obesity, alcoholism, trauma, etc. In the case of Prince, for instance, an old cardiac lesion, alcoholism, atheroma of the vessels, trauma. In the case reported by Seitz, great physical strain, obesity, alcoholism, and syphilis.

In a number of cases the cause for the hemorrhage cannot be given, partly on account of defective data, as in the cases of Löschner, Oppolzer, Amidon, Osler and Hughes, Birch-Hirschfeld, Hudson Rugg, Maynard and Fitz, Harris, Paul, Dieckhoff, and McPhedran.

Dieckhoff's first case was that of a cachectic man, sixty-three years old, with hypertrophy of the prostate and paresis of the bladder, who died with symptoms of increasing collapse on the third day after being under observation. At the autopsy, the pancreas formed a dark, brownish-red tumor, smooth on section. The lobules of the gland and small portions of the fat tissue in the immediate vicinity of the hemorrhage were necrotic.

The second case was a middle-aged woman who had suffered for years from diabetes mellitus. In the last year no sugar was found in the urine on repeated examination. At the autopsy there was an extensive extravasation of blood in the abdomen, which had destroyed also a portion of the pancreas.

A case reported by McPhedran is of especial interest, as it concerned a boy nine months old, on whom laparotomy was performed.

During the first three months of life there was frequent colic. Coagulated milk often was found in the stools. Intestines sluggish, stools soft and yellow. In the ninth month the stools became more fluid and contained numerous small, yellow, fatty particles. On November 13, 1895, vomiting suddenly occurred. On November 15th, temporary improvement, vomiting returned, followed by collapse. In the evening, colic for an hour, tenderness in the epigastrium, no dejection in spite of the use of purgatives. On November 16th, feeble and apathetic. Vomiting after taking food, no movement of the bowels in spite of laxatives. Abdomen slightly distended. An oblong mass as large round as the middle finger in the region of the ascending colon. It was hard, movable with respiration, dull on percussion. Intussusception was thought of. Operation. After the abdomen was opened, the resistance proved to be an accessory lobe of the liver. Intestine normal. Death the next morning. In making the diagnosis, the possibility of a hemorrhagic pancreatitis also was thought of. Autopsy: The middle third of the pancreas and its immediate vicinity were deeply infiltrated with blood.

PATHOLOGIC ANATOMY.

Klebs presents the following picture in his work published in 1870: " The pancreas is dark-red or violet, the meshes of the interstitial tissue are filled with fresh or altered blood, the acini dull gray, usually diffusely tinged with blood-pigment. The hemorrhagic masses extend also into the vicinity of the gland, and especially into the retroperitoneal connective tissue. Moreover, the whole gland appears softened, friable, the serous covering of the anterior surface is partially destroyed, and the ichorous, hemorrhagic material escapes into the omental bursa."

The following statements are derived from reports in recent literature:

The pancreas affected by hemorrhage appears, as a rule, enlarged, and only exceptionally of normal size (Draper). Fearnside states that in his case the gland was enlarged fourfold, while La Fleur, Putnam, and Whitney report that it was doubled in size.

The hemorrhage may arise within the gland and affect the whole organ or certain parts of it, or it may have its main seat in the peripancreatic tissue and from there penetrate into the gland.

The consistency of the gland varies. It appears somewhat increased in those cases in which inflammatory processes have already been established, but, as a rule, the gland is softer than normal. The softening may affect either the whole or certain parts of the organ. In the most advanced cases the tissue is completely disintegrated and discontinuous. A gangrenous, dark-red, discolored pulp replaces the pancreas (Prince).

Very frequently the gland is surrounded by a compact layer of tissue, infiltrated with blood, which must be cut through before the gland is exposed.

The surface of the organ is generally smooth. In Rugg's case a relatively large opening, resembling an ulcer, and containing a clot of blood as large as a walnut, was found on the anterior surface of the pancreas.

The color varies according to the intensity of the hemorrhage. Often only circumscribed spots of blood are visible, while in other cases the entire organ is changed into a dark-red or dark-brown mass, in which no structure is recognizable when the hemorrhage is extreme. These variations in color are seen also on section of the gland. In consequence of the frequent combination of hemorrhage and fatty changes the section appears marbled, from the alternation of hemorrhagic and fatty portions. The fatty alterations are especially marked in the interlobular tissue, and it appears traversed by opaque, white, broad or narrow patches which surround the darker portions infiltrated with blood. At times, although rarely, the hemorrhage affects only a portion of the gland, the rest of the organ appearing entirely free and showing normal structure (Putnam and Whitney).

Pigmented areas are found at times as the result of former hemorrhages; for instance, in the vicinity of fat necrosis.

When the hemorrhage occurs merely as the accompaniment of other conditions, or in death from suffocation, the extravasations, as a rule, are distributed through a part or the whole organ.

The ductus Wirsungianus is either dilated or it is occluded in places; at times filled with blood, which escapes through it from the lacerated gland into the intestine.

Hemorrhage is not, as a rule, limited to the pancreas, but generally extends into the surrounding tissue and infiltrates it more or less extensively. Moderate hemorrhages may be found in the adjacent mesentery and in the subperitoneal and retroperitoneal tissue. The hemorrhage takes place at times also into the general peritoneal cavity. In other cases a peritonitis is present (Prince, Bauer, Fearnside, Hirschberg) or the peritoneum may be normal. Death may have occurred too early, perhaps, for inflammation to have taken place, since blood may remain for a long time in the abdominal cavity without producing signs of irritation, as is shown by the observations of Dieckhoff.

The liver is stated in many cases to have been very fatty, a condition not to be surprised at when the usual etiologic factors are considered. In Kötschau's case the fatty liver appeared as one of the features of a general, excessive obesity. The serosa of the intestine showed numerous white deposits of calcium salts. Among the other changes of the abdominal organs, Kötschau mentions multiple ecchymoses in the mucous membrane of the stomach, Gerhardt-Kollmann ecchymoses in the mucosa of the cecum, Williams a small hemorrhage in the mesentery, Birch-Hirschfeld hemorrhagic contents in the duodenum.

There are other anatomic conditions allied to the hemorrhage, as fatty heart, atheroma of the coronary arteries, mitral stenosis (Prince), cardiac aneurysm (Zenker), aortic insufficiency, and emphysema (post-mortem records of the Vienna General Hospital).

Fearnside found the kidneys abnormally small and indurated. The venous hyperemia of the solar plexus noted by Zenker in two cases should be mentioned, because he regarded it as intimately connected with the hemorrhage.

The minute alterations of the gland structure can be investigated only in those cases in which there is no complete destruction of the tissue. The results of microscopic examination with regard to this point have been given by various authors. Each of the two following examples represents a different type. In the first (Putnam and Whitney), death occurred three days after the beginning of the illness, while in the second (Dieckhoff), the disease certainly lasted more than three weeks.

Putnam and Whitney found three sharply defined zones in the pancreas. In the middle zone was the interlobular fat tissue, continuous with the fat tissue surrounding the pancreas; it was extensively infiltrated with blood, and frequently made porous by the destruction of fat-cells. In other places it contained a fibrillated meshwork, finely granular material, bacteria, and numerous acicular fat crystals. In addition, foci of round-celled infiltration were found in this fat tissue between the relatively normal portions of the pancreas and the hemorrhagic and necrotic interlobular fat tissue.

On one side of this middle zone the acini were sharply defined and the nuclei stained easily. Many lobules contained granular epithelium and indistinct nuclei. Intralobular and interlobular infiltration with blood-corpuscles and numerous collections of round cells were seen in places. On the other side of the hemorrhagic zone, although the lobules were distinct, the outlines of the acini were frequently confused. The cells were granular, often not sharply defined, and the nuclei did not stain. In places the lobules were replaced by granular detritus and the cells were widely separated. Here and there between these necrotic acini, stained islands were found, evidently colonies of bacteria, thrombosed veins, and more rarely small collections of round cells (Fitz).

The changes which occur at a later stage of the hemorrhage are described by Dieckhoff in both his cases:

Dieckhoff found "the extravasated blood permeated in part by immature connective tissue proceeding from the living tissue in the neighborhood. The latter contained clusters of young connective-tissue cells, between which were polynuclear and single giant cells in addition to the wandering round cells; from this point the capillaries grew into the blood-clot, of which it inclosed large portions, and proceeded far into the tissue of the gland, and especially into the fat tissue. The gland-lobules and isolated small portions of the fat tissue in the immediate vicinity of the blood-clot were necrotic. The connective tissue also between the lobules and acini was dead."

The microscopic appearances of other inflammatory conditions and their relation to hemorrhage have already been mentioned in the cases of hemorrhagic pancreatitis (Zahn, Kraft, Haidlen, Dittrich).

Osler and Hughes, in a case of hemorrhage in the pancreas, found an increase of round cells in the semilunar ganglion, cloudy swelling of this ganglion, and edema of the Pacinian bodies lying behind the duodenum and pancreas. In the two following experiments on animals the occurrence of hemorrhage into the pancreas was shown by us:

EXPERIMENT OF JANUARY 17, 1895.—Injection of 5% chlorid of zinc into the tissue of the pancreas; 0.2 c.c. of a 5% zinc chlorid solution was injected into four different places. A hematoma resulted in one place at the middle portion of the pancreas, elsewhere there was no alteration from the injection. Abdominal wound closed. On January 18th the animal was found dead in the morning.

Autopsy: The abdominal cavity contained a moderate hemorrhagic exudation.

Pancreas appeared enlarged and infiltrated with blood except a place about as large as a kreuzer in the free descending portion. On section the structure in the duodenal portion was not recognizable. Elsewhere evidences of a lobular structure were seen in places. In the descending portion the structure of the normal pancreas appeared more distinct. Duodenum deeply injected; intestinal contents somewhat colored with blood. Liver of normal size and consistency, somewhat anemic in places.

EXPERIMENT OF FEBRUARY 17, 1895.—Injection of $\frac{1}{10}$ normal sulphuric acid into the ductus Wirsungianus. Dog of medium size; without food for thirty-six hours. The ductus Wirsungianus was opened at the point of entrance into the intestine and 4 c.c. of sulphuric acid were injected by means of a Pravaz syringe. The injection was easily made. As the fluid penetrated the tissue, the splenic portion of the pancreas became somewhat more succulent, the lobules stood out more distinctly, and the venous injection of the previously pale organ, became more pronounced. Ligation of the duct and section between the ligatures. On February

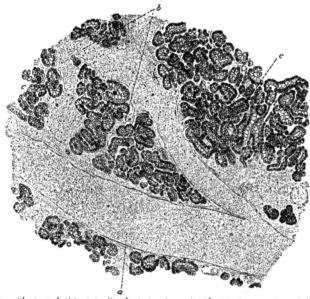

FIG. 13.—*a,* Blood-vessel distended with blood; *b,* extravasated blood in the parenchyma between the lobules; *c,* normal pancreatic tissue.

18th the animal was found dead in the morning. Life lasted about twenty hours after the operation. Urine and stools evacuated; vomiting of mucous fluid. Urine brownish-yellow, about 150 c.c. Sugar 2.2%. Acetone in small amount (shown in the distillate). Indican in small amount.

Autopsy: Peritoneum pale, intestine contracted, empty, pale; the duodenum only somewhat more strongly injected. In the stomach about 20 c.c. of brownish, turbid, slimy fluid of neutral reaction. Pancreas of normal size, with a hemorrhage as large as a pea in the duodenal part corresponding to the ductus Wirsungianus. The tissue here is degenerated and the structure indistinct. In the splenic portion the tissue is more succulent, the lobules are indistinct and blurred. Tissue appears opaque. The remaining portion of the pancreas is of normal appearance and consistency. Spleen small and shows nothing abnormal. Liver appears normal.

A microscopic preparation obtained from the experiment first described is shown in figure 13.

Résumé.—In the first experiment a hematoma occurred in one place as the immediate result of the injection. Both animals died within twenty-four hours. In the second experiment, glycosuria was present. At the autopsy on the first animal there was a hemorrhagic exudation in the abdominal cavity and an extensive destruction of the tissue of the whole pancreas in consequence of the hemorrhage, except of a portion of the size of a kreuzer in the free descending portion. On microscopic examination distinctly enlarged blood-vessels are seen engorged with blood, and there is hemorrhage into the parenchyma of the gland, which is forced apart in different places. The parenchyma appeared normal without any signs of inflammatory changes. In the second case these changes could be seen only in circumscribed spots near the ductus Wirsungianus.

SYMPTOMS.

Pancreatic hemorrhage is never wholly free from symptoms except in those cases in which small hemorrhages are found incidentally at the autopsy.

A great variety of symptoms are mentioned in the cases of non-traumatic hemorrhages hitherto reported. It is scarcely to be assumed that years of constipation, disturbed appetite or digestion, have any thing to do with the later occurrences, but it may be that these are due to gradually developing changes in the pancreas, which afterward may become the cause of the hemorrhage. Likewise colic and attacks of cramps also which have occurred years before the hemorrhage can scarcely be considered as having any relation. It is different with the transient colicky pains in the region of the stomach, which occur without definite cause during the weeks or months preceding the hemorrhage. Although it is not easy to bring forward positive proof that they are perhaps related to the small hemorrhages in the gland, yet it is quite probable that the fatal hemorrhage is preceded by smaller hemorrhages which may be manifested by the appearance of such pains. It certainly is to be assumed that slight hemorrhages may be recovered from. In many cases, however, there are no prodromal symptoms. The attack occurs quite suddenly during the best of health and not infrequently causes sudden death. Violent pain is the most frequent and constant symptom. As a rule, it dominates the picture of the disease and lasts until death.

The seat of the pain is not always the same. It is limited, as a rule, to the abdomen, although in a case reported by Hooper the disease began with severe pain below the left breast, and in that of Rugg there was pain in the left lumbar region. The point of most intense pain varies: at times it is in the region of the stomach, the left hypochondrium, the region of the right colon, and again the most intense pain is felt in the lower abdomen. The pain is generally colic-like in character and may abate at times or entirely disappear, and then return with increased severity. The degree of the pain also may vary. As a rule, it is very violent and almost unendurable. Exceptionally there is only a dull, painful sensitiveness throughout the abdomen. Stojanovics divides this somewhat too categorically into two varieties:

(a) Epigastric pains with a sense of warmth; they occur especially when the stomach is empty, increase gradually, recur at shorter and shorter intervals, and are often accompanied by vomiting of a fluid resembling saliva, sometimes acid and sometimes tasteless, and which is evacuated with the sensation of burning pains along the esophagus.

(b) Pains above the umbilicus. These are said to occur at a later stage. They radiate toward the spine, have a dull, intermittent character, and occur with the greatest severity a few hours after eating. Opiates, as a rule, give no special relief. The development of these severe pains is explained by the close relationship between the pancreas and the sympathetic nerve apparatus. An enlargement of the gland must result in pressure on the semilunar ganglion, while, on the other hand, the mesenteric plexus is woven around the blood-vessels of the gland (Nimier).

Vomiting naturally occurs very frequently in this as in every acute pathologic process in the abdomen. A mere inclination to vomit or the absence of vomiting is exceptional. The vomiting as a rule is cumulative. At times it intermits for a few hours or for a day or two; then it returns, perhaps with a fresh exacerbation of the hemorrhage or with a beginning peritonitis, and increases in severity toward the end of life. The vomited substance is often greenish, stained with bile. A dark brown fluid (Fearnside) or actual blood (Hooper) are relatively rare.

Hemoptysis was observed in a case reported by Draper. Fecaloid vomiting has been observed in several cases, for instance, those of Hovenden, Simon, and Stanley. Hiccough has occurred under certain circumstances, both with and before the vomiting. Jaundice was very rare.

The abdomen is often distended and tympanitic. The meteorism is either extended uniformly over the whole abdomen and increases toward the end of life (Hooper), or it is limited to the upper part of the abdomen (Hilty).

A tumor on palpation of the abdomen is extremely rare in pure hemorrhage. Fearnside was able to feel a deep transverse tumor between the ensiform process and the umbilicus. Hirschberg was able to show on the right only a larger coil of intestine. McPhedran found in the region of the ascending colon an oblong mass as thick as the middle finger. This proved at the operation to be an accessory lobe of the liver. When there are hemorrhages in cysts or neoplasms or the formation of cysts from hemorrhage, a tumor can be palpated. Fever rarely occurs in consequence of the rapid progress. Birch-Hirschfeld noted the presence of high fever in his two cases, and in some of the histories reported a moderate fever is noted. Morton Prince notes the occurrence of repeated chills. Subnormal temperatures are easily understood in a disease in which collapse is so frequent. The pulse is usually small, weak, feeble, corresponding to the rapid diminution of strength, and collapse.

The sensorium is, as a rule, well preserved. Loss of consciousness is noted among the exceptions (Kotschau); also delirium (Birch-Hirschfeld, Hilty).

Few changes in the urine are observed in the short course of the disease. As a rule, the urine was not examined or there was complete anuria. Whitney mentions the presence of albuminuria, and Gerhardi the lack of indican. In the case observed by Dieckhoff, diabetes had existed earlier, but the urine was free from sugar at the time of the hemorrhage. Cutler found 6.1% sugar in his patient. Sarfert found 1% of sugar in the urine removed after death.

The condition of the bowels varies; constipation is more frequent than diarrhea. The disease not infrequently develops with the symptoms of intestinal obstruction, as, for instance, in the cases of Gerhardi, Fitz, Hirschberg, Hovenden, McPhedran, Parry, Dunn and Pitt, Simon and Stanley, Sarfert, Allina. When cysts form, the intestine may be obstructed by pressure.

Attacks of fainting were observed by Fearnside three days before death. Collapse is an extremely frequent occurrence, and forms one of the essential features of the disease. In the fulminating cases it develops quite suddenly after the patient has been perfectly well, or it appears a few hours after the first pain. In the cases progressing more slowly it occurs also somewhat independently two or three days after the existence of the symptoms. It is the forerunner of impending death, and it has never been overcome.

COURSE.

Hemorrhages may be divided into those with acute and those with chronic course, apart from the cases in which slight hemorrhages occur without disturbance, and which it is probable may be wholly recovered from. The former are the more frequent, and Nimier makes three subdivisions: (*a*) the fulminating; (*b*) the very acute; (*c*) the acute.

The cases are most numerous in which there is an interval of twenty-four to thirty-six hours between the first symptoms of the disease and death. The chronic cases include those in which the hemorrhage takes place at intervals and which, under certain circumstances, may recover, a part of the whole gland being sequestrated and discharged. Among the chronic cases also are those in which hemorrhagic cysts eventually form. These chronic cases may last for weeks or even months.

In the fulminating cases, death occurs suddenly or in the course of an hour. What is the cause of this sudden death?* Undoubtedly in a number of cases it is not the quantity of blood lost and the resulting anemia. A series of cases have already been referred to in which the quantity of extravasated blood was much too small to permit the death to be regarded as the result of hemorrhage. It is also improbable that the sudden disturbance of function of a part or of the whole gland should be regarded as the cause of death. This is contraindicated, in the first place, by the results of experiments on animals, which show that animals survive the sudden removal of the entire organ.

Other factors must be presented in explanation. Mention has already been made of two hypotheses. Zenker believes death to be due to shock, analogous to Goltz's experiment, and supports his view by his autopsies. In two cases he was able to show a very marked venous hyperemia of the celiac plexus; the heart was relaxed, the cavities distended, and contained no blood. The abdominal vessels also were hyperdistended, a condition analogous to that found in Goltz's experiment.

Sarfert found a similar condition in his second case: flabby, empty heart, abdominal vessels hyperdistended, venous hyperemia of the solar plexus. Friedreich considers it more justifiable to regard the death as due to the irritation of the semilunar ganglion by the pressure of the rapidly distended pancreas and a consequent disturbance of the movements of the heart.

* The publication of Greiselius of 1672 is worthy of note: "Observatio de repentina suavi morte ex pancreate sphacelato." (Death of a man forty-two years old in an attack of colic, eighteen to nineteen hours after the beginning of the illness.)

There are no new hypotheses advanced since the communications of Zenker and Friedreich, but Seitz remarked: "The future must decide whether the disturbed function of the pancreas lacerated by the hemorrhage may not play a part." Doubtless there are cases in which death is wholly the result of hemorrhage, as in that reported by Seitz.

The explanation of those cases in which the course is mild at first and becomes violent only in the last days or hours may be sought in the fact that the hemorrhage was periodic in its occurrence and only finally became intense enough to cause death.

The chronic course may be brought about in different ways: by periodic occurrence of the hemorrhage, or by the subsequent development of a peritonitis, sepsis, necrosis, or suppuration of the pancreas, escape of the fluid into the peritoneal cavity or into the stomach and intestine. It has already been mentioned that in certain cases at such a stage recovery may take place by sequestration and discharge of the gland.

DIAGNOSIS.

It is perhaps impossible with our present means to diagnosticate positively a pancreatic hemorrhage or a "hemorrhagic pancreatitis." Even under the most favorable circumstances it may be suspected that there is perhaps such a condition. To be sure, in the case observed by them, Fitz and Williams made the diagnosis of acute pancreatitis or pancreatic hemorrhage. This was of course only a diagnosis based on probability.

In the case of Williams, a man seventy years of age was suddenly seized with colicky pain in the region of the stomach which lasted five hours and radiated toward the left and toward the navel; the region of the stomach was not sensitive, there was vomiting, the pulse was regular and small, six hours later collapse occurred and sixteen hours afterward death took place. It must be admitted that in this case various diseases were to be thought of, and that it was not necessary to regard pancreatic hemorrhage or hemorrhagic inflammation as the only possibility.

In fact, in most of the cases of pancreatic hemorrhage there was either no diagnosis or the affection was regarded as something quite different. Intestinal obstruction, peritonitis from perforation, perforating ulcer of the stomach or intestine, pyosepticemia arising from the intestine, purulent peritonitis, etc., have been suspected.

The diagnosis is made relatively most easily in traumatic hemorrhage. A pancreatic cyst from trauma may be thought of when after injury to the abdomen there are sudden violent pain and prostration and afterward a tumor appears more or less distinctly fluctuating behind the stomach between the navel and the costal cartilages.

As a matter of fact, the diagnosis of a traumatic pancreatic cyst has been definitely established in certain cases by means of an exploratory puncture, and a successful operation has resulted.

In the present state of our knowledge, in certain cases the possibility of a pancreatic hemorrhage also, with or without inflammation, may be thought of with many other possibilities, when there are no further indications for diagnosis, if an individual who in consequence of his constitution, as in atheromatosis, syphilis, obesity, alcoholism, etc., is liable to diseases of the pancreas is suddenly seized in the midst of health by a violent attack of pain in the epigastrium with vomiting and collapse, and speedy death occurs in a few hours or days.

Even in the chronic cases in which there are manifestations of peritonitis or gangrene of the pancreas and rupture of ichorous cavities the nature of the disease is hardly more than to be suspected, and the condition must be made clear by an operation or the discharge in the feces of the sequestrated pancreas. Even then, as in Chiari's case, it will be doubtful whether the sequestration of the gland was the result of inflammation or of hemorrhage.

TREATMENT.

There can be no question of a rational treatment in an affection of so rapid a course, the correct diagnosis of which is so difficult. Nothing further need be said of the insufficiency of internal treatment. Simon and Stanley propose the prophylactic use of intestinal antiseptics, especially salol; based on the assumption of the etiologic importance of a bacillary infection from the duodenum, and because they regard the prolonged retention of chyme in the duodenum, especially in fat people, as increasing the danger of infecting the pancreas.

Surgical treatment also is probably useless in the acute cases. A number of successful results show that an operation is indicated only in the cases in which cysts or abscesses develop.

VII. PANCREATIC CALCULI.

THE formation of concretions in the pancreas has been recognized for a long time. According to the thorough study of Giudiceandrea, the first communication dates from the middle of the seventeenth century. Graaf (1667) mentions two cases observed by Panarol and Gaeia. These were followed by the publications of Bonetus (1700), Galeati (1757), Morgagni (1765), Greding (1769), and Cowley (1788).

In the beginning of the nineteenth century, Merklin and Baillie reported two cases of pancreatic calculi. After a long interval appeared the publications of Elliotson (1832), Gould (1847), and Fauconneau-Dufresne (1851). Soon afterward Virchow reported two cases (1852), and in 1864 v. Recklinghausen published his important communication. Publications have appeared more frequently since 1875, and especially in recent years a large number of very instructive observations have been communicated by Freyhan (2 cases), Fleiner, Lichtheim, Minnich and Holzmann, and the comprehensive publications of Nimier and Giudiceandrea. The last-mentioned author collected 48 cases, to which two original cases were added.*

There is no doubt that only a small percentage of calculi of the

* Besides these the cases should be mentioned of Clayton, Crowden, Dieckhoff (2 cases), Fleiner, Frerichs, Gille, Gagliard, Leichtenstern (2 cases), Michailow, Moore (3 cases), Müller, Munk and Klebs, Nicolas and Mollière, Rörig, Shattock. A case of pancreatic calculus is reported among the autopsies of the Vienna General Hospital in 1894, in a man sixty years old, with fatty degeneration of the substance of the gland and fibrous induration. Thus, in all there are 70 known cases.

pancreas found at autopsies is published. It is not very rare to find small concretions or sand in the pancreas or in the pancreatic ducts. Statements with reference to this condition are to be found in the text-books on pathologic anatomy by Ziegler, Birch-Hirschfeld, and Orth.

Number of Calculi.—As a rule, several calculi are found. In the collection made by Ancelet (1860) in only three cases was there a solitary calculus; in individual patients 4, 7, or 8 and in two 12 calculi were found, while in eight other cases the occurrence of numerous concretions is noted.

Not infrequently the main duct or the smaller excretory ducts are actually incrusted with sand. Sottas, for example, found numerous small calculi in the main duct and in the small adjoining ducts in addition to a calculus as large as a bean near the outlet of the duct in the duodenum. Numerous concretions were found in small, newly formed cavities in the sclerosed substance of the gland. Baumel also saw numerous calculi both in the excretory ducts and in the canals of the gland, in shape wholly adapted to the cavities in which they lay. In Curnow's case, likewise, the smallest excretory ducts of the gland were entirely filled with calculi. Lancereaux found both excretory ducts occluded by large calculi, and, in addition, an extensive incrustation of the excretory ducts of the second order.

Seat of the Calculi.—According to the cases thus far reported, the calculi are oftenest to be found in the excretory ducts near the duodenal opening, at times in the diverticulæ of the duct, as mentioned by Freyhan and Giudiceandrea. Concretions are rarely met in the caudal portion of the duct. The calculi are found also in the small and smallest excretory ducts in the parenchyma, even in sacculations of the ducts, and are either freely movable, enveloped in slimy fluid, or attached to the wall.

Pancreatic calculi have been found at times in cysts (Giudiceandrea, Shattock) and in abscesses, as in the cases of Fauconneau-Dufresne, Fournier, Leichtenstern, Moore, Portal, and Salmade.

Size.—As a rule, the size of the pancreatic calculi is not great; it is compared with that of a bean, pea, lentil, hemp-seed, hazelnut, or large cherry, in addition to the previously mentioned gravel-like concretions which incrust the pancratic canals like fine sand. The largest calculus on record was $2\frac{1}{2}$ inches long and $\frac{1}{2}$ inch in diameter (Schupmann).

Weight.—The weight corresponds with the size, and is usually small. Matani and Schupmann found the heaviest calculi; the weight reported by the former was 2 ounces, while that by the latter was 200 grains.

The *shapes* of the calculi may vary exceedingly. They are spherical, ovoid, with smooth or rough surface, at times also are arborescent. The calculus described by Schupmann resembled the crystalline formations which are found on and around the frames at salt-refining works. Various pointed elevations—outgrowths, as it were—project like branches of a tree some lines above the surface; these are processes of the calculus which, proceeding from the body, have continued into the branches of the main excretory duct and have filled them.

The *color* of the calculi is white, whitish-gray, or yellowish. Exceptionally, dark and even black stones are described (Bonetus, Merklin). .

The *consistency* is either hard or soft, very friable.

Chemical Composition.—Virchow found in the excretory ducts of the pancreas two small, microscopic, concentrically striated, somewhat firm concretions, with the microscope showing concentric lamellæ, and composed of an insoluble coagulated proteid substance; statements of the other authors agree that the pancreatic calculi most frequently consist of calcium carbonate and calcium phosphate. In addition to these, inorganic substances, as sodium phosphate, magnesium phosphate, and sodium chlorid, were found; and of organic constituents, cholesterin, leucin, tyrosin, xanthin, and the above-mentioned coagulated proteid substance found by Virchow. Henry analyzed a concretion which weighed 9 gm., was of the size of a nut, and was also interesting because of its external form. Projections from one surface extended into the tissue of the gland; the entire surface was surrounded by a hard, resistant membrane, the removal of which permitted the recognition of a system of hollow spaces which were filled with yellowish concretions and powdery sand. All these spaces were filled with a white, milky fluid, which held in suspension a calcium salt. Two-thirds of the concretion were composed of calcium phosphate; the remainder was composed of equal parts of calcium carbonate and organic material. In addition, traces of sodium phosphate and sodium chlorid were demonstrable. The small bodies resembling grapeseeds consisted of calcium carbonate and organic matter.

The occurrence of calcium phosphate in the concretions is mentioned also by more recent authors. Generally calcium carbonate also is found, and in rare cases the latter is present alone (Freyhan). In one of Freyhan's cases the calculus, as large as a plum-stone, had a nucleus of pure calcium carbonate and a soft envelope of organic substance in which cholesterin especially was found. The calculi found by Minnich in the feces also consisted of calcium carbonate and calcium phosphate. The results of chemical analysis show that in the formation of the calculi there is not a simple precipitation from the secretion of a normal gland, as the normal pancreatic juice contains only a small amount of calcium phosphate and is entirely free from calcium carbonate.

One of Shattock's observations appears unique. Small calculi consisting of pure oxalate of lime were found in the contents of a pancreatic cyst. Shattock thought that the oxalic acid had been produced by microorganisms. According to present knowledge, only Aspergillus niger in anaerobic growth can produce this acid.

PATHOGENESIS.

The causation of calculi in the pancreas is at present obscure. The material for investigation is rare, and therefore insufficiently studied to justify too positive assertions. In general, the assumption appears plausible that there are the same determining factors as in the formation of gallstones. The simple stagnation of the secretion is certainly one of the most important factors, but it is not the only decisive one. From anatomic reasons the secretion of the pancreas becomes much more rarely stagnant than is the case with the bile. If only one excretory duct is obstructed, the second duct can assume the function and permit the evacuation of the secretion into the intestine. In order to cause a complete retention, either both ducts must be obstructed, or, what is oftener the case, the second duct must be obliterated, either congenitally or from some acquired affection, or numerous intrapancreatic ducts must have become impermeable.

That stagnant secretion alone does not cause the formation of concretions is supported by the clinical fact that in many cases of closure of the

15

excretory ducts, whatever may be the cause, no calculi could be found. Calculi could not be produced, as a rule, in experiments on animals, either by tying the Wirsungian duct or by injection into it (Pawloff, Mouret). Thiroloix alone was successful in one instance. He injected sterilized soot into the ductus Wirsungianus. At the autopsy the gland was found atrophied, and in the splenic portion surrounded by dense connective tissue, there was a cystic cavity, containing a fluid as clear as water, in which were numerous very dense, irregularly shaped calculi of the size of a pinhead. The ductus Wirsungianus also was filled with small calculi.

The fact already mentioned that there is no calcic carbonate in the normal pancreatic secretion, while pancreatic calculi very often are composed of this material, is in favor of the view that pathologic changes in the pancreatic juice precede the formation of the calculi; that is, that the stagnation first causes formation of calculi, when it is composed of a pathologic pancreatic secretion.

Analogous to the pathogenesis of gall-stones, it may be assumed that a catarrh in the pancreatic ducts—a *sialangitis catarrhalis*—causes such changes in the pancreatic secretion that the resulting stagnation leads to the formation of calculi. An ascending duodenal catarrh in most cases is the probable origin of such a catarrh, and if both excretory ducts are simultaneously affected, a sufficient explanation is offered for the stagnation and also for the alteration of the pancreatic juice, which leads to the formation of the calculi.

Changes in the pancreatic secretion and disturbances in the outflow of the secretion may be accomplished also by other causes. An abnormal secretion may be formed by morbid, especially indurative processes in the gland, and the resulting hindered outflow of secretion may give rise to the formation of concretions. In one of the cases of Lancereaux, syphilis and, in that of Baumel, chronic alcoholism, are mentioned as etiologic factors. It is conceivable that these processes leading toward the production of chronic indurative inflammation of the pancreas might cause stagnation of a pathologic secretion and thus give rise to the formation of calculi.

Pathologic processes in the vicinity of the pancreas which limit the outflow of the secretion from the gland may, together with stagnation, cause such changes of the secretion as to give the conditions necessary for the formation of calculi. Gall-stones which press on or are wedged in the ductus Wirsungianus, peripancreatic indurations, and neoplasms— although these are rare conditions—thus may cause lithiasis in the pancreatic ducts.

In the presence of a stagnant secretion *sialangitis pancreatica* must play the most important part in the formation of calculi in the pancreas, analogous to the condition of cholangitis in cholelithiasis. A lithogenic importance is ascribed by many authors to the immigration of bacteria from the intestine, a condition which is easily possible. Nimier supports this view by the positive results of the examination by Galippe of salivary calculi which are chemically and nosologically analogous to pancreatic calculi. In one of his cases Giudiceandrea found, in the midst of numerous calcium crystals and detritus, a large number of similar bacilli of the shape of Bacterium coli, and, in addition to these, a considerable number of long, delicate bacilli, which he was unable to identify. In a second case investigated bacteriologically he saw numerous forms of cocci and bacilli of various kind and size, but, on the whole, in much smaller numbers than in the first case. The normal pancreatic secretion was free from micro-organisms.

Giudiceandrea considered it questionable what importance should be attached to the discovery of the colon bacillus in the nucleus of a pancreatic calculus, but thinks it can hardly be denied that its presence may contribute to the progress of calculus formation. Farther investigations are needed to decide whether this assumption can account for the development of pancreatic calculi or whether there is a direct bacterial influence.

It is well known that Naunyn has established the frequent occurrence of Bacterium coli commune in the biliary passages and inclines to the view that the invasion of this bacterium gives rise to a catarrh of the mucous membrane and thus to the formation of calculi. Further investigations must decide whether this view applies also to the origin of pancreatic calculi or whether there is a direct bacterial influence. The immigration of pathogenic bacteria from the intestine might have considerable importance in the causation of an infectious sialangitis, which would lead to the formation of an abscess if there were calculi in the pancreas. Unfortunately there are no investigations at present tending to the solution of this question.

PATHOLOGIC ANATOMY.

The pathologic changes which have been found in the gland when calculi are present may be primary or secondary; that is, they may be the cause or the result of their formation. The presence of calculi in the gland gives rise to secondary changes of the parenchyma which may lead to the complete destruction of the secreting tissue. Fatty degeneration of the parenchyma may occur; this was true, for instance, in v. Recklinghausen's case, in which the pancreas was changed into a mass consisting of fat lobules, resembling the normal organ only in form and size, but showing no gland tissue. In Freyhan's cases, also, only fat and connective tissue were present in place of the normal gland tissue.

In other cases either induration or atrophy occurred. In one of Moore's cases, in which the stone compressed the ductus Wirsungianus near its mouth and caused distinct dilatation, marked increase of connective tissue was clearly visible to the naked eye. On microscopic examination the interstitial growth of connective tissue was especially distinct and occasional bands of round cells showed that in certain parts of the gland the process was still advancing. The new-formation of connective tissue followed the marked dilatation of the pancreatic ducts and caused a pancreatic cirrhosis, as disease of the bile-ducts in the liver causes a growth of connective tissue with the eventual result of cirrhosis. Similar conditions were shown by Lichtheim, Fleiner, Sottas (combined with fatty degeneration), and Lancereaux (associated with atrophy of the gland), and Baumel found the growth of connective tissue especially connected with the vessels and excretory ducts. Hansemann notes two cases of pancreatic calculi in which there was atrophy of the whole organ. Curnow also reports a case with marked atrophy of the pancreas.

The occurrence of abscesses in consequence of calculus formation is relatively rare (Fournier, Salmade, Portal, Roddick, Moore, Fauconneau-Dufresne, Leichtenstern, Galeati). As a result of the obstruction from the calculus there is naturally a dilatation of the pancreatic ducts, which may attain considerable dimensions, according to the size and number of the incarcerated calculi and the quantity of stagnant secretion. In v. Recklinghausen's case a partial ectasia thus attained the size of a child's head. The dilatation is in many cases to be regarded as the result of the atrophy and shrinkage of the gland lobules.

As has been previously described, the dilatation may extend to the smallest ducts. Diverticula may occur and incrustations may cover the entire wall of the small and smallest ducts as well as of the sacculi proceeding from them. In rare cases cysts may form in consequence of this dilatation (Clark, Curnow, Dieckhoff, Goodmann, Gould, v. Recklinghausen, Tricomi). The necrosis of fat tissue also at times is associated (Giudiceandrea). Cancer in rare cases also accompanies the calculus, and, according to Schupmann, may cause the latter by stenosis of the excretory duct.

Calculi in the biliary passages not infrequently accompany those in the pancreas. Ancelet has collected eight such cases; this concurrence was found also in the cases of Curnow, Phulpin, and Dieckhoff. Renal calculi also may be found at the same time. In the earlier literature such a case is noted by Merklin. A woman thirty-six years old suffering for twelve years from renal colic, evacuated calculi with the urine, and a concretion as large as a nut was discharged in the feces. At the autopsy a calculus as large as a nut was found in the pancreas and there was a large abscess in the mesentery, which contained three calculi of the size of almonds and several smaller calculi. In the kidney there were none.

In the small intestine there is at times a diffuse catarrh (Lichtheim), or hypertrophy of the duodenal glands (Lancereaux).

STATISTICS.

There are only a few statements concerning the frequency of pancreatic calculi. Giudiceandrea states that in 122 bodies which were examined after death within three months, calculi were found in the pancreas twice. This may be regarded as a relatively high ratio. According to Naunyn, the proportion of gall-stones, judging from results of postmortem examinations in the different pathologic institutes, is between 5% and 12%. The ratio given by Giudiceandrea is 1.64%. Further observations are necessary in order to make more definite statements.

AGE.

In 32 cases the age is as follows:

	MEN.	WOMEN.
5 to 10 years	1	0
11 to 15 "	1	0
16 to 20 "	0	0
21 to 25 "	2	1
26 to 30 "	2	0
31 to 35 "	2	2
36 to 40 "	6	1
41 to 45 "	4	0
46 to 50 "	2	0
51 to 55 "	2	0
56 to 60 "	1	2
61 to 65 "	1	0
66 to 70 "	0	0
71 to 75 "	2	0
Total	26	6

This table shows that calculi occur oftenest between the ages of thirty-six and forty-five years and are much more frequent in men than in women.

SYMPTOMS.

Pancreatic calculi without doubt frequently cause no symptoms, especially when they lie quietly in the place where they arise. Decided symptoms first appear when the calculi begin to move or when the secondary changes in the gland give rise to especially prominent symptoms of disease. The picture of the disease can be most clearly presented if a well-observed case is briefly reproduced, such as that described by Minnich:

A man sixty-eight years old was attacked in his fortieth year by very severe biliary colic. Typical pigmented gall-stones were found in the stools by the physician. After ten years there was a recurrence of the attacks with the discharge of pigmented cholesterin calculi during a period of six months. Quiescence followed. In the summer of 1893 the patient had several attacks of cramps which he regarded as biliary colic. In November, 1893, there were feelings of pressure and tension over the region of the stomach. The difficulty lasted for one month without the occurrence of an attack of colic. Toward the end of the month there was diarrhea without pain for three days. On the third of December, Minnich saw the patient during an attack of colic. There were severe, cramp-like, writhing pains in the left hypochondrium. The patient makes the following statement regarding the pains: There was first a dull sensation of pressure and constriction over the epigastrium and under the left border of the ribs, which caused him now to inspire deeply and again to press the painful places with his fist and to walk restlessly about the room. The pains soon became stronger and increased to actual paroxysms. They were localized especially in one spot, deep in the abdomen, close to the left border of the ribs within the mammillary line. At the height of the attack the pains proceed in circles along the edge of the costal cartilages to the spine and dart violently beneath the left shoulder-blade. When the pains abate, they return to the above-mentioned spot beneath the left costal cartilage, and which the patient states that he could cover with a 5-franc piece. There is a slight tenderness to pressure in the place mentioned. The attack stopped suddenly after two hours. Neither albumin, sugar, nor bile pigment were to be found in the urine. The attacks were of almost daily occurrence. The temperature was normal; pulse regular, 76. Liver not enlarged, gall-bladder not palpable, stomach not dilated. The examination of the feces showed round or flat concretions varying in size from a lentil to a cherry-stone; small crumbs and gravel also were found. The concretions consisted of a tough, semi-solid mass which could be crushed with the finger. The surface was smooth, the color light yellowish-gray. The cut surface was perfectly white and was similar to that of a fruit-seed. Lamination and a central nucleus were not recognized. Microscopically the substance of the calculus appeared perfectly amorphous. The calculi were very readily soluble in chloroform which became opaque-white. On heating in a test-tube dense fumes of strongly aromatic odor arose; in the upper part there was some yellow water of condensation, and a perfectly white calculus which gave the reaction of calcium carbonate, and phosphate appeared in the residue. The attacks were repeated in the further course of the disease, but no more concretions were found. About three weeks after Minnich's observation, Holzmann saw the patient in Eichhorst's clinic. The attacks of colic occurred in the way above described, but some noteworthy symptoms had developed. During the attack the patient had a marked flow of saliva, over a liter of nearly clear viscid fluid, mixed with a few fragments of food, being discharged. The examination of the salivary fluid showed a weak potassium-sulphocyanid reaction, and it very actively changed starch into sugar. In the examination of the urine sugar was found, all tests being positive: Amount, 1100 c.c.; specific gravity, 1022; no maltose was found. In the later attacks there was a moderate flow of saliva, but no sugar was found in the urine. Later there was a fever reaching 38.2° C. (100.8° F.). The feces contained here and there undigested muscle-fibers, no fat crystals; concretions were no longer found.

Only a few of the cases which have been reported have had so typical a course as that just described.

The pains or unpleasant sensations may be of different kinds. There may be an almost continuous feeling of pressure or dull sensation of pain in the epigastrium, or there may be temporary attacks of more or less pronounced colic varying in intensity and duration. In the case of Minnich-Holzmann they were centered under the border of the left ribs. This may perhaps rarely be the case. They are generally concentrated in the epigastrium, radiate to both sides, and are in no way distinguishable from atypical biliary colic or gastralgia. These pains, as all violent abdominal colic, may be accompanied by nausea, retching, vomiting, and collapse.

Salivation is not a frequent occurrence, in cases of pancreatic calculi. Capparelli, Holzmann, and Giudiceandrea alone have observed it. Diarrheas are noted by Fleiner and Lichtheim. In the case described by the latter, the diarrhea lasted for a year and resisted all treatment.

The occurrence of fatty stools is of great importance. They were present in the cases described by Clark, Gould, Reeves, Capparelli, Chopart, and Lancereaux. Lichtheim found fat crystals very abundant in the stools. Faulty digestion of meat also was found at times. Holzmann occasionally saw a few undigested muscle-fibers.

The presence in the stools of concretions originating from the pancreas is the most important and most decisive symptom. There are two such observations up to the present time, those of Minnich and Leichtenstern. In Merklin's case a calculus was found in the feces, but it was not proved that it came from the pancreas, although after death a calculus was found in the pancreas.

The frequent occurrence of diabetes is of great importance, and was noted by Baumel, Capparelli, Chopart, Cowley, Elliotson, Fleiner, Frerichs, Freyhan (2 cases), Gille, Lancereaux (in 4 cases), Lichtheim, Lusk, Moore, Müller, Munk and Klebs, Nicolas and Mollière, v. Recklinghausen, Rörig, and Seegen. Holzmann saw transient glycosuria. Diabetes, or at least transient glycosuria, was found 24 times in 70 cases examined with reference to this condition, giving the striking ratio of 34 per cent. The diabetes, if not regarded as an accidental associate of the calculus, is probably in most instances to be considered as the result of the changes developed in the gland in consequence of the lithiasis. Under such an assumption the diabetes can occur only late after the onset of the symptoms of lithiasis. It may, however, be imagined that the same changes in the pancreatic tissue which lead to diabetes may also cause the formation of calculi, since dilatation of the pancreatic ducts, alterations of the secretion, and its stagnation may develop in consequence of induration of the tissue.

The various disturbances of digestion which are frequently found in patients with stone in the pancreas may be regarded as a consequence of the changes in the gland substance. The emaciation so often mentioned may be considered as a result of these digestive disturbances or the diabetes.

Jaundice belongs to the rare occurrences. In Galeati's case it may, perhaps, have arisen from the simultaneous cholelithiasis. Minnich mentions only a slight discoloration of the conjunctiva. In a case described by Giudiceandrea there was marked jaundice resulting from the compression of the common duct.

Fever is mentioned as a rare symptom. Holzmann regards it as analogous to the elevation of temperature so often observed in biliary and renal colic. The observations hitherto made on this point are too few to determine the importance of this symptom. Bonetus and Galeati speak of a tertian type of fever. In cases of infectious sialangitis with the formation of abscess an atypical fever with chills may develop (Roddick).

DIAGNOSIS.

The correct recognition of calculous disease of the pancreas is one of ' the most difficult tasks of the clinician, as may be illustrated by the fact that in the accessible literature of the subject the correct diagnosis was made only five times, and then by Lancereaux, Capparelli, Lichtheim, Minnich, and Leichtenstern. The last two found pancreatic calculi in the feces. Capparelli observed the passage of the stones from an abscess, and Lancereaux and Lichtheim based their diagnosis on the occurrence of diabetes, preceded by attacks of colic.

Among the cardinal symptoms, which may lead to the correct diagnosis are pancreatic colic, the passage of characteristic concretions with the stools, diabetes, steatorrhea, and azotorrhea. The concurrence of the first two symptoms or the demonstration of characteristic concretions in the stools alone can render possible a correct diagnosis in the early stages of the disease. The occurrence of fatty stools, diabetes, and the disturbed digestion of proteids belong generally to a later stage of the disease, when there has been such deep-seated destruction of the gland, in consequence of the lithiasis, that the characteristic symptoms of disturbed pancreatic function become manifest. The above symptoms only can become prominent before the symptoms due to the stone when a rare diffused disease of the pancreas gives rise to the formation of the calculus. The diagnosis of calculus in the pancreas can never be made from the pain alone. The pancreas cannot be regarded as the unquestioned place of origin of the pain even if it has a colicky character and shows also the paroxysmal type centering in the left hypochondrium, as described by Minnich and Holzmann. Such a localization may be found in biliary or renal colic, in beginning pericolitis in the region of the splenic flexure, even in colic originating in the appendix.

Even if the attacks of colic are accompanied by salivation, the pancreatic origin is not indicated, as paroxysmal pains from other sources may be accompanied by salivation. Generally, however, the latter have by no means the same localization as those in the case described by Minnich. There are merely paroxysmal pains in the epigastrium radiating into both hypochondria and in no way to be distinguished from atypical biliary colic, gastralgia, and lead-colic. There are also certain negative signs, as absence of jaundice, tenderness and swelling in the hepatic region, which by no means justify the exclusion of biliary colic.

The second of the cardinal symptoms mentioned is alone pathognomonic. If characteristic concretions are found in the stools, the diagnosis may be made with absolute certainty. But this happens very rarely; up to the present time, only in two cases. The soft, small, mortar-like concretions may easily be overlooked.

The distinction between pancreatic and biliary calculi will, in most cases, present no difficulties. The demonstration of bile pigment indicates gall-stones; the pancreatic calculi are generally whitish or yellowish-white, and contain no bile pigment. They consist mostly of calcium carbonate and calcium phosphate, and only occasionally contain small amounts of cholesterin, while the translucent gall-stones consist largely of cholesterin. Calcium carbonate occurs frequently in gall-stones, but biliary concretions consisting largely of calcium carbonate are very rare (Naunyn). As a rule, bile pigment also will be present in these concretions.

It is most frequently the case that the two cardinal symptoms, colic and diabetes, develop either in sequence or at a certain stage exist together. Pancreatic calculi certainly are to be suspected, and perhaps regarded as somewhat probable, if attacks of colic which do not have the pronounced type of biliary colic with its associated symptoms precede for years the occurrence of diabetes. Such evidence, however, is not absolute proof, for the diabetes may have arisen from other causes than an affection of the pancreas, and the colic may depend on an atypical cholelithiasis or be of other origin. Diabetes and cholelithiasis are so frequently associated that it may easily be assumed that the two conditions coexist without any causal relation. When attacks of colic precede diabetes and are followed by other pancreatic symptoms, as fatty stools or faulty digestion of proteids, the probability that pancreatic concretions are present is materially greater; even then the proof is not incontestable, because a severe pancreatic affection with its consequences and irregular cholelithiasis may accidentally occur at the same time.

No diagnostic importance can be ascribed to the symptoms made prominent by many authors, as obstinate diarrhea, the occurrence of glycosuria rapidly disappearing after the attacks, emaciation, and fever. These aid in diagnosis only when they occur in connection with the cardinal symptoms.

The physician is oftenest concerned with the question whether gall-stones or pancreatic calculi are the cause of the colic. From the frequency of gall-stones and the rarity of pancreatic calculi in all doubtful cases cholelithiasis should first be thought of, and lithiasis of the pancreas should only be considered as at all probable when the above-mentioned symptoms corresponding to the failure of pancreatic function are present. Absolute certainty can be reached only by finding characteristic pancreatic concretions in the stools.

The diagnosis of infectious sialangitis which accompanies the lithiasis will be possible only when atypical high fever with chills, tenderness in the region of the pancreas, and eventually a demonstrable tumor in this situation, with the characteristic symptoms of abscess, are joined to the characteristic symptoms of lithiasis of the pancreas.

TREATMENT.

The difficulty of diagnosis renders the rational treatment of this affection rarely possible. There is, however, a single instance. At Eichhorst's clinic ½ to 1 c.c. of a 1% solution of pilocarpin was injected subcutaneously into a patient suffering from an undoubted pancreatic lithiasis in consequence of the experimental observations of Kühne and Lea, Heidenhain and Landau, and Gottleib, that pilocarpin increased the secretion of the pancreas. There was no result during the stay of the patient in the hospital, but after he had left it 1 c.c. of the 1% solution was injected three times a week. "The attacks of colic were said to have entirely disappeared and the patient had not felt so well for a long time as after this treatment."

Abundant food is the best means of exciting pancreatic secretion, according to the experiments on animals. The investigations of Dolinski show that hydrochloric acid and some other acids, also acid drinks and foods, when taken into the stomach promote an abundant secretion of the pancreatic juice. An investigation by Becker has shown that alkaline salts, given with or without food, check the secretion of the pancreatic juice. Perhaps some therapeutic indications may be gained from the results of these experiments.

As a rule, the treatment is wholly symptomatic, the colic being treated by narcotics and any disturbances of digestion or diabetes by a dietetic treatment. In the present stage of our knowledge surgical treatment is indicated only when an abscess or a cyst has developed in consequence of the lithiasis.

VIII. NECROSIS.

THE death of a part or of the whole of the pancreas may occur in the course of various processes which affect the pancreas or its surroundings. Necrosis begins when portions of the gland or the entire organ are deprived of nourishment by any diseased process.

CLASSIFICATION.

There are two groups, according to the etiologic factors: (1) Necrosis caused by diseases of the pancreas; (2) necrosis caused by diseases of the surrounding tissues. There is a third series of cases in which the cause cannot be ascertained, but it undoubtedly belongs in the two above-mentioned groups.

(A) NECROSIS FROM DISEASES OF THE PANCREAS.

The diseases are as follows: *

(a) **Necrotic Inflammations.**—Various forms of inflammation, especially the suppurative, may lead to necrosis. In the section on this subject reference has been made to the necrosis of large or small portions of the pancreas.

In Gendrin's case a large cavity communicating with the jejunum was found in the region of the pancreas. The pancreatic tissue was degenerated into a dense mass streaked with red, which formed the walls of the cavity. Habershon found a purulent, gangrenous inflammation of the head and middle of the pancreas and peripancreatic abscesses in the region of the duodenum and in the lesser omentum. Moore saw the pancreas destroyed to a great extent by suppuration and the tail infiltrated with pus and in shreds.

In a case of traumatic suppuration reported by Hansemann the se-

---

* The separation of these different factors is purely arbitrary, since there are numerous combinations between inflammation, hemorrhage, and fat necrosis, and each of these combinations may be connected with necrosis of the gland.

questrated pancreas lay in a cavity filled with pus. Dieckhoff reports
a similar case.   The middle and tail of the pancreas were entirely destroyed and changed into a mass filled with greenish and yellow fragments
and the tail was almost entirely detached.   In the pancreatic abscess
operated upon by Körte necrotic bits of tissue also were found in the
evacuated pus, and on microscopic examination contained acinous structures.   In chronic inflammations also the necrosis of small portions may
develop from the growth of the intima and the obliteration of the blood-
vessels (Dieckhoff).   In 1891 a case in point was examined after death in
the Vienna General Hospital.   Chronic pancreatitis with partial necrosis
of the tail of the pancreas was found in a man forty-one years old with
diabetes insipidus.

(b) **Hemorrhages within and around the pancreas** cause necrosis
of small portions or of the entire organ.   Such cases are reported by
Haller and Klob, Prince and Gannett, Whitney and Harris, Homans and
Gannett, Rosenbach, and Dieckhoff.   The following case may briefly be
mentioned as an example of the course of the disease:

Homans and Gannett (quoted from Fitz): A woman forty years old had an
umbilical hernia for two years after lifting a heavy weight; for the last two weeks
it was irreducible and painful.   On the day after entering the hospital there were
vomiting, violent colic, small, fluttering pulse; the next day persistent vomiting,
anxious expression, pulse 100, at times imperceptible; normal temperature.   The
day afterward the pulse was 140, temperature 38.2° C. (100.8° F.), vomiting ceased,
coma, dyspnea, death on the fourth day.   At the autopsy were found: Hemorrhagic infiltration and gangrene of the pancreas, circumscribed peritonitis, gangrene of the diaphragm, acute pleuritis and pericarditis.   Thrombosis of the
splenic vein.

Circumscribed necrosis of the pancreas may likewise be caused by
hemorrhages in consequence of arteriosclerotic changes in the blood-
vessels.   I had the opportunity of observing in the hospital such a case
which also was clinically noteworthy.

M. P., forty-four years old, admitted July 28, 1896: For two and a half months
violent pains in the region of the stomach, loss of appetite, constipation, gradually
increasing jaundice, and for four weeks considerable emaciation.   At the time of
admission there was a high degree of jaundice, cachectic appearance, great sensitiveness to pressure, also pain under the edge of the right ribs, liver dulness reaches
two finger-breadths below the border of the ribs, abdomen flat, no distinct tumor
palpable, no ascites, edema of the lower part of the thigh, urine contained much
bile pigment, but no sugar or albumin.   Temperature 37.2° C. (98.96° F.).   The
patient complained of unusually violent, continuous pain in the epigastrium, radiating over the abdomen, and was very weak.   Later, the weakness gradually increased;
there was dizziness on sitting up in bed, and the cachexia was marked.   The patient
almost refused to take any food on account of the pain.   Nourishment by enemata.
With marked exhaustion, death occurred November 7, 1896

The autopsy, conducted by Prosector Dr. Zemann, gave the following
result:

The body, much emaciated, showed a high degree of jaundice.   Thorax much
arched, abdominal walls slightly distended and of a dirty green color in the hypogastrium.   Lungs of diminished substance and collapsed.   Heart small, contracted.
Valves showed yellowish spots and were opaque.   The liver scarcely projected
beyond the border of the ribs, small and flabby; its surface smooth, capsule easily
torn.   On section, the liver dark green, the acinous structure distinct, the acini
very small.   The bile-ducts slightly distended, a small amount of dark, greenish-
yellow bile escaping.   The gall-bladder flaccid, about as large as a goose-egg,
contained a considerable quantity of uniformly colored, slimy bile.   Spleen somewhat enlarged, rich in blood, and soft.

The intestinal coils and the stomach were distended with gas. The great omentum was spread like an apron over the intestinal coils, to which it was agglutinated. The coils also were adherent by means of purulent fibrinous plates. Thin pus was to be found here and there inclosed in small spaces between the intestinal loops. The stomach contained gas and a little viscid, opaque, pale-gray, watery fluid. The mucous membrane was pale, covered with whitish mucus. Large amounts of dark-green bile in the duodenum, especially in the descending portion. The mucosa was stained of a bile-green color.

Near the mouth of the common duct a slightly prominent portion of the intestinal wall for about 2 or 3 cm. formed a soft, disintegrated mass of tissue, stained dark yellow, within which the opening of the bile-duct at first was not to be found. The large bile-ducts were thin-walled, dilated, and collapsed, and contained a small quantity of bile. The wall of the common duct immediately beyond its mouth was replaced by a whitish, moderately soft, succulent neoplasm, which was continued into the above-mentioned disintegrated tissue of the duodenal wall. The common duct was rather narrow at this point, but easily penetrated. The adjacent head of the pancreas was formed of large lobes, and was easily separated from the duodenum. The pancreas, somewhat narrower and thinner than normal, was closely adherent to the posterior wall of the stomach. On the anterior surface of the tail of the pancreas, bounded in front by the stomach and transverse colon and at the side by the spleen, was a spherical cavity about the size of a man's fist, with a pocket as large as a plum on the upper edge of the tail of the pancreas. This cavity, filled with thin pus, was surrounded on all sides by a thin membrane, coated superficially with pus. Careful investigation showed that this membrane also separated the pancreas from the cavity. On the lower border of the body of the pancreas was a group of pancreatic lobules about the size of peas, softened almost to the consistency of pap, and of a dark reddish-black color. These were surrounded by lobules which appeared as usual. The pancreatic artery and its traceable branches were thick-walled and frequently calcified. The splenic, renal, and intestinal arteries were similarly altered. There were thin masses very darkly stained with bile in the small intestine and bile-stained fecal matter in the large intestine. The kidneys were somewhat smaller than normal, capsule stripped off easily, surface smooth. Bladder contracted.

Diagnosis: Medullary carcinoma of the common duct extending to the duodenum with stenosis of the bile-duct. Ulceration of the cancer with relief of the stenosis by means of the destruction of the neoplasm. Recent diffuse peritonitis with fibrinopurulent exudation and with cyst-like encapsulation in the region of the tail of the pancreas. Circumscribed necrosis of the pancreas with hemorrhagic infiltration of the necrotic portion and chronic endarteritis and calcification of the pancreatic artery. Marasmus. General jaundice.

The microscopic examination of the necrotic mass in the pancreas showed a transformation of the cells into a fatty detritus mixed with numerous red blood-corpuscles. The walls of the capillaries everywhere had undergone fatty degeneration. Outside of the necrotic area also there were spots of fatty degeneration of gland cells and of capillaries.

The possibility of a cancer of the pancreas was thought of by me on account of the gradual development of a completely obstructing jaundice, the rapid progress of cachexia with extreme debility, the peculiar, violent pains, and the great sensitiveness to pressure under the right border of the ribs, as far as the middle line.

At the autopsy it was shown that two processes were going on at the same time: (1) A cancer of the common duct extending to the duodenum and causing a stenosis of the bile-duct, which was somewhat relieved by the degeneration of the neoplasm. Recent peritonitis. (2) A circumscribed necrosis of the pancreas with hemorrhagic infiltration of the necrotic portion in consequence of chronic endarteritis and calcification of the pancreatic artery.

It is probable that the picture of disease resembling that of cancer of the pancreas was developed by the combination of cancer of the common duct with the changes in the pancreas due to arteriosclerosis.

(c) **Fat necrosis** is frequently stated to be the cause of the necrosis of the gland. The hemorrhage caused by the fat necrosis or the extensive fat necrosis itself may lead to necrosis of the gland to a greater or less extent. It is not yet clear whether the same factor which has caused the fat necrosis may not lead also to necrosis of the pancreas, or whether the fat necrosis is to be regarded as a result of the necrosis of the gland.

Experiments on animals, as will be shown, permit the assumption that the fat necrosis may be caused by the action of the pancreatic secretion. Chiari's observations also, which will be mentioned later, show that multiple, circumscribed necroses of the gland-parenchyma probably may be caused by the same factor—autodigestion. It is, therefore, quite conceivable that in man also fat necrosis and necrosis of the gland-parenchyma may be attributed to the same cause. The relation between fat necrosis and gangrene of the gland will be considered later in the section on Fat Necrosis.

There are numerous communications on the subject of gangrene with or in consequence of fat necrosis: Balser, Mader-Weichselbaum, Farge, Whittier and Fitz, Gerhardi, Foster and Fitz, Langerhans, Hansemann, König, Caspersohn-Hansen, Körte, Simon and Stanley, Sarfert, Elliott, v. Bonsdorff. E. Fraenkel, Sievers, etc. Several of these cases will be mentioned in the section on Fat Necrosis. A brief sketch only of a few especially striking and clinically interesting examples follows:

Mader-Weichselbaum: Coachman's wife, forty-two years old, who four years before had suffered from jaundice due to gall-stones, was attacked with distention of the stomach, vomiting, and abdominal pain. On the next day jaundice developed. Two or three times a day there was a chill with subsequent fever and sweating.

Present condition: Moderate jaundice, temperature 38° C. (100.4° F.). Pulse scarcely accelerated. Splenic tumor. Liver normal. In both lumbar regions there was circumscribed, pronounced edema of the skin. Vomiting. Two days later there was a chill, temperature 40.2° C. (104.4° F.), loss of consciousness, and on the next day symptoms of a beginning (metastatic) meningitis. Two days later, temperature 37.4° C. (99.3° F.), with almost constant unconsciousness. Exploratory puncture in the region of the spleen produced a dirty, reddish fluid. Death on the next day

The autopsy showed purulent meningitis, enlargement of the spleen, thrombosis of the splenic vein, marked softening of the tail and a portion of the body of the pancreas, which was grayish-black in color and infiltrated with a thin, ichorous fluid. The tissue around the pancreas presented the same appearances. The head was quite intact and contained several yellow patches, from the size of a pea to that of hemp-seed, consisting of a thick, greasy pulp. Microscopically the latter consisted of numerous fat granular corpuscles, very small fat-drops, and numerous fat-crystals. Similar foci also were found quite abundantly in the transverse mesocolon and in the upper portion of the great omentum, at times surrounded by a hemorrhagic zone. Occasional pancreatic veins opening into the splenic vein were obstructed by grayish-red thrombi.

Weichselbaum concluded that gangrene of the pancreas resulting in pyemia had followed fat necrosis of the gland.

Caspersohn-Hansen: A very fat woman, thirty-six years old, was attacked with vomiting and severe pain in the region of the stomach; improvement after fourteen days' treatment. Then renewed vomiting, pain, slight distention of the abdomen.

Diagnosis: Circumscribed peritonitis in consequence of ulcer of the stomach. Resistance in the left upper half of the abdomen, small rapid pulse; exploratory laparotomy. After section of the abdominal walls a tumor-like mass was seen which had become firmly united to the peritoneum and proved to be fat tissue which had undergone diffuse fibrous induration. The abdominal cavity was opened and an opaque ascitic fluid evacuated. There was no inflammatory focus. At the autopsy a large cyst was found behind the liver, filled with a clear, odorless, dark, coffee-brown fluid. The following conditions were apparent: (1) Total necrosis and partial separation of the pancreas; (2) remains of hemorrhage into the pancreas; (3) circumscribed chronic peritonitis of the omental bursa, the exudation containing hematin; (4) disseminated fat necrosis.

Caspersohn regarded the fat necrosis as the cause of the hemorrhage. Necrosis of the pancreatic tissue resulted from the effusion of blood. An active dissecting inflammation developed for the elimination of the degenerated portions and extended toward the peritoneum. The foramen of Winslow became occluded and a cyst of the omental bursa was formed. The increasing distention of the cyst caused pressure upon the nervous apparatus and consequent collapse followed by death.

Körte * : Tinker twenty-two years old suffered for five years with attacks of pain in the stomach and vomiting. Was suddenly seized with violent abdominal pain, vomiting, and headache. Temperature 39.2° C. (102.6° F.). Pulse 140. Slight cyanosis, pain in the left lower abdomen and loin, serous pleurisy on the left side. Edema of the skin of the abdomen on the left side between the borders of the ribs and the pelvis. Puncture caused the escape of a brownish-red, turbid fluid, with crumbling fragments, in which were numerous long rod-like bacteria and fatty degenerated pus-corpuscles. Urine free from albumin and sugar. The skin was incised longitudinally along the anterior axillary line, from the border of the ribs to the brim of the pelvis. The retroperitoneal tissue was laid open and a large amount of the fluid described, containing numerous yellowish-brown crumbling shreds, was evacuated from a considerable depth. Drainage. The fever continued. Aspiration of the pleuritic exudation. An indistinct, fluctuating swelling was felt below the xiphoid cartilage. Laparotomy. Yellow, cheesy pus escaped on puncture. The gastrocolic ligament was divided, the wall of the abscess was torn in suturing, and a thick, brownish-yellow pus poured out, mingled with necrotic bits of tissue and fat-drops. Drainage; soon after the operation, collapse and death.

Autopsy: Pancreas about one-half its normal size, infiltrated with blood, and the head changed into a greasy, light-gray mass of clayey consistency. Gall-bladder filled with small concretions; fat necrosis in the omentum; a section of the left adrenal shows bright yellow masses similar to those in the omentum. The yellow material evacuated from the abscess consists microscopically of fat, fat-crystals, and yellow pigment, but contains no pus-corpuscles.

Sarfert: An extremely fat woman twenty-four years old was attacked fourteen days before death with sudden abdominal pain, abundant bilious but not fecal vomiting; pronounced meteorism, great sensitiveness to pressure, fever and dyspnea. Stools were obtained by enemata of oil; there was temporary benefit, followed by a renewal of obstruction. The temperature became elevated, there were cyanosis, vomiting, rapid pulse, collapse.

At the autopsy the abdominal cavity was filled with a yellow purulent mass in which floated numerous brittle, granular fragments of the color of yellow wax. The pancreas formed behind the stomach a dark-brown, shreddy mass surrounded by pus, the tail floating free. Foci of fat necrosis as large as beans were found in the mesentery, in the omentum, and in the preperitoneal fat.

(d) Chiari recently has called attention to a peculiar form of pancreatic necrosis. In 1891 " an autopsy was performed, twelve hours after death, on a man twenty-five years old who had died three days after the extirpation of a sarcoma of the left side of the neck, which had developed from the lymph-glands, from rupture of the left external carotid with consequent hemorrhage. In the left half of the body of the pancreas, which otherwise had the usual structure, although pale, there was a dark-green mass, about 1 cm. in size, irregularly formed and sharply limited from its surroundings, which immediately gave the impression of a circumscribed necrosis of the gland." The microscopic examination confirmed the diagnosis. "The mass consisted of necrotic pancreatic tissue, in which the acini were still to be distinguished. Neither in the cells of the acini, nor in the interstitial tissue, which did not appear thickened, was a nuclear stain to be obtained. Everything had become necrotic."

* This case (No. III of his series) is regarded by Körte as one of acute pancreatitis, with consecutive necrosis of the gland and fat necrosis, previously mentioned on page 126.

The pancreatic tissue surrounding the necrotic portions showed quite a considerable increase of interstitial connective tissue, which generally appeared extensively infiltrated with small cells. It was, therefore, as Chiari suggests, a case of circumscribed necrosis of the pancreatic tissue, with resulting reactive inflammation around it. There was no doubt that the circumscribed necrosis came first and the reactive inflammation in the vicinity afterward. There was no evidence that the necrosis was caused by a disturbance of the circulation, interstitial inflammation, or injury. Chiari thought it most probable that a chemical agent had caused the necrosis of the acini and the interstitial tissue several days before death, in time for the development of a reactive inflammation. He regards the pancreatic juice as such an agent which had caused an autodigestion of the organ analogous to the method of origin of the peptic ulcer of the stomach.

Two years later Chiari found a similar case. An autopsy was held on the body of a woman thirty-two years old who had suffered from diffuse bronchitis and erythema exsudativum multiforme. The pancreas was found somewhat larger than normal, of dense consistency and paler color. It contained numerous sharply defined, irregular foci, some as large as 1 cm., but most of them much smaller, yellowish-white, homogeneous, quite firm, and surrounded by a red zone. On microscopic examination, Chiari could distinguish three varieties: (1) Those in which the necrotic acini were not completely destroyed; (2) those in which the dead acini were destroyed in places; (3) those in which all the necrotic acini were more or less extensively destroyed. Elsewhere the pancreas showed throughout an increase of the connective tissue between the lobules and acini, in which there was a greater or less infiltration with small cells and moderate lipomatosis. There was, therefore, in this case also a reactive inflammation in the vicinity of the necrotic portion. There were also neither disturbance of the circulation, trauma, nor a precedent interstitial pancreatitis, hence Chiari considered it probable here likewise that the digestive action of the pancreatic juice had caused the necrosis.

(B) NECROSIS DUE TO DISEASE IN THE VICINITY OF THE PANCREAS.

There are several observations of this sort. The gangrene is most frequently produced by the passage of gall-stones, which cause inflammatory and ichorous processes.

Chiari and Schossberger: A man, thirty-eight years old, who had formerly suffered very little from sickness, had an attack of cholelithiasis; he was afterward well for one year. After an illness of twelve days occasional attacks of pain in the stomach appeared; then suddenly there were vomiting, severe colic, symptoms of intestinal obstruction, and collapse. On the next day there was no fever and the general condition was good. Two days later renewed symptoms of intestinal obstruction, pronounced meteorism, and vomiting which could not be relieved. After calomel and irrigation, there was a passage of very offensive stools, and the next day the condition was improved. Sixteen days later there was high fever, lasting three days, with renewed symptoms of intestinal obstruction; after passage of stools, the fever was again relieved, and for eighteen days free passage and obstruction alternated. A piece of tissue was found in the stools which Chiari diagnosticated as pancreatic tissue. For some time the patient noticed some sensitiveness on the left side of the abdomen, but some years later he was still perfectly well.

The piece of pancreas which escaped with the feces was about 13 cm. long, quite uniformly cylindric, and of the thickness of the index-finger; on longitudinal section it showed a piece of a canal about 3 cm. long, which appeared exactly like the ductus Wirsungianus. On microscopic examination, remains of acini could be recognized.

The following course of the affection could easily be imagined: A gall-stone perforated (probably from the common duct) and caused inflammation and suppuration of the tissue surrounding the pancreas, which opened into the duodenum or some other portion of the intestine, and the detached pancreas passed through this opening and was evacuated with the feces.

Rokitansky-Trafoyer (museum preparation): *A* wine-dealer fifty-two years old was suddenly attacked with severe colic two months after there had been disturbances of digestion. Diagnosis: Cholelithiasis. *After* a very severe attack, 18 gallstones were found in the stools, and three days later there was another severe attack of colic. The next day a large discolored mass of tissue was passed, which Rokitansky recognized as the sequestrated pancreas. Complete recovery after three weeks. Seven years later the patient was still in perfect health.

Chiari reports an interesting case of gangrene of the pancreas in consequence of perforation of the stomach by a round ulcer.

An inebriate fifty-four years old suffered for seven years from pains in the stomach and vomiting; the stools were frequently black. In the latter part of this period, the pains in the stomach became much more severe. At the time of admission the patient was fat and slightly jaundiced. Examination of the lungs showed dulness and bronchial breathing; the heart-sounds were clear but weak, the epigastrium painful, otherwise nothing abnormal. Temperature 37.7° C. (99.86° F.). In the third week of the stay at the hospital, bed-sores; in the fourth, parotitis on the left side, which disappeared after some days. Anorexia, progressive weakness, death after the patient had been in the hospital for six weeks.
    Autopsy: Extensive panniculus adiposus; cardiac muscle fatty degenerated; liver large, pale, infiltrated with fat; gall-bladder adherent to the duodenum and containing numerous concretions; in the stomach a fluid of offensive odor. In the posterior wall of the stomach, about half-way between the cardia and the pylorus, was a perforating ulcer, 1 cm. in diameter, through which a probe passed into the omental bursa; 3 cm. distant was a second round ulcer. Omental bursa transformed into a large ichorous cavity, entirely separated from the general peritoneal cavity by occlusion of the foramen of Winslow by adhesions; five perforations, some as large as the little finger, into the uppermost portion of the jejunum. Lying across the ichorous cavity was a cylindric shreddy mass of tissue, about 12 cm. long, of the thickness of the little finger at its left end and somewhat thicker at the right, entirely isolated and brownish-black in color. Near the descending portion of the duodenum, the central end of the ductus Wirsungianus was found embedded in indurated tissue; it was about 3 cm. long and opened freely into the ichorous cavity.

(C) NECROSIS OF THE PANCREAS FROM INDEFINITE CAUSES.

Chiari: In a woman forty-six years old for some days there were severe pain in the abdomen, vomiting, diffuse peritonitis; seven hours before death, chill and vomiting of a black mass of offensive odor. At the autopsy the body was found very corpulent and there was a recent, diffuse, purulent peritonitis. Sequestration of the blackish-brown pancreas, which was attached merely by remains of connective tissue, easily torn. On longitudinal incision of the pancreas the duct was easily recognized. Putrefaction in the omental bursa. Perforation of the duodenum and transverse mesocolon, opening in the pancreatico-duodenal artery. The gall-bladder contained 60 polyhedral stones.

In this case the sequestration of the pancreas might have been caused by a primary pancreatitis or peripancreatitis or by hemorrhage into the pancreas; on the other hand, "the possibility cannot be entirely excluded that the opening in the duodenum, which at the autopsy presented the characteristics of a perforation from without inward, in part, at least, originated in the intestine, perhaps from injury of the intestinal wall by a small foreign body with perforation into the omental bursa, the opening later being enlarged by the ichorous process. It would not be difficult to understand the sequestration of the pancreas in consequence of a traumatic peripancreatitis and pancreatitis caused by such a foreign body, since, according to Bruckmüller ('Lehrbuch der pathologischen Zootomie'), this occurrence is said to take place frequently in dogs" (Chiari).

Körte: Woman thirty years old; has borne three children; five days after the last confinement there was violent pain in the epigastrium with feeling of weakness; afterward fairly good condition. Six weeks later violent pains radiating from the upper abdomen over the body. She was admitted to the hospital on account of the severe pain. Slight jaundice, collapse, remittent fever up to 40° C. (104° F.). Sensitiveness of the abdomen, slight albuminuria, resistance in the left epigastric region extending to the kidney. Colon lies in front of the tumor; irregular variations of temperature for a month. The tumor remained at the left. Repeated puncture never caused the appearance of pus, but gave a brownish-yellow fluid in which were cells showing extensive fatty degeneration, yellowish-brown pigment, and some bacteria. Renewed high fever, poor general condition. Operation: Horizontal incision in the lumbar region, exposure of the lower end of the kidney; a yellowish-gray mass as large as a walnut was exposed in which were fatty contents; drainage; the condition continued bad. Fourteen days later, the wound was enlarged downward and a retroperitoneal cavity was reached which contained a brownish fluid and yellow necrotic fragments. Curettage. A sequestrated piece of tissue 11 cm. long and 2 to 2.5 cm. wide was removed; the fever abated. A week later there was severe hemorrhage from the depths of the wound, which was repeated; death. Autopsy: Large, ichorous, encapsulated abscess between stomach, spleen, diaphragm, and kidney. Only the head and a small piece of the tail of the pancreas were found, Parietal thrombosis of the splenic artery. Numerous calculi in the gall-bladder.

It is not to be determined in this case that the gall-stones were in any causal relation with the process. It certainly would be possible that the inflammation caused by the cholelithiasis in the bile-passages might have been continued into the pancreatic duct. In the cases of gangrene of Middleton, Garzia, and Israel also, no definite cause of the necrosis could be assigned.

Among reports of autopsies at the Vienna General Hospital for the last ten years there was likewise found a case of circumscribed necrosis in the tail of the pancreas of a diabetic, fifty-two years old, but no further information is given concerning the cause.

PATHOLOGIC ANATOMY.

The occurrence of partial or total necrosis as observed at operations and at autopsies is mentioned in the preceding statement. The appearances vary according to the duration and cause of the development of the process. Fitz suggests the following scheme, based on the duration of the process:

After a period of four days, the pancreas is doubled in size, dark red, consistency diminished, the section red or mixed gray and red. The cut surface is shreddy or the whole gland is transformed into a dark-colored mass of offensive odor. After ten days the pancreas is dark-brown, hard, firm, surrounded by hemorrhagic masses or embedded in spongy, dark green masses. Toward the end of the second week the gland is changed into a soft, dark, ragged, gangrenous mass. After three weeks the pancreas, dark-brown, lies almost free in the cavity of the omentum, connected with the wall only by a few bands that are easily broken or by fibrous tissue. During the fourth and fifth weeks the pancreas may become sequestrated and evacuated with the feces. Toward the end of the seventh week it may appear changed into a ragged, cylindric, dark-brown mass. This mass lies in the cavity of the omentum, which is filled with dark fluid and communicates with the stomach and intestine. General peritonitis does not occur frequently, since adhesions form, which prevent the escape of the pus into the abdominal cavity. Adhesive peritonitis is not rare. Pleuritis, pericarditis, acute leptomeningitis, and hypostatic pneumonia are found at times.

In the case reported by Dieckhoff the necrotic portion was transformed into a mass containing numerous green and yellow fragments. The microscopic examination showed:

"Scarcely any indication of pancreatic structure in the sequestrated portion of the gland, but there were merely large or small areas of necrotic tissue extensively infiltrated with pus-corpuscles, the nuclei of which were indented or fragmentary, and, in addition, often stained with difficulty. There was an enormous accumulation of micro-organisms in this portion. On staining by Weigert's method, there were found only lance-shaped diplococci and streptococci, which were sometimes within and sometimes between the cells. On staining with borax-methylene-blue, a few quite large, thick bacilli were found (probably Bacterium coli commune)."

Chiari, as above mentioned, could recognize microscopically three different foci in his cases of multiple, circumscribed necrosis, probably due to autodigestion.

(*a*) In the places where the necrotic acini were not entirely degenerated he could readily observe individual acini, although the epithelial nuclei did not stain. The interstitial tissue was not thickened. Its nuclei were either stained or unstained. The focus was surrounded by a zone of thick, fibrous tissue, infiltrated with small cells.

(*b*) In a second variety, as a rule, by far the larger portions of the necrotic acini were disintegrated into a finely granular mass. The interstitial tissue frequently showed slight nuclear increase and often contained clumps of brown granular pigment. The indurated tissue about these foci was generally more extensive than around those of the first variety.

(*c*) Foci in which all the necrotic acini were destroyed. Usually the boundaries between the acini were no longer distinct, but were replaced by a granular detritus of which the septa between the individual acini at times formed a part. There was an extensive development of connective tissue forming thick capsules around these foci. The anatomic condition in gangrene of the pancreas as it occurs in fat necrosis is considered in the section on Fat Necrosis.

Experiments on Animals.—In one case necrosis of the pancreas was produced after the injection of olive oil into the parenchyma and ligation of the body of the gland.

November 2, 1896: Small dog. Pancreas drawn forward. In the body and head of the gland 0.2 gm. Ol. olivarum were injected in three places. The middle portion of the organ was ligated in three places, the blood-vessels being spared. During the operation digestion was at its height; the chyle-vessels were distended; the pancreas was very large and of a rose-red color. The operation lasted about three-quarters of an hour.

November 3, 1896: The dog was quite lively and drank water. Urine 65 c.c., golden-yellow. Amount of sugar 2.4%. No acetone.

November 4, 1896: Dog very weak.

16

November 5, 1896: Refused food. No sugar in the urine. Bile pigment was present.

November 6, 1896: Dog found dead.

Autopsy: Slight suppuration of the abdominal wall. The peritoneum smooth and somewhat redder than usual. No fluid in the peritoneal cavity. Pancreas as a whole somewhat enlarged. Upon the surface were pale red spots and yellowish-white patches, elsewhere the color was either bright or dark red. The structure of the gland is everywhere recognizable, and between the individual lobules the blood-vessels are hyperdistended with blood. On the border between the head and tail there is a part as large as a bean, its surface dark red, in which the glandular structure is not to be recognized and which is surrounded by a yellowish-white zone. Immediately adjoining it, toward the tail, is a hemorrhage as large as a pea. Near the tail and separated by a ligature is a glistening chalk-like lobule in which no structure is to be recognized. The tissue everywhere feels denser and firmer than normal. The tail appears pale, dense, in places infiltrated with blood, but otherwise quite normal. The body shows the most marked changes and is dense. On section the

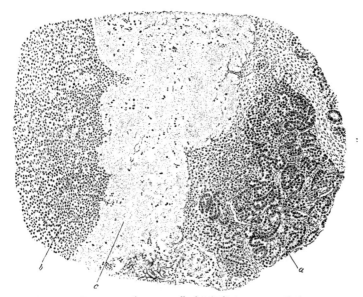

FIG. 14.—*a*, Normal gland tissue; *b*, small-celled infiltration; *c*, necrotic tissue.

gland structure is in part indistinct. There are dense portions as large as peas, yellowish-white or green in color, sharply limited from the reddened tissue, in which the details are indistinct. There is a lobule as large as a pea infiltrated with blood at the point of transition from the body into the tail. On section of the head the structure of the gland is to be recognized, the lobules project as granules, and in places, especially toward the surface of the gland, there are glistening yellowish-white, dense portions of the size of the head of a pin or larger. Toward the body is a portion as large as a pea, infiltrated with blood and surrounded by glistening white points as large as pinheads.

The microscopic examination gave the result shown in figure 14. There was an extensive small-celled infiltration around the necrotic focus, which extended also into the normal structure as far as the surface.

SYMPTOMS.

Many processes which are active within or around the pancreas may result in necrosis. Such are acute and chronic inflammations of the pancreas, moderate or circumscribed hemorrhage, trauma resulting in hemorrhage or inflammation, fat necrosis causing necrosis either directly or through hemorrhage, if perhaps it is not due to the same cause as the gangrene of the gland, autodigestive processes due to unknown causes, during life suppurative and ichorous conditions due to perforating ulcers of the stomach or to perforating gall-stones and all other factors which lead to an abscess of the omental bursa. It is certainly to be considered in a number of cases, as has repeatedly been stated, that infectious organisms entering from the intestine under certain conditions may be the cause of suppuration, putrefaction, and necrosis.

The numerous causes produce a varied course and a differing picture of disease. Moderate pancreatic hemorrhage, pancreatic abscess, extensive fat necrosis, perforating gastric ulcer, resulting in a retroventricular gangrenous condition, inflammation due to the passage of gall-stones, must produce pictures of disease varying in their beginning, their development, and their course up to a certain point, at which the peculiar necrosis of the gland, with all the secondary changes due to it, is established. Sometimes the development of this condition is preceded by years of suffering, as in case of gastric ulcer or cholelithiasis, while at other times the severe disease, with the group of symptoms described in the sections on Pancreatic Abscess and Pancreatic Hemorrhage, appears in the midst of perfect health, or at least when the condition is relatively good. It is obviously impossible that symptoms characteristic of the necrosis should become prominent when it is considered that the necrosis is the result of various processes, and when it occurs gives rise to new alterations in addition to the persistence and increase of those caused by the original disease. A pathologic condition thus arises not limited to the pancreas, but involving the neighboring structures, often for a considerable distance. Bursal abscess, retroperitoneal suppuration, the formation of a large gangrenous cavity which contains the necrotic pancreas, are then the prominent features.

In all cases from the beginning there are violent pains, at first limited to the epigastrium, but later radiating in all directions over the abdomen, toward the back, and often only into the left hypochondrium. These are soon followed by vomiting, persistent nausea, meteorism, tenderness, prostration, progressive collapse, accelerated pulse, dry tongue, irregular fever sometimes with chills. An apparent, temporary improvement may occur in some cases, until another and much more violent attack indicates a new stage in the progress of the disease. Besides these symptoms, intestinal obstruction is occasionally observed. In the cases of Gerhardi, Balser, Rosenbach, Hirschberg, Caspersohn, v. Bonsdorff, Allina, etc., the diagnosis of an internal constriction was made, and in several of the cases laparotomy was undertaken without any success in discovering the obstruction.

When a bursal abscess or a retroperitoneal collection of pus forms, a tumor may be recognized or there is a diffused or circumscribed resistance. Thus, Rosenbach felt behind and below the stomach a tumor the size of a child's head, König found a resistance and dulness as large as the surface of the hand, Caspersohn showed a resistance in the left upper half of the abdomen, and Körte felt a resistance, perhaps a tumor, in the upper abdomen. The tumor corresponds to the collection of pus which has developed in the omental bursa or in a retroperitoneal cavity. The sequestrated pancreas is sometimes found at the bottom of the pus cavity, as in the cases reported by Langerhans, Hansemann, Caspersohn, Rosenbach, Chiari, Israel, etc.

The abscess may rupture into the intestine, as has already been mentioned, and the sequestrated pancreas also may pass off with the stools, as in the cases reported by Rokitansky and Chiari.

Death occurs with the symptoms of rapid and continuous collapse or pyemia, peritonitis, fatal hemorrhage, embolism of the pulmonary artery, or metastatic pleurisy, pericarditis, or leptomeningitis—if the extremely rare event does not happen that the necrotic pancreas is discharged with the feces with resulting recovery, or if the latter event does not take place by the discharge of necrotic tissue and pus from a successful operation, as in Körte's case.

DIAGNOSIS.

The diagnosis of gangrene of the pancreas can only be made when the sequestrated pancreas passes off with the stools or when necrotic portions of the pancreas are found at an operation upon a pancreatic or bursal abscess or a retroperitoneal collection of pus. In favorable cases the diagnosis can be made of a bursal abscess or suppuration proceeding from the pancreas. The section on Pancreatic Abscess contains what is to be said on this point.

Successful treatment is possible only by means of an operation, and the section on Suppurative Pancreatitis states what is worthy of mention in regard to this subject.

IX. FAT NECROSIS (Balser); NECROSIS OF FAT TISSUE (Langerhans, Chiari).

Necrosis of fat tissue represents a peculiar disease of the pancreas, in many respects still mysterious, and of equal interest and importance in its origin, course, and results. Balser, in 1882, first called attention to this condition, which is by no means a rare pathologic change. Ten years before, Ponfick had described the presence, in the fat-marrow of the cylindric bones of a cachectic girl twenty-one years old, of small white foci consisting of very large fat-granular corpuscles which resulted in complete necrosis of the marrow tissue. There is no doubt that Klob had earlier observed the condition described by Balser, but had not recognized the importance of the change. In cases of atrophied pancreas caused by passive congestion in valvular disease, Klob saw, within the interstitial tissue, small clear white spots of almost tendinous appearance, from which material resembling an emulsion could be expressed, consisting in part of chalk molecules and gland-cells and in part of clumps of radiating crystals, probably calcium margarate.

Balser gave a minute description of the process in his fundamental work. There were found not infrequently—5 times in 25 bodies of adults selected indiscriminately—between the lobules of the pancreas opaque, yellowish-white, punctate foci, at times larger than pinheads and as a rule oval on section. The larger of these were peculiar in that the cut surface was not uniformly smooth, but the center was more or less completely detached from the periphery. In other foci the center was filled with a tallow-like material. These peculiar foci were often found not only between the lobules of the pancreas, but also in the fat tissue around the pancreas. Balser also found similar changes in four other cases. Once in the fatty bone-marrow, again in the very abundant subpericardial fat tissue, on both occasions in elderly men. In the other two cases there were very extensive and very numerous areas of fat necrosis in the vicinity of the pancreas and in the mesenteric fat tissue.

Balser regarded the fat necrosis as the probable cause of death in these cases. He summarizes the results of his observations as follows: "Opaque, yellowish-white foci may be found, in the interacinous tissue of the pancreas, and more rarely in the surrounding fat tissue in the bodies of many adults, whether fat or lean. In the rarer cases their extent, number, and size, with an associated necrosis of the central portion, are increased to a serious extent. Occasionally similar foci are found in the fat tissue of the bone-marrow and of the heart. Infiltration of the tissue adjoining the necroses indicating old or fresh hemorrhages is found rarely where the changes are few, but extensively where the changes are abundant. The necrotic areas may become confluent and prove a cause of death by their extent and by the simultaneous sequestration of large portions of the fat tissue in which they lie."

Balser came to the conclusion that an increase of the fat-cells in the vicinity of the pancreas was at the foundation of the process, "that this increase exceptionally, especially in very corpulent people, may reach such an extent that the death of large portions of the abdominal fat occurs, and in consequence gives rise to death, either through its extent alone or from the associated hemorrhages. Chiari next investigated this peculiar pathologic change. He confirmed the observation of Balser in individuals who were very marantic, especially as a result of tuberculosis, syphilis, progressive paralysis, cancer, alcoholism, etc., and also in five cases of severe disease of the pancreas.

Chiari came to another conclusion regarding the development of the process on the basis of his histologic investigations. According to him, this fat necrosis is a degenerative process, parallel with the retrograde metamorphoses so often occurring in other tissues, and to be designated fatty degeneration and simple necrosis.

The divergence of the views advanced by Balser and Chiari caused Langerhans to undertake an extensive histologic and experimental investigation, the results of which rendered the anatomic conditions quite clear, but offered merely an hypothesis concerning the etiology the soundness of which is still to be shown.

Fitz, in his frequently quoted article published in 1889, takes another view. He considers that there are necrobiotic and inflammatory forms of fat necrosis, the latter showing a tendency to gangrene; both varieties occur in the pancreas or in its vicinity. The inflammatory and the gangrenous forms are of especial importance, and in most cases are the result of an acute inflammation of the gland.

A large number of authors have studied the question of the necrosis of fat tissue, and have added to the statistics or have contributed anatomic and experimental investigations. Without attempting to give a complete list, the following names may be mentioned: Benda, Bruckmeyer, Caspersohn, Curschmann, Dettmer, Dieckhoff, Farge, Fitz, E. Fraenkel, von Gieson, Hansemann, Hawkins, Hildebrand, Hlava, Jackson and Ernst, Jung, v. Kahlden, König, Körte, Lubarsch, Mader and Weichselbaum, Marchand, Pinkham and Whitney, Ponfick, Rolleston, Sarfert, Sievers, Stadelmann, Lindsay Steven, Whittier and Fitz.

PATHOLOGIC ANATOMY.

The necrosis of fat tissue occurs in the form of small areas, the most of which are the size of a millet-seed or of a hemp-seed. Very large necroses may arise through the confluence of numerous neighboring foci. The color is usually pure white, intensely opaque, sometimes yellowish- or grayish-white. Many of the foci have a hemorrhagic or pigmented center, and most of them are found separated from the surrounding tissue. They are seated between the lobules of the pancreas and in its immediate vicinity. These alterations are found isolated in the pancreas and are very frequent in its vicinity (according to Balser, in about 20% of the bodies examined). Large numbers of fat necroses are found much more rarely at a greater distance from the pancreas, in the omentum and mesentery and in the paranephric fat. They are found at times also in the subpericardial fat, in the bone-marrow, and in the subcutaneous fat (Chiari, Hansemann). In Balser's first case there were numerous bright, sulphur-yellow, opaque depositions in the fat tissue, as a rule of the size of lentils, more rarely of the size of cherry-stones. They were disseminated in the subperitoneal fat tissue of the abdominal wall, omentum, and mesentery. In a case recently reported by E. Fraenkel, "the fat tissue of the great omentum and the mesentery of the small intestine contained a number of foci, at times as large as beans, isolated and in groups sharply defined from the normal tissue, with the luster of stearin, at times somewhat depressed, and remarkable for their dense consistency." The transverse mesocolon in the region of the splenic flexure, also the mesentery of the descending colon, were necrotic and perforated in numerous places. The foci were most abundant in the region of the pancreas, although the necrosis of the fat tissue was distributed extensively in the fat tissue of the abdomen. According to Balser, the small disseminated foci, either limited to the pancreas or its immediate neighborhood or distributed extensively throughout the fat of the entire abdomen, form the early stage of a process which is not at all uncommon in fat individuals. Similar necrotic conditions were found also by Balser in fat animals, especially in Hungarian and Algerian swine. He found almost constantly in them numerous foci of fat necrosis in the pancreas and its immediate vicinity, either punctate or at times as large as peas. Heller also has not infrequently seen fat necrosis in the fat of swine.

In the further course of the process the small necrotic foci become confluent and then other anatomic changes develop. The fat necrosis may, as many authors believe, give rise to inflammation, suppuration, hemorrhage, and necrosis of tissue. Thus the changes which are at first of little importance often prove deleterious. Many combinations occur.

PLATE 2.

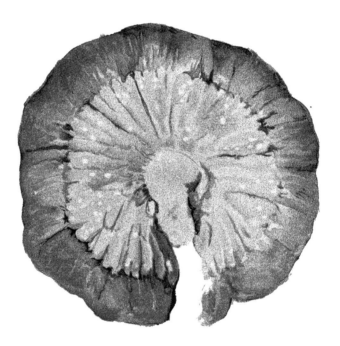

DISSEMINATED NECROSIS OF THE MESENTERIC FAT TISSUE IN ACUTE HEMORRHAGIC
PANCREATITIS.
(From the Warren Anatomical Museum of Harvard Medical School, Boston.)

Fat necrosis not infrequently occurs in acute and chronic inflammations, and it is an open question whether the fat necrosis has caused the inflammation, or whether, according to Fitz, Körte, and others, the inflammation has caused the fat necrosis, or whether both these conditions are attributable to the same cause.

The characteristic anatomic conditions which have been thoroughly described in previous sections develop when the necrosis of the fat tissue has led to more or less extensive hemorrhage in the pancreas or its vicinity, and when, either in consequence of these hemorrhages or directly, necrosis of portions of the gland or of the entire organ have formed.

The morbid process which is scarcely to be recognized at the outset, according to the view of those writers who maintain the idiopathic nature of fat necrosis, may lead to total destruction of the entire gland, which is to be found in a cavity filled with ichorous fluid and containing other shreds of necrotic tissue, either wholly sequestrated or loosely attached to its walls. In describing the microscopic appearances Balser, Chiari, and Langerhans, who first made extensive investigations of the subject, differ materially from each other.

Balser observed in fresh sections from the vicinity of definite fat necroses that the fat-cells were pressed apart by more or less broad bands which contained the minutest fat-granules, also large and small fat-drops, and wholly concealed all other structures—namely, cells of connective tissue, capillaries, and fibers. After extraction of the fat the oil drops were found to be contained in thin membrane. Balser regarded these small cells containing fat as young cells of fat tissue. In many sections he saw places which he regarded as the beginning of fat necrosis, and which were characterized by the occurrence of an amorphous, nearly hyaline mass, generally in the form of rings or spherical shells. These hyaline shells wholly corresponded in size to normal fat-cells; they were separated from each other by sharp lines and contained in the center a granular mass and a few formations resembling nuclei. According to Balser, in a later stage the spherical shells broke into smaller flakes, and thus a complete disintegration of the fatty portions occurs. In the change of fat-cells into granular balls Chiari observed small glistening bodies resembling chalk molecules, and, in addition, in the older foci peculiar flakes of the size and form of ordinary fat-cells. Neither Balser nor Chiari could establish the composition and significance of these flakes. Langerhans, however, succeeded in demonstrating by microchemic and chemical analyses that these masses consisted of a combination of fat acids and chalk. Sarfert showed combinations of sodium with fat acids in his investigation on fat necrosis.

Langerhans, who introduced the term fat-tissue necrosis, obtained a clear picture of the process by study of the smallest foci, even those scarcely visible to the naked eye. He presented the following explanation of the microscopic appearances: The smallest foci are not as large as a fat-lobule, and are not bounded everywhere by connective tissue, but in places by intact fat-cells. Broad bands filled with fatty detritus (the bands of Balser) lie between the unchanged fat-cells. The fat-drops lie quite free, and are not surrounded by protoplasm, as Balser stated. Along the edge there is found at times cellular proliferation, but always corresponding to the position of the vessels and the accompanying connective tissue. The growth of young fat-cells, described by Balser, could not be shown. The old fat-cells contain fat and ovoid nuclei, and there were chalk molecules between the fat-cells and within the broad bands. More marked growths at the borders of the necrotic foci were to be seen only where the fat-lobules were bordered by connective tissue. Genuine granular corpuscles were formed in the latter in consequence of the fatty degeneration of spindle and stellate cells. A short distance within the necrotic area the bands between the fat-cells have almost entirely disappeared and the latter are more or less completely filled, not with a finely granular material, but with very fine needles, which have the faint luster and the small curve of crystals of palmitic and stearic acids. These needles do not always entirely fill the fat-cell, but often lie upon the periphery as clumps or rings or spherical shells. The remaining space is then filled with fat-drops of various size. Nearer the center are yellowish-brown clumps with a faint luster, of very irregular shape and size. They are round, angular, jagged, star-shaped, or at times form distinct, broad rings (Balser's bits of spherical shells), which, especially at the center of the focus, may occupy the entire space of the pre-existing fat-cell. All these round and angular clumps, rings, and large flakes consist of a combination of lime and fat acids. When the necrosis is so extensive that several adjoining fat-cells are involved, the fibrous septa between them die, but remain as band-like strips projecting in a tongue-shaped fashion into the interior of the area of fat necrosis. If large blood-vessels lie within the necrotic foci, they constantly appear to have died; cells in the walls are frequently to be recognized, but the nuclei are no longer colored by any stain. If the blood-vessels are traced to the edge of the necrotic focus, a growth of the intima may be found at times, also thrombosis with a proliferation of cells and diffuse blood pigment in the vicinity. At the border of many foci granular and diffuse blood pigment is found, of bright yellow or brownish-yellow color, which on the addition of concentrated sulphuric acid gives the changes of color mentioned by Virchow.

Langerhans thus summarizes his observations: "The multiple necrosis of fat tissue begins with the decomposition of the neutral fat contained in the cells; the fluid constituents are eliminated and the solid fatty acids remain. The latter then unite with the calcium salts to form calcium salts of fatty acids. The entire lobule or several neighboring lobules then form a dead mass which is separated from the living tissue by a dissecting inflammation proceeding from the surrounding tissue. The multiple necrosis of fat tissue has nothing in common with ordinary fatty degeneration (Chiari's view) or with a growth of fat-cells (Balser), which always leads to the formation of a lipoma, the occurrence of which in the mesentery is not so very common."

ETIOLOGY.

The etiology of fat necrosis is not yet satisfactorily explained. A number of authors (Balser, Langerhans, Fitz, Jackson and Ernst, Hildebrand, Dettmer, Jung, Ponfick, Lubarsch, Dieckhoff, Körte, E. Fraenkel) have sought an explanation by means of bacteriologic and experimental studies. We also have sought for information by means of experiments on animals. Hypotheses alone have been offered, the proof of which is lacking. Balser in his first communication looked for micro-organisms as the cause of the disease, but with entirely negative results. "With the means now at our disposal," he says, "no formations foreign to the human organism can be demonstrated in fat necrosis."

In his address before the Eleventh Congress of Internal Medicine, in 1892, Balser reported positive results. He examined the necrotic foci from a "Pagunerschweine" which macroscopically resembled abscesses, and succeeded, after careful fixation in a concentrated aqueous solution of picric acid, hardening in graded alcohol, and staining with the Ehrlich and the Ehrlich-Biondi tri-color mixture, in finding "numerous gland-like formations of dark yellow or coffee-brown color, which bore a great similarity to the flower of a full aster These formations consist of oblong clubs, quite similar to those of actinomyces, but somewhat smaller. They generally are arranged as rays around a point, but now and then are found isolated in the tissues."

The objection was raised that these bodies, on account of their partial staining, might be crystalloid formations. Balser believes that this objection was invalid, because he also saw them in preparations which were carried through alcohol and water into concentrated acetic acid, and then, after boiling in alcohol and ether and preservation in alcohol and water, were stained with the same dyes. He also made bacteriologic experiments, but unfortunately his report was merely preliminary, and permits no definite conclusions. He found bacilli which caused no essential changes when implanted into the anterior chamber of the eye of two rabbits and one pig. "The injection of the cultures of these bacilli into the abdominal cavity of animals also had not caused at the time any especial sickness." Lubarsch found numerous cocci and bacilli in the necrotic portions of a case of necrosis of fat tissue examined a few hours after death. Dieckhoff, who reported the case, gives no further information.

The results of the bacteriologic examination already mentioned (page 125) as made by Jackson and confirmed by Ernst also were obtained by the investigation of a focus of fat necrosis.

Ponfick very recently has made a bacteriologic study, and is forced to the conclusion "that the fat necrosis as such can by no means be the nucleus and essence of so severe a general disease as is observed in such mysterious cases. On the contrary, the conviction is forced upon us that it offers merely the predisposition by furnishing certain points of attack in consequence of the peculiar instability of all necrotic tissue which is more receptive, and hence in greater danger of attack."

He cultivated a bacillus regarded by him as possibly allied to Bacterium coli commune or at least belonging to this genus. It was obtained from the blood infiltrated beneath the peritoneum covering the posterior wall of the abdominal cavity, in front of the body of the second lumbar vertebra, of a man who had died soon after being attacked with the symptoms of intestinal obstruction. Ponfick, however, considers it an open question whether this micro-organism in the retroperitoneal tissue can be regarded as a constant and essential accompaniment of fat necrosis.

E. Fraenkel made thorough microscopic and cultural investigations, but with wholly negative results, and concluded "that the investigations hitherto made are not calculated to give thorough support to the micro-parasitic etiology of the necrosis of fat tissue.

Another method of obtaining light upon the pathogenetic factor was attempted. In his first work Langerhans had suggested "that during the metabolism within or around the cell some injurious substance appears and causes the decomposition of the oil." He attempted to find by experiments this external injurious substance. With strict antiseptic precautions he crushed the pancreas of a freshly killed rabbit in a mortar containing distilled water and finely splintered glass, filtered the mixture, and injected it into the fat tissue of other rabbits. He succeeded in causing necrosis of the fat tissue in one only of the 12 experiments (9 in rabbits and 3 in dogs). At the autopsy there was seen at the place of injection, at the upper end of the left kidney, just under the peritoneum, an opaque, yellowish-white, very dense mass about 4 mm. in diameter, which was sharply limited from the surrounding fat tissue. "From the microscopic appearances," says Langerhans, "there can scarcely be any doubt that the injection caused a circumscribed acute inflammation and necrosis of small portions of the fat tissue." He was able to distinguish three zones: The central resembled in most respects an inspissated abscess, the middle was composed of small, necrotic portions of fat tissue, and the outer zone corresponded to the fibrous septa between the individual fat-lobules and showed a decided cellular proliferation and the development of cells of higher order.

Langerhans does not believe that the splinters of glass alone are responsible for the formation of the abscess, but considers it more probable that the fat-ferment in the fresh pancreatic tissue caused purulent inflammation by immediate contact with the various tissues and cleavage of the oil drops in the living fat-cells and consequent necrosis of the fat tissue by mediate and weakened action.

When the above-mentioned communication was published, Langerhans had not finished his experiments, and, therefore, was very careful in stating his conclusions. He believes it possible " to produce fat necrosis by the action of fresh pancreatic juice on living fat tissue," but considers that still other etiologic factors must be present.

In his "Outlines of Pathologic Anatomy," which appeared later, Langerhans states definitely that the causes of multiple necrosis of fat tissue are merely hypothetic. Jung and Dettmer almost simultaneously produced fat-tissue necrosis by experimental methods. The former placed in the opened abdominal cavity of a rabbit a gelatin capsule filled with trypsin, and in that of each of three other rabbits several pieces of a dog's pancreas as large as the thumb. "Fat-tissue necrosis was produced in each animal by the action of pancreatic ferment, especially of fresh pancreatic tissue; at times it was superficial only, and again it was deeper seated. It seems fitting to ascribe this necrosis of fat tissue, partly to the fat-emulsifying and fat-decomposing ferments of the pancreatic juice, but in greater part to the enzyme which causes the decomposition of proteids."

Dettmer began with the assumption that the agent causing the necrosis of the fat tissue was either the normal pancreatic juice, the outflow of which was obstructed, and which, therefore, reached the surrounding tissue, causing necrosis, or that there escaped a product arising under pathologic conditions. He therefore tied the excretory ducts or the blood-vessels or both in cats and dogs. In a second series of experiments the pancreatic juice was conducted directly into the abdominal cavity. In order to find out which ferment in the pancreatic juice was active in the production of fat necrosis, he injected into the abdominal cavity in a third group of experiments pancreatic tissue, and in a fourth trypsin. Dettmer reached the following conclusions:

1. When the outflow of the pancreatic secretion from the gland is disturbed by closure of the pancreatic duct, with or without simultaneous interference of circulation, changes occur in the interpancreatic and parapancreatic fat, which resemble those described by Balser and Langerhans as multiple fat-tissue necrosis.

2. The changes in the fat tissue described as fat-tissue necroses are caused by the fat-ferment of the pancreatic juice and not by the trypsin.

The experiments were carried on under the direction of Hildebrand, who reported them at the Congress of the Surgical Association. He referred to twelve experiments in which he had succeeded in producing typical fat necrosis in the pancreas, omentum, and mesentery. The arrangement of the experiments is that described by Dettmer, as above reported.

The most careful and most instructive experiments were made by Körte. He operated on 24 cats and 6 dogs, and succeeded in causing typical fat necrosis in 10 out of 29 successful experiments. In the first series the pancreas or its blood-vessels were injured mechanically;

pieces of the gland were excised also and implanted in the abdominal cavity. In a second series he endeavored to cause inflammation of the gland by the injection of irritating or infectious substances at times associated with mechanical injury. In the third series he sought to determine the way in which the pancreas, previously inflamed by artificial means, bore its injuries.

In the first series of experiments fat necrosis occurred only when, in addition to the injuries inflicted, pieces of the gland were cut out and implanted in the abdominal cavity. "The animals generally died between the second and eleventh days after the operation; only one cat survived, and was killed a month later. At the postmortem examination necrosis of the fat tissue was found in four animals out of six; in two it was limited to the immediate vicinity of the pancreatic wound or of the implanted piece, while in the other two it was noticed in distant portions of the subperitoneal fat tissue; to be sure, the necrosis in these animals was not so extensive as usually is the case in the disseminated fat necrosis of man." In the second series of experiments Körte found necrosis of fat tissue in 6 out of 16 experiments in which pyogenic or chemical irritants were injected. In the third series fat necrosis never occurred.

Körte's conclusions with regard to necrosis of fat tissue artificially produced is as follows: "Necrosis of fat tissue may be produced by injuries and inflammations of the pancreas artificially produced, especially by solution of continuity and implantation of excised pieces of the glands. This result did not always occur, but only in a portion of the cases. The alterations obtained, however,—as Dettmer's experiments also teach,— have but a faint resemblance to the changes observed in man. The tendency to hemorrhage so frequently noticed in the latter was entirely lacking in the experimental fat necrosis."

"From the experiments on animals, as well as from experience in man, it seems very probable in many cases that the fat necroses associated with diseases of the pancreas are to be regarded as the consequence of the latter." We observed repeatedly the occurrence of fat necrosis in the course of various operations on the pancreas, especially after partial resection with implantation, and after injection into the tissues. Some of the experiments are here described:

FAT NECROSIS AFTER RESECTION AND IMPLANTATION OF PORTIONS OF THE PANCREAS.

January 8, 1896: Laparotomy on a small dog. The two portions of the pancreas which were not adherent to the intestine were removed and one part sewed into the subcutaneous fat tissue, the other into the great omentum.

January 9th: Dog very weak. No sugar in the urine.

January 10th: Dog found dead.

Autopsy: Peritoneum smooth and shining, spleen small. The dependent portions of the ileum and the omentum reddened, and in the latter are small hemorrhages in places. No further change in the fat tissue. The cut surface of the tail of the panceas appears infiltrated with blood and contains bright red points in the dark red tissue. Analogous changes are to be seen on the cut surface of the body of the pancreas, which also is spotted with bright red points and is softened throughout. The bit of pancreas sewed into the subcutaneous tissue is softened, greenish-gray, but injected in places with red. In the neighboring fat tissue are yellowish-white, shining, round spots of the size of a pinhead (fat necroses). The portion of the gland implanted in the omentum appears dark red, brown, soft, the acini not recognizable; round, yellowish-red, sharply defined foci as large as beans are seen in places.

FAT NECROSIS AFTER IMPLANTATION OF THE PANCREAS.

January 23, 1896: A dog of medium size, pancreas drawn forward and a ligature applied between its head and body, the former cut off and implanted in a fatty fold of the great omentum.

January 24th: Dog very weak. Bile-pigment and a small amount of sugar in the urine.

January 24th: In the afternoon the dog was found dead.

Autopsy: A large amount of bloody fluid in the abdominal cavity. The visceral peritoneum appears in places infiltrated with blood; there was a bright red extravasation of blood about a band's-breadth in size at the fundus of the stomach near the place where lay the portion of the omentum containing the implanted piece of pancreas; the blood-vessels of the intestinal mesentery were also markedly infiltrated with blood. The tail of the pancreas, which remained in position, appeared quite normal. In the portion of the body lying next to the duodenum were dull glistening round areas about the size of a pinhead, greenish-yellow in color, and surrounded by small, bright red extravasations of blood. Near the seat of the ligature was a hemorrhagic extravasation of the size of a hazelnut. The parenchyma of the pancreas was soft. The portion of the pancreas which was sewed into the omentum appeared very rotten and soft. Its structure was distinctly recognizable. On the surface lighter areas are found having a dull-white luster, and on cross-section forming distinct streaks. The great omentum is very full of blood. In places there were dense extravasations of blood as large as hazelnuts, generally dark brown, but in some parts smaller areas of a brighter red were seen. Certain portions of the fat were studded with bright red areas, and foci, some larger than pinheads, of a greenish-yellow color could be seen surrounded by a hemorrhagic zone. Spleen small, dense. Kidney bluish-red, with some lighter colored spots on the surface.

PANCREATIC HEMORRHAGE AND FAT NECROSIS AFTER INJECTION OF CHLORID OF ZINC.

November 8, 1896: A dog of medium size. Injection of 0.2 c.c. 5% solution of chlorid of zinc into each of three different places in the pancreas. A hematoma in the middle portion of the gland was formed at the operation.

November 10th: The dog was found dead in the morning.

Autopsy: The abdominal wound was infiltrated with blood. Hemorrhage into the abdominal cavity. Pancreas not essentially enlarged. The surface stained with blood in places, especially in the tail and the middle of the gland. These portions seemed somewhat swollen and enlarged. The head of the gland appeared quite normal. In the parts of the gland stained with blood are bright red areas about the size of the head of a pin (fat necrosis), and sharply and clearly distinguished from the surrounding dark, brownish-red tissue. A yellowish-white, glistening, dense area (fat necrosis), about the size of the head of a pin, projected above the surface of a portion of the body of the gland lying next to the intestine. Macroscopically, no signs of inflammation were visible. The microscopic examination of a portion which had undergone fat necrosis gave the appearances represented in figure 15, page 253.

FAT NECROSIS AFTER LIGATION OF THE BLOOD-VESSELS.

February 2, 1897: Very fat, old dog. Ligation of the afferent and efferent blood-vessels of the pancreas. The duodenal portion is isolated and the blood-vessels leading to the intestine are tied. At the operation a portion of the fat was resected.

February 3, 1897: After an attack of hematemesis the dog was found dead.

Autopsy: Several large and small yellowish-white areas, having a dull luster (fat necrosis), and surrounded by extravasations of blood of the size of a pea, are seen in the middle, and both lateral portions of the pancreas. Large and small whitish, necrotic areas, some as large as hazelnuts, having a faint luster, and often surrounded by large or small extravasations of blood, are found in the fat tissue of the great omentum. Ulcerations of the duodenum. The peritoneum over the greater curvature of the stomach was stained bright red.

The following conclusions were drawn from these experiments:

1. Resection of portions of the gland and their implantation caused fat necroses in the neighborhood of the cut surface and of the implanted part.

2. Ligation of the afferent and efferent blood-vessels of the pancreas, isolation of the duodenal portion, and ligation of the blood-vessels leading to the duodenum, were followed by fat necroses surrounded by large and small extravasations of blood in the pancreas and in the great omentum.

3. The injection of chlorid of zinc into the tissue gave rise to fat necroses and also to marked hemorrhage into the gland.

4. The transplantation into the subcutaneous connective tissue of a resected portion of the pancreas caused the development of foci of fat necrosis in the immediate neighborhood of the embedded piece.

5. The fat necrosis was always most extreme in the neighborhood of the injured or implanted portion of the gland.

In some cases the attempt was made to cause an outflow of the pancreatic secretion by numerous slight injuries of the pancreas, or by cutting into the ductus Wirsungianus and opening its canal. In one case a

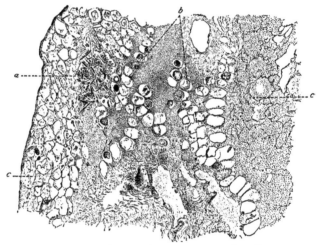

FIG. 15.—*a*, Needles of fat acids; *b*, flakes; *c*, necrotic fat tissue.

Pravaz needle was inserted into the gland in many places and the parenchyma torn. There was no development of fat necrosis. Neither did this occur in the experiments of February 12, 1896, which already have been mentioned, in which a solution of zymin was injected into the tissues of the gland in five different places, with the hope that fat necrosis might be caused by means of the known peptic quality of zymin. An indurative pancreatitis only developed.

It is evident on comparing the reported results of the many attempts to obtain a deeper insight into the etiology of fat necrosis that none of the hypotheses offered are entirely satisfactory. The view of Balser and Ponfick of the bacillary pathogenesis of the process is not established with sufficient certainty.

The suggestion first made by Langerhans, and later supported by Hildebrand, Dettmer, and Jung, is attractive and plausible; according to this, autodigestion, which perhaps plays a more important rôle in the pathology of the pancreas than is yet known, demands attention as an etiologic factor. Although this view satisfactorily explains the alteration in the pancreas and its neighborhood by means of the contact with the escaped pancreatic secretion, yet it is scarcely sufficient to explain the extensive changes in quite distant portions of the abdominal fat, as often observed in man; the occurrence of fat necrosis in the subepicardial and subcutaneous fat and in the bone-marrow and the severe general disturbances, often of sudden occurrence and rapidly fatal, cannot thus be explained. Further, the possibility that microparasites play an important part in these experiments on animals, upon which this theory is based, cannot be denied.

The question regarding the cause of the fat necrosis is obviously of far-reaching importance for the entire pathology of the pancreas. The relation of fat necrosis to the various processes, as " pancreatitis hemorrhagica," abscess, hemorrhage, and necrosis, has been mentioned in divers places in this section, and the relation of these processes to each other are often wholly obscure. As a rule, nothing is known of the cause or method of action, and it is uncertain whether both are not concurrent effects of the same cause. There is no agreement on this question among the authors. Some (Fitz, Körte) regard the fat necrosis ("in many cases very probably," Körte) as the result of inflammation, necrosis, and hemorrhage, while others (Balser, Langerhans, Seitz, E. Fraenkel) regard it as the cause. Ponfick, Dieckhoff, Lindsay Steven, and Rolleston hold a different view. Ponfick believes that the fat necrosis merely creates the predisposition to the severe processes; Dieckhoff assumes that the fat necrosis may give rise to diseases of an inflammatory nature, but considers it possible that the same cause (bacillary) which excites inflammation and suppuration also produces fat necrosis. Lindsay Steven regards the fat necrosis and the pancreatic necrosis as independent diseases, although he admits that extensive fat necrosis may lead to necrosis of the gland. Rolleston considers that the process is explained by changes in the sympathetic nervous system, especially in the solar plexus.

There is no doubt that wide-spread, rapidly fatal fat necroses may occur without other affection of the pancreas, as is shown by the case reported by E. Fraenkel, which will later be mentioned. Many other obscure points in the pathology of the pancreas will be made clear with the perfect understanding of the multiform process of fat necrosis, which is now apparently a wholly inconspicuous and irrelevant observation at a postmortem examination and again a very complicated disease producing extensive and wide-spread ravages, often rapidly causing death like a stroke of lightning, but usually with severe affections of the pancreas.

After our experiments were ended, Katz and Winkler continued an independent study of fat necrosis. The following results have been derived from the 26 experiments on animals previous to January 24, 1898:

1. Fat necrosis may certainly be produced by the following methods: The abdominal cavity is opened, the pancreas drawn forward, the main excretory duct tied in two places and cut between them; ligatures are then tied around the entire gland in different places, the blood-vessels being spared as much as possible. The abdominal cavity is closed by layers of stitches, and the wound is sealed with collodion. In every one

of the twenty dogs thus operated upon, fat necrosis to a greater or less extent occurred without exception.

The following experiment is reported as an illustration:

EXPERIMENT OF JUNE 26, 1897.—Dog of medium size. At the operation the chyle-vessels of the intestine appeared injected. The pancreas was rose-red. Ligation of the ductus Wirsungianus. Seven ligatures were tied about the entire gland, the blood-vessels being spared as much as possible.

June 28th, dog found dead.

Results of autopsy: Great omentum appears quite rich in fat. Numerous foci of fat necrosis as large as pinheads, confluent in places and surrounded by thickened fat tissue infiltrated with blood, are seen especially in the portion adjacent to the

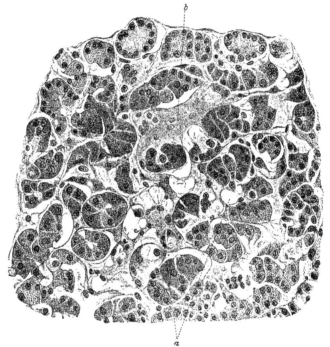

FIG. 16.—*a*, Clumps of fat; *b*, increased connective tissue.

duodenum. Just under these are found marked alterations of the pancreas; dark red discolorations with brighter colored ecchymoses as large as pinheads and obliterated gland-structure. The fat necrosis in the gland appears especially marked in those places cut into by the ligature, and is frequently continued into the neighboring fat tissue. The pancreas appears less reddened toward the spleen. The surface is softened in places and studded with foci of fat necrosis, like splashes of plaster. The fat necrosis is most marked near the entrance of the ductus Wirsungianus into the intestine. The gland here appears as if eroded, and there are distinct gaps filled with mortar-like material. Suffused spots with beginning necrosis are found near the knot in the ligature. In the splenic portion and in the adjoining fat tissue are solitary necrotic foci as large as peas and numerous miliary fat necroses, in part distributed throughout the tissue, and in part forming long lines. On section of the gland the tissue in the duodenal portion is soft, infiltrated with much blood, and containing a yellowish center; near the mouth of the ductus Wirsungianus the necrosis extends through the entire thickness of the pancreas, while near the surface in this region is a hemorrhagic nodule as large as a pea. There are numerous fat necroses, in part confluent, lying in the tissue infiltrated with blood, in a space about 4 cm., at the attachment of the great omentum to the greater curvature of the stomach.

Reference has already been made to a second experiment performed in the same manner (page 144). In this case the animal survived the operation, and about ten weeks later laparotomy was performed and the pancreas was extirpated. On microscopic examination, besides the existing induration, the changes in the gland lobules produced by the fat necrosis and the associated induration are represented in figure 16.

2. A very considerable leucocytosis in the animals experimented upon accompanied the fat necrosis. This was found in all cases (11) in which it was sought for and where there was extensive fat necrosis. The leucocytosis was present on the day after the operation.

The following experiments serve as examples:

EXPERIMENT OF NOVEMBER 17, 1897.—Dog of medium size. After the abdominal cavity is opened, the pancreas is drawn forward, the main excretory duct tied, and ligatures placed around the middle, head, and tail of the gland, sparing the blood-vessels as much as possible. The number of white blood-corpuscles at the beginning of the operation was 12,500.

November 19th: The dog was narcotized and blood withdrawn from the paw as at the operation. Number of the white blood-corpuscles, 310,000.

November 26th: Dog found dead, after having refused food for a number of days, without any apparent reason.

Autopsy: Cutaneous wound healed. No suppuration in the layers of the abdominal wall. Peritoneum smooth and shining. In the great omentum, especially along the blood-vessels, a hemorrhagic infiltration in which were numerous yellowish-white points as large as pinheads (fat necrosis). Pancreas pale red. In the middle, especially in the neighborhood of the mouth of the ductus Wirsungianus, the tissue is somewhat more red and dense and contains numerous small, yellowish-white spots (fat necroses). The gland-tissue appears as if forced apart by much enlarged bands of connective tissue. The two lateral portions of the pancreas show no additional changes. Spleen very small, of normal consistency. Liver normal.

EXPERIMENT OF JANUARY 3, 1898.—Small dog. Pancreas is drawn forward, the main excretory duct is tied, cut across, and eight ligatures are placed around the gland. Number of white blood-corpuscles, 30,000.

January 4th: In counting the white blood-corpuscles there is an unusually rapid coagulation of the blood. Number of the white blood-corpuscles, 135,000. The dog appears quite lively. Toward evening he becomes weaker, and dies at about ten o'clock in the evening.

January 5th: Autopsy: Peritoneum smooth and shining. No exudation in the abdominal cavity; pancreas of normal size; areas of normal color alternate with those which are much infiltrated with blood, and in which the gland structure is partly obliterated. At the beginning of the body of the gland there is an area of normal structure about the size of a hazelnut, adjoining which and between two ligatures is a dark violet portion of the gland containing several areas of a brighter red, with the structure obliterated. In the body of the gland the lobules are distinct, and toward the tail are some hemorrhages about as large as peas. Confluent foci of fat necrosis are found near the ligated duct, especially on the posterior surface. At the beginning of the tail the entire substance of the gland for about 4 cm. in length is in part dark violet and in part bright red, and the structure is wholly obliterated, especially in the violet portion; on the posterior surface there are foci of fat necrosis of silvery luster and confluent in places. The tip of the tail is normal except for a hemorrhage as large as a bean at the site of the last ligature. There are several foci of fat necrosis in the fat tissue and adjacent to the intestine, also on the surface of two neighboring lymph-glands. Spleen small, tissue firm, no evidence of sepsis.

Microscopic examination: (1) The areas of fat necrosis show numerous fat-cells filled with acicular fat-acid crystals and others with hyaline flakes. (2) The lobules in the necrotic portion of the pancreas are beset with acicular fat-acid crystals and numerous very minute granules. After the addition of acetic acid, the nuclei of the cells are distinct and granular. (3) The areas which were infiltrated with blood but showed macroscopically no fat necrosis are largely filled with very minute granules and are traversed by numerous capillaries distended with blood. (4) The portion of the pancreas which had not been tied and which is of normal appearance shows likewise very numerous minute granules, which, however, are found only within the lobules.

The following control experiments were undertaken in order to make clear the relation between the fat necrosis and leucocytosis

1. A blood count was taken before each operation, since a considerable leucocytosis is at times found in dogs. It resulted that a very decided increase in the number of white corpuscles took place after the operation even in those animals in which a definite leucocytosis was present before the operation: in one case an increase from 30,000 to 135,000 in the cubic millimeter; an increase from 35,000 to 118,500 in the cubic millimeter in another.

2. Narcosis (with morphin or chloroform) produced no essential influence, merely causing an increase from 5000 to 11,000 in a cubic millimeter. In a second case there was no modification.

3. The laparotomy caused no essential increase, as has previously been stated by Tarchanow, Emelianow, and Jacoby: before the operation, 7500; after the operation, 10,500 in the cubic millimeter; before the operation, 65,000; after the operation, 75,000 in the cubic millimeter.

4. Laparotomy and extirpation of the omentum caused no hyperleucocytosis.

5. After the injection of turpentine into the tissues of the pancreas and the production of an abscess there was a slight increase (from 11,000 to 15,000).

6. In total extirpation, 31,200 in the cubic millimeter were found before the operation, on the day after the operation 90,000, and on the following day 27,500.

It would be premature to draw any conclusions from this preliminary communication of facts requiring further confirmation. It must first be proved that the alteration of the blood stands in any relation to the fat necrosis. It is to be hoped that further investigation will advance the solution of the question concerning the true causes both of the local changes and the severe general symptoms.

[Subsequent investigations have confirmed the observations of Langerhans that fat necrosis can be produced by the contact of the constituents of the pancreas with fat tissue, and his hypothesis that the fat-splitting ferment of the pancreatic juice causes the necrosis by separating the fat into fatty acids and glycerin.

Abundant experimental evidence in support of the first statement has been furnished not only by the observers above mentioned, but also by H. U. Williams * and Flexner,† and the latter observer also has demonstrated by chemical methods the presence of the fat-splitting ferment in the areas of necrosis in a patient and in animals.

Flexner ‡ has shown also that hemorrhagic pancreatitis and fat necrosis may be produced by injections of hydrochloric acid, sodium hydroxid, and formalin into the pancreatic duct of dogs. Opie § was alike successful with bile, and Flexner and Pearce‖ conclude from their

---

* *Boston Med. and Surg. Jour.*, 1897, cxxxvi, 345; *Jour. Exp. Med.*, 1898, iii, 585.   † *Jour. Exp. Med.*, 1897, ii, 413.
‡ "Contributions to the Science of Medicine," dedicated to Wm. H. Welch, M.D., 1900, 743.
§ *Trans. Assoc. Am. Physicians*, 1901, xvi, 329.
‖ *Trans. Assoc. Am. Physicians*, 1901, xvi, 348.

experimental studies that the entrance into the pancreas of gastric juice and of bile are efficient causes of pancreatitis with hemorrhage and fat necrosis.

The summary by Körte * with regard to the relation between fat necrosis and disease of the pancreas needs but little modification in consequence of recent investigations:

"A slight degree of necrosis of fat tissue is not infrequently found in the pancreas and in the peritoneal fat in the absence of other alterations of the gland and without the production of morbid symptoms.

"It has been seen during life also without evident disease of the gland, and after a time has disappeared (personal observation).

"It is usually associated with hemorrhagic affections of the pancreas and their consequences (necrosis), and more rarely accompanies suppurative inflammation.

"Experiments on animals have shown that fat necrosis can result from injuries to the gland and from the stagnation of blood and secretion and from inflammation artificially produced in it. In man also fat necrosis has so immediately followed injury to the organ as to be regarded with a high degree of probability as the result of the injury to the pancreas (Warren).

"In accordance with such experiments and experience it is highly probable, in many instances at least, that the alterations of the peritoneal fat tissue associated with diseases of the pancreas are to be regarded as the result of the latter.

"It is possible that, at times, disseminated necrosis of fat tissue may promote the origin of inflammation, hemorrhage, and gangrene of the gland, since thereby the tissues are made less capable of resistance.

"The necrosis of fat tissue in rare instances is found without accompanying hemorrhage or inflammatory changes in the pancreas.

"Bacteria, especially intestinal bacteria, are not infrequently found in the foci of fat necrosis. Ponfick's hypothesis that the microbes are the cause both of the fat necrosis and of the subsequent pancreatic hemorrhage is not yet proved. It seems to me more probable that bacteria and irritants proceed from the inflamed, hemorrhagic or necrotic organ through the lymph-vessels into the surrounding fat tissue and produce in it the necrotic areas. It may be, as a third possibility, that bacilli advance from the diseased pancreas to the necrotic foci in the fat tissue and find in them a suitable soil for further development."—Ed.]

STATISTICS.

There are no satisfactory statistics regarding the frequency of fat necrosis. As already mentioned, it was found by Balser 5 times in 25 bodies taken indifferently as small, punctate foci or as areas of the size of a pinhead between the lobules of the pancreas. The foci are found less frequently in the fat tissue surrounding the organ. In the reports of the autopsies at the Vienna General Hospital from 1885 to 1895, 11 cases are recorded, of whom 6 were men and 4 women (in one case the sex was not stated); in 8 of these cases there was no diabetes. In 1891 chronic pancreatitis following fat necrosis was noted in a man forty years old. In 1893 in a woman nineteen years old there was a partial

* " Die Chirurg. Krankheiten u. d. Verletz des Pankreas," 1898, 198.

fatty degeneration of the pancreas and disseminated fat necrosis with beginning suppuration, and in a woman twenty-seven years old fat necrosis of the pancreas and mesentery. In 1894 in an individual aged fifty-five years (sex not stated), fat necrosis of the pancreas and hemorrhages in the superficial portions were present. The pancreas is uniformly much increased in size, the lobes on the surface appearing large, the cut surface studded with bright yellow points; man, fifty-four years old, beginning fat necrosis; man, fifty-three years old, fat necrosis of the pancreas, deposits of calcium salts in the parenchyma; man, forty-six years old, fat necrosis of the pancreas and mesentery; in 1895, man, sixty-three years old (inebriate), fat necrosis of the pancreas.

In three cases there was diabetes: 1889, in a woman, nineteen years old, fat necrosis in the region of the pancreas; 1890, an inebriate, forty-nine years old, beginning fat necrosis; 1895, fat necrosis in the pancreas with suppurative pancreatitis.

SYMPTOMS.

A clinical description of the morbid process just described, apart from the fact that it is justified only when the fat necrosis is regarded as an idiopathic process, is difficult in so far as it affects the pancreas, because the fat necrosis is usually not limited to the pancreas in all the cases productive of symptoms, but is diffused more or less over a large part of the abdominal fat.

The earliest anatomic changes, which not infrequently can be found at the autopsy, cause no symptoms during life, and it is only the later stages which produce the extensive disturbances which, as a rule, do not concern the pancreas alone, but also other portions of the digestive tract. As concerns the pancreas, the fat necrosis is a cause or accompaniment or result of severe inflammation, hemorrhage, and gangrene. The symptoms are caused by these severe processes only and not by the causal, concurrent, or consequent factor, the fat necrosis. The symptoms are the same whether the inflammation, hemorrhage, or pancreatic necrosis is caused by fat necrosis or by other conditions, and it is therefore necessary only to refer to the descriptions given in the sections on Inflammation, Hemorrhage, and Necrosis. Cases are there reported in detail which allow the assumption that fat necrosis is the cause of these processes. The disease is manifold, complicated, and severe when the fat necrosis is situated not merely in the pancreas and the surrounding fat tissue, but is spread over a large portion of the abdominal fat and there is a destruction of larger portions, with or without hemorrhage.

Types of the disease are furnished by some of the cases extracted from the literature and compared with the analogous reports given in previous sections.

Von Kahlden: Woman sixty years old, very fat; a few days before death there were severe abdominal pains, vomiting, constipation, meteorism, no tenderness; the vomiting persisting, the stomach was washed out, after which the general condition was improved; a small amount of fecal matter was passed, with some flatus. Death occurred in about eight days with symptoms of collapse.

Autopsy: Intestinal peritoneum much injected, intestines adherent, in the omentum and mesentery whitish nodules as large as a ten-cent piece; the omentum contained so many that it appeared like a tumor. Similar nodules in the parietal peritoneum; pancreas enlarged and contained large and small yellow and gray nodules projecting above the surface.

E. Fraenkel: (a) Woman forty-eight years old, brought to the hospital with the diagnosis of intestinal occlusion. Meteorism, jaundice, vomiting, pulse scarcely perceptible. On the next day, persistent collapse, passage of stools, death. Autopsy: Abundant fat in the abdominal wall, numerous foci of fat necrosis in the large and small omenta and in each of the epiploic appendices of the large intestines, all of which contained abundant fat. The splenic flexure was firmly united to the fat tissue behind it, in which were numerous foci of fat necrosis, and to the anterior surface of the left kidney and to the tail of the pancreas. The gastrocolic ligament contained numerous foci of fat necrosis. This was cut through and the omental bursa opened and the fat tissue surrounding the pancreas was found transformed into a dark brown mass filled with fat necroses. The pancreas is of satisfactory consistency and only a few areas of fat necrosis were to be recognized in the interstitial tissue.

(b) Woman fifty-two years old; about fourteen days before her admission to the hospital cholelithiasis was diagnosticated. Frequent nausea, vomiting, diarrhea, metorism, sensitiveness to pressure. When anesthetized and examined, a deep-seated, retroperitoneal tumor was felt. Laparotomy. Numerous small areas of fat necrosis were seen in the parietal and visceral layers of the peritoneum; therefore the operation was ended. Two days later there was hematemesis and the passage of bloody stools. Death eleven days after admission. At the autopsy, besides the necrotic portions of the transverse and descending mesocolon, which were infiltrated with blood, multiple perforations were found in the jejunum and on the posterior wall of the stomach, and there was almost an entire absence of the pancreas. The fat tissue around the left kidney also showed many areas of fat necrosis.

The manifestations of disease, whether consequences or complications of fat necrosis, are various. They sometimes resemble intestinal obstruction, bursal abscess, retroperitoneal tumor, or perforative peritonitis, or, in consequence of the temporary violent colic, with collapse, they suggest gall-stones, poisoning, or a severe infection.

Fraenkel communicates an interesting case: A patient was brought into the hospital with the suspicion of cholera and died. At the autopsy there was found an extensive necrosis of the greater portion of the abdominal fat, complicated with hemorrhage.

At the session of the Society for Internal Medicine in Berlin, April 27, 1896, Stadelmann reported the case of an individual twenty-three years old who formerly had been perfectly healthy, but was attacked within a few days by severe abdominal pains and quickly became comatose. On entrance the patient was in deep coma. The urine contained albumin, 3.4% of sugar, and there was a positive ferric chlorid reaction. Death occurred with increasing cyanosis. Benda demonstrated the specimen from this case. There was multiple fat necrosis of the peritoneum, associated with extensive disease of the pancreas. Nearly the entire gland was changed into hemorrhagic tumor, only a part of the head being preserved.

DIAGNOSIS.

The diagnosis of fat necrosis can be made with certainty only at an operation, as occurred in the cases reported by Körte and Fraenkel. The latter considers the diagnosis of fat necrosis possible when in obese persons there is a fluctuating tumor in the epigastrium, which disappears after preceding, very severe colic and with subsequent profuse diarrhea, to return after some time. The diagnosis is absolutely certain if necrotic fat tissue or pancreatic structure is found in the feces. The objection is to be raised that the eventual demonstration in the feces of such shreds of fat tissue or necrotic portions of the pancreas does not always prove that the necrosis of fat tissue is the cause of the process. The necrosis may just as well be the consequence of a gangrene which has developed in some other way.

The only treatment is surgical. Langerhans states that he had been informed by Fitz and Welsh that recovery from multiple fat necrosis and sequestration of the pancreas had resulted from the removal of the gland at an operation. Langerhans gives no further information. [This case is that mentioned by Osler.* The patient was supposed to have acute intestinal obstruction; the abdomen was opened by Halsted, who found a thick, dense mass in the region of the pancreas and foci of fat necrosis in the omentum and mesentery. The exploratory incision was closed, and the patient recovered. Four years later he suffered from similar symptoms, but refused an operation.—Ed.] In Thayer's patient with pancreatic abscess and disseminated fat necrosis recovery took place after the operation.

Spontaneous recovery is to be thought of only when fat necrosis is associated with sequestration of the pancreas and the latter is discharged with the feces.

[The surgical treatment of fat necrosis is so intimately connected with that of acute, non-suppurative pancreatitis that the treatment of the former condition is usually considered to include that of the latter. The exploratory incision reveals the foci of fat necrosis, and the discovery of an indurated, perhaps hemorrhagic mass in the region of the pancreas, in connection with the symptoms, is regarded as a sufficient justification for the diagnosis of acute pancreatitis. The latter diagnosis under these circumstances has repeatedly been confirmed by the postmortem examination of the fatal cases, and seems warranted in those which recover.

The following are to be added to the two cases above mentioned: That reported by Körte,† a combination of gangrenous pancreatitis and fat necrosis. This patient was in fairly good condition, although diabetic, four and a half years later.‡ The case of omental fat necrosis and large nodular mass behind the stomach operated upon by Gerster and reported by Manges.§ Munro's case of fat necrosis and mass in the region of the pancreas, reported by Lund‖ and Munro.** The case of hemorrhagic pancreatitis mentioned by Fowler †† and that of fat necrosis and greatly enlarged pancreas reported by Mayo.‡‡—Ed.]

* "Principles and Practice of Medicine," 4th Edition, 1901, 591.

† *Arch. f. klin. Chir.*, 1894, xlviii, 721.

‡ "Die chir. Krankh. u. d. Verletz. d. Pankreas," 1898, 187.

§ *Phila. Med. Jour.*, 1899, iii, 724.

‖ *Boston City Hospital Report*, 1900, 43.

** *Boston Med. and Surg. Jour.*, 1900, cxliii, 543.

†† *Trans Am. Surg. Assoc.*, 1901, xix, 180.

‡‡ *Jour. Am. Med. Assoc.*, 1902, xxxviii, 107.

X. ATROPHY, FATTY DEGENERATION, LIPOMATOSIS, AND AMYLOID DEGENERATION.

(a) ATROPHY.

IT can readily be understood that atrophy is among the most common affections of the pancreas. Marantic or senile atrophy is found as a manifestation of old age, and is then usually the consequence of arteriosclerotic processes or of general cachexia (cachectic atrophy). Lobstein has stated that the former is one of the frequent conditions in advanced years, and the following report of an autopsy performed by Dr. Zemann at the Rothschild Hospital is an example of the not infrequent senile atrophy: In a man eighty-four years old the aorta was found dilated, its walls flaccid, the intima of the arch markedly thickened; the peripheral arteries were large, very tortuous, and the intima thickened in places; the pancreas was grayish-red, the lobules very small, the branches of the pancreatic artery were narrowed in many places by the thickened intima; there was gangrene of the left great toe and of the tips of the second and fourth toes.

In simple atrophy the entire pancreas is diminished in size, the weight is often reduced to 1 to 1¼ ounces, while that of a normal pancreas, according to Vierordt, averages 3 to 3½ ounces. In the section on Diabetes as a Symptom of Diseases of the Pancreas, Hansemann's distinction between cachectic and diabetic atrophy is described (page 77). He states that the two varieties are to be distinguished macroscopically and microscopically. Diabetic atrophy belongs to the series of interstitial inflammations, and there is a marked similarity between it and granular atrophy of the kidney. Granular atrophy of the pancreas, according to Hansemann, leads very rarely to complete destruction of the organ, and it is surprising how much gland-substance, as a rule, is still present in this variety of atrophy. If, however, the gland-substance is exceptionally reduced to a minimum, the organ is transformed into a thin, flabby, fibrous body of less volume than the normal pancreas, at first sight giving the impression far more of atrophy than of inflammation.

It has already been stated that atrophy of the pancreas is no rare condition in diabetes. In 40 cases of diabetes in which there was disease of the pancreas Hansemann found simple atrophy in 36. Dieckhoff collected 53 cases of severe disease of the pancreas with diabetes, in 21 of which were atrophy and lipomatosis.

In the reports of autopsies at the General Hospital in Vienna from 1885 to 1895, atrophy was recorded 8 times in 12 cases of diabetes. Atrophy was found 78 times in the 188 cases of diabetes with disease of the pancreas mentioned under General Considerations.

I have seen several cases of atrophy of the pancreas in diabetes. Three of these, with the results of the autopsies by Dr. Zemann, are previously mentioned (page 60). Secondary atrophy of the pancreas may occur in consequence of pressure from without, by tumors (aneurysms, neoplasms, degenerated lymph-gland), or in consequence of some internal cause, as calculus-formation in the duct with dilatation of the excretory duct, cyst-formation, hemorrhage, abscess, chronic interstitial inflammation, lipomatosis, new-formations. Atrophy from pressure may reach such a high degree that the glandular substance may almost wholly disappear and the organ be changed to a thin, flabby body. Its course may be run with or without diabetes.

(b) FATTY DEGENERATION.

Fatty degeneration of the parenchyma of the gland frequently occurs in the course of infections and intoxications. This process was earlier regarded as acute parenchymatous inflammation. It occurs as cloudy swelling in the parenchyma of the pancreas in various infectious diseases, as typhoid fever, variola, puerperal fever, yellow fever, plague, etc., analogous to the similar changes in the liver, kidney, and muscles which generally occur at the same time. Friedreich saw such a parenchymatous degeneration in the course of a wandering, erysipelatous, double pneumonia in a strong young man.

Macroscopically the gland appears enlarged, at first reddened on account of hyperemia, but later whitish or grayish-yellow on account of the advanced degeneration of the epithelium and the edema of the interstitial connective tissue. The microscope shows that the changes affect only or chiefly the parenchyma, the cells of which are in a condition of cloudy swelling, ending in fatty degeneration and destruction; they appear very granular, opaque, somewhat enlarged, the granules dissolving in acetic acid and caustic potash. Each cell contains two or three, even five, large round nuclei and nucleoli (Dieckhoff, Friedreich).

The diagnosis of cloudy swelling is at present impossible. According to Friedreich, its existence may be suspected when the clinical signs of acute parenchymatous degeneration of the liver (acute swelling) and of the kidney (albuminuria), in addition to a considerable splenic enlargement and high fever are present in a severe case of acute infectious disease. Friedreich thinks that many cases of jaundice developing in the course of severe infectious diseases may be due to pressure of the swollen head of the pancreas on the ductus choledochus.

Fatty degeneration of the gland-cells occurs also in inflammation whether caused by pressure from within (stagnant secretion) or from without, or by other causes (phosphorus-poisoning). The tissue of the gland assumes in consequence a brighter, more yellowish color, the excretory ducts are filled with fat detritus and therefrom may be dilated. Such contents are to be found in the pancreatic duct even in complete fatty degeneration (Orth).

Fatty degeneration is found also in general obesity, especially in inebriates, analogous to fatty degeneration of the heart and blood-vessels. It may lead to hemorrhage, as has already been mentioned in the section on this subject (Friedreich).

Fatty degeneration of the gland is recorded twice in the reports of the autopsies at the Vienna General Hospital from 1885 to 1895. In 1893 the case is mentioned of a woman nineteen years old who suffered from the excessive vomiting of pregnancy and died in collapse. At the autopsy the condition was as follows: Metamorphosis adiposa pancreatis partialis et necrosis textus adiposi disseminata cum suppuratione incipiente. Urocystitis chronica. Ruptura cervicis uteri. In 1894 the autopsy of a man sixty-six years old showed confluent lobular pneumonia, pancreatic

calculus, fatty degeneration of the gland parenchyma and fibrous induration.

The interstitial growth of fat which occurs in the course of simple,
especially marantic atrophy, is the transition to genuine lipomatosis.
The atrophy of the gland-cells is the primary affection and the resulting
empty space is filled with the growth of fat tissue. The following case
examined after death at the Rothschild Hospital by Dr. Zemann is an
example: A man seventy years old was treated for emphysema, arteriosclerosis, and general dropsy; at the autopsy the pancreas was found
embedded in abundant fat tissue, very flabby, thin, speckled with red;
on section, lobules (small, pale grayish-yellow) were forced apart by
abundant flabby, edematous, dirty yellow fat tissue; the small branches
of the pancreatic artery were very narrow on account of thickening
of the intima, and at times almost completely closed by dense nodules.

This condition is often combined with fatty degeneration and is
represented by a new-formation of fat tissue, which gradually infiltrates
the entire gland, the structure of which is replaced by fat. The pancreas
becomes somewhat larger than normal, soft, and in extreme degrees the
entire organ is transformed into a yellow or yellowish-white mass of
fat.

(c) LIPOMATOSIS.

Lipomatosis is frequently combined with the formation of concretions. The
instructive case reported by Dieckhoff is given as an example: A woman thirty-five
years old two years before her admission into the Rostock Hospital suffered from a
pneumonia of the left side, on account of which she was treated for eight weeks.
Since then there have been persistent cough, expectoration, emaciation. At the time
of admission the diagnosis was pyopneumothorax. An exploratory puncture made
later showed a purulent exudation, in which were tubercle bacilli. Tubercle bacilli
were found also in the sputum. There were irregular fever with evening exacerbations, fetid sputum, albumin in the urine at times, but no sugar. The ribs were
resected and a large amount of very offensive pus was evacuated; there was at first
improvement, but soon afterward the condition became worse, there were cardiac
weakness, cyanosis, and death.

At the autopsy Lubarsch found the pancreas large, very flabby, almost fluc-
tuant. On section the substance was almost wholly transformed into a lobulated
mass with the luster of fat, containing here and there whitish streaks, and large, dilated ducts filled with calcium concretions. On chemical examination these concretions were found to consist predominantly of carbonate of lime and traces of phosphate of lime. On microscopic examination the extraordinary increase of fat tissue
was very noticeable. In many places there were also small necrotic foci, each of
which contained but a few cells.

In the section on Pancreas and Diabetes several cases of lipomatosis
are mentioned (page 62).

The formation of lipomata may be a feature of general obesity,
especially in drunkards. It occurs, however, in emaciated individuals
also, as is shown in the case mentioned before and by the following case,
reported by Lépine and Cornil:

A man fifty-seven years old, formerly a hard drinker, had lost flesh for about
six months, suffered alternately from constipation and diarrhea, had neither fever
nor vomiting. For two months slight edema of the legs. Marked emaciation. Internal organs showed no essential change. Autopsy: Pancreas of normal size and
shape, fatty degenerated throughout resembling a lipoma, gland tissue wholly absent. Between the lobules there is only fat tissue; the chief duct and accessory ducts
contain a thick, white, slimy fluid and small concretions.

(d) AMYLOID DEGENERATION.

This occurs in connection with the same process in numerous other organs, and involves, as Friedreich has shown, only the small arteries and capillaries. This author could not confirm the statement of Rokitansky concerning the occurrence of localized amyloid disease exclusively limited to the pancreas, and also of the amyloid degeneration of the gland-cells. On the other hand, he was able to show in the body of a phthisical patient twenty years old both amyloid degeneration of the vessels of the pancreas and pronounced fatty degeneration of the gland-cells. The pancreas in this case was yellowish-white and of less than normal consistency; on section there was such extensive fatty degeneration of the gland-cells that the organ appeared almost everywhere filled with fatty detritus; amyloid degeneration was found especially in the arteries of small and medium size, which ran in the interlobular tissue, and in the capillaries surrounding the gland lobules.

Friedreich's statement was confirmed by Kyber. He also found the pancreas degenerated in cases of general amyloid disease. As a rule, he saw single arteries entirely degenerated, giving the characteristic reaction. In two cases he found degeneration of the membrana propria of the acini in addition to that of the capillaries which surrounded the narrow lobules. The epithelial cells in these cases were to a great extent filled with fat granules and fat-drops, in part disintegrated, and of a yellow color; there was an increased amount of interlobular connective tissue. The organ externally appeared merely dense and anemic. Increased density and abundant development of interlobular connective tissue were found in those cases also in which only individual arteries were degenerated.

Among 155 cases of general amyloid disease, Hennings found amyloid disease of the pancreas in 3.9% of the cases.

XI. RUPTURE, PROLAPSE, DISPLACEMENT, AND BULLET WOUNDS OF THE PANCREAS.

(a) RUPTURE OF THE PANCREAS.*

INJURIES of the pancreas are, on the whole, rather rare. The organ through its anatomic position is quite safely protected from injury. When the latter is applied to a limited part of the abdomen, it may, under certain conditions, affect the pancreas. The force of the blow, according to Leith, must be directed more or less toward the back, and not obliquely upward or downward, in order that the pancreas may be pressed against the resistant spinal column. The organ can be injured from the front only under especially favorable circumstances, because

---

*The following statement is based on the comprehensive monograph of Leith.

it is protected in front by the abdominal walls, the tension of the abdominal muscles, the stomach, the omental sac, the ascending portion of the transverse mesocolon; and from behind, but less easily, being protected by the vena portæ, the vena cava inferior, the two crura of the diaphragm on both sides of the aorta, the trunk of the superior mesenteric artery, the left adrenal and kidney, and especially by the spine and the powerful muscles of the back.   In order that rupture of the gland may follow even violence from the front, the force must be very considerable and the stomach and intestine empty.   For the occurrence of a more severe injury, the force must be directed not only toward the median line and from the front backward, but also must be very great.

Leith divides ruptures into two groups: (1) Those ending fatally; (2) those pursuing a less severe course.

He includes the following 9 cases in the first group: seven published previously, one of his own, and one reported by Goldmann.   In only two was the pancreas alone injured; in the remainder other organs also were affected: once the lungs were ruptured, once the spleen, once the duodenum, and four times the ribs were fractured in connection with other internal injuries, as rupture of the liver, kidney, or spleen.   The cases reported by Leith are, in brief, as follows:

1. Leith: Boy, four years old, kicked in the stomach by a horse, fell against the wheel of the wagon, but was able to get up.   In the afternoon he felt ill and was unable to use his left arm.   Annandale found, on examination, a transverse fracture of the lower third of the humerus, but no signs of any other injury.   Later in the afternoon he appeared worse; there were shock, pain, indistinct symptoms of abdominal disturbance.   In the evening he was in collapse, so that an exploratory laparotomy was impossible and he died ten hours after the injury.   The autopsy, fourteen hours after death, showed no evidence of injury except that of the left arm.   In the abdomen about 1 pint of clear, dark-brown, inoffensive fluid; peritoneum markedly injected, not so transparent as usual; no hemorrhage.   Rupture of the duodenum near the end of the upper third, affecting about two-thirds of the circumference; escape of the duodenal contents, which appeared like coagulated milk.   Deeper down in the mesentery of the jejunum was a small tear and a slight hemorrhage; transverse colon pushed down, pancreas lying free, the ascending part of the transverse mesocolon and the subjacent pancreas ruptured.   The injury to the pancreas was less extensive than that of the mesentery, and was vertical, extending somewhat to the right and involving the entire width of the upper edge, but only a portion of the lower part.   Main excretory duct and the splenic vessels were intact; a line drawn through the tear, if continued meets one drawn through the torn duodenum; the rupture was due probably to the direct influence of the kick and the pressure of the organ against the spine.   The ruptured portions show a small gap and are slightly infiltrated with blood.   There is some blood in the retroperitoneal connective tissue toward the hilum of the spleen and near the suprarenal capsule.   In comparison with the severity of the injury there was surprisingly little hemorrhage. The foramen of Winslow was open.   The fluid in the abdominal cavity was mixed with pancreatic juice; the aorta was uninjured; the liver, kidney, and lungs were very pale, as after a severe hemorrhage.

According to Leith, the following points are noteworthy in this case: The nature of the injury, the absence of severe symptoms immediately after it, their subsequent rapid onset and severity, the lack of external injury to the abdomen, the absence of pain, the large quantity of exudation in the peritoneum, the extent of the rupture of the pancreas, the slight hemorrhage.

2. Goldmann: A young man suffered a severe injury from the fall of a heavy box on his abdomen.   It was thought that a corner of this box had grazed the epigastrium.   Symptoms of hemorrhage, intestinal occlusion, appearance of a tumor in the epigastrium, similar to a pancreatic cyst.   Nothing abnormal in the skin of

the abdomen; death occurred some hours after the injury. At the autopsy a transverse rupture of the pancreas was found, also marked hemorrhage into the cavity of the lesser omentum and rupture of the spleen; the other organs were not injured.

3. Jaun: Man fifty years old. Results of an assault in which, after his knees and elbows were tied together, he was laid on his back, struck in the abdomen with a shoe, and pushed about; he then walked about a mile toward home, supported by two persons, and died about eighteen hours after his admission to the hospital. Autopsy: The pancreas ruptured on the right half-way through. At the place of rupture there were small clots of blood; the rest of the organ was injected and showed marked extravasation of blood in the gland-substance; hemorrhagic exudation in the peritoneal cavity; externally nothing abnormal.

4. Wilks and Moxon: An adult man was run over. Pancreas ruptured in the middle, and divided into two halves, which lay near the spine. Some other slight signs of injury of the abdominal organs.

5. Wandesleben: Pancreas and lungs were injured. A pancreatic abscess developed which was opened by Wandesleben (Körte).

The four following cases were reported by Senn:

6. Cooper: A man thirty-three years old was run over by a rapidly running light wagon. No external signs of injury, the left lower ribs were broken, the pancreas was literally crushed and embedded in half-coagulated blood. He died some days afterward.

7. Travers: A drunken woman was knocked down by the wheel of a post-wagon but was not run over. She lived only a few hours. Some ribs were broken, the pancreas was torn through transversely, likewise the liver, and much blood escaped.

8. Stork mentions the case of a woman who was run over by a coach and who lived only a short time after the injury. Pancreas torn in two and embedded in a large quantity of semi-fluid blood. The liver torn, a number of ribs broken

9. Le Gros-Clark observed a case of rupture of the pancreas in a boy who had suffered other severe injuries and died soon afterward.

The communications of Rose and Wagstaff are more recent:

In Rose's case a rupture of the posterior wall of the stomach, combined with laceration of the pancreas, occurred after a trauma. The meal last taken escaped into the omental bursa and became mixed with blood and pancreatic juice, in consequence of which inflammation of the bursa followed. There was probably closure of the foramen of Winslow. The case was operated upon (incision and drainage), after which a fistula formed, from which a fluid was evacuated which showed the characteristics of pancreatic juice.

Wagstaff: Fall from a wagon, contusion of the left side, fracture of the femur. On the third day symptoms of peritonitis developed and death occurred on the fifth day. Autopsy: No peritonitis, rupture of the pancreas, large retroperitoneal extravasation of blood.

Symptoms.—Shock and collapse seem, as Leith states, to be the most prominent symptoms; they are usually caused by internal hemorrhage. In some cases the collapse occurs only after a considerable interval, and is probably to be ascribed to the complications. In no patient have the symptoms pointed to the pancreas as the chief seat of the injury. According to Leith, the absence of all external signs of injury to the abdomen is surprising and noteworthy. From a medicolegal point of view this is especially to be borne in mind.

Diagnosis.—It is impossible to make the diagnosis without laparotomy. The nature of the force, its exact seat and direction, may at most lead to a suspicion of a pancreatic lesion. Leith has ascertained by examination of the cadaver that in the epigastrium, a little to the left, the anterior surface of the pancreas could be accurately outlined with the finger through a three-inch incision in the median line. The gland

and its peritoneal covering can thoroughly be seen with an electric light introduced in a Ferguson's speculum.

Course.—In all the cases hitherto reported, with the exception of that of Rose, death occurred quickly. In six cases it was caused by internal hemorrhage, but it is probable that the hemorrhage from the neighboring organs simultaneously injured was the main cause. It is not to be assumed that the hemorrhage alone from a ruptured pancreas is of importance, except when the splenic artery or vein is lacerated at the same time (Leith).

Treatment.—It appears from the statements of Leith that "injuries of the pancreas rarely occur alone, and, further, as a rule present no marked symptoms. Hence the treatment should be expectant, except in those cases in which exploratory laparotomy has been decided upon. If a rupture of the pancreas then is found, it should be appropriately treated. The hemorrhage is to be checked by pressure and the lacerated ends are to be sewed together. The stitches should be relatively superficial and carried through the peritoneal covering and the superficial layers of the gland." Senn had earlier stated the fundamental principles of surgical treatment on the basis of his experiments on animals. In Rose's case the operation resulted in recovery.

Leith's second group comprises the much more frequent cases which run a milder course and are either entirely cured or suffer more or less severe after-effects. Large ruptures may lead to the passage of the pancreatic juice with blood and bits of destroyed pancreas through the foramen of Winslow and cause the production of a general peritonitis which usually runs a fatal course. In other cases the injury of the tissues may be followed by inflammation which may be healed with the formation of cicatricial tissue. In a third group, as already repeatedly mentioned, the result is a cyst formation.

In the section on Cysts cases are mentioned as "traumatic,' being caused by an injury or a laceration of the pancreas. Leith mentions 17 cases: Kulenkampf, Senn, Küster, Fenger, Steele, Freiberg, Karewski (2 cases), Cathcart, Riegner, Pitt and Jacobson, Richardson, Littlewood, Lloyd (2 cases), Thomas Lynn, Brown; in the following 12 cases also there is the history of an injury: Ledentu, Fisher (2 cases), Michailow, Lindner, Barnett, Martin-Morison, Schnitzler, Tilger, Tobin, Eve, G. Hadra. There is no doubt, as Tilger has previously suggested, that in a number of the cases mentioned pseudo-cysts only are found, caused by hemorrhage into the omental bursa.

The clinical description of this variety corresponds to that of cysts, and is given in the section on the subject.

(b) PROLAPSE AND DISPLACEMENT OF THE PANCREAS.

Prolapse of the pancreas may arise in the course of penetrating wounds of the abdomen. Several communications have been made on this subject. Senn mentions first the case of Laborderie. The omentum, however, and not the pancreas, was concerned, as Laborderie stated some weeks after his first publication (Körte). Hyrtl has suspected that in such cases the pancreas may be confounded with fat tissue hardened and soaked with blood. Senn further reports the observations of Dargau, Caldwell; Kleberg and Wagner, Thompson and Cheever. Odevaine

(1866) reports a case of a penetrating wound of the abdomen with prolapse of a large part of the pancreas; removal by ligature; recovery. The
communication of Pareira-Guimaraes is most recent:

A man thirty-three years old received a bayonet-stab in the left hypochondrium.
The injury caused a hernia which the physician regarded as the prolapsed omentum.
Antiseptic dressing was applied. Milk diet. Opium pills. The examination, made
forty-eight hours later, showed an oblique wound, about 4 cm. long, 10 cm. to the
left of the linea alba and 8 cm. below the umbilical line. There was a bulging tumor
5 cm. long, dark-red, conical, and somewhat flattened. Diagnosis: Hernia of the
tail of the pancreas. The patient suffered also from beri-beri. Nevertheless, his
condition was satisfactory. Wound enlarged and the organ replaced. A suture was
applied. On the day of operation there was a slight fever, the temperature running
up to 38.2° C. (100.8° F.). Otherwise the course was afebrile and recovery took
place after twelve days.

Displacement of the pancreas, especially of the tail, is possible on
account of the anatomic relations. The tail is the least fixed portion, as
Zuckerkandl emphasizes in his anatomic introduction to this article. He
states that it is not infrequent for a piece of mesentery containing a
lymph-gland to be pushed in between the tail and the mesial surface of
the spleen, in consequence of which there is a certain mobility to this
portion of the pancreas. Klebs states that the pancreas may be pushed
downward by lacing, while it may be shoved upward and lifted away
from the vertebral column by retroperitoneal tumors and aneurysms of
the large blood-vessels. The pancreas, thus,—although in very rare
cases,—may be ranked with those organs which are affected in enteroptosis.

Dobrzycki in 1878 reported a case of movable pancreas:

A carpenter fifty-six years old fell from a height two years previously. Since
then he suffered from symptoms resembling those due to movable kidney; vomiting
of a fluid of the nature of pancreatic juice and having an alkaline reaction. There
was a tumor in the region of the stomach, corresponding in shape and position to the
pancreas.

Cecchini (1886) reported a case of congenital ectopia of the head of
the pancreas with subsequent gastrectasia.

The pancreas may be situated in diaphragmatic and umbilical hernias.
Several cases have been reported. The cases of Vecker, St. Andre, and
Cavalier, in which the pancreas, colon, and omentum were dislocated
into the thoracic cavity, through a rupture of the diaphragm due to a
powerful emetic, as mentioned by Ancelet and Claessen. The displacement of the pancreas in diaphragmatic hernia has not infrequently been
elsewhere noted.

Claessen states that in the cases of Marrigues and Howel the pancreas was contained in the sac of a congenital umbilical hernia. Invagination of the pancreas into the intestinal canal also may take place.
Claessen cites a case reported by Baud, in which a portion of the duodenum, with the pancreas, the beginning of the jejunum, the transverse
colon, and the right part of the great omentum, had been invaginated
into the descending colon and the rectum. Claessen reports also the case
observed by Guibert of invagination in a child three years old.

(c) BULLET WOUNDS.

Cases of this sort are reported by Otis and described in detail by Senn.
The clinical description of these injuries belongs to surgical text-books.

XII. FOREIGN BODIES IN THE PANCREAS.

ASCARIDES are the only foreign bodies except gall-stones which have been found in the pancreatic excretory ducts and their branches.

Mauchard and Lieutaud, as stated by Claessen, mention the obstruction of the ductus Wirsungianus by lumbrici. Engel reports a case in which several ascarides filled the pancreatic duct and its branches. Numerous lumbrici had invaded the bile-ducts even far in the liver. Davaine mentions four cases. The duct usually contains a single ascaris, but in one case (Hayner) seven were found. Klebs found in the slightly dilated duct of a corpse six specimens, three of which were males and three females. The first pair which entered went to the left end and turned half-way around; the other four turned their heads toward the left side of the pancreas. It is presumable in all these cases that the migration took place after the death of the patient.

The following observation of Durante is recent: A pancreatic cyst was caused by closure of the ductus Wirsungianus by an ascaris. Shea found in a pancreatic abscess an ascaris 17 cm. long partly in the duct and partly in the duodenum. Drasche likewise saw an ascaris in a pancreatic abscess. Nash also once found a lumbricus 6 inches long in the pancreas. In the three cases last named, the postmortem immigration cannot be excluded.

BIBLIOGRAPHY.*

Abbe: "Acute Biliary Colic and Jaundice Due to Tumor of Pancr.," "Practit. Soc. of New York," 5, 4, 1895.

Abelmann: "Ausnutzung der Nahrungsstoffe nach Pankreasexstirpation." Dissertation, 1890.

Abelous: "Action des antiseptiques sur les ferm. du pancréas," "Compt. rend.biol.," 1891, p. 215.

Abercrombie: "Pathol. of the Pancr.," "Edinburgh Med. and Surg. Jour.," 1824, p. 243 *et seq.*

— "Pathologische und praktische Untersuchungen über die Krankheiten des Magens." Uebersetzt von Busch. Bremen, 1843, S. 501.

Achard: "Diabète bronzé." Thèse, Paris, 1895.

v. Ackeren: "Ueber Zuckerausscheidung durch den Harn bei Pankreaserkrankungen," "Berliner klin. Wochenschr.," 1889, Nr. 14.

Afanassiew u. Pawlow: "Beitrag zur Physiologie des Pankreas," "Pflüger's Archiv," 1877, Bd. XVI, S. 173.

Agnew, D. Hayes: "Cancer of the Pancr. and Stomach," "Proc. Pathol. Soc. Philadelphia," 1860, vol. I, p. 84.

— "Pancreatic Cyst," "Brit. Med. Jour.," 1891, I, 1284. Ref. in "Gaz. hebdom. de med.," June, 1891.

* This list contains not merely the references of the authors mentioned in this book whose original articles have been examined, but refers also to such data as may be found in bibliographies, for example, the Index-Catalogue of the Surgeon-General's Office, United States Army, volume X, Washington, 1889, and in several volumes of the Index Medicus by John S. Billings. Only a part of the publications in 1897 are recorded in the following list. The earlier literature has thoroughly been reviewed in the works of Claessen and Friedreich.

Agricolansky: "Einfluss des Strychnins auf die Pankreassecretion." Ref. in "Méd. mod.," 1893, S. 102.

Aigner: "Vier Falle von Carcinom des Pankreas." Dissertation, München, 1896.

Aigre: ("Pankreascarcinom") "Bull. soc. anat.," 1889, S. 253, cited by Mirallié.

Albers: "Einfacher Krebs des Pankreas," "Medic. Correspondenzbl. rhein. Aerzte," 1843, Nr. 8, S. 131, 144–244.

Albert: ("Pancreatic Cysts, Two Cases") "Arbeiten aus der chirurg. Klinik," 1892, Wien.

Alberti: "De morbis mesenterii et ejus quod pancreas appelatur." Dissertation, Württemberg, 1578.

Albertoni: ("Behavior of Sugar in Organism") "Annali di Chim.," 1892, vol. xvi.

— "Ricerche sperimenteli," 1877.

— "Sui poteri digerenti del pancreas nella vita fetale," "Sperimentale," 1878, p. 16, 596.

Aldehoff: "Tritt auch bei Kaltbütlern nach Exstirpation des Pankreas Diabetes auf?" "Zeitschr. f. Biol.," Bd. xxviii, S. 293.

Aldibert: ("Pankreascarcinom") "Bull. soc. anat.," 1892, S. 35; see Mirallié.

Aldor: "Beiträge zur Casuistik der Pankreasgeschwülste," "Gyógyászat," 1895.

Allen: "Exsection of the Pancr.," "Amer. Weekly," 1876, p. 305.

— "Pancreotomy," *ibid.*, 1877, p. 56.

— ("Carcinoma of the Pancreas") "Philada. Med. Times," 1875.

— *Idem*, "Trans. N. Y. Path. Soc.," 1879, iii, S. 40.

— "Fatty Stools Due to Disease of Pancr.," "Trans. N. Y. Med. Assoc.," 1884–1885, vol. i, p. 286.

Allessandrini: "Descriptio veri pancreat. glandularis et parenchymatosi in accipensere et in esoce reperti," Bonn, 1855.

Allina: "Ein Fall von Pankreasnekrose," "Wiener med. Wochenschr.," 1896, Nr. 45.

Amidon: ("Pancreatitis hæmorrhag.") "Boston Med. and Surg. Jour.," 1886, p. 594.

Ancelet: "Etude sur les maladies du pancr.," Paris, 1866.

— "Essai analytique sur l'anat. pathol. du pancr.," Paris, 1856.

— "De l'indigestion des graisses au point de vue des affect. du pancr.," "Gaz. des hôp.," 1860, p. 463.

— "Sur les malád. du pancr.," "Gaz. méd. de Lyon," 1864, p. 81.

Anders: "Case of Cancer of the Pancreas," "Phila. Med. Times," 1880, p. 803.

Anderson: "Case of Malignant Disease of the Pancr.," "Glasgow Med. Jour.," 1884, p. 59.

Andral: "Cancer du pancr. simulant un aneurysma de l'aorte abdom.," "Gaz. des hôp.," 1831, p. 61.

— "Cancer du pancr.," "Arch des. sciences méd.," vol. xxvii, p. 117.

Anger: "Kyste sanguin du pancreas," "Bull. soc. anat.," Paris, 1865, p. 192.

Annandale: ("Pancreatic Cysts") "Brit. Med. Jour.," 1889, 1, 1, vol. i, p. 241.

Annesley: "Researches into the Causes and Treatment of the More Prevalent Diseases of India," 1828, "2· Sammlg. auserlesener Abhandlungen," Bd. xii, 1829.

Antrum: ("Cancer of Pancreas") "Assoc. Med. Jorum.," 1855, cited by Dieckhoff.

Aphel: "Caso di cancro al pancr.," "Gazz. di Torino," 1885, p. 179.

Apolionio: "Sopra un caso di pancr. e milza succenturiat," "Gazz. di Milano," 1887, p. 196.

Aran: "Observ. d'abcès tuberc. du pancr. et colorat. anormale de la peau," "Arch. gén. de méd.," Paris, 1846, iii, p. 61.

Armbruster: "Ueber Aetiologie der Pankreas-Hämorrhagien." Inaug.-Dissertation, Tübingen, 1896.

Armstrong: "Primary Cancer of Pancr.," "Canad. Med. Assoc.," 1885, p. 555.

Arnozan: *Vide* Bonnamy, cited by Mirallié.

Arnozan et Vaillard: "Pancréas du lapin,." "Jour. de méd. de Bord.," 1881, 3. April; "Arch. de physiol. norm. et path.," 1884, p. 287.

— "Assoc. med. jour.," 1855.

— "Cirrhose total du pancr.," "Jour. méd. Bordeaux," 1880, p. 584.

Arthaud et Butte: "Recherches sur la déterminaison du diabète pancr. expérimentale," "Compt. rend. soc. biol.," 1890, p. 59.

Arthus, Maurice: "Glykolyse dans le sang et ferment glycolytique," "Arch. physiol.," 1891, p. 425; 1892, p. 337.

— "Compt. rend. soc. biol.," 1892.

Ashhurst: "Suppurating Cyst of the Pancr.," "Med. News," 1894, p. 377.

Assmann: "Zur Kenntniss des Pankreas," "Virchow's Archiv," 1888, Bd. cxi, S. 269.

Atkinson: "Case of Suppurative Pancreatitis," "Med. News," 1895, xviii, 5.

Aucher: "Diab. bronzé," "Bull. soc. anat.," iii, 5, 1895.

Aufrecht: "Pathologische Mittheilungen," 1881, S. 126 (" Cancer of the Head of the Pancreas ").

Ausset: ("The Administration of Pancreatic Substance in Pancreatic Diabetes") "Sem. méd.," 1895, S. 377.

Auvray: ("Carcinoma of the Pancreas") "Bull. soc. anat.," 1893, xxiii, 6; see Mirallié.

Babington: "Extensive Cancer. Degenerat. of the Pancr.," "Dubl. Quart. Med. Jour.," 1855, p. 237.

Baer: "Pankreassteine bei einer Kuh," "Deutsche thierärztl. Wochenschr.," 1893, S. 347.

Baginsky: "Vorkommen von Guanin und Xanthin im Pankreas," "Zeitschr. f. phys. Chemie," 1883, Bd. viii, S. 396.

Bailey: "Cancer of the Pancr., Liver, and Mesentery," "Phila. Med. Times," 1873, p. 667.

Baillie: ("Acute Pancreatitis") "Morbid Anatomy," 1833, p. 221.

Baillie-Sömmering: "Anatomie des krankhaften Baues von einigen der wichtigsten Theile im menschlichen Körper," 1820; see Claessen.

Baines: "Diseased Pancr.," "Med. Times and Gazette," 1862, vol. i, p. 281.

Baldi: "Rapporto fra glicosuria ed acetonuria nel diabet. speriment.," "Rif. med.," 1892, IV., Bd. iv, p. 15.

— "Lo zucchero nel organismo animale," "Lo S erimentale," 1894, clviii, p. 1.

— ("Influence on the Digestion of Fats") "Archpdi farmacol. e terap.," 1894, Nr. 10.

— "Azione del Arsenico," "Arch. di farmacol.," 1893, p. 449.

Balser: "Fettnekrose des Pancreas," "Verhandl. des XI. Internisten-Congresses," 1892.

— "Ueber Fettnekrose, eine zuweilen tödtliche Krankheit des Menschen," "Virchow's Archiv," 1882, Bd. xc, S. 520.

Bamberger: ("Acute Pancreatitis") "Wiener klin. Wochenschr.," 1888, Nr. 33.

— "Krankheiten des chylopoetischen Systems," S. 626. P. Abscess.

— "Krankheiten des chylopoetischen Systems," S. 628. P. Cysts and Carcinoma.

Bandelier, Bruno: "Beiträg zur Casuistik der Pankreastumoren." Dissertation, Greifswald, 1895-96.

Banham: "Perihepatitis Causing Stricture of Bile and Pancreat. Ducts and Cystic Enlargement of Pancr.," "Med. Times and Gaz.," 1885, i, p. 314.

Barbillon: ("Carcinoma of the Pancreas") "Bull. soc. anat.," 1884, p. 86; see Mirallié.

Bard et Pic: "Contribution à l'étude clinique et anatomo-pathol. du cancer primitif du pancr.," "Revue de méd.," 1888, vol. viii, p. 257.

de Bary: "Diabetes mellitus bei einem 9jährigen Mädchen," "Archiv f. Kinderheilkunde," 1893.

Bardeleben: ("Carcinoma of the Pancreas") *Vide* Dissertation of Rosenthal, 1891.

Bardenheuer: "De insania cum morbis pancreat. conjuncta," Bonn, 1829.

Barfoth: "De morbis pancreat. affect.," Dissertation, Lund, 1779.

Barlow: "Case of Tubercle of the Pancr.," "Transact. Path. Soc.," 1876, p. 173.

Barnett: ("Pancreatic Cysts") "New Zealand Jour.," 1893; Ref. "Brit. Med. Jour.," Epit. 1894, No. 51.

Barth: ("Carcinoma of the Pancreas") "Gaz. des hôp.," 1848, S. 600; "Bull. de soc. anat.," 1856, S. 110, 174.

— "Diabète bronzé," "Soc. d'anat.," 1888, p. 50.

Bartley: "Malignant Tumor of Pancr.," "Ann. Anat. and Surg. Soc.," Brooklyn, 1880, p. 495.

Barton: "Tumor of Pancr. and Pylor.," "Trans. Path. Soc.," Phila., 1874, p. 71.

Bartrum: "Case of Scirrhus of Pancr. and Stomach," "Assoc. Med. Jour.," London, 1855, p. 564, cited by Friedreich.

Bas, Arsène: "Des kystes volumineux du pancr.," Thèse, 1897.

Bastian: "Cancer of Pancreas," "Med. Times," 1883.

Battersby: "Sur le diagnost. des malad. du pancr.," "Gaz. méd. de Paris," 1844, p. 219, 617.

— ("Cyst") "Arch. gén. de méd.," 1844.

— ("Acute Pancreatitis") "Dublin Med. Jour.," May, 1824.

— "Two Cases of Scirrhus of the Pancr.," "Dubl. Jour. of Med. Science," 1844, vol. xxv, p. 219.

Battistini: "Zwei Fälle von Diabetes mellitus mit Pankreassaft behandelt," "Therapeut. Monatshefte," 1893, Nr. 10.

Baudach: "Ueber Angioma myxomatosum des Pankreas." Dissertation, 1885.
Bauer: "Krankheiten des Peritoneum" in Ziemssen's "Handbuch d. spec. Pathologie," Bd. VIII, Th. 2, S. 360 ("Fat Necrosis of the Pancreas").
— "Scirrhus of Pancr.," "New Jersey Med. Rep.," 1855, p. 588.
Baumel: "Pancréas et diabète," "Montpell. méd.," 1881, Mai; 1894, No. 45.
Bayne: "Scirrhous State of the Duodenum and Pancr.," "Am. J. M. Sc.," Phila., 1830, p. 265.
Béchamp, A.: "Sur les parties du pancréas capables d'agir comme ferments," "Comptes rendus acad. d. science," 1881, vol. XCII, p. 142.
Béchamp: "Vorkommen von ptomainartigen Körpern bei Pankreasverdauung," "Bericht d. deutschen chem. Gesellsch.," 1882, S. 1584.
Béchamp u. Baltus: ("Pancreatin Injection") "Compt. rend. acad.," 1880, Bd. XC, Nr. 8.
Beck: "Scirrhus of the Pancreas," "Lancet," 1887, Bd. II, S. 113.
— "Congenitale luetische Erkrankung der Gallenblase und der grossen Gallenwege," "Prager med. Wochenschr.," 1884, Nr. 26.
Becker: "Contribut. à la physiol. et pharm. du pancr.," "Arch. des sciences biol. St. Petersbourg," 1893, vol. II, p, 433.
Becker, N.: "Beiträge zur Physiologie und Pharmakologie der Bauchspeicheldrüse," "Arch. d. sciences biologiques," Bd. II, S. 433–461, quoted from Gamgee.
Bécourt: "Recherches sur le pancr.," Strassburg, 1850.
Behr: "De pancreate ejusque liquore," "Argent.," 1730.
Behrends: "Pancreatitis acuta," "Vorlesungen über prakt. Arzneiwissenschaft," Bd. III, S. 332.
Bell: "Cancer of Pancr.," "Proc. Path. Soc.," Phila., 1871, S. 158.
Benda: "Multiple Fettnekrose des Pankreas," "Verein f. innere Medicin," XXVII, 4, 1896.
Beneke: ("Hypertrophy of the Head of the Pancreas") "Bericht d. med. Gesellsch.," Leipzig, XVI, 7, 1889; Schm. J. B. 224, S. 218.
Bennet: ("Pancreatic Cysts") "Clinical Lectures," 1857.
— "Case of Cancer of the Pancr. and Oment.," "Med. Record," XX, 6, 1884; "Lancet," 1891.
Bérard: "Vicariiren f. Pankreas," "Gaz. hebd. de méd.," 1857, S. 560.
— u. Colin, "Mémoire sur l'exstirp. du pancr.," "Bull. Acad. de méd.," 1856, p. 1049; 1857, p. 250; "Gaz. de méd.," 1857; 1858, p. 59.
Berends: "Pancreat. ulcerosa." Opera postum. Berlin, 1829, I, p. 263.
Bericht der k. k. Krankenanstalt Rudolfstiftung 1868–1869, S. 301 (Pancreat. suppur.).
Berlioz: "Mémoire sur les maladies chroniques," etc. Paris, 1816, p. 115, cited by Claessen, p. 156.
Berlyn: "Phthisis pancreat.," "Med. Corresp. rheinisch-westphäl. Aerzte," 1842, S. 321.
Bernard: "Mémoire sur le pancreas," etc. Paris, 1856.
Bernstein: "Zur Physiologie der Bauchspeichelabsonderung," "Arbeiten aus der. physiol. Anstalt," Leipzig, 1870, Bd. IV, S. 1.
Besson: "Sur quelques faits patholog. pour servir a l'étude du pancr." Thèse, Paris, 1864.
Bettelheim: "Fall von Pankreascarcinom," "Deutsches Archiv f. klin. Medicin," Bd. XLV, 1889, S. 181.
Biach: "Ueber Carcinom des Pankreas," "Wiener med. Blätter," 1883, Nr. 6.
Biernacki: "Verhalten der Verdauungsenzyme gegen Temperaturerhöhungen," "Zeitschr. f. Biol.," 1891, S. 49.
Bigsby: "On Diseases of the Pancr.," "Edinburgh Med. Jour.," 1835, p. 85.
Billings: "Cancer of the Pancr.," "Chicago Med. Rev.," 1893, p. 43.
Bimar: "Sur une disposit. anomale des conduits excreteurs du pancr.," "Gaz. hebd. Montpell.," 1887, p. 232.
Biondi: "Contributo alla chirurgia del pancr.," "Riforma med.," 1896, II, No. 9, p. 97.
— "Contributo clinico e sperimentale alle chirurg. del pancreas." Casa editrice Dr. Vallardi, 1896.
Birch-Hirschfeld: "Lehrbuch der pathologischen Anatomie," 1887, Bd. II, S. 639.
— "Beitrag zur pathologischen Anatomie der hereditären Syphilis," "Archiv d. Heilkunde," 1875, S. 166.
Blancard: "Anatom. pract. rat. Amst.," 1688, cited by Claessen.
Blind: "Sarcome de la queue du pancr.," "Bull. soc. anat.," XXI, 12, 1896.

Blodgett: ("Cancer of Pancreas") "Homeopath. Times," New York, July, 1879; see Hagenbach, Nimier.

Blumenthal: "Klinische Beobachtungen über Pentosurie," "Berliner klin. Wochenschr.," I, 7, 1895; 1897, Nr. 12.

Blumer: "Adenocarcinoma of Pancr.," "Johns Hopkins Hosp. Rep.," Sept., 1896.

Boas: (Pancreatin) "Magenkrankheiten," Bd. I, S. 295.

Boccardi: "Ricerche anat. pathol. sugli amm. privati del pancr.," "Rif. med.," 1890. IV; "Arch. ital. biol.," 1891, p. 50.

Bodinier: "Terminaison du canal pancr dans le duoden., à 4 cm. au-dessus du canal cholédoque," "Bull. soc. anat.," 1843, p. 262.

Boë-Sylvius: "Praxeos medicae idea nova," "Lugd. Batav.," 1667, Bd. III.

Boeckel: "Des kystes pancréat." Thèse, Paris, 1891.

— ("Cancer of Pancreas") "Cong. franc. de chirurg.," 1892; *vide* Nimier.

Bogdan: "Carcinom primitif de la totalité du pancr.," "Bull. soc. méd. natural," Jassy, 1894, VIII, p. 3.

Bohn: "Pankreascarcinom bei einem halbjährigen Kinde," "Jahrbuch f. Kinderheilkunde," 1885, Bd. XXIII.

Boldt: "Statistische Uebersicht der Erkrankungen des Pankreas nach Beobachtungen der letzten 40 Jahre." Dissertation, Berlin, 1882.

Bond and Windle: "Diabetes Terminating in Coma," "Brit. Med. Jour.," 1883.

Bonet ("Lithiasis pancreat.") "Sepulchretum," Bd. II, S. 576, cited by Giudice-andrea.

Bonetus: "Polyalthes s. Thesaurus medico practicus," Bd. II, Genf, 1691, S. 666, Friedreich.

Bonnamy: "Etude clinique sur les tumeurs du pancr.," Paris, 1879

v. Bonsdorff: "Pancreat. acuta gangraen. Finska handling.," "v. Boas' Archiv," 1896, II, S. 241.

Bonz: "Nova acta nat. curios.," 1791, VIII, cited by Claessen.

Bormann: "Therapeutische Anwendung des Pankreas," "Wiener med. Blätter," 1895, S. 665.

Boucaud: ("Carcinoma") "Gaz. des hôp.," 1866, No. 10.

Bouchard: "Maladies par rallentissement de la nutrition," p. 172, cited by Mirallié.

Bouchardat et Sandras: "Fonct. du pancr. et digestion des féculents," "Compt. rend. acad.," 1845, Bd. XX, p. 1085.

Bouillot: "Arch. gén. de méd.," II, p. 198. Cited by Claessen, p. 345.

Bourquelot et Gley: "Propriétés d'un liquide provenant d'une fistule pancr.," "Compt. rend. soc. biol.," XXX, 3, 1895, p. 238.

Boutilier: "Carcin. of the Pancr.," "New York Med. Rec.," 1893, p. 221.

Bowditch: ("Carcinoma pancreat.") "Boston Med. and Surg. Jour.," 1852, XXV, 8.

Bozeman: ("Cyst of the Pancreas") "New York Med. Rec.," 1882, S. 46

Brault-Galliard: "Diab. bronzé," "Arch. de méd.," 1888.

Brèchemin, Gille: ("Carcinoma pancreat.") "Bull. soc. anat.," 1879, p. 417; "Progr. méd.," 1880, p. 70.

Brera: Cited by Claessen, S. 155.

Bressler: "Krankheiten des Unterleibes," Bd. II, Berlin, 1841, S. 251.

Bret: ("Carcinoma pancreat.") "Province méd.," 1891, p. 222; see Mirallié.

Briggs: ("Sarcoma of the Pancreas.") "St. Louis Med. and Chir. Jour.," 1890, p. 154.

Bright: "Cases and Observations Connected with Diseases of the Pancr.," "Med. Assoc. Trans.," 1833, p. 18.

Brockmann: "Pancreat. Cyst," "Omaha Clinic," 1893, VI, p. 260.

Brown: ("Cyst of the Pancreas") "Lancet," VI, 1, 1894, p. 21.

— "Some Diseases of the Pancr." "Proc. Conn. Med. Soc.," 1894, p. 135.

Brown u. Heron: "Ueber die hydrolytische Wirkung des Pankreas und Dünndarms," "Annalen d. Chemie u. Pharmacie," 1880, S. 228.

Brown-Séquard et d'Arsonval: "Injection dans le sang des extraits du pancr.," "Arch. de physiol.," 1892, p. 148.

Bruckmeyer: "Ueber multiple Fettgewebsnekross." Dissertation, Freiburg.

Bruen: "Case of Tuberculous Disease of the Pancr.," "Phila. Polyclinic," 1885, p. 7.

— ("Carcinoma Pancreatis") "Boston Med and Surg. Jour.," 1883, p. 110, cited by Mirallié.

Brunet: ("Calculus") "Jour. de méd. de Bord.," cited by Nimier: "Lithiasis."

Brunner: "Experimenta nova circa pancreas," Amst., 1683.

Bruschini: "Sul diabete mellito," "Gazz. degli osped.," XXIV, 11, 1892.

Bruzelius u. Key: ("Carcinoma of the Pancreas") "Deutsche Zeitschr. f. prakt. Medicin," 1878, Nr. 32.

Bubnow: "Einfluss des $Fe_2 (OH)_6$ und FeO-Salzes auf Fäulniss mit Pankreas," "Zeitschr. f. phys. Chemie," 1883, S. 315.

Büchner: "De damnis ex male affecto pancreate in sanitat. redundantibus," Hal., 1759.

Buckingham: "Scirrhous Pancreas.," "Boston Med. and Surg. Jour.," 1859, p. 89.

Bufalini: "Sulla attivita digerente del pancr. negli animali smilzati," "Univers. di Siena," 1879, p. 35.

Bürger: ("Diagnosis of Diseases of the Pancreas") "Jour. f. prakt. Heilkunde," 1839, S. 104, 434.

Bull: "Report of a Case of Pancreas Cyst," "New York Med. Jour.," 1887, p. 376, cited by Senn.

Buss: "Fall von Diabetes mit Lebercirrhose und Pankreasatrophie." Dissertation, 1894.

Caldwell: ("Injury of the Pancreas") "Transylvanian Journal of Medicine," 1828, vol. I, p. 116; cited by Senn, S. 33.

Call: "Case of Chronic Pancreatitis Resembling Malignant Disease," "Boston Med. and Surg. Jour.," 1887, p. 567.

Cameron: "Case of Scirrhus of the Pancr.," "Med. Times and Gaz.," 1869, p. 491.

Campbell: "Scirrhous Degen. of Pancr.," "South. Med. and Surg. Jour.," 1848, p. 336.

Cane: ("Cancer of the Pancreas and Phlegmasia alba dolens") "Brit. Med. Jour.," 1883, XXIV, 2.

— "Cancer of Pancr.," "Brit. Med. Jour.," 1891, II, p. 1309.

Canfield: ("Carcinoma pancreat."), "Phila. Med. Rep.," XXV, 9, 1871.

Canstatt: "Specielle Pathologie und Therapie," 2. Aufl., Bd. IV, Abth. 2, S. 735, 1845.

Cantani e Ferraro: "Alterazioni istologiche dei diversi organi nel diabete," Morgagni, 1883.

Caplick: "Ueber Diabetes mellitus." Dissertation, 1882.

Capparelli; "Sul diabete pancr. sperimentale," V. Medical Congress, Rom.; "Atti di XI. congr. med.," 1894, Physiol., p. 15.

— "Pancreas e diabete," Morgagni, 1883, p. 459: "Arch. ital. de biol.," 1892, p. 240; 1894, p. 398.

— "Metodo per conservare il pancr.," "Boll. Acad. Roma," 1893, p. 114.

— "Zur Frage des experimentellen Pankreasdiabetes," "Biol. Centralbl.," 1893, S. 495.

Carbone, Tito: "Adenomgewebe im Dünndarm," "Ziegler's Beiträge," Bd. V, S. 225 ("Accessory Pancreas").

Carmichael: "Cancer. Degenerat. of the Head of Pancr.," "Dubl. Quart. Med. Jour.," 1846, p. 243.

Carnot: ("Diabetes after the Injection of Cultures of Bacteria in the Pancreatic Ducts") "Soc. de Biol.," 1894, XXVI, 5.

Caron: ("Pancreatic Carcinoma") Thèse, Paris, 1889; see Mirallié.

Carson: "Cancer of Pancr.," "St. Louis Cour. Med.," 1881, p. 342.

Cash: "Versuche über den Antheil des Magens und des Pankreas an der Verdauung der Fette," "Du Bois' Arch.," 1880, p. 323.

— ("Cancer of Pancreas and Hemorrhage") "Brit. Med. Jour.," 1888, p. 132.

Casper: "Einiges über den Krebs der Bauchspeicheldruse," "Wochenschr. f. d. ges. Heilkunde," 1836, S. 433.

Caspersohn: "Fall von Blutung, Nekrose und Fettnekrose," "Centralbl. f. Chirurgie," 1894, S. 1163.

Castelain: "Hypertrophie du pancr.," "Bull. med. du nord," Lille, 1863, p. 30.

Cathcart: ("Pancreatic Cyst") "Brit. Med. Jour.," XXII, 2, 1890.

Cavalier: "Observ. sur les lésions du diaphragme," Paris, 1804; see Claessen, S. 43.

Cavallo et Pachon: "Activité digestif du pancr.," "Compt. rend. soc. biol.," 1893, p. 641.

— — "Pouvoir digestif du pancr.," "Arch. de phys. norm.," 1893, No. 4, p. 633.

Cavazzani: "Veränderungen im Sympathicus nach Pankreasexstirpation," "Centralbl. f. allgem. Pathologie," I, 7, 1893.

— "Alteraz. consecutive alla estirpaz. del pancr.," "Arch. di clin. med.," 1893, p. 493.

Cayley: "Fatty Degenerat. of Pancr.," "Transact. Path. Soc. London," 1872, p. 121.

— "Acute Pancreatitis," "Brit. Med. Jour.," 1896, vol. II, p. 1.

Cecchini: "Ectopia congenita della testa del pancr. e consecutiva gastrectasia" "Rassegna di sc. med.," Modena, 1886, p. 314.

Cenni: "Storia di due affezioni pancreatiche," Raccoglitore, 1845, p. 357.

de Cérenville: "Effets de l'ingestion de substance pancr. dans le diabète," "Rev. méd. Suisse Romaine," 1895, vol. XII, p. 660.
— "Tumeur cancer. du pancr.," " Bull. soc. med. de la Suisse Romaine," 1880, p. 86.
Cesaris-Demel: "Adenoma acinose del pancr.," "Arch. per le scienze mediche," 1895, vol. XIX.
Challand u. Rabow: ("Pancreatic Hemorrhage") "Bull. de la soc. méd. de la Suisse Romaine," 1877, p. 345.
Chambers: "Post-mortem Specimen of Fatty Pancr.," "Maryland Med. Jour.," 1883, p. 656.
Chambon de Montaux: "Hydatiden im Pankreas," "Observat. cliniques," 1789, p. 99.
Chandelux: ("Pancreatic Carcinoma") Vide Bard and Pic.
Chantemesse et Griffon: "Hæmorrhagie peripancreat.," "Bull. soc. anat.," Paris, 1895, p. 578.
Charmeil: "Observat. anatomique," "Jour. du méd. milit.," 1783, p. 97.
Charrin et Carnot: "Infect. pancr. ascendant par expér.," "Soc. de biol.," XXVI, 5, 1894; "Compt. rend.," XLVI, p. 438.
— u. Gley: ("Infectivity in Pancreatic Diabetes") "Compt. rend. soc. biol.," 1894, p. 438.
Chatelain: "De l'inflammation du pancr." Thèse, Paris, 1841.
Chauveau et Kaufmann: "Le pancr. et les centres nerveux," "Compt. rend. acad. sciences," 1893, p. 463 et seq.; "Compt. rend. soc. biol.," 1893, p. 29.
— — "Pathogenie du diabète," "Compt. rend. acad, sciences," 1893, p. 226.
Cheever: ("Injury") Cited by Senn, "Surgery of the Pancreas," p. 34.
Chew and Cathcart: ("Cyst of the Pancreas") "Edinburgh Med. Jour.," July, 1890.
Chiari: "Sequestration des Pankreas," "Wiener med. Wochenschr.," 1876, Nr. 13; 1880, S. 140; "Prager med. Wochenschr.," 1883, S. 285.
— ("Melanotic Sarcoma of the Pancreas") "Prager med. Wochenschr.," 1883, Nr. 13.
— "Congenitale luetische Erkrankung der Gallenblase und grossen Gallenwege," "Prager med. Wochenschr.," 1884.
— "Ueber sogenannte Fettnekrose," "Prager med. Wochenschr.," 1883, Nr. 30, S. 285.
— "Ueber Selbstverdauung des menschlichen Pankreas," "Zeitschr. f. Heilkunde," · 1896, S. 69.
Chicoli: "Calcoli pancreatici." Ingrassia, Palermo, 1885, I, p. 321.
Chittenden: "Proteolysis by Trypsin," "Med. Record," v, 5, 1894.
— and Cummins: ("Influence of the Bile on the Proteolytic and Amylolytic Action") "Amer. Chem. Jour.," 1885, p. 319.
— — ("Einfluss therapeutischer und toxischer Substanzen auf das Pankreassecret") "Transact. Connect. Acad.," 1885, p. 7.
Chopart: "Mal. des voies urinaires." "Diabetes with Calculus Formation," cited by Klebs, 547.
Choupin u. Molle: ("Cancer of the Pancreas") "Loire méd.," XV, 3, 1893, S. 62, 141, Mirallié.
Churton: ("Cyst of Pancreas") "Brit. Med. Jour.," 1894, vol. I, p. 1191; "Lancet," 1894, vol. I, p. 1374.
Chvostek: "Fall von Syphilis des Pankreas," "Wiener med. Wochenschr.," 1877, Nr. 33.
— ("Diseases of the Panreas") "Wiener med. Blätter," 1879, S. 791.
Chvostek-Weichselbaum: ("Syphilis") "Allgem. Wiener med. Ztg.," 1877.
Cibert: "Gros kyste glandulaire de la queue du pancr.," "Gaz. méd. des hôp.," 1896, p. 347.
Cimbali: ("Primary Cancer of the Head of the Pancreas") "Sperimentale," 1889, Septembre, p. 282.
Claessen: "Krankheiten der Bauchspeicheldrüse," Köln, 1842.
Clark: "Disease of the Pancr. and Liver Accompanied by Fatty Discharge," "Lancet," 1851, vol. II, p. 152.
Clarke: ("Calculus and Carcinoma") Cited by Friedreich.
Clayton: "Calculi of the Pancreas," "Med. Times," 1849, XX, p. 37.
Clutton: ("Pancreatic Cyst") "Lancet," 1892, vol. II, p. 1273.
Cochez: "Les manifestations hepatique du cancer du pancr.," "Rev. de méd.," 1895, p. 545.
— et Ramos: "Deux cas de cirrhose biliaire par obstruction à la suite d'un cancer de pancr.," "Rev. de méd.," 1887.
Cohn: "Zur Kenntniss des der bei Pankreasverdauung entstehenden Leucins," "Zeitschr. f. phys. Chemie," 1894, S. 203.

Cohnstein: "Ueber innere Secretion," "Allg. med. Centralztg.," 1895, S. 85.
Colenbrander: "Glykolytisches Ferment," "Maly's Jahresb.," 1892.
Collard de Martigny: "Pankreasconcrement," cited by Klebs, S. 55.
Collier: ("Cancer of Pancreas") "Brit. Med. Jour.," IV, 10, 1890; II, p. 790.
Comby: "Pankreas," "Sem. méd.," 1893, No. 3.
— "Diabète maigre chez un garçon de 14 ans.," "Méd. infant.," 1895, II, p. 29.
Conradi: "Handbuch der pathologischen Anatomie," 1796, S. 219.
Coolen: "Action physiol. de la Phloridzine," "Arch. de Pharmacodynamie," 1894, V, 1.
Cooper: ("Rupture of Pancreas") "Lancet," 1839, Bd. I, S. 486, cited from Leith.
Copetta: "Brevi cenni sulla anatom. patologica del pancr.," Brescia, 1895.
Cornil: ("Cyst") "Bull soc. anat.," 1862, S. 584, see Tilger.
Corso: "Il pancreas degli animali smilzati digerisce?" "Imparziale Firenze," 1878, p. 193.
Corvisart: "Collection des mémoires sur une fonction peu connue du pancr.," Paris, 1857–1863.
Councilman: "Primary Tumor of the Pancr.," "Johns Hopkins Hosp. Rep.," 1889, I, p. 51.
Counnaille: "Pancréatite suppurée," "Monit. scient.," Paris, 1876, p. 375.
Courmont u. Bret: ("Pancreatic Carcinoma and Glycosuria") "Clinique," 1894, p. 621; "Prov. med.," 1894, 301.
Courvoisier: "Casuist. Statist.," "Beiträge z. Chir. der Gallenwege," 1890.
Cowley: "London Med. Jour.," 1788, cited by Claessen.
Crisp: "Scirrhous Enlargement of Pancr.," "Trans. Path. Soc. London," 1861, p. 124.
Crompton: "Scirrhus of the Pancr.," "Prov. Med. and Surg. Jour.," 1842, p. 234.
— ("Cysts of Pancreas") "Birmingh. Pathol. Soc.," December, 1842.
Crowden: "Concretions in the Pancr.," "Brit. Med. Jour.," 1884, vol. II, p. 966.
Cruppi: "Ueber Diabetes." Dissertation, 1879.
Cruveilhier: ("Pancreatic Cyst") "Traité d'anat.," 1856, vol. III, p. 366; "Atlas d'anat. pathol."
Cuffer: "Cancer of the Pancr. Modified by Transfusion of Blood," "South. Med. Rec.," 1874, p. 12.
Curnow: "Pancr. with Numerous Calculi in its Ducts," "Trans. Path. Society London," 1873, vol. XXIV, p. 136.
Curschmann: ("Fat Necrosis"). Internistencongress, 1892.
Cutler: ("Hæmorrhag. Pancreat.") "Boston Med. Jour.," XI, 4, 1895; Virchow-Hirsch "Jahresbericht."

Da Costa: ("Cancer of Pancreas") "North American Med. and Surg. Rev.," 1858, p. 883.
Dahl: "Pankreasfermente bei Rinder- und Schafsföten." Dissertation, 1890.
Dallemagne: ("Parenchymat. Infectious Pancreatitis") "Jour. méd. de Bruxelles," 1892, No. 18.
Dalton: "Cancer of Pancr. and Duoden.," "Med. Chir. Rev.," London, 1840, p. 590.
Daraignez: "Abscès du pancr.," "Jour. méd de Bordeaux," 1887, p. 479.
Dargau: ("Injury of Pancreas") "Med. and Surg. Reporter," Aug. 22, 1874, cited by Senn, S. 33.
Dastre: ("Influence of the Bile on Fat Digestion") "Compt. rend. soc. biol.," 1887, p. 782.
— ("Absorption of Fats in the Intestine") "Arch. de physiol.," 1891, vol. III, p. 711.
—.("Pancreatic Ferments") "Soc. de biol.," XVII, 6, 1893; "Compt. rend. soc. biol.," 1893, p. 818; "Arch. de physiol. norm. et pathol.," 1893, p. 117; "Compt. rend.," 1895, CXXI, p. 899; "Soc. de biol.," XI, 5, 1895.
Davidsohn: "Ueber Krebs der Bauchspeicheldrüse." Dissertation, Berlin, 1872.
Dawidoff: "De morb. pancreat. observation. quaedam." Dorpat, 1833.
Day: "Case of Pancreat. and Hæmorrh.," "Bost. Med. and Surg. Jour.," 1892, p. 569.
Dechamps: "Cancer du pancr.," "Arch. méd. Belge," 1878, p. 257.
Deetjen: "Fall von primarem Krebs des Ductus choledochus," "Archiv f. klin. Medicin," Bd. LV, S. 211.
Defresne: "La pancréatine dans l'économie," "L'union méd.," 1886, No. 143.
— "Sur le mécanisme du diabète maigre," "Gaz. des hôp.," 1890, No. 57.
Déjerine: "Sclérose du pancr.," "Bull. soc. anat.," Paris, 1876, p. 165; "Progrès méd.," 1876, p. 460; "Gaz. hebdom.," 1877, V, 1.

Demel, Cesaris: "*Adenoma acinoso del pancr.,*" "R. *Accad.* di Torino," 1895, xviii, 3; "Rif. med.," i, 725.

Demme: "Medullary Cancer of Pancr.," "Med. and Surg. Reporter," 1858, i, p. 77.

— "Affectionen des Pankreas im Kindesalter," "Wiener med. Blätter," 1884, Nr. 51.

Denis: "Phlegmasie chronique du pancr.," "Ann. de méd. et physiol.," 1826, p. 56.

Dethier: "Deux cas d'affections du pancr.," "Jour. de soc. méd. de Lorrain," 1880, p. 577.

Dettmer: "Beitrag zur Lehre von der Fettgewebsnekrose." Dissertation, 1895.

Dickinson: "Cancer of the Head of Pancr.," "Liverpool Med. and Chir. Jour.," 1888, p. 85.

Dickson: "Case of Chron. Inflammation of Pylorus and Pancr. with Scirrhus," "Med. and Chir. Rev.," 1840, p. 590.

Dieckhoff: "Beiträge zur pathologischen Anatomie des Pankreas," Leipzig, 1896.

Di Mattei: "Degli effetti della irritazione sugli elementi glandulari del pancr.," "Giorn. di Acad. Torino," 1885, p. 76.

Dittrich: "Fall von genuiner acuter Pankreasentzundung," "Vierteljahrsschr. f. gerichtl. Medicin," 1890, S. 43.

— "Zur forensischen Bedeutung der Pankreasblutung," "Wiener med. Blätter," 1890, S. 405.

Dixon: ("Cyst of Pancreas") "New York Med. Record," xv, 3, 1884.

— "Primary Cancer of the Head of Pancr.," "New York Med. Jour.," 1884, p. 333.

Dobrzycki: "Fall von beweglicher Bauchspeicheldruse," "Medycyna," 1878.

Döring: ("Abscess") "Altenberger Journal," 1817, see Claessen.

v. Doeveren: "De pancreate carcinomatoso," "Observ. path. anat.," 1789, p. 35.

Doglioni e Gianelli: "Cancro della testa del pancreas," Bologna, 1895.

Dolinski: ("The Action of Acids on the Pancreas") "Compt. rend. soc. biol. Petersbourg," 1895, Nr. 5.

— "Ueber den Einfluss der Säuren auf die Pankreasverdauung." Inaugurations-Dissertation, Petersburg, 1894, cited from Gamgee.

de Dominicis: "Exstirpation expér. du pancr.," "Gaz. hebd. de méd.," 1890; "Münchner med. Wochenschr.," 1891, Nr. 41.

— "Ancora sul diabete pancreatico," "Giorn. intern. delle scienze med.," Anno 15, 1891.

— "Legatura del dotto di Wirsung," "Riv. clin. e therap.," 1894, p. 60.

— ("Pathogenes. of Diabetes") "Soc. de biol.," xxv, 5, 1893; "Arch. de med. exp.," 1893, p. 469.

Donkin and Wills: "Treatment of Diab. by Feeding with Raw Pancr.," "Brit. Med. Jour.," 1893, i, p. 1265.

Dorset: "Case of Scirrhous Disease," "New Jersey Med. Rep.," 1851, p. 91.

D'Orville: "De fabrica et usu pancreat," "Lugd. Bat.," 1745.

Draper: "Pancreatic Hemorrhage and Sudden Death," "Transact. of the Med. Assoc. of Amer. Physicians," 1886, 1; "Boston Med. and Surg. Jour.," 1886, No. 17, cited by Seitz.

Drasche: ("Pancreatitis acuta") "Bericht der k. k. Krankenanstalt Rudolfsstiftung," 1868, p. 301.

Drechsel: "Abbau d. Eiweiss," "Du Bois' Archiv," 1891, S. 254.

Dreschfeld: "Acute Diabetes Due to Cancer of Pancr.," "Med. Chron.," 1895, April.

Dreyfus: ("Cancer of the Pancreas") "Bull. soc. d'anat.," 1876, p. 381.

Dreyzehner: "Ein Fall von Pankreascyste und Nierendrehung," "Archiv f. klin. Chirurgie," 1895, Bd. i., S. 261.

Driver and Holt: ("Hemorrhage") From Fitz, S. 200, Case 15.

Drozda: "Klinische Beiträge zur Casuistik der Pankreaskrankheiten," "Wiener med. Presse," 1880, Nr. 31 ff.

Duclaux: "Sur la digestion pancréatique," "Compt. rend. acad.," 1882, xciv, p. 808; 1894, p. 808.

Duffey: "Connexion of Acute Diabetes with Disease of Pancr.," "Dubl. Med. Jour.," May, 1884.

Dumenil: "Induration du pancr.," "Compt. rend. soc. biol.," 1850, p. 65.

Duncan: ("Cancer of Pancreas") "Brit. Med. Jour.," vi, 6, 1891.

Duplay: "Induration du pancr.," "Arch. gén. méd.," 1834, p. 411.

Duponchel: ("Cysts of the Pancr.") "Méd. Rép.," vol. xxii, p. 162.

Dupré: "Cancer of the Pancr.," "Bull. soc. anat.," 1830, 1846, p. 44.

Durand: "De la maladie dite hémorrhag. pancréat." Paris, 1896; see Boas, vol. i, 465.

Durante: ("Pancreatic Cyst") Congr. d'italien Chirurg., 1893; "Rif. med.," 1893, iv, p. 359.

Durante: ("Pancreatic Carcinoma") "Bull. soc. anat.," xix, 5, 1893.
Dutil: "Cas de cancer primitif du pancr.," "Gaz. méd. de Paris," 1888, No. 38.
Dutournier: "Diab. bronzé." Thèse, Paris, 1895.
Dutto: ("Pancreatic Diabetes") "Acad. di Roma," 1893, xxviii, 3; "Boll. di accad. di Roma," 1892, xix, p. 307.
Dyson: "Malignant Disease of Pancr.," "Brit. Med. Jour.," 1887, vol. i, p. 115.

Earle: "Two Cases of Cirrhosis of Pancr.," "Chicago Med. Jour.," 1882, p. 254; "New York Med. Record," 1884, p. 505.
Ecke, van: "Cellules pancréat pendant l'activ. secret.," "Arch. biolog.," 1895, xiii, p. 61.
Ecker: "Bildungsfehler des Pankreas und des Herzens," "Zeitschr. f. prakt. Medicin," 1862, S. 354.
Eden, Paul: "Ein Fall von doppelter Zerreissung des Pankreas." Dissertation, Kiel, 1895–96.
Edinger: "Reaction der lebenden Magenschleimhaut," "Pflüger's Archiv," Bd. xxix, S. 247.
Edkins, Sidney: ("Changes Produced in Caseïn by the Action of Pancreatic and Rennet Extracts") "Jour. of Physiol.," 1891, Bd. xii, S. 193.
Edler: "Traumatische Verletzungen der parenchymatösen Unterleibsorgane," "Archiv f. klin. Chirurgie," 1887, Bd. xxxiv, S. 173.
Edwards: "Cases of Cancer of the Pancr.," "Ohio Med. Rec.," 1879, iv, p. 402.
Eichhorst: "Bauchspeicheldrüse" in "Eulenburg's Realencyklopädie," Bd. ii.
— "Neuritis diabetica," "Virchow's Archiv," 1892, Bd. cxxvii, S. 6.
Eisenmann: "Zur Pathologie des Pankreas," "Vierteljahrsschr. d. Heilkunde," 1853, S. 73.
Elliot: "Surgical Treatment of Pancreatitis, with a Case," "Boston Med. Jour.," vol. cxxxii, 11, 4, 1895.
Elliotson: "On the Discharge of Fatty Matter from the Alimentary Canal," "Med. Chir. Transact.," 1833, vol. xviii, p. 67, cited by Friedreich.
Ellis: "Obstruction of the Common Duct," "Boston Med. Jour.," 1877, p. 531.
Eloy: "Le diabète pancréatique," "Rev. gén. de clin. et therap.," 1893, p. 718.
Ely: ("Carcinoma in the Head of the Pancreas") "Med. Rec.," July, 1894.
Emelianow: ("Leukocytosis after Operations") Cited by Löwy and Richter, "Berl. klin. Wochenschr.," 1897, Nr. 47.
Emiliani: "Dello scirro del pancr.," "Bull. soc. med. Bologna," 1857, p. 161.
Emmert: "Panc. Tub.," "Jour. compt.," Bd. v, S. 126 (Claessen, S. 345).
Engel: "Krankheiten des Pankreas," "Med. Jahrbuch d. österr. Staates," 1840, S. 411; 1841, S. 193.
v. Engel: "Zur Diagnose des Pankreascarcinoms," "Prager med. Wochenschr.," 1894, Nr. 48, S. 609.
Engesser: "Das Pankreas," Stuttgart, 1877.
Eppinger: "Prager Vierteljahrsschr. f. Heilkunde," Bd. cxiv.
Estes: "Displacement of the Spleen and Pancr.," "Med. News," 1882, p. 119.
Eve: "Surgery of the Pancr., with Report of a Case," "Med. and Surg. Rep.," 1896, p. 19.
Ewald: "Einfluss der Milz auf die Pankreasverdauung," "Arch. f. Physiol.," 1878, Bd. ii, S. 537.
— ("Pancreatic Carcinoma") "Deutsche med. Wochenschr.," 1889.
Eyting: "Pancreatitis chronica," "Hufeland's Jour. d. prakt. Heilkunde," Bd. liv, 1822, S. 3, cited by Friedreich.

Fähndrich: "Carcinom des Pankreas." Dissertation, Freiburg, 1891.
Farge: "Haemorrhagie du pancr.," "Bull. soc. méd. d'Angers," 1883, x, p. 188.
Fauconneau-Dufrèsne: "Pancreatologie," "Union méd.," 1847, p. 2.
— "Précis des maladies du foie et pancréas," Paris, 1856.
Fearnside: ("Inflammation and Hemorrhage of Pancreas"). Illustrations of Pancreatic Disease. "London Med. Gaz.," 1850, p. 967; see Seitz.
Fenger: ("Pancreatic Cyst") "Chirurg. Westnik," 1890.
de Filippi: "Cisti ematica del pancr.," "Clin. chirurg. Milano," 1894, ii, p. 557.
Finger: "Krebs der Drüsen um das Pankreas," etc., "Prager Vierteljahrsschr. f. Heilkunde," 1861, S. 98.
Finnel: "Specim. of Pancreas, the Seat of Primary Cancer," "New York Med. Rec.," 1873, viii, p. 344.
Finotti: "Zwei Fälle von Pankreascyste," "Wiener klin. Wochenschr.," 1896, S. 266.

280   *BIBLIOGRAPHY.*

Fisher: ("Cyst of Pancreas") "Lancet," xxvii, 1, 1894; Bd. i, S. 201.
— "Case of Sanguineous Cyst Connected with the Pancr.," "Brit. Med. Jour.," xv,
    12, 1894; Bd. ii, p. 1362.
— "Peritoneal Sanguineous Cysts and Their Relation to Cysts of the Pancr.," "Guy's
    Hosp. Rep.," 1892; Virchow-Hirsch, "Jahresb.," Bd. ii, S. 508.
Fitz: "Acute Pancreatitis," "New York Med. Rec.," 1889, Nos. 8–10; "Boston Med.
    and Surg. Jour.," 1892.
— and Welsh: ("Fat Necrosis") See Langerhans: "Ueber Fettgewebsnekrose."
Flaischlen: "Fall von Pankreascyste," "Zeitschr. f. Gynäk. u. Geburtshilfe," 1893,
    S. 93.
Fleckles: "Pancreatitis chronica mit beginnender Induration des Magens," "Zeit-
    schr. f. die ges. Medicin," 1845, S. 102.
Fleiner: "Zur Pathologie der calculösen und arteriosklerotischen Pankreascirrhose
    und der entsprechenden Diabetesformen," "Berliner klin. Wochenschr.," 1894,
    S. 5 ff.
Fleischmann: "Leichenöffnungen," Erlangen, 1815.
Fles: ("Fall von Diabetes mellitus mit Atrophie der Leber und des Pankreas")
    "Holländ. Arch.," 1864, Bd. iii, S. 187; see Friedreich.
Fletcher: "Carcinoma of the Pancr.," "Med. and Surg. Jour.," 1843, p. 318; 1847,
    p. 552.
— "Abscess of the Pancr.," "Proc. Med. and Surg. Soc. London," 1848, p. 20, cited
    by Fitz, Case 36.
La Fleur: "Multiple Capillary Hemorrhage and Fatty Degeneration of the Pancr.,"
    "Med. News," 1888, p. 80, cited by Seitz.
Flexner: "Carcinoma of Pancr.," "Johns Hopkins Hosp. Rep.," 1892, p. 54; 1894,
    p. 16.
— ("Fat Necrosis") "Journal of Experim. Med.," July, 1897, p. 413.
Foà: "Micosi del pancr.," "Giorn. internat. de sc. mediche," 1881, p. 1032; see Orth,
    S. 907.
Formad: "Chronic Pancreatit. with Fat Necr.," "Univ. Med. Magaz.," Phila., 1891,
    p. 49.
Förster: "Handbuch der speciellen pathologischen Anatomie," 2. Aufl., 1863, S. 213.
Forwood: "Case of Cancer of the Pancr. and Stomach," "Med. and Surg. Rep.,"
    1858, vol. i, p. 125.
Fossion: "Sur les fonct. du pancr.," "Bull. d'acad. belge," Bruxelles, 1877, p. 378.
Foster and Fitz: ("Gangrene of Pancreas") See Fitz: "Med. Record," 1889.
Fothergill: "Case of Malignant Disease of the Pancr.," "Brit. Med. Jour.," 1896,
    vol. i, p. 1323.
Fournier: "Jour. de méd. chir. et pharm.," 1776, see Claessen.
Frank, Josef: "Praxeos medicæ universæ præcepta," vol. ii, 1843.
Fränkel, E.: "Fall subacuter Pankreasentzündung," "Zeitschr. f. klin. Medicin,"
    1882, S. 277.
— "Ueber Fettnekrose," "Münchner med. Wochenschr.," 1. u. 8. September, 1896.
Frerichs: "Leberkrankheiten," 1858, 1, S. 146, 153 (Carcinom).
— "Ueber den Diabetes," 1884.
Freyhan: "Diebetès und Steinbildung im Pankreas," "Berliner klin. Wochenschr.,"
    1893, Nr. 6.
Friedreich: "Krankheiten des Pankreas," Ziemssen's "Handbuch der spec. Patho-
    logie u. Therapie," Bd. viii, 2. Aufl., 1878; "Virchow's Archiv," 1857, Bd. xi,
    S. 389.
Frison: "Pancreatite suppurée," "Diabète sucrée," "Marseille méd.," 1875, p. 262.
— "Diabèt. pancréat.," "Marseille méd.," 1875, p. 257.
Fry: "Dislocations and Malformations of the Pancr.," "Texas Med. and Surg. Rec.,"
    1881, p. 325.
Fürbringer: "Behandlung mit Gewebsflüssigkeiten," "Deutsche med. Wochen-
    schr.," 1894, S. 293.
Fürstenberg: "Pankreasconcrement," cited by Klebs, S. 544.

Gabritschewsky: "Glykogenreaction im Blute," "Archiv f. experiment. Pathologie,"
    1892.
Gade: "Apoplexia pancreat.," "Norsk. Mag. Christiania," 1892, p. 903.
— "Carcin. giganto-cellul. caudae pancr.," "Heiberg's Festschr.," 1895, November.
Gaeia: ("Calculus") See Graaf: "De succo pancreat.," 1667, cited by Giudicean-
    drea.
Gaglio: "Sul diabete, che segue all'estirpazione del pancr.," "Riforma med.," 1891,
    i, p. 543.

Gairdner: "Case of Atrophied Pancr.," "Month. Jour. Med. Soc.," 1850, p. 184.
Galeati: "Commentar. ac. Bon.," 1757, xxiv; see Claessen.
— ("Calculi") "Commentar. de rebus in scientia natural. et medicin. gestis," 1758, p. 389.
Galliard: "Calcul du pancr. se déversant dans l'estomac," "Bull. soc. anat.," 1880, p. 191: "Progr. méd.," 1880, p. 796.
Gallois: "Diabète pancr.," "Bull. méd.," 1891, p. 625.
Galloupe: "Cancer of the Pancr.," "Boston Med. and Surg. Jour.," 1881, p. 592.
Galvagni: ("Pancreatic Carcinoma") "Gazz. di Torino," 1891, p. 181.
— "Sul carcinoma della testa del pancr.," "Gazz. degli osped.," 1894.
— "Carcinoma del pancr.," "Riform. med.," 1896, iii, p. 847.
— e Bassi: "Contributo alla diagnosi del carcinom. del. pancr.," "Riv. clin. e terap.," 1891, p. 613.
Gamgee: "Physiologische Chemie der Verdauung," Leipzig, 1897.
Garnier: ("Carcinoma pancreat.") "Progr. méd.," 1886, p. 1037; see Mirallié.
Garrigues: "Report on the Anat. and Hist. of Cysts of Pancr.," "New York Med. Rec.," 1882, p. 286.
Gaultier: "Dissert. de irritabilit. notione," Halle, 1793; see Claessen.
Gaumbault: "De la pancréatine," "Gaz. des hôp.," 1894, lxvii, p. 1328.
Gavoy: "Gastro-enteralg. symptom.," "Jour. de méd. d'Algérie," 1879, p. 144.
Gegenbauer: "Fall von Nebenpankreas in der Magenwand," "Virchow's Archiv," 1863, S. 163.
Gendrin: ("Pancreat. suppurat.") "Hist. anat. des inflammations," 1826, ii, p. 239'
Genersich: ("Pancr. annulaire") "Verhandlungen des X. intern. med. Congresses,". 1890.
Gerhardi: "Pankreaskrankheiten und Ileus," "Virchow's Archiv," 1886, S. 303. Dissertation, Zürich, 1886.
Gerhardt: "Handbuch der Kinderkrankheiten," 4, Bd. ii, S, 753 (Birch-Hirschfeld: Syphilis und Pankreas).
Gibbons: "Enormous Encephaloid Cancer of Pancr.," "Pacif. Med. and Surg. Jour.," 1862, p. 216.
— "Cancer of Pancreas," "Pacif. Med. and Surg. Jour.," 1866, p. 24.
v. Gieson: "Fat Necrosis in the Pancreas," "New York Med. Record," 1888, p. 477.
Giffen: "Cyst of Pancr.," "Med. News," Phila., 1893, p. 626.
Gillar: "Primärer Krebs der Bauchspeicheldrüse," "Med.-chirurg. Centralbl.," 1883, S. 239.
Gille: ("Calculus") "Soc. d. anat.," 1878, cited by Lapierre.
Gillet: ("Pancreatic Secretion in Childhood") "Verhandl. d. X. internat. Congresses," 1891.
— "Sur quelques digest. pancr. artif.," "Ann. de la policlin.," 1890, i, p. 56.
Giorgi: ("Diabetes"). Thèse de Lyon, 1890.
Girode: ("Effect of Comma Bacilli") "Societé de biologie," xv, 10, 1892.
Giudiceandrea: "Sulla calcolosi del pancr.," "Policlin.," 1896, pp. 33, 126.
Glatigny: ("Pancreastbc.") "Ancien jour. de méd.," vii, p. 38. Claessen, p. 353.
Gley: "Sur le diabète alimentaire chez les animaux privées du pancr.," "Compt. rend. soc. biol.," 1891, p. 752.
— ("Destruction of the Pancreas") "Compt. rend. soc. biol.," 1892, p. 841.
— ("Decomposition of Salol") *Ibid.*, ix, 4, 1892.
— "Action d'un liquide extrait du pancr. sur les chiens diabet.," "Arch. de physiol.," 1892, p. 753.
Gley and Charrin: "Diabète expériment.," "Compt. rend. soc. biol.," 1893, p. 836.
Godart: "Cancer du pancr.," "Bull. soc. anat.," 1847, p. 287.
Goiffey: "Cyst of Pancreas," "Amer. News," x, 6, 1893: Virchow-Hirsch, "Jahresbericht," Bd. ii, S. 508.
Goldmann: ("Rupture") See Leith: "Rupture of Pancreas."
Goldscheider: ("Treatment of Diabetes") "Deutsche med. Wochenschr.," 1894.
Goldsmith: "On Diagnosis of Cancer of Stomach and Cancer of Pancr.," "Med. Record," Nov., 1884.
Gonzales, Hernandez: "Diab. bronzé." Thèse, 1892.
Goodmann: ("Cyst of the Pancreas") "Phila. Med. Times," xxii, 6, 1878.
Gorbatowski, W. K.: "Ein Fall von primärem Pankreascarcinom," "Medic.," iii, 1896.
Gorter: "De pancreatitide," "Lugd. Batav.," 1840.
Gottlieb: "Zur Physiologie des Pankreas," "Archiv f. experiment. Pathologie," 1894, Bd. xxxiii, S. 261; "Verhandl. d. med. Vereins zu Heidelberg," 1894, S. 203.

Gougenheim: ("Carcinoma pancreat.") "Soc. des hôp.," 1878; see Mirallié.
Gould, Pearce: ("Cyst of the Pancreas") Soc. for Med. Improvement, 1847, p. 217; "Lancet," 8, 8, 1891, Bd. II, p. 290; "Brit. Med. Jour.," 1894, vol. I, p. 1191.
— ("Calculus") Anat. Museum of Boston, 1847, p. 147.
Graaf, Regnerus de: "Opera omnia," 1667; see Claessen.
Graeve: "Pancreat. suppurat.," Upsala Forhandl. Referat., "Centralbl. f. klin. Medicin," 1893, S. 285.
Grandmaison: "Le diabète maigre," "Méd. mod.," 1892, p. 221.
— "Les pancréatites," "Méd. mod.," 1893, p 1154.
de Grazia: "Studio clinico e anatomico su alcuni stati del pancr.," "Rif. med.," 1894, II, p. 855.
Greding: "Adversaria medic. practica," II, 135; III, 86; 1769.
Greene: "Malignant Disease of the Pancr.," "Dubl. Jour. of Med. Scienc.," 1846, p. 250.
Greiselius: ("Gangrene of the Pancreas") "Misc. Acad. curios.," 1672, 1673, S. 74, cited by Claessen.
Griscom: "Transact. of the Med. Association," vol. XIV, Phila., 1864.
Griesinger: ("Diabetes") "Archiv f. Heilkunde," 1859, S. 44.
Gross: "Elements of Pathol. Anat.," Philadelphia, 1857.
— ("Pancreatic Cyst") "Arch. gén. de Paris," 1847, p. 215.
— ("Carcinoma of the Pancreas") "Phila. Med. Times," 1872, p. 354.
Grutzner: "Ueber einige ungeformate Fermente," "Du Bois' Arch.," 1876, S. 285.
Guelliot: "Glycosurie et inositurie," "Gaz. méd. de Paris," 1881, Nos. 6 and 7.
Guignard: "Rapport sur le traité de l'affect. calculeuse du foie et du pancr.," "Bull. soc. méd. Poitiers," 1852, 54.
Guillery: "Entzündungen des Pankreas," Berlin, 1879.
Gussenbauer: "Zur operat. Behandlung der Pankreascysten," "Langenbeck's Archiv f. Chirurgie," 1883, S 355.
— "Zur Casuistik der Pankreascysten," "Prager med. Wochenschr.," 1891, Nr. 32.
— "Zur Casuistik der Pankreascysten," "Prager med. Wochenschr.," 1894, S. 15.
— u. Winiwarter: ("Statistics Concerning Carcinoma") Cited by Biach.

Habershon: ("Gangrene of the Pancreas.") "On Diseases of Abdom.," 1892, Case 114.
Hadden: "Cirrhosis of Pancr. in Diabet.," "Path. Soc. Lond.," 1887, p. 163; 1890, p. 184.
Hadra: ("Rupture of the Pancreas") "Med. Record," 1896, xv, 7; "Centralbl. f. Gynäkologie."
de Haen: Opusc. T. I, S. 217; see Claessen, S. 155.
Hagenbach: "Complicirte Pankreaskrankheiten und deren chirurgische Beband-lung," "Deutsche Zeitschr. f. Chirurgie," 1887, Bd. XXVII, S. 110.
Haggarth: "Transact. of the College of Physicians of Ireland," vol. II, cited by Senn, p. 52.
Hahn: "Fall von Pancreascyste," "Centralbl. f. Chirurgie," 1886.
Haidlen: "Acute Pankreatitis im Wochenbette," "Centralbl. f. Gynäkologie," 1884, Nr. 39.
Haldane: "Cancer of Pancreas," "Assoc. M. J.," May, 1854.
Hale-White: ("Treatment with Pancreatic Extract") "Brit. Med. Jour.," IV, 3, 1893.
— "Carcinoma of the Pancr.," "Lancet," 1896, vol. II, p. 1805.
Haller u. Klob: "Pankreasgangrän nach Blutung," "Schmidt's Jahrb.," Bd. CV, 1860, S. 306.
— — ("Pancreatit. acuta") "Zeitschr. d. Gesellsch. d. Aerzte in Wien," 1859, Nr. 37.
Halliburton: "Case of Cancer of the Pancr.," "Med. Times and Gaz.," XX, 1, 1883.
Hamburger: "Untersuchungen über Einwirkung des Pankreassaftes auf Stärkek-leister," "Pflüger's Archiv," 1895, Bd. LX, S. 543.
Hammarsten: "Zur Kenntniss der Nucleoproteide," "Zeitschr. f. phys. Chem.," 1894, Bd. XIX, S. 20.
Hamilton: "Scirrhus of Panc.," "Dubl. Quarter. Med. Jour.," 1870, p. 476.
— "Cancer of Stomach and Pancr.," "Jour. Amer. Med. Assoc.," 1887, p. 630.
Hamon: "Cancer du pancr.," "Bull. clinique," Paris, 1836, 129.
Hanau: "Entstehung der eitrigen Entzündung der Speicheldrüsen," "Ziegler's Beitr. zur path. Anat.," IV, 1889, S. 487.
Handfield-Jones: "Observation Respect. Degeneration of the Pancr.," "Med. and Chir. Transact.," 1855, vol. XXXVIII, p. 195.

Hanot u. Chauffard: "Cirrhose hypertrop.," "Rev. de méd.," 1882.
— u. Schachmann: "Diab. bronzé," "Arch. de physiol.," 1886.
— et Gilbert: ("Carcinoma pancreat.") "Mal. du foie," 1888, p. 214.
Hanriot: "Lipase," "Sem. médicale," 1896, p. 463, 479.
Hansemann: "Die Beziehungen des Pankreas zum Diabetes," "Zeitschr. f. klin. Medicin," 1894, S. 191; Internat. Med. Congress, 1894.
Hansemann: "Traumatische Gangran und Eiterung des Pankreas," "Berliner klin. Wochenschr.," 1889, S. 1115.
Hansen: ("Abscess.") Dissertation, 1893.
Harder: "Obs. anat. practic.," cited by Claessen, S. 155.
Harris: "Degenerat. of Pancreas," "N. Amer. Med. and Chir. Rev.," 1858, vol. II, p. 515.
— ("Pancreatic Hemorrhage") "Boston Med. and Surg. Jour.," 1881, p. 593; 1889, p. 606; 1890.
— and Gow: "Comparative Histol. of the Pancr.," "Jour. of Physiol.," 1893, p. 349; vol. XIII, p. 469.
Harris and Grace-Calvert: "Human Pancreat. Ferment in Diseases," "St. Barth. Hosp. Rep.," 1894, p. 125.
— and Gow: "Ferment Actions of the Pancr.," "Jour. of Physiol.," 1892, p. 469.
— and Tooth: "Relations of Microorganisms to Pancr. Digestion," "Jour. of Physiol.," vol. IX, p. 220.
Harless: "Krankheiten des Pankreas, mit besonderer Berücksichtigung der Phthisis pancr.," Nürnberg, 1812.
Harley: "Jaundice," London, 1863 (Carcinoma pancr.).
— ("Diabetes") "Transact. Path. Soc. London," 1862, p. 118.
— "Absorption and Metabolism in Obstruction of Pancreat. Duct," "Jour. of Pathol. and Bact.," July, 1895.
— "Experiments Proving the Exist. of Pancr. Diabetes," "Jour. of Anat. and Phys.," 1891, p. 201.
— "Pathogen. of Pancr. Diabet.," "Brit. Med. Jour.," XXVII, 8, 1892.
— "Resorpt. of Fat," "Jour. of Physiol.," 1895, vol. XVIII, p. 1.
Harnack: ("Verfettung des Pankreas bei Diabetes") "Archiv f. klin. Medicin," Bd. XIII, 1874, S. 615.
Harrison: "Carcinoma pancreat.," "Phila. Med. Times," 1875.
Hartmann: "Tuberculose des Pankreas"; see Chvostek.
— ("Pancreatic Cyst") Congr. franc. de chir., 1891, bei Nimier, S. 758.
Hartsen: "Ueber Diabetes mellitus," "Archiv f. holländ. Beiträge zur Naturheilkunde," 1864, Bd. III, S. 319.
Hasfeld: "De pancreat. morbis," Berol, 1851.
v. Hauff: "Primäres Pankreascarcinom," "Wurttemberger Correspondenzbl.," 1876.
Hawkins: "Case of Pancreat. Hemorrhage and Fat Necrosis," "Lancet," 1893, vol. II, p. 358.
Hecker: "Syphilis congenita innerer Organe," "Monatsschr. f. Geburtshilfe u. Frauenkrankheiten," Berlin, 1869, S. 22.
Hedin, cited by Drechsel: "Abbau d. Eiweiss," "Du Bois' Archiv," 1891.
Hédon: "Exstirpation du pancr.," "Arch. de méd. expér.," 1891, Nos. 3, 4; "Compt. rend.," 1891, vol. CXII.
— "Pathogénie du diabète maigre," "Arch. de physiol.," 1892, p. 617; "Arch. de méd. exp.," 1893, p. 695.
— "Greffe souscutanée du pancr.," "Arch. de physiol.," 1892, p. 617; "Compt. rend. Acad.," XXVI, 7, 1892.
— "Effets de la destruction du pancr.," "Compt. rend. acad. scienc.," August, 1893; "Compt. rend. soc. biol.," 1893, p. 238.
— "Piqûre chez les anim. rendus diabet.," "Compt. rend. soc. biol.," 1894, p. 26.
— et Ville: "Digestion des graisses," "Soc. biol.," IX, 4, 1892; "Compt. rend. soc. biol.," 1892, p. 308.
Heidenhain: "Pankreassecret pflanzenfressender Thiere," "Pflüger's Archiv," 1876, S. 457.
Heinricius: ("Cyst of the Pancreas") Congrès des chirurg. du Nord, II, 1, 1896; vide Bas: Kystes du pancr.
Heller: "Echinococcus," Ziemssen's "Handbuch f. spec. Pathologie," Bd. III, S. 292.
Henning: "Merkwürdige Kranken- und Sectionsgeschichten," "Jour. d. prakt. Arzneikunde," 1799, S. 35.
Hennige: "Ueber Indicanausscheidung," "Deutsches Archiv f. klin. Medicin," Bd. XXIII, S. 285.

Hennigs: "Zur Statistik und Aetiologie der amyloiden Entartung." Dissertation, 1880.

Henry: "Sur les concret. que présente le pancr.," "France méd.," 1856, p. 42.

— ("Calculi") "Journal de chim. méd.," 1855, S. 273; see Giudiceandrea.

Herbst: "Unterbindung des Wirsungianischen Ganges," "Zeitschr. f. rat. Med.," 1853, Bd. III, S. 389.

Herczel: "Operirter Fall von Pankreascyste," "Pester med.-chirurg. Presse," 1894, S. 474. "Orvosi hétilap," 1895, Nr. 37.

Heritsch: "Spaltung von Essigather," "Centralbl. f. med. Wissensch.," 1875, Nr. 28.

Hernandez: "Contribucion al estudio de los pseudoplasmas del pancr.," Buenos Ayres, 1884.

Herringham: "Case of Primary Cancer of Pancr.," "Brit. Med. Jour.," XVI, 3, 1889; "St. Barth. Hosp. Rep.," 1894, vol. XXX, p. 5.

Herrmann: "Zur Diagnose des Pankreaskrebses," "Petersburger med. Wochenschr.," 1880, S. 61.

— "Zur Casuistik der Pankreascysten," "Deutsche militärärztl. Zeitschr.," 1895, S. 473.

Hersche: "Operation einer Pankreascyste mit seltener Lagerung," "Wiener klin. Wochenschr.," 1892, Nr. 51.

Herter: "Pankreassecret beim Menschen," "Zeitschr. f. phys. Chemie," 1880, Bd. IV, S. 160.

Hertodius a Totenfeld: "Cancrosum ulcus pancreat," Misc. Acad. natur. curios., 1670, I. p 230.

Herzen: "Einfluss der Milz auf Bildung des eiweissverdauenden pankreatischen Saftes," "Centralbl. f. med. Wissensch.," 1877, Nr. 24; "Arch. de phys. norm.," 1877, p. 792; "Pflüger's Archiv," 1883, S. 295; "Compt. rend. soc. biol.," vol. XLV, p. 814.

Herzog: "Verhärtetes Pankreas," "Wochenschr. f. d. ges. Heilkunde," 1839, S. 786.

Hess: "Beiträge zur Lehre von der Verdauung und Resorption der Kohlehydrate." Dissertation, 1892.

Hesse, G. T.: "De morbis pancreatis," Berol, 1838.

— "Tumor of Pancr.," "Proc. Med. Soc. of Brooklyn," 1879, p. 94.

Heubel: "Ueber ein mit dem Duct. Wirsungianus communicirendes Tractionsdivertikel des Oesophagus," "Archiv f. klin. Medicin," Bd. LV.

Heubner: "Ein Fall von Diabetes im Kindesalter," "Jahrbuch f. Kinderheilkunde," 1880; "Deutsches Archiv f. klin. Medicin," 1895, Bd. LV.

— "Syphilis des Kindesalters," 1896, S. 319.

Heurnius: "De morbis mesenterii et pancreatis," "Lugd. Batav.," 1599.

Hilderbrand: "Ueber Experimente am Pankreas zur Erregung von Fettnekrose," "Centralbl. f. Chirurgie," 1895, Bd. XXII, S. 297.

Hilty: "Fall von acuter hämorrhagischer Pankreatitis," "Corrbl. f. schw. Aerzte," 1877, Nr. 22.

Hinrichs: "Ueber Pankreascysten." Dissertation, 1889.

Hirschberg: "Zur operativen Behandlung des Ileus und der Peritonitis (Pankreasblutung)," "Berliner klin. Wochenschr.," 1887, Nr. 16, Fall 7.

Hirschfeld: "Acetonurie und Coma diabeticum," "Zeitschr. f. klin. Medicin," 1896, Bd. XXXI, S. 212; Bd. XIX, 1891, S. 249.

Hirschler: "Bildung von Ammoniak bei der Pankreasverdauung," "Zeitschr. f. phys. Chemie," 1886, S. 302.

— "Drei Falle von Pankreaskrebs," "Pester med.-chir. Presse," 1885, S. 665.

Hjelt: "Fall von Icterus auf Bindegewebswucherung beruhend." Cited by Schmidt, J. B. 1873, S. 132.

Hlava: "Pancréatit. haemorrhag. et la nécrose du tissu adipeuse," "Arch bohem.," 1890, Bd. IV, S 139.

Hochenegg: "Ueber cystische Mesenterialtumoren," "Wiener klin. Rundschau," 1895.

Hoffmann: ("Pancreatitis acuta.") "Untersuchungen über die pathologisch-anatomischen Veranderungen der Organe bei Abdominaltyphus," 1869, S. 191.

— "De pancreate ejusque morbis," Altdorf, 1807.

Hofmeister: "Ueber Resorption und Assimilation der Nährstoffe," "Klebs' Archiv f. experiment. Pathol.," 1889, S. 240.

— "Organ. Sauren und diastatische Wirkung des Pankreas," "Maly's Jahresb.," 1896, S. 267.

Hohnbaum: "Zur Diagnostik der Krankheiten der Bauchspeicheldrüse," "Wochenschr. f. d. ges Heilkunde," 1834, S. 241.

Holdefreund: "De pancreat. morbis," Halæ Magdeb., 1713.

Holley: "Carcinoma of the Pancr.," "Penna. Med. Jour.," 1855, S. 293.

Holmes: ("Pancreatic Cyst") "Brit. Med. Jour.," XIII, 7, 1895.

Holscher: "Langjähriges Leiden des Pankreas und Tod durch Perforation des Duodenum," "Hannov. Annalen d. ges. Heilkunde," 1840, S. 354.

Holzmann: "Zur Diagnose der Pankreassteinkolik," "Münchner med. Wochenschr.," 1894, Nr. 20.

Homans and Gannet: ("Gangrenous Pancreatitis following Hemorrhage") Vide Fitz, Case 66.

Hooper: "Diseased Pancr.," "Arch. of Med.," 1861, p. 282, cited by Seitz.

Hoppe: "Ueber einen abnormen, Harnstoff enthaltenden pankreatischen Saft des Menschen," "Virchow's Archiv," 1857, Bd. XI, S. 96.

Hoppe-Seyler, G.: "Beziehungen der Pankreaserkrankungen zu Diabetes," "Deutsches Archiv f. klin. Medicin," 1893, Bd. LII, S. 171.

Horrocks and Morton: "A Case of Pancreatic Cyst," "Lancet," XXIII, 1, 1897; vol. I, p. 242.

Horwitz: "Carcinoma of the Pancr.," "Coll. and Clin. Rep.," Phila., 1884, p. 166.

Hovenden: "Acute Pancreatitis," "Lancet," 1897, vol. I, p. 104.

Huber: "Syphilis des Pankreas," "Archiv d. Heilkunde," 1878, S. 430.

— "Plötzlicher Tod bei Pankreaserkrankung," "Deutsches Archiv f. klin. Medicin," 1875, Bd. XV, S. 455.

Huchard: "De l'emploi du pancréatine," "Union méd.," 1878.

— "Cancer du pancr.," "Bull. méd.," 1895, p. 15.

Hugounenq and Doyon: ("Pancreatic Treatment of Diabetes") "Lyon. méd.," 1897, Nr. 45.

Hulke: ("Cyst of Pancreas") "Lancet," 1892, Bd. II, S. 1273.

Hultgren: "Scirrhi pancreat. casus," Lundæ, 1837.

Hyrtl: "Pancr. accessorium u. Pancr. divisum," "Sitzungsber. d. Akademie d. Wissensch.," 1866, Bd. LII, S. 275.

Irwin: "Case of Cancer. Duoden. and Scirrhus of Pancr.," "Phila. Jour. Med. and Phys. Soc.," 1824, p. 406.

Isch-Wall: "Cancer du pancr.," "Progr. méd.," 1888, p. 423; "Bull. soc. anat.," 1889, p. 728.

Isham: "Chondrosarcoma of Pancreas," "The Clinique," X, 1876. Abstract "Schmidt's Jahrbuch," Bd. CLXXXIII, S. 90.

Israel: "Nekrose des Pankreas bei Diabetes," "Virchow's Archiv," 1881, Bd. LXXXIII, S. 181.

Jablonsky: "Glande pancr. dans le regime pano-lacté," "Arch. de scienc. biol. St. Petersbourg," 1896, IV, S. 377.

Jaccoud: "Sur le cancer du pancr.," "Jour. méd. et chir. prat.," 1885, p. 394.

Jacoby: ("Hyperleukocytosis") "Berl. klin. Wochenschr.," 1897, Nr. 47.

Jaffitte: "Diabète pancréat.," "Gaz. des hôp.," 1892, p. 2.

v. Jaksch: ("Diabetes") "Prager med. Wochenschr.," 1880, S. 193.

James: "Pancreatic Digestion," "Brit. Med. Jour.," 1885, vol. II, p. 1012.

Jamieson: "Cancer of the Pancr.," "China Med. Mission. Jour.," Shangai, 1887, p. 8.

Janeway: "Specimen of Pancr. Calculi," "New York Med. Rec.," 1872, p. 356.

— "Cystic Degeneration of Pancr.," "New York Med. Jour.," 1878, p. 523.

Janicke: "Zur Casuistik des Icterus in Folge von Carcinom des Pankreas," "Würzburger Verhandlungen," 1877. S. 125.

Jankelowitz: "Junger menschlicher Embryo und Entwicklung des Pankreas bei demselben," "Archiv f. mikrosk. Anatomie," Bd. XLVI, S. 702.

Jarvis: "Cancer of the Head of the Pancr.," "Proc. Connect. Med. Soc.," 1876, p. 37.

Jastrowitz and Salkowski: "Pentosurie," "Centralbl. f. med. Wissensch.," 1892, Nr. 19, 32.

Jaun: "Case of Laceration of the Pancr.," "Indian Annal. of Med. Sciences," 1855, p. 721, cited by Leith.

Jayaker: "Cancer of the Pancreas," "Ind. Med. Gaz.," 1870, p. 230.

Jeanselme: "Diabète bronzé," "Soc. dés. hôp.," V, 2, 1897; "Méd. mod.," p. 96.

Jenni: ("Carcinoma") "Schweizer Zeitschr.," 1850, Bd. II, "Schmidt's Jahrb.," Bd. LXIX, S. 38.

Jessner: "Zur Frage eines glykolytischen Fermentes," "Berl. klin. Wochenschr.," 1892, S. 417.

Johannson: "Exstirpation des Pankreas," "Hygiea," Stockholm, 1893, S. 309.

Johnson: "Primary Cancer of the Pancr.," "Med. Times and Gaz.," 1879, p. 591.

Johnston: "Calculous and other Affections in the Pancr.," "Amer. Jour. of Med. Sci.," Phila., 1883, p. 404.

Jones: "Fatty Degeneration of Pancr.," "Transact. Path. Soc.," 1854, p. 223.

— "Observation Respecting Degeneration of Pancr.," "Med.-chir. Transact.," 1855, p. 195.

Jung: "Beitrage zur Pathogenese der acuten Pankreatitis," Göttingen, 1895. Dissertation.

Kahlden: "Pankreas und Fettnekrose," Verein Freiburger Aerzte, I, 3, 1895; "Munch. med. Wochenschr.," S. 271.

Kappeller: "Die einzeitige Cholecystenterostomie," "Correspondenzbl. f. Schweizer Aerzte," 1887, S. 153; 1889, S. 97.

Karewski: "Zwei Falle von Pankreascysten," "Deutsche med. Wochenschr.," 1890, Nr. 46 f.

Kasahara: "Beziehungen zwischen Diabetes und Pankreasveränderungen," "Virchow's Archiv," 1896, J., Bd. CXLIII, S. 111.

Kaufmann: ("Pathogenesis of Diabetes") Soc. de biol., x, 2; xxiv, 3, 1894, S. 233, 254; Acad. de méd., xxvi, 3, 1894; "Compt. rend. acad.," 1895, p. 113; "Compt. rend. soc. biol.," 1895, p. 55; Soc. biol., xxix, 2, 1896; "Sem. méd.," xiv, 3, 1896, p. 92; "Arch. de physiol.," 1895, Bd. vii, S. 209, 287, 385, 1895; "Sem. méd.," Nr. 4, 1895.

— "Recherches expér. sur le diabète pancr.," "Arch. de phys.," 1895, Bd. vii, p. 209.

— "Mode d'action du système nerveux dans la production de l'hyperglycémie," *ibid.*, p. 266, 287, 385.

Kausch, W.: "Ueber den Diabetes mellitus der Vögel (Enten und Gänse) nach Pankreasexstirpation," "Archiv f. experiment. Pathologie und Pharmakologie," Bd. xxxvii, 1896, S. 274.

Keen: "Scirrhus of the Pancr.," "Transact. Pathol. Soc. Phila.," 1874, p. 69.

Kellermann: "Fall von Carcinom des Pankreas." Dissertation, 1894.

Kelly: "Two Cases of Carcinoma of the Pancr.," "Univers. Med. Magaz.," 1895, p. 98.

Kennan: "Acute pancreat.," "Brit. Med. Jour.," 1896, Bd. ii, p. 1442.

Kerckring: ("Carcinoma"). Spicilegium anatom., Abs. 42, 1717, cited by Claessen.

Kernig: "Fall von primärem Pankreascarcinom," "Petersburger med. Wochenschr.," 1881, S. 36.

Kesteren: "Case of Primary Cancer of Pancr.," "Pathol. Transact.," 1890, Bd. xi.

Kidd: "Primary Cancer of Pancr.," "Transact. of Pathol. Soc. London," 1882, p. 136.

Kilgour: "Case of Abscess of Pancr.," "London Jour. of Med.," 1850, p. 1052, cited by Fitz.

King: "Observ. sur un squirre du pancr.," "Répert. génerale d'anatomie," 1827, p. 43.

Kirmsee: "Zur Lehre von den Entzündungen des Pankreas," "Allg. med. Zeitung," 1838, Nr. 70.

Kissel: "Krankheiten des Pankreas," "Zeitschr. f. Erfahrungsheilkunde," 1848, S. 73; 1849, S. 241.

Kist: "De carcinome pancreat.," "Lugd. Batav.," 1855.

Kleberg: "Penetrirende Bauchwunde; Vorfall des Pankreas," "Archiv f. klin. Chirurgie," 1868, S. 523.

Klebs: "Handbuch der pathologischen Anatomie," 1870, Bd II, S. 533.

Klemperer: "Magenerweiterung durch Pankreaskrebs," "Deutsche med. Wochenschr.," 1889, S. 742.

Klob: "Pankreasanomalien," "Zeitschr. d. k. k. Gesellsch. d. Aerzte," 1859, S. 732.

— "Zur pathologischen Anatomie des Pankreas," "Oester. Zeitschr. f. Heilkunde," 1860, S. 529.

Knauer: "De pancreatitide ejusque sequelis," Jena, 1828, cited by Claessen.

Knieriem: "Asparaginsaure, Product der Verdauung von Pflanzenkleber durch die Pankreasdruse," "Zeitschr. f. Biologie," 1875, Bd. xi, S. 198.

Knowlton: "Scirrhus of the Pancr.," "Boston Med. and Surg. Jour.," 1843, p. 379; 1844, p. 233.

Kobler: "Typisches Fieber bei malignen Neubildungen des Unterleibes," "Wiener klin. Wochenschr.," 1892, Nr. 23.

Kofler: "Carcinoma pancreat.," "Riv. clin. e terap.," 1888, p. 620.

Köhler: "Die Krebs- und Scheinkrebskrankheit des Menschen," Stuttgart, 1853, S. 386.

Kollmann: "Zur Casuistik der Hämorrhagien ins Pankreas," "Aerztl. Intelligenzbl.," München, 1880, S. 421.

König: "Disquisitio morborum pancreat," Tübingen, 1829.

— "Fall von Pankreasnekrose." Dissertation, Kiel, 1889.

Kootz: "Operation einer Pankreascyste." Dissertation, 1886.

Kopp: "Denkwürdigkeiten aus der ärztlichen Praxis," i, 1830, S. 232; 1839, iv, S. 293.

Körte: "Abscess und Nekrose des Pankreas," XXIII. Chirurgencongress, April, 1894.

— "Pancreatit.hæmorrhag. et suppurat.," XXIV. Chirurgencongress, April, 1895.

— "Chirurgische Behandlung der Pankreaseiterung und Nekrose," "Deutsches Archiv f. klin. Chirurgie," Bd. xlviii, 1894, S. 721.

— "Beitrag zur chirurgischen Behandlung der Pankreasentzündungen," "Berliner Klinik," 1896, December.

Koskorozes: ("Carcinoma"). Galenos, 1882, S. 324.

Köster: ("Atrophy of the Pancreas.") Bericht d. Göteborger Spitales. Referat. Schmidt, J. B. 1894, Bd. ccxliv, S. 219.

Kotlar: "Einfluss des Pankreas auf das Wachsthum einiger pathogenenSpaltpilze," "Centralbl. f. Bakteriologie," 1895, Bd. xvii, S. 145.

Kötschau: "Hämorrhagie des Pankreas," "Centralbl. f. allgem. Pathologie u. path.-log. Anatomie," 1893, Nr. 12.

Kraft: "Merkwürdige Leichenöffnung," "Jour. d. prakt. Heilkunde," 1818, S. 68.

— ("Hemorrhagic Pancreatitis") "Hospitals Tidende," 1894, p. 805.

Kramer: "Pankreascyste," "Centralbl. f. Chirurgie," 1886, S. 23.

— "Primärer Pankreaskrebs," "Petersburger med. Wochenschr.," 1894, Nr. 48, S. 426.

Kraus: "Zuckerumsetzung im menschlichen Blute," "Zeitschr. f. klin. Medicin," 1892, Bd. xxi.

Krieger: "Beitrag zur Bauchchirurgie," "Deutsche med. Wochenschr.," 1888, S. 793.

Krönlein: "Ueber Pankreaschirurgie," XXIV. Chirurgencongress, April, 1895, "Wiener med. Wochenschr.," 1895, S. 1318.

— "Klinische und topographisch-anatomische Beiträge zur Chirurgie des Pankreas," "Beiträge zur klin. Chirurgie," 1895, S. 663.

Krüger-Hansen: "Ein Wort über Casper's Cur d. Scirrhus d. Pankreas," "Med. Argos," 1840, S. 628.

Kudrewetzky: "Pankreasabsonderung unter Nervenreizung," "Du Bois' Arch.," 1894, S. 83.

— "Tuberculose des Pankreas," "Prager Zeitschr. f. Heilkunde," 1892, S. 101.

Kühn: "Ueber primäres Pankreascarcinom im Kindesalter," "Berliner klin. Wochenschr.," 1887, S. 628.

Kühnast: "Ueber Pankreascysten." Dissertation, 1887.

Kühne: "Ueber das Trypsin," "Virch. Arch.," 1867, S. 130; "Verhandl. d. natur-histor. Vereines zu Heidelberg," 3, Bd. i, 1876; 4, Bd. i, 1876; "Untersuch. aus d. physiolog. Institut in Heidelberg," 1877; "Centralbl. f. med. Wissensch.," 1886, Nr. 35.

— and Lea: ("Chronic Pancreatitis") "Verhandlungen d. Heidelberger ärztl. Gesellsch.," 1876.

— — "Ueber die Absonderung d. Pankr.," "Unters. aus d. physiolog. Inst. in Heidelberg," 1882, Bd. ii, S. 448.

Kulenkampf: "Fall von Pankreasfistel," "Berliner klin. Wochenschr.," 1882, Nr. 7.

Külz u. Vogel: "Zur Kenntniss der Isomaltose," "Centralbl. f. med. Wissensch.," 1893, S. 817.

— — "Pentosen bei Diabetes," "Zeitschr. f. Biologie," Bd. xxxii, 1895.

Kuntzmann: ("Fatty Stools") "Hufeland's Journal," 1820, cited by Friedreich.

Küster: "Diagnose und Therapie der Pankreascysten," "Berliner klin. Wochenschr.," 1887, S. 154.

— "Zur Diagnose und Therapie der Pankreascysten," "Deutsche med. Wochenschr.," 1887, S. 189, u. 215.

Kyber: "Untersuchungen über amyloide Degeneration," "Virchow's Archiv," 1880, Bd. lxxxi, S. 421.

Labadie-Lagrave: ("Cancer of Pancreas.") Thèse de Dr. Salles, 1880, cited by Mirallié.

Labbé: ("Cancer of Pancreas") "Bull. soc. anat.," 1865, S. 267.

Labes: "Malum pancreat. ex obstruct. alvi," "Organ f. d. ges. Heilkunde," 1861, S. 17.

Laborde: "Cancer of Pancreas," "Gaz. méd. de Paris," 1860, Nr. 17.
— "Dégénération de la tête du pancr.," "Compt. rend. soc. biol.," 1860, Bd. I, S. 84.
Lachmann: ("Fall von primärem Pankreaskrebs.") Dissertation, 1889.
Laennec: ("Cancer of Pancreas") "Gaz. méd. de Nantes," 1892, S. 84, cited by Mirallié.
Laguesse: "Rech. sur l'histogénie du pancr. chez le mouton," "Jour. de l'anat.," 1895, p. 475; "Compt. rend. soc. biol.," xxvii, 1895, S. 602.
Lancereaux: "Diabète glycosurique," "Union méd.," 1890, p. 145.
— et Thiroloix: "Diab. pancr.," "Compt. rend.,"1892, p. 341.
— ("Gumma of Pancreas") "Bull. de la soc. d'anat.," 1855.
— "Traité de Syphilis," Paris, 1874, p. 251.
— ("Calculi of Pancreas, Diabetes") "Bull. acad. de méd.," 1877, S. 1224; 1888, viii, 5.
— "Diabète maigre," "Union méd.," 1880; "Gaz. méd. de Paris," 1891, p. 409.
— "Diabète sucrée avec altération du pancr.," "Bull. de l'acad.," 1888, No. 19; "Wiener med. Blätter," 1888, S. 716.
— ("Cancer of Pancreas.") Thèse de Thiroloix, 1892, S. 144, cited by Mirallié.
— "Ablation presque total du pancr. Diabet.," "Bull. acad. méd.," 1891, p. 367.
Landau: "Zur Physiologie der Bauchspeichelabsonderung," Breslau, 1873.
Landsberg: "Krankheiten des Pankreas," "Jour. f. prakt. Heilkunde," 1840, S. 15, 49.
Langdon-Down: "Transactions of the Clin. Soc.," vol. ii, 1869; "Centralbl. f. med. Wissensch.," 1869, Nr. 38.
Langerhans: "Acute Pancreatitis," "Deutsche med. Wochenschr.," 1889, S. 1030.
— "Präparat von Pankreasnekrose," "Berliner klin. Wochenschr.," 1889, Nr. 51, S. 1114.
— "Ueber multiple Fettgewebsnekrose," "Virchow's Archiv," 1890, Bd. cxxii, S. 252.
— "Ueber Fettgewebsnekrose." Festschr. zur Feier des 71. Geburtstages Virchow's, 1891.
Langendorff: "Versuche über Pankreasverdauung der Vögel," "Du Bois' Arch.," 1879, S. 1.
Le Gros, Clark: ("Rupture of the Pancreas") "Lect. of Surg. Diagn.," 1870, S. 298, cited by Senn.
Lapierre: "Diabète maigre dans ces rapports avec les altérat. du panc." Thèse, 1879.
Lappe: "De morbis pancr. quædam," Berlin, 1837, cited by Claessen.
Lardy: "Ueber Pankreascysten," "Corr. f. Schweizer Aerzte," 1888, S. 279.
Lauritzen: "On the Pancreas of Diabetes," "Hosp. Tid.," 1894.
Lawrence: "Pancreas Found in a State of Inflammation," "Med.-chir. Transact.," 1831, p. 367.
Lecorché: ("Atrophy of Pancreas in Diabetes") "Arch. gén. de méd.," 1861, Bd. xviii, S. 70.
Ledentu: ("Cyst of the Pancreas") "Bull. de la soc. d'anat.," 1865.
Lediberder: "Pemphigus foliacée, dégénérescence fibrokystique du pancr.," "Bull. soc. anat.," 1867, vol. xiii, p. 581.
Lee: "Disease of the Pancr.," "Nat. Med. Jour.," Washington, 1871, vol. ii, p. 430.
Lees: "Scirrhus of Pancreas," "Dubl. Med. Jour.," 1848, p. 188; 1854, p. 447.
Legendre: ("Cancer of Pancreas") "Bull. soc. anat.," 1881, S. 186.
Lehwess: "Krankheit des Pankreas," "Wochenschr. f. d. ges. Heilkunde," 1844, S. 802.
Leichtenstern: "Behandlung der Krankheiten der Bauchspeicheldrüse," "Handb. d. spec. Therapie von Penzoldt-Stintzing, Bd. iv, S. 203, 1896.
Leith: "Rupture of Pancr.," "Edinburgh Med. Jour.," November, 1895.
— "Abscesses in the Head of Pancr.," Soc. of Edinburgh, New Series, 1894-95, p. 242.
Lemoine et Lannois: "Contribution à l'étude des lésions du pancr. dans le diabète," "Arch. méd. expér.," 1891, iii, S. 1.
Lenander: ("Cancer of Pancreas") "Sem. méd.," 1893.
Leo: "Schicksal des Pepsins und Trypsins im Organismus," "Pflüger's Archiv," 1885, Bd. xxxvii, S. 223.
Lépine et Cornil: "Cas de lymphôme du pancr.," "Gaz. méd. Paris," 1874, p. 624.
— — "Cas d'altérat. graissense du pancr.," "Compt. rend. soc. de biol.," 1874, p. 372.
— "Exstirpat. du pancr. et diabète," "Lyon méd.," 1889, No. 48, 52.

Lépine: "Beziehungen des Diabetes zu Pankreaserkrankungen," "Wiener med. Presse," 1892, Nr. 27.
— "Sur l'action du bain froid," "Lyon méd.," 1892, p. 92.
— ("Glycolytic Action of the Blood") "Acad. des sciences," 1893, xvi, 1.
— "Production du ferment glycolytique," "Compt. rend. acad. soc.," 1895, p. 139.
— "Sur la glycosurie conséc. à l'ablat. du pancr.," "Compt. rend.," vol. cxxi, p 457.
— "Sur l'hyperglycémie conséc. à lablat. du pancr.," *ibid.*, p. 486.
— "Etiologie et pathogénie du diabète sucré," "Arch. méd. exp.," 1891, p. 222; 1892, p. 1; "Ann. de méd.," 1891.
— "Nouveau traitement du diabète," "Sem. méd.," 1895, p. 169.
— et Barral: "Sur le ferment glycolytique," Soc. de biol., xxv, 4, 1891; "Compt. rend. acad.," 112, Bd. vi, p 604; "Lyon méd.," 1892, p. 189.
— et Martz: "Ferment glycolytique," "Arch. de méd. exp.," vol. vii, p. 219.
— et Metzos: "Glycolyse dans le pancr.," "Compt. rend. acad. sciences," xvii, 7, 1893.
— ("Diabète Maigre without Pancreatic Lesion.") *Abstract.* "Rif. med.," 1891, p. 304; "Lyon méd.," 1892, No. 52, p. 591.
— "Pancreatite hæmorrhagique," "Lyon méd.," 1892, p. 303.
— "Etiologie et pathol. du diabète," "Rev. de méd.," 1894, p. 876.
Lerche: "De pancreatitide," Hallæ, 1827.
Leroux: "Etude sur le diabète chez les enfants," "Gaz. des hôpit.," 1881.
Letulle: ("Bronzed Diabetes") "Semaine méd.," 1885, p. 408.
Leube: "Bestimmungen des Fettgehaltes der Fäces bei Diabetikern." Dissertation, 1891.
— "Specielle Diagnose der inneren Krankheiten," 1889.
Leva: "Klinische Beiträge zur Lehre vom Diabetes mellitus," "Deutsches Archiv f. klin. Medicin," 1891, Bd. xlviii, S. 186.
Levier: "Leucin im Darm," "Schweiz. Zeitschr. f. Heilk.," 1864, Bd. iii, S. 140, cited by Friedreich.
Levère: "Studies in Phloridzin Glycosuria," "Jour. of Physiol.," 1894.
Lewaschew: "Bildung des Trypsins und Bedeutung der Bernard'schen Körperchen," "Pflüger's Archiv," 1885, Bd. xxxvii, S. 32.
v. Lichtenfels: "Icterus e carcinomat. pancreat.," "Bericht d. k. k. Krankenanstalt Rudolfsstiftung," 1867–1868, S. 277.
Lichtheim: "Zur Diagnose der Pankreasatrophie durch Steinbildung," "Berliner klin. Wochenschr.," 1894, Nr. 8.
Lietaud: "Hist. anat. méd. ed. Schlegel," vol. i, 1786, p. 296.
de Lignerolles: "Cancer du pancr.," "Bull. soc. anat.," 1866, p. 38, 62.
Lilienhain: "Beiträge zu den Krankheiten des Pankreas," "Jour. f. d. prakt. Heilkunde," 1825, Supplement. S. 78.
Lilly: "Case of Cancer of the Pancr.," "Med. and Surg. Rep.," Phila., 1884, p. 422.
Lindberger: "Trypsinwirkung bei Gegenwart freier Sauren," "Maly's Jahresb.," 1883, S. 280.
Lindner: "Fall von Pankreascyste," "Internat. klin. Rundschau," 1889, Nr. 8.
Lisser: "Pankreasklysmen b. Diabetes," "Méd. gaz. (Russ.)," 1895; "Therap. Wochenschr.," 1895, S. 133.
Litten: "Drei Fälle totaler Degeneration des Pankreas," "Charité-Annalen," 1877, 1878, S. 181.
— "Primäres Sarkom des Pankreas bei einem 4jährigen Knaben," "Deutsche med. Wochenschr.," 1888, Nr. 44.
Littlewood: ("Traumatic Cyst of Pancreas") "Clinic. Soc. of London," viii, 4, 1892; "Lancet," April 16, 1892, p. 871, cited by Nimier.
Lloyd: "Case of Jaundice with Discharge of Fatty Matters from the Bowel," "Med.-Chir. Transact.," 1833, vol. xviii, p. 57.
Lloyd-Jordan: ("Cancer of Pancreas") "Brit. Med. Jour.," 1888.
— "Injury of the Pancr.," "Lancet," November, 1892; "Brit. Med. Jour.," 1892, vol. ii, p. 1051.
Lobstein: ("Cyst") "Lehrb. der pathol. Anat.," 1834, cited by Tilger.
Lockridge: "Disease of Pancreas," "Amer. Pract.," 1876, p. 193.
Löffler: "Induratio pancreatis," "Zeitschr. f. Erfahrungsheilkunde," 1848, S. 363.
Loomis: "Necrosis of Pancr.," "New York Med. Rec.," 1890, p. 105.
Lösch: "Primäres Pankreascarcinom," "Petersburger med. Wochenschr.," 1883, S. 205.
Löschner: "Pankreashämorrhagie," "Wiener med. Zeitung," 1858, Nr. 45.
— "Zur Pankreatitis," "Weitenweber's Beitrage zur Medicin," 1842, Juli.

19

Löw: "Ueber die chemische Natur der ungeformten Fermente," "Pflüger's Archiv," 1882, Bd. xxvii, S. 203.
Löwenhardt: "Fall von Degeneration des Mesenterium und des Pankreas," "Wochenschr. f. d. ges. Heilkunde," 1845, S. 638.
Lubarsch, cited by Dieckhoff: "Beitr. z. pathol. Anat. d. Pankreas."
Lücke u. Klebs: ("Carcinoma") "Virchow's Archiv," Bd. xli, 1867, S. 9.
Ludolph: "Ueber operativ behandelte Pankreascysten." Dissertation, 1890.
Ludwig, Christian: "Adversaria med. practica," Leipzig, 1769, iii, S. 135 (Calculi).
Luithlen: "Carcinoma pancreatis," "Mem. aus d. arztl. Praxis," 1872, Bd. xvii, S. 309.
Lusk, cited by de Grazia: "Rif. med.," 1894, Bd. ii, S. 856 (Calculi); cited by Giudiceandrea.
Lussana: "Il pancreas," "Gazz. med. Ital. Lomb. Milano," 1852, p. 297; "Annali univers. Milano," 1868, p. 416.
— "Pancreatitis," "Gazz. med. Ital. Lomb.," 1851, p. 237.
Lütkemüller: "Carc. medull. pancreat.," "Jahrb. d. k. k. Krankenanstalten," 3. Jahrg.; "Med. Presse," xliii, 1896.
Lynah: "Cancer of Liver, Absence of Pancr.," "Charleston Med. Jour.," 1852, p. 325.
Lynn, Thomas: "Traumatic Pancreat. Effusion," "Lancet," xxxi, 3, 1894, p. 799.

Macaigne: "Abcès du pancr.," "Bull. soc. anat.," 1894.
— "Carcinom du pancréas," cited by Thiroloix.
McBurney: "Cyst of the Pancr.," "Ann. Surg.," Phila., 1894, p. 492.
McChupp: "Case of Scirrhus of Pancr.," "Med. Examiner," 1851, p. 640.
McClurg: ("Cancer") "Med. Examiner," Phila., 1851.
McCollom: "Cancer of Pancr.," "Boston Med. and Surg. Jour.," 1872, p. 371.
McCready: "Concretions from the Pancr.," "New York Med. Jour.," 1856, p. 78.
McDowel: "Cancer of the Pancreas," "Dubl. Quarterly Med. Jour.," 1850, p. 468.
McPhail: "Scirrhus of Pancr.," "New York Med. Jour.," 1854, p. 227.
McPhedran: "Hemorrhagic Pancreatitis," "Canad. Practit.," September, 1896; "Lancet," 1896, vol. ii, p 1324.
Machado: ("Sarcoma") "Correio medico Lisb.," 1883, p. 61.
Mackenzie: "Treatment of Diabet. by Pancr. Juice," "Brit. Med. Jour.," 14, 1; 1893, vol. i, p 63.
— "Cancer of Pancreas," "Med. Examiner," 1878, p. 126.
Mackintosh, Malcolm: "Case of Pancreat. Glycosuria," "Lancet," 24, 10; 1896, vol. ii, p. 1149.
Madelung: ("Surgery") In "Penzoldt-Stintzing's Handb.," Bd. iv, 1896.
Mader-Weichselbaum: "Gangrän des Pankreas," "Bericht d. k. k. Krankenanstalt Rudolfsstiftung," 1884; 1885, S. 371, 435.
Madre: "Etude clinique cur le cancer primitif et second. du pancr.," Paris, 1883.
Maercker: "De pancreate," Berol, 1830.
Maier: "Fall von Verfettung des Pankreas," "Archiv d. Heilkunde," 1865, S. 168.
Maigre: "Des phénomènes cliniques de la digestion à propos d'un tumeur du pancréas," Paris, 1866.
Mairet and Bosc: ("Experiments with Pancreatic Juice") Soc. biol., xxviii, 3, 1896.
Malassez: ("Digestive Power of the Pancreas of Splenectomized Dogs") "Gaz. méd.," 1881, S. 145.
Maly: "Pankreassaft" in "Hermann's Handbuch," Bd. v, 2. Theil.
Manley: "Case of the Pancr. Being a Solid Mass of Scirrhus," "Trans. Wisconsin Med. Soc.," 1874, p. 13.
Maragliano: ("Cancer of Pancreas") "Rif. med.," 1894, Bd. i, S. 355.
Marchand: "Pankreasblutung," "Berliner klin. Wochenschr.," 1890, Nr. 23.
Marchifaava: "Necrosi del pancr.," Soc. Lancisiania Roma, 11, 5, 1895; "Gaz. degli osped.," 1895, p. 670.
Marcuse: "Bedeutung der Leber für das Zustandekommen des Diabetes," "Zeitschr. f. klin. Medicin," 1894, Bd. xxvi, S 225.
Mariani: ("Cancer of Pancreas") "Revue de méd.," 1889, p. 7
Marie: "Diab. bronzé," "Sem. méd.," 1895, p. 229.
Marquet: "Gänzliche Verknorpelung des Antrum pylori und des Pankreas," "Magazin f. d. ges. Heilkunde," 1819, S. 147.
Marshall: "Treatment of Diabet. by Pancr. Extr.," "Brit. Med. Jour.," 1893, p. 743.
Marston: ("Cancer of Pancreas") "Amer. Jour. of Med.," 1854, p. 212, July (Mirallié).
Martin: ("Cyst of Pancreas") "Virchow's Archiv," Bd. cxx, S. 230. 1890.

Martin and Morison: ("Cyst of Pancreas") "Edinburgh Med. Jour.," July, 1893.
— and Williams: ("Influence of the Bile on the Pancreas") "Proc. of the Roy. Soc.," 1890, p. 160.
Martinotti: "Sulla estirpazione del pancr.," "Giorn. della R. Acad. di med.," 1888, No. 7.
Martland: "Tubercles of Liver and Pancr.," "Edinb. Med. and Surg. Jour.," 1825, p. 73.
Martsen cited by Giorgi: "Thèse de Lyon (Ca. pancr.)," 1890.
Masing: "Fall von Krebs," "Petersburger med. Wochenschr.," 1879, Nr. 28.
de Massary: "Cancer primit. du pancr.," "Bull. soc. anat.," xxx, 11, 1895.
— et Potier: "Diabète bronzé," "Bull. soc. anat.," xxvi, 4, 1895.
Masters: "Cancer of the Pancr.," "Med. and Surg. Rep.," 1891, p. 91.
Matani: ("Calculus") "Giorn. di med. Venezia," vol. iv, p. 174, Giudiceandrea.
Mathieu: "Malad. du pancr." in "Traité de médecine," 1892, vol. iii, p. 399.
Mauchart: "De lumbrico terete in ductu pancreat. reperto." Dissertation, 1738, by Friedreich.
Maxson: "Cancer of Pancr.," "New York Med. Jour.," xxi, 9, 1895.
May: "Casuistischer Beitrag zur Lehre vom Pankreasdiabetes," "Annalen d. städt. Krankenhauses zu München," 1894, S. 289.
Mayet: "Cancer primit. du pancr.," "Lyon méd ," 1885, p. 31.
Maynard and Fitz: ("Hemorrhage") See Fitz, S. 189, 203, Fall 5.
Mayo: ("Tubercles of Pancreas") "Outlines of Human Pathology," cited by Senn.
— ("Cyst of Pancreas") "Méd. Record," 1894, S. 168.
Mayo-Robson: ("Cancer of Pancreas") "Brit. Med. Jour.," 1889.
Mazzoni: ("Cyst of Pancreas") "Rif. med.." 1894, Bd. iii, S. 296.
Medicus: "Nonnulla de morb. pancreat.," Berol, 1835.
Meigs: "Cancer of Pancreas," "The Med. and Surg. Rep.," 1862, p. 107, cited by Mirallié.
Melion: "Beiträge zur Erkenntniss und Behandlung der Bauchspeicheldrüsenkrankheiten," "Oesterr. med. Wochenschr.," 1844, S. 449.
Ménétrier, cited by Hanot and Gilbert: "Maladies du foie," 1888, p. 214.
Mering and Minkowski: "Diabetes mellitus nach Pankreasexstirpation," "Klebs' Archiv," 1889, Bd. xxvi, S. 371.
— and Musculus: "Einwirkung von Pankreasferment auf Glykogenstärke," "Zeitschr. f. phys. Chemie," Bd. i, S. 359.
Merklin: "Ephem. cur. nat.," 8, S. 78 (Lithiasis), cited by Nimier.
Mery: ("Cancer of Pancreas") "Bull. soc. anat.," 1885, S 743, cited by Mirallié.
Mett: "Innervation der Bauchspeicheldrüse," "Archiv f. Physiol.," 1894, S. 58.
Michailow: ("Pancreatic Cyst") from "Wratsch," "Bull. med.," No. 1, 1895, p. 1081.
Michelsohn: "Fall von primärem Sarcocarcinom." Dissertation, Würzburg, 1894.
Middleton: "Necrosis of the Pancreas with Cyst-formation and Fat Necrosis," "Glasgow Med. Jour.," 1894, p. 90.
Miller: "Primary Carcin. of the Pancr.," "Med. Record," xxxi, 8, 1895, p. 301.
Milner: "Krebs der Gekrösdrüsen," Tübingen, 1856.
Minkowski: "Untersuchungen über den Diabetes mellitus nach Exstirpation des Pankreas," 1893, "Berliner klin Wochenschr.," 1890, Nr. 8.
— "Diabetes nach Pankreasexstirpation," "Centralbl. f. Pathologie," 1892.
— "Störung der Pankreasfunction als Krankheitsursache," "Ergebnisse der allgemeinen Aetiologie der Menschen- und Thierkrankheiten," von Lubarsch und Ostertag, 1896.
Minnich: "Fall von Pankreaskolik," "Berliner klin. Wochenschr.," 1894, S. 187.
Mirallié: "Cancer primitif du pancr.," "Gaz. des hôp.," xix, 8, 1893, p. 889.
Mitivié: ("Pancreatic Tubercle.") Dissert. sur l'hydrocephale aigu 1820. (Tuberc.) Claessen, p. 345.
Molander et Blix: "Cancer capitis pancr.," "Hygiea," 1876.
Mollard: "Sclérose du pancr.," "Lyon méd.," 1891, p. 299.
— "Pancr. sain chez un diabèt. maigre," *ibid.*, p. 239.
Mollière: "Pankreasblutung," *vide* Eichhorst: "Eulenburg's Realencyklopädie," Bd. ii, S. 435.
Monari: "Carcin. del pancr.," "Gazz. med. lomb.," 1894, p. 443.
Monastyrski: ("Cancer"): Thèse, 1890, cited by Nimier.
Moncorgé: ("Carcinoma of the Pancreas") "Progr. méd.," 1889, Nr. 48.
Mondière: "Recherches pour servir à l'histoire pathol. du pancr." (Carcinoma, Acute Pancreatitis.) "Arch. gén. de méd.," 1836, p. 36, 265.
Montgomery: "Two Specimens of Accessory Pancr.," "Transact. Path. Soc. Lond.," 1860, p. 130; "Lancet," 1861, 7.

Montuori: "Sull' azione glico-inibitrice del secreto pancr.," "Riforma med.," 1895, vol. i, p. 220.

Moore: "Pathol. Observat. of the Pancr.," "St. Barthol. Hosp. Rep.," 1882, p. 207.

— "Abscess of the Pancreas," "Brit. Med. Jour.," 1882, vol. i, p. 88.

— ("Calculi of Pancreas") Path. Soc. of London; "Lancet," 1884, vol. i, p. 69.

Morache: "Induration hypertroph. du pancr.," "Jour. méd de Bord.," 1881, p. 154.

Morat: ("Secretory Nerves of the Pancreas") Soc. de biol., xxvi, 5, 1894, S. 440; "Gaz. des hôp. Toulouse," 1894, p. 371.

Moret: "Pancreas graisseuse avec calculs," "Bull. soc. anat.," 1835, p. 30.

Morgagni: "Opera omnia," vol. iii, Epist. 68, 1, Lithiasis, cited by Giudiceandrea.

Morgan: "Disease of the Pancr.," "Madras Jour. of Med. Soc.," 1867, p. 161.

Moritz: ("Carcinoma of the Pancreas") "Petersburger med. Wochenschr.," 1888, S. 116

Morner: "Analyse des Inhaltes einer Pankreascyste," "Skand. Archiv f. Physiol.," 1895, Bd. v, S. 274.

Mosler: "Fall von Gallertkrebs des Pankreas," "Deutsches Archiv f. klin. Medicin," 1881, Bd. xxviii, S. 493.

Mossé et Daunic: "Diabète bronzé," "Gaz. hebdom.," xiii, 7, 1895.

Mouret: "Dégénérescence du pancr. chez le lapin consecut. à la ligature du canal de Wirsung," "Compt. rend. soc. biol.," xix, 1, 1895, S. 33.

— "Modific. de la cellule pancr. pendant la sécrétion," *ibid.*, p. 35.

— "Lésions du pancr. produites par l'injection d'huile dans le canal de Wirsung," *ibid.*, xxii, 2, 1895, p. 132.

— "Sclérose des greffes du pancr. chez le chien," *ibid.*, xxiii, 3, 1895, p. 201.

Moussons: "Intégrité du pancr. chez une fille diabétique," "Med. soc. Bordeaux," 1894, p. 344

Moutard, Martin: ("Cancer of the Pancreas") "Bull. anatom.," 1887, S. 342, cited by Mirallié.

Moyse: "Etude sur les fonctions et les maladies du pancr.," Paris, 1852.

Mugnai; ("Experiments on the Pancreas") "Collez. Italian. di lett. sulla med.," Ser. 5.

— "Pathol. e terap. chirurg. del pancr.," "Collez. Italian. di lett. sulla med. Milano," 1889, p. 383.

Muir, Robert: "A Case of Pancreatitis with Hemorrhage and Necrosis," "Edinb. Hosp. Rep.," Nos. 4 and 6, 1896.

Muhry: "Markschwammbildung im Pankreas," "Casper's Wochenschr.," 1835, Nr. 10, cited by Friedreich.

Mulert: "Pankreascyste." Dissertation, 1894.

Müller: "Beiträge zur pathologischen Anatomie der hereditären Syphilis bei Nengebornen," "Virchow's Archiv," Bd. xcii, S. 537.

— "Ueber Icterus," "Zeitschr. f. klin. Medicin," 1887, Bd. xii, S. 45.

Mumford: ("Cyst of Pancreas") "Brit. Med. Jour.," 1892.

Munk: "Bauchspeichel," "Eulenburg's Realencyklopädie," Bd. ii, S. 415.

— "Atrophie bei Diabetes," "Tagebl. der 43. Naturforscherversammlung," 1869, S. 112.

Munkenbeck: "Pankreascarcinom." Inaugurations-Dissertation, 1890.

Murchison: ("Cancer of Pancreas") "Maladies du foie," 1878, p. 125.

Musculus u. Mering: "Umwandlung von Starke durch Diastase," "Zeitschr. f. phys. Chemie," Bd. ii, S. 403, 1879.

Musmeci: ("Cancer of Pancreas") "Gazz. delgi osped.," xv, 10, 1890, S. 642.

Musser: "Abscess of Pancr.," "Amer. Jour. of Med. Sciences," April, 1886, p. 449, cited by Fitz, Case 53; "University Med. Magazine," March, 1895.

Nancrede: "Cancer of Pancr.," "Amer. Jour. of Med. Sciences," 1870, p. 150

Nash: "Lumbricus in Pancr.," "Brit. Med. Jour.," 1883, vol. ii, p. 770.

Nasse, Otto: "Untersuchungen über die ungeformten Fermente," "Pflüger's Archiv," 1875, Bd. xi, S 139.

— ("Pancreatic Tuberculosis") "Leichenöffnungen," S. 194 (Claessen, S. 345).

Nathan: "Total Obstruction of Intestine from Disease of the Pancreas," "Med. Times and Gaz.," 1870, ii, p. 238.

Naumann, Ulrich: "Ueber Pankreasveränderungen bei Diabetes." Dissertation, 1895–96.

Naunyn: "Klinik der Cholelithiasis," Leipzig, 1892.

Nauwerck: "Nebenpankreas," "Ziegler's Beiträge," 1892, Bd. xii, S. 29.

Nencki: "Spaltung der Säureester der Fettreihe und der aromatischen Verbindungen im Organismus und durch das Pankreas," "Klebs' Archiv," 1886, Bd. xx, S 367.

Nencki: "Zur Kenntniss der pankreatischen Verdauungsproducte des Eiweiss," "Ber. d. deutschen chem. Gesellsch.," 1895, Bd. xxviii, S 560.
Neumann, J.: "Syphilis" in Nothnagel's "Handb. der speciell. Pathol. u. Therap.," S. 390.
— "Nebenpankreas," "Archiv d. Heilkunde," 1870, S. 200.
Neumeister: "Physiologische Chemie," Jena, 1895, Bd. i.
Neve: ("Sarcoma of Pancreas") "Lancet," 1891, xix, 9.
— "Pancr. Disease," "Indian Med. Record," 1892, p. 208.
Newton, Pitt and Jacobson: ("Traumatic Cyst") "Lancet," 1891, Bd. i, S. 1315.
— "Fat Necrosis of the Oment. with Carcin. of the Pancr.," "Path. Transact.,' 1895, Bd. xlv, p. 91.
Nichols: "Case of Pancreat. Cyst," "New York Med. Jour.," May 26, 1888.
Nicolas et Mollière: "Lithiase pancréat.," "Bull. méd.," xxxi, 1, 1897, S. 97.
Nimier: "L'intervention opératoire dans les affect. du pancr.," "Arch. gén. de méd.," 1887, p. 309.
— "Hæmorrhag. du pancr.," "Rev. de méd.," 1894, p. 353.
— "Lithiase pancréatique," "Rev. de méd.," 1894, x, 9.
— "Chirurgie du pancr.," "Rev. de chirurg.," 1893, Nos. 8, 9, 12; 1894, No. 7.
Nobel, Le: "Fettentleerung mit dem Stuhle und Glykosurie," abstract, "Maly's Jahresb.," 1886, S. 449.
Noltenius: "Beiträge zur Statistik und pathologischen Anatomie des Diabetes mellitus." Dissertation, 1888.
Nommès: "Etude sur le pancr." Thèse, Lyon, 1891.
v. Noorden: "Die Zuckerkrankheit und ihre Behandlung," 1895.
Nothnagel: "Erkrankungen d. Darms u. Peritoneum," 1895, im "Handb. d. spec. Pathologie."
Notta: "Observat. du diabète maigre," "Union méd.," 1881, No. 25.
Noyes: "Disease of the Pancr.," "Trans. Rhode Island Med Soc.," 1892, Providence, 1893, p. 454.

Obici: ("Diabetes Mellitus and the Pancreas") "Boll. d. scienc. mediche," 1893, November; "Soc. med. chir. Bologna," xix, 5, 1893, p 727; "Boll. del Soc. di Bologna," 1896, iv.
Ochsner-Parkes: ("Pancreatic Cyst") "Archiv f. klin. Chirurgie," 1889, Bd. xxxix, S. 446.
Odevaine: "Protrusion of Large Portion of the Pancr ," "Indian. Med. Gaz.," Calcutta, 1866, p. 183.
Oedmansson: "Syphilis," Virchow-Hirsch, "Jahr. Ber.," 1869, Bd. ii, S. 561.
Oestreich: "Gallenblasenkrebs und multiple Pankreasnekrose," Verein f. innere Medicin, xix, 11, 1894; "Deutsche med. Wochenschr.," 1895, 5. Blg , S. 11.
Ogle: ("Cancer of Pancreas") "St. George's Hosp. Report," 1874, p. 223.
O'Hara: "Soft Cancer of Pancr.," "Transact. Pathol. Soc. Phila.," 1877, p. 12.
— ("Cancer of Pancreas") "Phila. Med. Times," 1875, p. 206.
Olivier: "Etude sur le développement du cancer pancréat.," "Beitr. z. pathol. Anatomie," 1894, Bd. xv, S. 351.
Oppolzer: "Pankreasblutung," "Med. Neuigkeiten," 1859, S. 105.
— "Krankheiten des Pankreas," "Wiener med. Wochenschr.," 1867, S. 5.
O'Rourke: "Specimen of Cancer of the Pancr.," "Amer. Med. Monthly," 1855, p. 139.
Orth: "Lehrbuch der pathologischen Anatomie," 1887, S. 901.
Orths: "Ueber Diabetes pancreaticus," Bonn, 1883.
Osler: "Scirrhus of Pancreas," "Med. News," Phila., 1883, p. 694.
— ("Cyst of Pancreas") "Med. Jour.," New York, v, 5, 1894.
— "Principles of Medicine," 1892.
— and Hughes: "Pancreatic Hemorrhage," vide Fitz., S. 226, "Transact. Phila. Path. Soc.," 1888, p. 80.
Osterloh: ("Syphilis") "Mittheil. aus dem k. sächs. Entbindungsinstitute" (Dresden), von Müller, S. 538.
Otis: "The Med. and Surg. History of the War of the Rebellion," part ii, vol. ii, Surg. Hist., p. 159, cited by Senn.
Otto: "Beiträge zur Kenntniss der Umwandlung von Eiweissstoffen durch das Pankreasferment," "Zeitschr. f. phys. Chemie," 1883, Bd. viii, S. 129.
Oulmont: ("Cancer of Pancreas.") Thèse de Lucron, Paris, 1891, cited by Mirallié.

Paderi: ("Concerning the Reputed Glycolytic Action of the Blood, the Kidneys, the Spleen, and the Pancreas") "Rif. med.," 1893, Bd. iv, S. 783.

Pal: "Zur Kenntniss der Pankreasfunction," "Wiener klin. Wochenschr.," 1891, S. 64.

Paldamus: "De damnis ex male affecto pancreate in sanitat. redundantibus," Halæ, 1759.

Palma: ("Diab. bronzé") "Berliner klin. Wochenschr.," 1893, xxi, 8.

Paltauf: ("Cyst") "Ergebnisse der allgemeinen Pathologie und pathologischen Anatomie," Lubarsch-Ostertag, 1896, S. 344.

Panarolus: ("Pankreas lapidosum") "Jatrologismorum," Rom, 1652, S. 51.

Panoff, Anna: "Zerlegung der aromatischen Säureester im Organismus und durch das Pankreas," Bern, 1887.

Parisot: ("Cancer of Pancreas.") Thèse, Paris, 1891, cited by Mirallié.

Parry, Dunn, and Pitt: "Case of Acute Hemorrhag. Pancreat.," "Lancet," 1897, vol. i, p. 36.

Parsons: "Case of Pancr. Cyst," "Brit. Med. Jour.," 1857, vol. i, p. 475.

Paul: ("Pancreatic Hemorrhage") "Boston Med. and Surg. Jour.," iv, 1, 1894, p. 8.
— "Case of Acute Pancreatitis," "Transact. of Clinic. Soc. London," 1895, p. 10; "Lancet," 1894, vol. ii, p. 914.

Pauli: "Krebs der Bauchspeicheldrüse," "Corr.-Bl. bayer. Aerzte," 1849, S. 553.

Paulicki: "Sarkom im Kopfe des Pankreas," "Allgem. med. Centralztg.," 1868, Nr. 90.

Pautz: "Zur Kenntniss des Stoffwechsels Zuckerkranker," "Zeitschr. f. Biologie," Bd. xxxii, S. 197, 1895.

Paviot: "Cancer de la tête du pancr.," "Prov. méd.," 1893, p. 147.

Pawlow: "Folgen der Unterbindung des Pankreasganges beim Kaninchen," "Pflüger's Archiv," Bd. xvi, S 123.
— "Beitrag zur Physiologie der Absonderungen," "Du Bois' Arch.," 1893, Suppl., S. 176.
— "Sur les nerfs secrétoires du pancr.," "Arch. d. scienc. biol. Petersbourg," 1894, vol. iii, p. 189.

Peabody: ("Rupture of Pancreas") "New York Med. Record," 1882.

Pemberton: "Abhandlungen über verschiedene Krankheiten des Unterleibes," Bremen, 1817, S. 71.

Pepper: "Cancer of Stomach and Pancr.," "Med. Examiner," Phila., 1842, p. 723.
— "Tumor of the Head of Pancr.," "Amer. Jour. of Med. Sciences," 1871, p. 159.
— "Hämatom des Pankreas," "Centralbl. f. med. Wissenschaften," 1871, S. 156.
— ("Calculi") "Amer. Jour.," 1857, cited by Giudiceandrea.

Percival: "Two Cases of Inflammation of the Pancr.," "Transact. Associat. King's College of Ireland," 1818, p. 128.

Pereira-Guimaraes: "Hernie traumatique du pancr.," "Progrès méd.," 1896, p. 236.

Perle: "De pancreate ejusque morbis," 1837. Dissertation.

Petit, A.: ("Pancreatic Tuberc.") "Jour. de Leroux," Boyer et Corvisart, xxii, S. 406 (Claessen, S. 345).

v. Petrykowski: "Cystom d. Pankreas." Dissertation, 1889.

Phulpin: ("Cyst of Pancreas") "Bull. soc. anat.," 1892, p. 9.

Pilliet: "Sclérose du pancr. et diabète," "Progr. méd.," 1889, No. 21.
— "Epithéliome de la tête du pancr.," "Bull. soc. anat.," 1889, p. 245.

Pinkham and Whitney: ("Pancreat. hemorrhag.") Vide Fitz.

Pischinger, Oskar: "Beiträge zur Kenntniss des Pankreas." Inaugural-Dissertation, Munchen, 1895 (numerous references concerning the comparative histology of the pancreas).

Pisenti: "Quantitá di indicano," "Arch. per le sc. med.," 1888, p. 87.

Polack: "De pancreate ejusque inflammatione," Prag, 1835.

Ponfick: "Sympathische Erkrankungen des Knochenmarkes bei inneren Krankheiten," "Virchow's Archiv," Bd. lvi, S. 591; 1872, S. 15; 1893, S. 35.
— "Zur Pathologie des Pankreas," "Verhandlungen d. med. Sect. schles. Gesellsch f. vaterland. Cultur," 1890.
— "Fettnekrose," "Verhandlungen d. Congresses f. innere Medicin," 1892, S. 549.
— "Zur Pathogenese d. abdom. Fettnekrose," "Berl. klin. Wochenschr.," 1896, Nr. 17.

Pop: "Carcinoma pancreat.," "Geneesk. Tijdschr.," 1866, p. 310.

Popper: ("Diabetes") "Oesterr. Zeitschr. f. prakt. Heilkunde," 1868, Nr. 11.

Portal: ("Pancreatic Calculi and Necrosis") "Observations sur la nat des malad. du foie," 1813.
— ("Abscess of the Pancreas") "Anat. méd.," 1804, 5, S. 353, bei Seitz.
— "Traité de l'apopléxie," Paris, 1811.
— "Cours d'anatom. médicale," v, S. 356, cited by Giudiceandrea.

Pott: "Fall von primärem Pankreascarcinom," "Deutsche Zeitschr. f. prakt. Medicin," 1878, Nr. 16.
Prince: "Pancreatic Apoplexy," "Boston Med. and Surg. Jour.," 1882, p. 28.
Putnam and Whitney: ("Pancreatic Hemorrhage") Vide Fitz, S. 202.

Quénu: "Pancreas " in "Traité de Chirurgie," vol. vi, 1892.

Rabère: "Carcinoma." Thèse de Bonamy, 1879, cited by Mirallié.
Rachford: "Influence of the Bile on the Fat-splitting Properties of Pancreatic Juice," "Jour. of Physiol.," 1891, p. 72.
Rachmaninow: ("Case of Pancreatic Hemorrhage with Fat Necrosis") "Medicinsk obrosenje," 1895, Nr. 21. Rf. Canstatt, J. B., 1895, Bd. ii, S. 380.
Radziejewski: "Asparaginsäure bei Pankreasverdauung," "Ber. d. deutschen chem. Gesellsch.," 1874, S. 1050.
Rahn: "Scirrh. Pancreat. Diagnosis," Göttingen, 1796.
Railton: "Pancreatic Cyst in an Infant," "Brit. Med. Jour.," 1896, vol. ii, p. 1318.
Ramey: "Carcin. du pancr.," "Jour. de Bord.," 1883, S. 24, cited by Mirallié.
Ramos et Cochez: "Cancer du pancr.," "Rev. de méd.," 1887, p. 770.
Rankin: "Malignant Disease of the Pancr.," "Brit. Med. Jour.," 1895, vol. i, p. 1033.
v. Rátz: "Erweiterung des Pankreasganges bei Thieren," "Monatshefte f. Thierheilkunde," Bd. v, S. 1.
Raynaud: ("Pancreatic Tuberc.") "Arch. gén. de méd.," vol. xxv, p. 165 (Claessen, S. 345).
Reale: "Ursprung und Behandlung des Diabetes mellitus," "Verhandl. d. X. Internisten-Congresses," 1891.
Récamier: ("Carcinoma") "Revue méd.," 1830.
Reclus: "Cancer of Pancreas," "Bull. soc. de chir.," 1892.
Reddingius: ("Cyst of Pancreas") "Nederl. Tydschr.," 1892, Nr. 10; s. Canstatt, "Jahresber.," 1892, Bd. ii, S. 443.
Reece: "Cancer of Pancr.," "Med. and Surg. Reporter," 1871, p. 6.
Reeve: ("Degeneration of the Pancreas") "Ann. of Surg.," August, 1893.
Reeves: ("Presence of Fat in the Feces") "Monthly Journal," March, 1854.
Regnier de Graaf: "Tractat. anatom. medicius de succ. pancreatic. natura et usu," 1671.
Rehm: "Aus der gerichtsärztl. Praxis," "Friedreich's Blätter f. gerichtl. Medicin," 1883.
Reinhard: "Carcinom des Pankreas." Dissertation, Würzburg, 1878.
v. Recklinghausen: "Concretionen, Ektasie des Ductus, Diabetes," "Virchow's Archiv," 1864, Bd. xxx, S. 362
Reichmann: "Anwendung der Pankreaspräparate bei atrophischem Magenkatarrh," "Deutsche med. Wochenschr.," 1889.
Rémond: "Contribution à l'étude du diabète pancr.," "Gaz. des hôp.," 1892.
— and Rispal: ("Treatment of Diabetes with Pancreatic Juice") "Compt. rend.," April, 1893.
— "Diabét. pancreat.," "Gaz. des hôp.," 1890, p. 776.
Remy et Shaw: "Expériences à propos des lésions du pancr. chez les diabet.," "Compt. rend. Soc. biol.," 1880; 1882, p. 599
Renant: ("Chron. Pancreat.") "Compt. rend. acad. des sciences," 1879, p. 247.
Rendu: ("Pancreatic Diabetes") "Sem. méd.," 1891 .
— et Massary: "Diab. bronzé," "Soc. des hôp.," v, 2, 1897.
Renvers: ("Diabetesbehandlung") "Deutsche med. Wochenschr.," 1894.
de Renzi and Reale: "Experimentelles und Klinisches zur Lehre vom Diabetes," "Berliner klin. Wochenschr.," 1892, Nr. 23; "Verhandl. d. Internisten-Congresses," 1891.
Reubold: "Ueber Pankreasblutung vom gerichtsärztlichen Standpunkt." Festschr. f. A. v. Kölliker, 1887.
Reynier: ("Cancer of Pancreas") "Bull. soc. chirurg.," 1892, cited by Nimier: "Chirurg. du pancr."
Reynolds and Gannet: ("Pancreatic Hemorrhage") "Boston Med. and Surg. Jour.," 1885, p. 275.
Rhode: "De syphilide neonatorum," 1825.
— "Ueber Diabetes mellitus," Würzburg, 1880.
Ria: "Carcinoma della testa del pancr.," "Alcune lez. di. clin. med.," 1884, p. 359.
Ribbert: "Folgezustände der Unterbindung des Pankreasganges," "Centralbl. f. klin. Medicin," 1880, S. 385.
Riboli: "Pancreat. acuta," "Gazz. Sardin," 1858.

Richardson: ("Pancreatic Cyst") "Boston Med. and Surg. Jour.," xxix, 1, 1891;
     v, 5, 1892; "Bull. med.," vii, 9, 1892.
— "Case of Pancr. Cyst," "Boston Med. Jour.," xxi, 3, 1895.
Richmond: "Carcin. of the Pancr.," "Buffalo Med. and Surg. Jour.," 1889, p. 728.
Riedel: ("Pankreascyste") "Langenbeck's Archiv f. Chirurgie," 1885, S. 994.
— ("Pankreasstörungen bei Cholelithiasis") "Penzoldt u. Stintzing's Handb. d.
     spec. Therapie," Bd. iv.
— "Ueber entzundliche, der Rückbildung fähige Vergrösserungen des Pankreas-
     kopfes," "Berliner klin. Wochenschr.," 1896, S. 1.
Riegner: "Cyste des Pankreas," "Berliner klin. Wochenschr.," 1890, Nr. 42.
Rigal: "Hypertrophie du pancr.," Soc. méd. d'obst. Paris, 1866, ii, 310; "Wiener
     med. Wochenschr.," 1870, S. 173; "Gaz. des hôp.," 1869, No. 142.
Riolan: "Commentar ad Fernel," 1588, cited by Claessen.
Riva-Rocci: ("Cancer of Pancreas") "Rivist. chir. e therap.," Nov., 1891; "Gazz.
     di Torino," 1892, No. 18.
Roberts: "On the Existence of a Milk-curdling Ferment in Pancr.," "Proceed.
     Royal Soc.," 1879, p. 157.
— ("Cancer") "Brit. Med. Jour.," September, 1865.
Robin: "Sur les propriétés émulsives du pancr.," "Jour. de l'anat.," 1885, p. 455.
Roboica: ("Parotitis and Pancreatitis") Cited by Friedreich, S. 249.
Rocque, Devic and Hugounenq: ("Diabet. and Pancreatic Disease.") "Rev. de
     méd.," 1892, S. 995.
Rocques: ("Cancer") Soc. d'anatom., 1857, S. 247, cited by Mirallié.
Roddick: "Pancreatic Abscess," "Canada Med. Jour.," 1869, p. 385, cited by Fitz,
     Case 41.
Rohde: "Zur Pathol. d. Pankr." Dissertation, 1890.
Rohrer: "Case of Scirrhosit. of the Pancr.," "Med. and Surg. Reporter," 1862, p.
     201.
Rokitansky: "Lehrbuch der pathologischen Anatomie," 1861, Bd. iii, S. 254.
Rolleston: "Fatal Case of Pancreatit. with Hemorrhage," "Lancet," 1896, vol. i,
     p. 705.
— "Fat Necrosis with Disease of the Pancr.," "Brit. Med. Jour.," 1892, vol. ii,
     p. 894.
Rörig: "Ein Beitrag zur Diabetesfrage," "Zeitschr. d. Vereins f. homoöp. Aerzte,"
     Bd. xiii.
Rosborg: "Pancreatit. suppurat. et indurat.," "Hygiea," 1885, p. 274.
Rose: "Beitrage zur inneren Chirurgie," "Deutsche Zeitschr. f. Chirurgie," 1892,
     Bd. xxxiv, S. 12 (Rhexis).
Rosenbach: "Einige bemerkenswerthe Laparotomien," "Centralbl. f. Chirurgie,"
     1882, Nr. 29, Beilage; "Verhandl. des XXIV. Congresses d. deutschen Gesellsch.
     f. Chirurgie," 1, S. 115, 1895.
Rosenberg: "Ausnutzung der Nahrunug," "Sitzungsberichte d. physiolog. Ge-
     sellsch. du Berlin," 23, 6, 1896; "Du Bois' Arch.," 1896, S. 535.
Rosenthal: "Fall von chronischer interstitieller Pankreasentzündung," "Zeitschr.
     f. klin. Medicin," 1892, S. 401.
— "Zur operativen Behandlung der Pankreasgeschwülste," Berlin, 1891.
Röser: ("Tuberc. of the Pancr.") "Schmidt's Jahrb.," Spplbd. iv, 184 (bei Kudre-
     wetzky, S. 103).
Rostan: ("Lues") "Bull. de la soc. anat.," 1855, p. 26.
Rotch: "Case of Cancer of the Head of Pancr.," "Boston Med. and Surg. Jour.,"
     1885, p. 175.
Rotgans: ("Cyst of Pancreas") "Nederl. Tijdschr.," 1892; s. "Canstatt. Jahres-
     ber.," 1892, Bd. ii, S. 443.
Rotter: "Pankreascyste," "Centralbl. f. Gynäkologie," 1893, S. 657.
Roussel: "Cancer du pancr.," "Loire méd.," 1888, p. 146.
Routier: "Tumeur ganglion, de la region du pancr.," "Bull. mens. soc. chir.,"
     1891.
Roux: "Cancer et kystes du pancr.," Paris, 1891.
Rowland: "Cancer of Pancr.; Diabet.," "Brit. Med. Jour.," 1893, vol. i, p. 13.
Rufus, Hall: ("Cancer of Pancreas") "New York Med. Record," 1892.
Ruge: "Beiträge zur Chirurgie der Nieren und des Pankreas," "Deutsche med.
     Wochenschr.," 1890, S. 426.
Rugg-Hudson: ("Pancreatic Hemorrhage") "Lancet," May, 1850.
Ruggi: "Intorno ad un cancro primitivo del pancr.," "Giorn. intern. delle scienz.
     med.," 1890.
Rühle: ("Pancreatitis") Cited by Dieckhoff.

Rumbold: "Glykosurie und ihre Beziehungen zu Diabetes," "Wiener klin. Wochen-schr.," 1894, Nr. 4–8.

Russel: "Cancer Degenerat. of the Pancr.," "Prov. Med. and Surg. Jour ," London, 1851, p. 153.

Russel, W.: "Treatment of Jaundice from Malignant Obstruction," "Edinb. Med. Jour.," July, 1895.

Saguet: ("Cancer"). Thèse de Lucron, Paris, 1892, cited by Mirallié.

Sahli: "Vorkommen von Trypsin im Harn," "Pfl. Arch.," 1885, Bd. xxxvi, S. 209.

de Saint Laurent: "Hypertrophie du pancr.," "Gaz. des hôp.," 1869, p. 562.

Salkowski: "Verhalten des Pankreasfermentes beim Erhitzen," "Virchow's Archiv," 1877, Bd. lxx, S. 158.

— ("Pankreasverdauung") "Du Bois' Arch.," 1878, S. 575; "Zeitschr. f. physiol. Chem.," 1878, Bd. ii, S. 420.

— "Ueber Pentosurie, eine neue Erkrankung des Stoffwechsels," "Berliner klin. Wochenschr.," 29, 4, 1895.

Salles: "Cancer primitif du pancr.," Paris, 1880.

Salmade: "Lithiasis u. Abscess d. Pancr.," *vide* Senn, S. 74.

Salomon: "Carcinom des Pankreas," "Charité-Annalen," 1877, S. 144.

Salzer: "Zur Diagnostik der Pankreascyste," "Zeitschr. f. Heilkunde," 1886, Bd. vii, S. 11.

Samberger: "Entzündung und Vereiterung des Pankreas," "Sanit.-Ber. d. k. med. Colleg. zu Posen," 1832, S. 26.

Sandmeyer: "Ueber die Folgen der Pankreasexstirpation beim Hunde," "Zeitschr. f. Biologie," 1891, Bd. xxix, S. 86; 1892, Bd. xxxi, S 86.

— "Folgen der partiellen Pankreasexstirpation," "Zeitschr. f. Biologie," S. 13.

— "Beiträge zur pathologischen Anatomie des Diabetes mellitus," "Deutsches Archiv f. klin. Medicin," 1892, S. 381.

Sandras: "Observ. des tubercules dans le pancr.," "Rev. méd. franç.," 1848, p. 279.

Sandwith: "Case of Scirrhous Pancr.," "Edinburgh Med. and Surg. Jour.," 1820, p. 380.

Sansoni: "Sul fermento glicolitico del sangue," "Acad. di Torino," 19, 6, 1891; "Riform. med.," 1892, vol. i, p. 146.

Santi: "Carcinoma pancreat.," "Gazz. degli osped.," 8, 2, 1891.

Sarfert: "Die Apoplexie des Pankreas," "Deutsche Zeitschr. f. Chirurgie," 1895, Bd. xlii, S. 125.

Satterthwaite: "Hæmatoma of the Pancr.," "New York Med. Record," 1875, p. 541.

— "Carcinoma of Pancr.," "Bull. New York Path. Soc.," 1881, p. 67.

Saundby: "Morbid Anatomy of Diabet. Mellit.," "Lancet," 1890, vol. ii, p. 383.

Sauter: "Zwei Fälle von Carcinom des Pankreas." Dissertation, Berlin, 1874.

Savill: "Spontan. Rupture of Pancr. Cyst," "Lancet," 1891, vol. ii, p. 666.

Schabad: "Phloridzindiabetes bei künstlich hervorgerufener Nephritis," "Wiener med. Wochenschr.," 1894, Nr. 24.

— "Ueber den klinischen und experimentellen Diabetes mellitus pancreaticus," "Zeitschrift f. klin. Medicin," 1894, Bd. xxiv, S. 108.

Schaper: ("Diabetes.") Dissertation, 1873.

Schenkius a Graefenberg: "Observ. med. tom. unus. Francof.," 1600, Obs. 291, p. 742.

Scheube: "Atrophie des Pankreas und Diabetes," "Archiv f. Heilkunde," 1877, Bd. xviii, S. 389.

Schiff: "Zur Physiologie des Pankreas," "Archiv d. Heilkunde," 1862, S. 271; "Pflüger's Arch.," 1870, S. 622.

Schirlitz: "Melaena in Folge einer Verhärtung des Pankreas," "Magazin d. ges. Heilkunde," 1829, S. 545.

Schirokikh: ("Pancreatic Secretion") "Arch. sciences biol.," St. Petersburg, 1895, No. 5.

Schlagenhaufer: "Fall von Pancreatit. syphilitica," "Archiv f. Dermatologie u. Syphilis," 1895, Bd. xxxi, S. 43.

Schlesier: "Zur Lehre vom Scirrhus der Bauchspeicheldrüse," "Med. Ztg.," 1843, S. 41.

Schmackpfeffer: "Observat. de quibusdam pancreat. morbis." Dissertation, Halle, 1817.

Schmidt: ("Pancreatic Tuberc.") "Hufeland's Jour.," Bd. xxv, S.179 (Claessen, S. 345).

Schmitz: "Zur Pathogenese des Diabetes," "Berliner klin. Wochenschr.," 1891, S. 672.

Schnitzler: "Zur Casuistik der Pankreascysten," "Klin. Rundschau," 1893, Nr. 5.

Scholz: "Carcinoma pancreat.," "Bericht d. k. k. allgem. Krankenhauses," 1881, S. 32.

Schossberger: ("Calculus") Cited by de Grazia, "Rif. med.," 1894, Bd. II, S. 856.

Schroeder: ("Pankreascyste.") Dissertation, 1892.

Schueler: "Fall von Sarcoma pancreat. hæmorrhag." Dissertation, 1894.

Schupmann: "Carcinom," "Hufeland's Jour.," 1841, Bd. XCII, S. 41.

Schwartz: "Cas de kyste pancr.," "Sem. méd.," 1893, No. 36; "Bull. de la soc. anat.," 1885.

Schwerdt: "Carcinom des Pankreas," "Correspondenzbl. d. ärztl. Vereines zu Thüringen," 1888, S. 374.

Sebire: "Observat. sur le pancr. cartilagineux," "Jour. méd. chir.," 1783, p. 548.

Sée, M.: "Anomalies des canaux pancréat.," "Compt. rend. soc. biol.," 1857, 4, S. 1.

Seebohm: "Zwei Fälle von primärem Pankreascarcinom," "Deutsche med. Wochenschr.," 1888, S. 777.

Seegen: "Der Diabetes mellitus," Berlin, 1893, 3. Aufl.

— "Umsetzung von Zucker im Blute," "Centralbl. f. Phys.," 1892, 12, 3; 22, 9, 1894; 20, 10; 3, 11, 1894.

— "Die Zuckerumsetzung im Blute mit Rücksicht auf Diabetes," "Wiener klin. Wochenschr.," 1892, Nr. 14.

Seelig: "Beitrag zum Diabetes pancreaticus," "Berliner klin Wochenschr.," 1893, S. 1013.

Segré: "Studio clinico dei tumori del pancr.," "Annal. univ. di med. e chir.," 1888, p 3.

Seidel: "Echinococcus im Pankreas," "Jena. Zeitschr. f. Medicin," 1864, S. 289.

Seitz: "Blutung, Entzündung und brandiges Absterben der Bauchspeicheldrüse," "Zeitschr. f. klin. Medicin," 1892, S. 1.

Senator: "Diabetes mellitus," Ziemssen's "Handbuch der spec. Pathologie u. Therapie," 1876, Bd. XIII

— "Zur Kenntniss der Pankreasverdauung," "Virch. Arch.," 1868, Bd. XVIII, S. 358.

— "Erkrankungen der Nieren," 1896, in Nothnagel's "Handb. d. spec. Pathologie."

— ("Diabetesbehandlung") "Deutsche med. Wochenschr.," 1894.

Sendler: "Zur Pathologie und Chirurgie des Pankreas," "Münchner med. Wochenschr.," 1, 12, 1896; "Deutsche Zeitschr. f. Chirurgie," Bd. XLIV, 1896.

Senn: "The Surgery of the Pancr," "Transact. of the Amer. Med. Assoc.," 1886.

— "Surgical Treatment of Cyst of Pancreas," "Amer. Jour. of Med. Sciences," July, 1885.

— "Die Chirurgie des Pankreas," "Volkmann's Sammlung klin. Vorträge," Nr. 313.

Servaes: "Fall von Pankreascarcinom," Allgem. ärztl. Verein zu Köln, "Berliner klin. Wochenschr.," 1878, S. 716.

Setschenow: "Neue Trypsinprobe," "Centralbl. f. med. Wissensch.," 1887, Nr. 27, S. 497.

Severi: "Carcinoma della testa del pancr.," "Gaz. degli osped.," 8, 12, 1894.

Sgobbo: "Sul midollo spinali di cani spancreatici e diabet.," Morgagni, 1892, p. 392.

Sharkey and Clutton: "Pancreatic Cyst," "St. Thomas' Hosp. Rep.," 1893, p. 271.

Shattock: "Calculi of Calcium Oxalate from a Pancr. Cyst," Path. Soc. of London, 21, 4, 1896; "Brit. Med. Jour.," 1896, vol. I, p. 1034.

Shea: "Abscess of Pancr.," "Lancet," 1881, vol. II, p. 791.

Sibley: "Treatment of Diabet. by Feeding of Raw Pancr.," "Brit. Med. Jour.," 1893, vol I, pp. 452, 579

Siebert: "Ueber Melliturie," "Deutsche Klinik," 1852.

— "Krankheiten des Pankreas," "Archiv f. d. ges. Medicin," 1849, S. 29.

Siebold: "Dissert. systematis salivalis," Jenæ, 1797.

Siegfried: "Ueber Phosphorfleischsäure," "Zeitschr. f phys. Chem.," Bd. XXI, S. 360

Sievers: "Pankreatit. acuta gangrænosa," Finska handlingar, "Boas' Archiv," 1896, vol. II, p. 241.

Signorini: ("Glycolytic Action of Certain Organic Fluids and Organs") Acad. med. fisica Fiorent, 1892.

Silver: "Fatty Degeneration of Pancr," "Transact. of Path. Soc. of London," 1873, vol. XXIV.

— and Irving: ("Atrophy of the Pancreas and Diabetes") "Transact. of Path. Soc. of London," 1878, vol. XXIX.

Simon: "Pankreascarcinom bei 13jährigem Knaben." Dissertation, Greifswald, 1889.

Simon and Stanley: ("Pancreatitis") "Lancet," 1897, vol. I, p. 1325.
Smith, Bisset: ("Scirrhus of the Pancreas") "Lancet," 5, 8, 193, p. 306.
Smith, Greig: "Chirurgie abdominale," Trad. de Vallin et Duret. 1894.
Smith, Walter: ("Abscess of the Pancreas") "Dublin Jour.," 1870, S. 201, cited by Fitz, Fall 43.
Smith: "Scirrh of the Pancreas," "Dublin Jour. of Med. Science," 1844, p. 175.
Socin: "Pankreascarcinom," "Jahresb. d. chirurg. Abth. zu Basel," 1887.
Sottas: ("Calculus of Pancreas") "Bull. soc. anat.," Bd. v, S. 635, cited by Nimier.
Sourrouille: "Pancréat. aiguë passée à l'état chronique," "Gaz. des hôp.," 1885, p. 1091.
Soyka: "Primäres Pankreascarcinom," "Prager med. Wochenschr.," 1876, Nr. 42.
Spiess: "Pankreasblutung," Rf. "Schm. Jahrb.," 1867, Bd. cxxxiv, S. 270.
Spitzer: "Zuckerzerstörende Kraft des Blutes und der Gewebe," "Pflüger's Archiv," 1895, S. 303; "Berliner klin. Wochenschr.," 1894, Nr. 42.
Stadelmann: "Ueber einen bei der Pankreasverdauung entstehenden Bromkörper," "Petersburger med. Wochenschr.," 1889, S. 452.
— "Multiple Fettnekrose," Verein f. innere Medicin, 27, 4, 1896.
Standthartner: "Carcinom des Pankreas," "Aerztl. Bericht d. k. k. Krankenhäuser," 1893, S. 77.
Stansfield: ("Cancer of Pancreas") "Brit. Med. Jour.," 1890, 6, 2
Stapper: "Beitrag zur Diagnose der Pankreascysten." Dissertation, 1892.
Starr: "Diseases of the Pancr.," "Syst. Pract.," Phila., 1885, p. 1112.
Steele: "Cyst of Pancreas," "Chicago Med. Jour.," 1888, p. 205.
— "Cancer of Pancreas," "Lancet," 1893, vol. II, p. 131.
Stefanini: ("Case of Suppurative Pancreatitis") "Gazz. degli osped.," 1896, p. 848.
Stein: "Ueber primäres Carcinom des Pankreas," Jena, 1882.
Steven, Lindsay: "Necros. of the Pancr.," "Lancet," 1894, vol. I, p. 963.
Sticker: "Todesfälle durch Pankreasapoplexie bei Fettleibigen," "Deutsche med. Wochenschr.," 1894, Nr. 12, S. 274.
Stieda: "Pankreascyste," "Centralbl f. allgem. Pathologie," 1893, Nr. 12.
Stillé: "Enlargement and Induration of the Pancr.," "Trans Path. Soc. of Phila ," 1857, p. 34.
Stiller: "Zur Diagnose des Pankreaskrebses," "Wiener med. Wochenschr.," 1895, Nr. 45.
— "Fall von Pankreascyste," "Wiener med. Zeitung," 1892, S. 283; "Med.-chirurg. Presse," Pest, 1892, S. 548.
Stintzing: "Carcinom des Pankreas," "Aerztl. Intelligenzbl.," München, 1883, S. 185.
Stockton and Williams: "Two Cases of Fat Necrosis," "Amer. Jour. of Med. Sc.," Sept., 1895.
— "Carcin. of the Pancr.," "Intern. Clin.," Phila., 1892, pp. 14, 17.
Stokvis-Hofmann: "Zur Pathologie und Therapie des Diabetes mellitus," V. Internistencongress, 1886.
Stolnikow: "Lehre von der Function des Pankreas im Fieber," "Virchow's Archiv," 1882, Bd. xc, S. 389.
Störck: ("Rupture") "Arch. gén. de Paris," 1836, cited by Leith.
Störk, A.: "Annus medicus secund.," 1762, p. 245 (Cyste), cited by Friedreich.
Strauss: "Ueber Magengährungen und deren diagnostische Bedeutung," "Zeitschr. f. klin. Medicin," Bd. xxvi, 27.
Strümpell: "Primäres Carcinom des Pankreas," "Deutsches Archiv f. klin. Medicin," 1878, Bd. xxii, S. 226.
Strunck: "Cyst. Erweiterung des Pankreasganges." Dissertation, 1895.
Subotic: "Ein operirter Fall von Pankreascyste," "Wiener allgem. med. Zeitung," 1887, Bd. xxxii.
Suche: "De scirrho pancreat.," Berol, 1834.
Suckling: "Carcinom pancreat.," "Lancet," 1889, vol. I, p. 127.
Swain: ("Cyst of Pancreas") "Brit. Med. Jour.," 4, 3, 1893
Sweet, G. B.: "Carcinoma of the Pancreas Associated with Glycosuria," "Austral. Med. Gaz.," Sydney, 1896, 15.
Sym: "Medullary Tumor of Pancr.," "Edinburgh Med. and Surg. Jour.," 1835, p. 125.
Symington: "Case of a Rare Abnorm. of Pancr.," "Jour. of Anat.," 1885, vol. xix, p. 292.
Sympson: "The Glycolytic Ferment of the Pancr.," "Brit. Med. Jour.," 1893, vol. I, p. 113.

Tabor: "Autopsy," "Bost. Med. and Surg. Jour.," 1844, p. 450.
Tanner: ("Cancer") "Prov. Med. Jour.," 1842.

Tarchanoff: "Innervation d. Milz," "Pflüger's Arch.," Bd. viii, S. 74.
Tarulli: ("Pancreatic Ferment in Urine") *Acad. med. fisic. Fiorent.*, 28, 5, 1892.
Taylor: "Cirrhosis of Liver, Disease of Pancr.," "Lancet," 1841, p. 223.
— "Scirrhus of Pancreas," "Pacif. Med. and Surg. Jour.," 1866, p. 19.
Taylor, T. C.: "Carcinoma of Pancr.," "Boston Med. and Surg. Jour.," 1887, p. 503.
Teacher: "Diagnosis of Pancreatic Diseases," "New York Med. Jour.," 1892, 2, 4.
. Teissier: ("Cancer") "Jour. de méd. de Lyon," 1847, S. 801, cited by Mirallié.
Terrier: ("Cancer") "Rev. de chirurg.," 1892.
Thacher: ("Carcinoma") "New York Med. Review," 1891, p. 79; "Proc. Path. Soc. of New York," 1892, p. 21.
Thayer: ("Hemorrhagic Pancr.") "Boston Med. and Surg. Jour.," 1889.
— "Acute Pancreatitis," "Johns Hopkins Hospital Rep.," 1895; "Amer. Jour. of Med. Sciences," vol. xc, p. 396.
Thiersch: ("Cyste des Pankreas") "Berliner klin. Wochenschr.," 1881, S. 591.
Thiroloix: "Exstirpation und Transplantation des Pankreas," "Compt. rend. acad.," 1982, p. 966; Soc. d'anat., 1, 7, 1892; Soc. de biol., 1892, 22, 10; Soc. de biol., 16, 4, 1894, p. 297; "Gaz. des hôp.," 1894, p. 1333; "Arch. de physiol.," 1892, p. 716.
— "Le diabète pancréatique," 1892.
— et Pasquier: ("Cyst") "Bull. soc. anat.," 1892, p. 311.
Thomas and Morgan: "Diseases of Pancreas and their Homœopathic Treatment," Chicago, 1882.
Thompson: ("Carcinoma") "New York Med. Jour.," 1889, S. 407, cited by Mirallié.
— ("Verletzung") Cited by Senn, "Chirurgie des Pankreas," S. 34.
Thomson: "Disease of Pancr.," "Syst. Pract.," Phila., 1841, p. 295.
Thorén: ("Cyst") "Eira," 1893, S. 99; "Centralbl. f. Gynäkologie," 1893.
Thorn: "Case of Scirrhus of Pancr.," "Lancet," 1855, vol. ii, p. 437.
Thornberry: "Case of Disease of Pancr.," "Amer. Practit.," 1877, p. 30.
Thou, Di: ("Calculus") Cited by Verardini, "Malattie del pancr.," S. 44, cited by Giudiceandrea.
Tibaldi: "Cirrhosi della testa del pancr.," "Annal. univ. di med. e chir.," Milano, 1876, S. 545.
Tilger: "Beitrag zur pathologischen Anatomie und Aetiologie der Pankreascysten," "Virchow's Archiv," 1894, Bd. cxxxvii, S. 348.
Tillaux: ("Cancer of Pancreas") *Vide* Nimier.
Tisné: ("Carcinoma.") Thèse de Lucron, 1893, cited by Mirallié.
Tobin: ("Cyst of Pancreas") "Méd. mod.," 1895, p. 489.
Todd: ("Chron. Pankreat.") "Dublin Hosp. Reports," vol. i.
Tonnelé: ("Abscess of Pancreas") "Archiv generales de médecine," Bd. xxii, cited by Claessen.
Tott: "Pankreaskrankheit," "Zeitschr. d. deutschen Chirurg. Vereines," 1853, S. 86.
Trafoyer: "Lageveränderung," "Allgem. Wiener med. Zeitung," 1862, Nr. 29.
Travers: ("Rupture of Pancreas") "Lancet," 1827, S. 384, cited by Leith.
Tremaine: ("Cyst") "Transact. of Amer. Chir. Assoc.," 1888.
Treves: "Case of Cyst of the Pancr.," "Lancet," 1890, vol. ii, p. 655.
Tricomi: "Le cisti del pancr.," "Gazz. degli osped.," 1892, p. 894.
Trombetta: ("Cyst") "Arch. di Società Italian. di chirurg.," 1892.
Troupeau: "Cancer de pancr.," "France médicale," 1873, p. 613.
Trousseau: "Clinique médical" (Diabet. bronzé), cited by Marie.
Trumpy: "Cancer pancreat.," "Jour. d. prakt. Heilkunde," 1830, S. 35.
Tulpius: ("Acute Pankreatitis") "Observat. med.," 1672, p. 328.
Tylden and Miller: "Recent Research on Diabetes," "Barthol. Hosp. Reports," 1891, vol. xxvii.
Tyson: "Cancer of the Head of the Pancr.," "Phila. Med. Times," 1870, p. 365; 1881, p. 786.

Ulrich: "Ausbreitung des Pankreas," "Gen.-Ber. d. k. rhein. med. Colleg.," 1831, Koblenz, 1833, S. 53.
Unckel: "Conspectus nosograph. pancreat.," Bonn, 1836.
Urban: "Hufeland's Jour. der prakt. Heilkunde," 1830, S. 87.

Van der Byl: "Med. Cancer of the Pancr.," "Trans. Path. Soc. of London," 1857, p. 228.
Varnier: ("Pancreatic Tuberc.") "Ancien jour. de méd.," 3, S. 9 (Claessen, S. 345).
Vanni: "Effetti del estirpaz. del pancr.," "Archiv di clin. med.," 1894, p. 157.

Vassale: "Alterazioni del pancr. consecut. alla legatura del condotto di Wirsung," 1887, Modena.
Velich: "Zur Lehre von der experiment. Glykosurie," "Wiener med. Zeitung," 1895, Nr. 46.
Venable: ("Tuberc.") Cited by Bigsby (Claessen, S. 345).
Verardini: "Stud. sul malattie del pancr.," "Giorn. med. di Roma," 1869, p. 201; "Rivist. Italian. di terap.," 1882, p. 3.
— "Cancer del pancr.," "Rév. med. di Sevilla," 1886, p. 108.
— "Chirurg. del pancr.," "Memor. Acad. Bologna," 1888, p. 245.
Verga: "Conversione del pancr. nel adipe," "Gazz. med. lomb. Milano," 1850, p. 200.
Vernay: "Etude clinique et anatomique du cancer de pancr.," Thèse, Lyon, 1884.
Vesselle: "Du cancer du pancr.," Paris, 1852.
Vidal: "Cancer du pancr.," "Clinique," 1829, p. 234.
Villière: "Rupture traumatique du pancr.," "Bull. soc. anat.," 1895, p. 241.
Virchow: "Zur Chemie des Pankreas," "Virchow's Archiv," 1853, S. 580.
— "Ueber Ranula pancreatica," "Berliner klin. Wochenschr.," 1887, S. 248.
— ("Pankreascysten") "Würzburger Verhandlungen," 1852, 2, S. 53; 3, S. 368.
Vogel: "De pancreat. nosol. generali," Hal., 1819.
Voigtel: "Handbuch der pathologischen Anatomie," 1804, Bd. I, S. 543.
Vulpian: "Sur l'action des ferments digestifs," "Bull. de l'acad. de méd.,' 1879, p. 901.

Wagner: "Accessorisches Pankreas in der Magenwand," "Archiv f. Heilkunde," 1862, S. 283.
— "Fall von primärem Pankreaskrebs," "Archiv f. Heilkunde," 1861, S. 285.
Wagstaff: "Case of Traumat. Intraperit. Hemorrhage," "Lancet," 16, 2, 1895, vol. I, p. 404.
Waid: "Scirrhus of the Pancr.," "Buffalo Med. and Surg. Jour.," 1878, p. 121.
Walker: "Cyst of Pancr.," "Trans. New York Path. Soc.," 1879, p. 85.
— "Significance of Colorless Stools," "Med.-Chir. Transact.," 1890, vol. LXXII.
Walsh: "Celiotomy for Absc. of Pancr.," "Med. News," 1893, p. 737.
Walter: "Thätigkeit des Pankreas bei Fütterung mit Fleisch, Brot und Milch," "Gesellschaft d. russ. Aerzte," St. Petersbg., 26, 9, 1897; cited by Boas, "Archiv f. Verdauungskrankheiten," Bd. III, S. 271.
Wandesleben: "Pankreasruptur," "Wochenschr. f. d. ges. Heilkunde," 1845, S. 729, cited by Leith and Körte.
Ward: "Two Cases of Cancerous Disease of Pancr.," "Lancet," 1863, vol. II, p. 66.
Wardell: "Disease of Pancr.," "System Med.," Reynolds, London, 1871, 3, S. 407.
Warren: "Pancr. Indurated and Enlarged," "Boston Med. and Surg. Jour.," 1829, vol. I, p. 147.
Wassilieff: "Calomel bei Gährungsprocessen;" "Zeitschr. f. phys. Chemie," 1882, Bd. VI, S. 112.
— ("The Physiology of the Pancreas") "Arch. sc. biol. de St. Petersbourg," 1893, Bd. I, S. 1, 28; Bd. II, S. 219.
Watson: "Case of Jaundice with Disease of Pancr.," "London Med.-physic. Jour.," 1830, p. 499.
Webb: "Scirrhus of the Head of Pancr.," "Phila. Med. Jour.," 1871, vol. II, p. 86; 15, 6, 1892.
Wedekind: "Primitiver Krebs des Pankreas," Würzburg, 1863.
Wegeli: "Casuistische Beiträge zur Kenntniss des Diabetes mellitus im Kindesalter," "Archiv f. Kinderheilkunde," Bd. XIX, 1895, S. 1.
Wegner: "Hereditäre Syphilis," "Virchow's Archiv," Bd. L, S. 305.
Weichselbaum: "Nebenpankreas in der Wand des Magens," "Bericht der k. k. Krankenanstalt Rudolfsstiftung," 1883–1884, S. 379.
Weir: "Pancreat. Cyst from a Calculus," "New York Med. Rec.," 1893, p. 803.
Weinmann: "Absonderung des Bauchspeichels," "Zeitschr. f. rat. Medicin," 1853, S. 247.
Weintraud: "Pankreasdiabetes der Vögel," "Archiv f. experiment. Pathologie," 1894, Bd. XXXIV, S. 303.
— u. Laves: "Respiratorischer Stoffwechsel eines diabetischen Hundes nach Pankreasexstirpation," "Zeitschr. f. phys. Chemie," 1895, Bd. XIX, S. 629.
Welch: "Cancer of the Pancr.," "Transact. Med. Soc. New Jersey," 1886, p. 231.
Werigo: "Ueber das Vorkommen von Penthamethylendiamin in Pankreasinfusen," "Pflüger's Archiv," 1892, Bd. LI, S. 362.
Wesener: "Fall von Pankreascarcinom," "Virch. Arch.," 1883, Bd. XCIII, S. 386.

Westbroock: "Carcin. of the Pancr.," "Proc. Med. Soc. Kings County," Brooklyn, 1879, p. 16.
Wethered: "Carcin. Pancr.," "Path. Society of London," 4, 2, 1890, cited by Mirallié.
Weyer: "Fall von Gallertkrebs des Pankreas," Greifswald, 1881.
White: "Treatment of Diabet. by Feed. on Raw Pancr.," "Brit. Med. Jour.," 1893. vol. I, p. 402.
White, Hale: ("Cancer of Pancreas") "Brit. Med. Jour.," 4, 3, 1893.
— "A Clinical Lecture on Carcin. of the Pancreas," "Lancet," December 26, 1896.
Whitfield: "Disease of Pancr.," "Lancet," 1841, vol. II, p. 445.
Whitney: "Hemorrhage into the Pancr.," "Boston Med. and Surg. Jour.," 1894, p. 379.
— ("Pancreat. hemorrh.") "Boston Med. and Surg. Jour.," 1881, p. 592, cited by Fitz.
— and Harris: ("Gangrenous Pancreatitis") "Boston Med. and Surg. Jour.," 1881, No. 25, cited by Fitz.
— and Homans: ("Hemorrhagic Pancreatitis") Vide Fitz.
Whittier and Fitz: ("Necrosis") "Mass. General Hosp. Rec.," 1884, Bd. v, cited by Fitz, Case 67.
Whitton: "Abscess of the Pancr.," "Austral. Med. Gaz.," 1891, p. 276.
Wilcox: ("Concretions of Pancreas") "Med.-chir. Transact.," Bd. xxv, cited by Klebs, S. 545.
de Wildt: ("Cyst of the Pancreas") "Nederl. Tydschr.," 1892.
Wilks: "Colloid Cancer of the Pancr.," "Transact. Path. Soc. of London," 1854, p. 224.
— and Moxon: ("Rupture of Pancreas") "Patholog. Anatomy," S. 491, cited by Leith.
Wille, E.: "Ein Beitrag zur pathologischen Anatomie des Pankreas beim Diabetes mellitus," "Mittheil. aus den Hamburger Staatskrankenanstalten," Bd. I, 1897.
Williams: "Cancer of pancr.," "Med. Times and Gaz.," 1852, p. 131.
— "Scirrhous Tumor of Stomach. and Pancr.," "Med. and Surg. Rep.," Phila., 1868, p. 274.
— "On Diabetes," "Ther. Gaz.," 15, 10, 1894; "Brit. Med. Jour.," 1894, vol. II, p. 1303.
Williamson: ("Alterations of the Pancreas in Diabetes") "Med. Chron.," 1892, No. 3; "Brit. Med. Jour.," 24, 2, 1894; "Lancet," 1894, vol. I, p. 927.
— "Diabetes Mellitus and Lesions of the Pancreas," "Med. Chronicle," May, 1897.
Willigk: ("Carcinom des Pankreas") "Prager Vierteljahrsschr.," 1856.
Wilson: "Extensive Disease of Pancr.," "Lancet," 1841, vol. I, p. 594; "Med.-chir. Transact.," London, 1842, p. 42.
Windle: "The Morbid Anatomy of Diabetes," "Dubl. Jour. of Med. Sciences," 1883.
Witzel: ("Pankreascyste") "Centralbl. f. Chirurgie," 1887, S. 9.
Wolff: "Ossif. of the Arter. of Pancr.," "Lancet," 1836, vol. II, p. 825.
Wölfler: "Zur Diagnose der Pankreascysten," "Prager Zeitschr. d. Heilkunde," 1888, Bd. IX, S. 119.
Wood: "Scirrhus of Duodenum and of the Head of Pancr.," "Med. and Surg. Rep.," Phila., 1866, p. 228.
— ("Treatment of Diabetes with Pancreas") "Brit. Med. Jour.," 1893, vol. I, p. 64.
Worthmann: "Disease of the Pancr.," "Glasgow Med. Jour.," 1892, p. 385.
Wrany: "Sectionsergebnisse der Prager pathologisch-anatomischen Anstalt," "Prager Vierteljahrsschr.," 1867, S. 8.
Wyss: "Zur Aetiologie des Stauungsicterus," "Virchow's Archiv," 1866, S. 454; 1860, S. 1.

Yeo: "Atrophy of the Pancr.," "Brit. Med. Jour.," 1874, S. 519.

Zahn: "Ueber drei Falle von Blutungen in die Bursa oment.," "Virch. Arch.," Bd. cxxiv, S. 238, 252.
Zawadzki: "Chemische Analyse des Pankreassaftes beim Menschen," "Oesterr.-ungar. Centralbl. f. med. Wissensch.," 1891, 9, S. 73.
— ("Cyst of Pancreas") "Lancet," 1891, 25, 4, Bd. I, S. 948.
Zenker: "Nebenpankreas in der Darmwand," "Virchow's Archiv," 1861, Bd. xxi, S. 369.
— "Hämorrhagien des Pankreas," "Berliner klin. Wochenschr.," 1874, Nr. 48; Breslauer Naturforscherversamml., 1874; "Schmidt's Jahrbuch," Bd. cLxxiii, S. 299.

Zeri: "Carcinoma primitivo del corpo del pancr.," Congr. med. int., 1892, p. 447.
— "Ueber tödtliche Pankreasblutung," "Deutsche Zeitschr. f. prakt. Medicin," 1874, Nr. 41.
Ziegler: "Lehrbuch der pathologischen Anatomie," 1895, 8. Auflage.
Ziehl: "Fall von Carcinom des Pankreas," "Deutsche med. Wochenschr.," 1883, Nr. 37.
Zielewicz: "Zur Chirurgie der Bauchhöhle," "Berliner klin. Wochenschr.," 1888, S. 294.
Zielstorff: "Fall von Unterleibscyste." Dissertation, Greifswald, 1887.
Zimmer: "Zur Lehre vom Diabetes mellitus," 1867.
Zoja: "Rare varietà dei condotti pancreat.," "R. Ist. Lomb. di scienz." Rendicont Milano, 1883, vol. xvi, p. 364.
Zukowski: "Grosse Cyste de. Pankr.," "Wiener med. Presse," 1881, Nr. 45.
Zweifel: ("Pankreascyste") "Centralbl. f. Gynäkologie," 1894, Nr. 27.

DISEASES OF THE SUPRA-RENAL CAPSULES.

BY

EDMUND NEUSSER, M.D.

20

DISEASES OF THE SUPRARENAL CAPSULES.

ANATOMY AND HISTOLOGY OF THE SUPRARENAL CAPSULES.

THE suprarenal capsules are a pair of small organs, each of which is situated, like a helmet or cap, upon the upper extremity of the corresponding kidney. Although in such close proximity, the suprarenal capsules and kidneys are almost entirely independent of one another; thus in the majority of cases the suprarenal capsule does not accompany the kidney when dislocated.

As a rule, these organs are not symmetrically situated. The right capsule (as also the right kidney) lies a little lower than the left and does not fit so accurately upon the upper extremity of the kidney, while the left capsule is displaced slightly to the inner side of the corresponding kidney.

The suprarenal capsules are flattened bodies with two principal surfaces, directed approximately anteriorly and posteriorly and frequently grooved in the adult. The two surfaces meet above in a broad and strongly convex border, while below they are bounded by a concave edge and separated from one another by a narrow concave surface. Thus their shape corresponds approximately to a triangle, rounded off at the top and with a somewhat concave base. There is a slight difference in the shape of the organs upon the two sides of the body, the right capsule being noticeably narrower and higher than the left. This is caused by the varying pressure of surrounding organs.

The size of the suprarenal capsule presents marked individual differences. In the negro these organs are conspicuous for their large size and abundant pigment. There are no distinct differences in size in the sexes, but it undoubtedly varies considerably with the age of the individual. In the first few months of fetal life these bodies considerably exceed the kidneys in size, by the sixth month they are only half as large, at birth the ratio is as 1 to 3 and in the adult as 1 to 28. In advanced age the suprarenal capsules undergo further atrophy and their consistence becomes very firm.

According to Orth, the dimensions of the normal adult suprarenal capsule are as follows: width 40 to 55 mm., length 20 to 35 mm., thickness 2 to 6 mm.; while their weight is 4. 8 to 7.3 grams.

The suprarenal capsule is surrounded externally by a moderate layer of fat and possesses a tense fibrous capsule containing elastic fibers (tunica albuginea); radiating from this numerous fibrous septa penetrate the parenchyma of the organ. For this reason the capsule cannot be removed without injury to the parenchyma.

Near the base of the anterior surface of the organ there is a deep groove through which the principal blood-vessels, lymphatics, and nerves enter and emerge, and which has therefore been termed the hilum.   The color of the external surface is composed of various shades of yellowish-brown.

On cross-section it is at once apparent, from differences in color, that the gland is composed of two distinct portions, the peripheral or cortical and the central or medullary portion.   The cortex is of a yellow color, clearly shows radiating lines, and is of a firm consistence.   The medulla is of a grayish-red color and of a soft spongy consistence, easily crushed. The junction of these two layers is marked by a narrow band of tissue, the intermediary zone of Virchow, which is really a part of the cortex and is of a deep brown color in advanced age.

Entering now upon the consideration of the finer structure of the suprarenal capsules, two elements are to be differentiated: first, the fibrous stroma continuous with the capsule; and, secondly, the cellular parenchyma.

The stroma consists of relatively thick septa which traverse the cortex in a radial direction toward the medulla, where they break up into a very fine network.   Smaller septa are also given off in the cortex to form a coarse network inclosing large and small groups of parenchymatous cells. Immediately beneath the capsule the meshes and the inclosed groups of cells are small and circular; in the broad middle portion they form large long radii like the septa, while in the innermost division of the cortex they are once more small, round, and delicate, corresponding to the outer zone. With reference to these histologic appearances the cortex has been divided since the publication of Arnold into three zones, called from without inward the zona glomerulosa, the zona fasciculata, and the zona reticularis; however, there is no sharp line of demarcation between them.

Finally, an exceedingly delicate network arises from the coarser septa of the stroma and surrounds each cell of the parenchyma.

In the medulla the stroma breaks up more uniformly into its component fibers and surrounds with an exceedingly fine network the individual parenchymatous cell.

All the spaces of the stroma are filled with groups of parenchymal cells.   In the cortex these groups assume various shapes, corresponding to the stromal spaces which contain them; thus, they are rounded in the zona glomerulosa, elongated columns in the zona fasciculata, which comprises the greater part of the cortex, or they may be irregular.

A few observers have demonstrated also columns of cells with a delicate central fissure.   Small, colorless, glistening granules have been found repeatedly in the cells of these columns in both man and animals, and also in the blood of the suprarenal vein, in addition to brownish flakes.   Their importance will be discussed later.

The cells of the fasciculate zone are normally filled with fat-droplets of varying size (fatty infiltration), and the cells of the intermediary zone contain brown pigment-granules in abundance.

The parenchymal cells of the medullary portion are irregular in shape, being polygonal or even stellate; they are stained dark brown by chromic acid or chromates.

The rich blood-supply of the suprarenal capsules has been recognized and commented upon for a long period of time.   The arteries are derived in part directly from the aorta (central suprarenal artery, the principal branch which enters at the hilum); in part from the arteries of the diaphragm, descending branches (superior suprarenal arteries); in part from the vessels of the kidneys, ascending branches (inferior suprarenal arteries). These arteries, following the septa and finest ramifications of the stroma, subdivide into a dense capillary network which is best developed in the medullary portion. From this the blood is collected into venous branches, the largest of which (central suprarenal vein) empties on the right directly, on the left as a rule indirectly through the renal vein, into the inferior vena cava.

It has been proved by the most careful histologic investigation that the relation between the capillaries and the cells of the parenchyma is a very intimate one, the endothelium of the capillaries immediately overlying the cell-masses of the parenchyma. Indeed, in the medullary substance, according to Manasse, large columns of cells project directly into the capillaries and are immediately bathed in blood.

The lymphatic vessels of the suprarenal capsules are very numerous; they originate between the cells of the cortex and form in the medullary portion a network surrounding the vein and emerge with it and empty into the lymphatic vessels of the kidney.

The rich nerve-supply of the suprarenal capsules is equally striking. Some of these nerves are non-medullated sympathetic fibers from the solar plexus and other adjacent plexuses; others are medullated fibers from the splanchnic, vagus, and phrenic nerves. In the medullary portion, particularly, whole clusters of ganglion cells lie embedded in the exceedingly delicate plexus of nerve-fibers.

EMBRYOLOGY.

GREAT differences of opinion exist among investigators as to the development of the suprarenal capsules. Not only do most authors admit that the cortical and medullary substances arise separately, but there are at least two opinions held as to the origin of each of these.

According to the majority of authors, the medullary substance is derived from the anlages of the sympathetic ganglia. Rabl believes that the medullary cells represent detached ganglion cells which have remained at the embryonal stage of development. A small number of authors hold the opinion that the medullary cells are derived from the cortical cells, and that only a few ganglion cells and nerve-fibers have entered from the sympathetic.

It is thought by one group of authors that the cortical substance is derived from an accumulation of cells of connective tissue at the anterior extremity of the primitive kidney. Other observers derive the cortical cells from a growth of epithelial cells in the body-cavity, which belong either to the genital ridge or to the primitive kidney.

Michalkovic regards the suprarenal capsules as detached portions of the genital glands which have remained at an early stage of development before sexual differentiation has occurred, and which, after the separation, have acquired other physiologic functions. According to Rabl, the cortical substance in birds is derived from the canals of the primitive kidney.

The suprarenal capsules are developed at the same time as the sympathetic system, when the primitive kidney begins to disappear.

The two separate anlages soon unite. That from the sympathetic • (medullary substance) in the beginning at least forms a part of the outer layer. Later this relation is reversed, and the anlage of the cortical substance gradually grows around that from the sympathetic.

The discovery of the frequent occurrence of accessory suprarenal capsules is of the greatest importance for the whole pathology of these organs. Their presence has been demonstrated in animals as well as in man by a large number of observers. They consist of fragments of suprarenal structure, varying in size from a pin's head to a pea or bean, scattered throughout the entire retroperitoneal space, but showing a special predilection for the region of the genital organs.

They are said to occur very frequently at the hilum of the suprarenal body and in its immediate neighborhood, and when thus situated they probably represent lobes which have become separated from the main organ. They occur also in the solar plexus, in the celiac ganglion, beneath the capsule of the kidney, and in the cortex of this organ, opposite the sacro-iliac articulation, but particularly often along the course of the spermatic cord and internal spermatic vessels from the retroperitoneal space to the epididymis; in the female they may be found in the broad ligament close to the parovarium. They are said to occur more frequently upon the right than upon the left side.

These accessory suprarenal glands occur frequently in man, being present, according to Schmorl, in 92% of all bodies examined. They occur also in animals, but, strange to say, they are very rarely found in certain species, notably never in guinea-pigs. Ordinarily these bodies consist of cortical substance only, though of late several cases have been observed where the medullary substance also was plainly developed (Dagonnet, Pilliet).

Their occurrence is important for two reasons: first, after destruction or impairment of function of the true suprarenal bodies, these accessory organs may hypertrophy and assume their function, so that, in spite of complete destruction of the suprarenal capsules, the symptoms characteristic of that condition may not appear; secondly, these rudimentary organs not infrequently degenerate and become the seat of malignant neoplasms.

PATHOLOGIC ANATOMY OF THE SUPRARENAL CAPSULES.

1. ABNORMALITIES OF DEVELOPMENT.

COMPLETE absence of the suprarenal bodies in individuals otherwise healthy has been demonstrated by recent as well as early investigators. Some of these cases are not above the suspicion that a displaced hypoplastic organ may have been overlooked, yet the most recent observers have proved that complete aplasia of the suprarenal capsules is not only possible, but in rare instances has actually occurred.

Cases of arrested development (hypoplasia) have been observed more frequently, occurring, however, exclusively in certain monstrosities which are characterized by defects of the cerebrum; as, for example, hemicephalus, cyclops, encephalocele, microcephalus, and syncephalus. Other malformations, especially of the genital organs, were frequently associated. Hypoplasia of the suprarenal bodies was found to occur only when there was absence of portions of the anterior cerebral lobes, which are known to originate at the very earliest period of fetal life. Hydrocephalus, which does not develop until a later period of fetal life, and defects of the posterior lobes, have no effect upon the development of the suprarenal bodies. [Ad. Czerny,* however, recently examined the suprarenal capsules of five cases of various degrees of hydrocephalus, and found them alike altered in all. The cortex was normally developed, but there was no medullary portion. This alteration of the capsules was regarded as representing a much earlier period of development than was indicated by the excess of ventricular fluid.—ED.]

Zander, who has lately devoted considerable attention to this subject, concludes from these facts that only the anlage and the differentiation of the suprarenal capsules depend upon the functional integrity of the anterior cerebral lobes. If the anlage has been completely differentiated, its further development is independent of the central nervous system, and is no longer influenced by injuries to the latter. The tracts which transmit this influence of the cerebrum upon the developing suprarenal anlage are wholly unknown.

Displacements of one or both of the suprarenal bodies are of the rarest occurrence. It is also worthy of note that this organ practically never participates in dislocations of the corresponding kidney, but is always to be found in its normal situation.

In a single case the two suprarenal glands were found fused, forming a horseshoe-shaped organ.

2. HYPERTROPHY AND ATROPHY.

In many cases it is quite difficult to decide whether the suprarenal is hypertrophied or not, for even under normal conditions these organs present wide variations in size. In well-developed, well-nourished individuals they are larger and richer in fat than in the weakly and emaciated. Also, we must bear in mind their relatively greater size in children and in negroes.

However, we are justified in speaking of hypertrophy of these organs when we have to deal with a definite unilateral increase in size resulting from impairment of function of the opposite organ by disease or removal. This is termed compensatory hypertrophy, and both substances of the gland take part in the process. [Simmonds † reports such a case in which the left capsule was extremely atrophied while the right capsule was seven times as heavy and ten to fifteen times as thick as its fellow. All portions, especially the central, were enlarged. The atrophied capsule was regarded as tubercular.—ED.] Similarly, any accessory suprarenal capsules which are present may hypertrophy and assume the function of the normal organ.

* *Centralbl. f. allg. Path. und path. Anat.*, 1899, x, 281.
† *Virch. Arch.*, 1898, CLIII, 138.

Marchand reports a very peculiar case of hyperplasia of the suprarenal capsule. He found both organs enormously enlarged and an accessory organ situated in the broad ligament. The subject was a pseudohermaphroditic female with atrophied ovaries. Marchand's theory in explanation of this case is that an abnormally large part of the undifferentiated body epithelium (from which suprarenal capsules and reproductive organs are both developed) was utilized in the formation of the suprarenal bodies at the expense of the embryonic ovaries.

Atrophy of the suprarenal capsules occurs normally in advanced age. The organs become smaller, thinner, and more flaccid. The fat disappears from the parenchymal cells and a considerable deposit of pigment usually occurs. Likewise in the various cachexias, the organ parts with more or less of its intracellular fat and becomes smaller. Thees atrophies possess no pathologic significance.

In certain rare cases a true pathologic atrophy has been observed without any apparent cause.

3. DEGENERATIONS.

(a) Cloudy swelling of the suprarenal parenchyma occurs quite frequently in the acute infectious diseases, such as typhoid fever, pneumonia, septic infection, erysipelas, and scarlatina. This condition is identical with that occurring in the liver, heart, and kidneys. The cells appear crowded with granules; the outlines of the former and its nucleus are indistinct. This form of degeneration is found particularly in the cortex.

(b) Fatty degeneration is difficult to diagnosticate, because the cells of the cortex are normally infiltrated with fat, even in the new-born. It has been observed in hereditary syphilis, circulatory disturbances, phosphorus-poisoning, and as an advanced stage of cloudy swelling. Fatty degeneration is differentiated microscopically from the normal fatty infiltration by the smaller size of the fat-drops and by simultaneous diminution of the cells and atrophy of their nuclei.

(c) Hyaline and dropsical degeneration may be mentioned simply as curiosities.

(d) Amyloid degeneration, on the contrary, is very common and pronounced, occurring in as marked a degree as in spleen, kidney, or intestine, and dependent upon the same causes as in amyloid degeneration of these organs. The capsules become large, dense, gray, and present a lardaceous appearance. The cortical and intermediary zones are affected chiefly, the medulla being involved to a lesser degree. The degenerative process is confined primarily and principally to the walls of the blood-vessels; subsequently the connective-tissue septa are involved, but not the parenchymal cells. The latter are compressed rather by the swollen intervening tissue, lose their fat, and atrophy after long continuance of the disease. Large homogeneous flakes of amyloid connective tissue are observed, particularly in the medulla.

4. CIRCULATORY DISTURBANCES.

(a) Congestion of the suprarenal capsules is very common, but it is usually the passive variety. The general stagnation of the blood in all diseases of the kidneys, heart, and lungs is very pronounced in the supra-renal capsules by reason of their rich blood-supply. Venous hyperemia is of comparatively frequent occurrence in new-born infants with or without coincident syphilis. After this congestion has lasted for a considerable period of time the organ becomes indurated and the capillaries and veins distinctly dilated.

Active hyperemia frequently occurs in acute infections, particularly profound septicemia. Capillary hemorrhages occur not infrequently during its course. In the guinea-pig these two conditions—active hyper-emia and punctiform hemorrhages—are invariably found postmortem after experimental inoculation with diphtheritic, typhoid, or pyocyaneus organisms.

(b) Anemia and anemic necrosis practically do not occur, the vascular network of the organ being too dense.

(c) Hemorrhages are not unusual. In addition to the above-mentioned capillary hemorrhages, larger—indeed, often very extensive—hemorrhages occur as the result of trauma, especially in the new-born; or after venous hyperemia, hemorrhagic diathesis, leukemia, or malignant neoplasms. Such hemorrhages may be the immediate cause of death if rupture of the gland occurs. As a rule, however, they remain encapsulated, sur-rounded by suprarenal substance, forming the so-called hematomata, which may attain the size of a man's head. When of long duration the blood undergoes the same changes here as in other situations. Coagula-tion occurs at the periphery, the blood-pigment is converted into methe-moglobin and hematin, giving a yellowish-brown color to the mass. Finally, most of the fluid is absorbed, the surrounding tissues contract, and lime salts may be deposited. Or this condition may terminate in the formation of a cyst, analogous to the apoplectic cysts of the brain.

(d) Thrombosis of the smaller veins or even of the principal vein, some-times continued from the vena cava, has repeatedly been observed. No considerable anatomic alterations are produced in the organ, as an ade-quate collateral circulation is established at once. Such thromboses have been found to contain lime salts; in other words, pheboliths were formed.

Emboli occur in the form of capillary bacterial emboli complicating septic processes and giving rise to microscopic necroses and punctiform hemorrhages.

5. INFLAMMATIONS.

As acute inflammation Virchow described a form of "hemorrhagic inflammation" in which he found the suprarenal capsule swollen, ex-tremely hyperemic, and studded with hemorrhagic infiltrations. This condition was observed in profound general infections of a septic nature (septicemia, scarlatina, etc.), and is doubtless identical with the above-mentioned form of active hyperemia with bacterial emboli and hemor-rhages.

Cellular infiltration and suppuration, whether metastatic or continued, are of relatively rare occurrence. Exceptionally abscesses have been ob-served to arise apparently spontaneously in one or both suprarenal cap-sules. Such abscesses may perforate into the surrounding connective tissue or into the intestine.

Chronic productive inflammation characterized by new-formation of connective tissue and partial atrophy of the parenchyma has been observed as a manifestation of syphilis. A marked proliferation of connective tissue is almost constantly present in chronic tuberculosis, and was, therefore, in former years frequently spoken of as an independent affection.

6. INFECTIOUS GRANULATION TUMORS.

These comprise syphilis and tuberculosis.

Syphilis occurs occasionally in the form of a typical gumma composed of granulation tissue terminating in central necrosis and peripheral cicatrization. As mentioned above, it may be manifested atypically in the form of a cirrhotic inflammation. Sometimes it is with difficulty differentiated from tuberculosis. Syphilitic thickening of the vessels is also observed.

Tuberculosis of the suprarenal capsules derives especial interest from its relation to Addison's disease.

Acute and subacute miliary tuberculosis are of rare occurrence. In the vast majority of cases we have to deal with a form of chronic tuberculosis characterized by an unusually protracted course and by the abundant formation of granulation and scar tissue, together with a well-marked tendency to calcification or at least inspissation of the caseous mass.

One or, more frequently, both organs may be affected; in the latter case the process is apt to be further advanced on one or the other side. In most cases it proceeds from the medullary portion, although the observations are by no means rare in which it commences in the cortex or even in the capsule and pericapsular connective tissue.

The typical form is the conglomerate tubercle, which is composed of a group of miliary nodules. Caseation begins at the center of the mass, while at the periphery there is abundant formation of granulation tissue containing fresh groups of miliary tubercles which in turn become confluent and cheesy. A large part of the granulation tissue is converted into a firm, fibrous callus. After several years' duration the whole organ becomes gradually involved, and it is not unusual to find absolutely no remains of normal suprarenal substance. Occasionally the new-formation of connective tissue extends beyond the capsule (and a dense callus is formed around the suprarenal bodies which becomes united with the capsule of the kidney and the diaphragm) and in which a part of the solar plexus is embedded. As a result of this process, the suprarenal capsules become irregularly enlarged, nodular, and very dense. Amyloid degeneration is frequently present at the periphery of the caseous mass.

In the great majority of cases tuberculosis of the suprarenal capsules is secondary to tuberculosis of other organs, the primary growth occurring in the lymphatic glands, lungs, or genitals. Exceptionally a primary tuberculosis of the suprarenal capsule may occur, and form the point of origin of a general miliary tuberculosis, in which case the rupture of the tuberculous focus into the suprarenal vein is demonstrable.

7. NEOPLASMS.

Neoplasms may develop in the suprarenal capsules proper or in the accessory rudimentary bodies, the latter being especially prone to their formation.

Excessive proliferation of circumscribed portions of suprarenal substance gives rise in the first instance to small tumors resembling lipomata which have been termed suprarenal strumas or adenomata. These are situated in the cortex of the suprarenal capsule, or, more frequently, in accessory glands occurring in the kidney. In the latter situation the term of renal adenoma or " heterologous renal struma " has been applied. They are small masses varying in size from a pin's head to a pea, yellowish-white in color, sharply defined, and surrounded by a connective-tissue capsule. They are histologically identical with the suprarenal cortex, even the typical fatty infiltration of the parenchyma being present.

As a rule, these tumors give rise to no symptoms during life and are only encountered accidentally at autopsies. Although they thus appear as wholly benignant, they are capable of undergoing metastasis like strumas of the thyroid. Such metastases often become much larger than the primary tumor, and, since the latter present no symptoms, are suggestive of primary growths. They may readily be recognized by their structure and by the fatty infiltration of their cells.

In addition to this formation of metastases, in itself a manifestation of malignancy, suprarenal strumas, after existing for a long period of time, tend to become malignant. They break through their capsule, replace the surrounding tissue, and grow into the veins.

Histologically these tumors are composed chiefly of polymorphous cells, the arrangement of which may closely simulate adenocarcinoma; although, according to the latest views, they are to be considered sarcomata of the vascular perithelium (perithelioma). Formerly these tumors were described as carcinomata or sarcomata. They may develop apparently directly from displaced embryonic suprarenal bodies without the preceding formation of an adenoma.

These malignant growths are further characterized by their extraordinarily rich, almost telangiectatic, vascular network, and by the fatty infiltration of their cells. The glistening, hyaline granules normally present in the suprarenal cortex are ·found both in the tumors and in the metastases. After attaining a moderate size these tumors may be recognized macroscopically by their numerous blood-vessels and resulting spongy structure, their fibers floating in water.

The peritheliomata are characterized by a tendency to metastasis, especially in certain organs, as the osseous system (vertebræ, bones of skull, head of femur, clavicle, etc.) and the brain.

Moreover, they are subject to degenerative changes which are almost exclusively fatty; the cells being predisposed to this variety by their normal condition of fatty infiltration. The center of the tumor becomes converted into fatty detritus into which hemorrhages frequently take place, causing a dissection of the spongy tissue in all directions and giving rise to a large or small hemorrhagic cyst.

These cysts, like the original tumors, are frequently found in the kidney, and until recently their mode of origin was obscure. Grawitz was the first to throw any light upon the subject, and in his honor they have been called Grawitz's tumors.

Other primary tumors of the suprarenal capsules are rare. Angiosarcoma and melanosarcoma have been observed in the cortex, also single instances of lymphosarcoma, angioma, and lymphangioma have been reported. Fraenkel has described a sarcoma, Virchow a glioma, and Weichselbaum a ganglionic neuroma in the medullary portion. [Although malignant tumors of the suprarenal capsules are most commonly found in adult life, Orr * reports the occurrence of a sarcoma of the right adrenal with extensive metastases in the liver in a child of seven weeks. Brucha- . now † states that a child fourteen months old had a cancer of the capsule twice the size of a man's fist, with metastases in the lymph-glands and ovaries.—Ed.]

Primary sarcoma and carcinoma in other organs, particularly the thyroid gland, breast, and ovary, may give rise by metastasis to similar growths in the suprarenal capsules.

[Ramsay ‡ gives the following summary of the study of sixty-seven cases of primary malignant tumors of the suprarenal gland: "(1) That while malignant tumors of the suprarenal glands are rare, they should be considered as one of the factors to be eliminated in the presence of an abdominal tumor; (2) that they are somewhat more common in the male sex; (3) that while in a certain proportion the symptoms are fairly well marked, there are many in which no symptom points to the suprarenal origin; (4) that rapid loss of strength, debility, emaciation, digestive disturbances, and abdominal pain are the most prominent symptoms; (5) that skin changes are rather the exception than the rule; (6) that they run a rapid course, the duration being shorter than usual with a neoplasm in other organs; (7) that the diagnosis is impossible in many, and difficult in all, cases; (8) that a differential diagnosis must be made from other suprarenal diseases, from renal tumors, from hepatic tumors, from diseased retroperitoneal glands, and from cysts and new-growths of the pancreas; (9) that the prognosis is always serious, even following a successful operation, from the great frequency with which both glands are found involved, and the tendency to early metastases; (10) that operation gives the only hope of relief, and that it has been successful in two cases; (11) that the principal difficulties in the operation are the friability of the tumor, the great tendency to hemorrhage, and the frequency of the adhesions."—Ed.]

8. PARASITES.

Very exceptionally echinococcus cysts have been found in the suprarenal capsule, one case of multilocular cyst being reported.

PHYSIOLOGY OF THE SUPRARENAL CAPSULES.

THE suprarenal capsules were discovered by Eustachius in 1564, but no satisfactory theory as to their function was advanced until the investigations of Addison. He first called attention to the relation existing between disease of these organs and a peculiar group of symptoms, and expressed the opinion that their extensive destruction led to severe general disease and death.

Experiments on animals were at once begun, and an effort was made

* *Edinb. Med. Jour.*, 1900, 221.   † *Prager Zeitschr. f. Heilk.*, xx, 39.
‡ *Johns Hopkins Hosp. Bull.*, 1889, x, 21.

to determine, first, whether the suprarenal capsules are or are not essential to life.

The first investigator was Brown-Séquard, who, in 1856, sought to obtain some knowledge of the function of the suprarenal capsules by extirpating these organs from different animals and by studying the symptoms which followed. After removing both suprarenal bodies he found that all the animals died within one or two days with symptoms of general weakness, convulsions, delirium, and coma. By control experiments he excluded the possible cause of death by injury to adjacent organs (liver, sympathetic nerves) or by peritonitis or hemorrhage and determined that it was due solely to removal of the suprarenal bodies. Extirpation of one suprarenal capsule also resulted in death, but not until a much longer period of time had elapsed. Brown-Séquard reported as a cause of death the accumulation of pigment in the blood-vessels and numerous pigment-emboli. He concluded from these observations that the suprarenal capsules are absolutely essential to life.

Very soon Brown-Séquard's views were most positively contradicted by a whole group of observers as a result of their experiments.

Gratiolet and Philipeaux succeeded in keeping several animals alive for weeks and months after removal of both suprarenal capsules. In their opinion this operation is not necessarily fatal, although the majority of animals subjected to it die from unavoidable injury to surrounding organs, especially the sympathetic plexuses and ganglia, the liver, and the peritoneum, or from purulent inflammation of this membrane. Brown-Séquard again brought forward several groups of experiments in support of his original theory, which he modified only in one particular—namely, that in animals with but little pigment (albinos) the suprarenal bodies were not absolutely essential to life, but maintained that the reverse was the case in pigmented animals.

Practically all earlier observers joined the ranks of Gratiolet and Philipeaux. Harley, especially, contradicted Brown-Séquard in every particular, and mention should be made also of Berruti and Perusino, Chatelain, and Schiff, who succeeded in keeping several animals alive for months after removal of both suprarenal capsules, while they attributed the death of the other animals to injuries accompanying the operation or to subsequent accidents, for example, exposure to excessive cold. Nothnagel also soon agreed with them; he did not remove the suprarenal capsules, but exposed them and crushed them with forceps as completely as possible. He succeeded in keeping a number of animals alive for a year and a half without the occurrence of the symptoms mentioned by Brown-Séquard—namely, weakness, delirium, or convulsions.

No further observations were made upon the importance and function of the suprarenal bodies until Tizzoni resumed the experiments in 1889. The results obtained by him with reference to the vital importance of this organ practically coincide with those of Brown-Séquard. Some of his animals survived the extirpation of both suprarenal capsules for almost three years, but eventually all died. He maintains, therefore, that the earlier experimenters were led to oppose Brown-Séquard's views because their animals were not kept under observation long enough, but were killed before the pathologic processes initiated by the operation had caused the animal's death. ·

Accordingly his conclusions are as follows: After the removal of both suprarenal capsules all animals die, without reference to age or color.

Their death results from removal of the suprarenal capsules and not in consequence of injuries from the operation, because death may not occur for years afterward, therefore the suprarenal capsules are absolutely essential to life. At the postmortem examination of his animals, Tizzoni found extensive alterations in the brain, cerebellum, spinal cord, and peripheral nerves as the cause of death.

From 1891 to 1893 Abelous and Langlois carried on a series of careful experiments upon frogs, guinea-pigs, and dogs. They found that removal of one suprarenal body gave rise to no special symptoms, but that death generally resulted if the greater part of the remaining capsule also was removed. When large portions of suprarenal substance were left behind, the death of the animal was long delayed or might not occur at all; in such cases the function of the suprarenal body was maintained, although very inadequately, by the remaining portions. After complete extirpation of both capsules, summer-frogs died within forty-eight hours; winter-frogs lived considerably longer, even a fortnight. All the guinea-pigs and dogs died within a few hours. If a portion of suprarenal body was grafted into these animals before the operation, their death was prevented. If these fragments were subsequently removed, the animals invariably died. It is also possible, after removal of both suprarenal capsules, to keep the animals alive twice as long as usual by injections of suprarenal extract. From these experiments Abelous and Langlois conclude that their animals died because the function of their suprarenal capsules was lacking, having excluded, by control experiments, injury to the kidney as a cause of death.

Thiroloix, Albanese, de Domenicis, and Marino Zucco also came to the conclusion that removal of both suprarenal capsules is fatal. The only opponent of this theory is Pal, who kept a dog alive four months and twelve days after complete extirpation of both suprarenal capsules, and demonstrated the absence of supernumerary suprarenal bodies at the autopsy. Finally, Szymonowicz, experimenting upon dogs, obtained the same results as Abelous and Langlois. He believes the contradictory results of the earlier authors to be due to incomplete removal of the suprarenal bodies. Nothnagel even found remnants of normal tissue after several of his operations, and it seems very probable that some fragments were left behind in Tizzoni's cases also. It is possible for such fragments to regenerate, assume the suprarenal function to some extent, and delay the fatal issue. Likewise any accessory suprarenal capsules which are present may vicariously assume the suprarenal function.

Stilling's experiments upon young rabbits furnish additional support for this view. He found after removal of one suprarenal body that the remaining organ almost doubled its original size, and that the accessory suprarenal bodies, previously invisible or at least very small, became enormously hypertrophied. This increase in size was due to the regeneration of both medullary and cortical substances. [The results obtained by Huttgren and Andersson * can similarly be explained. They removed one suprarenal from rabbits, allowed an interval to elapse, and then removed the other. Rabbits survived, but similar experiments on cats and dogs were lethal.—Ed.] Stilling decided that the suprarenal capsules possess without doubt an extrauterine function which is essential to life. Thiroloix also found hypertrophy of the remaining organ several months after removal of one.

*Centralbl. f. Phys., 1899, xiii, 503.

This completes the review of the experimental physiology of the supra-renal capsules. It is evident that Brown-Séquard's view—that these organs are essential to life—is strongly upheld by the most recent experiments. A single dog experimented upon by Pal seems to contradict the universal opinion. This case is open to Tizzoni's objection that the period of observation was too short, or accessory capsules may have been present; for, according to Pal's report, search was made for these organs only at the site of operation on either side of the vena cava. Yet even if this case is admitted, a single exception is certainly not sufficient to overthrow the theory of the importance of these bodies. Goltz removed the entire brain from dogs and the animals subsequently lived without a brain, yet no one would believe that the brain was not important to life.

The second question for the physiologists to solve relates to the function of these organs. Three different ways have been proposed in order to answer this question.

The first method consisted in the "clinical" observation of animals after removal of one or both suprarenal capsules. The results of these observations may be summed up as follows:

1. *Nutrition.* Brown-Séquard—later Philipeaux, Foá, Nothnagel, Tizzoni, etc.—noticed extreme emaciation in animals dying sooner or later after removal of both suprarenal capsules. Tizzoni found in animals surviving the operation for a long period of time that the nutrition was maintained until shortly before death, when emaciation ensued. Transient emaciation was noted by Abelous and Langlois after removal of one suprarenal body. In similar cases Szymonowicz sometimes failed to detect this, and even noted considerable increase in weight some time after the operation. Pal's case above mentioned behaved similarly. When only very small portions of the suprarenal capsules were left behind, Thiroloix and Lancereaux observed extreme emaciation.

2. *Temperature.* On this point the statements of different authors are very contradictory. Tizzoni, Abelous, and Langlois report a fall of temperature which is greater when both organs are removed. Szymonowicz was unable to demonstrate any considerable variation in temperature in either case.

3. *Disturbances of the nervous system.* Brown-Séquard observed profound cerebral symptoms, such as epileptic convulsions, delirium, and vertigo; if only one organ was removed, the convulsions and contraction of the pupil were greater on the corresponding side. Tizzoni observed similar symptoms in rapidly fatal cases, and, in addition, diminished motor power and reflexes, opisthotonos with dilated and unresponsive pupils. In animals living a long time after removal of one suprarenal body he found weakness with contractures of the anterior extremities and impaired sensation upon the corresponding side.

Other authors, including Abelous and Langlois, noticed a preponderance of paralytic symptoms extending from the posterior extremities to the anterior, also the loss of faradic nervous irritability, while the direct muscular irritability was unimpaired; death resulted from paralysis of the muscles of respiration. After removing both bodies Albanese exhausted his animals with faradic current and then observed clonic spasms, loss of reflexes, paralysis extending to the muscles of respiration, and arrest of the heart in diastole. Szymonowicz never observed convulsions after this operation, but, on the contrary, apathy, rigidity, weakness of the extremities, and difficult breathing.

The anatomic alterations underlying these various nervous disturbances have carefully been investigated by Tizzoni, who finds them to be fundamentally different in animals dying soon after the operation and in those surviving for several months.   In the former case these alterations consist of circulatory disturbances, stagnation of lymph, and irregularly scattered hemorrhages, together with exudation and secondary degeneration throughout the central nervous system (especially in the central canal), gray matter, and pia mater.   In the brain and cerebellum these foci are irregularly distributed, while in the medulla oblongata they correspond closely to the nuclei of the eighth to the eleventh cranial nerves. The alterations are most intense in the medulla oblongata and in the cervical region of the cord, gradually diminishing toward the sacrum.   In the second group of cases—animals surviving the operation for a considerable period of time—the alterations in the central and peripheral nervous systems are primarily independent of circulatory disturbances.   They comprise degeneration of the posterior columns (especially the columns of Goll), extending even to the cerebellum, degeneration of the posterior roots, and atrophy of the posterior horns.   The latter changes begin in the posterior horn of the side operated upon, extending thence to the anterior horn of the opposite side, and finally involving the whole gray substance.   In the medulla oblongata the nuclei of the glosso-pharyngeal and vagus groups are atrophied, in the brain the changes are confined to the cortex.   Finally, Tizzoni found degeneration of the celiac and mesenteric plexuses of the sympathetic and of the peripheral nerves (sciatic). Tizzoni believes that these changes in the central nervous system are transmitted by the sympathetic, the degeneration extending from the abdominal plexuses of the latter, along the ganglionated cord to the spinal cord and brain.

4. *Disturbances of the digestive organs.*   Loss of appetite was reported by most observers after removal of one or both suprarenal capsules, in the former case as a transient symptom.   Nothnagel, Albanese, and Tizzoni observed increased peristalsis and diarrhea.   Jacoby believes that the suprarenal capsules contain an inhibitory center for intestinal peristalsis; he bases this opinion upon the above-mentioned observations and upon original experiments, in which, after removal of the suprarenal capsules, an irritable condition of the intestine was produced by vagus stimulation. Pal only exceptionally obtained results corresponding with Jacoby's view.

5. *Changes in the blood.*   Brown-Séquard found a large excess of pigment in the blood and numerous pigment-emboli, and therefore concluded that the suprarenal capsules belong to the hemo-vascular glands and that there is a certain substance present in the body which is readily converted into pigment, and that the function of the suprarenal capsule probably is to so alter this substance that its peculiar property is lost.   No subsequent investigator has succeeded in confirming this observation of Brown-Séquard.   There are conflicting reports as to the number of red and white corpuscles and percentage of hemoglobin, these being variously reported increased, diminished, or normal.   The views of different authors concerning the chemical alterations in the blood are more in harmony, and are of the utmost importance for the physiology and pathology of the suprarenal capsules.

Brown-Séquard had already discovered the following facts.   After removal of both suprarenal capsules life may be prolonged by injecting the blood of healthy animals. On the other hand, the blood of animals deprived of both suprarenal capsules, when injected, hastens the death of animals from which only one organ has been removed. He therefore attributes poisonous properties to the blood of animals deprived of their suprarenal bodies. Abelous and Langlois obtained similar results in frogs. Later Langlois repeated these experiments with dogs and confirmed the poisonous action of the blood of animals subjected to this operation upon other animals similarly operated upon, but was unable to demonstrate any effect upon healthy animals. Marino Zucco and Raphael Suppino found that the blood of rabbits deprived of their suprarenal capsules acted like curare. These authors conclude that certain substances accumulate in the blood of these animals which, like curare, paralyze the motor nerve-endings and in part the muscles themselves; and that the function of the suprarenal capsules is to neutralize or destroy these substances. According to this view, the suprarenal capsules are neutralizing organs.

Abelous, Langlois, and Albanese investigated the origin of these poisonous substances. In the course of their experiments they found that summer-frogs died much sooner than winter-frogs after removal of both suprarenal capsules; that frogs deprived of both suprarenal capsules die much sooner if their muscles are tetanized by the faradic current than if they are let alone; that the phenomena of exhaustion appear much earlier and last longer in animals subjected to this operation than in healthy animals; that the alcoholic muscle-extracts of exhausted but healthy animals when injected into frogs deprived of suprarenal bodies produce the same effect as the alcoholic muscle-extracts of animals similarly operated upon but not exhausted. They conclude, therefore, that the poisonous products of excessive muscular activity are identical with the poisons accumulating in the organism after removal of the suprarenal capsules. Normally these muscle-poisons are rendered harmless by the activity of the suprarenal bodies and only temporary exhaustion is noted, but as soon as the suprarenal capsules are extirpated these poisonous substances accumulate. These authors believe the neutralizing action consists in oxidation of the muscle-poison.

Albanese found that while ordinarily 4 mg. of neurin are required to kill a frog, 1 mg. suffices in animals deprived of their suprarenal capsules, and concludes that this is the substance which accumulates in the blood as the result of nervous and muscular activity and is neutralized by the suprarenal bodies.

Thiroloix reached an entirely different conclusion as to the function of these organs. Although believing that animals deprived of their suprarenal bodies perish from the accumulation of toxins in their blood, he holds that the suprarenal bodies are not neutralizing (antitoxic) organs, but are rather regulators of cell nutrition. In the absence of these organs the nutrition of the cells is interfered with, and the metabolism of the poorly nourished cells becomes abnormal, resulting in the formation of toxic substances which cause the animals death.

6. Szymonowicz investigated the *pulse, respiration, and blood-pressure* after extirpation of both suprarenal capsules, and found that the pulse and respiration were not constantly affected, but that a considerable fall of blood-pressure immediately followed the operation. [Strehl and Weiss * show that this same fall of blood-pressure follows section of the suprarenal

* *Pflüger's Archiv.* 1901, Bd. LXXXVI, S. 107.

vein, providing the other adrenal has been removed.   If the vein is simply clamped, the blood-pressure falls; when the clamp is released, the pressure rises even to a greater height than before.

Moore and Purinton * studied the results obtained by the removal in cats and kittens of one suprarenal capsule and at a later period the removal of the remaining suprarenal body.   In several instances the second operation was followed by death within a few hours.   In three such cases large clots were observed in the right auricle with processes extending into the ventricle and venæ cavæ.   These clots bore all the appearances of antemortem clots.   They therefore concluded that death was caused by cardiac thrombosis, which in turn was due to the lowering of blood-pressure following the total removal of the suprarenal capsules.—ED.]

7. *Changes in the skin and mucous membranes.*   A few observers report the development of abnormal pigmentation after extirpation of the suprarenal capsules.   Nothnagel several times found spots of pigment in the buccal mucous membrane of young rabbits, but does not claim that they were the result of the operation.   Tizzoni, however, found pigmentation in thirteen animals out of thirty which he had operated upon, independent of the mode of operation and color of the animal.   He attributes this condition to alterations in the nervous system resulting from the operation. The pigment was situated around the snout, upon the nasal and buccal mucous membranes, and was especially characteristic on the under surface of the tongue.   It never appeared earlier than two months after the operation, increased in intensity the longer its duration, and never disappeared.   The pigment was situated in the deepest layers of the epithelium or epidermis and in the migratory cells of the subepithelial connective tissue.

The second method for determining the function of the suprarenal bodies was the investigation of the action of suprarenal extracts.   It is remarkable that these experiments were not undertaken sooner.   Johannes Müller had already called attention to the method in his "Text-book of Physiology," asking (p. 491, chap. IV, vol. II): "Does the blood undergo a peculiar change in its passage through the vascular network of the cortex, escaping as altered blood through the suprarenal veins into the general venous system?   The left suprarenal vein should be ligated in the living animal and the fluid in the vein and suprarenal body should be examined."

Foa and Pellacani, in 1879 and 1883, were the first to investigate the physiologic action of extracts of suprarenal bodies.   They injected the extracts into frogs, guinea-pigs, rabbits, and dogs.   Symptoms of poisoning resulted, consisting of impairment of sensation and reflexes followed by general paralysis.

Guarnieri and Marino Zucco confirmed (1888) the poisonous properties of the aqueous extract of the suprarenal capsule.   They attribute this action to neurin and organic phosphoric acids which they found abundantly present.   Alzais and Arnaud experimented in the same direction. The most recent methodic and exhaustive investigations of the subject have been made by Schäfer and Oliver, Szymonowicz and Cybulski, Gluzinski, Velich and Biedl (1894–1896).

[One of the most interesting and important facts regarding the material which is yielded by the suprarenals is the minuteness of the dose which is necessary to produce the results.   As little as 0.0055 (5½ mg.) of dried

Amer. Jour. of Phys., 1900-1901, 4, p. 51.

suprarenal is sufficient to obtain a maximal effect upon the heart and arteries in a dog weighing ten kilos. For each kilogram of body-weight the necessary quantity to produce a maximal effect is 0.00055 gm., or little more than half a milligram. The active principle is, however, contained only in the medulla of the gland, not in the cortex, and the medulla in all probability does not form more than one-fourth of the capsule by weight. Of the dried medulla certainly not less than nine-tenths are composed of proteid and other material which is not dialyzable and which otherwise does not conform to the chemical properties which are associated with the active substance of the gland."*—ED.]

Oliver and Schäfer injected both a glycerin extract and an aqueous extract into various animals and observed the following three principal effects:

1. An enormous rise of blood-pressure, the result of excessive contraction of the blood-vessels. This rise of blood-pressure was increased by section of the vagi or by paralyzing their peripheral terminations with atropin. Destruction of the medulla oblongata and the entire spinal cord and section of the peripheral nerves caused a similar increase of blood-pressure. Stimulation of the depressor nerve during the administration of suprarenal extract failed to produce a fall of blood-pressure.

From these facts it follows that the rise of blood-pressure is the result of a direct action of the extract upon the muscular fibers of the heart and arteries.

2. Slowing and strengthening of the heart's action and pulse. These result from stimulation of the vagus centers. After destruction of the medulla oblongata, section of the vagi, or paralysis of their peripheral terminations by atropin, the heart's action was increased in frequency as well as in force. The increased frequency greatly exceeded that following section of the vagi alone, from which it is apparent that suprarenal extract increases the frequency of the heart's action. The authors observed a like result also when the extract was applied to the excised frog's heart.

3. In frogs and mammals the duration of muscular contraction was lengthened.

Its action upon respiration was inconstant. Large doses killed rabbits within twenty-four hours. The enormous rise of blood-pressure produced by this substance distinguishes it from digitalis and ergotin, which cause an inconsiderable rise. These authors deny that the active substance is neurin, because the latter diminishes blood-pressure. Extracts of the medullary portion of the capsules alone were active. Suprarenal extract from healthy human beings was very powerful, while the extract from two cases of Addison's disease was totally inert. Extirpation of the suprarenal capsules and ligation of the renal vessels apparently had no particular effect upon the result of the injection.

These authors conclude that the suprarenal bodies elaborate an internal secretion which maintains the physiologic tone of all the muscular tissues, especially of the heart and vessels.

Szymonowicz in Cracow carried on experiments independently of these other observers. He employed aqueous and alcoholic extracts from different animals with like results. Extracts from the medullary substance alone were active, but the effect occurred sooner if an extract of the entire gland was administered. Szymonowicz therefore believes that the cortical substance may in some way further the action of the medullary portion.

* "Text-book of Physiology," Schäfer, 898, vol. I, p. 1957.

The action of the extract was delayed in animals deprived of their suprarenal capsules, but lasted longer when once developed. The most striking action of suprarenal extract is a rise of blood-pressure greater than that produced by any other drug. The heart's action is diminished in frequency but increased in force, and the respirations are shallow. The rise of blood-pressure sometimes exceeded 300 mm. of mercury; it was invariably increased after section of the vagi, and the administration of atropin caused a rapid onset of the increased blood-pressure. On the other hand, section or partial destruction of the spinal cord very decidedly diminished this action of suprarenal extract, while complete destruction of the cervical and thoracic cord abolished it. Szymonowicz concludes that the vasomotor centers of the medulla oblongata principally, and to a lesser degree the centers in the spinal cord, are concerned with this rise of blood-pressure. The immediate cause is a contraction of the systemic blood-vessels which Szymonowicz demonstrated by direct measurements. After the slowing of the pulse had disappeared he repeatedly observed its increased frequency. When curare was administered very large doses of suprarenal extract were required to develop slowing of the pulse. After administration of atropin the rise of blood-pressure was invariably accompanied by increased frequency of the heart's action. Section of the vagi also accelerated the heart's action, which after the injection was greater and was associated with increased blood-pressure. This effect of suprarenin upon the action of the heart is due to stimulation of the vagus in the medulla oblongata; electric stimulation of the peripheral end of the cut vagus may cause still further slowing of the heart's action. Arrhythmia or allorhythmia was almost invariably noted after administering large doses of the extract, hence Szymonowicz concludes that the surparenal extract acts directly upon the nerve structures of the heart itself. Shallow respiration was the only constant respiratory symptom noted, yet Szymonowicz is convinced that the substances contained in the suprarenal extracts are capable of stimulating the respiratory center and, in large doses, of paralyzing it. He observed no poisonous action, healthy animals, indeed, bearing very large doses. None of the other organic extracts—as, for example, from the brain, spinal ganglia, testes, or thyroid gland—possess similar properties, although a moderate fall of blood-pressure and acceleration of the heart's action (*i. e.*, the opposite action to suprarenal extract) were noted in two cases after injecting an extract of the pineal gland.

The experiments of Szymonowicz were continued by Cybulski, who investigated the chemical properties of suprarenal extracts.

He demonstrated that strong solutions of the extracts proved fatal in rabbits. These animals are characterized by remarkably delicate blood-vessels, and in fatal cases he observed extravasations in the lungs, heart, brain, and medulla oblongata, and, in addition, infarctions and edema of the lungs. Weak solutions, on the contrary, were wholly harmless, even in considerable quantities. Large doses of suprarenal extract may completely suspend the activity of the vagi and may paralyze the vasomotor centers. Very rarely Cybulski observed paralysis of the respiratory centers. The reflexes of frogs were slightly impaired by suprarenal extract. In addition, he found that the active substance of suprarenal extract is elaborated in the suprarenal capsules, entering the blood by dialysis. Defibrinated blood of the suprarenal vein produces, when injected into animals, the same results as suprarenal extract but of less intensity.

The urine of animals after administration of suprarenin acted in like manner, though in less degree, proving, according to Cybulski, that suprarenin is in part excreted by the kidney.

Cybulski especially emphasizes that suprarenal extract, or more particularly its active principle, is very readily oxidizable, being rendered inert by a 1% solution of potassium permanganate.

This explains, on the one hand, the transient action of the extract under normal circumstances, since it is speedily oxidized in the metabolism of the tissues; and, on the other hand, the accumulation of this substance in the blood and the more decided production of its characteristic effects when the organism is poor in oxygen (for example, in asphyxia). With reference to the analogy existing betweeen the phenomena of asphyxia (increased blood-pressure, slowing of the pulse, etc.) and the symptoms produced by suprarenin, Cybulski believes that the toxicity of the blood in asphyxia results from the accumulation of suprarenin. This opinion is supported by certain experiments; thus, in the absence of suprarenin from the blood (after extirpation of the suprarenal capsules) the phenomena of asphyxia do not appear, but can be developed by injecting suprarenal extract; when the blood of asphyxiated animals is injected into healthy animals, its action is similar to though less powerful than that of suprarenal extract. Cybulski consequently believes that the suprarenal secretion is a physiologic tonic for the respiratory center, its function being to maintain the rhythmic activity of this center independently of all chemical or nervous stimuli.

As the result of their combined observations, Szymonowicz and Cybulski conclude as follows:

1. Extirpation of both suprarenal capsules causes a decided fall of blood-pressure; the pulse becomes small.

2. Intravenous injection of suprarenal extract causes a marked rise of blood-pressure with slowing and strengthening of the heart's action.

3. The same symptoms, although less intense, are produced by the injection into the circulation of the blood of the suprarenal vein.

4. The suprarenal body is an organ essential to life.

5. The function of the suprarenal capsules is to elaborate and add to the blood a substance which stimulates the activity of the vasomotor centers, the centers of the vagus and accelerator nerves, and the respiratory centers, and permanently preserves the tonic tension of these centers.

6. The theory of the neutralizing action of the suprarenal capsules can be dispensed with, for the loss of the above-mentioned tonic influence is sufficient to explain all symptoms occurring after their removal.

Gluzinski also confirms the rise of blood-pressure produced by suprarenal extract, but emphasizes, in contradistinction to Szymonowicz and Cybulski, the highly poisonous properties of the glycerin extract which he used; this is manifested, he states, by intense circulatory disturbances based upon the rise of blood-pressure which is brought about by injury to the medulla oblongata and spinal cord. Unless the death of the animals thus poisoned early followed the injection pulmonary edema and hemorrhages into the lungs, pleura, and pericardium occurred. Gluzinski believes these to be secondary results of the rise of blood-pressure and disturbance of the pulmonary circulation. Gourfein speaks similarly of the poisonous properties of suprarenal extracts.

Thus all investigators agree that suprarenal extracts raise blood-pressure, but there are marked differences of opinion as to whether the action is central or peripheral. While Szymonowicz and Cybulski attribute this effect to the action of the extracts upon the central apparatus in the medulla and cord, Oliver and Schäfer explain it by direct action upon the heart and blood-vessels. Velich and Biedl recently instituted control experiments in order to settle this point, and came independently to the same conclusion—that the suprarenal extracts act, as Oliver and Schäfer maintained, upon the peripheral apparatus of the blood-vessels. They found that a considerable rise of blood-pressure was produced by injections of suprarenal extract even after complete destruction of the spinal cord. This view was confirmed by Gottlieb, who injected suprarenal extracts into animals narcotized by chloral. Even then the injection was followed by a considerable rise of blood-pressure, although the vasomotor centers were completely paralyzed by chloral. It has thus been proved beyond doubt that the rise of blood-pressure is caused by a peripheral action upon the heart and blood-vessels, but while Oliver and Schäfer attribute this to a direct action upon the muscular fibers, Gottlieb believes it to result from the specific action of the poison upon the intracardial motor ganglia and upon the peripheral vascular ganglia which control the dilatation of the vessels.

The positive proof of the peripheral action of the extract was furnished by Biedl. He experimented with living, excised organs (kidneys, extremities) by flushing them with blood charged with suprarenal extract. Such an excessive contraction of the vessels was caused that the outflow from the vein ceased, although the pressure applied to the entering blood was increased threefold. (Personal statement.) [Bardier and Fraenkel have shown that a similar change in the kidney also takes place when the suprarenal extract is injected intravenously.*—Ed.]

Darier's experiments furnish further proof of the peripheral action of suprarenal extract. When cocain fails to produce anesthesia of the conjunctiva because of excessive hyperemia, it may be combined with suprarenal extract. A single drop of this mixture produces a striking pallor and complete anesthesia of the conjunctiva. The suprarenal extract, therefore, produces a contraction of the conjunctival blood-vessels.

[Mosse † found that the direct application of the extract to the nasal corpora cavernosa diminished their injection.

Blum ‡ showed that the subcutaneous or intravenous injection of suprarenal extract may cause a considerable degree of glycosuria in animals. This occurs not only when the diet is free from carbohydrates, but also in hunger even when all glycogen has disappeared from the liver. He ascribes the glycosuria to a toxic action upon one or more of the organs prominent in carbohydrate metabolism—the organ attacked most probably being the pancreas. The presence of acetone, diacetic acid, and β-oxybutyric acid was not noted.

Zuelzer § confirms Blum's results. He obtained glycosuria in an animal after fourteen days of starvation. Occasionally diacetic acid was detected, never acetone, but albumosuria frequently occurred. The glycosuria is the result of hyperglycemia and is not caused by a renal lesion. Levulose or lactose given at the same time as the suprarenal extract caused respectively levulosuria or lactosuria.—Ed.]

Soc de Biol., 1899, June 24, p. 544.   † *Therap. d. Gegenw.*, 1900.
‡*Deut. Arch. f. klin. Med.*, 1901, LXXI, Heft 2 u. 3.
§*Berl. klin. Wochen.*, 1901, p. 1209.

The third method of physiologic investigation is the chemical. Addison first called the attention of chemists to the suprarenal capsules. Vulpian, in 1856, was the first to investigate them. He found a substance in the juices of the suprarenal capsules which became dark colored, almost black, but with a tinge of blue or green, upon addition of chlorid of iron. Upon addition of oxidizing agents he obtained a beautiful rose color. Virchow and Vulpian showed that this substance was found only in the medullary juices, and believed it probably a sulphur compound. Virchow found, in addition, large quantities of leucin and myelin. Cloez and Vulpian succeeded in demonstrating hippuric and taurocholic acids in the suprarenal capsules of sheep. These substances for a while played a rôle in the pathology of Addison's disease. Their presence has recently been denied (Stadelmann and Beier).

A chromogenic substance was found in the suprarenal capsules by Seligsohn, Holm, and MacMunn. It was convertible by oxidation into a pigment and was believed by the last-named author to be hemochromogen. Arnold finally succeeded in isolating a pigment in the form of dark red, oily drops which crystallized upon drying. The crystals were soluble in water and alcohol, insoluble in ether, chloroform, or carbon disulphid. Krukenberg continued the investigation of this pigment and its colorless progenitor; he proved that both substances were dialyzable and recognized that they were neither albuminous, resinous, nor fatty, but that their chemical behavior closely resembled that of pyrocatechin. He was inclined to believe these substances identical. Brunner held the same view.

Other authors called attention to various other substances. Alexander demonstrated an enormous amount of lecithin in the suprarenal capsules, much more than in any other organ outside of the central nervous system. He concludes that the suprarenal capsules elaborate this substance, so indispensable to the nervous system, and furnish it to the latter. Lubarsch found glycogen in the suprarenal capsules of the embryos of rabbits and guinea-pigs. Marino Zucco and Dutto, as already mentioned, proved neurin to be a constant constituent of the suprarenal capsules and ascribe the physiologic effect on the blood-pressure to a combination of this material with glycero-phosphoric acid. This was disproved by Oliver and Schäfer. Manasse found a substance containing phosphorus and yielding sugar, closely related to jecorin. This probably was a combination of a carbohydrate with lecithin. In fresh blood from the suprarenal capsules of dogs he found small, hyaline, glistening, colorless granules which were stained by chromic acid and were soluble in alcohol. These presumably correspond to the glistening granules found by Gottschau and Pfaundler in the blood of the suprarenal vein. All three authors believe these homogeneous masses are a secretion of the medullary substance which enters the circulation through the suprarenal vein. According to Lubarsch, they are closely related to Russell's fuchsin bodies, the latter consisting, in his opinion, of lecithin or glycogen or a combination of these substances with proteids. Nebarro found globulin and small quantities of albumin; Külz found inosit.

Of late years considerable attention has been paid to the chemistry of the suprarenal capsules on account of the experiments with suprarenal extracts. Moore (the chemical collaborator of Oliver and Schäfer) and Cybulski almost entirely agree that the active substance is soluble in water, glycerin, and alcohol; insoluble in ether, chloroform, and amyl-alcohol (carbon disulphid, ligroin—Moore). The substance was not destroyed by boiling or by dilute acids, but was decomposed by alkalies, especially upon heating.   Its reducing property, already mentioned by Vulpian, was confirmed.

The substance is very susceptible to oxidizing agents, being decomposed by a small quantity of a 1 % solution of potassium permanganate.   It is dialyzable through animal membranes.   According to Moore, it is neither a proteid, a glucosid, nor a sugar.

Sigmund Fraenkel finally succeeded in isolating the active principle of suprarenal extract in the form of a syrupy, non-crystallizable substance, readily soluble in water and alcohol, soluble with difficulty in acetone. Even a trace of this substance produces the characteristic effect upon blood-pressure, and on account of this very conspicuous property it was termed sphygmogenin by Fraenkel.   When this substance is treated with an aqueous solution of chlorid of iron, a deep green color is produced; no ammonia is set free upon boiling it with lye; no red color is produced with Millon's reagent; it possesses strong reducing properties.

It immediately reduces an ammoniacal silver solution, sets iodin free from iodic acid, but does not reduce Fehling's solution.   Solutions of the free substance are acid, but neither form salts nor can they be converted into ethers by ethyl alcohol and hydrochloric acid.   This indicates, as Fraenkel says, that the acid reaction is due to hydroxyl.   The substance is readily oxidizable; its physiologic action is suspended by hydrogen dioxid or potassium permanganate.   It is not decomposed in the blood, but in the tissues the properties of this substance are impaired, since the rise of blood-pressure after subcutaneous or rectal injection is not so conspicuous as after venous injection.   Sphygmogenin is very susceptible to exposure to light, air, and prolonged boiling; by these means its solutions are rendered physiologically inert and no chlorid of iron reaction is produced.   According to Fraenkel, these two properties run a parallel course.

According to its reactions, sphygmogenin belongs to the group of ortho-dihydro-oxybenzol derivatives.   Krukenberg's view—that the substance is identical with pyrocatechin—is contradicted by its wealth in nitrogen, slight solubility in ether, and by its reaction with lime-water, with which it yields a red instead of a green color.   It might, however, be a derivative of pyrocatechin containing nitrogen, and Fraenkel calls attention to the striking fact that pure pyrocatechin produces a similar rise of blood-pressure.   The most recent chemical investigations of Mühlmann throw a new light upon this question.   He treated with water and a little acetic acid the fresh, pulverized suprarenal capsules of cows or calves.   The solution was filtered and evaporated, the brown syrupy residue was digested with alcohol, filtered, and the alcohol driven off.   The residue was readily soluble in alcohol and water, soluble with difficulty in ether, and gave a red color upon addition of sublimate to its neutral or faintly acid solution.   The solubility of this residue and its further chemical reactions, particularly the reaction with sublimate, prove that pyrocatechin was not contained in it.

Yet Mühlmann, upon boiling the residual substance with hydrochloric acid, succeeded in splitting it up and demonstrating pyrocatechin as a result.   He thus proved that pyrocatechin exists in combination in suprarenal extract.   Upon testing sections of fresh suprarenal capsules with chlorid of iron, the medullary substance alone yields the characteristic (ferric chlorid) pyrocatechin reaction, while the cortex remains unstained. From this fact, Mühlmann feels justified in concluding that pyrocatechin is formed in the medullary substance of the suprarenal capsules, while the cortical substance furnishes the material. Mühlmann believes that the protocatechuic acid of vegetable food is the mother-substance of pyrocatechin.

Although the chemical investigations have furnished much that is new, and have considerably extended our knowledge of the function of the suprarenal capsules, no definite results have been attained. The most striking constituents are sphygmogenin, pyrocatechin, neurin, and lecithin. Probably the next task will be to ascertain the nature of the residue containing nitrogen after the separation of the sphygmogenin.

[Abel and Crawford,[1] in 1897, showed that the constituent of the suprarenal capsule which raises the blood-pressure may be completely precipitated from an aqueous extract by benzoyl chlorid and sodium hydrate. On decomposing the resulting benzoyl products a residue is obtained which possesses great physiologic activity. This residue gives the color-reactions of Vulpian, reduces silver nitrate, and has the other specific qualities of suprarenal extracts. When contaminating substances are removed, the active principle is left as a highly active sulphate or hydrochlorate. It is therefore a basic substance. Abel, like v. Fürth,[2] did not obtain pyrocatechin from it, nor was the former able to agree with Moore[3] that pyridin was the active principle isolated.

In 1898 Abel[4] isolated the active principle in the form of a benzoate whose formula he expressed as $C_{17}H_{15}NO_4$, and named it epinephrin. The free base could not be isolated without a loss of the physiologically active qualities. Its active salts, however, when applied locally markedly constringe the blood-vessels, have a faintly bitter taste, and cause a slight loss of sensation on the tongue. When introduced into the circulation these salts produce a marked increase of blood-pressure of long duration. They at first stimulate, then paralyze, the respiratory centers, and if the dose is further increased the heart is paralyzed.

Von Fürth,[5] working independently, isolated from suprarenal capsules an iron compound which he named suprarenin. He considers it the constituent of the gland which raises the blood-pressure and holds that its presence in epinephrin accounts for the physiologic activity of the latter. Abel,[6] however, has been able to show conclusively that epinephrin and suprarenin are in reality the same substance and that epinephrin can be prepared from v. Fürth's product. Epinephrin as first described by Abel is actually a mono-benzoyl-reduced epinephrin, which is expressed by the formula $C_{17}H_{15}NO_4$. Subtracting the benzoyl group C_6H_5CO, one gets $C_{10}H_{11}NO_3$, which is the native or unreduced epinephrin. This is a very soluble, apparently very hygroscopic substance, which is quite unstable and does not reduce copper. It was at first isolated as a sulphate or bisulphate by Abel,[7] but he recently gives a new and simpler process by which the active principle can be isolated as a basic, minutely crystalline compound, easily converted by mineral acids into a physiologically active substance giving all the characteristic reactions of epinephrin.

Takamine[8] has recently isolated from suprarenal capsules a substance —adrenalin—which he claims is the principle of the gland which raises the blood-pressure. Aldrich,[9] working independently, has confirmed Takamine's work, but Abel[10] offers satisfactory proof to show that adrenalin is an impure product, closely related to epinephrin—being probably a mixture of native and reduced epinephrin with traces of foreign substances rich in nitrogen.

Hunt * isolated from the aqueous extract of suprarenal capsules from which Abel had removed epinephrin a crystalline body which, injected into an animal, caused a marked fall of blood-pressure. The body was soluble in cold water, insoluble in alcohol, and gave the odor of trimethylamine on heating. The chemical and physiologic properties of the substance agree with cholin.

Jacoby † has found a ferment in the medulla and cortex of the suprarenal capsule which oxidizes salicyl-aldehyde to salicylic acid. He did not determine its composition.

Mention has already been made of Croftan's diastatic ferment.

LITERATURE ON EPINEPHRIN, SUPRARENIN, ADRENALIN.

1. Abel and Crawford: "Johns Hopkins Hospital Bulletin," 1897, viii, p. 151.
2. v. Furth: "Zeits. f. phys. Chemie," 1898, 24, p. 142.
3. Moore: "Jour. of Phys.," 1897, xxi, p. 382.
   Moore and Purinton: "Amer. Jour. of Phys.," 1900–1901, iii, No. 8, p. xv.
4. Abel: "Johns Hopkins Hospital Bulletin," 1898, ix, 214.
5. v. Fürth: "Zeits. f. phys. Chemie," 1898, 26, p. 15.
6. Abel: "Zeits. f. phys. Chemie," 1899, 28, p. 318.
7. Abel: "Amer. Jour. of Phys.," 1899–1900, iii, No. 8, p. xvii.
   v. Fürth: "Zeits. f. phys. Chemie," 1900, 29, p. 105.
   Abel: "Johns Hopkins Hospital Bulletin," 1901, xii, p. 80.
   — "Johns Hopkins Hospital Bulletin," 1901, xii, p. 337.
8. Takamine: "Therapeutic Gazette," 1901, xxv, p. 221.
9. Aldrich: "Amer. Jour. of Phys.," 1901, v, p. 457.
10. Abel: "Johns Hopkins Hospital Bulletin," 1902, xiii, p. 29.

THERAPEUTIC PROPERTIES OF SUPRARENAL EXTRACT.

In consequence of the physiologic vasoconstrictor action of the suprarenal capsule, the attempt was made to make use of this property to diminish the blood-supply in diseased mucous membranes, especially of the eye and nose, and to arrest hemorrhage. The first to call attention to this action were Bates (eye), Hajek and Swain (nose and throat), Floersheim (heart and lungs), Grünbaum (alimentary tract), Churchill (uterus), Habgood and Heelas (prostate). Senator and others studied the influence of the extract on metabolism and Stölzner employed it in rickets.

At first the powdered capsules were employed, then aqueous solutions, but of late Takamine's adrenalin has displaced all other preparations in local use. (For a description of adrenalin see p. 329.)

Bates ‡ applied a small quantity of a 10% aqueous solution to the eye in numerous cases of congestion and observed an immediate pallor which lasted for some time. He found the extract useful in prolonged operations, for when repeatedly applied hemorrhage was prevented and cocain anesthesia indefinitely prolonged.

Hajek is mentioned by Königsten ⁊ as using suprarenal extract experimentally in the nose, but Swain ‖ was the first to publish a report on its extensive use in diseases of the nose and throat. It acted as a powerful local vasoconstrictor, contracted erectile tissue, and could be applied

---

* *Amer. Jour. of Phys.*, 1899–1900, vol. iii, No. 8, p. 18.

† *Zeits. f. phys. Chemie*, 1900, xxx, 135.

‡ *N. Y. Med. Jour.*, 1896, lxiii, 647.

§ *Wien. med. Presse*, 1897, Bd. xxvii, p. 857.

‖ *Trans. of the Amer. Laryngological Assoc.*, 1898, p. 165.

without danger. Its widest application was in acute congestions, but it was also helpful in chronic conditions of the hay-fever type.

Mandeville,* McKenzie, † and Reynolds ‡ all have found the local use of suprarenal extract of great value in epistaxis. Reynolds maintains that a 1 : 1000 solution of adrenalin in sodium chlorid may be relied upon to relieve any case of epistaxis. He does not believe that it predisposes to secondary hemorrhage. McKenzie's case was remarkable in that the patient had hemophilia. His experience is in contrast to that of Grün-baum,§ who found it of no use in such states. Solis-Cohen‖ used adrenalin 1 : 5000 with great relief in hay-fever.

The use of the extract in the eye and nose therapeutically and for purposes of diagnosis is now established, but elsewhere in the body and for other conditions its trial has not yet passed the experimental stage.

Floersheim ** has studied the effect of suprarenal capsule administered internally in 82 cases of heart disease. He administered 3 grains at a dose and found that it exerted little influence on the normal heart. The action of a weak and irregular heart became stronger and more regular and the diffused apex-beat was more sharply localized.

This observer†† also has employed suprarenal powder in a great variety of affections of the respiratory tract. He reports favorable results in acute and chronic bronchitis, bronchiectasis, asthma, congestion and edema of the lungs. In thirty-seven cases hemoptysis was checked by the internal administration of suprarenal capsule in three-grain doses.‡‡ Kenworthy §§ reports a similar experience in fourteen cases. Bates, in an excellent summary of the literature,‖‖ mentions six cases of edema of the glottis in which life appeared to be saved by the internal or local use of suprarenal extract.

Grünbaum *** mentions benefit from the use of one or two five-grain suprarenal tablets in hemorrhage of the gastro-intestinal tract.

Churchill is quoted by Bates ††† as having observed benefit from the internal use of suprarenal tablets in uterine hemorrhage. Floersheim ‡‡‡ adds 23 similar cases.

Habgood §§§ gave five grains of suprarenal capsule twice daily for prostatic hemorrhage. This lessened and after some days disappeared, but the use of the medicament was attended with palpitation, and was therefore stopped, but the hemorrhage returned. Heelas‖‖‖ in a similar case injected locally a few drops of suprarenal extract (five grains to the dram) through an india-rubber catheter three times a day. The hemorrhage ceased and there were no deleterious general effects.

* Cited by Bates, *Med. Rec.*, Feb. 9, 1901, p. 207.

† *Brit. Med. Jour.*, April 27, 1901, p. 1009.

‡ *Am. Med.*, July 6, 1901, p. 32.   § *Brit. Med. Jour.*, Nov., 1900, p. 1307.

‖ *Am. Med.*, Sept. 7, 1901, p. 376.

** *N. Y. Med. Jour.*, Oct. 6, 1900; also *ibid.*, May 4, 1901.

†† *Med. Rec.*, Nov. 17, 1900, p. 774.

‡‡ *Loc. cit.* and *Med. News*, Jan. 4, 1902, p. 17.

§§ *Med. Rec.*, Mar. 16, 1901, p. 415.

‖‖ *International Magazine*, Dec., 1900, p. 885.

*** *Brit. Med. Jour.*, Nov., 1900, p. 1307.

††† *Med. Rec.*, Feb. 9, 1901.   ‡‡‡ *Med. News*, Jan. 4, 1902, p. 17.

§§§ *Brit. Med. Jour.*, May 25, 1901, p. 1266.

‖‖‖ *Brit. Med. Jour.*, June 8, 1901, p. 1402.

Munro * claims benefit in acne rosacea from the combined use of the extract locally and internally.

Reynolds,† who has used adrenalin in 1222 cases, reports that in many instances prompt and sometimes lasting benefit follows the introduction of a drop of the adrenalin solution through the Eustachian catheter into the middle ear.

Stölzner ‡ treated 76 children suffering from rickets with suprarenal extract and observed remarkable and rapid improvement.   Neter § failed to confirm these observations.   Königsberger ‖ tested Stölzner's statements in a large number of cases with chiefly negative results.   There was no specific effect, but simply a slight improvement in the general condition, which he attributed to the effect on the circulatory apparatus and the respiratory center.

The influence of suprarenal extract on metabolism is not striking. Senator ** sums up his conclusions, based on the study of the metabolism of a patient with Addison's disease to whom he gave 34.8 gm. of tablets of fresh sheep's suprarenals in eighteen days, in these words: there is nothing further to say than that they were well borne without any disagreeable effects, and on the whole stimulated the appetite.

Pickardt †† studied a similar case and found a marked destruction of body albumin amounting in four days to 18.02 gm. nitrogen.   Such a single unfavorable result naturally allows no conclusion to be drawn.

Kaufmann ‡‡ investigated the question and came to the same conclusion as Senator.—ED.]

SYMPTOMATOLOGY OF DISEASES OF THE SUPRA-
RENAL CAPSULES.

IT is impossible to present any definite symptomatology of the suprarenal capsules until their function has been made wholly clear by physiology and experimental pathology.   The specific and characteristic symptoms afforded by impairment or loss of function are lacking.   In fact, numerous cases are recorded presenting at autopsy extensive alterations of the suprarenal capsules without a single symptom during life having aroused the suspicion of disease of these organs.   Apparently such cases have run their course without a single symptom, or at least no symptoms were produced which could not be explained by other coincident pathologic processes.

Another group of cases may produce local symptoms, such as a tumor, which eventually may cause effects of pressure upon adjacent organs, nerves, and blood-vessels, or may give rise to lumbar and sacral pain;

---

* Cited in Gould's "Year-Book," 1902, p. 566.

† *Am. Med.*, July 6, 1901, p. 32.   ‡ *Deut. med. Wochen.*, 1899, No. 37.

§ "Jahr f. Kinderheilkünde," 1900, 52, 600.

‖ *Münch. med. Wochen.*, 1901, No. 16.

** *Charité-Annalen*, 1897, Bd. xxii, 235.

†† *Berl. klin. Wochen.*, 1898, xxxv, 727.

‡‡ Cited in *Zeit. f. diatet. u. phys. Therapie*, 1901, 5, 508.

however, in the majority of cases the symptoms are not characteristic and the diagnosis can be made only by exclusion, and then only with a certain degree of probability.

In a third group of cases remote symptoms make their appearance, brought about by metastasis from a malignant suprarenal tumor.

In spite of the absence of any apparent connection, these symptoms may arouse the suspicion, or at least suggest the possibility, of a primary suprarenal affection.

Finally in a fourth group (by no means very small) local, remote, and general symptoms make their appearance in a combination which was first described as a type of disease by Addison, and has since been universally recognized as Addison's group of symptoms.

Although the occurrence of this group of symptoms permits the diagnosis of suprarenal disease with a certain degree of probability, there is no doubt that this probability is by no means a certainty. In some cases of well-marked disease of these organs this group may be entirely absent or only a few of the symptoms capable of very numerous explanations be present; on the other hand, this group of symptoms may be particularly well developed without a trace of pathologic alteration in the suprarenal capsules.

The conditions are still further extremely confused by the occurrence of numerous complications or by localization elsewhere of the lesion (tuberculosis, carcinoma) usually present in the suprarenal capsules in Addison's disease.

It is not only impossible to diagnosticate surely disease of the suprarenal capsules during life, but it is also exceedingly doubtful whether there are definite anatomic characteristics of such disease.

Under such circumstances it can readily be appreciated that Leube, in his work on diagnosis, dismisses the subject with the statement that diseases of the suprarenal capsules as yet are incapable of diagnosis.

It is therefore necessary, instead of discussing the clinical features of diseases of the suprarenal capsules, to describe in the first place Addison's disease, and to supplement this by briefly mentioning those symptoms which in the absence of Addison's group might possibly suggest disease of the suprarenal capsules as their origin.

ADDISON'S DISEASE.

PATHOLOGIC ANATOMY OF ADDISON'S DISEASE.

In discussing the pathologic anatomy of Addison's disease the changes in those organs which bear a causal relation to the disease will first be considered. The structures concerned are the suprarenal capsules and the sympathetic nervous apparatus.

The suprarenal capsules are the organs most regularly presenting anatomic alterations in Addison's disease. Lewin's extensive statistics show: Typical cases of Addison's disease with healthy suprarenal capsules, 12%; typical cases of Addison's disease with diseased suprarenal capsules, 88%; diseases of the suprarenal capsules without bronzing of the skin, 28%; diseases of the suprarenal capsules with bronzing of the skin, 72%.

In most cases of Addison's disease, tuberculosis of the suprarenal capsules is present in all its manifestations. As a rule, both organs are simultaneously affected, sometimes so completely that not a trace of normal tissue can be demonstrated. Both organs are not always alike affected by the disease. In some cases the two organs are only partially diseased; in others only one organ is affected and may be more or less completely destroyed. In the majority of cases the tubercular process runs an exceedingly chronic course, characterized by central caseation and peripheral cicatrization. The latter condition is not confined to the organ itself, but involves the capsule and pericapsular connective tissue, thence extending in all directions. Fibrous indurations thus form which may extend to the celiac ganglion, penetrating it and enveloping the nerve-fibers passing from it to the suprarenal capsules and other nerve-bundles; they may extend also to the liver and duodenum.

The bacilli of tuberculosis have been demonstrated repeatedly in the caseous suprarenal capsules. In but one case was the caseation caused by the bacillus of pseudo-tuberculosis of Hayem and Lesage.

Malignant tumors of the suprarenal capsules, primary as well as secondary, are next in frequency among the causes of Addison's disease. Both medullary and scirrhous cancers occur, and angiosarcoma and melanosarcoma are found as well as the usual varieties of sarcoma. In isolated cases various other tumors of the suprarenal capsules are regarded as the cause of Addison's disease—namely, adenoma (suprarenal struma), syphiloma, echinococcus cyst, and hematoma.

Formerly chronic interstitial inflammation of the suprarenal capsules played an important rôle in the etiology of Addison's disease, but in the majority of cases, if not in all, this condition should be considered as a form of tuberculosis.

In a considerable group of cases simple or inflammatory atrophy of the suprarenal capsules, in a few cases hypoplasia of otherwise healthy organs or even the absence of one or both suprarenal capsules, have been advanced as causes of Addison's disease.

In contradistinction to all these processes, which are characterized by a more or less chronic course, Virchow observed an acute hemorrhagic inflammation of the suprarenal capsules in a few instances of rapidly progressing Addison's disease.

Exact microscopic investigations of the changes in the sympathetic system have only recently been made. Lesions have been observed both in connection with, and in the absence of, diseases of the suprarenal capsules. They may affect, first, the sympathetic ganglia in the substance of the suprarenal capsules and the pericapsular ganglia occasionally present, then the nerve-fibers running from the suprarenal bodies to the celiac ganglion, the ganglion itself and the solar plexus, in addition the sympathetic tracts, extending from this point even as far as the cervical ganglion of the ganglionated cord, and finally the splanchnic nerve. Very often the changes in the ganglia of the suprarenal body, in the pericapsular ganglia, the fibers of the suprarenal and solar plexuses, and in the celiac ganglion itself are dependent upon tubercular disease of the suprarenal bodies and the resulting cicatrization; they may result also from a localization of the tubercular process in the abdominal lymphatic glands.

Compression by other kinds of glandular tumors (carcinoma, sarcoma, pseudo-leukemia, leukemia) or by aneurysm of the abdominal aorta is rare. Even simple inflammatory processes in the retroperitoneal space have been observed as the cause of such degenerations.

Minor alterations in various parts of the sympathetic system have repeatedly been considered by some authors as pathologic, while this is denied by others. Certain alterations, although admitted to be pathologic, occur not only in Addison's disease, but also in all other cachectic conditions, especially in pulmonary tuberculosis. For this reason, and also on account of their inconstant occurrence in typical Addison's disease, such lesions cannot be considered as the anatomic basis of this affection.

Extensive alterations of the sympathetic system are found in a comparatively small number of cases.

Kahlden, Fleiner, Ewald, and Brauer have made the most thorough histologic investigations of these conditions. The lesions of the ganglia comprise alterations in the ganglion cells, in the blood-vessels, and in the connective-tissue sheaths. The ganglion cells are more or less pigmented, the cells are often shrunken within their capsule, and the nuclei are disintegrated. Sometimes, indeed, the capsule contains only hyaline fragments. Hyaline degeneration of the walls of the blood-vessels and small-celled infiltration of the adventitia have been observed. Foci of small-celled infiltration, apparently originating in the blood-vessels, were repeatedly found in the connective-tissue sheaths of the ganglia. These alterations did not affect all or even a majority of the cells of the ganglia outside the suprarenal bodies, well-preserved cells being abundantly associated with degenerated ones.

The changes in the nerve-fibers were manifested by irregularities of outline, globular or spindle-shaped swellings alternating with abnormal thinness of the fiber (beaded appearance), fragmentation or transformation of the medullary sheath into flakes or minute granules, and in places almost complete destruction of the medullary fibers. Only occasional fibers as a rule were involved. Jurgens found complete gray degeneration of a splanchnic nerve from compression by an aortic aneurysm. Extreme atrophy of these nerves was found by Fleiner; moderate atrophy was noted by Ewald.

Fleiner believes that the spinal ganglia also bear a causal relation to Addison's disease. In two cases, in addition to changes in various portions of the sympathetic apparatus, he found degenerative changes in the spinal ganglia and the extramedullary portions of the posterior roots, in the vagus, and in a few peripheral spinal nerves.

Several investigators also have found alterations in the spinal cord. Demange, as early as 1877, reported a case of Addison's disease with tuberculosis of the suprarenal capsules in which he found also granular degeneration of the cells of the anterior horn and medullary destruction of the nerve-fibers in the lumbar cord. Burresi and Semmola also found alterations of the spinal cord which they considered of great importance; further, Abegg observed in one case small-celled infiltration of the pyramidal tracts of the dorsal cord; and, finally, Kalindero and Babes demonstrated a striking increase of neuroglia and thickening of the blood-vessels in the antero-lateral tracts and posterior horns, and atrophy and medullary degeneration of the nerve-fibers of the posterior roots. Vucetic found degenerative changes in the posterior roots, particularly of the lumbar cord. Kahlden found similar changes in several but not in all cases. He proved, however, that this was not a specific result of disease of the suprarenal capsules, because he found the same changes in the spinal cord of two phthisical patients without disease of the suprarenal bodies.

Pathologic alterations in a number of other organs have been demonstrated in Addison's disease; some of these are to be considered as sequels, others as complications. In the main, serous infiltration, anemia, hyperemia, or atrophy, with edema or thickening of the meninges, were repeatedly observed; in addition, though more rarely, cancerous nodules, tubercles, and multiple small areas of softening; several times tubercular meningitis, and in one case disease of the hypophysis.

The thyroid gland was often strikingly small and bloodless; in other cases it was enlarged, or the seat of cancerous metastases. Occasionally, persistence of the thymus gland was noted. In more than half of all cases tuberculosis of the lungs and mediastinal glands was found; frequently pleural adhesions and in a few cases metastatic cancer in the lungs and pleura; other changes were unimportant or accidental. Brown atrophy of the heart, sometimes extreme, was very often present; fatty degeneration also was observed, and hypertrophy in rare instances and only in the presence of complications. Atheromatous degeneration of the valves and blood-vessels, even in young people, was frequently observed.

In the digestive tract the following changes were found: injection, catarrhal swelling, and ecchymoses of the gastric mucosa; frequently a decided swelling of the solitary follicles and Peyer's patches often combined with ulceration, and, in addition, very extensive slate-colored pigmentation of the mucous membrane and follicles, and in a large number of cases tubercular ulcers. Tuberculosis and carcinoma were of frequent occurrence in the mesenteric and retroperitoneal glands. The abdominal wall, mesentery, and omentum contained in many cases large accumulations of fat, although the rest of the body might be emaciated. The liver has variously been reported as small or large, containing much or little blood, amyloid or fatty, infiltrated with cancerous nodules or with tubercles. The spleen was often simply enlarged or in a condition of amyloid degeneration. As a rule, the pancreas was found to be large, hyperemic, dense or cancerous. Carcinoma or tuberculosis of the genital tract was observed frequently; nephritis was an infrequent complication. In the osseous system, in addition to metastases of malignant growths and caries (especially of the vertebral column), a wine-colored staining of the marrow was observed by Gabbi in two cases. The muscles in many cases were described as thin or lacking ("geschwunden"). The histologic alterations in the skin will be more fully described elsewhere.

SYMPTOMS AND COURSE.

In the year 1855, Addison described the disease which has since been called by his name, and which he was the first to associate with alterations in the suprarenal capsules, as an idiopathic anemia, characterized by extreme loss of power and apathy, digestive and nervous disturbances, and bronzing of the skin. After running a chronic course with symptoms of progressive cachexia, it invariably ends in death, which may be attended by violent symptoms, such as uncontrollable diarrhea, coma, or convulsions.

After more than forty years, during which the disease has aroused the greatest interest, there is scarcely anything essential to be added to this description.

Addison's disease is, on the whole, rather rare. It occurs more frequently in men (60 to 67%). The majority of cases occur between the ages of fifteen and sixty; it rarely occurs in children and the aged, although it has been observed in them. The youngest case recorded was a child three years old, the oldest had already reached eighty years.

The following have been mentioned as causes of Addison's disease: malaria, alcoholism, exposure to cold, blows in the region of the kidney, malnutrition, mental worry, and pyschic disturbances—all of which have been regarded as important in the etiology of a great variety of diseases. A few of these may be of actual importance by weakening the organism and favoring the acquisition of tuberculosis, which is the most frequent anatomic lesion of Addison's disease.

[Interesting in this connection is the communication of Fleming and Miller,* who observed five cases—the mother and four children—of Addison's disease in the same family.—ED.]

In the vast majority of cases the onset is so insidious that the patient is unable to tell when the disease began. As a rule, the first symptom noticed is early fatigue in the performance of accustomed duties. This is intermittent at the outset, but gradually increases and develops into a permanent sense of weakness and exhaustion accompanied by a striking indisposition to work. In the beginning of uncomplicated cases the lack of power and debility frequently present a striking contrast to the relatively good general appearance of the patient and the abundance of abdominal fat. Indeed, the patient for a long time may be free from all other symptoms of disease.

Almost constantly the second cardinal group of symptoms—the disturbances of the digestive apparatus—gradually appear. The appetite little by little fails, the patient complains of a sense of pressure in the epigastrium, eructations, sometimes pyrosis, very often discomfort, nausea, and, as the disease progresses, more and more frequent vomiting, obstinate constipation, more rarely diarrhea, or an alternation of the last two conditions. There is very often intense epigastric pain radiating to the hypochondriac regions, and sometimes, by reason of its intensity, dominating all other features of the disease; or there may be similar fixed or radiating neuralgic pains in the lumbar and sacral regions. In other cases vague pains in the abdomen and extremities are complained of. Sometimes there are transient, severe pains in the various joints, apparently of a rheumatic nature, and occasionally accompanied by swelling.

Sooner or later the third and most striking cardinal symptom of Addison's disease is added—namely, a dark pigmentation of the skin.

As a rule, this begins very gradually and inconspicuously, so that the patient himself knows nothing of it and has his attention first called to it by other persons. At the outset the color is a dirty yellow, yellowish-brown, or smoky gray; later, the shade deepens until it is a pronounced bronze or black, as in the negro, presenting sometimes a peculiar greenish or bluish shimmer. The pigmentation generally begins in parts of the

* *Brit. Med. Jour.*, April 28, 1900, pp. 10-14.

22

skin exposed to the sun's rays, and in those naturally rich in pigment; the regions next affected are those which are considerably compressed by the clothing, and, finally (and very typically), the mucous membrane of the mouth, from the lips to the posterior pharyngeal wall, is involved, and more rarely other mucous membranes. The parts, therefore, which are first affected are the face, backs of the hands, genitals and nipples, axillary folds, and extensor surfaces of the joints, and these areas, as the pigmentation progresses, always present the deepest color. The pigment is never distributed uniformly over the whole surface of the body, but, as a rule, certain areas of the skin are very deeply colored, or the pigmentation may appear in the form of scattered, large, irregular, and faintly outlined spots interspersed with lighter areas of skin which are sometimes strikingly free from pigment (vitiligo). There may be quite often also, scattered over diffusely pigmented areas of skin, more sharply circumscribed, intensely dark spots varying in size from a poppy seed to a hemp-seed or lentil. Upon the mucous membranes the pigmentation is very rarely diffuse, but generally regularly arranged in fairly well-defined spots or stripes: conjunctivæ, nail-beds, and hair present only rarely conspicuous alterations.

Disturbances of other organs also are noted. In the nervous system there exist almost constantly very striking apathy, psychic depression, low spirits, and loss of energy. Very frequently, from the onset of the disease, the patient complains of insomnia, in rare cases somnolence; frequently there are headaches of varying intensity and duration, and in some cases loss of memory or impairment of intellect. In a few cases temporary delirium and mild cerebral disturbances have been observed. Dizziness, ringing in the ears, spots before the eyes, and a tendency to fainting are very frequent conditions. The symptoms of anemia, such as pallor of the skin and mucous membranes, murmurs in the veins of the neck and over the heart, may be absent for a while, but are, as a rule, always present in the later stages in addition to emaciation and cachexia. The intensity of these symptoms does not correspond to the extreme loss of strength or to the conditions observed in other cachexias (*e. g.,* tuberculosis or cancer). The pulse is almost invariably very small and compressible, as a rule rapid, rarely slow or irregular. Upon auscultation the heart-sounds are feeble.

Palpitation and dyspnea may occur even in uncomplicated cases; the former particularly upon exertion or mental excitement, attended as a rule by a very rapid, small, and irregular pulse. In uncomplicated cases the temperature is usually normal or, as the disease progresses, it may become subnormal, the latter condition often being attended by a feeling of cold. In the absence of renal complications no important urinary symptoms are noted. Disturbances of menstruation have repeatedly been observed. Dropsical swellings are of the rarest occurrence even with pronounced cachexia.

The course of this disease is essentially chronic. The symptoms may remain stationary for a time or may even be considerably improved, but eventually they become more and more severe. The loss of power and debility may become extreme, but are practically never accompanied by actual paralysis. Appetite is completely lost, but the thirst not infrequently is intense; vomiting becomes repeated, and hiccough often appears. With the continuance of these symptoms and increasing prostration, death may occur from cardiac weakness; more frequently the fatal issue is preceded by an acutely occurring violent termination. The temperature rises and may become very high. Diarrhea takes the place of constipation. Vomiting and diarrhea may be uncontrollable. Alarming cerebral symptoms appear, such as delirium, more rarely psychoses with motor excitement, frequently choreiform spasms or even epileptiform convulsions, finally collapse and coma; in some cases the condition is not unlike the terminal stage of typhoid fever. After it has lasted for several days, death as a rule ensues.

The duration of a typical case such as has just been described is at least a number of months, perhaps a few years. There are, however, many variations from the type both in symptoms, duration, and course.

In the first place, the disease may set in acutely with symptoms of digestive disturbance, after which it may pursue a chronic course. Such cases are really quite rare, although Averbeck believed they formed the majority. Further, the sequence of the individual symptoms and their intensity may widely vary. Not infrequently digestive disturbances, more rarely pigmentation of the skin, form the first feature. One or the other of the cardinal symptoms (even melanoderma) may be absent or appear very late and be only imperfectly developed.

The disease not only may begin suddenly with epigastric pain, diarrhea, headache, and fever, but also may terminate fatally in a short time, even in less than a month, with symptoms resembling an acute toxemia, cholera, or typhoid fever. Such cases are exceedingly rare. [Sergent and Bernard * report an interesting series of cases of sudden death occurring in acute and subacute Addison's disease. They consider it due to an acute or subacute functional insufficiency of the gland, superadded to the existing pathologic process and bearing the same relation to the latter that jaundice bears to acute or chronic hepatitis. Such adrenal insufficiency should be borne in mind in medicolegal cases as a possible explanation of sudden death.—ED.] On the other hand, the duration of the disease may be unusually prolonged. In such cases the symptoms remain quiescent even for several years, or may show considerable improvement, during which the patient feels almost entirely well and the physician even may hope that there is a permanent cure. As a rule, this improvement is suddenly interrupted by an acute exacerbation, speedily ending in death. The longest duration ever reported was ten to thirteen years.

Amid all these variations nothing but the fatal termination can be predicted with absolute certainty. The few published cases of recovery from Addison's disease are open to grave doubts as to the accuracy of the diagnosis.

The most striking deviations from the type of this disease are brought about, as has already been mentioned, by the remarkably frequent complications. Tuberculosis heads the list of these both in frequency and variety of manifestation, since the localization of this affection in the suprarenal capsules is the most common cause of Addison's disease.

Tuberculosis is rarely actually confined to the suprarenal capsules. Minor manifestations in other organs do not obscure the symptoms of Addison's disease.

If in addition to tuberculosis of the suprarenal capsules there is extensive bacillary disease of the lungs alone or of other organs in addition, especially the intestinal canal; or if a general miliary tuberculosis has

* *Arch. gen. de méd.*, 1899, II, 27.

been originated by the process in the suprarenal capsules, then the symptoms of Addison's disease may not only be strikingly modified and obscured, but they may be forced entirely into the background and the diagnosis rendered impossible. Under these circumstances marked emaciation, intermittent fever, cough, night-sweats, diarrhea, and digestive disturbances are present from the outset. The localization of the tuberculosis elsewhere may dominate the disease; for instance, meningeal symptoms or paralyses (vertebral caries).

Such symptoms as loss of power and vomiting, pain, and anemia, do not justify the diagnosis of a localization of the disease in the suprarenal capsules; nor does pigmentation even, for this may occur in ordinary tuberculosis. In like manner cancerous cachexia, and in rare cases syphilis, may influence the course of Addison's disease and may render its diagnosis difficult or impossible.

In addition to this general description of the disease, it will be necessary to consider in detail certain symptoms or groups of symptoms which are characterized by special variability or complexity.

CHANGES IN THE SKIN AND MUCOUS MEMBRANE.

Pathologic pigmentation is the only alteration with which we have to deal; it is the most striking sign of Addison's disease, in consequence of which this affection has frequently been termed suprarenal melasma, bronzed skin.

Pigmentation is only very rarely the initial symptom, but as a rule makes its appearance sooner or later after the occurrence of loss of power and disturbances of digestion. As the disease progresses the intensity of the pigmentation and the severity of the other symptoms run a fairly parallel course. There may be temporarily almost complete disappearance of the pigment during the occasional remissions of the disease. On the other hand, many cases have been observed where, in spite of remission of all other symptoms, the pigmentation of the skin remains unchanged. In one case reported by Labadie-Lagrave the melanoderma disappeared just before death.

In a few cases in which melanoderma was absent until the end of the disease, the diagnosis of Addison's disease was based upon the progressive loss of power and digestive disturbances for which there was no other explanation. The principal lesion found at autopsy was disease of the suprarenal capsules (Fenwick). To be historically accurate, we should, as Lewin actually did, exclude cases without bronzed skin from the group of Addison's disease. On the other hand, too strict adherence to the integrity of the three chief symptoms of Addison's disease would lead to an imperfect understanding of the deviating types. Such a classification is also justified by many analogies.

For example, were those cases only to be regarded as Basedow's disease which present all the characteristic symptoms, as tremor, exophthalmus, struma, and tachycardia in classic form, it would be necessary to exclude all those cases in which one or the other symptom was lacking. Yet such cases are sufficiently well known and recognized as "formes frustes" of the disease. In like manner scarlet fever may exist without a rash, and pellagra without eruption. It is probable, therefore, that cases of Addison's disease without melanoderma will maintain their place among the clinical types of the disease.

Nevertheless melanoderma is a very important lesion of Addison's disease, particularly from the standpoint of diagnosis, and for this reason its clinical peculiarities, especially of location, must carefully be considered.

Beginning with the head, attention first may be called to the different ways in which this pigmentation may occur upon the scalp. Cases have been reported in which the pigmentation ceased more or less abruptly at the border of the hair and the scalp remained entirely free from pigment. In others a uniform and even very intense pigmentation of the scalp was noted. As a rule, the hair itself is not pigmented, although in a few cases a change of color from light brown to dark brown or even black has been observed. The skin of the face is one of the most deeply pigmented regions, but otherwise presents little that is peculiar. Gerhardt described the frequent and characteristic occurrence of a very dark band of pigment along the margins of the lids.

The skin of the trunk as a whole is of a lighter shade, interspersed with relatively small areas of darker pigmentation. The distribution of the latter is dependent upon the normal excess of pigment in certain parts of the body and upon the constriction of clothing. The former manifests itself in an intense pigmentation of the areolæ of the nipples, especially in women who are or have been pregnant, of the anal folds, and of the genitals; the latter especially in men, in whom the penis and scrotum are frequently described as almost black. In women who have been pregnant the linea alba also shows a very dark color.

The effect of constricting clothing is most noticeable in thin people. In these there may be remarkably deep pigmentation, not only of the parts of the body affording support to the clothing, but also of all the bony ridges and prominences. Not only are the shoulders, axillary folds, and iliac crests very deeply pigmented, but also the skin over the clavicles, manubrium sterni, spines of the scapulæ, spinous processes of the vertebræ, and tuberosities of the ischia. In women and men who wear belts the waist is frequently encircled by a very intense brown ring corresponding to the position of the belt. The occurrence also of widely scattered, deeply pigmented spots over the whole surface of the trunk has already been mentioned.

In the extremities the pigmentation usually is deepest on surfaces exposed to the sun and on the extensor surfaces and prominences near the joints. On the palms and soles the pigmentation is faintest; in some cases there may be none at all, in others it may be faint or in spots or only on the crests of such folds as may be present. The absence of pigmentation from the bed of the nails is quite characteristic, although not without frequent exceptions. Yet even when the pigmentation of the matrix of the nails is present, it is rarely so intense as in the vicinity, and sometimes appears as distinct longitudinal stripes.

The effect of accidental cutaneous lesions upon the pigmentation finally should be mentioned. Every abnormal irritant acting upon a circumscribed area of skin produces some effect upon its color. Local parasitic diseases or eczema attended by itching and scratching cause a darker pigmentation; blisters and cupping usually produce a like effect. Cutaneous scars may be deeply pigmented or may be entirely free from pigment; in the latter instance, however, they are surrounded by a dark brown areola.

Areas completely devoid of pigment may arise without any apparent cause in the midst of this diffuse pigmentation. Such patches of vitiligo are inconstant, but when present in any number produce a very striking, often mottled appearance. One case is reported of the sudden appearance of vitiligo patches attaining a diameter of 5 cm.

So much for the typical pigmentation. Not every case of Addison's disease presents pigment in all these situations, or if present the intensity of the pigmentation may vary. Not infrequently the pigment is confined to certain parts of the body, as the upper extremities, or the face and neck; or a certain part of the body ordinarily pigmented may remain entirely free. It should again be stated that the occurrence of Addison's disease without pigmentation is recognized.

Pigmentation of the mucous membranes is of the greatest importance, particularly in differential diagnosis. In the majority of cases it appears here later than in the skin, and is only rarely diffuse. This pigmentation is of regular occurrence only in the mucous membrane of the mouth. Rarely the lips may present a diffuse, purplish or chocolate-brown coloration, much more frequently the pigment appears in the form of brown or black spots or lines, especially at the angles of the mouth. There is often a horizontal line of pigment on the mucous membrane of the cheeks, forming a continuation of the fissure of the lips. Upon the mucous membrane of the gums, hard and soft palate, and tongue, the pigment occurs almost exclusively in the form of spots. In very exceptional cases a smoky-gray coloration of the tongue and posterior pharyngeal wall has been observed. Pigment spots upon the larynx and small hemorrhages in the oral mucous membranes have been seen in rare instances.

. No constant changes are found in the other mucous membranes. It was stated for a long time that the ocular conjunctivæ, more particularly over the scleræ, never participated in the universal pigmentation, but, on the contrary, were conspicuous for their striking pearly-white color. Upon superficial examination this statement may still seem to hold good, but upon closer examination numerous deviations will be found. Although the whole conjunctiva is never pigmented to a noticeable degree, it is not unusual to find (as Leva particularly reports) small and not very dark spots of pigment upon both palpebral and ocular conjunctivæ.

Pigmentation of the mucous membranes of the genitals is now and then noted. The nymphæ and vaginal mucosa have been described as "black," and on the glans penis spots of brown pigment are quite frequently seen.

Exceptional cases of genuine Addison's disease may run their course and terminate fatally without any pigmentation of the mucous membranes. More rarely the mucous membranes are pigmented but the skin is not. It is evident that both groups of cases present considerable diagnostic difficulties.

Apart from the occurrence of pigmentation, the skin and mucous membranes very seldom present any other alterations. As a rule, the skin is smooth and elastic; in rare cases the onset of pigmentation is attended by itching; dryness and desquamation have been observed, and, on the other hand, excessive perspiration.

In several cases a very disagreeable odor from the skin has been noticed, and in one case it was described as fish-like. In a few instances the breath has had a similar unpleasant odor. In one case a scanty roseolous eruption was seen combined with disease of the joints; in another case an eruption resembling purpura. Among complications, molluscum contagiosum, very rarely furunculosis, and psoriasis have been observed.

The hair presents little that is abnormal beyond the occurrence of pigmentation which may affect both the hair of the head and the beard. In several cases loss of hair was reported with or without subsequent restoration; more rarely the hair has turned gray during the course of the disease; this took place in individuals of relatively advanced age. Alopecia areata is of rare occurrence.

DISTURBANCES OF THE NERVOUS SYSTEM.

The most frequent and, as a rule, the most constant symptom from the beginning to the end of Addison's disease is the extreme physical and psychic loss of power, which is the result, at least in part, of injury to the nervous system. This condition is first manifested by the striking rapidly occurring fatigue in the pursuit of customary duties formerly carried on without difficulty. At first the exhaustion is intermittent, but soon increases in frequency and finally becomes permanent. As the disease progresses the patients not only become incapable of performing even a very simple task, but show an increasing distaste for activity and movement of any kind. Finally this may go so far that the patients lie passive, and even eating and drinking are distasteful. Psychic symptoms develop simultaneously—for example, increasing apathy, indifference, and ill temper; there is often complete loss of energy, the patients are low-spirited and apathetic, drooping, or actually melancholic; other patients may be angry or morose, obstinate and sullen. This loss of power is also manifested by diminished resistance to external injuries. A slight excess (alcoholic), a mild infection, such as a simple sore-throat, otherwise speedily overcome, may be attended by serious sequels and may produce an aggravation of the condition ending in death.

Among the remaining nervous symptoms, cerebral symptoms must first be mentioned. Obstinate insomnia is one of the most frequent, and sometimes is an early symptom. Less often somnolence is observed, or the two conditions may alternate. In a few cases very frequent yawning has been reported.

Headaches are frequent, but vary extremely in intensity, duration, character, and location. Sometimes their great intensity renders them tormenting. Vertigo, ringing in the ears, specks before the eyes, and a tendency to fainting are frequent symptoms. Fainting may occur in well-nourished, not visibly anemic individuals upon the slightest provocation; *e. g.*, upon simply touching the epigastrium, sitting up in bed, or after prolonged standing. Coincidently the face becomes pale, the pulse almost disappears, and a cold sweat often breaks out.

The above-mentioned apathy may be accompanied by a progressive impairment of mental power, manifesting itself as loss of memory and intelligence, thoughtlessness, but in isolated cases as stupidity, dementia, or idiocy. In other cases periods of stimulation or excitement are observed consisting of anxiety, restlessness, or jactitation, all characterized by a certain feebleness of action. Muscular tremors and choreiform twitchings have been noted in a number of instances; severe general convulsions and epileptiform attacks very rarely occur before the terminal stage. Raving, transient delirium, paranoia, and religious insanity have all been observed a few times.

The organs of special sense are very rarely affected, and then only to a slight degree. Impairment of smell and taste, partial loss of hearing and vision, and in one case night-blindness are reported.

Although muscular weakness may be extreme, actual paralysis does not occur in Addison's disease unless complicated by vertebral caries, cerebral hemorrhage, etc. On the other hand, the sensory nerves are often affected, giving rise chiefly to pain, which not infrequently is an early symptom. The patient may complain of vague pains in all the extremities, or there may be neuralgic pains confined to particular regions, such as the epigastrium, hypochondria, sacral and lumbar regions, the extremities, and sometimes even the joints. The pain in the joints may be accompanied by transitory swelling, so that the condition has been correctly diagnosticated as articular rheumatism. Paresthesiæ are of rare occurrence, consisting of a sense of numbness or local death, itching of the fingers, and formication; these are combined with pallor and cyanosis, and are regarded as vasomotor neuroses. Diminished sensibility is still more rare.

As yet, very little attention has been paid to the reflexes. In the publications of the last few years numerous contradictory statements are found. Some of the reflexes are said to be normal or even increased, others are diminished or absent (especially the patellar reflex).

The pupillary reflexes also are not uniform; they are present as a rule; in a few cases they were observed to be sluggish.

In the last stage of the disease violent disturbances of the nervous system very often appear. They are manifested by delirium, hallucinations, periods of intense, even maniacal excitement; further, epileptiform convulsions followed by collapse, somnolence, and loss of consciousness, and finally complete coma. Irregular respiration, even Cheyne-Stokes' breathing, has been reported in several instances. In a few cases incoordination of the movements of the eye, rigidity of the neck, pinhead pupils or inequality of the pupils, spasms of the muscles of the back, and involuntary micturition have been observed without any meningitic lesions being discoverable at autopsy. However, the last stages of the disease may be complicated by actual tubercular meningitis or by solitary tubercles in the brain which may produce similar symptoms.

DISTURBANCES OF CIRCULATION.

These may be central or peripheral. There is often progressively increasing weakness of the heart. The cardiac impulse is feeble; the sounds of the heart are faint; the pulse is small, weak, and generally somewhat accelerated. In rare cases slowing of the pulse has been observed.

Even moderate physical exercise or excitement may cause extreme excitation of the heart's action associated with palpitation and irregularity. Leva observed stenocardial pain in the region of the heart, associated with palpitation and dyspnea. Rarely anemic murmurs are heard over the heart and blood-vessels. The complication with atheromatous changes repeatedly observed even in young persons would be manifested by the well-known symptoms referable to the heart and vessels. Forcible pulsation of the abdominal aorta is frequently seen, and is in striking contrast to the feebleness of the peripheral pulse. As the heart grows weaker in persons not anemic, more or less pronounced cyanosis also occurs.

CONDITION OF THE BLOOD.

As yet, the examinations of the blood in Addison's disease have yielded very contradictory results.

Addison himself regarded the disease as the result of a specific anemia, and reported an increase of white blood-corpuscles in one case. Averbeck also believes Addison's disease to be a special type of anemia which is invariably fatal, and which depends less upon alterations in the elements of the blood than upon a diminution of its total mass and alteration of its composition. Buhl observed a considerable diminution of red corpuscles without leucocytosis, and a great reduction or complete absence of fibrin. Averbeck, on the contrary, reports a case in which the blood was very readily coagulable and there was a great tendency to the formation of rouleaux without any leucocytosis. The observations of other authors are just as contradictory. Some report normal conditions; others, oligocythemia, occurrence of microcytes and poikilocytes with diminution of hemoglobin; and, finally, the leucocytes are reported as increased, diminished, or normal.

According to Nothnagel, anemia is not a primary symptom of Addison's disease. He was unable to demonstrate either leucocytosis, a diminution in number or disintegration of red corpuscles; or loss of hemoglobin or rouleaux formation; or, finally, the occurrence of free pigment in the blood. The recent examinations show no constant changes.

The number of red corpuscles and percentage of hemoglobin have repeatedly been proved to be normal or very slightly diminished. In a few cases they were increased, but this is readily explained by the concentration of the blood in consequence of profuse diarrhea. The quality and quantity of the leucocytes presented no material differences. An increase of eosinophiles was not observed (Kolisch and Pichler).

Tschirkoff carefully estimated the amount of hemoglobin. He found it but little changed even in late stages of the disease when the red corpuscles were moderately reduced in number. In severe cases he found a relative increase of reduced hemoglobin, and apparently methemoglobin also was present in considerable quantity.

These recent observations confirm Nothnagel's view that pronounced anemia does not form a part of Addison's disease. The abnormal blood-counts reported by several authors are explained by the occurrence of complicating tuberculosis or cancer of other organs or by the undue development of certain symptoms, as, for example, anorexia, obstinate vomiting, or severe diarrhea.

Very recently F. H. Mueller found in the blood of a patient with Addison's disease who was taking large quantities of milk, large numbers of actively motile and glistening granules in addition to poikilocytosis. These granules were not modified by several days' exposure to osmic acid and were not soluble in acetic acid. He found the same elements constantly in normal blood, although in diminished numbers.

In this connection the results of the examinations of the blood in two cases of Addison's disease under my observation are reported.

The first patient was a young girl who came from Mähren to my hospital in Vienna. In addition to pigmentation of the skin, particularly on the fingers, forehead, neck, and lower extremities, small spots of pigment were present also on the mucous membrane of the gums, tongue, and soft palate. The girl was pale, and anemic murmurs were detected over the veins and heart. She had taken iron for chlorosis, but without avail. Her chief complaints were general weakness, psychic and physical sluggishness. I made the diagnosis of Addison's disease and prescribed the internal administration of suprarenal extract. The patient continued this treatment at her home with temporary benefit. Several weeks later her relatives informed me that she had died, apparently of an intercurrent pleurisy. There was no autopsy.

On the day after the above examination was made, preparations of blood, stained by Ehrlich's method, showed practically no changes in the red corpuscles, especially no polychromatophilia in Ehrlich's sense, and no abnormal coloration of the plasma. The number of leucocytes was apparently normal. The differential count was as follows:

Polynuclear neutrophiles.. ....46.8%
Eosinophiles 4.0%
Transitional forms....................................... 4.6%
Large mononuclear 8.0%
Small mononuclear (lymphocytes) 36.6%

The considerable increase of mononuclear forms, especially of lymphocytes, in this case is striking.

The second patient was a middle-aged woman who came to me after the diagnosis of Addison's disease had already been made by Nothnagel. In addition to a faint, diffuse pigmentation of the face and hands this patient presented a few scattered spots on the mucous membrane of the cheeks and gums and a slight pallor of all the mucous membranes, but otherwise no abnormal appearances. The blood-pressure was diminished, measuring, according to Basch, 125 mm. in the radial artery. I first saw the patient in the spring of 1896. At that time the examination of the blood was as follows:

Red corpuscles................................4,425,000 ⎫ 1 : 637
White corpuscles .... 6,950 ⎭
Hemoglobin (Fleischl).......................................65%
Color-index 0.73

In the fresh preparation, blood-plates and fibrin present in normal quantity, rouleaux formation good; in the stained preparation, marked difference in the size of the red corpuscles, but no actual macrocytes or microcytes. No poikilocytosis, no nucleated red corpuscles. Differential count as follows:

Polynuclear neutrophiles.................................62.8%
Eosinophiles 3.5%
Transitional forms 4.1%
Large mononuclear 6.9%
Small mononuclear (lymphocytes) 22.7%

At this time an excess of lymphocytes was lacking. The patient went to Franzensbad, took a four weeks' cure, and again visited me. Her appearance was somewhat improved. Another examination of the blood resulted as follows:

Red corpuscles 4,550,000
White corpuscles 5,600
Hemoglobin (Fleischl) 80%
Color-index 0.88

Examination of the fresh specimen: rouleaux formation good, blood-plates abundant, fibrin formation very slight.

Examination of the stained preparation: no abnormalities of size or shape and no nucleation among the red corpuscles.

Differential count of leucocytes:

Polynuclear neutrophiles 57.14%
Eosinophiles.. 4.65%
Transitional forms .... 3.7 %
Large mononuclear....................................... 4.65%
Small mononuclear (lymphocytes).........................29.86%

In spite of the improvement of the anemia and the distinct increase of hemoglobin, there was found in the second examination of this patient's blood a moderate increase of lymphocytes; at least, a relative increase as compared with the polynuclear forms. This condition has never been observed in recovery from other anemias, and has already been reported by Ehrlich, in connection with the account of a case of posthemorrhagic, pernicious anemia, as of unfavorable prognostic significance, since it indicates an abnormal, regenerative action of the spleen and lymph-glands as opposed to the bone-marrow. Although no positive conclusions can be based upon these few observations, I should consider it advisable to investigate this subject further in suitable cases, and to give a guarded prognosis if the relative number of lymphocytes is found to be progressively increasing, even though the patient may feel comparatively well.

DISTURBANCES OF THE ABDOMINAL ORGANS.

In Addison's disease a large number of symptoms, both subjective and objective, are referable to the abdomen.

On inspection of the abdomen there may be two abnormal conditions recognized: on the one hand, the abdomen may be swollen and tympanitic; on the other, collapsed, or even hollowed.

In many cases upon palpation nothing abnormal is found. In another considerable group the abdomen is the seat of spontaneous pain and tenderness upon pressure. The former may be variously situated; sometimes only a slight, indefinite pain "all through the stomach" is complained of, or the pain may be intense and increased by movement. In the latter case the whole abdomen, as a rule, is extremely painful on pressure, and this symptom has repeatedly led to an incorrect diagnosis of peritonitis. The interpretation of this symptom becomes still more difficult if, as has actually been observed, an indefinite resistance, diffuse or circumscribed, is found upon palpation; for tubercular peritonitis has also been observed as a complication of Addison's disease.

Of more frequent occurrence are the sharply localized pains situated chiefly in the epigastrium and in the lumbar and sacral regions.

The epigastric pain is the most frequent, and is apt to be very severe and persistent, often intensified by pressure, and frequently relieved only by bending the body forward. The neuralgic character of this pain sometimes suggests lead colic or the gastric crises of tabes. The pain may radiate from the epigastrium in the form of a typical intercostal neuralgia, or may extend irregularly into the hypochondriac regions, toward the back, or into the shoulder and arm; so that hepatic colic may be simulated when on the right and gastric ulcer when on the left side.

Next in frequency are the lumbar and sacral pains. These, as a rule, are deep seated; although in some cases there may be well-marked cutaneous hyperesthesia. A. Fraenkel explains this hyperesthesia as the result of radiation such as occurs in other neuralgias. In like manner he regards the attacks of dyspnea and subjective sensation of air-hunger seen in Addison's disease as due to the abdominal neuralgia, analogous to the attacks of thoracic oppression and dyspnea occurring in ulcer of the stomach. According to Traube, these latter attacks are the equivalents of the neuralgic pains by transference of stimulation from the gastric to the pulmonary branches of the vagus nerve.

Among all the organs of the abdominal cavity, the digestive apparatus most frequently presents severe symptoms, which may temporarily wholly dominate the clinical picture of the disease. It is true that cases have been reported in which all, or at least a majority, of the other symptoms of the disease were well developed, yet the digestive organs continued normally to perform their function, and nutrition was maintained until the end and was extremely good, in contrast with the other severe symptoms. These cases are in the minority; in the great majority digestive disturbances are found, and these, together with the striking loss of power, are the most frequent early symptoms of the disease. They begin, as a rule, insidiously with impairment of appetite which the patient cannot account for. Often they immediately succeed some error in diet, and then become persistently worse.

The anorexia is followed by a sense of weight and fulness in the epigastrium, which is generally increased by eating. The tongue is moderately coated as a rule, rarely dry, and the breath is frequently fetid. As a result, the patient frequently acquires a profound distaste for food, particularly meats. To these symptoms are added eructations of gas, pyrosis, in other cases typical and not infrequently very violent attacks of gastralgia, uneasiness, nausea and vomiting, and in a few cases also paroxysms of obstinate hiccough.

The chief gastric symptom is vomiting. At the beginning of the disease it may be independent of the taking of food, occurring in the morning when the stomach is empty, the vomited matters being scanty and consisting of a colorless or bile-stained mucus, closely resembling the morning vomiting of alcoholics (Guermonprez). On the contrary, even from the very beginning, the vomiting may be associated with the taking of food, and this is always the case in the late stages of the disease. This symptom is subject to intermissions of weeks or months, which are followed by severe exacerbations, arising without any apparent cause, or as the result of a slight attack of indigestion. As a rule, however, the frequency, severity, and duration of vomiting are increased toward the end of the disease, nutrition is greatly interfered with, and the patient becomes very much reduced. In some cases there may be no gastric disturbances whatever, while in others a hearty appetite may continue, although the loss of power is extreme and the patient suffers from severe cardialgia and frequent vomiting. Cases with ravenous appetite have been reported by Peacock, Kussmaul, and Laureck; these are very rare, and in the last case mentioned, anorexia occurred at intervals and was complete in the terminal stage. During the frequent periods of remission all digestive disturbances disappear; the emaciated patient may again become well nourished and in every way improved.

In contrast to the loss of appetite, thirst may be excessive, independently of any apparent cause, *e. g.*, severe vomiting or diarrhea.

In the last stage of the disease the gastric symptoms are greatly intensified. Persistent, and in many cases uncontrollable, vomiting appears, and the resulting exhaustion alone may be the immediate cause of death. When vomiting is particularly severe, traces of blood may be mixed with the vomited matters or ecchymoses or hemorrhagic erosions of the gastric mucous membrane may be found after death. Vomiting of large quantities of blood does not occur in genuine Addison's disease, but is due to complications, as ulcer or cancer of the stomach.

The physical examination of the stomach yields little of value, with the exception of more or less sensitiveness to pressure and occasional splashing sounds. The chemical examination of the gastric contents and of the vomited matters is also negative, as a rule. Absence of free hydrochloric acid and of pepsin has been demonstrated in very few cases by Leichtenstern, Kahler, Minkel, and Brauer.

Intestinal disturbances are often although not always present. Constipation and diarrhea occur with almost equal frequency. According to Lewin's extensive statistics, diarrhea is the more common, but these statistics do not give a correct idea of these symptoms during the whole course of the disease. In my investigation of the literature of this subject constipation, sometimes indeed extremely obstinate, was found to be of more frequent occurrence at the beginning and during the further course of the disease with the exception of the terminal stage. In certain cases there was alternate constipation and diarrhea, and in a few instances after the administration of laxatives uncontrollable diarrhea supervened. In the terminal stage of the disease severe, profuse, and frequently uncontrollable diarrhea occurs in the majority of cases, while the persistence of constipation until the end is very rare. The diarrhea is seldom accompanied by colicky pains, and tenesmus is even more rare. Mucus is often present in the stools, blood very rarely and in mere traces.

The gastro-intestinal disturbances vary if the disease pursues an abnormal course or if intestinal complications are present. The disease rarely may be ushered in by an acute intestinal initial stage, which, after lasting one or two weeks, gradually subsides into the ordinary chronic course. The symptoms in these cases are usually rather violent, consisting of distress, anorexia, cardialgia, vomiting, and usually diarrhea. Further, those rare cases must not be forgotten in which the disease runs a rapid course with symptoms of an acute gastro-enteritis, terminating fatally with collapse and cramps in the legs, and strongly simulating acute arsenical poisoning or cholera.

Even in chronic cases the gastro-intestinal symptoms are very often decidedly and considerably influenced and altered by the occurrence of complications which result chiefly from tuberculosis. Tubercular ulcers of the intestine and tuberculosis elsewhere are of frequent occurrence. Dysentery and typhlitis are much rarer complications. Hayem and Lesage report a case of Addison's disease complicated by an enteritis due to the pseudo-tubercle bacillus.

The other organs of the peritoneal cavity very rarely give rise to symptoms. Enlargement of the liver and jaundice are caused by complications, and may be associated with enlargement of the spleen, or the latter condition may be present without the former.

Concerning the retroperitoneal organs there is little to say. Disease of the suprarenal capsules rarely gives rise to other local symptoms than lumbar and sacral pain, except perhaps the presence of a tumor.

The reproductive organs rarely give rise to symptoms although amenorrhea at times occurs, but dysmenorrhea is very rare. In male patients impotence has occasionally been observed. Complicating tuberculosis or cancer of the genitals is of more frequent occurrence. In women cancer of the uterus and ovaries is frequent, tuberculosis of the tubes and endometrium is rare. In men tuberculosis of the epididymis may occur.

CONDITION OF THE URINE.

Hitherto the examinations of the urine in Addison's disease have been incomplete and with but little method. The reaction was in most cases acid, the specific gravity somewhat diminished, the total quantity normal or diminished. The few cases of polyuria reported are of interest because Oliver and Schäfer made use of suprarenal extract in the treatment of diabetes insipidus with apparently good results. Among pathologic constituents, small quantities of albumin were found in the terminal stage; well-marked albuminuria occurred only in the presence of complicating renal disease. Small quantities of hippuric and taurocholic acids have been found. Marino Zucco, Dutto, and Albanese found neurin in the urine. Ewald found a hitherto unknown amin base with an elementary composition represented by the formula $C_5H_7NO_6$. Urobilin was observed in a few cases; in the majority the urinary coloringmatters were reduced. Thudichum found uromelanin in one case. According to previous analyses, the excretion of the normal constituents of the urine is not materially changed. The excretion of urea was diminished in many, that of uric acid in a few cases. Leva reports in one patient the diminished excretion of creatin. Indican was frequently increased. Leva and Rosenstirn found all the constituents of the urine equally diminished, with the exception, according to the latter author, of sulphuric acid. Leva reports the striking marked increase, sometimes even twenty-fold, of the volatile fatty acids (acetic and formic). Nothnagel and v. Jaksch found acetonuria in a comatose patient with Addison's disease. At a not very advanced stage of the disease, Kolisch and Pichler determined by careful quantitative analyses that the utilization of food and the destruction of albumin were normal.

In my second case, mentioned above, Dr. Kolisch made a quantitative analysis of the twenty-four hours' quantity of urine with the following results: Quantity 1000 c.c., specific gravity 1017, urine very cloudy from urates, dark yellow. No nucleo-albumin, no albumin, no sugar, no acetone, indican not increased. Total nitrogen 9.38 gm., ammonia 0.3, uric acid 0.42, uric acid nitrogen 0.14, xanthin basic nitrogen 0.12, total phosphoric acid 1.7, united to alkalies 1.3, united to earths 0.4. Acidity: 100 c.c. urine correspond to 12 c.c. decinormal alkaline solution.

Dr. Freund gave me the following analysis of the urine in another case of Addison's disease: Quantity 1100 c.c., specific gravity 1023, reaction acid; acidity 2.1 gm. hydrochloric acid; alkalinity 1.3 gm. sodium hydrate. Urine almost clear, amber-yellow; sediment containing mucus, numerous spermatozoa, crystals of uric acid, leucocytes. Total nitrogen 11.3; urea nitrogen 9.5; alloxuric bodies nitrogen 0.35, consisting of uric acid nitrogen 0.15 and xanthin basic nitrogen 0.20; ammoniacal nitrogen 0.12. Indoxyl and skatoxyl very abundant, oxalic acid increased. Oxyacids, somewhat increased. Ether sulphuric acid 0.27, total sulphuric acid 2.5, sulphuric acid from sulphates 1.98. Total phosphoric acid 2.40, united to alkalies 2.1, united to earths 0.3. Chlorids 9.8. Albumin, sugar, acetone, diacetic acid, urobilin wanting. Albumoses present, traces of peptone. Melanin reaction negative, reducing power of the urine increased (uric acid solvent power 0.48). Glycuronic acids plainly demonstrable.

DIFFERENTIAL DIAGNOSIS OF ADDISON'S DISEASE AND OF DISEASES OF THE SUPRARENAL CAPSULES IN GENERAL.

As the diagnosis of scarlet fever is usually determined by the presence of a typical rash, so in the absence of the latter the diagnosis of scarlet fever without rash is definitely established by other symptoms, therefore the differential diagnosis of Addison's disease must be differently reached according as the case is one with pronounced pigmentation or one in which this most prominent diagnostic sign is lacking.

It has already been stated that there are cases of Addison's disease without melanoderma. In our opinion the bronzing of the skin is a symptom of as conspicuous diagnostic importance as the scarlatinal rash in the diagnosis of scarlet fever. Nevertheless it cannot be regarded as an essential constituent of the picture of the disease. In the first-mentioned group of cases the pigment is obviously the starting-point in the differential diagnosis, and a large number of other affections must be considered which are characterized by a like pigmentation of the skin.

It is first to be borne in mind that there are different degrees of physiologic pigmentation dependent upon race and climatic conditions. The attention is much more attracted by the dark coloration of a northener than by the like pigmentation in a southerner, or a mulatto. What is physiologic for the one may be pathologic for the other. So that in southerners or in races other than the Caucasian it may be necessary to differentiate physiologic pigmentation from that of Addison's disease. For diseases of the suprarenal capsules may occur in any race, and Addison's disease has actually been observed in a Hindoo, a mulatto, an Armenian, and in a girl from Lebanon (Lewin). In such cases, in addition to the general symptoms of Addison's disease, pigmentation of the matrix of the nails or of the buccal mucous membrane perhaps may be valuable. It is well known that in negroes and mulattoes the matrix of the nails is of the same color as the rest of the skin, while in Addison's disease pigmentation in this situation is exceptional, or, if it does occur, is generally less intense than in the surrounding skin. Pigmentation of the mucous membrane of the mouth would speak strongly for Addison's disease, although not necessarily, especially if confined to the lips, for, according to Nothnagel, similar pigmentation of the lips may occur in perfectly healthy individuals. Pigmentation of the mucous membrane of the buccal cavity is more conclusive, although a few observers—*c. g.*, Eichhorst—have found physiologic pigmentation even here. Nothnagel described a case of idiopathic cardiac hypertrophy which should be mentioned in this connection. It presented, in addition to a moderate pigmentation of the skin, very conspicuous brownish-gray spots on the mucous membrane of the lips, cheeks, and tongue. There were no other symptoms of Addison's disease, and at autopsy the suprarenal capsules were found to be perfectly normal.

The age of the patient must also be considered, for in very old people there is sometimes a diffuse pigmentation of the whole surface of the body, but it is never very intense, does not present the typical localization of the pigment of Addison's disease, and never involves the mucous membranes. It is also important that Addison's disease is of the rarest occurrence in the aged, and is characterized, in addition to other symptoms, by apathy and depression of spirits, while old people are apt to be humorous and exceedingly talkative. Even in senile marasmus, the aged never present such intense asthenia as occurs in Addison's disease.

Among the pathologic pigmentations that occurring in malaria should first be considered. In this disease the differential diagnosis is based upon the history, the characteristic appearances in the blood (plasmodia and pigment), and upon the physical examination of the abdominal viscera. Malarial pigmentation does not occur in the form of circumscribed spots, but is rather diffuse, and of an ashen-gray or earthy hue. Pigmentation of the mucous membranes does not occur in malaria, and this sign is particularly valuable when Addison's disease develops in an individual who has already had malaria. Several such cases have been recorded.

In the last stages of pulmonary tuberculosis and in cancerous cachexia pigmentations are encountered similar to those in malaria. These may occur independently of any disease of the suprarenal capsules or of a lesion of the abdominal sympathetic. Such cases may present considerable difficulties, for all the characteristic symptoms of Addison's disease, loss of power, vomiting, diarrhea, etc., may result from the underlying disease. The diagnosis of this condition is based upon a careful consideration of the relation and succession of the individual symptoms and upon the appearance of the pigmentation, which, on the whole, resembles that occurring in malaria. Furthermore, a moderate "cachectic dropsy" of the skin is of frequent occurrence in these affections, while in the cachexia of uncomplicated Addison's disease this condition is exceedingly rare. If the tubercular or cancerous process has involved the abdominal glands (exclusive of the suprarenal capsules), the differential diagnosis cannot be made.

Pellagra is another disease in which there may be extensive pigmentation of the skin. I refer here less to the circumscribed pigmentations on the neck, backs of the hands and feet, and face remaining behind after the specific torpid and indolent erythemas of pellagra, than to the diffuse or rarely spotted pigmentation of the remaining skin. In my studies of pellagra I have observed this not only in the dark complexioned Italians and Roumanians, but also in the blond Hungarians (Czangos) in Roumania. The earlier students of pellagra (Strambio, Felix, Russel, Landouzy, and Billod) reported a similar pigmentation of the skin, often very intense, resembling the color of a Gipsy or of an Ethiopian. Their observations were confined exclusively to pellagra occurring in the Latin races, as Italians, Spaniards, and Roumanians, whose skin is naturally rich in pigment. I wish to emphasize particularly the occurrence of pellagrous pigmentation in the skin of the blond Hungarian also, because these cases prove beyond doubt that the pellagrous poison bears a causal relation to the pigmentation, and fully justify an opinion which I have already mentioned—that there is a form of pellagra which runs its course with symptoms of Addison's disease. If all the symptoms of the case are taken into consideration, these two diseases are not likely to be confounded.

In the first place, the erythemas already mentioned as occurring almost exclusively in the spring and fall are highly characteristic of pellagra. In cases uncomplicated by malaria, the mucous membranes are pale or livid and are unpigmented. There is frequently a very intense anemia, often suggesting pernicious anemia, but more frequently, to be sure, complicated with malaria or syphilis. Pellagra is very rarely associated with tuberculosis. Out of 500 cases of pellagra I found in only one instance a condition at the apex suggestive of tuberculosis. According to the report of the Mercy Hospital at Goerz, not a single case of tuberculosis occurred among their pellagrous insane patients during a period of several years, while almost all the other insane patients living in the same wards died of tuberculosis. It appears from this that pellagrous patients are, to a certain extent, immune from tuberculosis. This is valuable from a diagnostic standpoint, because the relation between Addison's disease and tuberculosis is sufficiently well known.

The contrast between pellagra and Addison's disease is very well shown by the blood-count. In every case of pellagra in which I examined the blood I found, both during and after the erythema, a fairly constant increase in the number of the eosinophilic cells even in those cases where the blood gave no evidence of a qualitative anemia.

I was able to demonstrate a similar increase of eosinophilic cells in the mucous stools by treating the dried preparation with eosin-glycerin and subsequent staining with Lugol's solution. This method also showed the abundant occurrence of clostridia, which were stained a deep violet by iodin. In the cases of Addison's disease which Kolisch and I examined there was no increase of eosinophilic cells in the blood; this is a valuable distinction from pellagra.

There are many analogies in the gastro-intestinal symptoms of the two diseases. Bulimia is more frequent in pellagra, anorexia is conspicuous in Addison's disease. Diarrhea predominates in the initial stage of pellagra, while in Addison's disease obstinate constipation is the rule in the beginning, followed by diarrhea in the terminal stage.

An important diagnostic sign of pellagra is the appearance of the tongue. In most cases there are deep indentations between the papillæ which may be regularly arranged like the squares on a chess-board or like alligator leather—the *gercures* of the French. Nothing of the kind is observed in Addison's disease.

The nervous symptoms of pellagra and Addison's disease likewise present many analogies. In pellagra the functional psychoses are of earlier and more frequent occurrence and comprise melancholia, mania, delirium, and tendency to suicide; while in Addison's disease pronounced psychic disturbances are rarely found and only in the terminal stage. Pellagrous insanity terminates, as a rule, in paralytic dementia; the latter is never observed in Addison's disease. Such symptoms as increased tendon-reflexes, facial reflex, contractures, and muscular atrophies are frequently observed in pellagra, but do not form a part of the clinical picture of Addison's disease. Pellagra occurs endemically, it is dependent upon a diet of maize, and pursues a regularly intermittent course with relapses in the spring and fall; while Addison's disease pursues a gradually progressive course independently of these circumstances.

Further, in many cases of pseudoleukemia a general pigmentation of the skin is observed. This may result from various causes. It may be caused by the pressure of enlarged retroperitoneal and mesenteric glands

23

upon the abdominal sympathetic and its appendages, as has been de-scribed by Marvin, Wright, and F. Raymond; or it may be due even to lymphomatous infiltration of the suprarenal capsules themselves. All such cases actually belong to true Addison's disease, and are mentioned in order to call attention to the fact that pseudoleukemia, and perhaps also leukemia, may present the clinical picture of Addison's disease. On the other hand, this pigmentation may result from scratching in conse-quence of itching of the skin, especially when due to chronic irritation. The melanoderma in this case does not corespond to the type of Addison's disease, being principally confined to the scratched areas, while the remain-ing symptoms of pseudoleukemia or leukemia will lead to the diagnosis of the underlying disease. A similar explanation answers for the pigmentation occurring in many other itching skin diseases; as, for example, prurigo, eczema, and the like.

Vogt described as "vagabond's disease" another form of melanoderma occurring in destitute individuals infected with lice and exposed to all sorts of inclement weather. When such persons are also cachectic, Addi-son's disease may be closely simulated, and just such cases led Hebra at one time to deny the existence of Addison's disease as a distinct affection. The diagnosis is based upon the effect of baths and care of the skin; upon the fact that the skin is dry and scaly and presents numerous scratch-marks (of extremely rare occurrence in Addison's disease); the pigmentation is confined to the covered parts of the body where the skin is immediately in contact with the clothing, while the hands and feet are but faintly pigmented, as a rule; finally, the mucous membranes are not affected, although there are exceptions. In many cases this differential diagnosis may be extremely difficult; patients with Addison's disease through indolence and apathy may become destitute and infected with lice, and may present themselves in this condition for examination.

In rare instances diffuse pigmentation may be caused by a primary melanosarcoma of the skin. A case of this kind was observed by Bamberger in the Rudolf Hospital at Vienna. A patient was ad-mitted to his wards who first gave the impression of Addison's disease. Her skin presented a diffuse brownish-black pigmentation, but at the same time a firm glandular tumor was detected in the left groin. The tumor was firmly adherent to the subjacent tissues, while the overlying skin contained a large number of bluish-black spots varying in size from a pinhead to a lentil, scarcely elevated to the touch, and connected by dark lines. In the skin of the abdomen, on the back, and in the axilla, bluish tumors as large as a kreuzer were found, which, taken in connection with the above-mentioned glandular tumors, led to a diagnosis of melanotic sarcoma. The dark urine gave a black color with chlorid of iron.

The autopsy showed a melanotic sarcoma of the skin of the trunk and extremities, with metastases in the internal organs and intact suprarenal capsules. Upon microscopic examination numerous nodules of melanotic sarcoma were found, and, in addition, large numbers of wandering cells which had taken up pigment from these melanotic growths and were carrying it elsewhere. The diffuse pigmentation of the skin then arose.

Pigmentation of the skin in Basedow's disease has been reported. Personally, I have never seen diffuse pigmentation in this affection, but have observed a partial pigmentation of the skin of the face resembling chloasma uterinum. Chvostek reports a very interesting case of severe Basedow's disease which presented, in addition to scattered dark brown spots, a diffuse bronzing of the skin which disappeared with subsidence of the symptoms of the Basedow's disease, reappeared with their recurrence, and disappeared permanently upon cure of the disease. The nails were white and there were no deposits of pigment in the oral mucous membrane. The cases of recovery from Basedow's disease with bronzed skin illustrate the diagnostic difficulties arising when cases of true Addison's disease (resulting from disease of the suprarenal capsules confirmed at autopsy) are associated with the symptoms of Basedow's disease, as have been reported by Fletcher and Greenhow.

Slight diffuse and spotted pigmentation of the skin is frequently observed in scleroderma and sclerodactylia. The pigmentation is rarely so intense as to suggest Addison's disease. Pigmentation of the mucous membranes is absent as a rule, although Nothnagel reports a patient who suffered from scleroderma but who did not have Addison's disease, and in whom a deep grayish smoke-colored pigmentation of the buccal mucous membrane was present. The diagnosis is based upon the characteristic features of these diseases. Several cases of scleroderma with very intense and wide-spread pigmentation of the skin have been reported as complicated with Addison's disease. At autopsy this statement was found to be incorrect, for no lesions of the suprarenal capsules or abdominal sympathetic were found.

Diseases of the female reproductive organs form a special group which may eventually lead to pigmentation of the skin. Reference is not here made to the frequently occurring pigmentation of the face, areolæ, and linea alba, but especially to a diffuse coloration of the skin which, upon first sight, may suggest Addison's disease. I recall a patient in whom there was a striking pigmentation of the extremities and trunk and extensive ascites. The gynecologists found a resistance on both sides of the uterus in the vicinity of the adnexa, but were unable to state positively whether an ovarian tumor was present or absent. A prominent surgeon in Vienna declined to operate, suspecting disease of the suprarenal capsules on account of the bronzing of the skin. I found in the blood no evidence of cachexia, no diminution of red corpuscles, but an increase of eosinophilic cells. The patient finally decided to submit to an operation and Professor Albert performed bilateral oophorectomy for cystic degeneration. The most interesting feature of the case was that the bronzing of the skin disappeared quite rapidly after the operation. The case, therefore, was one of apparent Addison's disease cured by removal of the ovaries. This case, in connection with a second observed by me in which a typical Basedow's disease appeared after extirpation of both ovaries, forms an interesting supplement to Chvostek's case mentioned above.

It may appear paradoxical to speak of the differential diagnosis between jaundice and Addison's disease. The ordinary forms of jaundice present scarcely any difficulty even when occurring in extremely cachectic individuals, as the cancerous and tubercular. Difficulty, on the contrary, may be afforded by those cases of Addison's disease in which the bronzed skin is accompanied by jaundice due to an affection of the glands in the portal fissure (cancer, tuberculosis) or to metastases in the liver or to complications with diseases of the biliary passages. In such cases the correct diagnosis can be made only by an exceedingly careful separation of the symptoms of Addison's disease from the clinical picture as a whole.

In uncomplicated cases of the acute and chronic varieties of icterus gravis diagnostic errors are not only possible, but have actually been made.

According to Cochran, in many cases of malignant yellow fever the skin is eventually of a bronze hue.   Leva reports an unusually interesting case from Eichhorst's clinic.   The patient was a strong man and presented a "peculiar light bronze pigmentation of the skin, most marked on the face, in both axillæ, on the backs of the hands, on the mons veneris, in the hollows of the knee, on the back, genitals, and anal folds.   Several spots of brown pigment were found on the mucous membrane of the lips, a series of brown spots of the size of peas were present on the mucous lining of the cheeks.   The conjunctivæ were stained a faint yellow, not in spots." The patient died in coma and the clinical diagnosis was morbus Addisonii comatosus.   At autopsy atrophic cirrhosis of the liver was found, while the suprarenal capsules were intact.   (Whether, as Leva believes, this was a case of simple melanotic jaundice must remain undecided in view of the existing cirrhotic degeneration of the liver.)

Diabetes mellitus should first be mentioned among the other affections in the course of which melanoderma has been observed.   French clinicians, particularly Trousseau, Hanot and Chauffard, Letulle, Brault and Gaillard, and most recently Marie, have described cases of so-called *diabète bronzé*.   This type of the disease is characterized by rapid course, diarrhea, meteorism, and finally by a diffuse pigmentation of the skin in addition to the usual diabetic symptoms (dryness of the mouth, polydipsia, polyphagia, polyuria, and glycosuria).   The pigmentation is distributed over the whole surface of the body, is most intense on the face, extremities, and genitals, and is distinguished from the melanoderma of Addison's disease only by the constant absence of circumscribed spots of pigment and of pigmentation of the mucous membranes.   In particularly well-marked cases the pigmentation presents a metallic luster and a peculiar, grayish-black hue, resembling the broken surface of cast-iron.   In these patients there is coincident enlargement and induration of the liver.   It is worthy of note that several days before death the excretion of sugar may almost entirely disappear, and that, during the whole course of the disease, the striking diabetic symptoms of polydipsia, polyphagia, polyuria, and glycosuria are not so conspicuous as in the ordinary forms of diabetes mellitus. Upon postmortem examination the anatomic basis of this disease is found to be a hypertrophic, pigmentary cirrhosis of the liver (*cirrhose hypertrophique pigmentaire*) with sclerosis of the pancreas and accumulation of pigment in various organs, particularly the heart and lymphatic glands. These observations are very suggestive of the "hemochromatosis" described by v. Recklinghausen.   The pigment found in the organs contained iron, and therefore must be regarded as a direct derivative of the coloring-matter of the blood.   Some authors consider this disease as diabetes mellitus complicated with hypertrophic pigmentary cirrhosis, while Marie regards it as a peculiar form of disease, and places it at the side of pancreatic diabetes.   This affection may easily be distinguished from genuine Addison's disease by the symptoms already described; the diagnosis could be difficult only in the terminal stage, after disappearance of sugar from the urine.

There is still another group of cases in which glycosuria and melanoderma may be combined—namely, where glycosuria is due to disease of the pancreas and at the same time the latter has involved the large abdominal sympathetic nerve structures.

In certain affections of the pancreas melanoderma may occur without glycosuria.   Such a case was reported by Aran as occurring in a woman twenty-five years of age whose skin was the color of a mulatto and who died from progressive marasmus accompanied by vomiting and epigastric pain. At autopsy, caseous degeneration and cavity-formation were found in the pancreas and enlargement and calcification of the celiac and splenico-pancreatic glands. The diagnosis of such conditions could be made only by determining the primary disease of the pancreas, either by the history (pancreatic colic), the discovery of a pancreatic tumor, the occurrence of maltose in the urine, under certain circumstances by a diminished excretion of indigo, or, finally, by demonstrating the occurrence of changes in the stools—steatorrhea, azotorrhea—brought about by an interference with the pancreatic secretion.

A special variety of melanoderma results from the accidental or medicinal administration of inorganic poisons. First among these is the arsenical melanosis, a form of disease which has only recently been well understood. This is most often observed during the administration of arsenic for medicinal purposes, and may make its appearance relatively soon, disappearing, as a rule, entirely or almost entirely after discontinuance of the drug. In certain cases a permanent discoloration of the skin has been observed. The cutaneous distribution and localization of the arsenical melanosis is identical with the melanoderma of Addison's disease, but in the former condition the mucous membranes are not involved. In some cases melanosis is the only symptom; in others further symptoms of chronic arsenical poisoning may appear—*e. g.*, disturbances of the digestive and respiratory organs and of the central and peripheral nervous system.

In some cases the diagnosis of arsenical melanosis can readily be made; under other circumstances it may be exceedingly difficult, particularly when the arsenic has been introduced into the system without the knowledge of the patient through the medium of wall-paper or furnishings. In such cases the diagnosis can be made only after a careful consideration of all the characteristic symptoms of arsenical poisoning, or by finding arsenic in the urine or feces. Even during the intentional medicinal administration of arsenic diagnostic difficulties may arise; for example, cutaneous pigmentation may appear in a tubercular patient for whom arsenic has been ordered. In such a case an incorrect diagnosis of Addison's disease might very easily be made.

The administration of silver also may produce a dark pigmentation of the skin. Reduced silver is deposited in the cutis and in the tunica propria of the sweat-glands. The pigmentation is deepest in parts exposed to the light. Silver is present in the form of minute granules of equal size, deposited outside of the cells. On the contrary, the pigment of Addison's disease lies within the cells.

In January, 1892, during a course in diagnosis at the Rudolf Hospital I presented a patient whose appearance was of interest in this connection. The patient's face was pigmented, the ocular conjunctiva was gray, likewise the matrix of the nails and a few scars; the penis was not pigmented. It was learned that the patient had been treated with silver nitrate for an affection of the stomach thought to be gastric crises; so the diagnosis lay between Addison's disease and argyria. In argyria the color of the skin is at first pale gray, as if it had been marked with a lead-pencil, and the pigmentation is equally distributed over the whole surface of the body. If the administration of silver is continued, the color eventually becomes dark blue, and has even been mistaken for cyanosis. Gerhardt calls attention to such cases in his text-book on "Auscultation and Percussion," and offers as a method of differentiation the disappearance on pressure of the color of the lips in cyanosis, while in argyria the color remains unchanged. It is also to be borne in mind that pigmentation of the visible mucous membranes, especially of the mouth, occurs in addition to pigmentation of the skin in workers in silver. Small blue spots may be present on different parts of the body, especially on the hands and forearms, although the color of the remaining skin may remain unchanged. The pigmentation thus may correspond in every particular to that of Addison's disease. In such cases there are still two aids in diagnosis: The first is excision and microscopic examination of a fragment of the pigmented skin; the other is examination of the urine for silver, although a positive result may not occur in actual argyria. In the above-mentioned patient the diagnosis was actually made by the discovery of silver in the urine.

In the preceding paragraphs the diagnostic features of all possible forms of melanoderma have been presented and the feasibility of a correct diagnosis in the majority of the cases noted. That this cannot always be made is well shown by a case brought before my clinic.

The patient was a man, thirty years of age, who presented a diffusely mottled pigmentation of the skin and pigmented spots upon the buccal mucous membrane. The conjunctiva and matrix of the nails were unstained. His appearance corresponded in every particular with the melanoderma of Addison's disease. The patient was an Italian, but did not eat polenta, and stated that his skin had been so brown since birth that he was frequently mistaken for a Gipsy. Some years before he had had intermittent fever which yielded to quinin. The physical examination showed splenic tumor and enlargement of the liver and of a gland in the left axilla. The patient had an attack of intermittent fever while in the hospital; no plasmodia were found, but leucocytosis was present. By occupation he was a gold-worker, and as such had a good deal to do with silver, but none was found in the urine. Finally, in addition to quinin, which now had no effect on his febrile attacks, the patient received arsenic for a considerable period of time. Although loss of power and gastro-intestinal symptoms were absent, the case was thought to be one of Addison's disease on account of the characteristic color and typical distribution of the pigment. In making the diagnosis I had to differentiate between no less than six forms of melanoderma; namely, congenital pigmentation, malarial cachexia, pseudoleukemia, argyria, arsenical melanosis, and Addison's disease. The clinical picture did not correspond entirely to any one of these conditions, but it was finally decided that the case was most probably a protracted pseudoleukemia, localized perhaps in the abdominal glands. Whether this view was correct or not I do not know to this day, for the patient improved and left the hospital, and I have never seen him since.

If the diagnosis of Addison's disease is difficult in the presence of melanoderma, in the absence of this symptom it is often rendered quite impossible. Difficulties then can arise in all directions. Such a case of concealed Addison's disease may possibly be suspected if the other cardinal symptoms, loss of power and gastro-intestinal disturbances with pain in the epigastrium and back, are typically developed without any apparent cause. It is impossible to formulate any general rules for the diagnosis of these cases; it is also impossible to discuss in detail the differential diagnosis of every pathologic condition simulating this form of Addison's disease. Such cases may be encountered in numerous disguises, for instance, in the beginning and subsequent course as neurasthenia, hysterias, hyperemesis gravidarum, aneurysm of the abdominal aorta, ulcer or cancer of the stomach, circumscribed peritonitis, etc.; in the terminal stage as meningitis, typhoid fever, acute general peritonitis, internal strangulation, uremia, acute arsenical poisoning, or even cholera. The endless reports of cases of Addison's disease give numerous examples of the occurrence of such usually unrecognized cases. This polymorphism of the disease is largely based on the multiformity of the causes.

It is, to say the least, strange that in the classic cases of Addison's disease with melanoderma very little attention is paid to the anatomic basis of the disease; while as soon as the bronzed skin is lacking we cling to the suprarenal capsules, not venturing to diagnosticate a given set of symptoms as "Addison's disease without melanoderma" unless the suprarenal capsules are found to be diseased, either accidentally at operation or after death. In the latter event we are perfectly willing to admit that the essential diagnostic feature is afforded by the suprarenal capsules, while in the classic cases with melanoderma we are still inclined to attribute the chief rôle to the sympathetic system. One thus unconsciously proves how intimately connected melanoderma and the sympathetic system are, on the one hand, and the remaining symptoms of Addison's disease and the suprarenal capsules, on the other; and thus also unconsciously admits that nevertheless the fundamental lesion of Addison's disease is found in the suprarenal capsules.

This being admitted, it remains to search for the diagnostic features by means of which pathologic changes in the suprarenal capsules may be recognized during life, particularly when the symptoms of Addison's disease are absent. The means at our disposal for the solution of this problem are very insufficient, for there are only a few uncertain signs capable of calling our attention to the suprarenal capsules in the diagnosis of difficult cases.

In the first place, the local symptoms should be considered: severe lumbar pain causing difficulty in walking, sometimes relieved by bending the body forward, often radiating to the epigastrium. Further, the occurrence of a tumor in the hepatic or splenic region which may extend downward almost to the iliac crest. In such cases all the means should be employed which are in use for the differential diagnosis of abdominal tumors. By thus excluding the connection of the tumor with the liver, spleen, kidney, pancreas, or retroperitoneal glands, its relation to the suprarenal capsules may be considered probable. A positive diagnosis can sometimes be made by exploratory puncture, particularly when the tumor is cystic or consists of soft, loose tissue. If scolices are found in the fluid obtained by puncture, the presence of an echinococcus cyst is proved. Fragments of the tumor perhaps may be obtained and the presence be demonstrated of the characteristic, large, flat, suprarenal cells containing numerous fat-drops and glycogen. If the cells are arranged in double rows about very numerous blood-vessels, the diagnosis of perithelioma may be possible. It must be borne in mind in such cases that accessory suprarenal capsules may be the origin of the tumors.

A similar exact diagnosis may at times be made when portions of such a tumor escape in the urine. Then, of course, the perithelioma has either extended from the suprarenal capsules to the kidney or may have developed primarily from an accessory suprarenal body in the kidney.

The possibility of such a diagnosis is demonstrated by a case observed in our clinic and diagnosticated by Professor Kolisko as suprarenal perithelioma by the microscopic examination of the clot containing fragments of the disintegrated neoplasm evacuated with the urine after preceding hematuria. The diagnosis was confirmed at autopsy. In the case of cystic tumors it might be possible to demonstrate the presence of suprarenal extract by injecting into animals the fluid obtained by exploratory puncture and observing its physiologic action in increasing blood-pressure.

It is probable that tumors of the suprarenal capsules which contain the typical gland cells of the suprarenal bodies typically arranged even in their metastases possess the property of secreting, perhaps even in excess, the physiologically active substance of the suprarenal body; as adenocarcinoma of the liver and its metastases may secrete bile, and as adenocarcinoma of the thyroid gland and its metastases contain thyreoiodin.

Two clinical observations recently made at the Vienna General Hospital support this theory. In the first case a moribund patient, twenty-five years of age, was admitted to the medical wards with symptoms of cerebral hemorrhage. The case was diagnosticated as Bright's disease owing to the wiry pulse. At the autopsy multiple hemorrhages were found in the brain identical with those resulting from the increased blood-pressure of contracted kidneys. One suprarenal capsule was cancerous. There was no disease of the kidneys or blood-vessels as a cause for the increased blood-pressure. A similar case occurred in an elderly individual. These observations certainly prove that the occurrence of cerebral hemorrhage with a pulse of high tension should suggest, particularly in young persons, the possibility of disease of the suprarenal capsules with pathologically increased secretion.

Fraenkel describes another case having an important bearing upon this subject, which, however, in the abstract at hand is not perfectly clear and free from criticism. A girl eighteen years old presented symptoms of weakness, headache, vomiting, pulse of high tension, hypertrophied left ventricle, albuminuric retinitis, large quantities of albumin, a few casts and epithelial cells in the urine, no edema, frequent epistaxis. Death occurred suddenly in collapse. At the autopsy a very vascular tumor, probably angiosarcoma, of the left suprarenal capsule was found. Both kidneys appeared normal, but there were hemorrhages in the renal pelves, the mucous membrane of the small intestine, the media and adventitia of the pulmonary artery, likewise into the endocardium and superficial muscular layers of the left ventricle.

The clinical picture was identical with that of chronic nephritis (contracted kidney), while at the autopsy none of the corresponding alterations in the kidney were found. If this observation is correct, it is a question whether all these symptoms, including the albuminuric retinitis, were not caused by the primary disease of the suprarenal capsules, and whether the albuminuria noticed during life should not be considered as the expression of a toxic irritation from the circulating products of the suprarenal bodies. The occurrence of multiple hemorrhages in this and in the two cases previously mentioned is noteworthy in connection with the fact that some authors (Gluzinski) observed similar hemorrhages into various organs (lungs, brain, pleura, pericardium, etc.) in animals after injections of suprarenal extract.

To this may be added the following communication from Professor Kolisko. In young patients with diseased suprarenal capsules he repeatedly observed endarteritic vascular disease for which no other cause was apparent. It is easily possible that this was not merely a coincidence, but that there was a close connection between the disease of the suprarenal capsules and that of the blood-vessels. Hereafter when thickened and tortuous blood-vessels are found in a young person and cardiac and renal disease, syphilis, and diabetes can be excluded as etiologic factors, the possibility of a disease of the suprarenal bodies should be borne in mind.

A clue to the existence of primary malignant tumors of the suprarenal bodies is afforded by the occurrence of metastases in especial organs. The prostate, thyroid, mammary gland, and suprarenal capsule are characterized by the tendency of their malignant growths to form metastases apart from regional infections in the bones, particularly in the vertebræ, long bones, and skull. If metastases are found in these places of predilection and the presence of a primary tumor in the breast, prostate, or thyroid gland can be excluded, the suprarenal capsule then should be thought of, especially if the metastases are soft and pulsating. Symptoms of cerebral tumor likewise should call to mind the fact that tumors of the suprarenal capsule are very prone to form metastases in the central nervous system, particularly in the brain (Kolisko).

Finally, hypothermia should be mentioned as a very important symptom directing attention to disease of the suprarenal capsules. It has been stated repeatedly that affections of the suprarenal capsules are often characterized by abnormally low temperatures; this is true not only of tumors and uncomplicated tuberculosis of the suprarenal capsules, but also of acute purulent inflammation of these organs. Chvostek's case is a classic instance in which a perinephritic abscess caused by calculus extended to the suprarenal capsules and was characterized in the final stage of the fever by temperatures of 36°, 34°, and even 32° C. (96.8°, 93.2°, and 89.6° F.). The occurrence of subnormal temperature in the course of acute suppuration instead of the expected fever is certainly very striking. Therefore, if hypothermia is observed in the course of an acute suppuration in the lumbar region, which has arisen either primarily or by extension from the renal pelvis, kidney, spleen, liver, or psoas, this fact should at once suggest the possibility of a primary or secondary participation of the suprarenal capsule in the suppurating process.

Finally, attention may be called to two diagnostic procedures furnished by the most recent physiologic investigations.

The experiments on animals by Brown-Séquard, Abelous, and Langlois showed that the blood of animals deprived of suprarenal capsules is poisonous, producing in healthy frogs symptoms similar to curare, while it hastens the death of animals whose suprarenal bodies have been removed. In cases of disease of the suprarenal capsule attended by suppression of function would not human blood possess similar poisonous properties, and would not frogs, both before and after removal of the suprarenal capsules, afford a sensitive diagnostic reaction for such blood? According to Cybulski, the urine of animals which have been injected with suprarenal extract increases the blood-pressure; might it not be possible that the urine of man with a disease of the suprarenal capsules associated with hypersecretion should contain the similar property of increasing the blood-pressure?

In the foregoing pages a few suggestions only have been offered for the diagnosis of Addison's disease in the absence of melanoderma; to apply these rightly at the bedside must be left to the judgment of the physician.

PROGNOSIS.

In general, the statement holds good that Addison's disease is fatal. The few cases reported as " cured" are either not above suspicion from the standpoint of diagnosis, or are to be explained by the fact that one of the well-known, lengthy periods of remission had been mistaken for recovery and reported as such. It is true that certain anatomic lesions do not absolutely preclude the possibility of cure. In the first place, this is true of syphilis; it also holds good for unilateral destructions of the suprarenal capsule which are accessible to operative treatment. This is conceivable in the case of an echinococcus cyst or in localized tuberculosis of one suprarenal capsule. A case of the latter kind was actually reported recently by Oestreich. There was Addison's disease without melanoderma; the symptoms disappeared entirely after an operation (removal of the diseased suprarenal capsule) performed under a mistaken diagnosis. Whether the cure in this case will be permanent or not cannot yet be determined, although this possibility is by no means excluded.

It is, as a rule, impossible to decide whether or not a given case is suitable for operation. In the majority of cases there is bilateral tuberculosis of the suprarenal capsules, or coincident advanced tuberculosis of other organs, or an extension of the process to the adjacent nerve-plexuses, or malignant tumors—in all of which the prognosis is certain.

The question as to the duration of life is based upon the diagnosis of the anatomic basis of the disease. Life lasts longest in uncomplicated tuberculosis of the suprarenal capsules; carcinoma here, as elsewhere, runs a more rapid course. The duration of the disease in most cases is one to three years. Exceptional instances are reported in which the disease terminated fatally within a few months, and others in which the duration was eight, ten, or even thirteen years. Even in these protracted and remittent cases the prognosis as to the duration of the disease must be very guarded, for even in the midst of relatively good health severe symptoms may suddenly appear to which the patient succumbs within a short time.

TREATMENT.

There is no causal treatment of Addison's disease. Perhaps in the future the fruits of physiology and chemistry will become available for therapeutic application in diseases of this organ, as is already the case with the thyroid gland. The first experiments in this direction have already been made. The internal administration of suprarenal substance or extract in diseases of the suprarenal capsules has been followed by only transient improvement or by none at all. Likewise the subcutaneous injection of the extract, as undertaken by French investigators, in two cases beyond increasing the diuresis produced only negative results. This should not deter from further trials, since it is known that the active principle of the suprarenal capsules is so very easily decomposed that when administered internally it probably produces no effect, and when administered subcutaneously only a partial effect. Perhaps intravenous injection in appropriate cases would yield better results.

The implantation of a dog's suprarenal capsule into a patient with Addison's disease for therapeutic purposes has already been attempted by Augagneur, with the result that the patient, who, however, was also in an advanced stage of phthisis, died within three days. [According to Poll,* in the transplantation of the suprarenal the medullary portion, considered by the physiologists as the chief seat of the active substance, is completely destroyed.

The effect of the treatment of Addison's disease with preparations of suprarenal capsules cannot be determined, at present, with any degree of accuracy, owing to the inability to decide upon the exact nature of the questionable cases. The clinical characteristics of this affection are often not so sharply defined as to permit the diagnosis without a reasonable doubt. If the patient continues to improve, and eventually recovers, the condition of the capsules must always remain unknown unless a post-mortem examination eventually is made. A number of cases have been reported in which temporary improvement has followed the use of suprarenal preparations and after death the capsules have been found diseased. Vollbracht † treated his patient for thirty-two days with suprarenal extract. Improvement occurred during this period, but the patient died a few weeks later with meninigitic symptoms, although evidences of meningeal infection were not found after death. The suprarenal bodies were almost completely destroyed, probably at a time when there were no clinical evidences of Addison's disease. Edel ‡ also used the extract and noticed improvement within a few days. The patient soon resumed his laborious occupation, and after five weeks the pigmentation had almost wholly disappeared. The remedy was discontinued with the onset of meningitic symptoms, and the discoloration of the skin soon became nearly as deep as before. Death took place after the meninigitis had continued for a week. There was a tubercular nodule of the size of a pea in the right suprarenal body, and the solar plexus and semilunar ganglion were embedded in dense fibrous tissue. Slight, transitory improvement from suprarenal extract was reported also by Foster.§ Trevithick, ‖ on the contrary, obtained no benefit from its use. W. W. Johnston ** has tabulated from various sources fifty cases of asserted Addison's disease treated with suprarenal preparations. Ten cases are stated to have recovered and sixteen to have improved. He adds one under his own observation who showed marked improvement with gain in flesh and strength during the five months' use of suprarenal tablets. Box †† states that of eight cases treated in St. Thomas' Hospital four died during the first week of treatment. Two lived ninety-five and one hundred and twenty-one days respectively, during which time 3255 and 7200 grains, largely of the medullary portion of sheeps' fresh capsules, were taken, chiefly by the mouth. No permanent improvement and no increased vascular tension were observed. Two other patients were treated with tablets by the mouth and with subcutaneous injections of the watery glycerin extract, which at first caused some discomfort. One patient did not improve; the other increased somewhat in strength and the pigmentation diminished.—Ed.]

In a certain sense the possibility of treatment based on etiology is afforded by syphilis, but unfortunately cases of Addison's disease thus caused are of rare occurrence. Finally, when symptoms of Addison's

* Cited in *Centralbl. f. Phys.*, 1898, xii, 321.
† *Wiener klin. Woch.*, 1899, xii, 736.
‡ *Münch. med. Woch.*, 1900, xlvii, 1821.
§ *Lancet*, 1899, i, 1561.   ‖ *Lancet*, 1900, ii. 105.
** *Trans. Assoc. Am Phys.*, 1900, xv, 65.   †† *Practitioner*, 1901, lxvi, 520.

disease arise from compression of certain portions of the abdominal sympathetic by tubercular or lymphomatous glands, intravenous injections of arsenic may cause a disappearance of these symptoms by reducing the size of the glands.

The further treatment is entirely symptomatic. Considerable temporary improvement in a number of cases has followed the administration of glycerin, nitroglycerin, amyl-nitrite, and strychnin, or the use of faradic or particularly galvanic electricity. Apart from the employment of these agents, the usual indications are for strengthening diet and the use of tonics.

Care must be observed in the treatment of the frequent constipation, for persistent and uncontrollable diarrhea may follow the administration of drastics.

PATHOGENESIS OF ADDISON'S DISEASE.

The difficulty in systematizing the various forms of Addison's disease is due chiefly to our imperfect knowledge of the function of the suprarenal capsules, in part to the great variety of anatomic lesions occurring in these organs, in part to the unequal development of the pathologic process, and, finally, to the fact that disease of the suprarenal capsules by contiguity produces disease of adjacent organs (particularly the nervous apparatus). The greatest confusion has arisen because there are typical cases of this affection in which the suprarenal capsules are found to be perfectly normal at autopsy.

Nevertheless the relation between Addison's disease and the suprarenal capsules is so constant that the relatively few exceptions are not capable of casting a doubt upon it. It is supported by the experience of the last forty years and Lewin's extensive statistics, which prove the occurrence of disease of the suprarenal capsules in 88% of the typical cases of Addison's disease.

The suprarenal capsules, analogous to the thyroid, are sometimes classed as glandular organs with an internal secretion and sometimes as nervous organs. Numerous hypotheses have been advanced in explanation of the symptoms of Addison's disease, among which two in particular deserve especial consideration. The first theory attributes the symptoms of Addison's disease to changes in the abdominal sympathetic and its ganglia; the second or humoral theory explains Addison's disease as an autointoxication resulting from disturbances of the function of the suprarenal capsules; this function is considered to render harmless or neutralize certain products of tissue change.

The former theory was insufficient for those cases of Addison's disease presenting no lesions in the sympathetic system and its tracts. The latter theory failed when cases were found presenting during life the symptoms of Addison's disease, while at autopsy the suprarenal capsules were found to be intact, and yet changes were present in the abdominal sympathetic nerve and celiac ganglion; furthermore, because the symptoms of Addison's disease were lacking when there were extensive lesions of the suprarenal capsules, even complete caseation of both organs or entire absence of them.

Jürgens reports a case of especial importance in which an aneurysm of the abdominal aorta with compression and consecutive atrophy of the splanchnic nerve ran its course under the typical clinical picture of Addison's disease.

Other cases presented during life the symptoms of Addison's disease while at autopsy there was found a combination of diseases, involving, on the one hand, the suprarenal capsules; on the other hand, the sympathetic and splanchinc nerves and, further, the spinal cord. These cases are too obscure to permit any positive conclusions to be drawn, and the same is true of those cases in which the suprarenal capsules are said to have been lacking but no symptoms of Addison's disease were present.

The supporters of the sympathetic theory claim that unless the sympathetic nerves also are involved the symptoms of Addison's disease do not make their appearance, although the destruction of the suprarenal capsules may be complete. It must also be borne in mind that accessory suprarenal capsules or other organs may exist which are capable of assuming vicariously the function of the suprarenal bodies.

With reference to the second group of cases,—those presenting the symptoms of Addison's disease, but with perfectly normal suprarenal bodies and sympathetic,—it must be observed that every case of " bronzed skin " does not justify the diagnosis of Addison's disease, and that even in cases terminating fatally with symptoms of cachexia and bronzed skin diagnostic errors have frequently been made.

It has been found necessary to classify as pseudo-Addison's disease those affections incidentally complicated by loss of power and bronzing of the skin.

On account of all these factors the greatest confusion has reigned with reference to Addison's disease. It was known that it had something to do with the suprarenal capsules, but it was not possible to explain the cases occurring in the absence of disease of these bodies; and yet it seemed, in spite of the anatomic polymorphism, that the uniformity of the clinical symptoms was such that some explanation must be sought.

The earlier physiologists regarded the suprarenal capsules as a part of the sympathetic nervous system. Brücke regarded this as probable " because, in proportion to the small size of the organ, a very large number of nerves enter into it, and because these nerves do not form peripheral end-organs, but rather such end-organs as are found in ganglia and in the central nervous system—namely, ganglionic bodies; these, as is already known from experience elsewhere, are to be considered not as the terminations but as the origin of nerves. There is no occasion for classifying these organs among the glands, because it is not known that they possess any secretory activity, and they do not even present a true adenoid structure, as is found in the spleen and thymus."

The more recent investigations of the physiologic action of suprarenal extracts have, as is already known, proved the suprarenal capsule to be an organ, analogous to the thyroid, which elaborates a physiologically active substance; in other words, this organ is really a gland with an internal secretion. It is perhaps remarkable that Funck and Grünhagen formerly expressed the opinion that the nerves of the suprarenal capsules were gland nerves bearing the same relation to gland cells as the nerves supplying the cells of the salivary glands (Pflüger). At the Sixty-sixth Congress of German Naturalists and Physicians, held in Vienna, Kölliker emphatically stated that the nerve-endings in the medullary substance abounding in nerves bore a peculiar relation to the individual cells, each of which was surrounded by a network or mesh of terminal fibrils; and that the cells of the medullary substance were not nerve-cells, but simple gland cells.

He further states that the cells of the medullary substance, under the influence of nerves, elaborate certain substances which are furnished to the blood. He believes that the cells of the cortex also possess this function, although to a lesser degree.

Although the final solution of the problems of Addison's disease must be left to the physiologists and experimental pathologists, I cannot but express at this point my personal view of the essential nature of Addison's disease.

This opinion conforms closely to an idea which I have already expressed in my work on pellagra, published in 1887. The results of my observations at that time were summed up in the following words: " Pellagra is a chronic systemic disease consisting in delicate nutritive disturbances in the sympathetic nervous system and in the central nerves and blood-vessels pertaining to it. It is caused by a poisonous principle, the harmless antecedents (mother-substances) of which are contained in decayed corn. This substance is decomposed in the intestinal canal of a susceptible individual with the formation of a poisonous, apparently volatile radical which produces intestinal autointoxication."

Elsewhere, while enumerating the various diseases which pellagra may simulate, Addison's disease was included, and the thought was added that in time, perhaps, a common theory might be forthcoming in explanation of the obscure etiology and nature of those diseases which are clinically so similar to pellagra.

In view of the latest physiologic investigations of the functions of the suprarenal capsules and of the changes occurring in the sympathetic system in Addison's disease, I believe the theory which I have already advanced in explanation of pellagra is equally applicable to Addison's disease; particularly in virtue of the following considerations.*

In his lecture on the sympathetic Kölliker considers the sympathetic nervous system to be a many-linked chain composed of contiguous and interlacing motor and perhaps also of sensory units which originate in the cerebrospinal nerves, and regards them merely as an offshoot of the cerebrospinal system, for the latter is composed also of many psychic and somatic, centrifugally or centripetally conducting units or neurons.

Waldeyer has shown that each neuron consists of three parts—the nerve-cell, the nerve-fiber, and the terminal filaments; and that impulses may be transmitted in either direction, from the cells to the filaments or in the reverse direction.

If the suprarenal capsules are to be considered an organ provided with these terminal filaments of Waldeyer (and such were actually observed by Kölliker!) and inserted into the sympathetic nervous system, it is readily conceivable that the splanchnic nerve, with its radiation in the solar plexus, may act as the secretory and trophic nerve of the suprarenal capsule, just as the sympathetic nerve acts in relation to the submaxillary gland. The suprarenal capsules would then be connected by centripetal and centrifugal tracts with the gray matter of the spinal cord and the centers of the splanchnic nerve in it.·

* Unfortunately I did not receive Ewald's paper upon this subject until after the following considerations and conclusions had been written; in this work he advances a theory similar to my own, assuming the disease to be of a system the centers of which lie in the suprarenal capsules and the celiac ganglion.

This idea of the splanchnic nerve as a trophic nerve is supported in Jürgens' case of Addison's disease above mentioned occurring in connection with an aneurysm of the abdominal aorta. In this there was, in addition to pressure-atrophy of the splanchnic nerve, atrophy of the corresponding suprarenal capsule.

It must be left for the experimental pathologists to furnish proof of the importance of the splanchnic nerve as a secretory nerve of the suprarenal capsules. Dr. Biedl has already undertaken experiments in this direction, from which it appears that upon stimulation of the splanchnic nerve the suprarenal capsule becomes hyperemic and the flow of blood from the suprarenal vein is increased; this shows at least that the splanchnic nerve exerts a positive vasodilating action upon the suprarenal capsules. The experimental pathologist can answer much more positively and more speedily than the clinician whether the hyperemia thus produced is attended by an increased secretion of the active suprarenal substance; or whether the same conditions prevail here as in the submaxillary gland upon stimulation of the chorda tympani and sympathetic, which, it is well known, possess an antagonistic action; whether the splanchnic nerve produces both vasodilation and increased secretion, as the chorda tympani does in the submaxillary gland; and, finally, whether the other nerves supplying the suprarenal capsules—*e. g.*, the vagus—have any determining action upon its function.

It is known that the tonic centers of the splanchnic nerves are situated at the junction of the cervical and dorsal cord; that their central ganglion cells are most abundant between the eighth cervical and second dorsal nerves; but that these cells also are present in gradually diminishing numbers both above and below these points, so that the entire center extends in the long axis of the spinal cord from the sixth cervical to the fifth dorsal nerve. The ganglion cells forming the center are situated in the motor areas of the gray matter of the cord. In the cervical cord they are situated in the lateral horns, in the dorsal cord in the lateral divisions of the anterior horns. These "sympathetic-motor" cells do not differ either in size or in structure from the voluntary motor cells of the anterior horns (Biedl).

Therefore if the trophic centers of the splanchnic nerve bear the same relation to its peripheral distribution in the abdominal viscera as the centers of a motor nerve bear to its peripheral distribution, it is readily conceived that Addison's disease may be the manifestation of such a systemic disease involving the central and peripheral tracts of the splanchnic nerve and also its intermediate and terminal organs (just as poliomyelitis, neuritis, and myositis all result in paralysis of the end-organ, the muscle).

According to this view, the location of the degenerative process is immaterial, whether in the spinal center, in the course of the splanchnic nerve, in the celiac ganglion, which is in part an intermediate organ, or in the end-organ, the suprarenal capsule itself.

In every case the result is a more or less complete suspension of the function of the end-organ—and this is to be sought for in every case as the cause of Addison's disease.

Although the latest physiologic investigations have not positively determined the function of the suprarenal capsules, they have furnished important data. At any rate, it is known that this organ is a gland with an internal secretion and produces a physiologically active substance which is important to life.

One group of physiologists claim that the production of this substance is the sole function of the suprarenal capsules; others maintain that these organs exert a neutralizing action, by means of which the toxic products of nervous and muscular activity are rendered harmless.

May not both views be correct? May not both functions be contained in the suprarenal capsules? From the standpoint of expediency this seems highly probable, and it is conceivable that the poisonous products of tissue changes in other organs may be carried to the suprarenal capsules and undergo various chemical processes (oxidation, reduction, decomposition, and reunion), and finally be synthetically elaborated into a secretion which is important to life.

The theory of such a double function is compatible with the existence of two histologically different substances in the suprarenal capsules, and, to my mind, is not without analogy. The theory of the function of the thyroid is cast upon perfectly similar lines.

It is assumed that out of the poisonous products (perhaps xanthin bases, Lindemann) of tissue change which are carried to the thyroid certain substances are synthetically produced which are essential to the nutrition and function of the brain. The function of the suprarenal capsules may similarly be explained, particularly since these organs are known to present many analogies. The suprarenal capsules may bear the same relation to the solar plexus as the thyroid capsule bears to the brain, and, indeed, the solar plexus has been called the abdominal brain.

According to this theory, when the suprarenal capsules are the seat of organic or functional disease, the absence of their peculiar secretion results in impairment of the nutrition and function of this abdominal brain, while at the same time the poisonous products of metabolic activity are not destroyed, but accumulate in the system, causing an autointoxication. As the result of these two factors, the entire organism suffers as well as the nerves and blood-vessels of the sympathetic system which are primarily involved.

Congenital imperfect development (tubercular) or acquired vulnerability of these nerves and blood-vessels predisposes to the early acquisition of these disturbances, which may be manifested merely by functional inefficiency or eventually also by anatomic alterations. No gross lesions of the sympathetic system will be found unless the underlying anatomic cause of the impairment of function of the suprarenal capsules is situated in the sympathetic tract primarily or has extended by contiguity from the suprarenal capsules to the adjacent sympathetic plexuses.

Does this theory correspond to the anatomic lesions which are actually found in Addison's disease?

Statistics furnish incontestable proof that the suprarenal capsules are of the utmost importance in the production of Addison's disease, pathologic alterations being present in these organs in 88% of all cases. That, on the contrary, the changes in the sympathetic system are too insignificant and inconstant to adequately explain all cases of Addison's disease is supported by the statements of Brauer, who, after a careful consideration of all previous histologic conditions in the sympathetic system, came to the following conclusions: "It has not yet been proved that the underlying cause of Addison's disease is an anatomically demonstrable affection of the sympathetic nervous system. The inconstant occurrence of such lesions, the questionable significance of some of the alterations described, the occurrence of similar lesions in the sympathetic system without coincident Addison's disease, and, finally, the entire absence of lesions occasionally reported render it highly probable that there is no constant relation between Addison's disease and changes in the sympathetic system. It seems more likely that the alterations in the sympathetic system are secondary to the as yet unknown cause of Addison's disease or to the profound cachexia, and thus, perhaps, may produce or influence certain symptoms of the disease.

If the fundamental cause of Addison's disease is considered to be a progressive impairment and finally a complete suspension of the function of the suprarenal capsules, two sets of questions must be answered:

1. What is the explanation of the symptoms of Addison's disease when both suprarenal capsules are diseased?

2. What is the explanation of those cases which present clinical or anatomic deviations from the type?

With reference to the first question, the most prominent symptoms from the outset in the clinical course of Addison's disease—asthenia and loss of power with its special manifestations in various organs—can be readily accounted for by this theory of the injury of the double function of the suprarenal capsules. The tone of the entire vascular system is impaired because of the deficient production of suprarenal secretion, which raises blood-pressure. This gives rise, in the first place, to atonic hyperemia of the abdominal viscera with anemia and impairment of function of all other organs. Thus is explained the frequent contrast between the pulsation of the abdominal aorta and the small, soft, peripheral pulse which, together with its rapidity, is a manifestation of the loss of tone of the vagus roots from cerebral anemia. At the same time the toxic products of the metabolic activity which are only imperfectly neutralized in the suprarenal capsules produce their general systemic effect and increase the action of the first-mentioned element. The combination of these two factors accounts for a large group of nervous symptoms (vertigo, ringing in the ears, fainting, headache, etc.) and also for the violent symptoms of the acute terminal stage following sudden complete suspension of the suprarenal function.

The gastro-intestinal symptoms are partly the result of these general systemic disturbances, but in the majority of cases they are due to the local pathologic process in the suprarenal capsules, whether through nervous influence or by direct extension to the gastro-intestinal sympathetic tracts.

The explanation of the third cardinal symptom, the melanoderma, requires a more detailed discussion, which I shall precede by a few remarks upon pigment formation in general.

Histologic investigations seem to prove that the mode of production of pigment in health and in a great many pathologic conditions is identical. This view is based chiefly upon the results of Karg's experiments. He grafted fragments of white skin upon a negro, excised portions of the graft at frequent intervals, and studied under the microscope the progressive formation of pigment in the grafts. These investigations led him to conclude that the pigment is formed in the cutis vera by peculiar cells, the so-called chromatophores. These are very numerous in the immediate neighborhood of the papillary blood-vessels, show many branches, and gradually penetrate upward to the lowest layers of the epidermis, the rete Malpighii, finally sending their projections, stuffed with pigment-granules, between the separate rete cells. By a kind of phagocytosis the pigment

24

contained in these projections is taken up by the cells of the rete. Karg succeeded in demonstrating the very same process in the pigmentation of Addison's disease, and concludes that all varieties of pigmentation arise in the following way: " Pigmented cells from the cutis vera penetrate to the epidermis, send out processes in all directions, and yield their pigment to the epithelial cells."

This view is shared by most of the recent investigators of this question, the only difference of opinion being as to whether the chromatophore cells originate from connective tissue or epithelium. This question is of minor interest to the clinician.

Karg demonstrated in like manner the process of absorption of pigment in the reverse direction after grafting a negro's skin upon a white person. After six weeks the rete Malpighii was entirely free from pigment, but the cutis vera contained numerous leucocytes and wandering cells, all richly laden with pigment. In this case also stellate cells were found at the junction of the cutis vera and the rete Malpighii, sending processes into the latter. These processes were not so plainly visible, because they no longer contained pigment. According to other observers, at least a part of the pigment is to be found in the lymphatic glands corresponding to the particular area of skin.

It is necessary to establish a second fact underlying the theory of melanoderma—namely, that the formation of pigment in the lower animals is directly controlled by the nervous system.

Vulpian showed that in frogs the changes in the color of the skin are governed by special nerves, which, although following the distribution of the vasomotor nerves, possess an entirely different function. The frog's skin contains large, branching pigment-cells, called chromoblasts, which are capable of contraction and expansion, producing alternately a light or dark coloration of the skin. The nerves which stimulate contraction of the chromatophores, thereby producing a lighter color of the skin, run in the tracts of the vasoconstrictor nerves, while those which cause expansion of the chromatophores and a darker color of the skin accompany the vasodilator nerves.

As has just been stated, similar branching pigment cells, chromatophores, have been found by Karg and many other observers in the pathologically pigmented and even in the normal human skin.

There are many other arguments in support of the theory that in man both production and absence of pigment are dependent upon nervous influences. One fact is the occurrence of abnormal pigmentation, not only in organic diseases of the central and peripheral nervous system,— *e. g.*, tabes, syringomyelia, and neuritis,—but also in functional neurosis and neuralgias. Doubtless the pigmentation developing during pregnancy and in diseases of the female genitals (ovarian cysts) belongs to this category.

The above-mentioned conditions observed in animals seem to justify the conclusion that the formation of pigment in man also is controlled by the vasomotor nerves, in other words, by the sympathetic nervous system, acting through the medium of chromatophore cells.

The origin of the pigment contained in the chromatophore cells is a question which cannot be answered so positively. The fact that the chromatophores are most abundant around the blood-vessels, particularly around the capillaries of the cutis, suggested at once the thought that their pigment was derived from the blood, either directly from the hemoglobin or indirectly from the colorless albuminous bodies of the blood-plasma. This view holds good in spite of the fact that the pigment-granules do not respond to the tests for iron, since it has repeatedly been shown that this reaction may be absent even from deposits of pigment positively derived from hemoglobin—*e. g.*, extravasations of blood. The pigment formed by plasmodia is also free from iron, yet this is without doubt a product of the digestion of hemoglobin.

It must frankly be admitted that no actual knowledge is possessed of the derivation of the pigment in Addison's disease; in the first place, because the chemical composition of this pigment is unknown, and yet it is known that there are several different varieties of melanin. It may be taken for granted that the pigment is originally derived from the blood, but whether from the decomposition of red blood-corpuscles or from some colorless antecedent contained in the plasma it is impossible to decide. The analogy with the above-mentioned conditions observed in animals leads to the belief that the pigment formation in Addison's disease also takes place under the control of the sympathetic system.

The pigmentation of Addison's disease may be compared with that observed in chronic arsenical poisoning, which may appear in some individuals after the administration of Fowler's solution of arsenic. Wyss investigated the microscopic appearances of the skin in this condition. He found an iron-free pigment situated primarily in the rete cells overlying the papillary layer and the interpapillary areas, the intensity of the pigmentation corresponding approximately to that observed in the Malpighian layer of a moderately dark mammary areola. Another favorite site of this pigment was the papillary layer of the skin, especially in the neighborhood of the blood-vessels. Finally, the pigment may be deposited in the perivascular lymph-spaces. In the latter situation the abundance of the pigmentary deposit depends upon the wealth of the corresponding cutaneous area in papillæ and upon the duration and intensity of the arsenical melanosis.

Wyss bases his views as to the origin of this pigment upon Stirling's examination of the blood in children during the internal administration of Fowler's solution. Stirling found that the number of red corpuscles and the percentage of hemoglobin were reduced one-half, and for this reason Wyss feels justified in assuming that the pigment present in arsenical melanosis is derived from decomposed blood-pigment.

The analogy between these conditions and those observed in Addison's disease is striking. Even the abundant deposit of pigment in the lymphatics of the papillæ is simulated by the occurrence of pigment in the peripheral lymph-glands in Addison's disease as observed by Schmorl, who interprets this as an evidence of the transference of granular pigment from the skin into the peripheral lymphatic vessels. He also explains the pigmentation of the cutaneous lymph-glands which he observed in two negroes and two mulattoes as a physiologic absorption of pigment from the skin into the corresponding lymphatic vessels.

The idea is perhaps not forced that the deposits of pigment observed in the cutaneous lymph-spaces in arsenical melanosis also is attributable to a reversed absorption of pigment.

According to this view, the cutaneous melanosis of arsenical poisoning and of Addison's disease would correspond in all important histologic details and in their manner of explanation.

This striking similarity is of especial importance because it is known that arsensic acts as a poison upon the sympathetic nervous system, paralyzing the terminations of the splanchnic nerves. The theory that this pigmentation occurs through the agency of the sympathetic nervous system would gain in probability if in future cases of arsenical poisoning after relatively small doses of arsenic no destructive changes in the blood, particularly in the red corpuscles, were to be found.

That an abnormal pigmentation of the skin also may arise during the course of other chronic poisonings characterized by delicate anatomic changes in the sympathetic nervous system is shown by those cases of pellagra which I and other authors have reported.

The following conclusions may be drawn:

1. Since all cases of pigment formation, whether normal or pathologic, present the same histologic alterations;

2. Since it must be taken for granted that the normal formation of pigment is controlled by the nervous system, particularly the sympathetic;

3. Since abnormal pigmentation has been observed as the direct result of a number of diseases of the nervous system;

4. Since some sympathetic nerve-poisons are capable of developing an abnormal pigmentation in susceptible individuals;

5. Finally, since a number of diseases having no connection with the suprarenal capsules (*e. g.*, *diabète bronzé*, ovarian cysts, Basedow's disease, scleroderma, etc.) may be attended by extensive melanosis:

The conclusion is justified that the pigmentation of Addison's disease also is due to the same cause; that is, to a disturbance of innervation in the sympathetic tract. Neither experiments on animals, nor clinical observation, nor postmortem examination, have furnished any evidence in support of the fact that the suprarenal capsules have anything directly to do with the formation or destruction of the antecedent of this pigment; on the contrary, these observations tend to prove that disease of the suprarenal capsules does not produce an abnormal pigmentation of the skin unless secondary involvement of the sympathetic system has occurred.

Therefore melanoderma is not of equal rank in the pathology of Addison's disease with, for example, loss of power. It is not a direct, but rather an indirect, suprarenal symptom; its frequent occurrence in disease of these organs being sufficiently explained by the intimate relation existing between the suprarenal capsules and the sympathetic nervous system and by the regular extension of the pathologic process to the latter; indeed, this symptom may be absent, even though the suprarenal capsules are entirely destroyed, as long as the sympathetic tracts controlling the formation of pigment remain intact.

The facts that the melanoderma by no means always runs a parallel course with the severity and progress of the other symptoms of Addison's disease; that in severe cases the melanoderma may be only partial or slight; that this symptom often may not appear until the terminal stage, or, on the other hand, may be one of the first symptoms of the disease—these facts still further tend to prove that "melanoderma and disease of the suprarenal capsules do not stand in the simple relation of cause and effect."

Neither does pigmentation of the mucous membranes, so important in the diagnosis of Addison's disease, furnish any fundamental distinction between this and other melanodermata, for similar deposits of pigment have been observed in other diseases having absolutely no connection with the suprarenal capsules, and even in perfectly healthy individuals.

The cases presenting clinical or anatomic deviations from the type must be considered under different heads.

1. How are those cases to be explained in which, in spite of complete destruction of both suprarenal capsules, the three cardinal symptoms of Addison's disease are entirely or in part lacking?

It is true that in some cases, in spite of extensive destruction of both suprarenal capsules, Addison's disease was not diagnosticated, but it must not be imagined that these cases presented no symptoms attributable to the suprarenal bodies. Small pulse, loss of power, disturbances of the nervous and digestive systems, apparently were present, but were attributed to the underlying disease (tuberculosis or cancer), simply because the conspicuous criterion for the diagnosis of Addison's disease, melanoderma, was not present. It has just been stated why this symptom may be absent in such cases.

2. How does it happen that tubercular disease of the suprarenal capsules is so generally accompanied by the typical symptoms of Addison's disease, while in other forms of disease, particularly in cancer, this group of symptoms is very often lacking, although both glands may be extensively involved?

The cause for this lies, in the first place, in the exquisitely destructive nature of the tubercular process, which completely destroys the specifically active cells of the organ either by caseation or by the frequently added fibrous degeneration; and, in the second place, in the well-marked tendency to extension manifested by the tubercular disease. Other affections which destroy the specific gland cells will be manifested by the same symptoms, as, for example, the simple sclerotic, chronic inflammations and the scirrhous forms of cancer.

Primary adenocarcinoma and perithelioma behave in an entirely different manner. In addition to the fact that these tumors are rarely bilateral, still another circumstance must be taken into consideration—namely, that the cells of these new-growths more or less completely maintain the character of the original gland cells, and are capable of continuing, at least in part, the function of the latter. This has also been observed in cancers of other organs,—*e. g.*, the liver,—for even the metastases from this organ are capable of secreting bile. That some forms of cancer lead rather to an increase than to a suspension of the glandular function seems to be shown by those cases which presented during life a wiry pulse and cerebral hemorrhages resulting from the rapid rise of blood-pressure. These cases were mentioned in the section on differential diagnosis; they form a supplement to those rare cases of carcinoma of the thyroid which run their course with symptoms of Basedow's disease, and which are generally regarded as an expression of the increased functional activity of the gland.

3. Why in severe cases of Addison's disease is only unilateral or incomplete bilateral disease of the suprarenal capsules present at autopsy?

When one suprarenal capsule is diseased, it must be borne in mind that the function of the other capsule may be suppressed through the agency of supposed trophic and secretory sympathetic nerve-fibers; this influence being transmitted to the abdominal ganglia of the sympathetic or to the centers of the splanchnic nerve in the spinal cord, which are connected by collaterals with those of the opposite side. The conditions may be similar to those observed in connection with the renal secretion, when the sudden arrest of the secretion of one kidney produces reflexly arrest of the functional activity of the healthy kidney also; or it may have to deal with a process which Charcot makes use of in the explanation of muscular atrophy following chronic articular rheumatism, and which he terms "*torpeur des cellules mortrices.*"

On the contrary, in some cases of unilateral suprarenal disease in which the symptoms of Addison's disease are absent it must be assumed that a vicarious activity of the intact suprarenal capsule exists; just as disease of one kidney may give rise reflexly to hypersecretion from the opposite kidney. Whether, in any given case, the function of the second organ will be suppressed or vicariously increased; and why at one time the one, at another time the opposite, occurs, it is entirely beyond our power to predict.

In explanation of those cases of fully developed Addison's disease in which both suprarenal capsules are found intact, it must be assumed that the tropho-secretory system of the capsules is injured in some place elsewhere, and that the function of the suprarenal capsules is consequently incomplete or arrested. As, for instance, a muscle, although anatomically intact, loses its function when its motor nerve is diseased.

Further, the theory that the splanchnic nerve is a trophic nerve for the suprarenal capsule would throw light upon those cases in which partial tubercular changes are found in the suprarenal capsules in the course of disease of some part of the splanchnic nerve. One could readily conceive how, in disease of the splanchnic nerves themselves or of their central tracts, secondary nutritive disturbances are set up in the suprarenal capsules, with the result that these organs furnish a *locus minoris resistentiæ* for the lodgment of the bacilli. There are plenty of analogies for this circumstance. One needs only to refer to the frequent occurrence of decubitus or arthritic inflammation upon the paralyzed side in hemiplegia, or to the occurrence of trophic affections of the fingers and toes in syringomyelia, etc.

A similar influence to that exerted by a diseased suprarenal capsule upon its healthy fellow is manifested by a focus of disease upon its healthy surroundings within the same organ; in other words, the function of the healthy part of the organ may be suppressed because of circulatory disturbances or because of the local irritation—*e. g.*, toxin (tuberculin)— proceeding from the focus of disease. This suppression of function may be permanent, in which case the Addison's disease leads progressively to its fatal issue; or it may temporarily disappear in case the adjacent diseased process is arrested. The intermissions and remissions so frequently observed in the course of Addison's disease are explained as soon as the action of the local poison is suspended by the recovery of those portions of the glands which still remain intact. The nature of the underlying tubercular process precludes the permanence of these remissions, for even after an arrest of several years this process may be lighted up anew, and may again exert its injurious influence upon its surroundings, leading either to temporary acute exacerbations or terminating, with violent symptoms, directly in death.

4. How is Addison's disease explained in the absence of disease of the suprarenal capsules?

The explanation of these cases has already been given, when in the development of our theory it was stated that if the suprarenal capsules were not actually diseased, the cause of their functional inactivity must be sought for in an injury to the nerve-tracts controlling their function—*i. e.*, in the spinal cord, in the splanchnic nerve, or in the celiac ganglion. An example of this type is the frequently cited case of Jürgens, in which aneurysm of the abdominal aorta running its course under symptoms of Addison's disease produced suppression of the function and secondary atrophy of the corresponding suprarenal capsule from compression of the splanchnic nerve.

5. Finally, how are those cases of Addison's disease to be explained without any pathologic changes in the entire apparatus?

This question is a very difficult one to answer. In the first place, there are certain cases presenting during life the typical symptoms of Addison's disease in which no alterations are found in the "apparatus" at autopsy, although extensive pathologic alterations in other organs are present. These cases cannot satisfactorily be explained by the existing methods of clinical diagnosis and pathologic technique. As the clinician is unable to decide, in a complicated case of this kind, whether the loss of power results from coincident disease of the suprarenal capsules or from the severe underlying disease,—*e. g.*, cavernous phthisis, endocarditis, etc.,—so the pathologist is unable to predict from the appearance of the cell whether it was capable of performing its function during life or not. If cases should be found, although none are certainly known at present, terminating fatally with the typical symptoms of Addison's disease although no lesion of the apparatus or any other severe disease is demonstrable postmortem, we could no more explain such cases than we now can explain the cases of chorea minor and hysteria which terminate fatally without any pathologic changes being found after death.

Finally, our views as to the nature of Addison's disease may be summed up briefly as follows:

The suprarenal capsule is a gland with an internal secretion. It possesses a double function: first, the neutralization of the toxic products of the metabolic activity of other organs; second, the synthetic production of a substance which is essential to the sympathetic system maintaining its nutrition and a normal tone.

In every case the symptoms of Addison's disease result from impairment, or eventually complete suppression, of these functions of the suprarenal capsules, brought about by disease of the capsules themselves or of the nerve-tracts controlling their function. These nerve-tracts extend from the spinal cord through the splanchnic nerve and the celiac ganglion. This impairment and eventual suppression of the function of the suprarenal capsules account for the nutritive and functional disturbance of the sympathetic system, on the one hand, and for the general autointoxication, on the other. In addition to these two principal factors, extension of the pathologic process in many cases to the abdominal sympathetic is responsible for the occurrence of some of the symptoms of Addison's disease.

Pigmentation of the skin and mucous membranes is not an integral part of Addison's disease, and, though of decided diagnostic significance, is not an essential feature. It is rather an indirect than a direct suprarenal symptom, arising only through the agency of local or general disease of the sympathetic system.

BIBLIOGRAPHY.

Abegg, H. B.: "Zur Kenntniss der Addison'schen Krankheit," Inang.-Dissert., Tubingen, 1889.

Abelous, J. E.: C. R. Soc. de Biol., 1892; "Arch. de Physiol.," 1893 Ser. v, Bd. v.

Abelous et Langlois: C. R. Soc. de Biol. 1891 und 1892; "Arch. de Physiol.," 1892, Ser. v, Bd. iv.

Abelous, Langlois et Charrin: C. R. Soc. de Biol. 1892; "Arch. de Physiol.," 1892, Ser. v, Bd. iv.

Addison, Th.: "On the Constitutional and Local Effects of Disease of the Suprarenal Capsules," London, 1855.

Albanese: "Atti delle R. Acc. dei Lincei," 1892.

Albu, Albert: "Ueber die Autointoxicationen des Intestinaltractus," Berlin, 1895.

Alexander: "Untersuchungen über die Nebennieren und ihre Beziehungen zum Nervensystem," "Beitr. z. pathol. Anat. u. allg. Pathol.," 1891, xi.

Alezais et Arnaud: "Marseille méd.," 1889 u. 1891; "Revue de méd.," Paris,1891, xi.

Aran: "Arch. génér. de méd.," 1846; cited by Friedreich, "Die Krankheiten des Pankreas," "Ziemssen's Handbuch," Leipzig, 1875, Bd. viii, 2. Hälfte.

Arnold, J.: "Ein Beitrag zur feineren Structur und dem Chemismus der Nebennieren," "Virchow's Archiv," 1866, Bd. xxxv.

Augagneur: Cited by Dufour (s. d.).

Averbeck, H.: "Die Addison'sche Krankheit," Erlangen, 1869.

Bamberger, E.: "Melanosarkom der Haut," etc., "Bericht der k. k. Krankenanstalt Rudolfstiftung in Wien vom Jahre 1891."

Bamberger, H.: "Krankheiten der Nebennieren" in: "Krankheiten des chylopoetischen Systems," Erlangen, 1864.

Baruch, F.: "Ein Fall von Morb. Addisonii," Inang.-Dissert., Prag, 1895.

Bartsch, H.: "De morbo Addisonii," Inaug.-Dissert., Königsberg, 1867.

Beier: "Untersuchungen über das Vorkommen von Gallensäuren und Hippursäure in den Nebennieren," Inang.-Dissert., Dorpat, 1891.

Beneke: "Pathologische Anatomie der Nebennieren" in "Zülzer's klin. Handbuch der Harn- und Sexualorgane," Leipzig, 1894.

Berdach, K.: "Ein Fall von primärem Sarkom der Nebenniere," etc., "Wiener klin. Wochenschr.," 1899, Nos. 10 and 11.

Berruti u. Perusino: "Giornale dell' Accad. med.-chirurg. di Torino," 1857 and 1863.

Biedl, A.: "Ueber die centra der Splanchnici," "Wiener klin. Wochenschr.,"1895, No. 52; "Zur Wirkung der Nebennierenextracte," "Wiener klin. Wochenschrift," 1896, No. 9.

Biehler, R.: "Ein eigenthümlicher Fall von Morb. Addisonii," Inaug.-Dissert., Rudolfstadt, 1892.

Billod: "Traité de la pellagre," Paris, 1865.

Brauer, L.: "Beitrag zur Lehre von den anat. Veränderungen des Nervensystems bei Morb. Addisonii," "Deutsche Zeitschr. f. Nervenheilkunde," 1895, Bd. vii, 5. u. 6. Heft.

Brault, A.: "Maladies du Rein et des capsul. surrénales," "Traité de méd.," Paris, 1893, T. v.

Brown-Séquard: "Recherches expérimentales sur la physiol. et la pathologie des capsules surrénales," "Arch. génér. de méd.," Paris, 1856; "Nouvelles recherches," etc., C. R. xliii, xliv, xlv, and "Journ. de physiol.," 1858, T. i; "Influenze de l'extrait aqueux de caps. surrén. sur des cobayes" . . . C. R. Soc. de Biol. 1892; "Influence heureuse de la transfusion de sang" . . . C. R. Soc. de Biol. 1893.

Bruhn, J.: "Ein Fall von Addison'scher Krankheit," Inaug.-Dissert., Kiel, 1869.

Brunner: "Schweiz. Wochenschr. f. Pharmak.," 30.

Buhl: "Wiener med. Wochenschr.," 1860, No. 2.

Burresi: "Lo sperimentale," 1880, Bd. lxvi.

Chassevant et Langlois: C. R. de la Soc. de Biol. Paris, 1893.

Chatelain: "De la peau bronzée ou maladie d'Addison," Thèse, Strassbourg, 1859.

Chauffard: "Maladies du foie," etc., "Traité de méd.," Paris, 1892, T. iii.

Chvostek, Jr., F.: "Störungen der Nebennierenfunction als Krankheitsursache (Morb. Addisonii)" in: "Ergebnisse d. allg. Pathol. u. pathol. Anat.," von Lubarsch und Ostertag, Wiesbaden, 1895.

Chvostek, Sr., F.: "Ein Fall von suppurativer Entzündung der linken Nebenniere," "Wiener med. Presse," 1880, Nos. 45–47.
Cybulski, N.: "Weitere Untersuchungen uber die Function der Nebenniere," "Anzeiger der Akad. d. Wissench." in Krakau vom. 4 Marz 1895; "Gazetta lekarska," 1895, xv.
Dagonnet: "Beiträge z. pathol. Anat. d. Nebennieren," "Zeitschr. f. Heilkunde," 1885, Bd. vi.
Darier: "Ophthalmolog. Gesellschaft in Heidelberg," August 7, 1896; Referat in "Wiener klin. Wochenschr.," 1896, No. 40.
De Dominicis: "Atti delle R. Accad. med.-chir. di Napoli," 1892; "Giornale Assoc. Napol. de med. e natur," 1894; "Arch. de physiol.," 1894, Ser. v, Bd. vi.
Dejean: "Sur l'Etiologie de la pellagre," Thèse, Paris, 1868.
Demange: "Revue médicale de l'Est," 1877.
Demiéville: "Deux cas de mal. d'Addison," "Rev. méd. de la suisse romande," 1884, iv. Jahrg., No. 9.
Dornhöfer: "Ueber die Addison'sche Krankheit," Inaug.-Dissert., Würzburg, 1879.
Dufour: "La Pathogenie capsulaire de la mal. bronzée," Thèse, Paris, 1894.
Dungern, E. v.: "Beitrag zur Histologie der Nebennieren bei Morb. Addisonii," Inaug.-Dissert., Freiburg i. B., 1892.
Engelbertz, L.: "Morb. Addisonii," Inaug.-Dissert., Bonn, 1892.
Ewald, C. A.: "Ein Fall von Morb. Addisonii," "Dermatol. Zeitschr.," Bd. i, Heft 4.
Feldkirchner, J.: "Zwei Fälle von Morb. Addisonii," Inaug.-Dissert., Landau, 1871.
Fenwick: "Brit. Medical Journal," 1886.
Fliener, W.: "Ueber die Veranderungen des sympathischen und cerebrospinalen Nervensystems bei 2 Fällen von Addison'scher Krankheit," "Deutsche Zeitschr. f. Nervenheilkunde," 4. Februar, 1892; "Ueber den heutigen Stand der Lehre von der Addison'schen Krankheit," "Volkmann's Vorträge," Leipzig, 1892, N. F. No. 38.
Foà: "Rivista clin. di Bologna," 1879.
Foà und Pellacani: "Arch. per le scienze med.," 1879, Bd. iii, and 1883, Bd. vii; "Rivista clin. de Bologna," 1880.
Fraenkel, Albert: "Ein Fall von Addison'scher Krankheit," Inaug.-Dissert., Berlin, 1870.
Fraenkel: "Ein Fall von doppelseitigem, völlig latent verlaufenem Nebennierentumor," Inaug.-Dissert., Freiburg i. B., 1886.
Fraenkel, Sigmund: "Beiträge zur Physiologie und physiol. Chemie der Nebenniere," "Wiener med. Blätter," 1896, No. 14.
Funck u. Grünhagen: Cited by Lewin, "Charité-Annalen," Bd. ix.
Gabbi: "Rivista clinica di Bologna," 1886.
Gerhardt: "Bronzekrankheit," "Jenaische Zeitschr. f. Med.," ii; "Lehrbuch der Auscultation u. Percussion."
Gottlieb: "Ueber die Wirkung der Nebennierenextracte auf Herz und Blutdruck," "Archiv für exper. Pathol. u. Pharmakol.," 1896.
Gottschau: "Arch. f. Anat. u. Physiol.," 1893, and "Biol. Centralbl.," 1883, Bd. iii.
Gluzinski, W. A.: "Ueber die physiol. Wirkung der Nebennierenextracte," "Przeglad lekarski," Krakau, 1895, No. 9; "Einige Worte zur Frage der Nebennierenextracte," "Gazetta lekarska," Warschau, 1895, No. 12.
Goldstein, L.: "Die Krankheiten der Nebennieren" in: "Zülzer's Handbuch," 1894.
Gourfein, C. R.: Paris, 1895.
Gratiolet: "Note sur les effets qui suivent l'ablation des capsules surrénales," C. R. Paris, 1856, xliii.
Grawitz: "Die Entstehung von Nierentumoren aus Nebennierengewebe," "Langenbeck's Archiv," Bd. xxx.
Greenhow, E. H.: "On Addison's Disease," London, 1866.
Guarnieri u. Marino Zucco: "Experimentelle Untersuchungen über die toxische Wirkung des wässerigen Extractes der Nebennieren," "Chem. Centralbl.," 1888.
Guay: "Sur la pathogénie de la maladie d'Addison," Thèse, Paris, 1893.
Guermonprez: "Contribution à l'étude de la maladie bronzée d'Addison," Thèse, Paris, 1875.
Guttmann, M.: "Ueber die Addison'sche Krankheit," Inaug.-Dissert., Berlin, 1868.
Haas, L.: "Ueber die Addison'sche Krankheit," Inaug.-Dissert., Würzburg, 1862.
Hackert, H.: "Morb. Addisonii," Inaug.-Dissert., Jena, 1884.
Harley: "Brit. and Foreign Med.-chirurg. Review," 1858, xxi.
Hayem u. Lesage: "Bulletin et mém. de la soc. méd. des hôp. Paris," 1891.

Hertwig, O.: "Lehrbuch der Entwicklungsgeschichte des Menschen und der Wirbel-thiere," Jena, 1890, 3. Aufl.

Heschl: "Drei Falle von Addison'scher Krankheit," "Wiener med. Wochenschr.," 1873, No. 33.

Hirzel, E.: "Beitrag zur Casuistik der Addison'schen Krankheit," Inaug.-Dissert., Zürich, 1860.

Holm: Cited by Sigmund Fraenkel.

Jaccoud, S.: "Traité de pathologie interne," Paris, 1879, T. II.

Jakoby: "Arch. f. exper. Pathol. u. Pharmakol.," 1892, Bd. XXIX.

Jores, L.: "Specielle pathol. Anat. u. Physiol. der Harn- u. männl. Geschlechts-organe" in: Lubarsch-Ostertag, Wiesbaden, 1896, III. Abth.

Jürgens: "Berliner klin. Wochenschr.," 1884; "Deutsche med. Wochenschr.," 1885.

Kahlden, C. v.: "Beiträge zur pathol. Anat. der Addison'schen Krankheit," "Arch. f. pathol. Anat.," Berlin, 1888; "Ueber Addison'sche Krankheit," "Zeigler's Beitrage zur pathol. Anat. u. allgem. Pathol.," 1891, Bd. X; "Ueber Addison'-sche Krankheit und über die Function der Nebennieren," "Zusammenfassendes Referat," Centralbl. f. allgem. Pathol. und pathol. Anat.," Jena, 1896, Bd. VII, Nos. 32 and 33.

Kahler, O.: "Prager med. Wochenschr.," XII, Nos. 32 and 33.

Kalindero u. Babes: "Un cas de maladie d'Addison," Paris, 1890.

Karg: "Anatomischer Anzeiger," 1887, No. 12.

Kinzler, G.: "Ueber den Causalzusammenhang zwischen Zerstörung der Neben-nieren und Bronzed-skin," Inaug.-Dissert., Tübingen, 1895.

Klebs: "Handbuch der pathologischen Anatomie," Berlin, 1870.

Koelliker: "Ueber die Nerven der Nebennieren" und "Ueber die feinere Anatomie und die physiologische Bedeutung des sympathischen Nervensystems," Vor-träge, Referat in "Neurolog. Centralbl.," 1894, No. 20.

Kolisch u. Pichler: "Ein Fall von Morb. Addisonii mit Stoffwechseluntersuchung," "Centralbl. für klin. Medicin," 1893, No. 12.

Krukenberg: Cited by Sigmund Fraenkel.

Külz: "Sitzungsberichte der Marburger Gesellschalft," etc., 1876, No. 4.

Kussmaul: Cited by Laureck.

Labadie-Lagrave: "Maladie bronzée ou maladie d'Addison," "Traité des maladies du sang," Paris, 1893.

Lancereaux: "Arch. génér. de méd.," Paris, 1890, XXV.

Landerer, P.: "Zur Casuistik der Addison'schen Krankheit," Inaug.-Dissert., Tüb-ingen, 1878.

Langlois: C. R. Soc. de Biol., 1893, and "Arch. de physiol.," Ser. V, Bd. V.

Langlois et Charrin: "Lésions des capsules surrénales dans l'infection," etc., "La Semaine médicale," 1893, No. 46

Laureck, P.: "Zur Casuistik des Morb. Addisonii," Inaug.-Dissert., Bonn, 1889.

Leichtenstern: "Ueber Morb. Addisonii," "Deutsche med. Wochenschr.," 1891.

Leva, J.: "Zur Lehre des Morb. Addisonii," "Virchow's Archiv," 1891, Bd. CXV.

Lewin, G.: "Studien über die bei halbseitigen Atrophien und Hypertrophien, namentlich des Gesichtes vorkommenden Erscheinungen, mit besonderer Berucksichtigung der Pigmentation," "Charité-Annalen," Berlin, 1884, IX. Jahrg.; "Ueber Morb. Addisonii mit besonderer Berücksichtigung der eigen-thümlichen abnormen Pigmentation der Haut," "Charité-Annalen," Berlin, 1885, X. Jahrg.; "Ueber Morb. Addisonii," II. Theil," "Charité-Annalen," 1892, XVII. Jahrg.

Lindemann: "Ueber die antitoxische Wirkung der Schilddrüse," "Centralbl. für allgem. Pathol. und pathol. Anat.," 1891.

Lubarsch, O.: "Die albuminösen Degenerationen," Lubarsch-Ostertag, Wiesbaden, 1895, II. Abth.

MacMunn: "Il Morgagni," 1889, II, No. 9.

Manasse, P.: "Virchow's Archiv," 1893 and 1894, Bd. CXXXV; "Zeitschr. f. physiol. Chemie," 1895, Bd. XX, Heft 3.

Mankiewicz, O.: "Ueber die bösartigen Tumoren der Nebenniere," Inaug.-Dissert., Strassburg, 1888.

Mann, Fr.: "Ueber Bronzehaut," etc., Inaug.-Dissert., Greifswald, 1893.

Marchand: "Intern. Beitr. z. wissenschaftl. Med.," 1885, Bd. I; "Virchow's Archiv," Bd. XCII.

Marie, P.: "Sur un cas de diabète bronzée," "Leçons de clinique médicale," Paris, 1896.

Marino, Zucco: "Chemische Untersuchungen über die Nebennieren," "Chem.

Centralbl.," 1888, und Dutto (Chem.)," Unters. über die *Addison*'sche Krankheit," "Unters. zur Naturl. d. Menschen," xiv u. xv.

Marischler, J.: "Ein Fall von lymphat. Leukamie und einem Grawitz'schen Tumor der rechten Niere," "Wiener klin. Wochenschr.," 1896, No. 30.

Marwin: Cited by Eichhorst, "Handbuch der spec. Pathol. u. Ther.," 1887, Bd. iv.

Merkel, G.: "Die Krankheiten der Nebennieren" in "Ziemssen's Handb.," Leipzig, 1875, Bd. viii, 2. Hälfte.

Michalkovic, G. v.: "Intern. Mon. f. Anat. u. Histol.," 1885, Bd. ii.

Minkel, Ad.: "Beitrag zur Kenntniss der *Addison*'schen Krankheit," Inaug.-Dissert., Bonn, 1883.

Minot, Ch. S.: "Lehrbuch der Entwicklungsgeschichte des Menschen," German Ed. by Kästner, Leipzig, 1894.

Moore: "Proceed. of the Physiol. Soc.," 1895.

Mühlmann: "Zur Physiologie der Nebenniere," "Deutsche med. Wochenschr.," 1896, No. 26.

Müller, H. F.: "Ueber einen bisher nicht beachteten Formbestandtheil des Blutes," "Centralbl. f. allgem. Pathol. und pathol. Anat.," 1896, Bd. vii.

Müller, Johannes: "Handbuch der Physiologie des Menschen," Koblenz, 1844, ii Buch.

Nabarro: "Proceed. of the Physiol. Soc.," 1895.

Neusser, E.: "Die Pellagra in Oesterreich und Rumänien," Wien, 1887.

Nothnagel, H.: "Experimentelle Untersuchungen über die *Addison*'sche Krankheit," "Zeitschr. f. klin. Med.," 1879–1880, Bd. i; "Zur Pathologie des Morb. Addisonii," "Zeitschr. f. klin. Med.," 1885, Bd. ix; "Morb. Addisonii," Vortrag. Allgem., "Wiener med. Zeitung," 1890, Nos. 2–4.

Oestreich, R.: "Operative Heilung eines Falles von Morb. Addisonii," "Zeitschr. f. klin. Med.," Berlin, 1896, Bd. xxxi, 1. u. 2. Heft.

Oliver and Schäfer: "Proceed. of the Physiol. Soc.," 1894; "Jour. of Physiol.," 1895, xviii, 3.

Orth, J.: "Lehrbuch d. spec. pathol. Anat.," Berlin, 1889.

Pal, J.: "Nebennierenexstirpation bei Hunden," "Wiener klin. Wochenschr.," 1894, No. 48.

Peacock: Cited by Laureck (s. d.).

Pfaundler: "Zur Anatomie der Nebenniere," "Sitzungsber. d. kais. Akad. d. Wissench. in Wien," 1892, Bd. cl, Abth. 3.

Philipeaux: C. R. 1856–1858, xliii, xliv, xlvi.

Pilliet: "Capsules surrén. dans le plexus solaire," "Bullet. de la soc. anat. de Paris," 1891.

Posselt, A.: "Bericht über fünf zur Obduction gelangte Fälle von Morb. Addisonii," "Wiener klin. Wochenschr.," 1894, Nos. 34–38.

Pottien, W.: "Beitr. zur Addison'schen Krankheit," Inang.-Dissert., Göttingen, 1889.

Quain-Hofmann: "Lehrbuch der Anatomie," 1870.

Rabl, H.: "Die Entwicklung und Structur der Nebennieren bei den Vögeln," "Arch. f. mikroskop. Anat.," xxxviii.

Rawitz, B.: "Grundriss der Histologie," Berlin, 1894.

Raymond, F.: "Morb. Addisonii mit Integrität der Nebennieren," "Bericht in der Société médicale des hôpitaux," 11. März, 1892. Referat in: "Wiener med. Presse," 1892, No. 15.

v. Recklinghausen: "Ueber Hämochromatose," "Tageblatt der Heidelberger Naturforschversammlung"; cited by Dieckhoff, "Beiträge z. pathol. Anat. des Pankreas."

Rosenstirn: "Die Harnbestandtheile bei Morb. Addisonii," "Virchow's Archiv," Bd. lvi.

Roth, P.: "Ein Fall von Morb. Addisonii," Inaug.-Dissert., Würzburg, 1888.

Schenk, S.: "Lehrbuch der Embryologie des Menschen und der Wirbelthiere," 1896, 2. Aufl.

Schiff: "Sull'exstirpatione delle capsule surrenali," Imparziale, 1863.

Schmalz, Rich.: "Zur Casuistik des Morb. Addisonii," "Deutsche med. Wochenschrift," 1890, No. 36.

Schmidt, M. B.: "Hämorrhagie und Pigmentbildung" in: Lubarsch-Ostertag, 1895, ii. Abth.

Schmorl, G.: "Zur Kenntniss der accessor. Nebennieren," "Ziegler's Beiträge," 1891, ix.

Seligsohn: Cited by Sigmund Fraenkel.

Semmola: "Gazette hebdomad. de méd. et de chir.," 1881.

Solger, B.: "Anatomie der Nebenniere," "Zülzer's Handbuch," Leipzig, 1894.
Stadelmann: "Zeitschr. f. physiol. Chemie," XVIII.
Steffann, P.: "Ein Fall von Morb. Addisonii," Inaug.-Dissert., Würzburg, 1881.
Stierling: Cited by O. Wyss.
Stilling: "Ueber die compensatorische Hypertrophie der Nebennieren," "Virchow's Archiv," 1889, Bd. CXVIII.
Strübing, P.: "Die Neubildungen der Niere," "Zulzer's Handbuch," Leipzig, 1894.
Suppino: "Riforma medica," 1892, Bd. III.
Szymonowicz, L.: "Ueber die Erscheinungen nach der Nebennierenexstirpation bei Hunden und über die Wirkung der Nebennierenextracte," "Anzeiger der Akad. der Wissensch." in Krakau, 1895; "Die Nebennieren vom Standpunkte der Morphologie und Physiologie," Krakau, 1895 (Polish); "Die Function der Nebenniere," "Pflüger's Archiv," 1896, Bd. LXIV, 3.-4. Heft.
Thiroloix: "Bullet. de la société anat. de Paris," 1892 and 1893.
Thudichum: Cited by Eichhorst, "Handbuch d. spec. Pathol. und Therapie."
Tizzoni, G.: "Ueber die Wirkungen der Exstirpation der Nebennieren auf Kaninchen," "Beiträge z. path. Anat." (Ziegler), 1889, VI.
Tschirkoff: "Ueber die Blutveränderungen bei der Addison'schen Krankheit," cited by Grawitz, "Klinische Pathologie des Blutes," Berlin, 1896.
Velich, Al.: "Ueber die Einwirkung des Nebenierensaftes auf den Blutkreislauf," "Wiener med. Blatter.," 1896, No. 15.
Virchow: "Zur Chemie der Nebennieren," "Virchow's Archiv," 1857, Bd. XII; "Berliner klin. Wochenschr.," 1864, No. 9.
Vulpian: C. R. Paris, 1856; "Gaz. méd.," 1856–1857.
Vulpian et Cloez: C. R. Paris, 1857.
Weichselbaum: "Grundriss der pathol. Histologie," 1892.
Willrich, E.: "Ein Fall von Sklerodermie in Verbindung mit Morb. Addisonii," Inaug.-Dissert., Göttingen, 1892.
Wright: "Case of Lymphadenoma," "Dublin Journ.," 1888.
Wyss, O.: "Ueber Arsenmelanose," "Correspondenzblatt für Schweizer Aerzte," 1890, XX. Jahrg.
Zander, R.: "Ueber functionelle und genetische Beziehungen der Nebennieren zu anderen Organen, speciell zum Gehirn," "Ziegler's Beitrage," 1890, VII.

Extensive bibliographies are given in the works of Kahlden, Lewin, and Szymonowicz.

DISEASES OF THE LIVER.

BY

PROF. DR. H. QUINCKE

AND

PROF. DR. G. HOPPE-SEYLER.

Edited, with Additions,

BY

FREDERICK A. PACKARD, M.D.

DISEASES OF THE LIVER.

INTRODUCTION.

(Quincke.)

1. TOPOGRAPHIC ANATOMY AND DIAGNOSIS.

POSITION; SIZE.

THE liver is situated in the lower part of the thorax closely wedged against the concavity of the diaphragm. The larger portion lies to the right of the median line, but a small portion extends beyond it to the left. Both anteriorly and posteriorly the greater part of its convex surface is directed toward the parietes and is covered by the ribs. It is in direct contact with the muscular walls of the abdomen only in the upper half of the epigastrium in the angle formed by the two costal arches. Above, it is bounded by the lower surface of the right lung, a small part of the left lung, and the heart.

The lower surface of the liver, concave and irregular in outline, is in contact with the anterior and posterior surfaces of the stomach in the region of the lesser curvature, the upper part of the duodenum, the transverse colon, and the hepatic flexure of the colon, as well as with the right kidney and adrenal. Only when it is enlarged does the left lobe of the liver extend as far as the spleen. The right and left lobes are separated on the convex surface of the organ by the suspensory ligament, and on the lower surface by the ligamentum teres. The hepatic artery, the portal vein, and the bile-ducts enter the liver through a short, transverse fissure (the porta hepatis) situated in the middle of the lower surface. The gall-bladder is situated in a longitudinal fissure to the right of the porta, below and anteriorly, while the inferior vena cava occupies the posterior part of the fissure. The ligamentum teres (the obliterated umbilical vein) is seen in the longitudinal fissure to the left of the porta. This, together with the ductus venosus Arantii, is directed toward the inferior vena cava.

The shape of the liver is considerably modified by the shape of adjacent organs, and varies in different individuals. The weight, too, is different. In a healthy adult the average weight of the liver is about 1500 gm. (3 pounds).

According to the investigations of Frerichs,* the weight of the liver fluctuates between one-seventeenth and one-fiftieth of the body-weight in people of different ages (in adults between one-twenty-fourth and one-fortieth of the body-weight), its absolute weight being from 0.82 to 2.1 kg. In children the liver is relatively larger, in the aged relatively smaller, than in middle-aged persons. In children, too, the left lobe is not so small in comparison with the right as it is in adults.

* "Leberkrankheiten," 2, Hefte 1, p. 18.

H. Vierordt * calculates that the average weight of the organ in an adult man is 1579 kg., in a woman 1526 kg. Assuming the average body-weight to be figured as 100 (in male subjects), then the liver weighs (according to Vierordt):

In the new-born... 4.57
From one to nine months................................... 2.9
From ten to eleven months................................. 4.9
From one to fifteen years................................. 3.4
From sixteen to twenty-five years......................... 2.7

These figures, of course, refer to the liver after death and after the removal of all the blood. During life the organ is much larger, owing to the large quantity of blood that it contains. In the course of laparotomies this observation has frequently been made. According to an experiment by Sappey, a liver weighing 1450 grams could contain 550 c.c. of fluid within its vessels.

Monneret † found that a liver weighing 1600 gm. when its vessels were ligated, lost 360 gm. of blood in twenty-four hours, and was able, on the other hand, to take up 1200 gm. of fluid if a forcible injection was used.

PERCUSSION.

The liver is examined during life by percussion, palpation, auscultation, and inspection. The first method is the most frequently employed. The so-called **absolute liver dulness**—*i. e.*, the dulness over that part of the convex surface of the liver that is not covered by the lung—is first determined. It is not possible by percussion to determine the exact outlines of the part of the liver in immediate contact with the dome of the diaphragm and the concave lower surface of the lung; for this reason this area of so-called relative liver dulness is, with few exceptions, of slight clinical value.

The upper boundary of absolute liver dulness corresponds to the lower margin of the right lung. It intersects at the spinal column, the eleventh rib; in the scapular line, the lower margin of the ninth rib; in the axillary line, the lower margin of the seventh rib; in the mammillary line, the sixth intercostal space; in the parasternal line, the sixth rib.

The extent of the absolute liver dulness, according to Bamberger, is as follows:

In the axillary line, in men, 12 cm.; in women, 10.5 cm.
In the mammillary line, in men, 11 cm.; in women, 9 cm.
In the parasternal line, in men, 10 cm.; in women, 8 cm.
Width of the left lobe, in men, 7 cm.; in women, 6.5 cm.‡

As a matter of fact, these measurements are only of limited utility, because they fluctuate greatly even in perfectly healthy persons of an average size, depending on the shape of the costal arch and of the lower thoracic aperture. In the case of the heart and the spleen it is possible to give normal measurements; but in the case of the liver the outlines of the organ itself and of the area of percussion dulness are determined by the relation of its margins to the margin of the thorax. Normally, the lower margin of the liver extends a little above the costal arch in the axillary line, crosses the costal arch in the mammillary line, cuts the median line half-way between the umbilicus and the ensiform cartilage, and extends from this point to the region of the apex-beat. Even these topographic relations fluctuate within wide limits, particularly in females. In them the lower margin of the liver may extend from 1 to 2 cm. further down-

* "Anatom.-physiolog. Tabellen," Jena, 1893, pp. 20 to 23.
† *Archives générales de médecine,* 1861, i, p. 561.
‡ Tables with many individual measurements are given by Frerichs, loc. cit., pp. 37–40.

ward. In children this is the rule, because the liver is larger and the ribs are less developed and run more horizontally.

From a practical point of view it is of some value to measure the extent of the hepatic dulness in an individual case and to express it in figures, because in this way it is often possible to determine changes in these dimensions that may occur in the course of disease.

In order to determine the location of the lower margin of the liver it is best to percuss gently, beginning below and progressing upward. The first modification of the percussion sound should be noted. On account of the thinness of the margin this modification will be very slight. The tympanitic sound of the stomach and of the intestines, situated underneath this sharp margin, frequently renders percussion of this part very uncertain. As we progress upward the tympanitic sound grows weaker. In some cases, however, it does not disappear entirely, but may persist even to the upper margin of absolute dulness.

In order to percuss successfully, the abdominal muscles should be completely relaxed. The absence of a large amount of subcutaneous fat renders the proceeding more exact. If the stomach and intestines are distended with gas, percussion is rendered difficult, as it is also if any air is present in these parts.

In enlargement of the liver the lower margin usually moves downward, so that, in general, an extension of the absolute dulness downward occurs. If the liver is smaller and less thick than normal, the lower percussion boundary will move upward, the dull sound will be mixed with the tympanitic sound, or, in some cases, absolute dulness will disappear.

At the same time, it must be remembered that, even if the liver is of normal size, the areas of percussion dulness may be changed owing to abnormalities in the shape of the thorax or of the abdominal cavity. An increase of the antero-posterior diameter of the thorax produces a decrease in the hepatic dulness for the reason that the anterior part of the organ (in the erect position of the body) occupies a more horizontal position, and, consequently, is in contact with a smaller area of the anterior parietes below the lung.

This change in the position of the liver has been called **retroversion** or "marginal position" of the liver, for reasons which, by the way, are not quite clear. The liver must be imagined as standing on its posterior dull margin when the body is in the horizontal position.

This diminution in the area of percussion dulness, even when the liver is normal, is seen in the barrel-shaped emphysematous thorax, in the kyphosis of old age, and in spondylitic kyphosis of the lower dorsal vertebræ, as well as in slowly developing ascites in young persons whose thorax is still sufficiently pliable to permit of a barrel-shaped distention.

. On the other hand, the area of dulness may be enlarged, even when the liver is normal, if the antero-posterior diameter of the thorax is diminished. This may occur in paralytic thorax or in cylindric corset-thorax, owing to the fact that the ribs are pressed downward, and are situated near to the spinal column, thus coming in contact with a larger portion of the anterior surface of the liver. In these cases the whole organ, particularly its anterior margin, occupies a more vertical position. This condition has been called "**anteversion**" of the liver.

If the enlarged gall-bladder extends below the hepatic margin, it can usually be detected by percussion, the area of dulness so produced being directly continuous with the hepatic dulness.

25

PALPATION.

If the abdominal walls are normal, a normal liver cannot be palpated, since its thick right edge is hidden behind the costal margin, and the edge toward the left is so thin that it does not offer sufficient resistance to be felt. The liver is only palpable if the abdominal walls are abnormally relaxed, or if the resistance of the organ is abnormally increased. The former is found in great emaciation, and in relaxation of the muscles following distention, either as a result of pregnancy or of pathologic increase of the abdominal contents. Palpation is made particularly easy by separation of the abdominal muscles. The consistency of the substance of the liver is most frequently increased by fatty infiltration, passive congestion, and pressure from lacing. In the latter case the liver is, as a rule, enlarged and its lower margin forced downward. It is also possible to palpate large irregularities on the surface of the liver, such as carcinomatous nodules and gummata. If the abdominal walls are thin, even nodular irregularities of the surface, such as those present in cirrhosis of the liver, may be capable of detection by palpation. In addition to the consistency and outline of the anterior surface, thickening and indentations on the lower margin may occasionally be distinguished by palpation.

Exceptional thickness of the abdominal walls renders palpation impossible. Even when the abdominal walls are of medium thickness it is necessary that the muscles should be completely relaxed and that the patient be placed in the horizontal position, and preferably be instructed to bend forward a little. The physician should place himself to the right of the patient, place the right hand flat upon the abdomen, and, following the respiratory rhythm, press downward with the tips of the fingers at the beginning of each respiration. Palpation may be aided, particularly in thin females, by pressing the kidney and the liver forward from the lumbar region with the left hand. If the abdominal walls are stretched and relaxed, as in many women, or immediately after aspiration of ascitic fluid, it is sometimes possible to palpate the lower surface of the liver. To accomplish this, the four fingers of the left hand should be placed in the lumbar region and the thumb of the left hand in front below the costal arch. In this way the liver is grasped from above, fixed, and, if possible, forced forward and downward. In some cases the right hand can now feel the sharp margin and grasp it between the fingers and the thumb.[*] Landau-Rheinstein [†] recommends in performing this method of examination to have the patient in the erect position, as then the liver is forced forward and downward by its own weight. In some cases, according to Wijnhoff,[‡] it is practicable to instruct the patient to sit on a chair and bend the body forward with his hands on his knees while the physician examines from behind and to the right of the patient.

Normally, the gall-bladder can neither be felt nor percussed, because it never extends much below the margin of the liver. Even when it does protrude, it is impossible to palpate it, because its walls are not sufficiently tense as long as the bile-passages are permeable. It becomes palpable, however, as soon as the tension of its walls increases and it protrudes below the margin of the liver. Thickening of its walls and concretions within the organ can frequently be felt. The gall-bladder is situated slightly

[*] Glénard, *Lyon méd.*, 1892, ii, p. 191; 1890, ii, p. 345.
[†] *Berlin. klin. Woch.*, 1891.   [‡] *Nederland. Tijdschrift*, 1889, No. 2.

within the mammillary line, approximately where the margin of the liver crosses the costal arch. When the liver is enlarged or in an abnormal position, or when its outline is changed, the gall-bladder may be found in different locations. It is most frequently displaced downward, occasionally, however, laterally, particularly outward. In ascites and meteorism it is often useful to perform palpation by giving a sudden jog, by which the fluid or the coils of intestine are rapidly pushed away, making it easier to feel the liver.

The liver is moved downward by the diaphragm with each inspiration, a circumstance that facilitates palpation of the organ. When the warmed hand is placed upon the abdominal wall and the patient instructed to inspire deeply, the liver is alternately approximated to the finger-tips and removed. Owing to the fact that the liver is in contact with the diaphragm over so large a surface, its respiratory motility is greater than that of other organs only indirectly in contact with it, as, for instance, the kidneys, the colon, and the mesentery. Sometimes it is possible to fix one of these latter organs in their inspiratory position with the left hand, the liver then alone moving upward with the ascending diaphragm. Only if the neighboring organs are adherent to the liver will they participate in its inspiratory and expiratory motility. This movement is not only palpable, but•can also be demonstrated by percussion—an important feature in the interpretation of dulness in the region of the liver, as it gives us the means of determining whether it is produced by that organ.

Even on deep inspiration the lower margin of the liver rarely extends more than 1 or 2 cm. further downward. The upper margin of the absolute liver dulness may be moved downward from 1 to 5 cm., owing to the entrance of the sharp lower margin of the lung into the pleural sinus during inspiration. The area of the absolute liver dulness is therefore increased during each inspiration.

If the liver is adherent to the anterior abdominal wall by peritoneal adhesions, the respiratory motility of the lower margin of the liver may be absent. If pleural adhesions fix the diaphragm or the lungs to the thoracic walls, the upper margin of the absolute liver dulness is only very slightly changed by respiration or does not move at all.

Whenever we are in doubt whether we are dealing with a tumor of the liver or of some other abdominal organ, we may have recourse to alternate filling and emptying of the intestinal tract in addition to the determination of respiratory motility. This distention may occur physiologically, but it is better produced artificially by inflating the stomach with gas, or filling the intestine with water. In the former case the liver is pushed upward and to the right, in the latter only upward. In this manner the organ may be pressed upward against the abdominal wall, and thus the margin of the liver and the gall-bladder become more accessible to palpation. A tumor of the kidney, on the other hand, would be pressed backward by these proceedings.*

INSPECTION; AUSCULTATION.

In rare cases inspection will give us information in regard to changes in the consistency and the form of the liver. If the volume of the liver is greatly increased, asymmetry of the thorax will be seen both anteriorly and posteriorly in the erect position of the body. If, on the other hand,

* O. Minkowski, "Die Diagnostik der Abdominaltumoren," *Berliner klin. Wochenschr.*, 1888, No. 31.

the liver is normal in size, or only slightly increased in volume, and the abdominal walls are very thin and relaxed, the same will be observed. In these cases the outline of the liver or the gall-bladder may sometimes be more clearly perceptible to the eye than to the hand, particularly during forced respiration. [Inspection may also show a shadow ascending and descending with the movements of the diaphragm corresponding in its position with the margin of the liver and analogous to Litten's diaphragm phenomenon.—ED.]

Finally, we must consider a few special signs that are observed during examinations of the liver.

A *systolic pulsation* combined with a systolic enlargement is found in tricuspid insufficiency when the liver is hyperemic from venous congestion. This pulsation is caused by a transmission of the blood-wave backward from the right heart, and is analogous to the venous pulse felt in the jugular vein. It is differentiated from simple transmitted pulsations by the fact that it can be felt over the whole liver, and that the liver simultaneously increases in size and consistency. Much more rarely a systolic pulsation is transmitted through the arteries in aortic insufficiency.

Systolic blowing sounds over the vessels have been heard in aneurysm of the hepatic artery and in malignant neoplasms (Leopold, Martin, Rovighi) as well as in cholelithiasis (Gabbi, Martini). In a few cases these sounds were apparently caused by compression of the hepatic artery.*

Friction sounds caused by fibrinous exudations from the peritoneum are occasionally heard over the liver as well as over other abdominal organs. These sounds can be perceived better by the sense of touch than by the ear. In the case of the liver they are caused by the respiratory movements of the organ, and can be differentiated from pleuritic friction sounds by their location. [In hydatid cyst of the liver the so-called "hydatid fremitus" may be felt; while "gall-stone crepitus" has been claimed by some authors to be of diagnostic value in cholelithiasis.—ED.]

CHANGES IN SIZE.

By one or the other of the above-mentioned methods it is possible in the majority of healthy and of sick subjects to outline approximately the part of the liver in contact with the parietes of the body. The interpretation of the findings made by these methods must, of course, as we have already mentioned, frequently be modified, for the reason that in different individuals the formation of the body, and with it the formation of the liver, is different, and because changes in the position of neighboring organs can exercise an influence on the position of the liver relative to the parietes. As a rule, changes in the shape and size of the liver are determinable in that part of the organ that is accessible to palpation. The palpatory findings are more valuable and more positive than those of percussion; and wherever palpation can be performed, the results from it should be valued more highly than those obtained from percussion.

An enlargement of the organ usually produces a dislocation of the lower margin downward. This is caused, on the one hand, by the effect of gravity; on the other, by the greater resistance offered by the diaphragm

* Leopold, *Archiv der Heilkunde*, Bd. xvii, p. 395. Martini, *Riv. clin. ital.*, 1891, No. 3. Gabbi, *Riv. clin. ital.*, 1889, No. 1. Rovighi, *Riv. clin. di Bologna*, 1886, No. 5.

as compared to the slight resistance offered by the gastro-intestinal tract. Tumors that develop on the convexity of the liver rarely produce a decrease in the volume of the lung. Such a result is seen only in those cases where the lesion causes at the same time a reduced contractility of the right side of the diaphragm; and here we are usually dealing, not with a simple dislocation of the diaphragm, but with anatomic changes of its tissue following inflammation or the development of a neoplasm. Simple enlargement of the liver is found in hyperemia, hypertrophy, fatty and amyloid degeneration, leukemia, hypertrophic cirrhosis, and multilocular echinococcus. Enlargement of the liver with changes in its outline is found in carcinoma, echinococcus, and abscess. In corset liver, and in lobulation of the organ following syphilitic hepatitis, the change in the outline of the organ is more conspicuous than the increase in its volume; the latter change, in fact, may be completely absent.

A decrease in the size of the liver is found in the atrophy of old age, in that form of chronic inflammation called atrophic cirrhosis, and, in the most conspicuous manner, in acute atrophy. As a rule, in these conditions the posterior dull margin of the liver remains unchanged, so that the decrease in the size of the organ usually produces a movement upward of the lower margin, and, in this manner, a decrease in the absolute liver dulness. In acute atrophy the organ collapses and seems to be folded upon itself.* The latter accident is prevented if the liver is adherent to the anterior abdominal wall, the liver in this case growing thinner while its surface area does not decrease.

There can be no doubt that the size of the liver can be influenced by the relative filling of its vessels with blood. We will discuss this at some length in the section on hyperemia of the liver. Normally such a change is not perceptible. Heitler † is the only one who makes the statement that the liver dulness may thus increase by 3 cm. within a few minutes.

A change in the size of the liver may be simulated by changes that occur in neighboring organs, and by dislocations of the liver produced by such changes, particularly if the liver is by them approximated to or removed from the abdominal walls. Enlargement of the liver dulness may be simulated by the presence of inflammatory exudates or of tumors in the right pleural cavity, or by thickening of the lower margin of the lung. Large exudates on the right side force the diaphragm and the liver downward, the right lobe of the liver being dislocated more than the left. Left-sided exudates change the position of the left lobe, though to a lesser degree, the lower margin of the liver in this case running horizontally instead of diagonally across the abdomen. Pneumothorax, also, can produce a dislocation of the liver downward. At first the area of dulness is reduced in size; later, when the distention with air assumes greater proportions it is increased. In emphysema the liver also occupies a lower position than normal, but, owing to the retroversion which frequently occurs at the same time, the area of dulness is smaller than normal. In shrinkage of the right lung the liver is drawn upward and the area of dulness is somewhat enlarged.

Large pericardial exudates, and enlargement of the heart itself, may force the left lobe of the liver downward. As a rule, these lesions are

* Gerhardt, *Zeitschr. für klin. Medicin*, Bd. xxi, 1892, p. 374.
† Heitler, "Die Schwankungen der normalen Leber- und Milzdämpfung," *Wiener med. Wochenschr.*, 1892, No. 14.

accompanied by passive congestion of the liver, and in this manner produce an enlargement of the whole organ.

Inflammatory exudates occurring between the liver and the diaphragm (subphrenic abscess) force the liver downward and the diaphragm upward, and in this way may simulate either enlargement of the liver or pleuritic exudates.

The liver is more frequently dislocated downward than upward. The muscle of the diaphragm offers considerable resistance, and usually does not yield at all until increase of pressure within the abdominal cavity occurs, with distention of the whole abdomen as a result. The latter occurrence is usually combined with dilatation and change in the form of the lower thoracic aperture, so that the liver is placed more horizontally, and the area of absolute dulness is diminished. As a rule, this area is rather difficult to determine. In the case of ascites this difficulty is due to the general dulness; in the case of meteorism, to the loud tympanitic sound.

Finally, a decrease in the liver dulness can be produced by the (rather rare) entrance of air between the liver and the anterior abdominal wall, or by the intervention of the transverse colon or loops of small intestine between the liver and the abdominal wall. The latter accident occurs chiefly in enteroptosis and in general relaxation of the abdominal walls. As a rule, the true shape of the liver can still be determined by repeated examinations, particularly if the patient be placed on the right side or flat on his back, with depressed shoulders.

CHANGES IN FORM. (CORSET LIVER.)

The substance of the liver is ordinarily soft and plastic during life, although we usually see the organ after death, when postmortem changes have hardened it. The physiologic shape of the organ, therefore, is largely determined by the mould of neighboring organs, particularly of the muscular and bony tissues. In the case of the liver more than in the case of any other organ the general outline is dependent in each individual on the shape of the thorax and the body generally. All pathologic changes in its surroundings produce considerable deviations from its normal form. For instance, scoliosis, tumors, or exudates that press upon the organ from above, from the side, or from below, may change its shape. As a rule, these deforming influences are permanent; where they are only transitory, —as, for instance, in large pleuritic exudates or in subphrenic abscesses,— the plasticity of the liver tissue favors the establishment of the original shape. Tumors within the liver that do not change its substance but act mechanically—as, for instance, echinoccocus—may also produce displacement of liver-substance and a change in the normal form of the organ.

In the opposite sense, the relaxation of pressure normally exercised on the surface of the liver may produce extensions of the liver-substance, so-called ectases of the liver. For instance, a hole in the diaphragm (Klebs *) or a hernial opening of the linea alba (Kusmin) may permit of such protrusions.

For completeness' sake the change of form that is seen in transposition of the viscera must be mentioned. In this anomaly the shape of the liver is the reverse of the normal.

Furrows are occasionally found upon the convex surface of the liver, which are produced by pressure of the ribs. Frequently the serous mem-

* *Virchow's Archiv,* Bd. XXXIII, p. 446.

brane over these furrows is slightly thickened. On the convex surface of the right lobe of the liver deep, narrow furrows, called longitudinal or expiration furrows, are occasionally found running parallel to the suspensory ligament. They probably owe their origin to a lateral compression of the liver which occurs when the diaphragm is contracted and the abdominal muscles (particularly when the clothing is too tight) compress the organ. These changes in the form of the liver are not recognizable during life.

Of the acquired changes of form, that variety which is called **" corset liver"** is of considerable pathologic and clinical· importance. This deformity is not produced by lacing alone, but may be the result of wearing various kinds of tight-fitting clothing, particularly at a time of life when the body is not yet developed and the thorax is soft and pliable. In order to exercise their effect, these influences must, of course, act for a long time. Among the causes of the condition there may be mentioned here the use of corsets of various degrees of stiffness, softer bodies made of cloth, tight waists, either buttoned or laced, skirt-bands, belts, and straps. These articles of apparel influence the shape of the liver only in small part through the abdominal walls. In much greater part they act through pressure on the ribs and cartilages, by modifying the relative position of these parts and retarding their growth. In this way these irrational methods of dressing continue to exercise a pernicious effect for a long time after they have been discarded, and consequently produce permanent, irreparable, and sometimes progressive damage.

Corset liver is naturally found chiefly in women, not only in those who wear corsets, but also in peasant women who wear waists and skirt-bands.

According to the conventional custom, artificial deformation of the body begins with confirmation; that is, at about the fourteenth year, rarely sooner.

According to the tabulations of Leue, based upon 3484 autopsies on subjects above sixteen years of age, corset liver was found in 1.9% of male bodies and 25.3% of female bodies. If changes of high degree are not considered alone, but also those changes that are barely recognizable, but can unquestionably be attributed to the effect of lacing upon the liver, it will be found that 5.7% occur in men, 56.3% in women. The percentage increases, with the increasing age of the subject, from 2% to 73%.

The deformities of the thorax and the liver that result from irrational clothing show wide variations. A great deal will depend on whether the pressure was exercised in a narrow or a wide zone, high up or low down. In the same individuals, in addition, the pressure may be exercised in different parts of the body in the course of many years, as the subjects change the style of their clothing with the changes of fashion. It is possible to distinguish four types, which, it is true, may merge into one another.

First, *low waist,* a very narrow ring underneath the costal arch; in still more marked cases a slight change of the costal angle and a slight inversion of the lower margin of the thorax. Here the liver is contracted only near the lower margin of the right lobe, and its sharp edge is somewhat atrophic and the serous covering thickened.

Second, *medium waist.* The narrowest place is found below the xiphoid process; the costal arches are somewhat ectopic.

Third, *high waist.* The narrowest point is at the level of the xiphoid process. Owing to the ectopic position of the costal arches the thorax assumes an hour-glass form.

Fourth, *cylindric-paralytic contracted thorax.* This form is produced by tight waists or cylindric corsets without any waist-line.

In the last form the lower part of the thoracic aperture is uniformly narrowed, the thoracic walls are thus pressed against the liver, and the organ is uniformly elongated so that the right lobe assumes a tongue-shaped form. On the other hand, in the narrow high waist (third type) only the upper part of the liver is compressed, so that the upper part of the growing organ is, so to speak, pressed into the substance of the lower part of the right lobe. In this manner the lower portion of the liver grows longer, wider, and thicker, really hypertrophic, assuming in some cases a cake-shaped or hemispheric outline. In the medium waist (second type) the greatest pressure is exercised lower down, so that the portion of the liver that is pressed downward is not so bulky. It is frequently separated from the upper part by a broad furrow running horizontally or diagonally across the organ.

The liver, elongated from narrowing of the thorax, usually protrudes considerably below the costal arch, so that, as a rule, the organ can be readily percussed and palpated, and its form determined. This is particularly easy because the muscular walls and the adipose tissue become somewhat atrophic from the pressure.

If pressure is continued for a long time the costal arch may be so forced into the liver-substance as to cause it to atrophy. In the same manner narrow and very tight skirt-bands act on the elongated lobe of the liver so that the bridge between the main mass of the liver and the lower part of the right lobe becomes thinner than the lobe. Ultimately this connecting band may become so attenuated that it forms merely a thin strip containing no liver-substance whatever, but only blood-vessels and bile-ducts. Frequently, before attenuation occurs to such a degree, pressure on the most contracted part of the liver has caused stasis of blood or of bile in the separated lobe, and so causes the latter to increase in size.

Those portions of the liver that are exposed to permanent pressure usually show changes of the serous covering ranging from a slight clouding to fibrous thickening. As a rule, the callosities run horizontally or approximately so, but they may bisect the anterior surface of the liver in different places from the lower margin of the right lobe up to the middle of the left. Rarely, a piece of the lower margin of the left lobe may become separated from lacing.

We see, therefore, that the changes in the form of the liver that may be produced by the pressure of the clothing are of varying kind and of varying degree. Diffuse pressure produces an elongation of the liver and a folding inward of its convex surface; local pressure (frequently transmitted by the costal arch) produces local atrophy from pressure, and perihepatitis.

Frequently inflammatory processes that originate in the serous part of the compressed surface may extend, and lead to adhesions with the abdominal wall or to thickening of the capsule.

With elongation of the right lobe the biliary channels situated on the lower surface, particularly the gall-bladder, are also elongated, so that, frequently, by indirect compression of the cystic duct, the flow of bile is prevented, and dilatation or catarrh of the gall-bladder results, or, later, concretions may form.

Symptoms.—A corset liver may exist without causing any symptoms, and usually the condition is discovered only when the abdomen is examined for some other reason. In rare cases the separated lobe causes symptoms through its volume, through pressure upon neighboring organs, or through its motility. Such symptoms may be transitory if the separated lobe becomes swollen or painful through stasis or inflammation. The rare cases of separation of a portion of the left lobe are said by Langenbuch to cause more marked symptoms.

Elongation of the liver frequently simulates enlargement of the organ. The preponderating elongation of the right lobe in corset liver is of value in differentiating the two conditions. At the same time one should remember that it is more difficult to form a precise opinion in regard to the degree of enlargement of the liver in women than in men.

In addition to being changed in form, the corset liver is of increased consistency. This is due in part to a local increase in the hepatic parenchyma, in part also to the perihepatitis and passive hyperemia often observed in the separated lobe. If the separation is very marked, the lobe will appear like a tumor that has no connection with the liver, but seems to be connected with some other organ, such as the intestine, the kidney, the ovary, or the mesentery. If the separation is not so far advanced, and if there are no adhesions, the movements of the tumor with the phases of respiration will usually facilitate the recognition of its hepatic origin.

The **diagnosis** is most difficult in those cases in which the separated lobe is joined to the liver by a narrow bridge of connective tissue. In such instances the lobe may be movable toward both sides as well as anteroposteriorly, or it may drop downward and become covered by the intestine. To arrive at a positive conclusion as to its nature, the growth must be examined several times and under different conditions (for instance, after distention of the stomach and intestine with gas). In a case of this kind the swelling may be confounded with floating kidney. It is well to remember that, notwithstanding the motility of the lobe of the liver, this can be palpated better through the anterior abdominal wall, whereas the kidney can be reached much more readily through the lumbar region; and, further, that the distended ascending and the transverse colon are situated between these two organs.

The diagnosis is particularly difficult if other pathologic conditions develop on the basis of a corset liver. This occurs quite frequently, for the reason that the primary cause,—*i. e.*, lacing,—in addition to producing deformities of the liver, causes a large number of disturbances in other organs, so that we are almost justified in speaking of a corset disease. Some of the lesions of this condition are the formation of gall-stones, with colic, inflammation and carcinoma of the gall-bladder, distention of the gall-bladder, and perihepatitis. The latter may originate partly from the gall-bladder, partly from the lacing furrow. The effect of lacing on the thoracic organs is to produce moderate degrees of passive congestion, and as a result enlargement of the whole organ.

Other organs of the upper part of the abdominal cavity may be affected by lacing as follows: Abnormal motility and dislocation of the right kidney, ptosis of the stomach and of the transverse colon, cardialgia, ulcer of the stomach, diffuse stasis in the portal system as a result of the compression of the liver, and, following this portal stasis, intestinal catarrh, hemorrhoids, attacks of colic, and constipation. The latter is particularly favored by the direct pressure that is exercised on the ascending and descending colon, particularly in the type of low waists. Compression of the upper part of the abdominal cavity causes a dislocation of its entire contents. This results in an abnormal distention of the abdominal walls below the umbilicus, and, if certain other conditions prevail, may lead to pendulous abdomen.

It is true that of all these possible consequences of lacing only one may develop fully, so that it may happen that while pronounced changes are present in other organs, no lesion of the liver is discoverable during life. It is important, however, from a clinical and diagnostic point of view to remember the common cause of all these disturbances. An abnormal shape of the liver and deformity of the thorax, even though other symptoms are not present, frequently give us valuable clues in diagnosticating and treating abdominal diseases. This obtains even when tight clothing has been discarded long before.

A corset liver, no longer in an active stage of development, or secondarily involved, may lead to confusion in the presence of other pathologic conditions and render the diagnosis more difficult. Among such conditions might be mentioned tumors of the kidney and of the suprarenals, psoas abscess, typhlitis, coprostasis, and inflammations in the region of the hepatic flexure of the colon. It is frequently impossible to arrive at a definite conclusion in regard to the presence or absence of one or the other of these diseases or in regard to the presence or absence of contracted liver, until the sensitiveness and inflammation in the region of the liver have so decreased that the different parts of the tumor may be palpated and differentiated.

As mentioned above, the right lobe of the liver is usually considerably elongated downward. If a certain portion of the lower margin should be isolated by indentation, this may become still more elongated, and extend downward in the shape of a tongue; such tongue-shaped processes are found with great frequency in the region of the gall-bladder, particularly toward the right. If the gall-bladder also enlarges, such a process becomes still more elongated, and, if it becomes inflamed, will become enlarged. A number of surgeons, particularly Riedel, have called attention to the difficulty that such a tongue-shaped process may cause in the diagnosis of gall-bladder diseases, and in operative procedures in diseases of this organ. [It is rather remarkable that such tongue-like processes are seldom felt in routine examinations of cases unless hepatic trouble calls particular attention to the liver.—Ed.]

The milder degrees of the stationary corset liver do not call for any **treatment.** The complications arising from this condition, however, must be attended to, particularly perihepatitis, passive congestion, and the various troubles due to gall-stones. In practice it is frequently impossible to differentiate between these conditions and the other sequels of lacing, and the whole complex picture must therefore be treated together. The measures of treatment that are to be considered in this connection are a simple and non-irritating diet, a daily evacuation, courses of saline mineral water or of those containing chlorids, and the support of the relaxed abdominal walls and the displaced intestine by a bandage or a band applied below the umbilicus. If the separated lobe of the liver extends very far downward and is very sensitive, it is impossible to apply any but a soft elastic bandage. In such cases a supporting pad (Landau) is more agreeable, and is very appropriate, for the reason that such an appliance exercises pressure which is more firm and is limited to the lower half of the abdomen.

In cases in which indirect support of a corset liver did not relieve the disturbances. Billroth and others have opened the abdominal cavity, and have attached the•separated lobe to the anterior abdominal wall by sutures passed through the calloused part of the lobe. Langenbuch in one case ablated a separated lobe of the left side that was causing much disturbance. Such a procedure will be found to be easy if much of the liver-substance has disappeared from the contracted furrow.

The most important duty of the physician in regard to the condition under discussion is its prevention. However great the fear of tradition and of fashion, the chances of success in this direction are not bad. Formerly physicians believed deformities of the liver alone were the result of lacing, but nowadays we know that numerous diseases involving other abdominal organs, in addition to the liver, may be the result of tight clothing. This knowledge has only been acquired within the last decade and will have to be gradually communicated to the laity by physicians. Even now many women follow the advice given, and the number will increase as the good effect of rational clothing becomes more apparent.

It is necessary not only to combat the corset, but all forms of tight clothing, such as waist- and skirt-bands. Such articles of clothing are particularly detrimental while the body is in the stage of development, especially if the muscles are weak and the bones soft. The powers of resistance against the damages of lacing are not dependent on a definite age, but on the period of life in which development of the body is completed, which, as we know, varies in different individuals.

Particular attention should be paid, primarily, to the size of the waist that is worn. This should permit free respiratory movements. Further, a decrease in the weight of the clothing worn on the lower half of the body should be insisted upon (bloomers instead of skirts, and loose, adaptable materials), or the clothing should be attached to the shoulders by broad or conical straps.*

The various articles of clothing that have been recommended by physicians and manufacturers, so-called "health corsets," etc., only in part comply with the demands. The American corset seems the most practical, as it consists of a well-modeled underwaist made of some resisting material, with broad shoulder-pieces, to which the garments of the lower half of the body are attached by buttons. These corsets have a few flexible whalebones that are to be removed in laundering.

CHANGES IN POSITION.

We have already mentioned some of the moderate changes in the position of the liver that may occur: viz., rotation around the horizontal axis (retroversion and anteversion) and dislocation produced by diseases of neighboring organs. The latter usually occur downward, and may in some instances be remedied; it will depend on the primary cause of the trouble whether this is possible or not.

FLOATING LIVER.

Hepar mobilis s. migrans; Hepatoptosis; Descensus hepatis; Foie flottant; Wanderleber.

This consists of a marked displacement of the liver, together with abnormal mobility. The liver is anchored in its normal position in the concavity of the diaphragm by several peritoneal folds: viz., (1) The

* Spener, "Die jetzige Frauenkleidung," Berlin, Walther, 1897, und *Deutsche med. Wochenschr.*, 1897, No. 1.

coronary ligament, originating from two flat peritoneal folds on the posterior surface of the liver that are occasionally in contact with each other, forming a very short and tense mesentery, or, more frequently, leaving uncovered a portion of the liver surface, as broad as several fingers. To the right and left these ligaments separate and form the so-called triangular ligaments.   (2) The suspensory ligament, a long reduplication of the peritoneum running from the diaphragm to the convex surface of the liver.   It is attached at the porta hepatis and, together with the ligamentum teres, extends to the umbilicus.   The liver is further attached to the spinal column and the diaphragm by the inferior vena cava, which is usually embedded in the posterior margin of the liver, but is often completely surrounded by liver-substance.

The connective-tissue strands that run through these ligaments would alone not be capable of supporting the large gland weighing 1500 gm. They in fact chiefly fulfil the purpose of preventing lateral displacement. The liver is really supported by the elasticity and tone of the abdominal walls, assisted by the stomach and intestine, which support it from below like air-cushions.   In addition, the elastic traction of the lungs that maintains the vault of the diaphragm, and the cohesion of the convexity of the liver with the diaphragm (preventing the separation of the two serous surfaces and still permitting a gliding movement), are factors in supporting the liver.   The ligaments simply circumscribe lateral movements.   (Atmospheric pressure has as little to do with the support of the liver as it has with the fixation of the femur in the hip-joint.)

All these factors combine to prevent the separation of the liver and the diaphragm, so that they nearly always remain in contact.   If they are separated at all, it is only by a small space.   Slight degrees of descent of the liver occur in ascites, in which a layer of fluid, that may be several centimeters thick, may force its way between the liver, on the one hand, and the diaphragm and the abdominal wall, on the other.   Greater degrees of descent are possible only if the above-mentioned suspensory ligaments become elongated.   When this occurs, the liver may sink below the costal arch, even as far as the symphysis pubis, and fluid, tumors, or coils of intestine, particularly of the transverse colon, may occupy the place of the liver in the right vault of the diaphragm.   Owing to the attachment of the ligamentum teres to the umbilicus, descent of the liver is usually combined with rotation of the organ, the right lobe thereby occupying the lowest position. Usually ptosis of the liver is combined with great motility of the organ, so that by pressure from without and changes in the position of the body it may be possible, in part or completely, to replace it in its normal position.

Frequency of Occurrence and Causes.—The highest degree of abnormal motility, floating liver proper, is not frequently seen.   Cantani first described it in 1866, and since then it has been more frequently observed. It is found principally in women (approximately in the proportion of ten to one as compared with men).   The chief cause is the relaxation and attenuation of the abdominal walls, so-called pendulous abdomen, usually following repeated pregnancies, particularly if the patient has gotten up too soon.   The condition is usually combined with separation of the abdominal muscles.   As a result of these causes the intestines drop forward and downward, and in this manner the liver is deprived of one of its normal supports.   Large hernias may act similarly, even without stretching of the abdominal walls, particularly if the hernial sac incloses many coils of intestine.   Another mechanical factor must be considered in pendulous abdomen—*i. e.*, the direct traction that the abdominal walls exercise on the liver through the umbilicus and the ligamentum teres (Landau, Langenbuch).

Other favoring circumstances are the following: Violent exertion, persistent vomiting (Rosenkranz), coughing or sneezing (Landau), and acute mechanical influences, such as a fall or sudden violent exertion. In a case described by Leube distention of the inferior vena cava following tricuspid insufficiency seems to have loosened the attachments of the liver. Stretching of the ligaments of the liver from a swelling of the organ that later recedes may also in some instances permit greater excursions of the liver.   Lacing and rapid emaciation are only occasionally mentioned as causes; but they certainly have some influence, particularly when they are responsible for the relaxation of the abdominal walls.

As the rare occurrence of floating liver is in contrast to the frequency with which the above-mentioned etiologic factors are present, we must conclude that in certain individuals some particular conditions must assist.   Most probably a congenital tendency to relaxation and stretching of the ligaments of the liver must exist, of the same kind as that which makes the formation of a true mesohepar possible.   It has not been demonstrated so far whether the latter is congenital or preformed.

Symptoms.—A floating liver forms a tumor in the right side of the abdomen, sometimes extending as far as the symphysis.   Its convex surface is directed forward.   It is usually possible to determine the hepatic outline by palpation, and this is facilitated further by the flaccid character of the abdominal walls.   If lacing has been indulged in the form of the liver is frequently changed.   In the erect and semi-recumbent positions the liver is low down in the abdomen, while in the dorsal position it is usually possible to replace the liver by manual pressure.   In doing this the previously sunken epigastrium becomes filled out and the normal area of hepatic dulness is restored.   When the liver is absent from its normal place, the percussion sound of the lung merges directly into that of the intestine.   It is rare to find a dislocated liver attached in an abnormal position by adhesions (Richelot).   If this is the case, it can, of course, only partly be replaced.

Pressure exercised over the dislocated liver is usually not painful, but frequently produces sensations in remote parts.   A floating liver may also cause spontaneous pain, particularly when its weight exercises a great degree of traction or when the traction that existed is suddenly increased, as, for instance, in jumping, walking, raising the arms (particularly the right one), sneezing, coughing, and yawning. Sometimes the pain becomes paroxysmally exacerbated without any visible cause. Pain is usually relieved by manual or other fixation of the tumor, by sitting down, or by assuming the dorsal position or a position on the right side. · The pain is felt in the right hypochondriac region and the epigastrium, and frequently radiates toward the right shoulder and the lumbar region.   A feeling of bearing-down and of colicky pains may arise, while occasionally intestinal disturbances, or a feeling of fulness or of some living thing in the abdomen, may be complained of.   Fainting spells may occur.

In addition, numerous disturbances of the digestive tract are noticed, such as various gastric disturbances, belching, meteorism, and constipation.   These are explained by traction upon and temporary occlusion of the intestine. Respiratory disturbances and palpitation must be attributed to dragging upon the diaphragm. Occasionally symptoms of portal stasis are noticed, such as ascites, hemorrhoids, metrorrhagia, or, as a result of the twisting of the vena cava, edema of the lower extremities. [Albuminuria, increase in the quantity of the urine, and purpura are also seen at times.—Ed.] Icterus is rare, although this symptom might be expected as a result of the traction exercised on the biliary passages. A slight sub-icteric color is sometimes observed. [Mac-Naughton Jones has reported a case of recurring hemorrhage from the stomach apparently due to ptosis of the liver.—Ed.]

Diagnosis.—The diagnosis of floating liver may be difficult at first, as the unusual size of the palpable tumor is startling. In general, however, the relaxation of the abdominal walls permits an accurate determination of the outline of the tumor by bimanual palpation, and the area of hepatic dulness is not found in the normal place. The most important diagnostic sign is the possibility of replacing the tumor into the region where the liver normally belongs; this is particularly easy if the patient is placed in the horizontal position. If the manœuver succeeds, the normal area of hepatic dulness will return.

The descended liver will always appear larger than normal, even though no pathologic enlargement exists. This is due to the fact that it presents for palpation a larger surface than normal.

The diagnosis of floating liver is particularly difficult if ascites exists. At the same time, the presence of fluid within the abdomen makes palpation very difficult and, in addition, we are deprived of the knowledge derived from the area of hepatic dulness. In such cases puncture may be necessary in order to assist the diagnosis.

In an oft-quoted case reported by P. Müller, a peculiarly shaped and thickened mesentery was erroneously taken for a floating liver. In this case ascites existed and the liver was forced upward considerably, so that hepatic dulness was absent from the normal place. The fact that the apparently dislocated liver could not be replaced in its normal position had not been considered. It is also possible for the dislocated liver to become adherent, and in this way the diagnosis may be made very uncertain. [The misplaced liver has been mistaken for hydronephrosis (Peters), floating kidney (Terrier and Baudonin), renal tumor, and typhlitis (Richelot), the error being discovered at operation.—Ed.]

Treatment.—Replacement of the liver in its normal position can never be performed directly, but only indirectly through the agency of the abdominal organs. It may be brought about by applying an elastic abdominal bandage which replaces the tone of the abdominal wall, or by shortening the stretched abdominal wall by excising a wedge-shaped piece in the region of the linea alba and sewing the abdominal walls together. Kispert proposed fixation of the liver by stitching, and tried it several times. Langenbuch has selected the lower costal cartilages as the line of fixation. All the other accompanying symptoms and sequels of floating liver must of course be treated.

Prophylaxis can accomplish a great deal. The chief indication is to prevent the development of a pendulous abdomen and pathologic enlargement of the abdominal cavity immediately after pregnancy by the employment of faradization, massage, and douches. On the other hand, a re-establishment of normal abdominal dimensions and tone may be temporarily aided by the application of a suitable abdominal bandage [and by abdominal exercises. The "straight-faced corset," advocated for the relief of floating kidney, is usually more convenient and effectual than the elastic bandage. The production of adhesions between the convexity of the liver and the dome of the diaphragm by irritation of their surfaces, as in Talma's operation for the relief of ascites, might be of value in conjunction with the other methods mentioned. It has been suggested that the liver may be held in position by suturing the fundus of the gall-bladder to the parietal peritoneum.—ED.]

LITERATURE.

GENERAL WORKS ON DISEASES OF THE LIVER.

Budd, G.: "On Diseases of the Liver," London, 1845.
Charcot, F. M.: "Leçons sur les maladies des foie," Paris, 1877.
Chauffard, A.: in Charcot, Bouchard et Brissaud's "Traité de médecine," 1892, tome III, p. 663.
Dupré, F., in "Manuel de médecine" of Debove und Achard, 1895, tome VI.
Frerichs: "Klinik der Leberkrankheiten," 2 Aufl., 1861.
Harley, G.: "Diseases of the Liver."
Langenbuch, C.: "Chirurgie der Leber und Gallenwege," Stuttgart, 1894, 1897.
Leichtenstern in Penzoldt und Stintzing's "Handbuch der speciellen Therapie," Bd. IV, Abtheilung 6b, p. 138.
Murchison: "Clinical Lectures on Diseases of the Liver," London, 1877.
Thierfelder, Ponfick, Leichtenstern und Schüppel in v. Ziemssen's "Handbuch der speciellen Pathologie," Bd. VIII, 1880.
Text-books on Pathologic Anatomy by Birch-Hirschfeld, Klebs, Orth, and Ziegler.

CORSET LIVER.

Böttcher: "Virchow's Archiv," Bd. XXXIV, 1865, Taf. II.
Frerichs: loc. cit., I, p. 47, with illustrations.
Hackmann, K.: "Schnürwirkungen," Dissertation, Kiel, 1894.
Hayem: "Maladie du Corset," "Archives générales de médecine," II, p. 169, 1895.
Hertz: "Abnormitäten in der Lage und Form der Bauchorgane, etc.," Berlin, 1894.
Langenbuch: loc. cit., II, p. 107; "Berliner klin. Wochenschr.," No. 3, 1888.
Lene, E.: "Ueber die Häufigkeit der Schnürleber," Dissertation, Kiel, 1891.
Riedel: "Ueber den zungenförmigen Fortsatz des Leberlappens," etc., "Berliner klin. Wochenschrift," 1888, pp. 577, 602.
Spener: "Die jetzige Frauenkleidung," Berlin, Walther, 1897.
— "Deutsche med. Wochenschr.," No. 1, 1897.
Thierfelder, p. 37. Klebs, p. 361.
"Mittheilungen des Vereines für Verbesserung der Frauenkleidung," Berlin, 1897.

FLOATING LIVER.

Cantani: "Schmidt's Jahrbücher," Bd. CXLI, p. 107, 1866.
Curtius: "Symptome und Aetiologie der Wanderleber," Dissertation, Halle, 1889.
Dolozynski: "Virchow-Hirsch's Jahresbericht," II, p. 218, 1894.
Faure: "L'appareil suspenseur du foie," etc., Thèse, Paris, 1892.
Kispert: "Berliner klin. Wochenschr.," p. 372, 1884.
Kranold: "Württemberger med. Correspondenzblatt," Nos. 21, 22, Bericht II, p. 200, 1884 (Section).
Landau, L.: "Die Wanderleber und der Hängebauch der Frauen," Berlin, 1885 (45 Fälle, Literatur), "Deutsche med. Wochenschr.," p. 754, 1885.
Langenbuch: loc. cit., p. 119.
— "Berliner klin. Wochenschr.," No. 13, 1889.
— "Deutsche med. Wochenschr.," No. 52, 1890.
Leube: "Würzburger Sitzungsberichte," p. 100, 1893.
— "Münchener med. Wochenschr.," No. 4, 1894 (Postmortem).
Müller, P.: "Zur Diagnose der Wanderleber," "Deutsches Archiv für klin. Medicin," Bd. XIV, 1875.
Richelot: "Fixation d'un foie déplacé," "Gazette des hôpitaux," No. 22, 1893, Bericht II, 261.
Rosenkranz: Ibid., . 714. 1887.
Thierfelder: loc. citp p. 42.
Wolff, G.: "Enteroptose und Wanderleber," Dissertation, Leipzig, 1896 (Literature).

2. GENERAL PATHOLOGY AND PHYSIOLOGY OF THE LIVER.

Our knowledge of the normal function of the liver has been increased by the study of a number of morbid conditions of this organ. The liver is larger than the other abdominal organs, and consequently any abnormality in its consistency is the more readily detected. Considerable pathologic significance has always been attached to such changes, and the exact interpretation of these various lesions was for a long time very inaccurate. In many instances an explanation was artificially constructed and based on preconceived ideas. Above all, the more apparent changes in the amount of blood and of fat that the organ contained were credited with an exaggerated significance. The liver was looked upon as the organ in which blood was formed from the chyme, in which the veins originated, and in which the body-heat was generated.

These various assumptions as to the significance of the liver in pathology were disproved by closer criticism, and, following the example of Bartholinus, it was supposed that the only function of the liver was the manufacture of bile, disturbance of that function causing the conspicuous symptom of jaundice. The same confusion in regard to function that existed in the case of the liver obtained in the case of the bile. All diseases that were complicated by jaundice were declared to be "bilious" in character and due to some deep-seated lesion. These "bilious" disturbances with participation of the liver are, even nowadays, a part of the pathologic teachings and views of many physicians, and in particular of the laity; more so in England and America than in Germany.* Such views, however unfounded, fantastic, and entirely wrong they may have been, at the same time incorporated a correct idea. They signified that so important, so large, and so peculiarly constructed an organ as the liver, at all events had some other function besides the excretion of bile. Magendie and Tiedemann experimentally determined its function of assimilating certain constituents of the food. Claude Bernard and Hensen discovered glycogen in the liver and thereby established its relation to carbohydrate metabolism. Other observations, such as the occurrence of fatty liver after forced feeding, had previously made it probable that the liver had something to do with metabolism, but the discovery of the glycogenic function of the liver was the first exact demonstration of the fact that a gland, aside from forming an external secretion, could also manufacture a number of substances that returned into the general circulation and might play an important rôle in the nutrition of the general organism. The researches of the last few years have demonstrated that a number of other glands have the function of producing both internal and external secretions.

It must be remembered, at the same time, that the function we designate by these terms was not completely unknown and unrecognized up to that time. It was known of every organ that it not only absorbed substances from the tissue-juices, but also poured substances into them. As a rule, it is true, these substances were regarded as excretions, and were not credited with any further significance in the economy. I will only mention the muscles, among other parenchymatous

* This statement can hardly be considered entirely justified at the present time.—ED.

organs, that secrete lactic acid, and carcinomata, that pour into the general circulation substances capable of influencing metabolism.

It is probable that the internal secretion of no other organ is of such importance for the body as is that of the liver, and even to-day we are not able to estimate the true extent of its significance. There can be no doubt that its pathologic significance is far-reaching, more so than we can now appreciate. Particularly in the case of the liver is the close interdependence of internal and external secretion apparent, and we can readily observe in many lesions that an impediment in the outflow of the latter seriously interferes with the former.

ANATOMY AND HISTOLOGY.

We will limit ourselves to a brief review of the internal structure of the liver. The arrangement of the parenchyma is, to a large extent, dependent on the course of the numerous blood-vessels contained in the organ.* The large portal vein enters through the porta hepatis and ramifies into numerous branches and capillaries that are ultimately reunited to form the numerous hepatic veins which leave the organ at its posterior margin and empty directly into the inferior vena cava, while the branches of the hepatic vein of the liver are separated from the adjacent parenchyma by a very thin wall. The portal vein and its branches, on the other hand, are accompanied along their whole course by a connective-tissue sheath called Glisson's capsule. Within this capsule are also found the hepatic artery, the bile-ducts, the lymph-vessels, and the nerves corresponding to the course of the vessels. Certain areas are visibly outlined within the liver, forming the lobules. These measure from 1 to 1.5 mm. in diameter. Seen in sections, it will be found that each lobule has a small venous radicle in its center and that several branches of the portal vein and the hepatic artery enter it from the periphery. The capillary network within the lobule is arranged in such a manner that the different capillaries seem to radiate from the center and inclose the hepatic cells within its meshes, the latter thus also being arranged in radiating lines. These rows or columns of glandular tissue are unicellular in many animals (for example, the rabbit), but multicellular in man. From the interlobular biliary passages, with their gradually lessening wall of glandular tissue and cubical epithelium, the biliary capillaries originate and penetrate the lobules, dividing in such a manner that each one is separated from the corresponding blood-capillary by at least one liver-cell. According to older views, these form an anastomosing network; but according to Retzius, they do not anastomose, but run a tortuous course and give off many branches. Each of these finest passages seems to terminate within a liver-cell in a knob-shaped opening (the "secretion-vacuole" of Kupffer). In this way each liver-cell is in contact on one side with a bile-capillary, on the other with a blood-capillary.

According to Nauwerck † and others, the intracellular continuations of the bile-capillaries are in connection with an anastomosing network of capillaries surrounding the nucleus. This is particularly apparent in biliary stasis and after staining with saffranin. According to Fraser and Nauwerck, an intracellular network can also be demonstrated by injection of the artery. I am inclined to consider the

* A good diagram of the portal tree after Rix is given by Langenbuch, pp. 12, 13.

† Nauwerck, "Leberzellen und Gelbsucht," *Münchener med. Wochenschr.*, 1897, No. 2.

26

former network as more probably physiologic than the latter, and I think that it has not been clearly demonstrated that the two are not identical.

[Schaefer* has recently found in the protoplasm of the cells varicose canaliculi filled with material injected into the portal vein. Houser† has found and more definitely described the intracellular capillary network.—Ed.]

The nerve-fibers of the hepatic plexus are derived partly from the celiac plexus, partly from the vagus. They penetrate the liver together with the hepatic artery and ramify with it. Nothing definite is known in regard to their terminations.

According to Disse,‡ lymphatic vessels lined with endothelium can be seen after injection. They are seen both in Glisson's capsule, following the ramifications of the portal vein, and within the adventitia of the hepatic veins. They anastomose directly with one another, and are, furthermore, connected by lymph-channels that have no endothelial lining. The latter form sheaths around the blood-capillaries in the liver lobules, so that they are situated between the capillary walls and the liver-cells. They possess a membranous wall that is in direct contact with the liver-cells. These cells contain a relatively large, round nucleus, and, according to Disse, are identical with the stellate cells of Kupffer. Fibrillæ extend from these membranes and enter the rows of liver-cells, in this manner connecting the sheaths of the capillaries.

The liver-cells proper are constructed on the general type of epithelial cells. They have a long polygonal shape, varying during life. Their diameter is about 15 to 40 μ. They have a round nucleus from 4 to 12 μ in diameter. The appearance of the cells changes with the exercise of their physiologic function.§ During fasting each cell, like the whole liver, is smaller, the protoplasmic reticulum is narrower, and the granules embedded within it much finer. During digestion the appearance of the liver and of its individual cells changes in a different manner according to the kind of food that is ingested. After the ingestion of albuminous food the liver becomes more vascular, but remains hard and resistant, while its cells are larger than during fasting and the fine granules within the protoplasm are more numerous. After carbohydrate feeding the liver enlarges more than after proteid ingestion, while at the same time it grows softer, more friable, and grayish-yellow, and its capillaries become compressed owing to the enlargement of the liver-cells. The latter contain, inclosed in the meshes of their protoplasm, large masses of amorphous glycogen, staining with iodin. With both kinds of diet the changes in the liver-cells occur uniformly and in the same manner in the lobules of all portions.

On a fatty diet the liver also enlarges and assumes a whitish-yellow color. The fat is primarily deposited in the periphery of the lobules, and as a result the outlines of the different lobules become more clearly visible. Each cell contains the fat in the shape of minute droplets that later coalesce to form larger drops.

Sometimes the liver-cells, particularly those that are more centrally situated, contain a finely granular pigment of unknown constitution. A normal liver never contains bile-pigment.

According to Cavazzani,‖ experimental irritation of the celiac plexus causes a diminution in the size of the liver-cells and reduction of their glycogen. His experiments were made on dogs and rabbits. After the operation a decrease of the glycogen and an increase of the sugar within the liver can be chemically determined.

* *Anatom. Anzeiger*, 1902, Bd. xxi, pp. 18–20.
† *Science*, May 30, 1902, p. 874.
‡ J. Disse, "Ueber die Lymphbahnen der Säugethierleber," *Archiv für mikroskopische Anatomie*, 1890, Bd. xxxvi, p. 203. (Gives the earlier literature.)
§ Heidenhain, Hermann's "Handbuch der Physiologie," Bd. v, 1, p. 221. Affanassiew, *Pflüger's Archiv*, 1883, Bd. xxx, p. 385.
‖ Cavazzani, *Pflüger's Archiv*, 1894, Bd. lvii, p. 181.

Changes in the liver-cells have also been observed after the administration of certain drugs. Thus Iwanow * found an enlargement, later a diminution, in the size of the nucleus in frogs after the administration of antipyrin, the enlargement being accompanied by a loss of chromatin and changèd staining qualities of the protoplasm. Neumann † found in mice the cells very small after phloridzin, very large after administering cocain, cumarin, and in mouse septicemia. (For the influence of various poisons on the glycogen and fat in the liver see below.)

The circulation of the blood within the liver is remarkable because of certain peculiarities in the arrangement of the blood-vessels and the enormous development of the capillary network. The blood-pressure in the main vessel that carries the blood to the liver, the portal vein, is less than in the arteries of the organ. Thus, v. Basch ‡ found the blood-pressure in a dog whose splanchnic nerve had been severed to be from 7 to 16 mm. Hg; Heidenhain § found 5.2 to 7.2 mm. ($\frac{1}{2}$ to $\frac{1}{3}$ of the bile-pressure); while J. Munk ‖ found 26 to 30 mm. if he allowed a soap solution to flow into the liver at the same time. The pressure will vary much according to the amount of blood present, the state of the portal capillaries, and the resistance within the liver itself.

[Sérégé,** by an interesting series of experimental, clinical, and patho.ogic observations, as well as by certain facts derived from comparative anatomy, has shown that there are two distinct currents going to the right and to the left lobes of the liver through the portal vein, the one current being derived from the territory drained by the large mesenteric vein and proceeding to the right lobe of the liver; the other current representing the flow from the splenic and small mesenteric veins and going to the left lobe of the liver. Experimental investigation in animals by the injection of India ink into the two mesenteric veins confirmed the evidence of comparative and pathologic anatomy, while the freezing-point and specific gravity of the blood from the large mesenteric vein and the small mesenteric vein with the splenic differed sufficiently to agree with the view that there is a more or less complete separation of the two currents after their entrance into the portal trunk.—ED.]

I have succeeded in finding only an isolated statement in regard to the rapidity of the blood-flow. Cybulski †† found it to be from 2.4 to 2.7 c.c. per second in a small dog.

It is impossible to state, at present, what is the effect of the mixing of the arterial and portal blood upon the rapidity of the blood-flow in the capillaries. It is conceivable that the one might hinder or accelerate the other.‡‡

The action of the heart and the respiration are of great significance in

* Iwanow, *du Bois Reymond's Archiv,* 1887.
† A. Neumann, "Ueber den Einfluss von Giften auf die Grösse der Leberzellen," Dissertation, Berlin, 1888.
‡ v. Basch, "Arbeiten der physiologischen Anstalt in Leipzig," 1875, x, p. 253.
§ Heidenhain, Hermann's "Handbuch der Physiologie," v, p. 269.
‖ J. Munk, *Archiv für Anatomie und Physiologie,* physiologische Abtheilung, 1890, Supplement, p. 131.
** *Jour. de méd. de Bordeaux,* April 12, 1901.
†† Cybulski, quoted by Nencki, *Archiv für experimentelle Pathologie,* 1895, Bd. xxxvii, p. 39.
‡‡ Compare Gad, "Studien über die Beziehungen des Blutstroms in der Pfortader zum Blutstrom in der Leberarterie," Dissertation, Berlin, 1873. See also the section on Hyperemia of the Liver.

regard to the blood-current in the liver. The hepatic veins are, by these functions, subjected to a continuous and rhythmic suction that is increased by the pressure exercised upon the convex surface of the liver by the diaphragm during each inspiration.

It is probable (even if we cannot prove the assumption positively by measurement) that the blood flows more slowly through the capillaries of the liver than through the capillaries of any other region of the body. This is probably one of the reasons, though not the only one, why a large number of leucocytes are always found within the hepatic capillaries. It also explains why fine particles, like grains of cinnabar, malarial pigment, etc., are found either free or within the leucocytes in the hepatic capillaries. The same phenomenon is seen in the bone-marrow and in the spleen. Micro-organisms suspended in the blood are arrested in the liver in the same manner. From the capillaries, the fine granules enter Kupffer's stellate cells and the connective-tissue corpuscles of the periportal tissues.

The blood-current within the liver varies with the width of the afferent vessels and the nervous influences that govern this.

Köppe * has demonstrated in dogs that a well-developed muscular layer, that is found not only in the arteries but also in the portal vein, is responsible for these changes. The main branch has no valves and is equipped with an internal circular musculature and an external longitudinal layer of muscle-fibers. The branches within the liver have more of the longitudinal fibers, while in the extrahepatic branches coming from the intestine the circular fibers predominate. The latter are also found in the long and short intestinal veins that have no valves, while in the submucosa the veins have neither valves nor muscular fiber.

The vasoconstrictor nerves of the liver are derived from the celiac plexus through the splanchnic nerve. From the cord they enter the sympathetic in the region of the sixth dorsal to the second lumbar vertebræ on both the right and the left sides.

Section of the nerves of the liver produces hyperemia and enlargement of the organ, as well as edematous swelling of its interstitial tissue (Affanassiew †). Faradic irritation of the splanchnic nerve ‡ causes a diminution in the size of the organ from the influence upon the intrahepatic branches of both the portal vein and the hepatic artery as manifested by an increase of the blood-pressure within these vessels. Vasodilator fibers reach the hepatic vessels from the vagus.

That the smallest vessels of the liver are capable of independent contractions can be demonstrated by the fact that gently stroking the surface of the liver produces a fine, pale line, as happens in the skin under similar irritation (Vulpian §).

It is probable that the nerves derived from the splanchnic act not only on the vessels, but also on the liver-cells and the biliary secretion. (See Cavazzani above.)

The effect of Bernard's piqure is transmitted to the liver through nerves that pass through the cord and the sympathetic and reach the liver through the splanchnic nerves. The piqure produces hyperemia by an acceleration of the blood-current in the liver. It is probable that the liver-cells are directly influenced by this operation. ‖

It may be well in this place to discuss the remarkable power of regeneration possessed by the liver after removal of portions of the organ by operation. Ponfick instituted experiments in this direction on rabbits and dogs, and found that after

* Köppe, "Muskeln und Klappen in den Wurzeln der Pfortader," *Archiv für Anatomie und Physiologie*, physiologische Abtheilung, 1890, Supplement, p. 168.

† Affanassiew, *Pflüger's Archiv*, Bd. xxx, S. 419.

‡ François-Franck und Hallion, "Recherches expér. sur l'innervation vasoconstrictive du foie," *Archives de physiologie*, 1896, p. 908.

§ Cited by François-Franck.

‖ Langendorff, *Archiv für Anatomie und Physiologie*, physiologische Abtheilung, 1886, S. 274. Morat and Dufour, "Les nerfs glycosécréteurs," *Archives de physiologie*, 1894, p. 371

removal of one-fourth to one-half of the total mass, the remaining portion began to increase in size at the expiration of only a few days, at the same time growing more fragile, softer, and more vascular, resembling in the latter respect the spleen. The parenchyma itself, if empty of blood, appears lighter than normal, shiny, moist, and the outline of the lobules is not very distinct. The liver remnant increases for several weeks, so that finally the original bulk of the liver is attained, while in some cases an overcompensation occurs. This compensatory growth and enlargement occurs even after repeated ablation of pieces of the organ. The original shape of the liver, of course, does not return. The regenerated organ has a more plump shape which otherwise depends upon the location of the piece removed. The presence of other diseases does not seem to interfere with the regeneration of the liver.

Microscopic examination reveals that the increase in size is due to a swelling of the liver-cells followed by cell-division. The new cells are distributed diffusely but irregularly throughout the whole of each lobule, and by the end of the second week may outnumber the normal liver-cells. They are distinguished from the latter by their rounder form, by a larger nucleus and stronger affinity for stains. Some of them contain two nuclei, so that the division of their protoplasm seems to occur later. A proliferation of blood-capillaries proceeds with the cellular proliferation, the new capillaries varying in diameter and the lymph-channels surrounding them being in many places dilated. Owing to the proliferation of the hepatic cells and capillaries, the normal radiating type of vascularization within the individual lobules is converted into a cavernous one. Each individual lobule is increased, even to double its normal size, frequently altered in its structure, and furnishes small processes that, in their turn, possess their own central vein. Even the larger bile-vessels show proliferation in their epithelium and connective-tissue layer, but at no place lateral offshoots. The bile-capillaries no longer show the normal regular polygonal arrangement, but take an irregular, tortuous course corresponding to the new-formation of glandular cells.

The whole process constitutes a process of regeneration of such unusual extent that Ponfick has proposed the name re-creation for it. It is probably brought about by the reaction of the body to the functional disturbances following removal of parts of the liver, and is a conservative process.

A similar process seems to occur in human disease, as in multilocular echinococcus and in extensive localized syphilitic lesions.* It is possible, too, that the same obtains for the "nodular hepatitis" described by Sabourin and others. Hochhaus could not discover similar regenerative processes following local necroses of limited extent from cold. After a few hours, however, there occurred a determination of leucocytes into the marginal zone with a mitosis of the nuclei of the connective tissue structures in that region. [Similar attempts at regeneration are seen in certain cases of atrophy of the liver (Meder and Ibrahim). See the section on Atrophy of the Liver.—ED.]

[In spite of considerable discussion the significance and nature of the newly formed "bile-capillaries" seen in certain forms of hepatic cirrhosis are not as yet clearly determined.—ED.]

FUNCTIONS OF THE LIVER.

The most radical procedure advised for determining the hepatic function is—

Excluding the Action of the Liver.—The results of this procedure are complicated and not readily interpreted. Three experimental methods are possible: viz., extirpation, injury to the parenchyma by chemicals injected through the bile-passages, and interruption of the blood-supply. The last method is the oldest. In the earliest experiments the portal vein was ligated, and it was found that the animals rapidly died with a great decrease in the blood-pressure. Formerly it was thought that this was due to "bleeding to death into the portal vein" as a result of the excessive filling of the intestinal vessels with blood (Tappeiner). This view has never been proved, nor has the real cause of the phenomenon been discovered. Gradual occlusion of the portal vein did not lead to the desired goal, for the

---

* Virchow, *Virchow's Archiv*, Bd. xv, S. 281.

reason that the liver received blood from collateral paths (Oré). Von Schröder, later, combined ligation of the portal vein with conduction of its blood into the renal vein, and succeeded in keeping the animals alive in this manner for from one hour to an hour and a half.

Ligation of the hepatic artery also led to necrosis of the whole organ and the rapid death of the animal (Cohnheim and Litten). Ligation of the aorta below the diaphragm and occlusion of the vena cava above the hepatic vein (Bock and Hoffmann) caused death within less than an hour. Ligation of the celiac and mesenteric arteries (Slosse) permitted the animals to live for from five to fourteen hours, but did not completely exclude the establishment of a collateral circulation to the liver (in this case from the colon), nor did it exclude the possibility that decomposition within the intestine and its walls was in part responsible for some of the symptoms. Kaufmann, in order to do away with the latter possibility and thus remove any objections to the whole procedure that might be made on that score, at the same time extirpated the intestines tributary to the portal system.

All these procedures bring about the death of the animal within a few hours. Their life can be preserved for a longer period of time by making what is called an Eck fistula, by which the blood of the portal vein is carried through a permanent fistula into the inferior vena cava. Even after the establishment of such a fistula violent nervous manifestations, especially with a meat diet, endanger the life of the animal and may lead to its early death (Hahn, Massen, Nencki, Pawlow).

The first method of disconnecting the liver (by extirpation) frequently fails, because this proceeding is followed by the same complications as simple ligation of the portal vein. In amphibious animals and in birds this difficulty is not so great, because a communication between the portal and renal veins permits the flow of blood from the former to the vena cava. Extirpation of the liver, for this reason, has been frequently performed in frogs (J. Müller and others), pigeons (Stern), and ducks and geese (Naunyn and Minkowski). The frogs could be kept alive for days, the birds as long as twenty hours. Nencki and Pawlow finally performed extirpation of the liver in dogs after making an Eck's fistula and kept the animals alive for six hours.

The second method, chemical destruction of the hepatic parenchyma, consists in the injection of dilute acids into the bile-passages. E. Pick employed $\frac{1}{25}$ normal sulphuric acid solution with simultaneous ligation of the bile-duct; Denys and Stubbe used 2% to 5% acetic acid, which they injected into the bile-duct from the duodenum, thus allowing the bile-duct to remain patent afterward. Following these injections, wide-spread necrosis occurs, followed in from six to forty-eight hours by the death of the animal.

The results of these different procedures appear in a different manner and after varying periods of time on account of the various secondary results that are produced, particularly in regard to disturbances of circulation. As a rule, the length of life varies inversely with the degree of the exclusion of the liver. Severe nervous disturbances appear, such as apathy, increasing somnolence, and, frequently, premortal spasms. In animals with an Eck's fistula these symptoms are preceded by a period of excitation. Occasionally it is found that after the removal of the liver the formation of bile-pigment and of bile-acids stops, the blood loses its sugar, and less urea is formed and excreted than normally. Most investigators seem to be in doubt whether to attribute death to these perversions of metabolism or to poisons that are produced by other metabolic disturbances.

The organism can well tolerate the loss of part of the liver, as is shown by a variety of diseases in which parts of the liver are destroyed. Ponfick, in his experiments on rabbits, has demonstrated how far this tolerance goes. He was enabled to remove even half of the liver without permanently injuring the animals, which recovered completely and seemed to prosper. In favorable cases even two-thirds of the liver could be removed with impunity, particularly if the whole amount removed was not taken away at one sitting. Ablation of four-fifths of the organ caused death in less than sixteen hours. In one animal partial extirpation was performed at three sittings, the second one month, the third four months, after the first. The animal survived the last operation by two days and a half, although only 15% of the normal liver was left.

This tolerance is probably due to a compensatory increase of function in the remaining portion of the liver and is manifested by an enlargement of the remnant which occurs a few days after the operation. At the end of three weeks the enlargement is always quite pronounced, and in many cases progresses so far that the normal weight of the liver is reached or even exceeded (by as much as 29%). In one case the remnant had increased to double its size within five days (the remnant amounted to about 25%). We have already described the anatomy of this wonderful compensatory growth.

In those cases where the animals died and no direct results of the operation proper (embolus, inflammation, hemorrhage, etc.) caused death, the fatal issue must be attributed to a cessation of the hepatic function and the contraction of the vascular area. The latter effect also manifests itself in partial removals of hepatic tissue by the occurrence of hyperemia and hemorrhages within the intestine and stomach, particularly in their mucous membrane, and, further, by hemorrhagic exudation into the abdominal cavity. The colon never grows hyperemic, but the spleen, on the other hand, becomes very hyperemic and swells to twice its normal bulk. As a rule, these symptoms of stasis are most pronounced in larger extirpations, varying in degree, however, in different cases. They are most pronounced on the first day after the operation, much less so on the days following, and finally disappear altogether.

Diseases of the liver characterized by a slow or rapid destruction of parenchyma (acute atrophy or atrophic cirrhosis) corroborate, as we shall see below, the results of these experimental studies. In fact, these diseases were the direct incitement to the performing of experiments along these lines.

Extirpation of the liver gives us a general picture of the significance of the organ in general metabolism. Its true rôle can, however, be discovered only by analyzing the participation of the liver in the catabolism of the different groups of the constituents of the body. In the following a brief review of these processes is given.

Nitrogen Metabolism.—We know in regard to the part that the liver plays in nitrogen metabolism that it converts ammonia and allied substances into urea. This occurs on a large scale if ammonia in combination with carbon dioxid or oxidizable acids is artificially introduced (Hallervorden, Coranda, v. Schröder). Physiologically a large quantity of ammonia is carried to the liver by the portal vein. This ammonia is generated partly in the intestine, particularly after a meat diet, partly in the stomach and intestine from chemical processes that occur within the mucosa during the secretion of gastric and enteric juice (Nencki, Pawlow, and Zaleski). Disconnection of the liver increases the ammonia in the blood and the urine and decreases the excretion of urea in the urine (Slosse, Nencki, and Pawlow). According to Nencki, the material for the formation of urea is ammonium carbaminate, which is normally carried to the

liver.   In dogs with an Eck's fistula it is said to exercise a toxic effect and
to produce the spasms and other nervous phenomena (the latter is doubted
by Lieblein).   Nencki calls attention to the fact that the liver is probably
not the only place in which urea is formed.

In birds uric acid, which is the end-product of their nitrogen metab-
,olism and corresponds to urea in mammals, is also formed in the liver.
Following extirpation of the liver birds excrete only a small amount of
uric acid, and in its place a considerable quantity of ammonium lactate
(from 50% to 60% of the total nitrogen) (Minkowski).

The same thing occurs after the administration of urea, which normally increases
the formation of uric acid in birds.   Horbaczewski's synthetic production of uric
acid from ammonia and trichlorlactic acid makes it probable that uric acid is formed
within the body from lactic acid and ammonia.

The separation of ammonia from amido-acids that are administered can, at
all events, occur elsewhere than in the liver.   The excretion of urea is not markedly
changed in birds by extirpation of the liver.   Lieblein's observation on dogs, that
obliteration of liver-tissue is followed by an increased excretion of uric acid, can be
attributed to an excessive catabolism of the nuclei of the liver-cells.

In man a relative increase of the ammonia and a decrease of the urea (in
proportion to the total nitrogen) is occasionally found in acute and chronic
atrophy of the liver.   It seems natural to attribute this to a disturbance
of the urea-forming function of the liver.   According to Weintraud, however, this power seems to be preserved for a long time even in advanced
cirrhosis, and it is probable that some of the ammonia remains untrans-
formed only for the reason that it is needed to neutralize the abnormally
formed acids.

In a case of phosphorus-intoxication, Munzer could decrease the am-
monia-nitrogen from 16.6% to 6.2% by administering bicarbonate of
sodium.   Engelmann and Minkowski also succeeded in decreasing the
excretion of ammonia in geese whose livers had been extirpated, by giving
bicarbonate of sodium.   As, however, the quantity of uric acid was not
increased, the disturbance of uric acid formation following the extirpation
cannot be attributed to a binding of the necessary ammonia by lactic
acid.

Carbohydrate Metabolism.—When a quantity of carbohydrate in
excess of the immediate needs of the body is ingested, the excess is stored
in the liver and in the muscles in the form of glycogen.   From these storage places the glycogen is gradually poured into the blood to be utilized
by the different organs.   In long-continued starvation glycogen is, therefore, absent from the liver or present only in traces.   The dextrose and
the levulose of the food are, according to C. Voit, the only direct sources
of the hepatic glycogen.   In the absence of these substances glycogen can
be formed from fat and proteid, and be deposited in the organ, this formation, according to Seegen, apparently taking place in the liver itself.

The glycogen stored in the liver regulates the percentage of sugar in
the blood.   If the liver is disconnected by extirpation (Minkowski) or by
interruption of its circulation (Bock and Hoffmann), the sugar rapidly
disappears from the blood.

A decrease of the hepatic glycogen is found in starvation, in fever
(Manassein, Hergenhahn), in artificial elevation of the body-temperature
(Paton, May, Schulte-Overberg), after injections of acid into the bile-ducts
(F. Pick), in diabetes mellitus of man, and after extirpation of the pan-
creas in birds (Kausch).   This decrease of glycogen is, in part, due to the

decreased ability of the liver to retain the glycogen, so that more sugar enters the blood; in part, to an increased consumption of sugar.

The interrelationship between hepatic activity and glycosuria is remarkable, and has been frequently studied. That the liver is the source of the blood-sugar is demonstrated by the following observations: (1) Glycosuria does not occur after piqure, strychnin-poisoning, or carbon monoxid intoxication, if the liver has been extirpated, or if it has been previously rendered free from glycogen by ligation of the bile-ducts (Wickham-Legg, Schiff, Gürtler, Langendorff). (2) In frogs pancreatic diabetes does not occur if the liver has been previously extirpated (Marcuse). After extirpation of the pancreas the glycogen stored in the liver is more rapidly poured into the blood, as is demonstrated by the course of the excretion of sugar (Minkowski).

Transitory glycosuria may, therefore, depend upon perversion of the function of the liver. Such perversion cannot, however, be made alone responsible for the persistent excretion of sugar that is seen in diabetes mellitus. The latter can only be caused by a diminution of the normal consumption of sugar in the organism. Clinical experience, moreover, reveals no relationship between diabetes and hepatic lesions.* If the two conditions are found at the same time, this must be considered as a coincidence, and no significance can be attached to it. The only thing that has been positively determined is a reduction of the hepatic glycogen in human diabetes and in experimental pancreatic diabetes, and this is probably a secondary occurrence.

Owing to the fact that the liver is recognized as a reservoir for glycogen, a number of French investigators have followed in the footsteps of Claude Bernard, who looked for alimentary glycosuria in diseases of the liver. Bernard found it in dogs after gradual obliteration of the portal vein, and explained the phenomenon by assuming that through the formation of a collateral circulation with parts surrounding the liver, the sugar ingested could circumvent the portal vein and enter directly into the systemic blood-vessels. In fact, Naunyn, Schöpfer, and Seelig found that injection of sugar into the systemic veins produced glycosuria, whereas the same result did not follow the same injection into the mesenteric veins. Clinical observations on cases of disease of the liver have, however, led to very conflicting results. Even in the healthy the power of assimilating sugar varies considerably, ranging, according to Hoffmann, between 100 and 250 grams. In atrophic cirrhosis this limit is occasionally somewhat reduced, but such a reduction is not observed in diseases of the liver in general.† According to v. Jaksch, it is reduced in phosphorus-poisoning, particularly in the stage of marked swelling of the liver. [Strauss‡ examined 38 cases of various hepatic troubles and failed to find alimentary glycosuria except for a brief time in two cases of trauma in the hepatic region. Brault§ has also studied the preservation of the glycogenic function in atrophic cirrhosis.—ED.] Very little is known in regard to the quantity of glycogen stored in the liver in disease (excepting in diabetes). This is due to the fact that postmortem changes can rarely be excluded. Still less is known about the process of glycogen formation in man.

* Glénard, "Des resultats obj. de l'exploration du foie chez les diabetiques," *Lyon médical*, 1890, No. 16-25.
† Minkowski, Ergebnisse der allgemeinen Pathologie von Lubarsch und Ostertag, 1897, p. 720.
‡ *Berlin. klin. Woch.*, December 19, 1898.   § *Presse méd.*, May 29, 1901.

Experimental investigation has taught us that the glycogen is reduced in poisoning by phosphorus, arsenic, and antimony,[*] and after the administration of strychnin, morphin, chloroform,[†] and various other poisons. Kunkel believes that the most important in this respect are those forms of poisons that change the constitution of the blood entering the liver by the production of violent disturbances in the intestinal tract.[‡] According to E. Neisser's [||] experiments on mice, glycogen cannot be found microchemically after administering phloridzin, papain, asparagin, coniferin, and cumarin, while after giving morphin, amygdalin, and mytilotoxin it is found, the latter substances exercising an inhibiting effect upon its conversion.

Metabolism of Fat.—The liver stores up fats as well as carbohydrates. The fat ingested is deposited here within a few hours after eating (more rapidly than in the connective tissue), and it is also readily given up again. This is the physiologic fatty liver which is particularly striking in suckling animals. The fat reaches the liver chiefly through the chyle vessels and the thoracic duct, so that it has to pass into the blood-current before it arrives at the liver. Within the chyle a little of the fat is in solution, either as fat or (as much as 2%) as soap, but the greater portion is seen in the form of neutral fat in fine emulsion (according to J. Munk, even after feeding with fatty acids). Probably some fat also reaches the liver directly by way of the portal vein in solution as soap, and is then changed by the liver (J. Munk). After feeding with fat the blood in the portal vein contains no more free fat than the blood in the carotid (Heidenhain).

Feeding experiments show that fat can also be formed from carbohydrates and can be deposited in the liver (as is seen in the purposeful fattening of livers of geese). It is not known where this conversion occurs.

We know still less in regard to the participation of the liver in the conversion of proteid into fat. It is certain, however, that under certain pathologic conditions such a conversion occurs within the liver itself.

The liver is probably concerned not only with the storing of fat, but also with its further elaboration, as during starvation the deposit of fat in the liver decreases more rapidly than in other organs that store it. A certain proportion of fat, however, always remains in the liver even after long periods of hunger.

In dogs, according to Rosenfeld, the fat of the liver is reduced to about 10% of the dry residue by a total abstinence of five days. It is immaterial whether the animals are fat or lean. Rosenfeld could hardly ever reduce it to less than 10%, even after long periods of starvation. That fat plays a very important rôle in the nutrition of the liver-cells is shown by Spee's observation that in the embryos of rabbits and guinea-pigs the cells of the endoblast, and later only those cells that were to form the liver-cells, contained numerous droplets of fat, this being particularly true for that half of the cells directed toward the mesoblast. This fat could not have come from the vitelline membrane.

According to O. Nasse, the glycogen required for combustion is derived from the fat. This for the present is pure hypothesis. Under certain conditions, however, there is a migration of fat from other places of deposit into the liver. This becomes particularly manifest after the exhibition of phloridzin (Rosenfeld). If the percentage of fat in the liver of a

[*] Salkowski, *Virchow's Archiv*, Bd. xxxiv, p. 79.

[†] Böhm, *Archiv für experimentelle Pathologie*, Bd. xv, p. 450.

[‡] Kunkel, "Einfluss von Giften auf den Glykogengehalt der Leber," *Würzburger Sitzungsbericht*, 1893, p. 135.

[||] E. Neisser, "Beiträge zur Kenntniss der Glykogens," Dissertation, Berlin, 1888.

dog is reduced by a fast of five days, and if the animal receives a fairly large dose of phloridzin (2 to 3 grams for each kilo of weight) on the sixth and the seventh days, a large deposit of fat will, after forty to forty-eight hours, be found within the liver, and the organ will, moreover, be seen to be very much enlarged. The fat deposits are principally found in the center and in a narrow peripheral zone, later in the whole extent of the lobule. The quantity found amounts to about 25% to 75% of the dry residue. This fat has not been formed in the location where it was found, for the percentage of albumin in the liver is hardly changed. In addition, this deposit of fat disappears within twenty-four hours if the animal is starved further. That the fat is carried to the liver through the blood is made manifest by the milky appearance of the serum and the percentage of fat found in the blood. The adipose tissue of the animal's body furnishes this fat, as Rosenfeld proved by using dogs that had been fattened with mutton fat and showing that after five days of starvation the liver contained about 10% of dog fat, whereas after poisoning by phloridzin the liver of such animals contained from 50% to 60% of mutton fat in addition.

It is a peculiar fact that phloridzin does not produce a fatty liver in animals that are fed on carbohydrate and meat, while feeding with fat increases the deposit of fat in the liver. It seems, therefore, that the storing of glycogen interferes with the storing of fat. The fat also disappears more rapidly after phloridzin-poisoning if meat alone, or meat and sugar, are given, than on starving; so the fat may even be reduced to from 3% to 4% below normal.

Human pathology also teaches us that, particularly in phosphorus-poisoning, such a migration of fat to the liver can occur.

According to F. Hoffmann, the fat of the liver, even after feeding with neutral fat, contains more free fatty acids than the fat of any other organ (according to J. Munk, 5% to 10% of the neutral fat of the liver). This also demonstrates that the liver plays a peculiar rôle in the metabolism of fat.

In disease the fat of the liver varies in quantity owing to a number of causes. Sometimes the liver itself may be the seat of changes which are characterized by necrobiotic fatty degeneration of albumin or by a deficient elaboration of the fat entering the liver, sometimes general disturbances of metabolism may be present and occupy the foreground of the disease-picture. These may cause either a deficient or an excessive supply of fat to the liver. Sometimes the fat of the liver is so excessive that it determines the pathology of the disease. We will discuss fatty liver among the special diseases of the organ, and will recur to some of the details bearing on the question in that place.

Detoxicating Function.—Carbohydrates and fats are not the only substances that are stored in the liver. Some of the heavy metals, such as iron, copper, mercury, arsenic, and antimony, suffer the same fate. This property of the liver has a certain toxicologic significance. That the liver plays an important rôle in intoxication by many other poisons has been known for a long time; but it is only within the last decade that this subject has received particular attention. The liver exercises a protective function either by storing or by excreting poisons circulating through the body.

The protective action of the liver may be exerted in three ways: (1) The poison may be rapidly excreted with the bile; (2) the poison may be stored in the liver, in which manner the poison is removed from the general circulation, and thus, instead of producing acute poisoning, causes a more mild and protracted form; (3) the poison may be chemically transformed into a less harmful substance.

The starting-point for all these investigations was the discovery made in Ludwig's laboratory by Heger that nicotin added to the blood disappeared if the blood was allowed to pass through the liver. After Heger, a number of investigators made experiments in different directions. Some compared the toxicologic action of different substances when they were introduced into the intestinal canal and into the subcutaneous connective tissues, or into a mesenteric and a systemic vein; while others attempted to identify the substance chemically or to test its toxicologic action after it had been allowed to flow with the blood through the liver or had been mixed with hepatic pulp. Thus, in addition to nicotin, hyoscyamin, strychnin, atropin, quinin, and morphin were tested in this manner. Heger states that one-fourth to one-fifth of the poisonous substance is retained by the liver, while Roger says that this amount varies from 50% to 100%. While Heger, Jaques, and others assume a simple storing, and explain the reduced toxic action from the more gradual entrance of the poison into the general circulation; others, again, as Lautenbach and Schiff, demonstrated a chemical transformation of the alkaloids.

According to Buys and Heger, hyoscyamin is so changed by liver-pulp or filtered liver-juice that its presence can no longer be demonstrated physiologically or chemically.* The liver of a frog and of a rabbit acts more powerfully in this respect than does that of a dog.

In the case of curare the protective action of the liver, according to Lussana, consists in the excretion of the poison through the bile. Other authors (for example, Zuntz and Sauer in regard to curare, and René regarding nicotin) claim not to have found this action. Roger concludes from his experiments that the protective action or the detoxicating power of the liver is proportionate to the amount of glycogen that it contains, and that the various poisons enter into combination with this substance.

Kobert assumes that certain very insoluble compounds of the alkaloids with the bile-acids are formed. These were described by de l'Arbre.† He calls attention to the fact that, according to Anthen,‡ the formation of the bile-acids is dependent on the glycogen contained in the liver.

In the same manner as in the case of the alkaloidal poisons already mentioned, it has been shown that there exists a protective action of the liver against antipyrin, cocain, peptone,§ the poisons produced by putrefaction, bacterial poisons, and the toxins of putrefaction that originate within the intestine.

The blood from the portal vein of a dog is more poisonous to rabbits than is the blood from the hepatic and systemic vessels (Roger). Egg-albumen (Cl. Bernard), casein (Bouchard), and soap (J. Munk), if injected into the mesenteric veins, are changed in their passage through the liver. Sodium soaps injected into a systemic

---

* Quoted from Hanot, p. 448, and Minkowski.
† de l'Arbre, "Ueber die Verbindung einzelner Alkaloide mit Gallensäuren," Dissertation, Dorpat, 1871.
‡ Anthen, "Ueber die Wirkung der Leberzelle auf das Hämoglobin," Dissertation, Dorpat, 1889.
§ Questioned by J. Munk (loc. cit., p. 137).

vein produce narcosis and death from paralysis of the heart (in doses of 0.29 gram per kilo of animal), whereas, when injected into a mesenteric vein, death occurs only after a dose from two and a half to five times as large. The liver has no detoxicating power, in regard to digitalin, glycerin, acetone, or potassium and sodium salts, and a very slight action on alcohol.

Bouchard has attempted to determine the toxicity of certain substances found in the urine by injecting them into rabbits intravenously. He found certain differences in the urinary toxicity in healthy subjects and in persons afflicted with certain diseases. As the toxicity of the urine is increased in certain diseases of the liver, Bouchard's pupil, Roger, concluded that the detoxicating power of the liver was reduced, a view borne out by the observation that in cases in which the toxicity of the urine was very high a mild glycosuria occurred, showing that the power of the liver to store glycogen had been reduced. Other authors, particularly in France, found the toxicity of the urine frequently, though not constantly, increased in diseases of the liver, and Bellati found the same in experiments on dogs. On the other hand, Queirolo found no excessive toxicity of the urine in cases of cirrhosis of the liver in dogs with an Eck fistula between the portal vein and the inferior cava.

The conversion of carbaminate of ammonia and of other organic ammonia compounds into urea may be considered as a physiologic example of the protective action of the liver. We are, however, not justified in declaring this to be the main purpose of this conversion.

The history of the bile-acids furnishes another example of physiologic protective action. They are absorbed from the intestine by the intestinal mucosa, enter the liver, and are poured back into the intestine by the way of the bile-ducts. In this manner they circulate in the intestine and the portal system and are prevented from entering the systemic circulation in large quantities.

The questions under discussion have only recently been subjected to careful examination, and are so complicated that we are for the present still far from having solved them. While suggestive, the teleologic point of view, which starts with the protective action of the liver, is perhaps unfavorable to a true solution of the problem. The conception of a "poison" is indefinite and one-sided. The specific character of the circulation and of the chemism of the liver, that causes the storing of important nutritive substances, probably has the same action in regard to other substances. An elective power is, moreover, found in the case of other organs than the liver (for example, the kidneys, and the ganglion-cells), and we must agree with Queirolo, who attributes a greater protective power to the epithelium and the walls of the intestine than to the liver. Quite a number of examples can be quoted of the formation of double compounds or of synthesis in the liver by which the original substances are changed, as is true, for instance, of phenyl-sulphuric acid (Kochs), while the liver has no monopoly in regard to these chemical processes, and it is equally conceivable that it may increase as well as decrease the toxicity of different substances. Our aim must be to examine each substance individually and to determine the changes that it undergoes. The mere determination of toxicity considers only the coarser properties in a very summary manner, and it is quite possible that the so-called "urinary poisons" found in certain diseases of the liver may have been formed within the liver itself instead of being formed outside of the liver and passing through the deranged hepatic filter.

Some authors attribute the detoxicating power of the liver to the fact that poisons are excreted in the bile. The quantity of poison excreted in the bile is, however, very small, and, in addition, it would be readily reabsorbed in the intestine; so that, both teleologically and in fact, the liver plays only a very insignificant rôle in the elimination of poisons from the body.

[In 1898* Adami described a minute diplococcus, resembling that present in Pictou's cattle disease, which he had discovered in specimens of cirrhosis of the liver. Later the same organism was found by him in the normal liver, but in smaller number and staining with less intensity than in cases of cirrhosis. On injection of pure cultures of this diplococcoid or of the ordinary form of colon bacillus into the ear-vein of rabbits these organisms were found in large numbers in the hepatic cells, while the bile of the animal remained sterile. Within fifteen minutes after the injection some bacilli were found in the endothelial cells of the liver, and within two hours they were found in the hepatic cells themselves. It is probable, therefore, that the liver has a protective and bactericidal function in addition to its detoxicating power.—Ed.]

The Formation of Bile.—The most important constituents of the bile are the bile-pigments, the salts of the bile-acids, and cholesterin.

Bile-pigment is excreted by the liver in the form of bilirubin, "bile-yellow," but is readily converted into substances of different color (biliverdin, biliprassin, bilifuscin, and bilihumin). These conversions, that are in part surely oxidative, may in part be due to other chemical processes. They sometimes begin, if stasis of bile occurs, within the bile-passages, but they usually begin only where the bile has reached the gastro-intestinal tract or as a pathologic process in other tissues. In the intestine the greater part of the bilirubin is converted into hydrobilirubin by the action of bacteria. The significance and the genesis of this substance will be discussed under icterus.

We frequently see bilirubin formed from the hemoglobin of extravasated blood, partly in the form of crystals (hematoidin), partly in the form of diffuse imbibition of the connective tissue and of elastic fibers (Langhans, Quincke). We also know from experiments and from pathologic findings that the hepatic cells possess particular powers of attraction for the bilirubin circulating in the blood, and seem to direct it toward the bile-passages. The bilirubin normally found in the bile is, however, not formed in other parts of the body to be later excreted by the liver, but is manufactured within this organ by a specific action of its cells.

The material from which these pigments are formed is hemoglobin; for, as Tarchanoff, and later in a more exact manner Stadelmann, have shown, the injection into the blood of hemoglobin in solution is followed by an increased excretion of bilirubin. Of the hemoglobin so injected, however, no more than 1.9% is converted into bile-pigment. Numerous pathologic facts point in the same direction. The more bilirubin there is in the bile, the darker is the color and the greater the consistency of the latter (Stadelmann).

With the exception of Baum, no one has so far ever been able to demonstrate directly the presence of bilirubin within the liver-cells under normal conditions. It is also very doubtful whether Anthen's † observation that macerated liver-cells

* *Montreal Medical Journal*, July, p. 485.
† E. Anthen, "Ueber die Wirkung der Leberzellen auf das Hämoglobin," Dissertation, Dorpat, 1889.

can destroy hemoglobin outside of the body will permit us to draw any conclusions in regard to their having this power as a vital process. For the present, therefore, the manner in which blood-pigment is elaborated within the liver-cells is altogether obscure, and the same obscurity surrounds the question as to how the hemoglobin reaches these cells. It can hardly be assumed that blood-corpuscles or debris of corpuscles are taken up by these cells. It is probable that hemoglobin (possibly in a changed form) enters the liver-cells by diffusion from its solution in the plasma, or, as is less probable, that it comes from leucocytes containing red blood-corpuscles and clinging to the walls of the hepatic capillaries. Although Naunyn and Minkowski in birds poisoned with arseniuretted hydrogen saw bile-pigment formed in the cells containing blood-corpuscles within the hepatic capillaries, this discovery does not necessarily apply to mammals and to normal conditions.

As bilirubin contains no iron, this element must be separated from hemoglobin in the formation of the bile-pigment. Iron is, in fact, found in larger quantities in the liver than in any other organ. It seems that the hemoglobin molecule in another way can be split and lose iron without forming bile-pigment.

The bile always contains small quantities of iron. In man, according to Hoppe-Seyler and Young, bile from the gall-bladder contains about 6 mg. in 100 c.c. Kunkel * found the same quantity in the bile from a gall-bladder fistula in a dog. This, however, corresponded only to about one-seventh of the amount of hemoglobin used for the formation of the bile-pigment. In the gall-bladder, according to Tissier, D. Gerhardt, and Fr. Muller, urobilin is also always present. Tissier, Hayem, and others regard the latter, as well as the indefinite substance "bilirubidin," as a product of the secretion of the liver formed in excess in diseased conditions of the organ. It could possibly be reabsorbed from the intestine and excreted by the liver (see page 421), or it might have originated as a product of the function of the walls of the gall-bladder.

It is possible that hematoporphyrin (isomeric with bilirubin) is formed by the liver under certain pathologic conditions and is then excreted in the urine.†

The bile-acids, glycocholic and taurocholic acids, are found in the bile in the form of their sodium salts, and are also formed by a specific action of the liver-cells.

Older statements in regard to their presence in the suprarenals (Vulpian ‡) must be considered doubtful. We know nothing definite in regard to the mother-substance or the method of formation of the bile-acids. It is stated that they are also formed more freely even outside of the body when the liver contains much glycogen.§ The formation of the bile-acids and that of bile-pigments, at all events, occur quite independently of one another (Stadelmann).

When the salts of the bile-acid enter the blood, they are in great part excreted by the liver and the bile, in small part by the kidneys,‖ while a third portion is probably decomposed. They normally reach the blood through reabsorption from the intestine.**

* Kunkel, *Pflüger's Archiv*, Bd. x, p. 359.

† Schulte, "Ueber Hämatoporphyrinurie," *Deutsches Archiv für klin. Medicin*, 1879, Bd. LVIII, p. 313.

‡ Vulpian, cited by Virchow, "Zur Chemie der Nebennieren," *Virchow's Archiv*, Bd. XII, 1857, p. 481

§ Kallmeyer, "Ueber die Entstehung der Gallensäuren," Dissertation, Dorpat, 1889. Klein, "Ueber die Function der Leberzellen," Dissertation, Dorpat, 1890.

‖ Naunyn, "Beiträge zur Lehre von Icterus," *Archiv für Anatomie und Physiologie*, 1868. Vogel, "Maly's Jahresbericht," 1872, S. 243. Höne, J. (and Dragendorff), "Ueber die Anwesenheit der Gallensäuren im normalen Harn" (about 0.07 gm. in 1 liter), Dissertation, Dorpat, 1873.

** The absorption does not take place in the duodenum; but glycocholic acid is absorbed from the jejunum and ileum, taurocholic acid and cholic acid exclusively from the ileum. Tappeiner, "Sitzungsbericht der Wiener Akademie," 1878, III. Abtheilung, April.

If an excessive formation of bilirubin is experimentally produced, the excretion of the bile-acids in the bile decreases (Stadelmann). In the same manner a reduction is observed in fever (Paton and Balfour *) and in long-lasting stasis of bile (Yeo and Herroun *). Nothing is known in regard to the conditions that govern increased excretion.

Cholesterin forms about 1% of the solid constituents of normal bile. It is of subordinate importance in general metabolism and in physiology, and only important because it is a factor in the formation of biliary concretions. According to the researches of Naunyn and his pupils,† it cannot be regarded as a product of the hepatic secretion for the reason that an increased introduction of cholesterin either from the intestine or by subcutaneous injections exerts no influence on the excretion of cholesterin in the bile (Jankau). The quantity of cholesterin found in the bile is independent of the diet (Thomas), and, except in cholelithiasis, not increased in disease (Kausch). Cholesterin, when found in the bile-ducts as well as in other locations, as in atheromatous cysts, must be considered as a disintegration product of the epithelium. It is quite probable that the presence of bile within the bile-ducts exercises a deleterious influence on the lining epithelial cells and causes an excessive disintegration of them beyond that of other mucous membranes. Possibly disintegrating liver-cells also furnish a part of the cholesterin. Austin Flint's and Müller's cholesteremia (an increase of the cholesterin in the blood) can no longer be considered a valid and justifiable clinical conception.

The quantity of bile excreted has been carefully studied in animals, and has been found to be much greater in rabbits and guinea-pigs than in dogs and cats. In sheep the conditions are similar to those in the latter class of animals. The figures given for man are very indefinite, as they are chiefly obtained from cases with fistula, and usually after stasis had existed for some time. According to v. Wittich, the quantity of bile excreted in twenty-four hours is said to be 530; according to Westphalen, 453 to 566 c.c.; according to Ranke, 14 gm. per diem per kilo.‡ Hammarsten found 600, Körte as much as 1200 c.c. excreted in the twenty-four hours.§

The exact quantity of bilirubin and of the bile-acids excreted in twenty-four hours is not known. As regards bilirubin, Kunkle states that a dog of 4.7 kg. excretes 0.307 grams, Vossius that a dog of 25 kg. excretes only 0.108 grams. Noel-Paton ‖ found in man an excretion of 0.2 to 0.7 gm. of bilirubin in twenty-four hours. Bidder and Schmidt calculate 4 gm. of bile-acids for a dog, while in man Voit estimates it at 11 gm., and Stadelmann at 8 to 10 gm. in the twenty-four hours.

The conditions under which bile is secreted are manifold, and the quantity varies in different animals with biliary fistula, as well as in accordance with the rapidity of the blood-stream, nervous influences, and the phase of digestion. The taking of food, particularly, increases the excretion, the time at which an increase of the flow of bile occurs being stated differently by different investigators. Heidenhain** assumes two maxima in

---

* Quoted by Minkowski, in " Ergebnisse der allgemeinen Pathologie," p. 697.
† Naunyn, "Klinik der Cholelithiasis," 1892, p. 12. Jankan, "Cholesterin-und Kalkausscheidung mit der Galle," *Archiv für experimentelle Pathologie*, 1892, Bd. xxix, p. 237. Kausch, "Ueber den Gehalt der Leber und Galle an Cholesterin," Dissertation, Strassburg, 1897. Thomas, "Ueber die Abhängigkeit der Absonderung und Zusammensetzung der Galle von der Nahrung," Dissertation, Strassburg, 1890.
‡ Heidenhain, loc. cit., p. 252.
§ Cited by Stadelmann, *Berliner klin. Wochenschrift*, 1896, p. 184.
‖ According to Hammarsten.
** Heidenhain, loc. cit., p. 269; see also Murchison, "Functional Derangements of the Liver," p. 34.

the excretion curve, the one in the third to the fifth hour, the other in the thirteenth to the fifteenth hour. It is probable that this varies according to the species of animal and the composition of the food. The increase is probably produced, on the one hand, by certain reflexes, particularly from the mucosa of the intestine; on the other, by the substances that are absorbed.

If the flow of bile is profuse, there is an increase in the quantity both of water and of solid constituents. According to Heidenhain, even the ratio of the latter is greater. If abstinence from food is persisted in for a period longer than twenty-four hours,. the bile is excreted less copiously and is more concentrated. A pure meat diet is most efficient in producing an increased flow of bile, a meat diet with carbohydrates acting to a lesser degree (Spiro). On a fat diet the excretion of bile, according to some authors, is small; according to Rosenberg and others, however, it is very copious.

The specific gravity of the bile varies greatly (1005 to 1030). The solids amount to from 3% to 10%. The bile in the gall-bladder, owing to the absorption of water that occurs there, is always more concentrated than is the bile obtained from fistulas. I observed a specific gravity of 1047 in man after a fast of several days. The bile from the gall-bladder, at the same time, is more viscid and frequently cloudy from the admixture of mucus and particles of pigment. It is not impossible that an absorption of water, and possibly of matters in solution, occurs in the bile-passages. The proportion of the different constituents of the bile varies, and the conditions that govern their excretion are only in small part known to us. Certain relations between the secretion of the bile and the other processes that occur in the liver must exist, and it has been stated that this is true particularly of the flow of bile and the formation of glycogen, but nothing exact has been demonstrated.

It is a remarkable fact that a part of the bile-acid salts are reabsorbed in the intestine, and that a part of them (according to Stadelmann, two-thirds or more) are again excreted with the bile. Possibly the same is true to a lesser degree in regard to the bile-pigments. These substances, therefore, in a way circulate between the liver and the intestine * (Schiff) and enter the general circulation in small quantities only. It is possible that their chemical power is better utilized in this manner and that a saving of useful material is secured.

The bile-acids are undoubtedly broken up within the intestine into taurin and glycocoll, on the one hand, and cholalic acid, on the other, the latter alone appearing in the feces. In the dog 0.5 gm. or one-eighth (Hoppe-Seyler), in man 3 gm. or one-fourth (Bischoff), of the secreted bile-acids are passed with the feces. Of the portion that is reabsorbed, a part is voided in the urine, a part is re-excreted in the bile, and a part is destroyed by combustion. It is possible that there are other substances that act in the same manner as do the salts of the bile-acids. Lussana claims that curare is such a body, and in this way attempts to explain its slight toxicity when taken by the mouth.

If it is difficult to demonstrate increase and decrease of the excretion of bile in animal experiments; it is still more difficult to arrive at definite conclusions from the observation of pathologic conditions. The color of the feces has been utilized as a standard; but, while it is true that the chief coloring-matters of the feces are the bile-pigments, still a number of other factors are concerned in this coloration. As these must all be

* Stadelmann, "Icterus," p. 95.

considered, it is very difficult to reach definite conclusions.* In addition to the peculiar color of different articles of food, the transparency of each substance must be considered. If finely divided substances of different refractive power (fat-crystals, air-bubbles) are abundantly distributed through the feces, the latter will appear lighter in color. Besides urobilin, the feces always contain other derivatives of the biliary pigments whose constitution is unknown. They also contain a chromogen of urobilin, which is formed from it by further reduction, and which, in the presence of oxygen and on extraction with acid alcohol, is reconverted into uro bilin. The quantity of other pigments and of the chromogenic substance is very varying, and probably depends upon the bacterial flora of the in testine. In individual cases, particularly if digestive disturbances exist, this may produce considerable change in the color of the feces.

Attempts to determine by extraction the quantity of bile-pigment derivatives present in the feces have been only partially successful so far, owing to the fact that these substances decompose so readily. G. Hoppe-Seyler † found 0.7% to 3.2% normally, and an average of 1.7% of impure urobilin per diem, while Boltz and Fr. Müller found 0.08% to 0.09%.

In addition to urobilin, Fr. Müller frequently found cholecyanin in the feces (frequently in direct proportion to urobilin). In diarrhea the feces usually contained unchanged urobilin.

Notwithstanding the lack of exact data in regard to the excretion of bile and its fluctuations in pathologic conditions, the assumption of such clinical entities as acholia, hypocholia, oligocholia, on the one hand, and of polycholia, on the other, is fully justified. Here the proportion of bile-pigment to bile-acids may aalso be changed, so that the French have created an "*acholie totale,*" n "*acholie pigmentaire,*" and an "*acholie des acides biliaires.*"

The observations reported in regard to (completely or almost) colorless bile ‡ are open to criticism. We can only say to-day that in fever § ex perimentally produced, and after Brown-Séquard's piqure, ‖ the excretion of bile is decreased, and that frequently in chronic cachexias, in the fatty liver of tuberculosis, and sometimes in atrophic cirrhosis of the liver, the bile and the feces are very pale.

Stadelmann ** found a decreased excretion of bile-acids in the ad vanced stage of phosphorus-poisoning and in icterus from poisoning by toluylenediamin and arseniuretted hydrogen. It is probable that their formation is also decreased in chronic biliary stasis and in fever.

Physicians have assumed the existence of polycholia from the dark color of the feces and the occurrence of icterus (see below) in many forms of

* Quincke, H., "Farbe der Fäces," *Münchener med. Wochenschr.,* 1896, No. 36. Hoppe-Seyler, G., "Ueber die Ausscheidung des Urobilins in Krankheiten," *Virchow's Archiv,* 1891, Bd. cxxiv, p. 47.

† Hoppe-Seyler, G., "Ueber die Einwirkung des Tuberculin auf die Gallen farbstoffbildung," *Virchow's Archiv,* 1892, Bd. cxxviii, p. 43.

‡ Ritter, M. E., "Quelques observations de bile incolore," *Journal d'Anatomie et de Physiolog. (de Robin),* 1872, p. 181. Hanot, "Contribut. à l'état de l'acholie," *Archives générales de médecine,* 1885, i, p. 12. Létienne, "De la bile à l'état patholog.," Thèse de Paris, 1891, p. 17.

§ Pisenti, *Archiv fur experimentelle Pathologie,* 1886, Bd. xxi, p. 219.

‖ Naunyn, "Beiträge zur Lehre vom Diabetes," *Archiv für experimentelle Pathologie,* 1874, Bd. iii.

** Stadelmann, *Archiv für experimentelle Pathologie,* Bd. xv, xvi; Bd. xxiii p. 433.

dyspepsia as well as in the gastro-intestinal infections and intoxications. Affanassiew* experimentally produced this deeper color by section of the nerves of the liver. An increased formation of bile-pigment has been positively demonstrated only after poisoning with toluylenediamin and arseniuretted hydrogen (*pleiochromia, polycholie pigmentaire*). The same presumably occurs in those forms of intoxication coming under clinical observation in which a destruction of red blood-corpuscles takes place. In the beginning of phosphorus-poisoning, according to Stadelmann, an increase in the formation of bile-pigment is said to occur.

Blumreich and Jacobi found the gall-bladder very much dilated by bile in rabbits some time after extirpation of the thyroid, and conclude that an increased formation of bile had occurred as a result of the procedure.† [Ligature of the bile-duct is, on the other hand, said to have caused an excess of secretion (Murray). —Ed.]

As the assumption of disturbances in the flow of bile has occupied a large place in medical thought, attempts have been made to influence the flow of bile by therapeutic means. A large number of drugs were considered cholagogues and were employed not only where a decreased secretion of bile was assumed, but also where obstacles to the outflow of the bile existed. A more careful analysis has shown that the conclusions reached were in many instances wrong, and that the error was caused both by the increased evacuation of the intestine that followed the administration of many of these drugs and by the coloration of the feces by other substances.

By employing dogs with biliary fistulæ, Prévost and Binet found on introducing different drugs, either subcutaneously or by the mouth, the following results:

INCREASE OF SECRETION.	INCREASE SLIGHT, INCONSTANT OR DOUBTFUL.
Bile.	Sodium bicarbonate. ⎫ ‡
Salts of bile-acids.	Sodium sulphate. ⎭
Urea.	Sodium chlorid, Carlsbad salts
Oil of turpentine (? Stadelmann).	Propylamin, Antipyrin.
Potassium chlorate.	Aloes, Cathartic acid.
Sodium salicylate.	Rhubarb.
Salol.	Hydrastis Canadensis.
Sodium benzoate.	Boldo.
Euonymin.	Antifebrin ⎫
Muscarin.	Diuretin ⎬ (Stadelmann).
Sodium oleinate (Blum, see below).	Santonin ⎭

DECREASE OF THE SECRETION.	EXERCISING NO INFLUENCE.
Potassium iodid.	Sodium phosphate.
Calomel.	Potassium bromid.
Iron, Copper (subcutaneously).	Lithium chlorid.
Atropin (subcutaneously).	Corrosive sublimate.
Strychnin in toxic doses.	Sodium arseniate.
	Alcohol, Ether, Glycerin.
	Quinin.
	Caffein (? Stadelmann).
	Pilocarpin (according to Stadelmann reducing, according to Affanassiew increasing).
	Kairin, Cytisin.
	Senna, Colombo.

* *Pflüger's Archiv.* Bd. xxx, p. 418.
† *Pflüger's Archiv,* 1896, Bd. LXIV, p. 27.
‡ According to Lewaschew, quite effective, according to Stadelmann, ineffective.

EXCRETED WITH THE BILE.

Bilirubin.

Urobilin.

Salts of bile-acids.

Hemoglobin.*

Turpentine.

Salicylic acid.

Potassium iodid and bromid.

Potassium chlorate.

Arsenic.

Iron, lead, mercury in traces.

Caffein (?).

Fuchsin, Cochineal.

Sodium indigo-sulphate.

Phyllocyanic acid from chlorophyl.†

Grape-sugar, still more readily cane-sugar.‡

NOT DEMONSTRABLE.

Antipyrin, Kairin.

Benzoic acid.

Quinin, Strychnin.

Copper, Lithium, Urea.

Stadelmann's experiments show that water by mouth or by rectum does not increase the flow of bile in the least. Practical experience, on the other hand, particularly with Carlsbad waters, seems to contradict his experiments.

The action of large quantities of oil as a cholagogue has been much discussed lately, since it appears to assist in the removal of gall-stones. While Rosenberg maintains that there is an increase in the excretion of bile in from thirty to forty minutes after the administration of the oil, Stadelmann and his pupils deny this effect. Blum § administered pure oleate of sodium (in doses of 2 to 5 grams) and noticed a marked increase in the flow of bile in dogs with biliary fistulæ, while in human beings he found his observation corroborated; a small quantity of the oleate seems to enter the bile. It is possible that the apparent contradiction in these experiments can be attributed to the varying quantities of fatty acids present in the oil. ‖

Different factors are concerned in the movements of the bile through the bile-passages: namely, the pressure exercised by the secretion itself, gravity, respiratory movements, and contraction of the walls of the bile-ducts.

The pressure of the biliary secretion is small in comparison to the pressure found in other glands (in the dog 110 to 220, an average of 200 mm. of soda solution),** but always greater than the pressure in the portal vein. In man this pressure has so far not been measured. Gravity must necessarily, to some extent, assist the flow of the bile from the liver, owing to the topography of the organ. Respiration helps from the fact that each movement of the diaphragm exercises pressure and a slight degree of compression on the convex surface of the liver.

Contractions of the walls of the bile-ducts, already described by Haller, Rudolph, and Johannes Müller in pigeons,†† have recently been

* When more than 0.02 per 1 kg. was injected into the rabbit, after the third hour. R. Stern, *Virchow's Archiv*, 1891, Bd. cxxxiii, p. 33

† Wertheimer, "Elimination de chlorophylle par le foie," *Archives de physiolog.*, 1893, p. 122.

‡ Mosler, according to Heidenhain, *loc. cit.*, v, 1, p. 275

§ Blum, F., "Ueber eine neue Methode zur Anregung des Gallenflusses," *Der ärztliche Pratiker*, 1897, x, No. 3.

‖ Prévost and Binet, "Einfluss von Medicamenten auf die Galle," *Revue de médecine de la Suisse romande*, 1888, No. 5. Stadelmann, "Ueber Cholagoga," *Berliner klin. Wochenschr.*, 1896, S. 180 und 212. Rosenberg, Discussion, *Berliner klin. Wochenschr.*, 1896, p. 216. (Also references to earlier literature.)

** Heidenhain, *loc. cit.*, v, 1, p. 269.

†† For literature bearing on this question, see Daraignez, "Ictère spasmodique," Thèse de Paris, 1890.

observed in a number of mammals by Doyon and Oddi,* by whom careful studies were made on rabbits, dogs, and cats by direct and graphic methods.

Peristaltic waves were observed running from the liver toward the ampulla and occurring about every fifteen to twenty seconds. In addition, there were slow fluctuations in the tension of the ductus choledochus and of the gall-bladder. These movements were still observed after the liver had been removed from the body, so that they are either purely muscular or due to the influence of peripheral ganglia. If the great splanchnic nerve is irritated, the bile-ducts contract along their whole length and the sphincter of the ductus choledochus at the duodenum may even close entirely (Oddi). If the central end of the cut splanchnic be irritated, a relaxation of the bile-ducts results (preceded, according to Oddi, by a brief but strong contraction). The tonus of the sphincter of the ductus choledochus, according to Oddi, equals the pressure of 675 mm. of water. Reflexly, the innervation of the bile-ducts may be influenced with the result of inhibition or excitation, and the nerves of the ducts may also be influenced by irritation of the central ends of the vagus and of the sciatic. Irritation of the mucosa of the stomach and intestine usually produces spasm of the gall-bladder, sometimes also relaxation of the sphincter of the common duct. The center for these irritations is situated at the level of the first lumbar nerve in the dog, the anterior root of this nerve containing the motor branch for the musculature of the bile-ducts.

Pathologically, this contraction of the bile-ducts is manifested particularly in gall-stone colic, possibly also in other painful spasms and in spasmodic closures of the bile-ducts with icterus.

If we briefly review the physiologic facts we have mentioned, we see that the function of the liver is manifold. Owing to its situation, it is in intimate relation with the gastro-intestinal tract and helps to assimilate and stores nutrient material that it later pours into the blood-current. This applies to proteids, carbohydrates, and fats. In addition, the liver receives metabolic products from the systemic blood, in part converting them into other substances, in part returning them into the blood-current unchanged. In this manner the liver forms a central point of metabolism, and in comparison with this function the secretion of the bile seems insignificant. The latter is, no doubt, intimately related to the other functions, but is not by any means the chief function of the liver.

In view of all this, we can understand that the function of the liver is important in numerous pathologic conditions, although we are able to appreciate only a small portion of these relations. In the clinical sense disturbances in the formation and the excretion of bile are of paramount importance, if for no other reason than that they lead to so conspicuous a symptom as the intense yellow discoloration of the skin called icterus. This symptom occurs so frequently and is so important that its origin and manifestations merit particular discussion.

LITERATURE.

GENERAL PATHOLOGY OF THE LIVER.

Cohnheim: "Allgemeine Pathologie," ii, p. 57, 1880.
Denys et Stubbe: (Loewen.) "Étude sur l'acholie ou cholémie expérimentale,"

*M. Doyon, "Etude de la contractilité des voies biliaires," *Archives de physiolog.*, 1893, pp, 678, 710; "Action du syst. nerveux sur l'appareil excréteur de la bile," ibid., 1894, p. 19. R. Oddi, *Archives ital. de biologie*, vol. viii, x. *Sperimentale*, 1894, p. 180, *Jahresbericht* ii, p. 215; "Di una disposizione a sfinctere alla sboca del coledoco," Lab. di Fisiol. di Perugia, 1887, cited by Dupré. Thèse de Paris, 1891, p. 27.

"La Cellule," 1893, p. 447. "Centralblatt für allgemeine Pathologie," Bd. iv, p. 102, 1893.

Hahn, Massen, Nencki u. Pawlow: "Die Eck'sche Fistel zwischen unterer Hohlvene und Pfortader," etc., "Archiv für experimentelle Pathologie," Bd. xxxii, p. 161.

Hanot, V.: "Rapports de l'intestin et du foie en pathologie. Revue critique," "Archives générales de médecine," 1895, ii, pp. 427, 580; 1896, i, pp. 65, 311.

Heidenhain: "Physiologie der Gallenabsonderung" in Hermann's "Handbuch der Physiologie," Bd. v, 1.

Hergenhahn: "Arbeiten aus dem städtischen Krankenhaus zu Frankfurt a. M.," 1896.

v. Jaksch: "Alimentäre Glykosurie bei Phosphorvergiftung," "Prager med. Wochenschr.," 1895.

Kaufmann, M.: "De l'influence du foie sur la glycémie," "Archives de physiolog.," viii, p. 151, 1896.

Krehl: "Pathologische Physiologie," Leipzig, 1898.

v. Lieblein: "Die Stickstoffausscheidung nach Leberverödung beim Säugethier," "Archiv für experimentelle Pathologie," Bd. xxxiii, p. 318, 1894.

Marcuse: "Bedeutung der Leber für das Zustandekommen des Pankreasdiabetes," "Zeitschrift für klin. Medicin," Bd. xxvi, p. 225, 1894.

Minkowski: "Ergebnisse der allgemeinen Pathologie. Lubarsch and Ostertag," 1897, p. 679 (Literaturbericht).

—"Untersuchungen über den Einfluss der Leberexstirpation auf den Stoffwechsel," "Archiv für experimentelle Pathologie," Bd. xxi, 1886.

— "Ueber die Ursachen der Milchsäureausscheidung nach Leberexstirpation," "Archiv für experimentelle Pathologie," Bd. xxxi, 1893.

Münzer:"Der Stoffwechsel des Menschen bei acuter Phosphorvergiftung,""Deutsches Archiv für klin. Medicin," Bd. lii, p. 199, 1892.

— "Die Erkrankungen der Leber in ihrer Beziehung zum Gesammtorganismus des Menschen," "Prager med. Wochenschr.," 1892, Nos. 34 and 35.

— "Die harnstoffbildende Function der Leber," "Archiv für experimentelle Pathologie," Bd. xxxii, p. 164, 1894.

Naunyn und Minkowski: "Ueber den Icterus durch Polycholie," "Archiv für experimentelle Pathologie," Bd. xxi, 1888.

Neisser, E.: "Beitrag zur Kenntniss des Glykogen," Dissertation, Berlin, 1888.

Nencki, Pawlow and Zaleski: "Ueber den Ammoniakgehalt des Blutes und der Organe und die Harnstoffbildung bei Säugethieren," "Archiv für experimentelle Pathologie," Bd. xxxvii, p. 26, 1895.

Nencki and Pawlow: "Zur Frage über die Art der Harnstoffbildung bei Säugethieren," "Archiv für experimentelle Pathologie," Bd. xxxviii, p. 215, 1897.

Nencki and Zaleski: "Archiv für experimentelle Pathologie," Bd. xxxvi.

Noorden, C. v.: "Pathologie des Stoffwechsels," 1893.

Ponfick, E.: "Experimentelle Beiträge zur Pathologie der Leber (Exstirpation)," "Virchow's Archiv," Bd. cxviii, p. 209, 1889; Bd. cxix, p. 193, 1890; Bd. cxxxviii. Supplement, p. 81, 1896.

Pick, E.: "Versuche über functionelle Ausschaltung der Leber bei Säugethieren," "Archiv für experimentelle Pathologie," Bd. xxxii, p. 382, 1893.

Pick, F.: "Ueber die Beziehungen der Leber zum Kohlehydratstoffwechsel," "Archiv für experimentelle Pathologie," Bd. xxxiii, p. 305, 1894.

Roger, F.: "Des Glycosuries d'origine hépatique," "Revue de médecine,' p. 935, 1886.

Schiff, M.: "Ueber das Verhältniss der Lebercirculation zur Gallenbildung," "Schweizer Zeitschrift für Heilkund," 1861.

Schulte-Overberg: "Ueber Einwirkung hoher Aussentemperaturen auf den Glykogenbestand der Leber," Dissertation, Würzburg, 1894.

Stern: "Ueber die normale Bildungsstätte des Gallenfarbstoffes," Dissertation, Königsberg, 1885.

Tappeiner, H.: "Ueber den Zustand des Blutstromes nach Unterbindung der Pfortader," "Arbeiten aus der physiologischen Anstalt zu Leipzig," vii, p. 11, 1892.

Weintraud: "Untersuchungen über den Stickstoffumsatz bei Lebercirrhose," "Archiv für experimentelle Pathologie," Bd. xxxi, p. 30, 1892.

FAT.

Heidenhain: "Pflüger's Archiv," Bd. xli, Supplement, p. 95, 1888.

Hofmann, F.: "Ueber die Reaction der Fette," etc., "Beitrag zur Anatomie und Physiologie als Festgabe für C. Ludwig," p. 173, 1874.

Munk, J.: "Zur Lehre von der Resorption, Bildung und Ablagerung der Fette im Thierkörper," "Virchow's Archiv," Bd. xcv, p. 407.
Nasse, O.: "Fettzersetzung und Fettanhäufung im thierischen Korper," "Biolog. Centralblatt," vi, 235, 1886.
Rosenfeld, G.: "Ueber Fettwanderung," "Verhandlungen des Congresses fur innere Medicin," 1895, p. 414.
— "Ueber Phlorizinwirkungen," "Verhandlungen des Congresses für innere Medicin," 1893, p. 359.
Seegen: "Ueber die Fähigkeit der Leber Zucker aus Fett zu bilden," "Pfluger's Archiv," Bd. xxxix, p. 132, 1886.

FATTY DEGENERATION IN PHOSPHORUS-POISONING.

Lebedeff: "Pflüger's Archiv," Bd. xxxi, p. 15, 1883.
Leo: "Zeitschr. für physiolog. Chemie," Bd. ix, p. 469, 1885.
v. Starck: "Deutsches Archiv für klin. Medicin," Bd. xxxv, p. 481, 1884.
Rosenfeld, G.: "Die Fettleber beim Phlorizindiabetes," "Zeitschr. für klin. Medicin," Bd. xxviii, p. 256, 1895.

DETOXICATING FUNCTION.

Bellati, L.: "Ueber die Giftigkeit des Harns bei Leberkrankheiten" (many references to Literature), Moleschott's "Untersuchungen zur Naturlehre," 1894, p. 299.
Hanot, V.: "Rapport de l'intestin et du foie en pathologie. Revue critique," "Archives générales de méd.," 1895, ii, pp. 427, 580; 1896, i, pp. 65, 311.
Héger: "Experiences sur la circulation du sang dans les organes isolés," Bruxelles, Thèse, 1873.
— "Notice sur l'absorption des alcaloides dans le foie," etc., "Journal de méd.," Bruxelles, 1877.
— "Sur le pouvoir fixateur de certains organes," etc., "Comptes-rendus de l'Académie des sciences," May, 1880, p. 1226.
Kobert: "Lehrbuch der Intoxicationen," p. 27, 1893.
Minkowski: "Ergebnisse der allgemeinen Pathologie," Bd. iv, p. 734, 1897.
Munk, J.: "Ueber die Wirkung der Seifen im Thierkörper," "Archiv für Anatomie und Physiologie," physiologische Abtheilung, Supplement, 1890, p. 116.
Queirolo, G. B.. "Ueber die Function der Leber als Schutz gegen Intoxication vom Darm," Moleschott's "Untersuchungen zur Naturlehre," 1894, p. 228.
Roger, G. H.: "Action du foie sur les poisons," Thèse de Paris, p. 228, 1887 (copious bibliography).

BACTERICIDAL FUNCTION.

Adami: "Montreal Med. Jour.," July, 1898, p. 485; "Transactions of Association of American Physicians," 1899, vol. xiv, p. 300.

ICTERUS, JAUNDICE.

*Gelbsucht; Morbus regius.**

The term icterus is applied to that peculiar discoloration of the tissues by bile-pigments, so conspicuous as a clinical manifestation of various diseases in Caucasian races. In the clinical picture of certain diseases of the liver icterus plays an important rôle. For this reason a detailed description of its origin and of some of its individual symptoms is appropriate in this place. The special pathology of icterus will be discussed in the section on diseases of the bile-ducts, and in the description of catarrhal icterus all other forms that are described as independent diseases will be discussed.

In a healthy body bile-pigment is found only in the bile—the secretion of the liver. This pigment might be primarily formed in the blood and only excreted by the liver (like urea from the kidneys), or it might be formed within the liver. In the former instance icterus would be due

* From color of gold, the *rex metallorum.*

to an interference of secretion (so-called "suppression icterus"), in the latter to a reabsorption of the pigment that had been formed in the liver. From the experiments on extirpation of the liver in birds, performed by Naunyn and Minkowski, it may be stated as a positive fact that bile-pigment is normally not formed outside of the liver, so that there is no such thing as a "suppression icterus."

While ligation of the ductus choledochus in birds was followed by the appearance of biliverdin in the urine in one and one-half hours, and in the blood in five hours, this pigment was absent from the blood and present only in traces in the urine after removal of the liver. Though inhalation of arseniuretted hydrogen in normal geese produced polycholia and icterus (with biliverdin and bile-acids in the urine), the polycholia ceased upon removal of the liver, and both polycholia and icterus failed to occur in animals from whom the liver had been removed.

It is possible that in certain pathologic conditions bile-pigment might be formed in other locations than the liver, and by entering the circulation produce a discoloration of the tissues. According to the different origin of the pigment, we might, therefore, speak of·a "hepatogenous" and an "anhepatogenous" icterus. In fact, we know to-day (Langhans, Quincke) that bile-pigment can be formed from extravasated blood-pigment in the connective tissues, partly imbibed by these tissues, and in part appearing in the form of crystals (crystals of hematoidin and of bilirubin). Moreover, von Recklinghausen * found that bile-pigment developed in the leucocytes of a frog's blood which had been kept in a moist chamber for from three to ten days. The quantity of bilirubin found in extravasations of blood is very small, and it seems to have little tendency to diffuse itself or to enter the circulation. We certainly know of no case in which general icterus arose from the formation of bilirubin in such abnormal foci. In other words, we know of the formation of bilirubin outside of the liver, but we do not know of an anhepatogenous icterus.

According to the formation of bilirubin in this or that organ or in this or that tissue (for example, the blood or the connective tissues), we would have to speak of an hematogenous or an inogenous † form of icterus. In accordance with certain theoretic considerations, a number of investigators several years ago thought that they were justified in assuming the occurrence of an "hematogenous icterus." They placed this form in juxtaposition to the hepatogenous form without considering that there are still other locations outside of the liver besides the blood in which the formation of bile-pigment can occur. This method of designating the different forms of icterus led to additional confusion because these authors attempted to designate by their new names not only the location in which icterus was supposed to originate, but also the material from which they thought the bile-pigment was formed. We know of no substance except hemoglobin from which bilirubin can be formed. The liver, therefore, can only form bile-pigment from the pigment of the blood. Therefore, the abnormal coloring-matter in every case of icterus, just as is the case with normal bile, must be of hematogenous origin as it is derived from hemoglobin. The term "hematogenous icterus" is therefore superficial. The same is true in regard to the term bemato-hepatogenous jaundice, by which Affanassiew would designate those forms of jaundice which are accompanied by increased disintegration of the red cells. For this condition the name of "cythemolytic," proposed by Senator, would be more appropriate. [In this connection a case recently reported by Bettmann ‡ is of interest. He reports the case of a man aged twenty-nine years who for years had been deeply tinged with icterus, and also had hemoglobinuria.—Ed.]

* v. Recklinghausen, "Allgemeine Pathologie," 1883, p. 434.
† From ἱς (plural ἱνες), connective tissue.
‡ *Münch. med. Woch.*, 1900, No. 23.

We are, therefore, not justified in assuming that jaundice can occur without some participation of the liver in the process; but at the same time the details of the origin of hepatogenic icterus are still quite obscure.

Icterus most frequently occurs as a result of the absorption of bile from the biliary passages. This happens whenever its exit into the intestine is impeded (obstructive icterus, mechanical icterus, resorption icterus). The secretion-pressure of bile is very small, being in guinea-pigs and dogs equal to only about 200 mm. of water (Heidenhain).* Very slight obstruction, therefore, is sufficient to stop the flow of bile. Even when such an obstruction occludes only a few of the biliary passages, or if only a partial obstruction exists in the main channel, at least a certain portion of the bile may be reabsorbed and cause icterus.

Obstruction to the flow of bile may be produced in various ways. Their anatomic recognition is usually easy if the occlusion was complete, as the intestinal contents are then colorless and the usual post-mortem discoloration of the mucous membrane of the duct is absent below the point of obstruction. Where a stone or some object producing compression caused occlusion of one of the ducts, the decision is of course simple. Occasionally, however, all anatomic evidence of an obstruction is absent, even though during life the clinical symptoms pointed positively to stasis of bile. This may be due to the fact that before death the obstruction really was removed or that the occlusion was due to a spasm that relaxed after death, or, finally, because the cessation of all blood-pressure and turgescence after death may have changed the mechanical conditions that caused an obstruction during life. In addition, a complete examination of all the finer biliary passages to their finest sub-divisions is manifestly impossible. The causes of an obstruction of the biliary passages may be compression from without from tumors, kinking of the ducts themselves, occlusion of their lumen by concretions or other foreign bodies, neoplasms or inflammatory swelling of their walls. All these causes of obstruction may be present either in the main duct or in a number of its branches, even of its smallest ramifications. Particularly in the latter, swelling from hyperemia or inflammatory infiltration, shedding of degenerated epithelium, viscid mucus, and finely granular precipitates play an important rôle.

Even if the mucous membranes are intact, so that no viscid mucus is exuded, the viscid consistency of the bile itself, as it is sometimes seen in poisoning from toluylenediamin (Stadelmann, Affanassiew), may constitute an obstruction to the flow of bile.

The smaller the bile-passage, the more occlusion is produced by even minute obstructions. We can readily understand the conditions prevailing in these cases by comparing them to similar conditions in the finer air-passages, where we can measure the degree of obstruction during life by auscultation. Catarrhal asthma and edema of the larynx should teach us how rapidly such obstructions can occur, and how rapidly again such swellings of the mucous surfaces can disappear, as well as how different the postmortem findings may be from the conditions that we knew existed during the life of the patient.

Other factors that are concerned in the narrowing of biliary capillaries are compression by dilated blood-capillaries (venous stasis), by newly formed connective tissue, by swollen liver-cells (which probably occurs in phosphorus-poisoning), by distortion of the trabeculæ of liver-cells

* Loc. cit., p. 268.

(Hanot), and in various interstitial and parenchymatous diseases of the liver. As a rule, all these agencies will involve only single and disseminated groups of capillaries. In view, however, of the diffuse nature of the primary lesions a great number of bile-passages may be affected.

Besides mechanical obstructions to the outflow of the bile, certain other mechanical factors seem to be concerned in the reabsorption of the bile. In dogs we almost invariably find bile-pigment in the urine during fasting, while during digestion these pigments are not found. This is best explained by assuming that during the period of rest of the digestive organs the bile-ducts also are at rest, so that no peristaltic movement occurs. As a result, the bile contained within them may be absorbed, particularly since, under these circumstances, the bile stagnates and undergoes thickening. Possibly the slight degree of icterus sometimes seen in the conjunctiva of human subjects during periods of inanition may be explained on the same grounds.

The compression produced by the respiratory movements of the diaphragm exercises the same effect on the flow of the bile in the liver as it does on the flow of blood. It is quite possible that the cessation or reduction of these movements, that frequently occurs in diseases of the respiratory organs (pleuritis, pneumonia), may be instrumental in producing a retardation in the outflow of bile. A portion of the bile-pigments that enter the intestine is reabsorbed, partly as urobilin, partly as bilirubin. The latter is, as a rule, again excreted by the liver. Only in the new-born does a part of the portal blood circumvent the liver and enter the systemic blood-vessels directly through the ductus venosus Arantii. In the new-born all the bile-pigments remain unchanged in the intestine, owing to the absence of a bacterial flora in that viscus, and they are abundant in the meconium formed during fetal life. The frequent occurrence of icterus neonatorum can be explained from a combination of these circumstances (Quincke). In adults, also, icterus may occasionally originate from reabsorption of bile-pigment from the intestine following polycholia (see page 493).

Just as an increase of the pressure in the biliary capillaries may change the normal relation between the pressure of the bile and the pressure of the portal blood, so a decrease of the pressure in the portal and hepatic vessels may cause similar disturbances and lead to icterus. Frerichs assumes that icterus originates in this manner in many cases of stenosis of the portal vein and after psychic disturbances.

While it is true that mechanical disturbances play a certain rôle in the causation of icterus, careful consideration will show that these need not necessarily be present, but that the bile may readily enter the blood as the result of purely functional disturbance of the liver-cells.

If these cells normally pour bile-pigment into the biliary capillaries and sugar and urea into the blood-capillaries, we can readily understand how a lesion of these cells may cause both quantitative changes in their function as well as perversion in the direction in which they give off their products. This is seen in many other kinds of cells and glands. For instance, diseased renal cells pour albumin into the urinary passages, changes in the vessel-walls cause changes in the constitution of the lymph and have a share in the production of inflammatory exudates. Thus, as Minkowski says, it is not at all inconceivable, and we have analogies to strengthen our view, that under certain circumstances the liver-cells may pour the bile-pigments formed by them into the blood-capillaries instead of into the bile-capillaries. Minkowski calls this process "parapedesis of bile." Liebermeister and Pick also have attempted to explain certain forms of icterus by assuming functional disturbances in the liver-cells, either with or without demonstrable anatomic alterations. Liebermann has called this form of icterus "diffusion icterus" or "akathectic icterus" (from χαθεχειν, "to hold fast"). E. Pick has called it "paracholia." The latter author, we believe, goes too far in his belittling of the importance of the mechanical factor in the causation of icterus.

The question arises as to where and how the bile enters the blood-current when its outflow is hindered. We must assume that absorption chiefly occurs at the center of the acini, because the greatest amount of staining by bile is found here. Heidenhain, it is true, was able to find indigo-sulphate of sodium, injected into the bile-ducts of living animals, only in the interlobular and not in the intra-acinous bile-passages. It is possible that his deduction, that absorption occurs only in the former, holds true for the particular stain he employed in his experiments; in the case of bile it is, however, certainly not true. Older investigators (for example, Frerichs, loc. cit., p. 98) have assumed that absorption occurs through the veins as well as through the lymphatics. In recent years the latter alone are considered as the channels through which absorption occurs, particularly since Fleischl and Kufferaht have shown that in a dog, after ligation of the main bile-duct, the lymph taken from a fistula in the thoracic duct contains bilirubin and bile-acids, whereas the blood does not. This finding corresponds with the statement that after ligation of the thoracic and the main bile-duct in dogs both the blood and the urine contain no trace of biliary constituents for several (as many as seventeen) days (v. Harley and v. Frey). The question as to what became of these remains unsolved. Moreover, bile still makes its appearance in the blood if the thoracic duct is ligated some days after the bile-duct. Microscopically, the livers of animals in whom such a stasis of both bile and lymph had been produced showed an enormous dilatation of the bile-capillaries and of the perivascular lymph-spaces. The liver-cells, owing to the pressure, were reduced to one-half their normal size and number, and were separated by fissures in which the two dilated systems of vessels communicated.

D. Gerhardt, as was to be expected, saw icterus follow ligation of both the thoracic and the common bile-duct. It seemed to appear as rapidly and to be as intense as it was when the thoracic duct remained open. We see, therefore, that if there is occlusion of the lymph-channels, which ordinarily carry the bile away in case of an obstruction to its flow, the bile can be absorbed through other channels, and that these can only be the blood-vessels. [Queirolo and Benvenuti * have recently confirmed Gerhardt's results. They, however, believe that the lymph-vessels play a very slight part in absorption of bile, which they believe is accomplished through the intra-hepatic venous system.—Ed.] In recent obstructive icterus of man (and of the dog and cat) the liver-cells in the beginning contain no bile-pigment, the latter being seen only in the biliary passages and capillaries and in the connective-tissue cells. After the stasis of bile has persisted for some time the liver-cells also become impregnated with pigment (in Gerhardt's experiments at the end

* *Il Policlinico*, 1900, No. 13; abs. in *Centralbl. f. innere Med.*, 1901, No. 9, p. 224.

of five to six days). The pigment, as we have already mentioned, is principally deposited in those cells that are situated near the center of the lobules, wherein yellowish lumps of different size and outline are seen. Nauwerck believes that he has demonstrated in these cells a fine capillary network surrounding their nuclei and anastomosing with the bile-capillaries. In chronic stasis the latter are frequently filled with brownish and yellowish masses, as in an incomplete artificial injection. In the beginning, therefore, of stasis of bile the liver-cells are capable of getting rid of the bile-pigment which they form, but if the stasis continues for too long a time, they are no longer able to do so. D. Gerhardt also saw within the area of greatest stagnation endothelial cells filled with granular masses resembling bile. These cells were derived not only from the lymphatic sheaths, but also from the blood-vessels themselves, into the lumen of which they protruded.

Other histologic changes frequently develop in the hepatic tissue, probably because other factors besides biliary stasis play a rôle. If the outflow of bile is impeded, the bile-passages are filled with secretion and distended, and the whole organ, as can be readily determined during life, is distended and enlarged in the same manner as after an artificial injection. Whether this distention is simply a concomitant feature of the stasis or is caused by it remains doubtful. This increase in size and tension, it is true, varies greatly, even though the degree of stasis at different times may be complete and equal. The color of the liver in recent stasis is very little changed; only after a duration of weeks does discoloration of the center of the lobules become apparent to the naked eye. Gradually discoloration increases in intensity and extent until in the course of months there is a dark yellow or even greenish shade within the lobules. The gall-bladder and bile-ducts, and also the biliary passages within the liver, may become greatly distended as a result of this long-continued stasis, so that their combined capacity may be equal to a liter. The substance of the liver in certain areas partly disappears under the influence of this pressure and the microscopic structure of the lobules may become changed.

In long-continued stasis of this kind the contents of the finer microscopic bile-passages may consist of clear colorless mucus. D. Gerhardt found the intra-acinous passages in great part colorless, so that only a part of these and the liver-cells contained notable quantities of bile-pigment.

As we can but rarely study in an early stage the anatomic changes produced in the liver by uncomplicated, complete stasis of bile in man, many investigators have attempted to study the subject experimentally. The results obtained vary, and are in many instances different from the conditions observed in human subjects. One of the principal reasons for this is the fact that the duration of the stasis and the time of observation differed in the different experimental series. As a rule, the latter was too short, as it rarely extended over three weeks and never reached more than five to six weeks. Another reason is the difference of the reaction in the different animals employed. Dogs and cats seem to be quite resistant, while guinea-pigs succumb in a few days, or at best after a week or two. Rabbits are not quite so susceptible, and occasionally survive the operation for five weeks. In all these animals death results, with loss of appetite and emaciation, and in acute cases coma and spasm may supervene.

The time at which icterus of the tissues is said to make its appearance varies greatly (from one to ten days). In cases of chronic stasis icterus is said to decrease gradually. Bile-pigment and bile-acids (not looked for by all authors) are present in the blood and urine (Lahousse), although, according to D. Gerhardt, Gmelin's reaction may not be demonstrable in the urine for days at a time.

The anatomic examination of the animals reveals that the liver is enlarged and vascular, and that necrotic areas are disseminated all through the organ. The latter may appear in the course of the first twelve hours, increase in size and number up to the third day, decrease from that time on, and disappear by the seventh to the tenth day. The smallest of these foci involve only a few of the liver-cells, the larger ones include several lobules. Lahousse states that the smallest foci are oval in outline ; Steinhaus, that they are cone-shaped with their bases pointing toward the periphery of the lobule and their apices toward the center. These areas are distinguished from their reddish-brown surroundings by their grayish-yellow or bile-pigment color. In the beginning they are surrounded by a hyperemic ring. Under the microscope it will be seen that these necrotic liver-cells have an icteric color, are swollen, are undergoing hyaline degeneration, and show the formation of vacuoles within them. The staining power of their nuclei is soon lost, and later also that of their protoplasm. In regard to the blood-capillaries in the necrotic areas, Beloussow states that they become occluded, Steinhaus that they are compressed by the swollen liver-cells, and D. Gerhardt that they remain patent. The lymph-channels are distended (Lahousse).

Around these areas there then follows round-cell infiltration. Later absorption of the necrotic foci is brought about through the formation of giant cells and the growth of connective tissue into and around the area. This connective tissue is at first rich in nuclei, but later becomes fibrous. Similar conditions were found in the case of pigeons examined by Stern up to the seventh day after ligation. While Steinhaus claims that the round-cell infiltration is limited to the immediate surroundings of the necrotic foci, and Foa and Salvioli state the same for the connective-tissue growth, nearly all other authors state that connective tissue, which in the beginning resembles embryonal tissue, and later shows oval nuclei and becomes fibrous, develops from the second to the third day in the interlobular spaces, and that this tissue is irregularly distributed, but altogether independent of the necrotic foci (D. Gerhardt, Pick). Soon this connective tissue begins to grow into the hepatic lobules from their periphery, advancing between the rows of liver-cells, but rarely reaching as far as the central vein.

The bile-ducts, after ligation of the ductus choledochus, are dilated throughout and are filled with bile, not only in their main branches, but even in their finer ramifications (according to Popoff, even in their finest intercellular capillaries). In the finer interlobular bile-passages there are masses of detached epithelial cells filling the lumen, and also proliferation of the epithelium. After a period of three to six days diverticula form. These diverticula are lined by low, broad cells with old nuclei instead of cubical and cylindric epithelium. With this formation of new bile-ducts the canaliculi pursue a tortuous course and form anastomoses. The branches penetrate into the lymphatic lobules, where they are lost among the rows of liver-cells. According to some authors, an increase in the length of the bile-channels takes place through the flattening and the increase in the number of the cells at the periphery.

The time at which the proliferation of the bile-capillaries begins is stated by Beloussow to be the fourth day, by Pick the third, by D. Gerhardt the second. Most authors agree in stating that the proliferation of the connective tissue and of the bile-capillaries occurs at the same time and in the same locations. D. Gerhardt assumes that the two processes in general are independent of one another; Charcot and Gombault, on the other hand, regard the proliferation of the bile-passages as the primary event, the proliferation of connective tissue in the inter-(later intra-) lobular tissue as the secondary event. At all events, the two processes are not in any way related to the formation or resolution of the necrotic foci, as they persist for a long time (as long as ten days) after these have disappeared. During the fifth or sixth week the lobules of the liver may be seen to be surrounded by connective tissue, so that the cell-masses in their center become considerably reduced. As a result of all these processes, the whole organ seems smaller and harder than normal and its cut surface resembles the liver of a pig.

In rabbits and guinea-pigs ligation of the bile-ducts leads in a comparatively short time to serious anatomic changes of the liver, and frequently causes death. The same experimenter may see different degrees and kinds of changes following this procedure. This is probably due to slight accidental variations in the operation, such as duration of the operation, struggles of the animal, or to individual peculiarities of the animal. In this manner some of the contradictory statements of different investigators may be explained. The occurrence of necrosis in a large number of liver-cells following the sudden obstruction to the outflow of bile can hardly be attributed to mechanical factors alone (according to the control experiments of D. Gerhardt with injections of salt solution into the bile-duct), but must be regarded as the result of chemical injuries inflicted on the liver-cells by the bile. Similar changes can be produced outside of the organism by allowing bile to act on liver-cells, and can be readily recognized microscopically (Chambard, Steinhaus). If death occurs within the first few days, it must be attributed to the general damage that has been done to the parenchyma of the liver and to the serious disturbances of metabolism resulting therefrom. In the later stages the bile no longer produces necrosis, possibly because it is carried off by the lymph-channels or because less is being secreted (according to Lahousse, icterus in these later stages decreases). At the same time the bile still stimulates the tissues to the formation of connective-tissue and to proliferation of the bile-passages; thus, it is possible that the animals can perish even after five weeks, convulsed from disturbances of the hepatic function.

Dogs and cats react entirely differently to the operation. In these animals ligation of the common duct is followed by a dilatation of the larger bile-passages and of the gall-bladder with a thickening of their walls. While Leyden at one time observed fatty changes in these cells, later observers (D. Gerhardt, Foa, and Salvioli in dogs) either found the hepatic cells unaltered or saw simple pressure atrophy in the peripheral parts of the lobules (Foa and Salvioli in cats, Popoff in dogs). Popoff alone reports an increase of the interlobular connective tissue in one case, and here only to a slight degree. Necrotic foci have never been observed. While it is true that the experiments performed on the latter class of animals are not so numerous by far as on the former, and while many of the experiments cannot be utilized for the reason that the bile-passages did not remain permanently imper-meable or that perforative peritonitis or abscesses occurred, still it may be said to be positively established that ligation of the bile-ducts produces much slighter anatomic changes in the liver and is less dangerous to life in dogs and cats than in rabbits and guinea-pigs.

Steinhaus attributes these differences to a greater secretion of bile and, as a result, to a greater increase in the pressure in the latter class of animals. Of the different animals, the following amount of bile per kilo of animal is secreted in twenty-four hours:

Guinea-pig ....175.8 gm. of bile.
Rabbit ....136.8 "   "
Dog .... 20.0 "   "
Cat .... 14.5 "   "

The difference might also be attributed to greater individual resistance of the liver-cells to the action of bile, or it might be due to the fact that in dogs and cats the bile can more readily escape into the lymph-channels. The experiments of V. Harley and of v. Frey, already mentioned, show that, if an obstruction is created both to the flow of bile and of lymph, distinctly visible communications are estab-lished between the two systems of vessels.

The presence of bile-pigment in the blood and urine of cats and dogs during starvation might also be explained from the fact that in these animals the bile can more readily find an exit into the lymph-channels (Naunyn).

As the slighter anatomic changes in dogs and cats as compared to guinea-pigs and rabbits coincide with the slighter vulnerability and greater resistance of the former animals to the operation, the conclusion seems justified that it is not the absorption of biliary constituents (that is equal in both classes of animals) into the general circulation that causes death after occlusion of the bile-ducts, but some other form of damage to which the liver is subjected.

It appears that human beings resemble dogs in their reaction to stasis of bile. Man can survive for years with stasis of bile and the function of his liver may con-tinue unimpaired. Again, an occlusion lasting for months may be removed and be followed by no impairment of health or functional activity of the liver. Anatomic examination, it is true, has in many instances revealed more serious changes than the clinical picture during life would lead us to suspect. Janowski, for instance, examined ten cases of stasis of a duration of from two weeks to more than a year (eight being cases with gall-stones), and found necrotic areas with inflammation and a proliferation of the bile-passages and of the connective tissue. The necrotic areas were, as a rule, seen in the peripheral portions of the lobules, and were most numerous in recent cases. They are said to originate from extravasation of bile which damages the liver-cells and at the same time compresses the blood-capillaries and in this manner induces anemic necrosis. In the marginal portions of these foci cell-infiltration and dilatation of capillaries are seen, followed by the formation of connective tissue. The bile-ducts, too, show desquamation of epithelium, cellular infiltration of the walls, and new-formation of connective tissue. The bile-capillaries themselves proliferate, and here and there they seem to originate from rows of liver-cells.

Raynaud and Sabourin also report thickening of the walls of the large bile-passages from connective-tissue proliferation in chronic stasis of bile, and in many cases, in addition, hyperplasia of the glands of the bile-duct. Sauerhering found necrotic areas in the human liver less diffuse than those described by Janowski, and resembling more the experimental foci, and surrounded by connective tissue. Under certain conditions stasis of bile due to gall-stones may produce so intense a proliferation of connective-tissue that (aside from the intense icterus) the picture of atrophic cirrhosis may be simulated both clinically and anatomically (see atrophic cirrhosis). Brissaud and Sabourin observed the final result of chronic biliary stasis in two cases where the stone occluded only the left hepatic duct. In these cases the left lobe of the liver had almost completely disappeared, being merely represented by connective tissue and fibrous blood- and bile-vessels. Such a stage can be reached only if the stasis of bile is but partial, so that a part of the liver remains intact and can perform the functions necessary for the maintenance of life. In one case the cirrhotic process had extended to the right lobe, in which no stasis of bile existed. I made a similar observation recently in an autopsy. In this case the left lobe was converted into a structure that was only as large as two adrenals and resembled these organs in shape. The right lobe was vicariously hypertrophied (total weight of the liver 3 kg.). A biliary concretion was embedded close to the gall-bladder and showed that at some time a gall-stone must have been impacted in the left hepatic duct and have caused the changes observed.

To judge from these considerations it seems that some analogy exists after all between human beings and rabbits and guinea-pigs.

What causes these differences in individual cases? In the first place, I attribute them to the differences in the rapidity with which the obstruction of the flow of bile occurs. With the exception of certain cases of gall-stone impaction, this never occurs so rapidly as in ligation of the ducts. The more gradual the increase in the pressure of the bile, the better the communication established between the bile- and the lymph-vessels. In the second place, certain complications usually coexist in the cases studied in human beings, particularly infection of the bile-ducts. For this reason the pathologic changes observed in man can only to a certain extent be compared with the findings in animals in which similar conditions have been produced experimentally, bacterial infections in the latter instance being almost invariably excluded. When we consider, finally, that in animals in which the biliary stasis is apparently equal in intensity and duration different degrees of swelling of the liver and of involvement of the general health are found, we will have to assume that, in the third place, possibly, individual differences in the rapidity of the outflow of the bile into the lymph-channels play a rôle in human beings.

If we summarize all these investigations, we see that in human beings in the beginning of the biliary stasis the liver-cells continue to secrete bile in a normal manner and to pour the excreted bile into the biliary capillaries. This bile is principally absorbed by the lymph-channels, but may in part and under certain conditions directly reach the blood-vessels. From anatomic investigation alone we are not able to state whether icterus is caused by stasis or by parapedesis of bile.

As a result of long-continued stasis of bile the liver-cells become functionally impaired, so that the quantity of the bile-acids (possibly also of the bilirubin) decreases. As an evidence of other metabolic disturbances, we find a decreased power on the part of the liver to store glycogen. Soon bilirubin is seen within the cells, being either formed here and not excreted, or produced in other portions of the liver and pressed into the cells from the dilated capillaries that surround them. The liver-cells are damaged chemically by the bile and directly by the mechanical pressure and by the obstacles that are created to the outflow of bile through the blood- and lymph-channels. Anatomically, these conditions are manifested in the cells by reduction of their size, changes in their outline and structure, and, finally, by fatty degeneration, necrosis, and imbibition of bile.

This picture is, in addition, not rarely affected by the action of micro-organisms that reach the bile-passages from the intestine. The effect of such an invasion is not always manifested in the same manner, and may be different in extent and rapidity of development. The width of the bile-passages varies considerably in different individuals, and on this account individual tolerance against biliary stasis may vary in different subjects. In some cases we see simple pressure-atrophy of the hepatic tissue; in others, in addition, reactive growth of connective tissue. According to the presence or absence of the one or the other effect, we see either simple intoxication from absorption of biliary substances or, in addition, a reduction and a perversion of other functions of the liver.

Other substances that are injected into the bile-ducts under a degree of pressure in excess of that of the bile are absorbed; for example, stains in solution (carmin, anilin-blue). Stains in suspension (India ink) penetrate the lymph-glands at the portal fissure by way of the lymph-channels and may even be carried beyond. If physiologic salt solution be allowed to flow into the ducts, the liver-cells are bleached out and sugar appears in the urine within a few minutes (Grützner).

Anatomico-histologic Changes in Other Organs.—The biliary con-stituents circulating in the blood soon penetrate the tissues. Very little is known in this respect in regard to the bile-acids, but bilirubin is, of course, readily recognized from the discoloration of the tissues that it produces. At first the latter enters the blood-stream and the plasma, where it can be recognized by the yellow color that it imparts to the plasma and by Gmelin's reaction. It is also readily found in serous transudates and exudates, and in the fluid within the ventricles of the brain and in serum from blisters. [It has also been detected in cerebro-spinal fluid obtained during life by lumbar puncture.—ED.]

The discoloration observed in dead bodies is, according to Minkowski, much modified by a postmortem imbibition of the tissues with blood-serum and lymph. There can, however, be no doubt that certain tissues have a particular selective affinity for bile-pigment, especially connective tissue. The yellow color is, therefore, particularly conspicuous in the intima of the vessels, the fasciæ, the connective-tissue layers of the skin and mucous membranes, and the subcutaneous tissues. Muscular and nervous tissue are only slightly colored by bile-pigment. The brain is slightly icteric only in the new-born; in adults it is colorless, and only the lymph in the perivascular spaces or the edematous fluid are colored slightly yellow. Gland-cells and epithelium, as a rule, absorb little bile-pigment, with the exception of the deepest layers of the rete Malpighii and the kidneys. In the former organs the pigment is seen diffusely all through the organ or in a granular form, as in all physiologic and patho-logic pigmentations. This massing of pigment, together with the im-bibition of the cutis, causes the relatively deep coloration of the external skin.

Bile-pigment is excreted by the kidneys. In the beginning of icterus and in mild cases it stains the cortex diffusely; later it assumes the form of yellowish granules that are also seen in the lumen of the canals. The epithelial cells of the tubuli contorti are still more deeply stained than are those of the cortex. Here, too, if the icterus persists for a long time, the yellow masses appear in the lumen in greater number and more closely packed. They are most numerous in the afferent tubules, which also show the greatest defects of the epithelium. In these tubes are seen cylindric casts colored yellow, green, or brown, formed in part by necrotic epithelial cells.* In addition to pigmentary infiltration, the epithelial cells of the uriniferous tubules show swelling, cloudiness, a loss of cilia, and necrotic disintegration (Moebius, Lorenz), changes which, according to Werner, are due to the action of the salts of the bile-acids. Macroscopically the cortex of the kidneys appears yellowish or even greenish in color, while the pyramids are streaked with dark green. More marked changes are seen only if complete stasis of bile has persisted for months. A few days after the stasis is relieved the cortex assumes its normal color, but the tubuli contorti and the parenchyma remain discolored for a longer period. Occlusion of the tubules and damage to the epithelial cells by constituents of the bile probably produce a diminution in the excretory power of the kidney, and may in this manner be detrimental to the whole organism.

The fetus of an icteric mother is also icteric, not, however, in proportion to the maternal icterus, the condition in the fetus being usually less marked.

The pus from cellular tissues is icteric, but mucus or mucopurulent secretions of mucous membranes, on the other hand, are not. Intestinal mucus occasionally forms an exception to this latter statement.

Symptoms of Icterus.—The presence of biliary materials in the general circulation produces a series of symptoms that are altogether independent of the primary cause of the trouble. These are of such significance that they merit separate discussion. They are most conspicuous in obstructive icterus, and are the more apparent the more complete the obstruction to the flow of bile. The prototype of the acute forms of this condition is found in simple cases of catarrhal icterus; that of the chronic forms, in occlusion of the ductus choledochus by a gallstone.

The most conspicuous symptom is the yellow discoloration of the skin and visible mucous membranes. By almost imperceptible degrees the color merges from a light sulphur yellow to a lemon yellow, then into a greenish and olive color, and finally a dirty yellowish-gray (Melas-Icterus). The shades last described are only seen in cases where icterus has persisted for months. As a rule, the discoloration is more intense on the trunk and the upper half of the body than on the lower half. It is frequently masked by the normal pigment of the skin and by its vascularity, the milder degrees of icterus being, therefore, more readily overlooked in brunettes and in full-blooded subjects than in blond or pale subjects. The yellow color is sooner and more readily observed in the sclera of the eyeball than it is in the skin; but it must be remembered that many people, in addition to showing a yellowish tinge where the muscles are inserted, normally have yellowish sclera both of the eyeball and of the conjunctiva. Icteric discoloration is not readily perceptible in the mucous membranes of the mouth and throat, owing to the blood-red color of these parts; but the paler lining of the gums occasionally shows it.

Very frequently patients with icterus complain of a feeling of itching, often causing them to scratch themselves severely. The scratched portions of the epidermis in these cases form dull whitish streaks that are clearly visible on the otherwise uniformly yellow skin. If the patients scratch themselves very vigorously, we see small papules and ulcers covered with scabs, or, if the skin be particularly delicate, the formations

* See Frerichs' "Atlas," Plate I, Figs. 8–11.

28

of blebs and of eczematous rashes. This form of pruritus must be classified as a symptom of intoxication analogous to the drug exanthems. It is impossible to state whether the deposit of bile-pigment in the skin has anything to do with its occurrence. It appears in different cases at various stages of icterus, in some cases in the beginning, in others if the disease has persisted for some length of time. Although sometimes it persists during the whole course of the affection, in others, again, it disappears before the icterus. This pruritus occurs chiefly in obstructive jaundice of considerable severity, and, as a rule, disappears as soon as the bile-passages become patent again, even though the icterus of the skin may persist. [Herter is inclined to attribute the pruritus to dryness of the skin, in view of its occasional appearance before pigmentation.—Ed.]

A peculiar skin lesion (not exclusively found in icterus) is seen in chronic icterus, called xanthelasma, or xanthoma. It consists in dirty, pale yellowish spots, that protrude very little beyond the level of the skin in the beginning, but later assume the tuberous form. They are chiefly found in the region of the eyelids. The pigmentation of these spots is not caused by bile-pigments, and, in fact, their connection with icterus is not definitely determined.* [In certain cases of long-standing jaundice peculiar areas of lighter yellow color are seen, looking as though the epidermis were raised by small quantities of serum. They are frequently linear in their arrangement.—Ed.]

The following secretions always contain bile-pigment in icterus: the urine, sweat, serous and inflammatory exudates, liquor amnii, pus from cellular tissues and from wound surfaces. Milk and pneumonic sputa are not constantly colored; while the tears, the saliva, and the mucus and mucopurulent secretions of the mucous membranes remain colorless.

The coloration of the urine is the most important, and has the greatest practical significance, since through the medium of the urine the constituents of the bile (the bile-pigments and the bile-acids) retained in the body are to be removed from the organism. If any considerable degree of stasis exists, the urine always contains bilirubin, and is consequently colored yellow even in very thin layers, so that the foam on the top of the urine also is discolored. In the vessel the urine is of a brownish-yellow to brown color, occasionally being mixed with red or with a dirty opalescent green or brown tint. The former is caused by urobilin, the latter by higher oxidation products of bilirubin. These pigments are usually formed only after exposure to the air, but, especially in chronic cases of icterus, may be seen immediately after the urine is voided.

Under the microscope hyaline cylinders are, as a rule, found in the urine (Nothnagel). If the icterus is of long duration, these casts contain yellowish renal epithelial cells. In the new-born these epithelial cells are not stained, but inclose the pigment in the form of granules and needles. While it is true that Litten † finds hyaline cylinders in every normal urine by means of the centrifuge, still they are more numerous in icteric urine, and indicate that the passage of biliary substances through the kidneys has produced an irritation of these organs.

Traces of albumin in solution may be found only after the icterus has persisted for a long time.

* Michel in Gräfe-Saemisch's "Handbuch der Augenheilkunde," Bd. iv, p. 425. Schwimmer und Babes, Ziemssen's "Handbuch der speciellen Pathologie," Bd. xiv, II, p. 446.
† Litten, *Berliner klin. Wochenschr.*, 1896, p. 263.

Bile-pigment is recognized chemically by methods which cause oxidation of bilirubin to green biliverdin. The most frequently employed method is to superpose the urine upon impure nitric acid, whereby oxidation goes beyond the formation of the green tint, and higher products of blue, orange, and reddish-brown shades are formed in successive layers until finally complete decoloration occurs. As nitric acid gives a dark color to a number of other pigments that are found in the urine, it is essential that the green shade should be clearly perceptible. Instead of superposing with nitric acid, the urine can be mixed with a few drops of a solution of nitrite of potassium and sulphuric acid be superposed. If the urine is mixed with only a few drops of impure nitric acid, a diffuse green color soon appears. This occurs more slowly if some other acid be added. Solutions of potassium iodid and chlorid of iron may also be employed as oxidizing agents by adding a few drops to the urine, when the green color appears gradually after one or several minutes.

These reactions do not all succeed equally well in every instance, and it is frequently necessary to test the exact quantities of the reagents and the reaction-time. This is apparently due to other urinary constituents, possibly modifications of the pigments themselves. Among these might be mentioned a colorless chromogen that is formed by reduction and a brown substance formed by oxidation of bilirubin. Occasionally the reaction is more distinct if the pigment is distributed over filter-paper either by dipping strips of the paper into the urine to be examined or by filtering the urine through filter-paper. If paper so impregnated be touched with fuming nitric acid, rings of different colors will be found. Sometimes the green color will appear if the paper be allowed to dry in the air. In case the urine contains albumin and is boiled, a part of the pigment is apt to be precipitated with the coagulate. If the quantity of pigment is very small or if other pigments are present, the test of Schwerdtfeger-Huppert is of value and is very delicate. It is performed as follows: The urine is mixed with lime-water and a stream of carbonic acid gas is passed through the mixture. The biliary coloring-matter is carried down with the calcium hydrate in the precipitate. The residue left on filtration is then washed with slightly warmed alcohol to which has been added a few drops of sulphuric acid. If bile-pigment is present, the fluid assumes a greenish color.

According to Gluzinski, icteric urine can be made green by boiling with a few drops of formalin solution, a test that is very delicate. On the addition of muriatic acid, the green color changes into violet.

If only very small quantities of bile-pigment are circulating in the blood, as in the beginning or toward the termination of an attack of icterus of considerable severity, no bilirubin, but urobilin alone, will be found in the urine, and hence the color will be yellowish-red. Urobilin is also frequently found in the urine together with bilirubin during icterus, as a rule in abundant quantities, but usually disappearing as soon as the bile is completely absent from the intestine (for details see below).

Urobilin can be detected directly with the spectroscope or after precipitation with ammonium sulphate. If bilirubin is present at the same time, it must first be precipitated with lime-water or baryta mixture, the urobilin being only in small part thrown down with these precipitates, the greater part remaining in solution. Hayem * recommends superposing the urine with water in a test-tube, urobilin diffusing upward more rapidly than bilirubin and being readily detected spectroscopically in the watery layer.

The liver itself produces no direct symptoms during life in the milder cases of icterus from stasis or from parapedesis. If the stasis of bile assumes more formidable proportions, the organ becomes distended and causes a feeling of fulness and discomfort, as well as tenderness on pressure by the fingers or by the overfull gastro-intestinal tract. Occasionally palpation seems to reveal an increased degree of resistance. Percussion shows an enlargement of the area of hepatic dulness. Sometimes the distended and full gall-bladder can be palpated and percussed. The degree of enlargement and resistance of the liver varies even where biliary obstruction is complete and occurs in a perfectly healthy organ. The anatomic findings in a liver affected in this manner may be perfectly negative. If the obstruction persists for many months, increase in the

* Chauffard, *loc. cit.*, p. 698.

size and consistence of the liver will be found. If the obstruction persists still longer, the size of the liver recedes in part or returns to normal, because of pressure atrophy or interstitial hepatitis.

No satisfactory explanation for this varying reaction of the liver can be given. It is probably due to differences in the width of the channels acting vicariously in carrying off the surplus of bile accumulated, these differences being founded on anatomic peculiarities. The presence or absence of infection of the bile-passages or of parenchymatous or interstitial hepatitis would have an important bearing upon the secondary effects of obstruction.

We might expect that increased pressure in the bile-capillaries would produce compression of blood-capillaries within the liver, particularly as the pressure in the portal vein is normally lower than it is in the bile-ducts. Betz has, in fact, noticed a lessening of the blood-stream in the portal system when the bile-ducts were filled. It is impossible to recognize such an occurrence clinically, as digestive disturbances and enlargement of the spleen may occur as the result of many conditions other than hyperemia from stasis. Even though increased transudation occurs from the serosa of the intestine as a result of the obstruction that exists to the outflow of this exudate, the parietal peritoneum may be stimulated to increased activity of its absorptive power, and in this manner the true condition may evade detection.

The spleen is often found enlarged in the diseases that are accompanied by icterus. As a rule, this is a result of causes other than those discussed above. It is usually due to infections or the excessive destruction of red blood-corpuscles producing a great accumulation of debris within the spleen. Even in simple acute obstructive jaundice (*icterus catarrhalis*) the spleen is occasionally, but not always, enlarged. Perhaps infection from the bile-ducts, only recently appreciated, plays a rôle; perhaps, too, venous stasis may be responsible. It is less probable that the swelling of the spleen is due to an accumulation of debris from the great destruction of red blood-corpuscles by the reabsorbed biliary acids (spodogenous tumor of the spleen).

The decrease in the normal quantity of bile poured into the intestine influences fat-absorption and putrefactive processes. In agreement with the findings of physiologic investigators, Fr. Müller found that the absorption of amylaceous substances was not at all interfered with and that of proteids only to a slight degree, but that the absorption of fats is greatly decreased. Of a given quantity of fat administered with the food, from 55% to 78% were recovered in the feces, as against 7% to 10% in normal subjects. J. Munk found a slightly better utilization of the fat, even as high as 64%, if abundant fat was ingested. In this case the waxy fats were not assimilated as well as the oily ones. The assimilation of the fatty acids was not changed by the absence of bile. The splitting of the fat within the intestine, according to J. Munk, is less active and occurs to a lesser degree. Fr. Müller found that the splitting of the fat was only perverted if the pancreatic duct was at the same time occluded.

Dastre's experiment is a fine demonstration of the significance of the bile in the absorption of fat. He ligated the ductus choledochus in dogs and established a fistula between the gall-bladder and a coil of the intestine below. Only in the region below this fistula was the chyle found to be milky, pancreatic juice alone being unable to induce absorption of fat.

It is not positively known what is the exact significance of the bile in the absorption of fat. It is possible that it acts purely physically by promoting the adhesion of the fat emulsion to the villi (Wistinghausen), or by exerting some influence on the vital activity of the intestinal wall.

The color of the feces, after exclusion of the bile from the intestine, is dependent only on the color of the ingesta. After a pure meat diet, for example, they are brownish-black. If the ingesta are colorless the feces are grayish-white or clay-colored. The pale color is increased by the mixture of large quantities of fat that is emulsified but not absorbed. In feces of this character the microscope frequently reveals long needles of fatty acids, and in particular a large quantity of needle-shaped, short crystals, arranged in sheaths. These consist of magnesium, potassium, and sodium soaps of the higher fatty acids. If they are very numerous, they may give the feces a shiny appearance. In partial stasis of bile the color of the feces may vary from a clay-colored, white, or brownish tint through all the different shades between this and the normal color. It is frequently possible by using acid-alcohol to extract urobilin from apparently colorless masses. In complete biliary obstruction traces of urobilin may be present, for intestinal mucus containing biliary coloring-matter may be mixed with the feces. Here, too, a reduction to chromogen may occur, so that the feces contain more pigment than would appear from inspection alone.

According to Bidder and Schmidt, the bile has antiputrefactive properties, and the feces of icteric patients are credited with a particularly bad odor. I cannot indorse this. The scale of malodorousness is, of course, altogether subjective.

Certain experiments show that the bile itself can readily putrefy, and that many bacterial species thrive exceedingly well in it (see page 472). The ethereal sulphates, that may be considered an index of intestinal putrefaction, were found increased in icterus by Brieger, Biernacki, and Eiger, not increased by Röhmann, Fr. Müller, Pott, and v. Noorden. [Lately Boehm* has found them greatly increased.—Ed.]

In view of the complicated bacterial fauna of the intestine, this question is not a simple one and cannot be readily decided. The antiputrefactive action of the bile is by no means demonstrated. It is possible that the action of the bile may be favorable to the growth of certain bacterial species or, on the other hand, that it may be unfavorable to their growth. In either instance the composition of the bacterial mixture and of its products would be changed.

Clinically the digestive disturbances following stasis of bile are very varying. As a rule, other disturbances of the stomach or intestine coexist, so that it is very difficult to decide how much is due to the absence of bile from the intestine. The frequent tendency to constipation may with some degree of certainty be ascribed to this factor, as may possibly, also, the tendency to flatulency. Disturbances of the appetite and an unpleasant bitter taste in the mouth are frequently complained of in icterus, as is also a distaste for certain foods, sometimes for fats and usually for meat.

It can hardly be assumed that the bile-acids circulating in the blood act directly on the nerves of taste and cause the bitter taste, since similar sensations are complained of in disturbances other than icterus (such as dyspepsia), and are, further, not proportionate to the degree of biliary stasis. According to Hayem, hyper-chlorhydria of the stomach usually coexists (?).

In many cases of simple chronic biliary stasis digestive disturbances and loss of appetite are singularly absent or very slight.

In addition to the yellow discoloration and the local disturbances produced by stasis, there are found in icterus a number of other symptoms affecting the circulatory and the nervous systems and the special senses.

* *Deutsches Arch. f. klin. Med.*, Bd. LXXI, Hft. 1.

The action of the heart is sometimes slower, the pulse usually smaller than normal.

Röhrig has shown that the salts of the bile-acids produce this effect from a paralysis of the intracardiac ganglia. Ranke, Traube, Feliz and Ritter, Löwit, and others ascribe it to their deleterious action on the heart-muscle. Löwit and Spalitta assume that, at the same time, the cardiac-inhibitory fibers of the vagus are irritated. That the latter certainly play an important rôle is demonstrated by the experiments of Weintraud, who, in one case, was able to increase the pulse-rate from 40 to 120 by an injection of atropin (1.2 mg.). [Mendez * found this accelerator action of atropin in only one out of five cases.—Ed.]

According to the animal experiments of Rywosch, small doses of the salts of the bile-acids dilate the vessels, whereas large ones contract them.

Herz † was enabled to determine a dilatation of the capillaries in icterus with the onychograph. It is also stated that a capillary pulse is seen (Drasche).

Over the heart systolic murmurs and a reduplication of the second pulmonary sound are occasionally heard. According to my observations, these signs are not more frequent in icterus than in many other conditions in which the general health is reduced. Potain, without sufficient proof, assumes that a spasm of the pulmonary capillaries occurs reflexly by stimulation from the bile-passages.‡

The body-temperature, as well as the pulse, are occasionally below normal (the former usually only a few tenths of a degree). Janssen § found such a reduction in 6 out of 18 cases of catarrhal jaundice.

Disturbances of sight, such as xanthopsia, hemeralopia, and nyctalopia, are quite frequent.

It was formerly assumed that the phenomenon of yellow vision was due directly to the yellow discoloration of the vitreous. This purely physical explanation has of late been again advocated by Hirschberg. Against this theory we can argue that, if it were correct, we should find this symptom more frequently, and that the degree of yellow vision should be in proportion to the degree of icterus. It is much more probable that a toxic nervous cause produces this symptom.

In five cases of chronic icterus Obermayer found changes in the bones—"drum-stick" fingers and toes—and painful periosteal swellings in the epiphyses of the arm and leg. [Similar "clubbing" of the extremities of the fingers and toes has recently been reported in a few cases of hepatic cirrhosis of different forms.—Ed.]

As the addition of the salts of the bile-acids to the blood outside of the body produces a liberation of hemoglobin, disintegration of red blood-corpuscles from this cause has been looked for in icterus. It is possible that it occurs, but it has not been demonstrated. A quantity of these bile-acid salts large enough to dissolve hemoglobin in the test-tube is never found circulating in the blood.

Hürthle has made the interesting observation that in dogs after ligation of the ductus choledochus or after poisoning with toluylenediamin, the cells of the thyroid show evidence of increased glandular activity, evidenced by a large quantity of colloid in the epithelial cells and in the lymph-spaces. Hürthle assumes that some chemical irritant is carried off by the blood. Lindemann in four cases of grave icterus in human subjects found the lymph-channels of the gland filled to a greater degree than normal, and therefore assumes an increased formation of colloid. He ascribes to this colloid an antitoxic action destined to replace or compensate the disturbed detoxicating function of the liver.

In addition to bile-pigment and urobilin mentioned above, the urine contains cholalic acid even in those forms of icterus that cannot positively be attributed to stasis of bile, as in pyemia.

In order to demonstrate the presence of this substance it is necessary to isolate it (by extraction with alcohol, precipitation with baryta-water, etc.) and then to perform Pettenkofer's reaction (the formation of a purple color on addition of a solution of cane-sugar and of concentrated sulphuric acid). The method of Strass-

* *Rivista de la Sociedad medica Argentina*, 1895, No. 22.

† "Verhandlungen des Congresses für innere Medicin," 1896, p. 467.

‡ Chauffard, *loc. cit.*, p. 692.

§ *Deutsches Archiv für klin. Medicin*, 1894, Bd. LIII, p. 262.

burger is shorter, but, even if a positive result is obtained, unreliable. It consists in the addition of a solution of cane-sugar and impregnation of a piece of filter-paper with the mixture, the paper being allowed to dry and being then touched with a drop of concentrated sulphuric acid. If cholalic acid be present, a violet spot appears.

The quantity of cholalic acid found in the urine is always small. Bischoff in one instance found 0.34 per diem, but as a rule much less will be found.

Cholalic acid is also responsible for the slight cloudiness that is occasionally seen on addition of acids to icteric urine.

According to Lépine, the quantity of that fraction of sulphur that is oxidized with difficulty is increased in the beginning of biliary stasis, but may drop back to below normal at the expiration of several days. Normally the "neutral" sulphur amounts to from 14% to 25% of the total sulphur, but in icterus as much as 43% may be present. It is probable that all or the greater part of this sulphur is derived from the taurin of the bile.*

In severe or long-continued icterus albumin is found in the urine in small quantities, but sugar is not found in icterus *per se*. Wyatt † saw the sugar disappear from the urine in a case of diabetes in which severe icterus supervened, but after the disappearance of the jaundice the sugar reappeared. According to Bouchard and his pupils, the toxicity of the urine is increased in icterus (see above).

Fr. Müller found that the urinary excretion of nitrogen was not increased in icterus. The finding of other authors (Wilischanin, R. Schmidt), who report an increase in the nitrogen excretion, must be explained by something other than the icterus.

As already stated, the ethereal sulphates are in some instances increased, in other instances not increased.

Icterus is usually followed by disturbances of the general health, with a diminution of the general physical and mental powers and a feeling of weakness, discomfort, and depression. These symptoms are particularly conspicuous in the acute forms, and may be due to the gastro-intestinal disturbances that usually coexist or to auto-intoxication.

In chronic biliary stasis these symptoms persist for a longer or shorter period of time. When they diminish, we can assume that a tolerance to the action of the poison becomes established. In complete obstruction of bile the general health is always impaired. General nutrition suffers greatly even though the patients may live for months or even years. Quite frequently a tendency to hemorrhages in the skin, in the connective-tissue structures, and from the free surfaces of the body develops. These hemorrhages are undoubtedly capillary, but may nevertheless lead to serious loss of blood from epistaxis, hematemesis, and hemorrhages from the intestine.

Finally, in chronic jaundice unfavorable symptoms may appear in a somewhat acute manner and lead to the death of the patient in the course of a few days. With increasing weakness and loss of appetite stupor may develop, and death may follow a slowly deepening coma, often preceded by a stage of excitation with loud delirium and spasms of indefinite type. This syndrome, often appearing unexpectedly, resembles an acute intoxication, and has been considered as such and called " cho-

---

* Noorden, *loc. cit.*, pp. 274, 282.   † *The Lancet*, May, 1886.

lemia." The poison was thought to be the bile-constituents circulating in the blood, and they were believed to exercise their deleterious effect as soon as the kidneys refused to excrete them vicariously.

In the light of our present knowledge such an explanation is inadequate, as we frequently see such a termination in other diseases of the liver not accompanied by icterus (atrophic cirrhosis), and animal experiments have shown that partial destruction (Denis and Stubbe) of the liver or disconnection of the organ by an Eck fistula (Nencki and Pawlow) can also produce serious nervous symptoms with spasms and be followed by a fatal issue without the presence of any disturbance in the outflow of bile. As we know that in chronic biliary stasis the parenchyma of the liver is always damaged in one way or the other and is reduced in bulk, we are justified in concluding that in these cases disturbances of the non-secretory functions of the liver may lead to death.

According to this view, we are dealing with an auto-intoxication of a very complicated character, for, besides the constituents of the bile, we have toxic effects from all those substances which the liver is no longer capable of elaborating and of converting. It is probable that carbaminate of ammonia, which Nencki particularly accuses of great toxicity, plays an important rôle in this connection. In addition to this, a number of other unknown substances are active, among these being putrefactive products from the intestine and disintegration products of the liver-cells themselves.

In favor of the mixed character of this self-intoxication is the varying picture of the symptoms, which here, as in other forms of auto-intoxication, such as diabetic coma and uremia, is very striking. It might be useful to designate these individually different processes as hepatargia (from ἀργία, "inactivity") or as hepatic intoxication. The name cholemia is not appropriate for the reason that the bile plays only a secondary rôle, while still more misleading and even less appropriate is the "acholia" of Frerichs.

Even though the symptoms of hepatic intoxication appear suddenly, it can hardly be assumed that they really begin when they first become perceptible. It is very probable that certain much earlier perversions of the internal secretion of the liver-cells exist and involve possibly only a portion of the cells, and consist not so much in qualitative disturbances of function, particularly in the beginning, as in quantitative ones. It is impossible to state at what period of the biliary stasis these disorders begin; but it is probable that, in those acute conditions in which the liver is distended and enlarged, they may appear very early, perhaps only a few days after the formation of the obstruction, and that often the early appearance of severe general disturbances may be attributed to these perversions.

We are not always justified in making a bad prognosis if serious nervous disturbances appear in the course of icterus, for in infectious icterus, and even in acute yellow atrophy, patients have recovered despite the presence of such symptoms. It is worthy of mention that Damsch has on several occasions observed cataleptic rigidity in children afflicted with epidemic icterus, and considers this symptom to be of toxic origin.

In order to explain the occurrence of symptoms appearing in parts other than the digestive organs in benign forms of icterus, earlier authors assumed that these were due to intoxication from constituents of the bile, and in fact they succeeded in finding that the salts of the bile-acids did possess toxic properties. It is definitely established by experiment (see above) that these salts act on the heart, the nerves of the blood-vessels, the kidneys, the central nervous system, and the blood, but it has not been determined whether the itching and the xanthopsia are caused by them. Within late years the toxicity of bilirubin has been investigated. Bouchard felt called upon to assume a poisonous action for bilirubin from the fact that bile is not as toxic if it has been previously decolorized by animal charcoal. While de Bruin found that bilirubin was more toxic, Plásterer and Rywosch found that it was much less toxic than the salts of bile-acids. The effect postulated by the former investigator is due, according to the latter authors, to the disturbances produced by the intravenous injections as such, and to the effect of the sodium hydrate used as a solvent. Plasterer observed the death of frogs after an injection of only 4 mg. of bilirubin, and attributes its action to the formation of insoluble compounds with the lime-salts of the tissue-fluids and the resulting formation of thrombi in the vessels.

Flint has credited cholesterin with the primary rôle in the production of the toxic symptoms in icterus, basing his view on the increase in cholesterin in the blood. Müller attempted to strengthen this view experimentally, but his experiments were not free from error (thrombosis of vessels, toxic action of glycerin). According to Jankau,* the organism has the power of destroying even considerable quantities of cholesterin. The hypothesis of a cholesteremia can, therefore, not be maintained.†

Even though we can hold certain constituents of the bile responsible for certain symptoms of the intoxication, this by no means excludes the share of other substances in their production. Itching of the skin occurs especially in icterus, but it is also occasionally observed in cirrhosis of the liver without icterus. The hemorrhagic diathesis is neither an exclusive result of icterus nor of hepatic diseases in general, but it is nevertheless possible that it is caused by the toxic action of the bile. This is illustrated by a case reported by Hayem, where no stasis of bile was present, but where the gall-bladder had ruptured and the bile was absorbed from the peritoneum.

The results of partial stasis of bile are less characteristic than are those of the complete form. The former occurs either as the result of a partial obstruction of the large bile-ducts, whereby only a portion of the bile is allowed to flow into the intestine and the pressure backward is only slightly increased, or as the result of the complete obstruction of the finer bile-passages while others are patent or are incompletely involved. It is of no significance for intestinal digestion which of these forms of partial obstruction is present, as the important point is the amount of bile poured into the intestine. To judge from clinical observation, it appears that even a small quantity is of the greatest value in comparison to complete absence of all bile.

The disturbances of the general health, too, are much less severe and characteristic in partial than in complete obstruction of the bile, and as a rule the degree of the disturbance is proportionate to the degree of stasis. This is true only in a general way and approximately, as the color of the feces, of the skin, and of the urine, as we have already stated, gives us only an approximate estimate of the percentage of the bile escaping in unnatural directions. On the other hand, it is necessarily important, in judging of general symptoms, to know whether only a relative obstruction exists in the large ducts causing the entrance of bile into the blood, or whether a part of the smaller ducts is completely occluded. In the former instance, when the obstruction is situated in one of the large ducts, all of the liver-cells are exposed to abnormal conditions of a slight degree, while in the latter a certain part of the liver-cells is seriously damaged, and though, in this case, other healthy liver-cells may act vicariously and assume the functions of the diseased ones, thus

* See Naunyn, "Cholelithiasis," p. 10.
† For further details, see Thierfelder, *loc. cit.*, p. 253.

compensating the loss of function, at the same time the diseased cells produce abnormal metabolic products that are absorbed and act as poisons. It cannot be stated in a general way which of the forms of stasis is capable of doing the most damage, as this varies in different cases, and probably the disturbances differ qualitatively.

During life it is much more difficult to determine which form of biliary stasis exists from the specific symptoms than it is from other clinical phenomena.

Compared with other organs, the first form of partial biliary stasis would resemble a stenosis of the larger air-passages, the second one a capillary bronchitis with atelectasis and lobular pneumonia; or, in the case of the kidneys, the first form would be like a stenosis of the ureters, the second would be analogous to a calcareous infarction of the straight uriniferous tubules.

It is, further, impossible to differentiate the form of icterus from parapedesis from that due to partial stasis.

The assumption pronounced at one time, that bile-acids are found in the urine only in icterus from stasis, has been shown to be erroneous.

Course.—The degree and the course of icterus vary according to the primary cause of the disease. It may last one day only and may simply cause a faint yellow discoloration of the skin, or it may produce deep green shades of discoloration and persist for months and even years. The average duration of an attack of icterus is several weeks, for the reason that the formation and the removal of the obstruction require a certain time, while the same applies to the staining of the tissues with pigment and the subsequent decoloration. Those forms of icterus that are not certainly due to biliary stasis act in the same way. Complete obstruction with absence of all bile from the intestine is found only in a small number of cases, and here only for a limited time. Before and after the time of complete obstruction relative degrees of stasis exist, gradually shading into the normal conditions. We are able, nevertheless, to distinguish acute forms of icterus, usually of only slight grade, developing in the course of a few days and disappearing in a few weeks, and chronic forms, persisting for a longer time and developing from acute forms or extending over a very long period of time and developing very slowly.

The intensity of icterus is not proportionate to its duration, as we see acute icterus of a severe degree and chronic icterus of a slight degree, and vice versa.

At first the bile-pigment enters the blood-serum and the tissue-juices; later the skin and the conjunctiva turn yellow and the urine contains urobilin. No bilirubin is present in the urine at this stage, but later bilirubin is also excreted. In cases in which the stasis of bile develops very rapidly the reverse picture may be seen, the appearance of bile-pigment in the urine preceding any yellow coloration of the skin or conjunctiva. Such an occurrence, however, is rare. Since sudden stoppage of the flow of bile is usually due to the impaction of a stone, and as this accident is always signalized by the appearance of severe pain, we have a measure for the time that must elapse between the occurrence of the obstruction and the appearance of icterus. Sometimes a yellow tint of the skin and the conjunctiva may be noticed after twelve hours,* but several days must elapse before the icterus reaches

* Schüppel, *loc. cit.*, p. 240; also personal observations.

its highest degree of intensity. Colorless feces are, of course, not passed until all the colored portions have been evacuated.

In dogs icteric discoloration of the tissues is not noticed for two or three days * after ligation of the ductus choledochus. As will be shown below, we are not justified in drawing conclusions in regard to human subjects from experiments of this kind on animals. The urine in these animals contains considerable quantities of bilirubin in from sixteen to twenty-four hours after the operation, and at the time of profuse secretion of bile (soon after eating) the urine may contain pigment as early as eight to ten hours after the operation (D. Gerhardt).

If bile is excluded from the intestine for long periods of time, urobilin may disappear from the urine and bilirubin alone be excreted.

If the obstruction is suddenly removed, as by the passage of the stone, a slighter degree of biliary discoloration of the urine will be noticed and colored feces will be found after the evacuation of the remains of the clay-colored matter. In the first days after the passage of the stone the stools will contain excessive quantities of pigment, owing to the emptying of the dilated bile-passages that occurs as soon as the obstacle is removed, while solid feces may even contain unchanged bilirubin. I once saw this continue for four weeks in a patient taking little nourishment. If the obstruction to the outflow of bile is completely removed, bilirubin will disappear from the urine within two days, and after this time only urobilin will be excreted. At the expiration of from three to eight days this too disappears, although the icteric color of the skin persists for a much longer time.

Skin.	Serum.	Urine.	Feces.
1. Very light yellow.	Bile-pigment $\bigcirc$.	Bile-pigment $\bigcirc$. Urobilin $\bigcirc$ or a little only.	Normal color.
2. Slightly yellow.	Bile-pigment +.	Bile-pigment $\bigcirc$. Urobilin +.	Colored.
3. Yellow.	Bile-pigment +.	Bile-pigment +. Urobilin +.	Usually somewhat paler than normal.
4. Deep yellow.	Bile-pigment +.	Bile-pigment +. Urobilin + or $\bigcirc$.	Very little color or colorless.

+ means presence, $\bigcirc$ absence, of the substance indicated. Hayem and Tissier arrange a scheme similar to this, with the exception that they find urobilin in the serum wherever it is present in the urine.

In the majority of cases, however, icterus does not appear so suddenly nor are the effects of the stasis of bile removed so speedily as in the examples quoted above. As a rule, several obstructions will be found in different divisions of the bile-duct system. The degree of obstruction, too, will vary, as is manifested by the varying coloration of the feces at different stages of the disease. The color of the stools, on the one hand, the quantity of urobilin and bilirubin excreted, on the other, are an index of the degree of stasis. In moderate degrees of biliary stasis considerable degrees of cutaneous icterus may be present and the urine at the same time contain no bile-pigment, but only a quantity

* Frerichs, *loc. cit.*, i, p. 99.

of urobilin larger than normal; yet in these cases bile-pigment may be present in the tissues and be readily found in serous exudates if any are present, or in a blister raised for the purpose of making such examinations. The tissue-juices may contain a small quantity of bile-pigment, sufficient to stain the tissues, and at the same time not enough to be excreted unaltered in the urine. In the mildest degrees of cutaneous icterus bilirubin is absent even from the serum. It is possible to distinguish four degrees of icterus, as shown in the table on page 443.

This scheme is purely diagrammatic, and presupposes a certain uniformity in the different degrees of icterus. If the stasis increases or decreases, however, variations in the above may occur; thus, if the degree of obstruction increases, the urine may contain bile-pigment while the skin is only slightly colored or not colored at all;* on the other hand, if the degree of obstruction decreases, the skin may still be quite yellow and the bile-pigment and even the urobilin be completely absent from the urine.

Even though the degree of stasis remains the same, the color of patients with icterus changes daily, probably because of the varying degrees of turgescence of the skin and amount of blood in the cutaneous capillaries at different times.

In long-continued obstruction it is probable that the formation of bilirubin decreases, and possibly the dirty yellowish color of such patients can be explained in that way.

In addition to those cases that have been designated as instances of icterus from diffusion, and in which biliary stasis cannot be demonstrated, there are a number of cases that do not correspond to the picture of icteric discoloration of tissues and excretions just described. Thus Andral,† for example, reports the case of a patient in whom the sweat and urine contained bile-pigment, but whose skin and conjunctiva were not colored yellow. I have observed a case of catarrhal icterus ‡ in which the stools were completely decolorized and in which the skin was colored intensely yellow, while the urine, which was darker than normal and of a brownish hue, at no time contained urobilin or bilirubin. Hayem reports the complete absence of bile-pigment or of urobilin in the urine of a case of icterus persisting with varying intensity for many months, and this in spite of the fact that both bile-pigment and urobilin were found in the blood-serum.§ Hanot and Gombault,‖ in a case of carcinoma of the pylorus and cirrhosis of the liver, found no icterus, although the ductus choledochus was occluded by cicatricial tissue. As in this case the hepatic artery was occluded (?) and the portal vein narrowed, it is possible that there was a decreased secretion of bile.

The symptoms of icterus from stasis are very different in animals and in man. This fact has not always been considered in drawing conclusions from animal experiments in regard to the phenomena observed in human subjects. In human beings occlusion of the bile-ducts leads to icterus of the urine and of the skin in from twelve to twenty-four hours, while ligation of the common bile-duct is not followed by icterus in dogs for two or three days (Tiedmann and Gmelin, Frerichs), in guinea-pigs for six days (Steinhaus), and in rabbits Stadelmann and Gerhardt saw it occur in two or three days, and occasionally slight icterus on the first day. Gmelin's reaction is not given by the urine for several days.

In one experiment by Kühne general tissue-icterus, and on certain days urinary icterus, were absent in a dog even after the bile-duct had been ligated for twenty-two days. The ramifications of the bile-passages were filled with crystalline and amor-

* Compare, for example, Courvoisier, *Correspondenzblatt für Schweizer Aerzte,* 1896, p. 691.
† *Clinique médicale,* iii, p. 373, cited by Frerichs, i, p. 109.
‡ Quincke, *Virchow's Archiv,* Bd. xcv, p. 139.
§ Soc. méd. des hôpitaux, May 14, 1897, cited in *Berliner klin. Wochenschr.,* 1897, p. 511.
‖ *Gazette méd. de Paris,* 1881, p. 270, cited by Mangelsdorff, *Deutsches Archiv für klin. Medicin,* Bd. xxxi, p. 603.

phous pigment, but none was seen in the liver-cells. V. Harley and v. Frey ligated both the bile-duct and the thoracic duct in a dog and found that even after many days (seventeen) the blood and the urine contained no bile-pigment. From these experiments we must conclude that icterus does not occur so readily in these animals as in human beings, either because they form less pigment or because their tissues are not so readily impregnated with bile-pigment.

In contradistinction to this, it is known that bile-pigment very readily and easily enters the urine of dogs, so that these animals frequently show a slight degree of choluria when in a perfectly normal state, or at all events when starving. Naunyn* observed this in the majority of dogs, particularly older animals, and in cats. The presence of a biliary fistula does not alter this occurrence. As bile-acids also were found in the urine in larger quantities, the phenomenon was not due to concentration of the urine. In these animals diminution of the peristaltic action of the bile-passages and a decrease in the portal pressure seem to cause an absorption of bile-acids and of bilirubin within the liver, and these small quantities are then excreted in the urine. Steiner makes a similar statement in regard to the urine of rabbits. According to Stadelmann, choluria in the latter animals occurs only during starvation, and not constantly then.

New-born children in this respect behave entirely differently from dogs. Here the most severe degree of tissue-icterus may exist and still the urine be clear and completely free from bile-pigment in solution. On the other hand, the renal epithelium found in the sediment contains crystals and needles of bilirubin. The latter are also found as bilirubin infarcts in the collecting tubules of the kidneys (Virchow), and the pigment is seen in a crystalline form in the blood of the heart, both in icterus (Neumann) and occasionally without icterus (v. Recklinghausen). In new-born children, therefore, the tissues and the urine possess very slight solvent properties for bilirubin. Adults seem to occupy an intermediate position between the new-born and dogs in regard to the relative facility with which bilirubin can enter the tissues and the urine. Possible individual differences exist, so that different subjects incline more in the one or in the other direction.

In man there is occasionally observed a condition analogous to the excretion of bile-pigment in the urine of dogs during starvation.

The relation of urobilin to icterus merits special discussion. We have already mentioned that in slight degrees of icterus, as well as after or preceding severe degrees of obstructive jaundice, urobilin is excreted in the urine and colors it reddish-brown. This clinical observation induced Gubler to differentiate "*ictère biliphéique,*" or ordinary bile icterus, and an "*ictère hémaphéique,*" in which the coloration of the tissues and the urine was due to a pigment other than the ordinary bile-pigments. This new pigment, *hémaphéin,* was said to color filter-paper reddish-brown or salmon-colored instead of brown-yellow, and to be characterized by the appearance of a brown-red ring when superimposed with nitric acid. He thought that it was formed in the liver in cases of an "*insuffisance hépatique*" in place of the ordinary bile-pigment.

When C. Gerhardt discovered urobilin in the reddish urine of icteric subjects, he substituted so-called "urobilin icterus" in the place of the indefinite "*ictère hémaphéique,*" for the nitric acid reaction may be due to a variety of different pigments.

Both forms are said to be different from ordinary icterus, not only in regard to the pigment excreted in the urine, but also in the shade of the discoloration of the skin. Other authors have not confirmed these observations and have not been able to discover urobilin in the skin by spectroscopic methods (Quincke). On the other hand, bilirubin is found in the blood-serum (Quincke) and in the sweat (Leube) of these patients, so that many of these cases are clearly aggravated instances of icterus from stasis of bile.

* *Loc. cit.*, p. 581.

Genuine urobilin icterus, in which bile-pigment is replaced by uro-bilin, therefore, does not seem to exist; at least its existence has so far never been demonstrated (Quincke, Kelsch and Kiener, Tissier, D. Gerhardt, Fr. Müller). The cases that have been designated by this name are nothing more than mild cases of bilirubin icterus. It appears to me, therefore, that the name "urobilin icterus" is not happily chosen, for the reason that it is misleading.

On the other hand, the cases designated with this name are of great importance in the understanding of the pathogenesis of icterus, for the reason that they give us a clear insight into the subsequent fate of the bile-pigment in the body. We know that urobilin ("hydrobilirubin" of Maly) is normally found in the urine (Jaffé) and in the feces ("sterco-bilin" of Vanlair and Masius). In the same manner as it can be formed in the test-tube by the action of nascent hydrogen on bilirubin (Maly), so is it formed within the intestine by the reducing action of certain bacteria in the colon. In the meconium, therefore, bilirubin is found alone, and it is only after the expiration of several days that urobilin is found in the feces of the new-born. In the urine, in pathologic states, urobilin is readily recognized by its reddish color. That a relationship exists between this reddish color of the urine and certain digestive dis-turbances was known a long time before the discovery of urobilin. The discoloration of the urine by urobilin is increased in febrile diseases, particularly the infectious diseases, in heart lesions, in pneumonia, in certain diseases of the liver with and without icterus, and, finally, after parenchymatous hemorrhages or hemorrhages into the body-cavities. It is particularly among these cases that the defenders of "hemato-genous icterus" formerly sought their chief evidence in support of their views.

G. Hoppe-Seyler, D. Gerhardt, and Fr. Müller have attempted to estimate urobilin quantitatively by weighing and by spectroscopic methods. The task is complicated by the presence of other pigments, the frequent occurrence of a chromogen, and, finally, by the fact that urobilin is so readily decomposed. The figures obtained, therefore, are only approximately correct

G. Hoppe-Seyler found (by weighing) normally in the total daily urine from 0.08 to 0.14 grams, an average of 0.123 grams.

It was increased in icterus with complete stasis (0.17 to 0.22 grams), in icterus immediately after the removal of complete obstruction (0.2 to 0.4 grams), in extrava-sation of blood (as much as 0.57 grams), as well as in pneumonia with icterus, in Basedow's disease, and in retention of feces.

It was decreased in complete exclusion of bile from the intestine (0.05 to 0.09 grams), sometimes after the disappearance of an attack of icterus (0.06 to 0.09 grams), and in inanition, anemia, and cachexia. In these latter cases a diminution in the formation of bilirubin had probably occurred.

Fr. Müller and D. Gerhardt estimated the urobilin by spectrophotometric methods. During fasting they found it much decreased (9 mg. instead of the normal 13 to 20 mg. in twenty-four hours). It was increased in pneumonia whether accom-panied by icterus or not, in plumbism, heart lesions, hemorrhagic infarction, sepsis, scarlatina, erysipelas, phthisis, hemorrhage, hepatic disease with or without jaun-dice, and in jaundice without reference to its intensity.

The determination of urobilin in the feces is still more inaccurate and uncertain (compare page 418).

Some authors do not consider urobilin a uniform substance. Mac-Munn differentiated several kinds, particularly those of the urine and those of the feces. Jolles differentiates certain forms of urobilin that are physiologic and are formed from the oxidation of bilirubin, and pathologic forms that are the product of the reduction of bilirubin, the former showing a diffuse absorption-band, the latter one that is sharply defined. For the present it is hardly possible to utilize these views in this place.

There can hardly be any doubt that a large part of the urobilin that appears in the urine is absorbed from the intestine. In favor of this view we have the fact that urobilin is increased in digestive disorders and in constipation, and that it is decreased or disappears altogether (not only from the urine, but also from the bile and transudates, according to Fr. Müller, as is seen below) in complete exclusion of bile from the intestine, and is subsequently increased if the obstruction be suddenly removed so that large quantities of bile reach the intestine.

Fr. Müller has also shown that in cases in which no bile can enter the intestine, and where consequently no urobilin is found in the urine, the latter can be made to appear if bile is given by the mouth. The administration of hemoglobin, on the other hand, does not cause it to appear. Traces of urobilin that are found in the feces and the urine even in complete obstruction of the bile-ducts may be derived from icteric mucus secreted by the mucous membrane of the intestine.

A number of other observations, however, do not coincide with the purely enterogenous origin of urobilin. Above all, the typical cases of so-called "urobilin icterus," in which less bile than normal enters the intestine, seem to contradict such an assumption. Moreover, this is still further proved by those cases in which hemorrhage with or without icterus is followed by urobilinuria (as, for example, the cases of Dick), where the only possible explanation would be to assume that the hemorrhage produced polycholia and that this was followed by icterus. Several authors have, therefore, claimed that urobilin can be formed in the tissues by reduction of bilirubin, and that icterus disappears in this manner, the bilirubin being first reduced to urobilin in the tissues and then this pigment, which is more readily diffusible, being excreted by the kidneys (Kunkel, Quincke). Leube assumes that the bilirubin, circulating in the blood, is reduced in the kidneys. Fr. Müller, on the other hand, was not able to demonstrate that such a reduction occurred when he caused blood containing bilirubin to flow artificially through the kidneys.

Bile-pigment is not necessarily the only source of urobilin. Hoppe-Seyler succeeded in making it from hematin by the action of nascent hydrogen, which makes it appear possible that urobilin can be formed directly from hemoglobin either in the liver or outside of that organ. In support of this view the occurrence of urobilinuria after blood-extravasation might be adduced. Here the explanation that it is formed after the occurrence of polycholia will not apply, particularly when the hemorrhage occurs in patients with icterus in whom there is present an obstruction to the outflow of bile (D. Gerhardt). This author found hematoporphyrin in addition to urobilin in the urine after extravasations of blood, and, as this is another derivative of hemoglobin, its presence under these circumstances speaks directly against the above theory and lends support to the theory that urobilin is formed directly from hemoglobin and not through polycholia. Finally, it is possible that the liver under pathologic conditions may form urobilin. This assumption forms the basis of Gubler and Dreyfuss-Brissac's "insufficiency of the liver." Hayem and Tissier have recently defended this view, but they undoubtedly go too far, as they claim that urobilin can be formed only in the liver, and that its appearance in the urine is an index of the degree of disturbance of the liver and of the destruction of the red blood-corpuscles.

As a matter of fact urobilin is usually found in the gall-bladder (Fr. Müller, Tissier) under conditions that make it improbable that it is a postmortem change (Tissier). D. Gerhardt and Beck claim that this urobilin is absorbed from the intestine and excreted by the liver, and base their statement on the observation that in dogs this urobilin was absent from the bile flowing from a fistula after ligation of the ductus choledochus and reappeared after the administration of bilirubin by the mouth.

D. Gerhardt and Fr. Müller found urobilin in the blood-serum with and without icterus, and in serous exudates.

Giarré adduces as evidence of the formation of urobilin outside of the intestinal tract the observation that in infants with fever this substance may be found in the urine although not in the intestine.

The facts quoted contain many contradictions and make it impossible to make definite statements in regard to the genesis of urobilin and its significance in icterus. We cannot expect much from animal experiments for the reason that urobilin, when found at all in the urine of animals, is present only in very small and varying amounts. The greater part of the urobilin found in the urine is derived from the intestine, but it must be remembered that the quantity of urobilin absorbed in this manner is dependent not only on the quantity of pigment present in the intestine, but also on the degree of absorption, which is subject to many fluctuations.

I consider it very probable that under certain circumstances urobilin can also be formed outside of the intestines, either from bilirubin or from hemoglobin directly. In case it is ever formed in the liver under pathologic conditions, it may travel along a path different from that traversed by bilirubin. For instance, it may enter the lymph- or blood-channels directly from the liver-cells, or it may first enter the bile-passages and later be reabsorbed.

Diagnosis.—The diagnosis of icterus is made from the yellow discoloration of visible parts of the body. The yellow color of the sclera is usually noticed first, but it is necessary to remember that in health these tissues are occasionally tinged with yellow. The yellow color of the hands and of the face is not so readily recognized as is the discoloration of the trunk. It is important to differentiate the strictly yellow shade from other possible tints, and it is of practical importance to remember that the yellow color of the skin can only be properly observed by daylight. By candle, lamp, or gaslight it cannot be seen, or is barely perceptible; while in electric light or Welsbach light it is more readily visible. It is sometimes useful to compare the color of the skin with that of white linen.

The dark color of the urine is of diagnostic importance, but it should never be forgotten that it may be due to pigments other than bilirubin. Many cases of icterus are accompanied, during a part or all of their course, by the presence of urobilin alone in the urine. Bilirubin is present only where more severe degrees of biliary absorption are present, and the demonstration of its presence by Gmelin's reaction is an index more of the degree and the stage of the absorption of bile than of its existence.

The color of the feces must always be observed. With the reservations made above, their color gives valuable information in regard to the existence of biliary stasis and of its intensity.

Of the other concomitant symptoms of icterus, itching of the skin is very frequent, slowing of the pulse is present only in a small number of cases, and visual disturbances are observed very rarely.

Whereas all other forms of pigmentation of the skin (sunburn, cachexia, morbus Addisonii) can be readily distinguished from icterus by their brownish shade, the administration of picric acid and of its salts produces a discoloration of the skin and sclera hardly distinguishable from icterus following biliary stasis. This form of discoloration follows, for instance, the administration of potassium picronitrate (0 5 to 1.0 per diem) in the treatment of tapeworm, and malingerers have occasionally used the drug for this purpose. The urine here is colored yellow in the beginning, later reddish-brown, but naturally does not give Gmelin's reaction for bilirubin. Large doses of picric acid cause hemolysis, albuminuria, and hematuria.*

LITERATURE ON ICTERUS.

Affanassiew: "Ueber anatomische Veränderungen der Leber während verschiedener Thätigkeitszustände," "Pflüger's Archiv," Bd. xxx, p. 424, 1883.

Biernacki: "Darmfäulniss bei Nierentzüundung und Icterus," "Deutsches Archiv für klin. Medicin," Bd. xlix, p. 87, 1891.

Brieger: "Einige Beziehungen der Fäulnissproducte zu Krankheiten," "Zeitschr. für klin. Medicin," Bd. iii, p. 465, 1881.

Brissaud, E., et Ch. Sabourin: "Deux cas d'atrophie du lobe gauche d. f. d'origine biliarie," "Archives de physiolog.," 1884, i, p. 345, 444.

Damsch und Cramer: "Ueber Katalepsie und Psychose bei Icterus," "Berliner klin. Wochenschr.," 1898, p. 277, 300.

Dastre: "Recherches sur la bile," "Archives de Physiolog.," 1890, p. 315.

Dick, R.: "Ueber den diagnostischen Werth der Urobilinurie für den Gynäkologen," "Archiv für Gynäkologie," Bd. xxiii.

Dreyfuss-Brissac: "De l'ictère hémaphéique." Thèse de Paris, 1878.

Gerhardt, C.: "Ueber Urobilinicterus," "Correspondenzblatt des allgemeinen ärztlichen Vereins in Thüringen," 1878, No. 11.

Gerhardt, D.: "Zur Pathogenese des Icterus," "Verhandlungen des Congresses für innere Medicin," 1898, p. 460.

— "Ueber Hydrobilirubin und seine Beziehungen zum Icterus." Dissertation, Berlin, 1889.

— "Ueber Urobilin," "Zeitschr. für klin. Medicin," Bd. xxxii, p. 305, 1897.

Gluzinski: "Formalinprobe des Harnes." "Wiener klin. Wochenschr.," 1897, No. 52.

Gorodecki, H.: "Ueber den Einfluss des Hämoglobins auf die Zusammensetzung der Galle." Dissertation, Dorpat, 1889.

Grimm, F.: "Ueber Urobilin im Harn," "Virchow's Archiv," Bd. cxxxii, p. 246. 1893.

Harley, V.: "Leber und Galle während dauernden Verschlusses von Gallen- und Brustgang," "Archiv für Anatomie und Physiologie," Physiologische Abtheilung, 1893, p. 290.

Hayem: "Ictère biliphéique: hémophilie," "Gazette des hôpitaux," 1889.

Hürthle: "Ueber den Secretionsvorgang in der Schilddrüse," "Deutsche med. Wochensch.," 1894, No. 12, p. 267.

Janowski: "Beiträge zur patholog. Anatomie der biliären Lebercirrhose," "Ziegler's Beiträge zur pathol. Anatomie." 1893, p. 79.

Jolles, A.: "Ueber das Auftreten und den Nachweis des Urobilins im normalen und pathologischen Harn," "Wiener klin. Rundschau." 1895, No. 46–48.

Kiener und Engel: "Sur les conditions pathogéniques de l'ictère et ses rapports avec l'urobilinurie," "Archives de Physiolog." 1887, p. 198.

Kühne, W.: "Beiträg zur Lehre vom Icterus." "Virchow's Archiv." Bd. xiv, p. 310. 1858.

Kunkel: "Ueber das Auftreten verschiedner Farbstoffe im Harn." "Virchow's Archiv," Bd. lxxix, p. 435, 1880.

Langhans: "Virchow's Archiv," Bd. xlix, p. 66.

* Kobert, "Lehrbuch der Intoxicationen," p. 496.

Lépine: "Sur un nouveau symptome de trouble de la fonction biliare," "Revue de Médecine," 1881, p. 27, 911.

Létienne, A.: "De la bile à l'état pathologique." Thèse de Paris, 1891.

Leyden, E.: "Beiträge zur Pathologie des Icterus," Berlin, 1886.

Liebermeister: "Zur Pathogenese des Icterus," "Deutsche med. Wochenschr.," 1893, No. 16.

Lindemann, W.: "Ueber das Verhalten der Schilddrüse beim Icterus," "Virchow's Archiv," Bd. cxlix, p. 202, 1897.

Lorenz, H.: "Ueber den Bürstenbesatz an pathologischen und normalen Nieren," "Zeitschr. für klin. Medicin," Bd. clii, p. 436, 1898.

Löwit: "Ueber den Einfluss der gallensauren Salze," "Prager Zeitschr. für Heilkunde," 1881, p. 459.

Minkowski: "Verhandlungen des XI. Congresses für innere Medicin," p. 127, 1892.

Möbius, P. L.: "Ueber die Nieren beim Icterus," "Archiv der Heilkunde," Bd. xviii, p. 83, 187.

Müller, Fr.: "Untersuchungen über Icterus," "Zeitschr. für klin. Medicin," Bd. xii, p. 45, 1887.

— "Ueber Icterus." Discussion in the Medical Section of the Silesian Gesselschaft für vaterländische Cultur, January, 1892; Sitzungsbericht des XI. Congresses für innere Medicin, 1892, p. 118

Müller, K.: "Ueber Cholesterämie," "Archiv für experimentelle Pathologie," Bd. i, p. 213, 1873.

Munk, J.: "Ueber die Resorption von Fetten, etc., nach Ausschluss der Galle vom Darmcanal," "Virchow's Archiv," Bd. cxxii, p. 302, 1890.

Nauwerck, C.: "Leberzellen und Gelbsucht," "Münchener med. Wochenschr.," 1897, No. 2.

Naunyn and Minkowski: "Ueber den Icterus durch Polycholie," "Archiv für experimentelle Pathologie," Bd. xxi, 1886.

Naunyn, B.: "Beiträge zur Lehre vom Icterus," "Reichert und du Bois' Archiv," 1868, p. 401; 1869, p. 579.

v. Noorden: "Pathologie des Stoffwechsels," 1893, p. 264.

Obermayer, F.: "Knochenveränderungen bei chronischem Icterus," "Wiener klin. Rundschau," 1897, Nos. 38, 39.

Pick, E.: "Ueber die Entstehung des Icterus," "Wiener klin. Wochenschr.," 1894, Nos. 26–29.

Plaesterer, R.: "Ueber die giftigen Wirkungen des Bilirubins." Dissertation, Würzburg, 1890.

Poncet: "De l'ictère hématique traumatique." Thèse de Paris, 1874.

Poth: "Stoffwechselanomalien in einem Falle von Stauungsicterus," "Pflüger's Archiv," Bd. xlvi, p. 509, 1890.

Quincke, H.: "Beiträge zur Lehre vom Icterus," "Virchow's Archiv," Bd. xcv, 1884.

Raynaud et Sabourin: "Note sur un cas d' énorme dilatation des voies biliaires," etc., "Archives de physiolog.," 1879, ii, p. 37.

v. Recklinghausen: "Allgemeine Pathologie," p. 434, 1883.

Rohrig: "Ueber den Einfluss der Galle auf die Herzthätigkeit." Dissertation, Würzburg, 1863.

Rywosch: "Ueber die giftigen Wirkungen der Gallensäuren," "Kobert's Arbeiten des pharmakologischen Institutes zu Dorpat," ii, p. 102, 1888.

— "Ueber die Giftigkeit der Gallenfarbstoffe," ibid., vii, p. 157, 1891.

Sauerhering: "Ueber multiple Nekrosen der Leber bei Stauungsicterus," "Virchow's Archiv," Bd. cxxxvii, p. 155, 1894.

Schmidt, R. (Neusser): "Zur Stoffwechselpathologie des Icterus catarrhalis," "Centralblatt für innere Medicin," 1898, No. 5.

Schrader: "Der hämatogene Icterus," "Schmidt's Jahrbücher," Bd. ccxvi, p. 73, 1887.

Senator: "Ueber Icterus," "Berliner Klinik," No. 1, 1888.

Spalitta: "Die Wirkung der Galle auf die Herzbewegung," "Moleschott's Untersuchungen zur Naturlehre," Bd. xiv, p. 44, 1889.

Stadelmann: "Ueber die Natur der Fettkrystalle in den Fäces," "Deutsches Archiv für klin. Medicin," Bd. xl, p. 372, 1887.

— "Der Icterus," Stuttgart, 1891, "Archiv für experimentelle Pathologie," Bd. xiv, p. 231; Bd. xv, p. 422; Bd. xvi, p. 118; Bd. xxiv.

— "Ueber den Kreislauf der Galle im Organismus," "Zeitschr. für Biologie," Bd. xxxiv, 1897.

Stern: "Ueber die normale Bildungsstäte des Gallenfarbstoffs." Dissertation, Königsberg, 1885.

Tissier, P.: "Essai sur la pathologie de la sécrétion biliaire." Thèse de Paris. 1889,
  Weintraud: "Ueber die Ursachen der Pulsverlangsamung im Icterus," "Archiv für
  experimentelle Pathologie," Bd. xxxiv, p. 37, 1894.
Werner: "Einwirkung der Galle und gallensauren Salze auf die Nieren," "Archiv für
  experimentelle Pathologie," Bd. xxiv, p. 31, 1888.
Wyss, O.: "Beitrage zur Histologie der ikter. Leber," "Virchow's Archiv," Bd.
  cccli, p. 553, 1866.

EXPERIMENTAL BILIARY OBSTRUCTION.

(D., Dog; C., Cat; R., Rabbit; G., Guinea-pig.)

Beloussow: "Ueber die Folgen der Unterbindung des Ductus choledochus" (G,. R.),
  "Archiv für experimentelle Pathologie und Pharmakologie," Bd. xiv, p. 200,
  1881.
Chambard: "Contribution à l'étude des lésions histologiques du foie consécutives à
  la ligature du canal choledoque" (G.), "Archives de Physiologie," etc., 1877.
Charcot et Gombault: "Note sur les altérations du foie consécutives à la ligature
  du canal choledoque" (G.), "Archives de Physiologie normale et pathologique,"
  1876, p. 271–299.
Foà e Salvioli: "Ricerche anatomiche experimentali sulla pattologia del Fegato
  (G., C., D., R.), "Archivio per le science mediche," vol. ii, 1878, and "Centralblatt für die medicinischen Wissenschaften," 1878, No. 33.
v. Frey: "Ueber Unterbindung des Gallenganges und des Milchbrustganges bei Hunden," "Verhandlungen des Congresses fur innere Medicin," 1892, p. 115.
Gerhardt, D.: "Ueber Leberveränderungen nach Gallengangsunterbindung" (R.,
  D.), "Archiv für experimentelle Pathologie," Bd. xxx, p . 1, 1892.
Lahousse: "Recherches expérimentales sur l'influence exercée sur la structure du foie
  par la ligature du canal choledoque" (G., R.), "Archives de Biologie," vol. vii,
  1, Fasc., 1887.
Legg, Wickham: "On the Changes in the Liver which follow Ligature of the Bile-
  ducts" (C.), "St. Bartholomew's Hospital Reports," vol. ix, London, 1873.
Leyden: "Beiträge zur Pathologie des Icterus" (D.), p. 83, Berlin, 1866.
Litten: "Klinische Beobachtungen, 1, "Ueber die biliäre Form der Lebercirrhose und
  den diagnostischen Werth des Icterus" (G.), "Charité-Annalen," 1880.
Mayer, H.: "Ueber Veränderung des Leberparenchyms bei dauerndem Verschluss
  des Ductus choledochus" (C., R.), "Medicinische Jahrbücher," Wien, 1872.
Pick: "Zur Kenntniss der Leberveränderungen nach Unterbindung des Ductus
  choledochus" (R.), "Zeitschrift für Heilkunde," Bd. xi, 1890.
Popoff, L.: "Ueber die natürliche pathologische Injection der Gallengänge und einige
  andere, bei der Unterbindung des Ductus choledochus bei Thieren beobachtete
  pathologische Erscheinungen" (D.), "Virchow's Archiv," Bd. lxxxi, 1880.
Simmonds: "Ueber chronische interstitielle Erkrankungen der Leber" (R.), "Archiv
  für klin. Medicin," Bd. xxvii, p. 85, 1880.
Steinhaus: "Ueber die Folgen des dauernden Verschlusses des Ductus choledochus"
  (G.), "Archiv für experimentelle Pathologie und Pharmakologie," Bd. xxviii,
  p. 432, ff., 1891.
Stern, H.: "Ueber die normale Bildungsstätte des Gallenfarbstoffes" (in pigeons).
  Dissertation, Königsberg, 1885.

3. GENERAL ETIOLOGY.

Diseases of the liver may be caused by mechanical, chemical, and nervous influences.

Among the mechanical causes traumata are rarely responsible for lesions. A more frequent cause is long-continued and slowly acting pressure from without, producing the corset liver. The pressure exerted upon the parenchyma of the liver by prolonged distention of the blood-capillaries (as in cardiac lesions) or of the bile-capillaries (as in biliary stasis) causes both disturbances in nutrition and atrophy.

Chemically, the liver can be damaged by substances that enter it either in solution or undissolved. They act primarily on the different systems of channels within the organ, either through the afferent blood-vessels (portal vein and hepatic artery, especially the former), through the bile-passages (as in stasis of bile and invasion by micro-organisms), or, more rarely, in a direction contrary to the blood-current, through the hepatic veins and the lymphatics.

The substances noxious to the liver are, as a rule, introduced from without with the nourishment, but may also be formed within the organism. Such substances are alcohol or phosphorus or arsenic, antimony, chloroform, etc., introduced experimentally. Probably included in this group are a whole series of substances which are partly introduced as such with the food and partly formed within the intestine by the action of bacteria. These latter bodies, in particular food-products and toxins, are very difficult to detect owing to their small quantity, yet they are very harmful. All these substances acting chemically enter the liver by the portal vein, so that they first affect the cells in the peripheral parts of the hepatic lobules. This may explain why so many diseases of the liver originate in this particular region.

It is further probable that many products of internal metabolism possessing toxic properties enter the liver.

Micro-organisms play a very important rôle in the pathology of the liver. The bacteria circulating in the blood-current accumulate within the hepatic capillaries from mechanical causes, or perhaps for other reasons, and may there be seen either free or within leucocytes. Among these must be mentioned the bacillus of typhoid, of tuberculosis, and of anthrax, actinomycosis fungus, and streptococci and staphylococci. The parasite of malaria belongs to the same group. [Adami's discovery of colon bacilli, especially in cirrhosis, is of great importance in this connection.—ED.]

We know comparatively little of the exact effect of these germs on the liver in acute diseases, but it can hardly be doubted that they act both mechanically and by the action of their specific toxins, producing the alterations in the parenchyma frequently seen in these diseases. Occasionally miliary abscesses (as in pyemia) or changes in the liver-cells (as in typhoid fever) with conglomerations of leucocytes are seen around these bacterial colonies. These little colonies are occasionally seen in enormous numbers, and may develop into larger foci in long-lasting diseases, as in tuberculosis and actinomycosis. Corresponding to the peculiar arrangement seen in the deposits of grains of cinnabar, these foci seem to show a certain predilection for the periphery of the lobules.

Micro-organisms may enter the liver by another channel: viz., the bile-passages. They do not follow the course of the bile, but enter the liver from the intestine. They probably begin to multiply within the larger bile-passages; in time, however, they penetrate and damage the smaller bile-passages and the parenchyma of the liver. The most important of these bacteria are Bacterium coli, staphylococci, and streptococci. Here the separation cannot be made between a local infection alone and a general infection with local manifestations.

Larger forms of parasites (echinococcus, distoma, and ameba) enter the liver from the intestine, entering the blood-vessels and being carried along in the blood of the portal vein. In the same manner large and small abscesses are formed in the liver when ulcerative processes or foci of suppuration are present in the intestine (as in dysentery); while carcinomatous infection of the liver may occur in the same way from cancer of the gastro-intestinal tract.

Abscesses and neoplasms rarely originate within the liver as a result of infection through the general circulation (by way of the hepatic arteries or veins). Still more rare is infection through the lymphatics from the stomach by way of the portal glands. From the peritoneum inflammation and formation of neoplasms extend only into the most superficial portions of the organ. In some diseases, such as typhoid fever, involvement of the liver may occur through several of these channels.

We see, therefore, that nearly all the infections of the liver occur from the intestine by way of the portal blood, or by way of the bile-passages, and that micro-organisms play an important rôle, partly mechanically, partly by the toxins which they produce.

It is difficult to form a correct estimate of the significance of nervous influences in the production of diseases of the liver. While we cannot always definitely state that they are the cause in a given instance, and while we frequently wrongly attribute certain lesions to their action, we are not justified in altogether ignoring their significance, since there can be no doubt that they can exercise an important predisposing influence, and we know positively that the blood- and bile-currents are influenced by the nervous system. Moreover, we have reason to believe that in all probability the functional activity of the liver-cells is affected by nervous influences. In addition, certain psychic and other nervous influences exercise an indirect effect on the liver through diminished cardiac activity and disturbance of digestion.

The frequency with which diseases of the liver occur varies in different countries and at different times. According to medical tradition, diseases of the liver are more frequent in tropic countries and during the warm seasons of the year. Exact proofs of these statements are lacking, and would be difficult to obtain. We can, of course, readily understand the localized occurrence of lesions caused by certain parasites, such as echinococcus, of the relative frequency of dysentery and amebic abscesses in tropic countries, and of malaria in southern Italy. These differences, particularly in regard to the geographic peculiarities, are also explainable by differences in the mode of life of different peoples, such as the quantity of alcohol consumed, perhaps the general character of the food, and the amount of exercise taken. These are all important determining factors. The statements made in regard to the influence of hot climates are based principally on observations made on Europeans that had immigrated into those countries. The appearance of "bilious" diarrheas accompanied by fever, so frequently noted, has led to the conclusion that the functional activity of the liver was increased. Even did these attacks signify an increase in the formation of bile, it would not necessarily indicate an increase in the metabolic functions of the liver. We are, it is true, justified in drawing such a conclusion indirectly from the fact that, owing to a smaller demand for the production of body-heat, less oxygen is absorbed and oxidation is reduced. As a result of this, we might expect that some of the intermediary products of metabolism would not be completely oxidized and would accumulate in the liver. In this manner both an excessive functional strain is imposed and qualitative changes in the function of the liver are produced. This condition will occur the more readily, the more food is ingested beyond that required for the needs of the body. Thus, the first few years of a sojourn in the tropics are particularly deleterious to Europeans for the reason that the adjustment of general metabolism to the new conditions is only slowly accomplished, and because the necessary reduction in the amount of food taken is not made at once. Among the natives, and among the women and children of the European residents, diseases of the liver (aside from the parasitic forms) are not more frequent than in other regions. In men the greater disposition to these diseases becomes less noticeable in proportion to the care they exercise in changing their accustomed mode of life by adopting a more moderate and less nitrogenous diet. According to the general consensus of opinion, the use of alcohol in even moderate doses is especially pernicious, just as in other countries similar quantities of alcohol act more unfavorably if less bodily exercise is taken or if the stomach is empty.

According to Cayley, the following proportion of diseases of the liver is seen among the British troops in India for each 1000 per annum:

	EUROPEAN SOLDIERS.	NATIVE SOLDIERS.
Cases of sickness	24.5 per mille.	1.6 per mille.
Mortality	1.43 per mille	0.11 per mille.

The predisposition to dysentery and malaria, on the other hand, is the same for both.

In India Europeans seem to suffer more from diseases of the liver than they do in Ceylon and in the West Indies. This is particularly the case in Madras, where the temperature is uniformly high during the whole year. In India residence in the mountainous districts is not favorable for patients with diseases of the liver because of the diarrheas and chillings to which they are subject in such localities.

The following table shows the influence of alcohol on diseases in general:

	IN THE WHOLE ARMY.	AMONG THE TEMPERATE.
Diseases	75 per mille	41 per mille.
Mortality	15 per mille	3 per mille.

Whenever the liver, for any of the reasons detailed above, is in a state of unbalanced equilibrium, it is readily seen that even slight external influences may produce actual diseases. Such a rôle is played by dyspepsia. Other agencies, also, that would not be considered important predisposing factors at home, such as the heat of the sun, fatigue, sudden chilling, particularly during sleep, are capable of doing much harm under these conditions.

The forms of hepatic lesions peculiar to warm climates are acute, parenchymatous, and suppurating hepatitis, chronic enlargement of the liver, and the complication of jaundice in all acute diseases.

The seasonal differences in the appearance of certain diseases of the liver, as shown by the frequent occurrence of icterus even in temperate climates, perhaps depend upon differences in the bacterial flora of the articles of diet and the consequent changes in the bacterial contents of the intestinal tract.

The relation between the action of the liver and disturbances of metabolism is probably very intimate, and at the same time is very little understood. French and English authors particularly, more instinctively than from any exact reasoning, attribute a great significance to the liver in the causation of gout (a term by them widely applied). There can be no doubt that the function of the liver is perverted in diabetes mellitus, and in many cases of obesity it is probable that some one of its many functions is overactive.

Such qualitative changes and perversions of its function may be followed by anatomic changes and permanent impairment of function.

A primary functional disturbance of the liver may often produce these metabolic perversions.

As in the majority of diseases, a combination of a variety of conditions and defects is almost always necessary to produce lesions of the liver; any one of the different factors alone would probably not have been able to cause the lesion.

LITERATURE.

Cayley, H.: "Tropical Diseases of the Liver," in A. Davidson, "Hygiene and Diseases of Warm Climates," Edinburgh and London, p. 612, 1893.
— "Tropical Affections of the Liver," Transactions of the Eighth International Congress for Hygiene in Budapest, p. 695, 1894.
Hirsch: "Histor.-geographische Pathologie," iii, p. 267, 1886.
Scheube: "Krankheiten der warmen Länder," p. 374, Jena, 1896.

4. GENERAL SYMPTOMATOLOGY.

In the clinical picture of diseases of the liver local symptoms, both subjective and objective, are inconspicuous. The same, as we have seen, applies to the study of the physiology of the liver, in which the local manifestations of functional activity are less apparent than, for example, in the case of the thoracic organs or even of the stomach and intestine. The shape and size of the liver are changed only in severe and in long-continued diseases. We have already discussed the method of determining these changes and the degree of accuracy of the results.

Pain is of subordinate importance as a symptom, as the parenchyma of the liver is non-sensitive, and consequently a great many diseases of the liver run their course without producing any pain. Among these we can mention fatty infiltration, amyloid degeneration, the various forms of cirrhosis, and echinococcus disease. Even great enlargement of the liver, if it progresses and develops slowly, may be painless and may only cause disagreeable subjective symptoms by impeding some of the movements of the body, by interfering with respiration, and by interfering with the function of neighboring organs, such as the heart, stomach, and intestine.

Pain proper in the hepatic region is caused by lesions of the serous covering of the organ and of the bile-passages.

Pain in the serous covering is most frequently caused by direct inflammation of this tissue or, less frequently, by distention of the capsule of the liver in very rapid enlargement of the organ. Consequently, a great many diseases of the liver are occasionally, though not constantly, painful. Examples of these are rapidly developing hyperemia, phosphorus-liver, abscess, and syphilitic hepatitis. Carcinoma and acute atrophy are also occasionally very painful. Sometimes the pain is distributed over the whole organ; in other cases, particularly in localized lesions, it is found only in the diseased area.

Pressure usually aggravates all forms of hepatic pain, as do movements and all forms of succussion, such as riding on horseback. If the patient lies on the left side or bends the body toward the left, pain originating from the serous covering of the liver is usually ameliorated, while, on the other hand, if the liver is very much enlarged, the position on the right side seems to afford more relief and to remove some of the pressure exercised on neighboring organs.

Pain in the right shoulder is a peculiar symptom that is found in many diseases of the liver, either in connection with or independent of localized pain. The pain may radiate from the shoulder to the side of the neck, to the scapula, or into the right arm. It may be either indefinite in character, or drawing, tugging, or burning, and is often aggravated by pressure over the liver or by movements of the arm. It is found chiefly in abscess and in hyperemia, but also in echinococcus disease and in carcinoma, and occasionally in syphilis and cholelithiasis. This pain seems to be present only in diseases that involve the convex surface of the liver. In abscess of the left lobe it may be occasionally felt in the left shoulder. It is a referred pain, and is explained by the anatomic distribution of the sensory nerves supplying the shoulder and the serous covering of the convex surface of the liver. The phrenic nerve sends sensory branches to the liver through the suspensory ligament. This nerve arises from the fourth cervical nerve, and from the same place come the sensory branches to the region of the right shoulder. Irritation traveling along the branches of the phrenic is transmitted along these fibers to the fourth spinal segment, and is there transmitted from ganglion cell to ganglion cell.

This shoulder pain is of clinical importance, inasmuch as it may, in certain stages of different diseases of the liver, be the only symptom pointing to an involvement of this organ.

The pain starting from the bile-passages does not originate in the mucous lining, but in the muscular wall of these ducts, and is caused directly by the stretching of their walls and by spasmodic contraction. The character of the pain is altogether different from that of the other just described, in that it is called a colicky pain, like all similar forms of pain emanating from hollow organs. It is usually observed in impaction of gall-stones, and will be described in a following section. It is distinguished from other forms of hepatic pain by its intensity, its periodic exacerbations, and the fact that it is comparatively independent of external pressure. This colicky pain usually radiates into remote parts of the body, into the epigastrium, and toward the back. It is frequently accompanied by reflex symptoms, such as vomiting, general pallor, collapse, and chills with elevation of temperature.

Some interesting information in regard to the origin of the pain was obtained from the study of a patient whose gall-bladder was opened under local anesthesia by Professor Bier, and a large number of gall-stones removed. Tugging at the gall-bladder produced violent pains similar to those that the patient had experienced during her attacks of gall-stone colic. Pain in the shoulder was absent during this manipulation, although the patient had complained of it six months previously to the time when she was admitted to the clinic with the diagnosis of perityphlitis, the pain in the shoulder then first directing attention to the liver as the seat of trouble.

Of all the disturbances of the hepatic functions, those concerned in the formation of bile-pigment would be the most readily recognizable were it not for the fact that the proportion of bile normally evacuated with the feces is so varying and changeable. We are altogether unable to control this, and, consequently, cannot determine fluctuations in the amount of pigment contained therein. It has been already shown above why the color of the feces is no index for the amount of bile-pigment secreted.

From a symptomatic point of view the reabsorption of bile is more important, as it is this which leads to .icterus. As this condition is readily recognized, it acquires a great clinical significance, but it has a very different significance in different cases.

Disturbances of the appetite and of the bowels are important, although in only a certain proportion of cases are these the direct result of the disturbed secretion of the liver, being more frequently manifestations of concomitant disturbances in the function of the stomach, the intestine, or the pancreas.

Changes in general metabolism as a result of diseases of the liver are clinically manifested by changes in the urine. This is frequently diminished in quantity, forms a sediment, and is darker in color, these changes being due partly to a greater concentration, partly to the presence of bilirubin, and partly to an increase in the quantity of urobilin and indoxyl. It is true that these changes in color may be due to still other causes, and that they cannot, as was formerly thought, be interpreted to signify in all cases that the liver is involved. Decrease in the excretion of urea, in the excretion of ammonia, alimentary glycosuria, and increased toxicity of the urine are all found in diseases of the liver, but the methods of determining these changes are too complicated and tedious for practical use, particularly as their significance is not positively determined. The French school of investigators especially emphasize and somewhat over-rate the significance of these urinary abnormalities. For the present they have a theoretic interest only.

The hemorrhagic diathesis may be considered an indication of perverted nutrition and of changes in metabolism. It is found after icterus has existed for some time, and occasionally before the appearance of other grave symptoms of hepatic disease. Hemorrhages into the retina make their appearance especially early (Litten).

The disturbances of the general health vary greatly in diseases of the liver. In localized lesions they may be slight or absent, but in diffuse diseases of the whole organ they are always present. This applies even to diffuse but transient forms, such as catarrhal icterus. These general disturbances consist in a change of disposition, the aspect of illness, loss of strength, and emaciation. According to various external conditions and the temperament of the patient, these different symptoms appear with varying prominence, and the physician should take them into consideration for both diagnosis and prognosis. As a rule, the disturbances are slowly developed, but they often suddenly and unexpectedly arise. They are found not only in pronounced icterus, but also when it is absent or when the skin is only slightly discolored. It appears that such patients are in a state of unstable equilibrium, so that small external causes may produce serious aggravations of their condition. One of the causes of these sudden exacerbations is a diminution in the excretory function of the kidneys, which, it would appear, can for a long time act vicariously.

Disturbances of circulation in the area of the radicles of the portal vein are frequently found, as a result either of primary disturbances of the circulation in the hepatic capillaries or intrahepatic branches of the portal vein (cirrhosis, syphilis), or of compression of the portal vein itself (more rarely, of the hepatic veins), or of diseases of its walls. If these circulatory disturbances reach a high grade, ascites and swelling of the spleen occur, the former being often so pronounced that it obscures all other evidences of disease.

The action of the heart and the respiration are impaired only as a result of the disturbance of the general health, mechanically by the ascites, or occasionally by contiguity. As symptoms of these conditions Labadie-Legrave names palpitation, intermittent cardiac action, a feeling of oppression, and attacks of angina pectoris. In icterus the action of the heart is usually slowed.

Disturbances of the nervous system are quite frequently observed, especially when jaundice is present. Pruritus, slowing of the heart, and disturbances of vision are those most frequently presented. If the icterus persists for a long time, but occasionally even without the existence of icterus, severe nervous symptoms are seen where chronic disease of the parenchyma of the liver has produced marked organic changes, especially if atrophy is pronounced. As in uremia, these may appear suddenly or develop gradually. In the more chronic cases they are usually preceded by loss of strength and disturbances of nutrition. The chief nervous disturbances observed are pruritus and changes in disposition and the amount of psychic energy. The mental disturbances may progress to drowsiness, unconsciousness, and coma. The more severe degrees of disturbances of the nervous system may be accompanied or interrupted by delirium and convulsions.

Those states that have been called *delirium* or *coma hepaticum* resemble, as previously explained, both the symptoms seen in animals after experimental removal of the liver and certain forms of intoxication. It is, in fact, probable that they are produced by an auto-intoxication with substances that are formed within the body; in other words, it is an hepatotoxemia.

The poisons may be of various origin. They may be either products of the diseased liver-cells themselves or substances which should normally be retained and excreted by the liver, but which, when the organ is diseased, enter the circulation. Among these toxic substances must be mentioned carbaminate of ammonia, which has been especially incriminated by Nencki. Other factors may consist of toxins produced by putrefactive processes within the intestine and intermediary products of general metabolism (among the latter, possibly certain acids). At times some of the constituents of the bile participate in this hepatotoxemia or hepatic auto-intoxication. (Compare page 440.)

It is possible that the sudden development of severe nervous symptoms occurs at a time when the vicarious excretory function usually assumed by the kidneys or other organs suddenly becomes insufficient, so that the body is suddenly exposed to the bad effects of an uncompensated insufficiency of the hepatic function. When the latter, which may be called hepatargia, is developing slowly, it is manifested clinically by less violent symptoms, such as slight changes in the general nutrition, slight loss of strength, and slight changes in the disposition of the patient.

The same is seen in uremic and diabetic forms of intoxication. Here, also, those cases that occur suddenly are the most striking, yet a great many cases develop less significant symptoms whose dependence upon the systemic poisoning can only be discovered on very careful examination. There are, also, all grades of transition between these two. All three forms of intoxication (hepatic, uremic, and diabetic) have specific symptoms, but they all resemble each other in that the nervous symptoms are rather vague and indefinite (appearing either as irritability or depression) and differ in almost every case. This variability in the intensity of the manifestations of toxemia is in all probability due to differences in the constitution of the toxic material and the rapidity of its accumulation.

As a rule, acute attacks of hepatic auto-intoxication appear within a few days before death, and are, therefore, premortal or terminal symptoms. This form of auto-intoxication terminates favorably much more rarely than does that of uremic and diabetic poisoning, and a patient hardly ever recovers after it is well developed. In the milder and more gradually developing forms of hepatargia a restitution to normal is possible, particularly in cases in which the disturbance of the hepatic function is due to removable biliary obstruction. These are the cases that formerly were wrongly called bile-intoxication or cholemia.

It is not possible in some cases to state definitely that a certain syndrome of nervous symptoms is due to hepatic toxemia, because a number of other diseases can produce similar states. Among those capable of producing coma should be mentioned chronic alcoholism, nephritis, meningitis, tuberculosis, and certain febrile complications. Chronic alcoholism and lead intoxication, also, may cause delirium and convulsions. Frequently there is a mixture of causes of nervous symptoms, such as the combination of alcoholism and chronic nephritis. The form that these nervous disturbances assume is manifold and but slightly characteristic, at times even simulating insanity. The diagnosis must be made from other symptoms pointing to an involvement of the liver. L. Levy, who has collected a number of these cases, is of the opinion that in hepatic coma mydriasis is more frequently seen, while in uremia myosis is usually present.

Ocular manifestations are seen only in severe cases of hepatic disease. They are xanthopsia, hemeralopia, retinal hemorrhages (particularly if a severe degree of icterus is present), retinitis pigmentosa, and, in cirrhosis, choroiditis atrophicans.

The temperature of the body is rarely changed in diseases of the liver, but in advanced stages of general disturbances of health as a result of disease of the liver and in icterus the temperature is sometimes subnormal.

In suppurative processes, involving either the parenchyma of the liver or the mucous membrane of the bile-passages, the temperature is usually raised. As the bile-passages are very narrow, suppurative processes within them, as a rule, lead to swelling of the mucous membrane, with retention of pus and fever from absorption. These forms of resorption fever are found in diseases of the liver, even when the suppuration is of very slight degree and extent, and even in those infections of the bile-passages in which only very small quantities of pus are formed. The fever sometimes assumes so irregular a type that it may be confounded with malaria, particularly as the attacks of fever occasionally run a course that resembles that of the tertian or the quartan type.

Those forms of febrile attacks ushered in by a chill and following the impaction of a gall-stone are especially peculiar. They may be only in part due to absorption.

Concretions of bile are frequently seen in combination with an infectious or suppurative form of cholangitis, so that the fever due to impaction may very well be combined with a fever from absorption. Following Charcot, French authors distinguish a definite type of fever, "*febris intermittens hepatica*." This is hardly justified, since in many other situations a purulent focus can exist whose source and nature may, as in this situation, remain often for a long time hidden from recognition and cause a similar "intermittent fever."

The fever under discussion may be distinguished from malaria (aside from the blood examination) by an evening exacerbation that is typical of all forms of fever from pus absorption, and that is particularly marked in hepatic suppuration owing to hyperemia of the liver during digestion. The taking of the temperature at short intervals will, in addition, show a very irregular type of fever.

LITERATURE.

Baas, K. L.: "Beziehungen zwischen Augenleiden und Leberkrankungen," "Münchner med. Wochenschr.," No. 32, 1894.

Charcot: "Maladies du foie," p. 95, 178 (Fever), 1877.

Chauffard: "De la guérison apparente et de la guérison réelle dans les affection hépatiques," "Archives générales de médecine," 1890, II, p. 399.

Labadie-Legrave: ("As to Symptoms in Connection with the Vascular System") "L'Union méd., 1891, No. 131.

Leopold, Levi: "Troubles nerveux hépatiques," "Archives générales de médecine," 1896, I, 58, 219, 535; II, 19, 157.

Litten: "Veränderungen des Augenhintergrundes," etc., "Zeitschr. für klin. Medicin," Bd. v, Heft 1.

Renvers: "Zur Pathologie des intermittirenden Gallenfiebers" (with Charts), "Charité-Annalen," vol. XVII, p. 174, 1892.

Wagner, E.: "Febris hepatica intermittens," "Deutsches Archiv für klin. Medicin," Bd. XXXIV, p. 529, 1884.

5. DIAGNOSIS IN GENERAL.

In view of the great number and the variety of the functions of the liver, it will usually be found that when the liver is diseased other organs also are involved. Sometimes the liver is primarily involved, sometimes secondarily, and occasionally the lesions of the liver and of the other organs are caused by the same agency. It is not always possible to decide, even at autopsy, into which category the lesions fall, and from the clinical picture the participation of the liver in a given syndrome is not always clearly indicated. We can distinguish four types, as follows:

I. The changes in the liver (anatomic or functional) are accompaniments of other diseases and are not recognizable in the symptom-complex, although they have a share in its production. To this class belong the changes in the hepatic parenchyma seen in the course of many infectious diseases, miliary pyemic abscesses, many cases of miliary tuberculosis and of secondary carcinoma of the liver, and probably, also, certain of the secretory anomalies observed in gastro-intestinal catarrhs.

II. The changes that occur in the liver are recognizable by certain symptoms and signs, but are insignificant in comparison to the symptoms of the primary disease. Such conditions are congestion of the liver in the course of certain cardiac lesions, fatty degeneration of the liver in general obesity, and those mild degrees of chronic hepatitis that occur in the course of those cases of alcoholism chiefly presenting manifestations of involvement of the heart or brain.

III. Diseases of the liver proper in the narrower sense, where the hepatic lesions dominate the picture. Examples of this class are catarrhal icterus, cholelithiasis, and many cases of abscess and echinococcus of the liver and of pronounced atrophic cirrhosis.

IV. Diseases in which the symptoms produced by the liver are conspicuous, but in which the liver is not really the organ primarily involved and is only affected as the result of a general intoxication or infection. To this group belong cases of acute phosphorus-poisoning, many cases of icterus gravis, many cases of "alcohol liver" and of syphilis of the liver. In all of these diseases other organs are damaged too, but not to such a marked degree as the liver. This relative preponderance of the symptoms attributable to the liver has to be kept in mind in forming a clinical judgment and arriving at a conclusion in many instances of disease.

From a practical point of view it is well, finally, to remember here, as in the case of other organs (as, for example, the lungs), that different diseases of the liver that have been discussed separately may occur in the organ at the same time and may exercise an influence on each other. As an illustration of this, we may see at the same time fatty infiltration, cirrhosis, hyperemia from stasis, catarrhal icterus, and, in addition, possibly in the same individual, gummata or concretions.

6. PROGNOSIS IN GENERAL.

In those cases in which a disease of the liver is only apparently the cause of illness (in the sense of the preceding section), but in which in reality some general disease is causing certain manifestations of hepatic involvement, the prognosis is naturally unfavorable. When jaundice is present, the course of the disease may be our only guide in determining whether the hepatic or the general disease is primary.

In case the liver alone is involved, it is important to determine whether the organ as a whole is affected, or whether the lesion or lesions are localized and the organ is only partially changed. Localized diseases (abscesses, echinococcus, gumma) are of themselves important because a certain portion of the organ remains capable of forming the internal and external secretions and can act vicariously for the diseased areas. *Ceteris paribus* all diffuse diseases of the liver offer a less favorable prognosis.

Diseases involving one or more of the large systems of vessels and ducts are especially important because they show a tendency to become diffuse. This applies most markedly to the bile-passages, and to a lesser degree to the blood-vessels. Purely mechanical lesions of these vessels and ducts are, as a rule, more favorable prognostically than are infectious lesions.

Toxic diseases are usually diffuse, and the prognosis depends on the removal of the primary toxic agent early in the disease. This is particularly the case in alcohol poisoning, perhaps in the lesions produced by digestive toxins, and, finally, in malarial infection.

In all diseases of the liver it is of paramount importance, from a prognostic point of view, to determine whether the liver-cells themselves are involved. It must be remembered, at the same time, that the degree of functional impairment is not necessarily proportionate to the degree of anatomic alteration.

Even when true degeneration of liver-cells occurs and when many cells perish, these changes, as a rule, progress gradually and in an irregular manner, so that the relatively intact portions can vicariously assume the rôle of those parts that are undergoing degeneration. In this manner the interruption of the hepatic functions is very gradual and the picture of hepatargia, or the hepatic insufficiency of the French authors, develops very slowly and imperceptibly. However, in these cases the picture of hepatic auto-intoxication may suddenly appear. We must consider the prognosis uncertain, therefore, in every case of icterus of long duration or obscure origin, as well as in those accompanied by pronounced general symptoms. The same applies to those cases in which, even without jaundice, there is reason to expect a high degree of parenchymatous change. As a rule, the clinical symptoms of these conditions are not very significant for prognostic purposes. The condition of the urine is important in the sense that a decreased excretion and a dark color are prognostically unfavorable, whereas a copious excretion and a light color (sometimes presenting the clinical picture of a urinary crisis) are prognostically favorable.

In many cases of icterus apparently running a mild course a sudden aggravation of the general condition, that may even terminate fatally, is sometimes seen. Both during the treatment of the disease in its active stages and in the after-treatment it is well to remember how uncertain the prognosis may be in such cases.

As in the case of many other diseases involving important organs, a cure in the clinical sense does not really constitute a cure. As a matter of fact, a certain degree of functional weakness of the affected organ usually remains, or a slow, latent progression of the disease continues.

7. GENERAL TREATMENT.

In view of the intimate relation of the liver to the processes of nutrition dietetic measures form an important portion of treatment. The liver may be rested, so to speak, by withdrawing all food for a time. This measure is not practical, however, for the reason that it can be carried out for so short a time, and because of all organs the liver, particularly, suffers from deficient nutrition. On account of the great significance of the liver in general metabolism, it is dangerous to allow its functional activity to sink below a certain point, and a certain amount of nourishment must be ingested to maintain its proper action.

Acute catarrhal icterus and acute parenchymatous hepatitis, in particular, call for the smallest possible amount of food, partly in order to spare the liver, partly also for other reasons. In all other cases it is only necessary to limit the amount and the kind of food. In the latter respect the general constitution of the patient must be considered as much as the general state of the liver; for example, the amount of fats and carbohydrates may have to be limited. In hot climates, it is said that a vegetarian diet best protects the liver. In febrile diseases, according to French authors, a meat diet is particularly bad, because the detoxicating function of the liver is said to be reduced. They recommend milk, starches, and sugars for the formation of glycogen. Such a diet corresponds essentially to the long-employed fever diet. There can be no doubt that it is indicated for many other reasons more important than the saving and protection of the hepatic function.

In general, it may be said that any limitation of the diet to any one class of food will be followed by an excessive strain on the liver in digestion of that one class. In the absence of special indications the following rules may be formulated for the regulation of the diet in diseases of the liver: viz., Restriction as to the quantity of the food, with a mixed diet of simple composition and preparation, and avoidance of all irritating articles of food. The three types of food, proteids, carbohydrates, and fats, should be represented in the food. The diet should be as free as possible from all indigestible residue and the composition of each meal should be as simple as possible, thus avoiding overloading of the gastro-intestinal tract, retardation of digestion, and the occurrence of putre-factive changes. The last point is particularly important because it seems that the bacteria of the intestine can produce toxic products capable of irritating the liver in the same manner as does alcohol. The latter article is to be particularly avoided, as it seems to be very harmful to the liver, especially when taken in concentrated form or on an empty stomach. Naturally, in the case of alcohol, as of other articles of food, the liver alone cannot be considered, and in patients that have been used to the taking of alcohol the stomach, heart, and nervous system must be considered, and it may be necessary to administer carefully graduated doses of certain alcoholic beverages. As a general rule, both the laity and physicians are in the habit of prescribing too large doses in cases of this kind. The same remark applies to spices, which, in addition to acting harmfully on the liver, are dangerous because they stimulate the patient's appetite and cause him to take too much food. Among this class of foods we would mention in particular mustard, the different kinds of pepper, radishes and horseradish, onions, celery, ginger, cinnamon, cloves, etc., also coffee, strong meat-broths, large quantities of salt, and the empyreumatic substances that are formed in baking and roasting. Because of the latter, white meat and boiled meat are preferable to red and roasted meat.

It is also well to remember that during digestion the demand upon all of the functions of the liver is increased, so that the quantity of food given at each meal should be small. It is well, therefore, to prescribe both the number of meals and the hours at which they should be taken, thus both regulating the amount of work that the liver has to do and obtaining certain periods of rest for the organ. Larger and less frequent meals are indicated only when one desires to produce a more copious outflow of bile for the purpose of flushing the bile-passages, as in certain diseases of the bile-ducts.

A milk diet is frequently prescribed for certain diseases of the liver, particularly cirrhosis. Milk, in fact, fulfils nearly all the indications in regard to dosage, simplicity, and absence of all irritating qualities. The ingestion of large quantities of fluid which is incidental to a milk diet is desirable. Besides milk, buttermilk and kefir should be mentioned as desirable articles. Glutinous articles of food are useful, as they are so readily assimilated. Sometimes a vegetable diet, so especially advocated by French authors, is indicated, particularly when torpidity of the intestine exists with a tendency to a putrefaction of proteids.

It is well to rest after meals, both for the sake of the liver and for other reasons, because by this precaution the functional hyperemia of the organ, so useful for digestion, is not disturbed.

As many chronic diseases of the liver (hyperemia, fatty degeneration, chronic hepatitis) are accompanied by a condition of general plethora and a general retardation of metabolic processes, it is necessary to pre-scribe a certain amount of physical exercise. By this circulation is increased and combustion is advanced, and the flow of blood through the liver, in particular, is accelerated, because with increased respiratory efforts the liver is rhythmically compressed and the venous blood is

made to flow more rapidly into the heart. The kind of exercises prescribed must be adapted to the general health of the patient and to
external circumstances.

It is well to avoid all compression by the clothing, in view of the
great influence that such compression exercises on the flow of blood and
of bile within the liver.

Different kinds of baths, particularly mud-baths, are useful in the
hyperemias and in hypertrophy from overingestion, chiefly because
they exercise a beneficial effect on the general circulation and on metabolism.

The regulation of the intestinal evacuation is very important in all
diseases of the liver, if for no other reason than that retention of feces
produces pressure on the organ, and a mild degree of catharsis is always
indicated in these cases. It is useful here, too, because it promotes a
more rapid elimination of the toxins that may have been formed. Salines
are particularly suitable, notably the sulphates of sodium and of magnesium, the tartrates, as well as rhubarb, aloes, and cascara.

It has been attempted to prevent the formation of intestinal toxins
by the administration of intestinal antiseptics. However seductive this
plan may appear on theoretic grounds, it is uncertain in practice, as a
disinfection of the intestine proper can hardly be produced. Just as
the bacterial flora of the intestine in health changes as regards its composition and products in accordance with the ingesta, so certain medicaments and foods may produce similar alterations in disease; yet this
subject is not at all understood, and what investigations are recorded
are tentative, incomplete, and chiefly based on an unconnected mass of
empiric observations. We can mention the following substances that
might be employed for the disinfection of the intestine: calomel (0.1 to
0.2 per diem) in small divided doses (Hanot recommends 0.01 to 0.02
in the morning on an empty stomach for a week, to be repeated after
a week, possibly several times); the subnitrate or salicylate of bismuth
(2.0 to 6.0 per diem); salol (2.0 to 6.0 per diem); naphthalin (2.0 to 4.0
per diem); resorcin (1.0 to 3.0 per diem); β-naphthol (1.0 to 3.0 per diem)..
Hydrochloric acid, by its influence on gastric digestion, acts indirectly.
I have employed pure cultures of brewers' yeast with great advantage
(dose 30 to 60 c.c. per diem).*

The excretion of the urine has to be considered in the treatment of
diseases of the liver as well as in the diagnosis. The indication is to
produce the excretion of a considerable quantity of moderately concentrated urine. In the first place, this is evidence that plenty of fluid
is circulating through the liver; in the second place, that the kidneys
are acting as a safety-valve for the removal of abnormal quantities of
biliary constituents and other noxious substances that may have
entered the circulation.

In icterus the regulation of the diet must be governed chiefly by the
condition of the gastric and intestinal mucosa, and, secondly, by the
diminution or the absence of the bile from the intestine. The latter
contingency demands a restriction in the amount of fat because this
would not be absorbed so well; for which reason the carbohydrates must
be given as a substitute for the fat, even though they are apt to produce
fermentation and meteorism. Meat, even in the absence of bile, is well

* "Verhandlungen des Congresses für innere Medicin," 1898.

digested. When there is much putrefaction in the intestine, the meat must be replaced by eggs or by vegetable albumin. In icterus with simple obstruction of bile it is necessary to individualize in regard to the diet. This is made apparent by the great differences observed in different patients in regard to the assimilation of fat, and the diet will have to be modified according to the degree of fermentation or putrefaction that happens to be going on in the intestine.

In every form of icterus it is well to give plenty of water in order to promote a copious secretion of urine. When sufficient water is not taken by the mouth, it is well to administer enemata or even to give hypodermic injections of normal salt solution. Frequent bathing also exercises a favorable influence on the urinary secretions.

Mosler and Krull have recommended the methodical use of enemata of water in icterus and in a number of other diseases of the liver. The former prescribes half a liter of lukewarm water three times daily, the latter orders from half to one liter of water, of a temperature of from fifteen to twenty-two degrees, given slowly and retained as long as possible. These enemata act by the water absorbed, by the flushing of the intestine, and by stimulating peristalsis, possibly even in the bile-ducts. The latter effect (increased peristalsis) is produced by the cool enemata, while absorption is greater after those that are warm. Their primary effect is on the blood and the blood-current in the portal vein, and in this way perhaps they improve the nutrition of the liver-cells and the secretion of the bile. Certain animal experiments by Stadelmann and others disprove such an action and do not show that the absorption of water is followed by such beneficial effect. Occasionally certain intestinal antiseptics, as salicylate of sodium and naphthol, are added to the enemata.

Among the drugs that are employed in the treatment of diseases of the liver, the so-called cholagogues have heretofore occupied a high place. Careful tests have, however, shown that a number of these remedies (such as calomel, rhubarb, and others) are not really cholagogues, although this does not diminish their therapeutic value, empirically discovered, but merely necessitates some other explanation of their action.

The following may be mentioned among the cholagogues that possess some clinical value:

The bile-acids (cholate of sodium in doses of 0.3 to 1.5 per diem), which act better than bile itself, are excreted by the liver and have a tendency to increase the quantity of bile-salts normally circulating through the liver.

Salicylate of sodium in doses of 2.0 to 4.0 per diem and salol in doses of 1.0 to 3.0 per diem (according to Lewascheff and others) were found by Lépine and Dufour to produce hyperemia of the liver. Benzoate of sodium belongs to the same class.

Oleate of sodium (advised by Blum in dose of 0.25, four to eight doses per diem) is a more rational prescription and seems to produce less injury than large doses of olive oil or of lipanin used as recommended by Kennedy.

In addition, oleum terebinthinæ, terpene hydrate, euonymin (0.1 once or twice daily or oftener), and podophyllin (0.02 from two to four times daily) have been with reason recommended as cholagogues. The cholagogic action of sodium bicarbonate, sodium sulphate, and sodium chlorate is not positively established. The most reliable physiologic cholagogue is a full meal consisting of meat, fat, and amylaceous material. All purgatives act as cholagogues in the sense of stimulating the peristaltic action of the bile-ducts.

A decrease in the excretion of bile always follows an increase as a
30

natural reaction. The flow of bile is also lessened directly by iodid of potassium and atropin.

In addition to producing quantitative changes in the secretion of the bile by dilution, the attempt has been made to modify it qualitatively by introducing certain substances that are excreted by the liver. These were expected to act partly upon the diseased mucous lining of the bile-ducts, and partly upon the bacteria present in these passages. As "biliary antiseptics" sodium salicylate and salol in particular have been employed. Oil of turpentine and chloric acid enter the bile in the same manner as does salicylate of sodium. This does not apply to the alkaline carbonates, according to Stadelmann and his pupils, although these salts have, for a long time, been administered for this purpose in the form of mineral waters.

With regard to the action of drugs upon the other functions of the liver-cells we know much less than we do in the matter of the secretion of bile. Among the drugs from which some such action is expected the following need mention: iodid of potassium and mercury (particularly in the form of calomel) in chronic inflammations, especially when interstitial proliferation is present; alkaline carbonates and sulphates, and sodium chlorid, particularly in fatty infiltration and in hyperemia from overeating.

It is said that oil of turpentine increases oxidative processes within the liver—a very doubtful point. We know that, in addition to mercury, other metals, such as iron and lead, are arrested in the liver and are therefore capable of exercising an influence on its function. So far no use has been made of this property in the therapy of diseases of the liver. The same applies to certain substances that are especially toxic for the liver, namely, phosphorus, antimony, and arsenic.

It was formerly believed that sulphuretted hydrogen and the alkaline sulphids in certain mineral waters could act as solvents (Roth), but it is probable that the action of these substances can be explained in a different manner.

It may be stated generally that the medicamentous treatment of diseases of the liver is based more on empiricism than on an exact experimental basis. When the attempt has been made to found a rational therapeusis on an experimental basis, the results obtained in many instances have not agreed with clinical observation. At the same time, it must be remembered that the functions of the liver are exceedingly complicated, so that the effects of medicaments influencing them must necessarily also be complicated and difficult to understand. In addition, the sphere of action of a certain drug may frequently be in a totally different region than is expected, while the functions of the liver are unquestionably in many instances modified indirectly either by the effect of a given drug on the heart, on the digestive tract, on respiration, or on the excretory function of the kidneys. In view of all this, the treatment of diseases of the liver must still rest upon clinical observation and experience, which can be controlled only by experiment.

Besides dietary regulations, the group of purgatives seem to play the most important rôle in the treatment of hepatic diseases; but it is not definitely determined that their beneficial effect can be attributed to their evacuating action alone.

The administration of mineral waters is very important in the treatment particularly of chronic diseases of the liver. The most important of the alkaline waters are Vichy, Neuenahr, Ems, Bilin, and Salzbrunn; of the alkaline-saline are Carlsbad, Bertrich, Marienbad, Franzensbad,

Elster, Rippoldsau, and Tarrasp; of the hot salt springs are Wiesbaden, Aix-la-Chapelle, Baden-Baden, Bourbonne, Kissingen, and Homburg.

It may be said that the hot waters mentioned act chiefly upon the parenchyma of the liver directly and on the secretion and composition of the bile, whereas the cold springs principally affect intestinal digestion and promote the peristalsis both of the intestine and of the bile-ducts. Of the latter less is probably absorbed. For the purpose of promoting peristalsis we can also employ the bitter waters.

The attempt has been made to influence the functions of the liver by certain local measures, such as local abstraction of blood, massage, and electricity.

Local bleeding by leeches applied to the region of the liver is of value in all forms of painful perihepatitis of whatever origin. As it is not possible to influence the blood-current within the liver by these means, from three to ten leeches have been applied to the region of the anus, for the purpose of relieving congestion in the portal system, just as occurs in spontaneous hemorrhoidal hemorrhages. This procedure was formerly very popular, but has lately fallen into disuse, probably without justification. Sacharjin recommends the application of leeches to the coccyx.

G. Harley attempted to withdraw blood from the liver directly (so-called "phlebotomy of the liver"). He anesthetized the patient and introduced a trocar having a diameter of $2\frac{1}{2}$ mm. from right to left to a distance of about twenty centimeters, and withdrew about six hundred cubic centimeters of blood. We can only warn against the employment of this measure. It is recommended particularly in "enlargement and inflammation" of the liver. In one case it produced a copious hemorrhage into the bile-passages.

The application of the ice-bag, of Priessnitz compresses, and of cataplasms has been proved to be useful in inflammatory and other pains originating from the serous covering of the liver and from the gall-bladder. It is very doubtful whether these measures can exercise any influence on diseases of the hepatic parenchyma itself.

Mechanical treatment of diseases of the liver can be carried out by breathing exercises and general gymnastics, particularly by such exercises as bring the abdominal muscles into play. Unless it is enlarged the liver is not accessible to manual massage, and these manipulations are, moreover, hardly indicated. It is, at the same time, not impossible that the lower surface of the liver, and possibly the bile-passages, may be influenced by general abdominal massage if the abdominal walls are considerably relaxed. C. Gerhardt has recommended direct massage of the gall-bladder, if possible combined with manual compression, in icterus simplex, in order to thus remove the obstructing plug of mucus. In case the gall-bladder cannot be reached, he recommends the application of a strong induced current with slow interruptions over the region of the gall-bladder. There is no doubt but that the good results claimed for this method of treatment must be attributed in large part to the increased peristaltic action of the intestine and of the bile-ducts that it produces reflexly.

The puncture of the abdomen for the removal of ascitic fluid also acts beneficially in a mechanical way by the removal of the excessive pressure and permitting normal circulation of the blood and of the bile to be re-established.

Surgical procedures are often crowned with success, and within late years are being employed more and more. They are usually directed toward the removal of biliary concretions and a correction of the lesion resulting from their impaction. In addition, abscesses of the liver, and echinococcus cysts are amenable to surgical treatment, and tumors can sometimes be removed. [In regard to the operative treatment of ascites see page 714.]

The injection of certain medicaments into the parenchyma of the liver has been attempted tentatively here and there; but the procedure promises very little. The injection of corrosive sublimate solution (1 : 1000) into echinococcus cysts has been successfully employed.

In conclusion, a few points in regard to the special treatment of icterus may be mentioned.

It is frequently necessary to relieve patients suffering from cutaneous pruritus, and measures directed toward an amelioration of this symptom are indicated in addition to the general measures that are being employed. Of greatest importance is the care of the skin by warm sponging and bathing. Washes containing dilute acetic acid, lemon juice, slippery-elm, or ammonia are beneficial, and baths containing bran, potash, or soda are recommended. The itching may be relieved also by powdering the skin with starch or lycopodium, to which salicylic acid or menthol may be added, or by washing with tar soap or solutions of carbolic acid (2%) or chloral hydrate (3%) in water or alcohol, or with chloroform, ichthyol, or menthol, or salicylic acid dissolved in alcohol, oil, or ether.

These different measures have to be tried to determine the most useful in the individual case, and if the icterus is of long duration it is frequently necessary to alternate them (see Leichtenstern, *loc. cit.*, p. 27). The best internal narcotic is amylene-hydrate in the dose of from one to two grams.

Stimulation of the secretion of bile is frequently advocated in icterus. This is indicated only in those cases in which an obstacle to the outflow of bile is situated in the larger bile-passages and where the obstacle does not produce a complete occlusion of the duct and is presumably removable. This may be the condition in certain catarrhal states and in small concretions. In one respect an increase in the secretion of bile must act harmfully in every case of icterus, for the reason that, as an increased amount of biliary constituents enters the blood-current, it produces certain toxic symptoms and perhaps acts deleteriously on the structure of the liver itself. This bad effect will increase with the degree of obstruction presented to the outflow of bile, a factor impossible to estimate during life.

Stimulation of the peristaltic action of the bile-ducts will cause an increased absorption during the time of the contraction of the ducts in case an obstruction exists in the common duct and the pressure is transmitted backward throughout the whole system of biliary canals. On the other hand, an increase in the peristaltic movements could act by shutting off the pressure-wave in the direction of the liver so that the increase of pressure would occur only in the direction of the bile-stream. We do not know in which direction the peristaltic wave is propagated. Mechanical compression of the gall-bladder is a more dangerous proceeding. If the external orifice of the bile-duct is occluded, this manipulation must necessarily produce a considerable increase of the bile-pressure even as far as the bile-capillaries, and in this manner might cause minute extravasations of bile and necrotic degeneration of portions of the hepatic parenchyma.

[In the original German edition the possibility of forming an external fistula of the gall-bladder in cases of chronic jaundice was discussed, and the possible advantages of such a procedure were considered. Since the appearance of the work this has earned a place among the well-recognized means of surgical relief of the condition. A consideration of this and the many other surgical measures employed at the present time in cases of more or less permanent biliary obstruction, would be out of place here and may be found in many of the more recent text-books on surgery and in numerous monographs and journals.—ED.]

The making of such an external gall-bladder fistula seems to me to possess certain advantages over a gall-bladder-duodenal fistula (cholecystenterostomy) for the reason that the latter is much more readily infected, both during the operation and subsequently, and in this way it may cause a general infection of the bile-passages.

In hepatic auto-intoxication the intestine should be emptied, diuresis should be stimulated, and the activity of the skin should be promoted by baths. In cases of severe coma, blood-letting may be of use (L. Levi).

LITERATURE.

Gerhardt, C.: "Volkmann's klin. Vorträge," No. 17, 1871.
Glass: "Ueber den Einfluss einiger Natronsalze auf Secretion und Alkaliengehalt der Galle," "Archiv für experimentelle Pathologie," Bd. xxx, p. 241.
Harley, G.: "Phlebotomie der Leber," "Münchner med. Wochenschr.," 1893, p. 887.
Hoffmann, F. A.: "Vorlesungen über allgemeine Therapie," p. 163, Leipzig, 1865.
Krull, J.: "Behandlung des Icterus catarrhalis," "Berliner klin. Wochenschr.," 1877, No. 12.
Leichtenstern in Penzoldt und Stintzing's "Handbuch der Therapie," Bd. iv, Abtheil. vi, p. 139.
Moritz, F.: "Grundzüge der Krankenernährung," pp. 187, 379, Stuttgart, 1898.
Mosler: "Zur localen Therapie der Leberkrankheiten," "Deutsches med. Wochenschr.," 1882, No. 16.
Sacharjin: "Klinische Abhandlungen," Berlin, 1890. (Calomel, bleeding.)
Stadelmann, E.: "Ueber Cholagoga" (with bibliography), "Berliner klin. Wochenschr.," 1896, No. 9.

DISEASES OF THE BILE-PASSAGES.

(Quincke.)

DISEASES of the bile-passages only rarely occur as the result of noxious influences affecting them through their external walls by continuity, although inflammation and neoplasms may so involve them. Diseases of their mucous lining are far more frequent, for the mucosa may suffer injury by substances coming from the liver-cells or the bile-capillaries and descending with the stream of bile, and also by substances from the intestine, which ascend in a direction contrary to the bile-current.

The first kind of injury may be inflicted by the bile itself as a result of a change in its normal composition or owing to an admixture of toxic substances. Instances of this kind are, for example, catarrh of the smaller bile-passages in acute phosphorus-poisoning, the experimental form of poisoning seen after the administration of toluylenediamin, the latter converting the bile into a viscid slimy substance and making it more difficult for the bile-ducts to excrete it.

Such descending forms of disease may play an important rôle in many acute and chronic forms of hepatitis, but these lesions cannot be separated clinically from the primary disease. The inner surfaces of the bile-passages may here be damaged either by the same noxious substances as are the liver-cells themselves or by the morbid excretions of the primarily diseased liver-cells.

It is further conceivable, although so far not demonstrated, that bacteria may gain an entrance into the bile-passages from the blood and may produce lesions of these tissues.

Experimentally various micro-organisms have been found to gain access to the bile. Thus, Bernabie found the bacillus of rinderpest, the bacillus of anthrax, Friedländer's and Fraenkel's pneumococcus; and Pernice and Scagliosi found staphylococci, anthrax bacilli, and Bacillus subtilis in the bile. Gilbert Dominici failed to find streptococci in the bile after injecting them into the blood. These authors, with Thomas and Sherrington, believed that microbes enter the bile only if foci of disease are present within the liver (Dominici, *loc. cit.*, p. 101). [For statements regarding contamination of bile within the gall-bladder see below.—Ed.]

The bile-passages are much more frequently involved in the second manner above mentioned, namely, by ascending from the intestine.

In order to understand the mechanism of this occurrence, it is necessary to recall the peculiar manner in which the main bile-duct enters the intestine. It passes obliquely through the wall of the intestine and terminates in a papilla or a fold of the mucous membrane of the duodenum, a strong muscular sphincter surrounding the orifice.

The pars intestinalis of the ductus chloedochus is 2.4 cm. long and about 0.5 cm. in diameter, being narrower than the rest of the duct. About 3 to 12 mm. before its entrance into the intestine it is joined by the pancreatic duct. The common funnel-shaped duct formed in this manner is called the diverticulum of Vater. Both the pancreatic and the bile-duct have at their orifice papillary excrescences which act like valves. The orifice of this common duct measures about 2.5 mm. in diameter but is capable of a great deal of stretching.*

The narrow orifice of this canal can very easily be occluded by a plug of mucus forming within it, as occurs, for example, in catarrhal swelling of the duodenal mucosa. The orifice may be either closed from pressure exercised from without or from an extension of inflammatory processes in its vicinity by direct continuity of tissue. Such an inflammation may extend for some distance into the main duct.

In view of the fact that the papilla of the ductus choledochus is continually dipping into the intestinal contents, it might be expected that some of this could readily penetrate the duct. As a matter of fact, however, intestinal contents very rarely enter the bile-duct. This is due to the small mucous fold at the orifice and to the oblique direction of the last portion of the duct, which form a sort of valvular protection. In addition to this, the periodic, automatic action of the sphincter closes the orifice and the periodic outflow of bile flushes the passage, these two factors together keeping it free from foreign material.

* Luschka, "Die Pars intestinalis des gemeinsamen Gallenganges," *Prager Vierteljahrsschr.*, 1869, Bd. CIII, p. 86 (with illustrations).

The normal bile and the bile-passages are sterile, and bacteria are only found in abnormal states. [For a further discussion of this point see the section upon cholelithiasis.—ED.] The species most frequently found are Bacterium coli, staphylococci and streptococci, the pneumococcus, the bacillus of typhoid, diplococci, and liquefying, putrefactive species. One or the other species may be seen sometimes alone, sometimes combined. This finding refutes the old theory that the bile always is antagonistic to all putrefactive processes and to bacteria. It is even possible to cultivate the above-named bacteria in the bile outside of the body. They enter the bile-passages in a direction contrary to that of the bile-current and probably adhere to the superficial layer of the mucous membrane (in exceptional cases being introduced by intestinal worms). The same conditions obtain in the case of the bile-ducts as in the case of the salivary glands and the urinary passages. Occasionally, in all these passages the protection afforded by the outflow of the secretion and by the muscular closure of the external orifice grows insufficient (as at the orifice of the urethra and the ureters), and the different bacterial species succeed in penetrating them either by the growth of the microbes or by their motility (Bacillus typhi, choleræ, coli). They may also succeed in gaining an entrance into the duct in case peristalsis or pressure from neighboring organs produces abnormal relative differences in pressure within the duodenum and the ductus choledochus. It is quite probable that here, as in other organs of the body, isolated bacteria may occasionally gain an entrance and do no harm because of their being speedily washed out again or of not finding conditions favorable to their development. In order that they may develop, there must be a number of favorable circumstances. Among these must be mentioned, as in the case of the urinary passages, the existence of mechanical obstructions to the outflow of the secretion (such as swelling of the mucosa in the region of the papilla, or impaction of concretions), partial or complete failure of the flushing process, or diminution in the nutrition and resisting powers of the mucous lining. These causes are all favored by an existing catarrh of the passages.

Other factors may be active in addition to those mentioned, such as a diminution in the quantity of the bile or changes in its constitution, perversions in the nutrition of the mucosa, disturbances of the innervation of the musculature of the bile-passages, etc. These different conditions may be the result of acute febrile and other diseases, or of acute digestive troubles and even of certain nervous disorders.

The consequences of the invasion of the biliary passages by bacteria differ according to the species and virulence of the invading microbe. Particularly in the case of Bacterium coli do we find these differences marked. Owing to these different conditions, we see all grades of inflammation of the mucous membranes. Beginning with an increased desquamation of epithelial cells and an increased secretion, the process may progress to suppuration and ulceration. Slight degrees of infection, particularly if they involve only the larger bile-passages or the main trunk, can presumably be overcome by the protective powers of the organism, so that the tissues again become sterile. On the other hand, we may occasionally find bacteria in the bile-passages without any symptoms that can be attributed to their presence and without any anatomic changes of the mucous membranes. This may be due to the fact that such a latent infection is very mild from the beginning or that it constitutes the remnant of a severe infection that is in process of cure. Such a condition is clinically important for the reason that the bacteria present may without evident cause suddenly increase in virulence and thus cause a renewed infection of the bile-passages.

The process of self-purification of the bile-passages is most difficult in the gall-bladder (which is practically a diverticulum of the ducts), chiefly on account of the narrowness of the cystic duct which constitutes a mechanical obstacle to the outflow of bile.

Our knowledge of the anatomy and of the genesis of the diseases of the mucous lining of the bile-passages is very incomplete because milder cases and cases in their incipiency rarely come to autopsy. In addition, it is impossible to examine the diseased secretion of the mucosa, as can be done in the case of similar inflammations of the urinary or the respiratory passages. The part that microbes play has been studied for a few years only. However important these "*infections biliaires*" may be, we must not overestimate their significance. I do not think, above all, that we are justified in following the example of many French authors, who teach that such infections alone can explain the pathology of all diseases of the bile-passages.

There is no justification in assuming that the bile has antiputrefactive properties, a view to which many investigators are inclined from the fact that feces containing no bile were particularly offensive. Bile itself readily undergoes putrefactive changes, and, according to Kossel and Limberg, it can exercise an inhibiting effect on putrefaction of the intestinal contents only when it is in great concentration. Staphylococcus aureus and Bacillus coli can be cultivated in bile as well as in bouillon (Létienne). Gilbert and Dominici injected microbes into the bile-passages of living animals and found Bacillus coli and typhi and the streptococcus and staphylococcus after from two to four weeks, the cholera bacillus and pneumococcus after from two to five days; all in an active and virulent state. [The length of time during which the typhoid bacillus may remain in the gall-bladder is further considered in the section on cholelithiasis.—ED.]

Normal bile removed from the gall-bladder during life or a few hours after death has in from fifty to seventy per cent. of the cases been found to be sterile. It cannot be determined positively whether the bacteria found in the remaining cases contaminated the bile as a result of defective technique in removing and examining the bile or as a result of postmortem immigration. It is not impossible that in some instances bacteria may have gained an entrance into the gall-bladder during the agonal stage. Duclaux and Netter found Bacterium coli and Staphylococcus aureus in the terminal portion of the ductus choledochus in normal animals. Girode found the cholera bacillus in the bile-passages fourteen times in twenty-eight cases of cholera. and among these cases he observed suppurative inflammation in only one instance. In case Bacillus typhi has gained an entrance into the bile-passages, inflammatory reaction is less rarely absent. This germ may remain in the bile-channels for from five to eight months after convalescence. The bacillus of typhoid, in particular, may gain an entrance into the bile-ducts by way of the liver, *i. e.*, by the descending path. Létienne, in one case, determined the same for Bacillus tuberculosis. Bacillus coli is the parasite most frequently found in these tissues. It is always present in the duodenum, and as it is favored by its motility, it may gain an entrance into the bile-passages in almost any primary disease of these parts, as, for example, in typhoid fever either alone (Dupré) or together with the typhoid bacillus (Gilbert and Dominici). As a rule, Bacillus coli produces an inflammation, but occasionally if the virulence of the germ is slight, no inflammation may result. It appears that this microbe may even participate in the formation of gall-stones. (For the literature on infection of the bile-ducts see the section on cholangitis suppurativa.)

The symptoms of disease of the bile-passages are, on the one hand, icterus; on the other, disturbances of the general health.

Icterus, in case it was not present before, is caused by the swelling of the mucous lining of the bile-passages. In this manner an obstruction is created to the outflow of the bile. In view of the narrowness of the bile-ducts such an obstruction is readily formed either by the swelling of the mucosa or by an increased desquamation of epithelial cells and an increased secretion of mucus. This is particularly the case in the finer passages. It is important to remember that the morbid products of a diseased mucous membrane may cause the precipitation of certain substances from the bile which gradually form masses and may form the nuclei of concretions. These, in their turn, keep up the catarrh and constitute an obstruction to the flow of bile, thus completing a vicious circle.

The general symptoms are either a result of the stasis of bile as such, or of the infection of the bile-passages, or of the absorption of the inflammatory products formed. We therefore have fever, and, in case the liver is secondarily involved, various perversions of the hepatic function.

As a rule, icterus and disturbances of the general health are seen together; yet it is possible for one or the other to be absent.

DISTURBANCES IN THE CANALIZATION OF THE BILE; NARROWING AND OCCLUSION OF THE BILIARY PASSAGES.

(Quincke.)

Whenever the lumen of the bile-passages is narrowed an obstruction to the outflow of bile is created, and dilatation of the passages above the narrowing is produced by the dammed-up bile. If the ductus choledochus is occluded, all the bile-passages are affected in this manner. If the ductus hepaticus or some of the smaller bile-ducts are occluded, their tributary branches alone become dilated. Occlusion of the cystic duct does not interfere with the circulation of the bile, but only stops the storing function of the gall-bladder. In this section we will discuss only those cases where the outflow of bile is impeded altogether, or at least in great part and for a long period of time.

CHRONIC OBSTRUCTIVE JAUNDICE.

Etiology.—Occlusion of the main duct may be produced either by the entrance of some foreign body that acts as an obturator, by some change in the walls of the duct, or by compression of the duct from without.

I. Gall-stones are the most frequent cause of obstruction. As a rule, they become impacted behind the narrow orifice into the duodenum and act as a plug or a ball-valve. In case inflammatory processes supervene as a result of the pressure of the stone on the walls of the duct, the narrowing may be still more increased.

Parasites are more rarely the cause of the obstruction. Of these, the echinococcus is the most frequent. In case the mother-cyst ruptures, daughter-cysts, whole or in fragments, may enter the bile-ducts. The much smaller cysts of the Echinococcus alveolaris can only occlude smaller bile-ducts, but, as a rule, they occlude many at a time. Echinococcus vulgaris rarely produces obstructive icterus by the pressure it exercises from without; in the case of Echinococcus alveolaris, on the other hand, both compression and inflammatory processes in the walls of the ducts may cause stasis and occlusion. Distomata and ascarides may penetrate the bile-ducts from the intestine, develop within these passages, and by growing produce occlusion and (chiefly owing to bacteria that they carry with them) inflammation of the walls of the ducts.

Blood-clots and plugs of mucus may also produce obstruction. The former are very rarely seen, the latter very frequently. Although they do not properly deserve to be classified among foreign bodies, they are capable of causing occlusion of the intestinal end of the common duct in the same manner as do the latter.

II. Inflammatory processes of the wall of the main bile-duct, in case the mucous membrane alone is involved, rarely produce complete occlusion for more than a few days, or at most a few weeks. A more persistent occlusion results if the connective-tissue structures of the wall or of the surrounding tissues are involved; for in such cases new-formation of connective tissue occurs, followed, as a rule, by the development of cicatricial tissue. Chronic phlegmonous inflammations of this kind can be caused by gall-stones impacted in the common duct, or, more rarely, by simple catarrhal inflammations (as a rule, bacterial in origin). In either instance cicatricial strictures of the passages are produced analogous to those seen in the urinary passages, notably the urethra. In exceptional cases the walls of the duct may grow together and a true atresia be the result.

Fibrous inflammations may also involve the duct from without by direct continuity of tissue, as from an ulcer of the stomach or duodenum, from cholecystitis, or from a perihepatic inflammation in the region of the porta hepatis developing as a result of cirrhosis, gummatous hepatitis, etc. The occlusion is produced either by the direct pressure of the cicatricial tissue or by traction or kinking following cicatricial contraction.

Occasionally the closure of the orifice of the bile-duct is congenital or develops shortly after birth, probably not as a congenital anomaly, but as the result of intra-uterine disease.

III. New-formations and tumors. Carcinoma of the ductus choledochus rapidly causes occlusion of its lumen. Obstruction is more frequently caused by carcinoma in the vicinity of the duct (stomach, duodenum, pancreas, gall-bladder), which may either compress the duct from without or grow into its walls and so occlude it. Even though such carcinomata are of small size, they may produce occlusion of the bile-ducts if they develop in their vicinity, particularly in the case of cancer of the stomach with metastases to the lymph-glands in the porta hepatis. The same mechanism may act in enlargement of the lymph-glands in the region of the porta due to tuberculosis, lymphoma, or secondary syphilis. Occasionally the enlargement of these glands causes compression of the portal vein with a resulting ascites from stasis.

Other agencies that can produce occlusion of the common duct by transmitted pressure, traction, or displacement are tumors of the right kidney or suprarenal, carcinomatous and tuberculous swellings of the mesenteric and retroperitoneal glands, aneurysms of the abdominal and of the superior mesenteric artery, the accumulation of masses of fecal matter in the hepatic flexure of the colon following prolonged constipation, the uterus when it is enlarged from pregnancy, and, finally, tumors of the ovary. Often many coexisting lesions occur to cause occlusion of the bile-duct, especially through the presence of slight peritoneal adhesions in the neighborhood of the porta.

Anatomy.—The bile-ducts are dilated above the obstruction. As a rule, the longer the duration of the stasis, the greater this dilatation. The main bile-ducts run a tortuous course and may become as large as a finger. On the surface of the liver there are areas in which even the smaller channels are dilated, forming net-like strands and resembling lymph-vessels. In certain portions of the liver great numbers of these dilated bile-channels are seen. The contents of the bile-passages may measure as much as a liter and the contents of the gall-bladder may be as much again. In the beginning the fluid contained in these vessels consists exclusively of bile; later the color disappears and the fluid grows colorless, mucous, or serous, and contains nothing but products of the mucous membrane and of its glands altered in character by the long-continued stretching and tension. It seems that under these conditions the production of bile decreases, and that what little bile is formed is not poured into the bile-passages and mixed with their secretions, but is directly absorbed into the general circulation. In the bile-capillaries numerous yellow plugs are seen under the microscope. We have already described the changes in the liver itself and have shown that they may either be atrophic or inflammatory in character.

In case the bile-ducts are infected with bacteria, we see, in addition to the changes just described, certain inflammatory lesions of the bile-passages and of the liver itself.

Symptoms; Diagnosis.—The symptoms of icterus that we have described above (see p. 433) are seen in a pure and uncomplicated form in the types of uncomplicated obstructive icterus that we are discussing. They occupy so prominent a part in the general morbid picture and make it so uniform that both the etiology and the prognosis are often for a long time difficult to determine. In order to solve the problem it is necessary to consider carefully the symptoms of lesions in other organs, the age and constitution of the patient, and the appearance and the course of the icterus itself. Sudden appearance of icterus, great fluctuations in its intensity, its sudden disappearance, and a repetition of the attack at long intervals, sometimes years apart, speak for gall-stones or the impaction of some other foreign body. This suspicion will be strengthened if, in addition, the attack of icterus begins with pain and an accession of fever. Compression and inflammation, as a rule, set in gradually and do not show such violent fluctuations in the intensity of the icterus. In addition, examination of the urine and the feces usually enables us to arrive at a diagnosis. At the same time, it must be remembered that compression may occasionally cause a sudden occlusion, and that, on the other hand, concretions may produce a gradual occlusion of the duct without other striking symptoms.

The condition of the gall-bladder sometimes gives valuable diagnostic clues. In compression and inflammatory occlusion of the bile-duct the bladder is frequently distended, in gall-stones it is usually contracted (Courvoisier). [Recent investigations would seem to permit an even stronger statement as to the value of this diagnostic point. Courvoisier's dictum is that in obstruction from causes other than gall-stones distention of the gall-bladder is the rule (Gewöhnliche). Cabot * has found only four exceptions to the "law" in 86 cases.—ED.]

Frequently the special diagnosis can be made only when the icterus is fully developed, or from its course, or even after it has subsided.

Prognosis; Duration.—The prognosis is dependent on the character

* *Med. News*, Nov. 30, 1901.

of the occluding agency. In many instances death occurs altogether independently of the existence of icterus, from cancer, suppurative inflammation, or gastric insufficiency. On the other hand, in certain cases of obstruction by stricture, concretions, or plugs of mucus death may occur from obstructive jaundice alone.

The prognosis is in general more unfavorable if icterus has persisted for more than two months, and grows worse as stasis continues beyond that time, not only because it becomes less probable that the obstacle will ever be removed, but also because the intoxication with bile becomes cumulative in its effect and the appearance of hepatargia with hepatic autointoxication may be expected at any time (see p. 440). Even in those cases where the stasis of bile is well borne for the first three or four months the strength and general nutrition will begin to suffer, and at the end of from eight to ten months, if icterus persists, serious nervous symptoms may suddenly develop, and in the course of a few days lead to death.

It is true that there are exceptional cases on record in which the condition of chronic biliary stasis was borne for a much longer time. Budd reports a case in which it persisted for four years, and Murchison, Barth, and Besnier speak of cases in which recovery occurred after six years.*

Hertz † describes a case of occlusion of the ductus choledochus by a gall-stone, in which the stools were of a light gray color for two years and a half and the skin was only slightly discolored to a dirty grayish-yellow. Eight times during this period attacks of icterus occurred that lasted, on an average, for six days and were accompanied by intermittent fever. The urine during the attacks was dark brown in color, but gave only a very slight Gmelin reaction. Hertz assumes that in this case the bile was completely absent from the intestine owing to the occlusion of the ductus choledochus, so that the only explanation for the non-appearance of icterus was the assumption that no bile was being formed. I believe that the obstruction (except during the attacks) was very slight, and that the greater part of the bile succeeded in entering the intestine through the bile-duct and a fistula that existed between the gall-bladder and the colon, and that the bile-pigment was here converted to the chromogen of urobilin by reduction.‡ [In many respects the case resembles some of the reported instances of "ball-valve stone."—ED.]

Legendre, Gailard, and Debove § describe cases in which icterus, resulting from complete occlusion, existed for twenty-five years without seriously interfering with the general health of the patient.

The treatment of biliary stasis is dependent on its cause; and at best is symptomatic. If the stasis persists for a long time, the establishment of a biliary fistula, even for a short time, seems indicated.

CATARRH OF THE BILE-DUCTS; CHOLANGITIS CATARRHALIS.

(Quincke.)

In the clinical sense, icterus catarrhalis and catarrh of the bile-duct are identical. From the anatomic point of view they are slightly different, since, on the one hand, we see catarrh of the bile-duct without icterus, and, on the other, we see attacks of so-called icterus catarrhalis that are not

* Cited by Schüppel, p. 127.

† Hertz: "Wie lange kann ein Mensch leben bei völligem Abschluss der Gallenwege nach dem Darme?" *Berliner klin. Wochenschr.*, 1877, pp. 76 and 91.

‡ Quincke, "Ueber die Farbe der Fäces," *"Münchner med. Wochenschr.*, 1896, No. 36.

§ *Berliner klin. Wochenschr.*, 1897, p. 371.

caused by catarrh of the bile-ducts. For the present we are unable, in individual cases, positively to localize the trouble in the large or the small bile-ducts, nor can we determine the exact pathogenesis in each case. For this reason we will first describe the clinical picture of catarrhal icterus and discuss the disease on this basis. After discussing this form in all its varieties, and after describing its mode of origin, we will proceed to a discussion of the other clinical forms of essential icterus. Some of the latter are certainly identical with catarrhal icterus, and should be classified with it; others probably originate in a particular manner and merit separate discussion.

ICTERUS CATARRHALIS.

Catarrhal Jaundice; Icterus gastro-duodenalis; Icterus simplex;
Icterus benignus.

Etiology.—The most frequent cause of catarrhal icterus being a gastro-intestinal catarrh, we frequently see it after overloading of the stomach, after eating very fatty, spoiled, or indigestible food, after taking much ice or drinking very cold beverages, and after the abuse of spirituous liquors. In many instances a slightly chronic condition, such as chronic alcoholism, exists and paves the way for the occurrence of an acute attack. Sometimes the attack of icterus is preceded by a chilling or a wetting. In some instances several of these predisposing factors coexist, and a number of persons are exposed to the same harmful influences, so that it appears as though icterus occurred epidemically.

The predisposition is increased by previous attacks of catarrhal jaundice, and by hyperemia or conditions of chronic enlargement of the liver.

In some instances no etiologic factor of any kind can be discovered, so that we are forced to assume a particular, individual predisposition to icterus.

Catarrh of the bile-passages is seen in the course of a variety of infectious diseases—among others, malaria, typhoid fever, and cholera; and in them icterus is at times seen. The jaundice seen in phosphorus-poisoning is also probably due to a catarrh of the smaller bile-ducts.

Concretions, by the mechanical pressure they exercise, sometimes produce a swelling of the mucous lining of the bile-passages. These concretions, however, are themselves usually the effect of a catarrh of the bile-passages, and are capable only of increasing the severity of the catarrh already existing.

Catarrhal icterus is a common disease and is seen more frequently in young subjects than in the old and the middle-aged. In view of its causes, it is more often seen in men than in women.

In children the disease is seen most frequently from the second to the seventh year, seldom during the first and second years of life.

Symptoms.—As a rule, following the different etiologic factors above enumerated, the symptoms of a gastric catarrh appear, with a feeling of pressure in the region of the stomach, loss of appetite, a coated tongue, nausea, and vomiting. In addition, headache, vertigo, depression, and, occasionally, fever are present. The bowels are, as a rule, constipated, rarely the opposite. The urine is scanty, reddish in color, and deposits a sediment. After the expiration of a few days icterus of the skin and a biliary discoloration of the urine are seen, and the feces grow light in color but are rarely altogether free from bile-pigment. After this condition has persisted for from one to two weeks the symptoms of the gastric catarrh diminish, the tongue becomes clean, and the appetite improves. Soon the signs of biliary stasis disappear, at first from the urine, later from the skin. As soon as the digestive organs begin to functionate normally, the general health seems to improve, not as rapidly, however, as might be expected from the reestablishment of normal digestion and the proper assimilation of food.

The duration of the whole disease until the complete disappearance of the jaundice usually is from three to four weeks. It takes several weeks more, however, before health is completely reestablished.

There are many exceptions to this usual course of an average case. The individual symptoms of an attack may vary and the duration of the disease may be longer or shorter.

The initial symptoms of a gastric catarrh are, as a rule, very pronounced, and precede the attack of icterus proper by three to four days, more rarely in a milder form by several weeks. In exceptional cases, icterus may develop before the appearance of gastric disturbances. Even in the cases where there is a complete obstruction to the entrance of bile into the intestine, this state exists for a few days only, so that varying quantities of bile are poured into the intestine at different times during the course of the disease, as is manifested by the varying color of the feces.

The symptoms of biliary stasis, as such, have been described above. In catarrhal icterus they are seen in their most typical form, varying, of course, in intensity and duration. Of the nervous symptoms, the itching of the skin is the most frequent, the slowing of the pulse less so. The milder and the shorter cases of catarrhal icterus, as well as the stage of convalescence from well-marked attacks, correspond to the picture of urobilin icterus described above.

The symptoms observed in the liver are varying and not characteristic. Sometimes a feeling of pressure is experienced in the region of the liver in addition to the feeling of oppression often complained of in the region of the stomach at the beginning of the attack. Increase in the size of the organ and in its consistency are found only in the very severe cases, probably in those only that are the result of infection.

In a certain proportion of cases (one-third to one-half) the spleen is enlarged.

The urine contains biliary constituents, or urobilin, hyaline casts (Nothnagel), rarely albumin.

Fever may be observed in the first few days of an attack of simple catarrhal icterus, but is not a frequent or conspicuous symptom. In the later course of the disease the temperature is sometimes subnormal.

Course.—The above description of catarrhal icterus applies to cases of medium severity. There are, however, other forms, as follows:

I. Abortive forms of slight degree, which are shorter in duration and in which the stasis of bile does not persist for so long a time. The mildest forms of this kind differ from a simple gastric or intestinal catarrh only in that the skin may be colored slightly yellow for a few days. As a rule, the severity of the disease corresponds to the duration and the severity of the biliary stasis.

II. Occasionally catarrhal icterus runs a protracted course and may persist for from two to five months. During this time it may be uniform or may fluctuate in intensity, the exacerbations being usually due to a repetition of the indiscretions that primarily led to the attack, the catarrh in process of cure being aggravated by a new acute attack. In those cases where febrile disturbances are seen with the recurrence of such an attack it is to be assumed that an infection of the bile-passages has occurred.

III. In the cases where the attack of catarrhal icterus persists for several weeks with the same intensity, the symptoms of gastric and intestinal catarrh as a rule recede and the symptoms of pure uncomplicated biliary stasis become more apparent (disturbances in the general health, depression, emaciation, a feeling of weakness, and, in a word, those symptoms described under the caption of Hepatic Autointoxication, page 440). It is, as a rule, impossible to decide whether the obstruction to the outflow of bile is situated in the main duct or in some of its branches.

The general clinical picture often so closely resembles the syndrome of biliary obstruction from some other cause, such as impacted gall-stones or some compressing neoplasm, that no definite decision can be arrived at until later in the course of the disease or until the permeability of the bile-ducts has been re-established. Recovery from these intense and long-lasting forms is slow, but generally complete.

IV. Occasionally it will be found that the symptoms of the initial gastric catarrh are very severe, resembling the initial stages of an attack of typhoid fever. Violent pain in the limbs with headache, great depression, insomnia, high fever with chills, swelling of the spleen, and gastric symptoms without any objective findings in any of the other organs, all point to a general infection. If icterus appears at the end of the first week, it is frequently mistaken for a secondary symptom or some complication. Occasionally, at this stage, tenderness over the liver and a slight degree of enlargement of the organ are found. The fever usually runs an intermittent course and fluctuates between 39° and 40° C. (102.2° and 104° F.). It may persist for several weeks and then disappear slowly, as do all the other symptoms. The whole course of this form resembles an attack of typhoid fever. This form is rare, but has been described for a long time. The attacks are usually, and probably correctly, attributed to a infection of the bile-ducts, and have been called infectious icterus (see below). Here, too, we encounter cases of different severity and duration resembling, on the one hand, simple catarrhal icterus, and, on the other, approaching in severity the fatal cases of icterus gravis. According to Chauffard, the toxic action of certain ptomains plays an important rôle in this form.

Sequels.—Catarrhal icterus is not infrequently followed by other disturbances, either following immediately in its train or not developing for several weeks after the attack. Among these must be mentioned the recurrence of attacks of icterus, which are analogous to the repeated occurrence of attacks of catarrh in other mucous membranes. It is probable that in these cases the swelling of the mucosa has not fully subsided, so that the latter reacts to some slight damaging agent, or, possibly, the orifice of the bile-duct was particularly narrow. In many instances the formation of concretions starts from catarrhal icterus, especially from the recurring form. Suppurative cholangitis may develop from a simple catarrh with or without concretions.

The catarrhal condition may subside in the main bile-ducts, but persist in the cystic duct and in the gall-bladder, so that we may see the development of hydrops of the gall-bladder or persistent inflammation follow such repeated attacks of catarrhal icterus.

Occasionally catarrhal icterus, and here again particularly the recurring form, is the starting-point for chronic inflammations of the hepatic parenchyma, such as Hanot's hypertrophic form and, possibly, of other forms of cirrhosis of the liver. In rare instances acute yellow atrophy of the liver has been known to develop after catarrhal icterus.

Anatomy.—The anatomic changes ordinarily seen in other catarrhs are occasionally seen in catarrhal icterus—namely, a loosening of the mucous membrane, desquamation of epithelial cells, and the secretion of mucus containing a varying number of leucocytes. All these changes may be seen at autopsy, even though the presence of a catarrh of the bile-passages was not suspected during life. On the other hand, the anatomic findings in a case of catarrhal icterus may be such that they do not at all explain the occurrence of icterus and of biliary stasis. As a rule, the presence of a plug of mucus in the intestinal portion of the bile-duct, absence of bile-staining of the ducts, and difficulty in emptying the gall-bladder by pressure, are considered evidence of its occlusion and impermeability during life. Both positive and negative findings in regard to these points are of only relative value, and must always be considered in connection with the color of the contents of the duodenum and the amount of material contained within the bile-passages. It can be seen that acute degrees of stenosis from swelling of the mucous membranes can be greatly changed after death if we study the conditions existing in such places as the larynx, which is much wider than the bile-ducts and consequently more easily examined. Opportunities for examining cases of recent catarrhal icterus postmortem rarely occur. It is probable that there are cases where we might expect to see the intestinal end of the ductus choledochus compressed by the swollen mucosa of the duodenum without its being itself diseased, others with catarrh of the bile-passages ascenting for varying distances into the duct, and others again that, as in phosphorus-poisoning and in hyperemia of the liver from stasis, involve the finer bile-passages alone. The latter cases would correspond to the so-called "capillary bronchitis," but would not in reality have anything to do with the bile-capillaries. Such a catarrh of the finer passages is developed in an irregular manner and does not involve all portions of the liver uniformly. Partial catarrh is seen in the intrahepatic bile-passages associated with concretions.

Whenever the terminal portion of the ductus choledochus is occluded by swelling or by a plug of mucus, the pancreatic duct also is usually occluded. This does not occur if the joint orifice of these two passages is abnormally constructed or if an auxiliary passage is present. Nothing definite is so far known in regard to the clinical significance of stasis of pancreatic juice occurring at the same time as stasis of bile.* (Salol is decomposed within the intestine, and, therefore,—whether the pancreatic juice be present or not,—cannot be employed for diagnostic purposes.)

Pathogenesis.—From the differences seen in the various clinical pictures of catarrhal icterus, and from the uncertainty of the anatomic findings, we are forced to the conclusion that this disease is not a clinical entity, but is composed of a group of different conditions varying with the anatomic seat of the trouble and the mode of origin.

For the present it is impossible to decide what rôle bacterial infection plays in this disease of the bile-passages. This point can be settled only

*Fr. Müller, "Untersuchungen über Icterus," *Zeitschr. für klin. Medicin,* 1887, vol. XII, p. 80.

by continued investigation of many cases. Exact conclusions are rendered particularly difficult by the possibility of secondary infection and of postmortem changes and microbic invasion. It is probable that bacterial infection forms the basis of many more cases than we suspect, and it is even possible that the majority of all cases are due to this factor. I think, however, that we are not justified in assuming such an origin for all cases of catarrhal icterus. Fever and disturbances of the general health in combination with icterus cannot be considered as diagnostic of bacterial infection of the bile-passages, for such an infection (as by Bacterium coli) may exist without producing any fever or even icterus. On the other hand, various serious disturbances of the general health may be caused by the absorption of toxins from the intestine or from simple stasis or bile or hepatargia.

Diagnosis.—The diagnosis of catarrhal icterus in those cases where it begins in a typical manner with the symptoms of a gastric catarrh is plain. In the cases, on the other hand, in which it begins less acutely, or in which the onset deviates from the typical course, the diagnosis is not so simple. In cases of the latter kind there is always danger of making the diagnosis of catarrhal icterus because of its greater frequency, the subsequent course making a revision of the diagnosis necessary. This is particularly the case in impaction of gall-stones, which may occur without causing any pain, and in cases of compression of the common duct by tumors—two conditions which may lead to the rapid development of icterus. For these reasons the only method of arriving at a diagnosis is by exclusion and by observing whether the disease runs a favorable course or not. In many instances, however, the youth of the patient, a knowledge of the primary cause of the trouble, such as a gastric catarrh, will assure the diagnosis. On the other hand, it must not be forgotten that, even though the icterus persists for many months, this does not exclude the catarrhal nature of the trouble.

Prognosis.—While the prognosis of this disease is favorable, as a rule, it can never be positively made, particularly in regard to the probable duration of the case and the length of convalescence. If the case begins acutely with fever, we can usually prognosticate that the disease will last for several weeks and will produce a considerable loss of strength and a reduction in the general nutrition of the patient. At the same time, a mild onset and incomplete stasis may be followed by a protracted attack. Those cases are particularly uncertain, especially as to the length of convalescence, in which a tendency to recurrence exists and in which errors of diet and hygiene have already been, or in all probability will be, committed by the patient. In old people an attack of simple catarrhal itcerus may end fatally from long-continued stasis of bile.[*] Toelg and Neusser have described the case of a strong well-nourished man who died within eight weeks with numerous hemorrhages into the cellular tissues and into the peritoneal cavity.

Treatment.—The treatment of acute catarrhal icterus is identical with that of acute gastric or intestinal catarrh. The only difference is that, owing to the complication with icterus, these cases need more time and greater care before a cure can be effected.

Only in those comparatively rare cases in which a chilling has preceded the attack is a course of sweating indicated. Wherever, with the appear-

---

[*] Leichtenstern, *loc. cit.*, p. 9. Fr. Müller, *Zeitschr. für klin. Medicin*, 1887, vol. XII, p. 80.

ance of icterus, a free evacuation of the bowels has not occurred, it is necessary to empty the bowels. Abstinence from all solid food, and limitation of the nourishment to tea, water, mineral waters, and thin soups will usually meet the patient's wants, and are indicated as long as the tongue is coated or fever exists and a feeling of pressure in the gastric region is present. The remedy indicated at this period is a solution of sodium bicarbonate (5 : 100). Hydrochloric acid is very popular, but not so appropriate. Large drafts of water, drunk as hot as the patient can tolerate, with dram doses of sodium phosphate three times daily have a beneficial effect upon the gastroduodenal catarrh.—ED.]

It is well to obtain a free evacuation of the bowels by drugs. For this purpose one or several doses of calomel (0.3 to 0.5) are indicated; later laxatives, such as Glauber's salts, Epsom salts, the tartrates, and rhubarb. The administration of castor oil is not so suitable, particularly for repeated use, and should not be used if much gastric disturbance exists. It is useful chiefly in the beginning of an attack where intestinal symptoms and colic predominate. [Sodium phosphate probably acts as well as any other laxative, and is unirritating.—ED.]

It is not necessary to combat existing diarrhea, especially at the outset. As a rule, it will disappear spontaneously if the patient observes the proper rules. In case it seems necessary to control it, hydrochloric acid, astringents, bismuth subnitrate, or tannigen (four doses of 1.0), may be used; but opium should only exceptionally be administered, and then only for the relief of violent colic.

The rules in regard to the general mode of life are important and should be carefully observed. Even in the absence of fever the patient should remain in bed as long, at least, as symptoms of acute dyspepsia are present. As soon as these symptoms disappear, and the patient begins to take a little nourishment, he may be permitted to leave the bed for a few hours at a time, and, where it is possible, stay in the open air, and may even be permitted to walk a few steps. All sustained bodily exertion and all exposure to chilling should be avoided as long as the flow of bile is not completely re-established. Particularly in protracted cases and during convalescence from dyspeptic disturbances careful regulations in these particulars should be made by the physician. The stage of the disease should, of course, not be judged from the color of the skin, but from the color of the feces and urine. With the return of appetite a little food can be administered, but all chemically and mechanically irritating articles of diet should be carefully avoided. Thickened soups, lean meat, white bread, and zwieback should be given first. Although theoretically milk is not a good article of diet because of its contained fat, practically it seems to be well borne; while meat, for no physiologic reason, is repugnant to patients, possibly because of the closure of the pancreatic duct. In regard to general principles of treatment, see page 462. The increase of the dietary should be governed by individual conditions in the same manner as in any other form of gastric catarrh. It is particularly important that each meal should be simple, that alcohol and narcotics should be avoided, and that little food should be given at each meal. The latter rule should also be observed during convalescence, when the appetite is frequently inordinately increased and its gratification may become dangerous to the patient.

In those cases that persist for several months the gastro-intestinal catarrh has usually ceased, and the general nutrition of the patient must be maintained and a more generous diet allowed, even though the stasis of bile persists. In such cases it is well to limit the amount of fat and to replace it by a corresponding amount of starchy food.

The administration of the remedies that are given during the time of the acute catarrhal attack should be stopped as soon as the dyspeptic disturbances are better or have disappeared. When the tongue is no longer coated, hydrochloric acid may be given with meals, and the administration of rhubarb may be continued, either alone or in combination with such bitters as gentian, calamus, or cascarilla in small doses.

As long as the stasis of bile persists wholly or in part, alkaline or alkaline-saline waters or the waters of different hot springs can be administered to advantage, especially the warm or hot waters, like Vichy, Neuenahr, or Carlsbad. The cold waters, such as Eger, Marienbad, Tarasp, and Rippoldsau, are indicated only in case there is a tendency to constipation.

The administration of enemata once or several times daily at the height of biliary stasis has been recommended in quantities of from one to one and a half liters (Mosler, Krull). The *rationale* of this method of treatment is based on the unsupported experimental finding of Stadelmann that the secretion of bile is increased by such injections. Possibly these injections, if they are retained for a long time, stimulate peristalsis, and in this manner promote the outflow of bile. I have occasionally employed injections with some success and other clinicians report the same. In view of the variable course of the disease it is a difficult matter to determine the true effect of the various remedies.

It has been the desire of physicians of all times to find remedies that would produce an increased flow of bile in biliary stasis. As a result, the action of certain drugs, such as calomel and rhubarb, whose beneficial effects in this disease were known, was explained on the idea that they were cholagogues. We know, however, particularly in the case of the two drugs named, that they do not possess this property. Where a large amount of mucus is present in the bile-passages and hinders the flow of bile, we would expect that a remedy that could dilute the bile or could exercise a solvent action on the mucus would aid in removing the obstacle to the outflow of bile. In this sense it is possible that the administration of much water by the intestine or by the stomach will act beneficially. The same applies to common salt, alkalies, and certain mineral waters, and to laxative remedies, and even food acts reflexly. As we have seen above, many theoretic objections could be formulated against the possibility of an increase of the secretion of bile by the administration of cholagogues.

Gerhardt: "Ueber Icterus gastroduodenalis," "Volkmann's Sammlung klin. Vorträge," No. 17, 1871.

Heitler: "Zur Klinik des Icterus catarrhalis," "Wiener med. Wochenschr.," Nos. 29 to 31, 1887.

Herzenstein, Helene (Dieulafoy): "Contrib. à l'étude de l'ictère catarrhal. prolongé." Thèse de Paris, 1890.

Senator: "Ueber Icterus; seine Entstehung und Behandlung," "Berliner Klinik," part 1, 1888.

Sommer, P.: "Ueber Icterus catarrhalis im Kindesalter." Dissertation, Kiel, 1896.

Toelg and Neusser: "Ein Fall von Icterus catarrhalis mit tödlichem Ausgang," "Zeitschr. für klin. Medicin," vol. vii, p. 321, 1884.

(See also Literature on Cholangitis, p. 514; on Icterus, p. 449; and on Icterus infectiosus, p. 507.)

ICTERUS EX EMOTIONE.

Icterus psychicus; Icterus spasticus.

In the eyes of the laity the secretion of bile and the hepatic functions in general are intimately connected with a disagreeable mood or a gloomy temperament. Such expressions as a "bilious temperament" and "his bile overflows" are illustrative of this idea. Jaundice, too, is usually attributed to an attack of anger, and in certain classes this idea is so deeply rooted that such an attack is postulated in every case of jaundice and the patient will try to remember when it occurred. It is not surprising that, as a rule, the patient will remember that he was angry a short or a long time before the occurrence of jaundice.

As examples of the dependence of jaundice upon psychic disturbances cases are adduced in which jaundice suddenly appeared a few hours or even a few moments after an attack of anger with a complete absence of all other predisposing factors or other symptoms of disease. Such examples, it is true, are rare and are transmitted by hearsay (see the summary by Daraignez). The causes given, besides anger, are sudden fright, mortal terror, and a gross insult. Besides jaundice, there may be seen, as a result of psychic injury, a feeling of great anxiety, pressure in the epigastric region, or violent diarrhea.

It is stated that emotional icterus does not persist for a long time, at most for a week, and that complete recovery rapidly ensues. In a few cases acute atrophy of the liver has been reported.

Different explanations of emotional icterus have been attempted, as follows:

I. Polycholia. The basis of this assumption is the theory that psychic disturbances are capable of causing an increased excretion of bile. This has not been proved, and even if it had it would not suffice for an explanation (see page 493).

II. A paralysis of the bile-passages (Laborde).

III. Disturbances in the circulation and particularly a sudden reduction in the tone of the abdominal vessels. In this way a diminution in the blood-pressure in the portal vein would be produced, and thereby bile from the bile-capillaries would be diffused into the blood-capillaries. In addition, fright might produce a sudden reduction in the strength of the heart-beat and of the respiratory movements, all factors that would tend to facilitate the above diffusion (Frerichs).

IV. Spasm of the bile-passages. It is said that a spasmodic closure of the ductus choledochus occurs and that stasis of bile is caused in this manner. It might even be that a general spasmodic contraction of other bile-passages supervened, and that in this manner still greater biliary pressure would be caused. [Débove* has supposed it possible that relaxation of the sphincter of the choledochus might occur from emotion and thus favor infection of the bile-passages.—ED.]

Of all these explanations, the last one seems to have the best foundation, because we know that the bile-passages are, in fact, capable of contraction, and that it is quite possible, to judge from analogous conditions observed in other organs, that disturbances in their normal movements can occur, and that these may be either spasmodic or paralytic in character.

* *Gaz. hebdom. de Méd. et de Chir.*, 1901, No. 33.

The older view, that biliary stasis must persist for several days in order to produce icterus, although based on animal experiments, has not been borne out by the facts observed. To judge from observations made in cases with impacted gall-stones, it seems that from six to twelve hours are sufficient (see page 444). An animal experiment (by Lépine and Douillet *) is worthy of mention, inasmuch as it shows that the constituents of the bile, which ordinarily enter the blood by way of the lymph-channels and the thoracic duct, can enter the hepatic veins directly in case the pressure within the bile-passages is suddenly increased.

It is true we do not know whether a spasm of the bile-passages lasting for several hours really occurs. We can concede, however, that such a thing is physiologically conceivable; so that we must agree that, hypothetically at least, icterus spasticus is possible. In many cases, in addition, the blood-pressure in the portal vein may be reduced, and in this manner a second factor be adduced that favors the entrance of bile into the blood.

A certain time, at all events, must elapse before a sufficient quantity of biliary constituents can enter the blood-serum, and after that a certain time must again elapse before the skin can become discolored. I am inclined to think that from three to four hours is the minimum time in which this can occur. We must seek another explanation for the cases of instantaneous jaundice that have been known to occur when persons were suddenly brought face to face with death, etc. In these cases either a slight degree of icterus existed at the time but was not noticeable until a sudden pallor of the skin occurred; or the skin of the patient was naturally yellow and the color did not appear until a sudden anemia supervened.

Those cases, too, in which from one to two days elapsed between the psychic disturbance and the appearance of jaundice can be explained in still a different manner. As a result of the fright a sudden stoppage of the functions of the stomach may occur with subsequent swelling of the mucous membrane. This would produce a simple catarrhal icterus. It is also conceivable that the psychic disturbance may lead to serious disturbances in the innervation and the peristalsis of the duodenum and the bile-passages, so that a paralysis of the sphincter of the ductus choledochus occurs, and in this manner some of the intestinal contents gains an entrance into the ducts and causes a bacterial infection of the bile-passages.

Chauffard: "*Archives générales de médecine*," 1890, ii, p. 410 (case 3, 1 hour).
Daraignez, J.: "Pathogénie de l'ictère emotif," Thèse de Paris, 1890.
Hardy: "De l'ictère émotionel," "Gazette des hôpitaux," 1882, No. 2.
Nagel: "Un cas d'ictère émotif, accompagné d'une éruption généralisée de lichen," "Progres méd.," 1886, No. 34, 14. Août.
Patoin: "Icterus from Emotions," "The Med. and Surg. Reporter," 1891, No. 114 ; "L'Union méd.," No. 70.
— "Ictère spasmodique immédiat," "Gazette des hôpitaux," No. 31, 1884.
Rendu: "Bulletin de la société clinique," p. 134, 1884 (¾ of an hour).

ICTERUS GRAVIDARUM.

Just as is the case with other individuals, pregnant women may become afflicted with simple, so-called catarrhal icterus. Toward the end of pregnancy an attack is favored by the pressure exercised on the lower surface of the liver by the enlarged uterus. In those cases where corset liver is present or where constipation with accumulation of fecal matter in the lower bowel exists the predisposition is still greater. As a rule, this simple form of icterus runs a benign course, in some instances not receding until after the child is born and the dislocation of the abdominal organs and

* "Thèse de Lyon," 1884.

the traction on the liver are corrected.   In rare cases the occurrence of
icterus during pregnancy causes the death of the fetus or a miscarriage.
[Benedict * has recently reported the cases of two sisters who had repeated
attacks of jaundice with enlargement of the liver synchronously with pregnancy and disappearing after abortion or premature delivery.—ED.]

In rare instances acute yellow atrophy of the liver may develop from
an apparently simple icterus.   A knowledge of this possibility should
induce us to be very guarded in our prognosis of icterus occurring during
pregnancy, and to treat such an attack with great care.

Frerichs: Loc. cit., I, p. 200.
Muller, P.: "Die Krankheiten des weiblichen Körpers," etc., Stuttgart, 1888, p. 119.
Spiegelberg: "Lehrbuch der Geburtshilfe," p. 246.

ICTERUS MENSTRUALIS.

Senator has described four cases of recurring icterus appearing immediately before or during menstruation.   As soon as the menstrual flow
became profuse the icterus disappeared.   In several of these attacks the
liver was found to be swollen, the feces to be decolorized, and the gastric
functions disturbed.   In the interim the general health was unimpaired.
Senator assumes that in these cases a hyperemic condition of the liver,
quite frequently observed during menstruation, was complicated by a
swelling of the mucous lining of the bile-passages.   According to Senator,
mild degrees of icterus are often seen during menstruation.

Frerichs † describes under the caption of "neuralgia of the liver"
a case in which for several years attacks of icterus accompanied by violent
pain and swelling of the liver immediately preceded menstruation.

Muller, P.: Loc. cit., p. 118.
Senator: "Berliner klin. Wochenschr.," 1872, No. 57.

ICTERUS EX INANITIONE (STARVATION JAUNDICE).

In cases of starvation lasting for a few days or for a longer period of
time (such as occurs in occlusion of the esophagus, or on refusal to take
food, etc.) a slight degree of icteric discoloration of the conjunctiva or of
the skin is occasionally observed.   Trendelenburg (quoted by Naunyn)
mentions one case of this kind in which he observed a slight reaction for
bile-pigment in the urine.

These cases are analogous to those that occur in dogs when they are
starved for experimental purposes; here also some bile-pigment is
usually found in the urine (see p. 445).   In both instances the peristaltic
action of the bile-passages is increased, and at the same time the blood-
pressure within the portal vein falls, so that absorption of bile is the
natural result.   In the case of human beings bilirubin, after absorption in
the liver, seems more easily to enter the tissues, whereas in the dog it is
more easily excreted in the urine.

Grimm ‡ reports the constant occurrence of urobilinuria in an opium-eater
who was on a restricted diet (milk and eggs).   Occasionally he would exhibit
a mild degree of icterus of the urine and of the skin.

It must be mentioned here that a great many persons, otherwise perfectly healthy, occasionally show a yellowish discoloration of the con-

* *Deutsche med. Woch.*, April 19, 1902.   † *Loc. cit.*, II, p. 528.
    ‡ *Virchow's Archiv*, 1893, vol. CXXXII, p. 265.

junctiva that can hardly be distinguished from a true icteric discoloration. These attacks may occur without causing any symptoms or they may be accompanied by a slight feeling of malaise. No definite statements in regard to the mode of origin and the significance of these attacks can be made.

ICTERUS SYPHILITICUS.

Aside from its occurrence as an accidental concomitant of syphilis, jaundice may be due to this infection and may originate in different ways. In the tertiary stage of the disease gummatous or diffuse hepatitis may lead to icterus (for examples of this form see Otto, *loc. cit.*). We are only interested in this place in that form of icterus seen in the earlier stages of syphilis which is called icterus syphiliticus and to which the prefix "precox" is occasionally added. This is a form of icterus from stasis and resembles simple catarrhal icterus as regards its duration, course, and degree. As a rule, too, it recedes in the same manner as does catarrhal icterus. Gubler (1854) was the first to call attention to the connection of this form of icterus with syphilis.

This form is not frequent in the secondary stage. Engel-Reimers states that it occurs in 1.4 % of all cases; later (according to Werner) in 0.3 % as studied in fifteen thousand cases of early syphilis. It seems that it occurs with varying frequency, as I observed six cases in four years, while in all the years before and after this period I saw only one other (see Otto, *loc. cit.*). Lasch has collected forty-six cases from the general literature and three of Neisser's. According to Fournier, syphilitic icterus is more frequent in women than in men. [Werner also found this preponderance in women.—ED.]

Jaundice appears usually with the first secondary symptoms on the skin and mucous membranes, sometimes not until a secondary exacerbation occurs. At the height of the disease the stools are, as a rule, but not in all instances, decolorized. Those cases of syphilis that are complicated by icterus usually run a severe course and develop serious secondary symptoms, usually with an initial rise of temperature and profuse eruptions in the skin and mucous membranes. In 80 % of the cases the lymph-glands are much swollen (Werner). Its duration varies, usually lasting, according to Werner, from three to four weeks. With appropriate and anti-syphilitic treatment the icterus usually disappears together with the other symptoms.

As catarrhal icterus is so frequently met with, it might be assumed that the combination of icterus and syphilis was a coincidence. The fact, however, that icterus is seen particularly during the stage of eruption speaks against the assumption that the simultaneous occurrence of the two conditions is a matter of chance. Further, the absence of the usual initial symptoms of simple catarrhal icterus (gastro-intestinal disturbances) and of the usual causative factors (errors in diet or taking cold) speaks distinctly against the identity of the form of icterus under discussion and catarrhal icterus. It is not surprising that the eruption of syphilis can bring about disturbances in the general health, and we know that stasis of bile produces similar disturbances. A leading argument in favor of the syphilitic origin of this icterus is the fact that it disappears under anti-syphilitic treatment, just as do all the other specific symptoms. In one case reported by Engel-Reimers icterus reappeared together with other symptoms of syphilis during a recurrent attack of the disease. In another case that I observed (Case 5 in Otto's series) ascites and swelling of the spleen developed simultaneously with icterus, all the symptoms disappearing again after a course of mercurial treatment had been instituted.

Sometimes acute yellow atrophy is seen to develop following the attack of icterus (Engel-Reimers, Senator, Neisser in Lasch's work). Engel-Reimers, in his three cases, observed a very considerable swelling of the lymph-glands in the region of the porta hepatis that is not, as a rule, seen in acute yellow atrophy.

Pathogenesis.—There can be no doubt that icterus syphiliticus is a form of obstructive jaundice.

A number of different explanations have been given for the occurrence of this stasis. The first theory, advanced by Rampold, was that it was due to the action of mercury. His position, however, is untenable, as this form of icterus is frequently seen before any treatment is instituted. Gubler assumed that the mucous membrane of the duodenum and of the bile-passages was swollen as a result of a specific involvement of these tissues, as is the case with the mucosa of the mouth, pharynx, and larynx; but such mucous lesions are never seen in the intestinal mucosa. Lanceraux's theory is much more probable. He assumes that the glands of the porta hepatis are swollen in the same manner as are so many other glands of the body, and that they occlude or compress the bile-duct from without. This idea is supported by the finding of Engel-Reimers reported above, and by my observation of the occurrence of ascites and enlargement of the spleen in one case, appearing and disappearing with the icterus. [In 41 out of Werner's 50 cases there was marked general glandular enlargement.—ED.] It is probable that in this condition the enlarged glands compress both the bile-duct and the portal vein, as they so often do in carcinomatous enlargement.

It can be readily understood why icterus syphiliticus is not seen more frequently when we consider that the same variation in regard to syphilitic enlargement probably exists in the case of the internal lymph-glands as of the external ones, and that, further, the anatomic relation of the portal lymph-glands to the bile-duct is different in different individuals.

Mauriac's theory must be regarded as altogether hypothetic. He states that an interstitial hepatitis, occurring at an exceptionally early stage of the disease, causes compression of the finer bile-ducts. Against the validity of this theory we can adduce the complete absence of anatomic foundation and the fact that the disease runs a short course in many instances, and, finally, that the stools are often completely colorless.

In addition to cases in which the syphilitic origin of the attack of jaundice is established beyond a doubt, there are many cases that are atypical and in which the mutual relations of the two diseases are not so distinct and definite. In cases where icterus appears alone and the symptoms of syphilis do not develop for some time, or, again, in cases in which icterus does not appear until after the disappearance of the secondary symptoms of syphilis, it is difficult to state whether they are independent or not. In the latter instance the icteric attack, in a way, takes the place of or is equivalent to a recurrence. Cases of this kind can be explained as well by the theory of mucous membrane involvement as by that of glandular swelling, because we often see glands and mucous membranes swollen as a result of constitutional lues some time before other localized manifestations of the disease appear. In all such doubtful cases it will be necessary carefully to consider the possibility of a non-syphilitic origin of the attack of icterus; and occasionally it will be impossible to arrive at a positive conclusion.

Bäumler; "Ziemssen's Handbuch der speciellen Pathologie," III, 1, p. 192.

Engel-Reimers: "Ueber acute gelbe Leberatrophie in der Frühperiode der Syphilis," "Jahrbuch der Hamburger Staatskrankenhäuser," I, 1889.

— "Ueber die visceralen Erkrankungen in der Frühperiode der Syphilis," "Monatshefte für praktische Dermatologie," XV, p. 478, 1892.

Gubler: "Mémoire sur l'ictère, qui accompagne quelques fois les éruptions syphilitiques précoces," "Mémoires de la société de Biologie," vol. V, p. 235, 1853.

Josef: "Ueber Icterus im Frühstadium der Syphilis," "Archiv für Dermatologie und Syphilis," vol. XXIX, 1894.

Lanceraux: "Traité historique et pratique de la Syphilis," II. édition, p. 146, 1866.

Lasch, O. (Neisser): "Icterus syphiliticus præcox," "Berliner klin. Wochenschr.," No. 40, p. 906, 1894 (3 cases). Mentions 49 cases from literature.

Otto, M.: "Ueber Icterus syphiliticus." Dissertation, Kiel, 1894 (7 cases, Quincke), Ref. in "Berliner klin. Wochenschr.," p. 1116, 1894.

Quincke: XII. Congress für innere Medicin, p. 180, 1893.

Senator: "Ueber Icterus und acute gelbe Leberatrophie bei Syphilis," ibid., p. 185.

Thümmel, K.: "Ueber Icterus in der Frühperiode der Syphilis." Dissertation, Berlin, 1894 (1 case, Senator).

Werner, S.: "Beitrag zur Pathologie des syphilitischen Icterus" (material of Engel-Reimers), "Münchener med. Wochenschr.," No. 27, 1897.

ICTERUS NEONATORUM.

The name icterus neonatorum is applied to a form of icterus that is very frequently seen in the new-born and that occurs independently of any other lesions and runs a favorable course.

This disease must not be confused (as it has been occasionally) with icterus occurring in the new-born and due to a variety of possible causes, such as septicemia or syphilis.

Jaundice is seen in about two-thirds of all new-born infants. Different investigators furnish various statistics (Cruse, 85%; Porak, 80%; Kehrer, 69%; Elsässer, 50%; Epstein, 42%; Seux, 16%). The disease is seen more frequently in boys than in girls, and occurs more often in small than in large children. It is frequently seen in the prematurely born, and also if the delivery was performed under chloroform (Hofmeier). It is more intense and more frequent in children whose skin is congested. The character of the food given has nothing to do with its occurrence.

It is probable that external conditions are in some way concerned in the appearance of the disease. Epstein states that it is rare in private families, whereas the statistics of different public institutions reveal varying degrees of frequency.

The icterus begins on the second or third day of life and, as is usual in adults, appears first on the face and the chest. The sclera becomes discolored later than in adults and becomes icteric only in the more severe cases. The yellow discoloration sometimes persists for a few days only, but as a rule remains visible until the middle of the second week, occasionally as long as the third and fourth weeks. Recurrence is rare. The general health and the functions of the infant seem to be undisturbed, although in very pronounced cases a little languor or sleepiness may be noticed. The urine is of a normal, light yellow color, but if it is very concentrated it may be a little darker and may contain a trace of albumin. This is more frequently seen in icteric than in other new-born children. Bile-pigment in solution is never seen;* but in the sediment bilirubin is

* Zweifel, Hofmeier; in exceptional cases, according to Cruse, *loc. cit.*

found within the desquamated renal cells either as a diffuse staining or in the form of yellowish granules or needle-shaped crystals. The stools have their ordinary golden yellow color. The pulse is not retarded. Hofmeier showed that in icteric children the initial decrease in weight is greater and the subsequent increase in weight is less than in normal infants. The excretion of urea and of uric acid is increased. These abnormalities are about in proportion to the intensity of the icterus. The prognosis as to life in infants with this form of icterus is the same as it is in normal babies.

The icterus gradually disappears spontaneously and requires no treatment other than a specially careful supervision of general hygiene.

Anatomic investigation reveals no typical changes that would explain the occurrence of this form of icterus. The liver, as in all new-born children, is very vascular, but not icteric. The bile within the gall-bladder is frequently thickened and contains much bile-pigment, but no obstruction is found in the bile-passages. Birch-Hirschfeld claims to have found an edematous swelling of the periportal connective tissue at the time of the development of the icterus. Orth states that there is constantly present an infarct of uric acid or of bilirubin in the medulla of the kidneys, most marked in the neighborhood of the apex of the papillæ. In addition, the latter author describes the finding at autopsy of numerous crystals of hematoidin and of bilirubin in the blood-clots of the heart and in all of the organs.

In the new-born obstructive icterus can of course also occur. Cases of this kind must, however, be distinguished from true cases of icterus neonatorum. Thus Virchow, and also Raudnitz, report cases of simple catarrhal icterus;* Kehrer describes a congenital narrowing of the common duct, and Birch-Hirschfeld reports the occurrence of congestive edema of the connective tissues surrounding the porta hepatis in cases of asphyxia following retarded labor. Pyemic icterus, too, is occasionally though rarely seen, but has nothing to do with icterus neonatorum [The occurrence of congenital narrowing or obliteration of the bile-ducts, especially described by Thomson, of Edinburgh, should here be mentioned as an additional and necessarily fatal cause of icterus in the new-born which should be held in mind as a cause of icterus not coming properly under the heading of icterus neonatorum.—Ed.]

Pathogenesis.—The frequency and the benign character of icterus neonatorum show that this condition is due to the great changes occurring in the child and its surroundings at birth, and that it may be almost regarded as a physiologic occurrence. As nearly all the functions of the body participate in this change, a great number of explanations of its occurrence have been offered.

The assumption that a stasis of bile produces this form of icterus is the least well founded of these, as the feces are never void of color. The occurrence of edema in the periportal connective tissue, as described by Birch-Hirschfeld, is not proved to be constant, although it is possible that now and then this condition may assist in the production of the icterus.

In view of this complete absence of all anatomic alterations in the bile-passages, icterus neonatorum was at one time looked upon as an example of jaundice of hematogenous origin. The yellow discoloration of the skin was genetically combined with the hyperemia of the skin present in the first days of life; but no proof could be adduced for the formation of the bile-pigment in the skin from extravasated blood (Zweifel) or imbibed blood-pigment (Porak). Hofmeier showed that soon after birth a great

* *Prager med. Wochenschr.*, 1884, No. 11.

many red blood-corpuscles were destroyed, and this discovery seemed to be a strong argument in favor of the hematogenous origin of this icterus, as was also the view that artificial plethora of the infant, produced by pressure on the placenta and a late ligation of the umbilical cord, intensified the icterus (Porak, Violet).* It is true that by these procedures the material for the formation of bile-pigment is increased, yet, here as in other forms of jaundice, we can assume that the conversion of blood into bile-pigment occurs in the liver alone, while the participation of this organ in the process is further demonstrated by the presence of bile-acids in the urine and in the pericardial fluid (Hofmeister, Halberstam and others).

Frerichs attempted to explain the origin of this icterus by circulatory disturbances in the liver, since the blood-pressure falls in the portal vein as soon as the blood no longer flows through the umbilical vein, and diffusion of the bile-constituents from the bile-capillaries into the capillaries of the portal vein could take place. It is true that this decrease in the portal pressure occurs, but it seems very probable that the differences in pressure would soon be equalized in the same manner as in ligation of vessels, where sudden changes in the blood-current are produced, but where the differences in the blood-pressure within the affected vessels are equalized within a few hours.

The theory, first pronounced by P. Franck, and later elaborated by the author, that icterus neonatorum is due to absorption of bile from the intestine has a surer foundation. Meconium contains much bile-pigment (according to Hoppe-Seyler, about 1 % in the meconium of a calf). As as soon as food is taken, both the secretion of bile and the absorptive powers of the intestinal mucosa are stimulated. In an adult the biliary constituents absorbed from the intestine are excreted in the bile after reaching the liver through the portal vein (intestinal hepatic circulation, see page 417); in the new-born, on the other hand, a part of the portal blood rich in biliary constituents flows directly into the vena cava by way of the ductus venosus Arantii, which remains patent for several days after birth. In this manner biliary constituents reach the general circulation and can produce icterus of the tissues.

The following additional factors must be considered: (1) The destruction of numerous red blood-corpuscles is followed in all probability by an increased formation of bile-pigment in the liver; (2) the formation of urobilin in the intestine as a result of bacterial action occurs in adults but is absent in the new-born; and is slight until after the end of the first week. We see, therefore, that a number of factors combine to increase the amount of bilirubin in the intestine and its absorption into the general circulation.

Another important factor is the difficulty with which the urine of a new-born child dissolves bile-pigments. As a result of this, the vicarious excertion by way of the kidneys is decreased. The observation of Orth, mentioned above, that crystals of bilirubin are found in the blood and tistues of the new-born shows, further, that the power of the tissue-fluids in general to dissolve bilirubin is less than it is in the adult. This factor, too, must therefore be considered favorable to the origin and the continuation of icterus neonatorum.

Orth and Neumann found that bilirubin also crystallizes from the blood in non-icteric new-born infants. Neumann, in particular, saw such crystals in the

* A. Schmidt, on the contrary, found the icterus more frequent and obstinate in children after immediate ligation of the cord.

fat-cells of the mesentery. This finding of Orth and Neumann must be interpreted to signify that probably in all new-born infants a certain amount of bile-pigment is found in all the tissues and in the general circulation, but that in only a few cases are sufficient quantities present to cause icterus.

Many authors conclude from the microscopic examination of the blood that red blood-corpuscles are simultaneously both destroyed and formed (Hayem, Hofmeier, Silbermann). Knöpfelmacher, it is true, could not verify these statements, nor did he discover any changes in the isotonia of the red blood-corpuscles. It is said that the red blood-corpuscles, when they are destroyed, furnish the material for the formation of abnormal bile-pigments. Silbermann assumes that, in addition, as a result of the destruction of red corpuscles, "fermentemia" with stasis and thrombosis supervenes in the portal capillaries, and that in this manner some of the intra- and inter-lobular bile-passages are occluded and obstructive jaundice results.

Rosenberg found droplets of fat on the epithelial cells of the gall-bladder in cats, dogs, mice, and rabbits, after feeding these animals with fat or after subjecting them to a long fast. He assumes that these droplets prevent the absorption of the bile from the gall-bladder. As in the new-born no fat is found on the gall-bladder epithelium before the first food is ingested, he assumes that this leads to absorption of bile and icterus. (Why not then also in the fetus?—Q.)

In the new-born two other diseases are seen that are accompanied by icterus—acute fatty degeneration and the epidemic form of hemoglobinuria described by Winckel.* It is possible that these diseases are in some way related to simple icterus neonatorum in the sense that the processes that lead to the "physiologic" form of icterus (icterus neonatorum) in a measure predispose to certain noxious agencies and prepare the ground for the other diseases and determine the characteristic features of these diseases.

v. Birch-Hirschfeld: "Virchow's Archiv," vol. LXXXVII, p. 1, 1882.
Cnopf: "Münchener med. Wochenschr.," p. 283.
Cruse, P.: "Archiv für Kinderheilkunde," 1880, I, p. 353.
Epstein. A.: "Ueber die Gelbsucht der Neugeborenen," "Volkmann's Sammlung klin. Vortráge," No. 180, 1880.
Frank, P.: "De curandis hominum morbis epitome," Tübingen, 1811, vol. VI, part 3, p. 333.
Halberstam: Dissertation, Dorpat, 1885.
Hofmeier, M.: "Virchow's Archiv," vol. LXXXIX, p. 493, 1882.
— "Zeitschrift für Geburtshilfe und Gynäkologie," vol. VIII, 1882.
Kehrer: "Oesterreichisches Jahrbuch für Padiatrik," 1861.
Knöpfelmacher, W.: "Das Verhalten der Blutkörper beim Neugeborenen," "Wiener klin. Wochenschr.," 1896, p. 976.
Neumann, E.: "Virchow's Archiv," vol. CXIV, p. 394, 1888.
Orth, J.: "Ueber das Vorkommen von Bilirubinkrystallen bei Neugeborenen," "Virchow's Archiv," vol. LXIII, p. 447, 1875.
Porak: "Revue mensuelle de médecine," 1878.
Quincke, H.: "Virchow's Archiv," vol. XCV, 1884.
— "Archiv für experimentelle Pathologie," vol. XIX, 1885.
Quisling, A.: "Archiv für Kinderheilkunde," vol. XVII, 1893.
Rosenberg, S.: "Ueber den intermediären Kreislauf des Fettes durch die Leber und seine Beziehungen zum Icterus neonatorum," "Virchow's Archiv," vol. CXXIII, p. 17, 1891.
Runge, M.: "Krankheiten der ersten Lebenstage," p. 216, 1893.
Schiff, E.: "Archiv für Kinderheilkunde," vol. XV, p. 191, 1893.
Schmidt, A.: "Archiv für Gynäkologie," vol. XLV, p. 283, 1894.
Schreiber, E.: "Berliner klin. Wochenschr.," No. XXV, 1895.
Silbermann, O.: "Archiv für Kinderheilkunde," vol. VIII (copious bibliography), 1887.
Stadelmann: Loc. cit., p. 220.
Violet: "Virchow's Archiv," vol. LXXX, p. 353, 1880.
Zweifel, P.: "Archiv für Gynäkologie," vol. XII.

* See also Baginski, "Lehrbuch der Kinderkrankheiten," 1892, pp. 59 and 61.

ICTERUS POLÝCHOLICUS.

The assumption that icterus can be produced by an excessive formation of bile is based on those cases of icterus in which, in addition to the yellow discoloration of the skin, the feces are not only not colorless, but, on the contrary, are more intensely stained with bile-pigments (urobilin), or in which profuse bile-colored diarrhœas are seen. The absorption of bile-pigment formed in excessive quantities could occur either in the intestine or directly in the liver. Certain experiments by Naunyn speak in favor of an absorption from the intestine. This investigator, after injecting 20 c.c. of pig's bile (or 0.1 of bilirubin) into the small intestine of a rabbit, found bile-pigment in the urine; but no icteric discoloration of the tissues was seen, probably owing to the short time during which an excess of bile-pigment was present.

An excess of bile might possibly be absorbed directly in the liver, because it might not be able to flow through the bile-ducts as rapidly as necessary. In fact, Stadelmann and others have demonstrated that bile containing a great deal of bile-pigment is viscous, as is seen after the injection of hemoglobin or of hemolytic poisons (toluylenediamin, arseniuretted hydrogen), whereby pleiochromia (an increase of pigment) is produced. As this bile is viscid and cannot be poured out as readily as normal bile, a relative degree of stasis is produced within the bile-passages, and, as a result, a jaundice from reabsorption of bile occurs. In this manner it is demonstrated experimentally that icterus polycholicus exists, caused by pleiochromia and the resulting viscidity of the bile. Grawitz* assumes that the icterus seen in certain cardiac lesions is due to polycholia, because, in this condition he found free hemoglobin in the blood-serum.

The only manner in which this question could be settled clinically would be by determining the quantity of bile-pigment or of urobilin excreted in the feces and the urine. G. Hoppe-Seyler attempted to do this in that form of icterus that occurs after the injection of tuberculin. This icterus is accompanied by an enlargement of the liver and of the gall-bladder. Normally 0.123 of urobilin is excreted in the urine, 1.7 in the feces. In the cases examined these figures rose to 0.89 and 4.7. G. Hoppe-Seyler further examined cases of icterus in exophthalmic goiter and in pneumonia (*loc. cit.*, p. 42) and found an increased excretion of urobilin, from which he concludes that the icterus seen in these cases is due to polycholia.

We are not justified in assuming from the dark color of the feces alone that we are dealing with a case of icterus from polycholia, as has been done by a number of authors—for example, Chauffard and Banti. At best, this is an assumption that is not based on solid grounds. Chauffard and others after him (for example, Girode) assumed that, particularly in icterus due to infections, the liver-cells are stimulated to increased activity by certain intestinal ptomains and other toxins, and that the bile-passages are unable to eliminate the excessive amount of bile. As opposing this idea we can only emphasize the fact that a considerable degree of partial stasis of bile can exist without causing a lighter color of the feces, and that normally the intensity of the color of the feces may vary within wide boundaries.

In many of those cases of icterus that are said to be due to polycholia we can venture an explanation on the basis of the hypothesis that diapede-

* *Deutsches Archiv für klin. Medicin*, vol. LIV, p. 611.

sis of bile occurs directly into the blood as a result of the disturbed function of the liver-cells (Minkowski, Liebermeister).

We shall have to recur to this icterus polycholicus, or, better, pleiochromicus, in subsequent sections.

Hoppe-Seyler, G.: "Ueber die Einwirkung des Tuberkulins auf die Gallenfarbstoffbildung," "Virchow's Archiv," 1892, vol. cxxviii, p. 43.
— "Ueber die Ausscheidung des Urobilins in Krankheiten," "Virchow's Archiv," 1891, vol. cxxiv, p. 42.
Naunyn: "Beiträge zur Lehre vom Icterus," Reichert and du Bois-Reymond's "Archiv," 1868, p. 432; 1869, p. 579.
Stadelmann: "Der Icterus," 1891, p. 242.

ICTERUS AFTER EXTRAVASATION OF BLOOD.

Icterus is frequently observed after large extravasations of blood. Although authors are sometimes guilty of careless interpretations of the causal connection between icterus and blood-extravasations, and have in some instances (Poncet, for example) failed to exclude the possibility of icterus neonatorum or of lesions of the liver, still we can hardly doubt that icterus may occur as a result of hemorrhage. Of course, the yellow color seen in the skin over hemorrhagic foci is not included under this caption.

Icterus following extravasation of blood has so far only been observed in man. It has been seen to occur after large traumatic or scorbutic hemorrhages occurring in the cellular tissues or into the body-cavities, as well as after spontaneous hemorrhages into the peritoneal cavity in lesions of the female sexual apparatus.

Icterus of the skin and of the conjunctivæ appears several days (three to eight, according to Dick, eight according to Poncet) after the hemorrhage and is very rarely intense. As a rule, it disappears after a few days or weeks. Urobilinuria is present at the same time, usually beginning a short time before the icterus becomes visible. The discoloration of the urine is frequently perceptible to the naked eye from the very beginning. Hoppe-Seyler made a quantitative determination of the urobilin in a case of hemorrhage into the uterine cavity and found it increased. Unchanged bile-pigment is rarely found in this form of icterus.

As both crystals of hematoidin (Langhans, Quincke) and a biliary imbibition of the connective tissues are seen after extravasation of blood, it might be assumed that all the bile-pigment that is found in different parts of the body might have been formed at the place where the extravasation of blood occurred. This, however, is not the case, for the bile-pigment formed here is generated much too slowly, and is not absorbed with sufficient rapidity to account for the general discoloration. Whatever bile-pigment is formed within the blood extravasation seems to have a tendency to adhere to the tissues in its immediate vicinity. The explanation of the process is that within the extravasation hemoglobin is liberated from the red blood-corpuscles and enters the circulation, and that on reaching the liver this blood-pigment is converted into bile-pigment, so that we are here dealing with an icterus pleiochromicus.

In hemorrhages of small extent no icterus of the skin is seen, but only urobilinuria. It is not decided whether all the urobilin is formed by the liver or whether a part is formed at the place of extravasation. An observation by D. Gerhardt seems to speak in favor of the latter supposition, inasmuch as he found that in icterus with occlusion of the bile-ducts extravasations of blood may lead to urobilinuria.

Different authors have at times emphasized the significance of uro-bilinuria in the diagnosis of blood extravasations not discoverable by other means. In view of the many interpretations that are possible for the appearance of urobilin in the urine such a connection must be carefully criticized before it is accepted (compare also Mandry).

In animals no one has so far positively demonstrated the occurrence of icterus or of urobilinuria following extravasation or injections of blood (Angerer, Quincke, and others). We are, therefore, not so fortunate as to possess an adequate and satisfactory explanation or experimental evidence of the conditions under which the formation of the substances under discussion occurs (compare pages 445 *et seq.*).

Angerer, O.: "Klinische und experimentelle Untersuchungen über die Resorption von Blutextravasaten," Würzburg, 1879.
Dick, R.: "Ueber den diagnostischen Werth der Urobilinurie für die Gnyäkologie," "Archiv für Gynäkologie," Bd. xxiii. Also Mandry, ibid., 1894, vol. xlv, p. 446.
v. Jacksch: "Zeitschr. für Heilkunde," p. 49 (icterus in scurvy), 1895.
Kunkel, A.: "Ueber das Auftreten verschiedener Farbstoffe im Harn," "Virchow's Archiv," 1880, vol. lxxix, p. 455.
Poncet, A.: "De l'ictère hématique traumatique." Thèse de Paris, 1874.
Quincke, H.: "Beiträge zur Lehre von Icterus," "Virchow's Archiv," vol. xcv, 1884. "Zur Physiologie und Pathologie des Blutes," "Deutsches Archiv für klin. Medicin," 1883, vol. xxxiii, p. 31.
Stadelmann: "Der Icterus," 1891, p. 242.

ICTERUS AFTER HEMOGLOBINEMIA.

The destruction of red blood-corpuscles within the blood-current is followed by the same results as the extravasation of blood. This is due either to a disintegration of red corpuscles or to the formation of "shadows" whereby the hemoglobin is dissolved and enters the blood-current. The most striking effects are seen in paroxysmal hemoglobinuria, in which, as a result of malaria, syphilis, or some other unknown predisposing factor, cold or excessive physical exertion brings on an attack. The attack begins with fever and usually produces hemoglobinuria, swelling of the spleen, and icterus of the skin. The urine, too, may contain bile-pigment but is always free from bile-acids.* In cases of this kind we must consider, in addition to the hemoglobin that produces the polycholia, the mechanical effect exercised by the stromata of the red blood-corpuscles, and possibly the toxic action of these and of other substances. In the kidneys this effect is particularly manifested by acute inflammation, a decrease in the quantity of urine voided, and the appearance of albumin and of casts.

The experiments of Schurig and v. Starck demonstrate that the large quantity of hemoglobin circulating in the blood is not alone responsible for the appearance of icterus. These investigators repeatedly injected large doses of hemoglobin into dogs and rabbits, and yet never witnessed the occurrence of icterus.

It appears that that form of icterus first described by Winckel in the new-born, and representing an epidemic form of hemoglobinuria with icterus, is due to some infectious agency of unknown origin. This disease is seen in children that are otherwise healthy. It appears at about the fourth day of life, beginning with cyanosis and followed by icterus and an acceleration of the pulse and of the respiration. The skin is cool and a very scanty amount of thick dark blood can be made to ooze from an inci-

* Leube, "Sitzungsbericht der physiologisch-medicinischen Gesellschaft zu Würzburg," 1886.

sion. Occasionally vomiting and diarrhea are seen. The urine contains hemoglobin, albumin, granular casts, and blood-corpuscles. The disease usually terminates fatally, in convulsions, at the expiration of from nine hours to two days. On autopsy, punctiform hemorrhages are seen throughout the internal organs. In addition, swelling of the spleen and fatty degeneration of the liver, heart, and kidneys are found. In the latter respect the disease corresponds to the picture of acute fatty degeneration described by Buhl. Icterus in this case is due in part, as in paroxysmal hemoglobinuria, to pleiochromia of the bile, in part to acute lesions of the parenchyma of the liver.

v. Birch-Hirschfeld: Loc. cit., p. 702.
Runge, M.: "Krankheiten der ersten Lebenstage," 1893, p. 172.
Hoffmann, F. A.: "Constitutionskrankheiten," 1893, p. 165.
Ponfick: "Ueber Hämoglobinämie und ihre Folgen," "Berliner klin. Wochenschr.," 1883, p. 389.
Schurig: "Ueber die Schicksale des Hämoglobins im Thierkörper," "Archiv für experimentelle Pathologie," vol. xxxix, 1898.
v. Starck: "Ueber Hämoglobininjectionen," "Münchner med. Wochenschr.," 1898, Nos. 3 and 4.
Winckel: "Deutsche med. Wochenschr.," 1879, Nos. 24–36.

ICTERUS TOXICUS.

Icterus is found in a number of intoxications. In the case of those poisons that produce a dissolution of red blood-corpuscles and hemoglobinemia the occurrence of icterus is readily understood. These forms of toxic icterus are closely related to the forms discussed above.

Among the poisons that can produce hemolysis are arseniuretted hydrogen and two mushroom poisons—helvellic acid from the truffle, and phallin, a toxic proteid substance from *Agaricus phalloides*. Occasionally cases of poisoning with the two latter substances have been studied in human beings. Experimental investigations have been made with toluylenediamin, glycerin, the bile-acids, and saponin substances. In addition to causing the separation of hemoglobin, some of these bodies, particularly toluylenediamin and phallin, cause destruction of red blood-corpuscles (rhestocytemia).

Another class of poisons, in addition to exercising the above effect on the red blood-corpuscles, act directly on hemoglobin and convert it within the corpuscles into methemoglobin. Among these poisons are the chlorates, pyrogallol, anilin and its derivatives (antifebrin, lactophenin, etc.), nitrobenzol, nitroglycerin, and the nitrites. In addition to these substances, which occasionally produce poisoning in man, there are a number of other substances that have only been investigated experimentally but are known to exercise a similar effect.

The results of the changes in the blood are the same in the case of poisoning with these drugs as in paroxysmal hemoglobinuria. The liberation of large quantities of hemoglobin causes pleiochromia and thickening of the bile (polycholia), which in its turn leads to obstructive icterus. These results have been made the object of careful experimental investigation in the case of arseniuretted hydrogen and of toluylenediamin (Stadelmann and Affanassiew). It is probable that each of these substances acts somewhat differently in regard to the injury they do to the red blood-corpuscles; while also it is very probable that they exercise individually different effects on certain organs, such as the liver and the kidneys. Whereas, therefore, the primary intoxication is the same in the case of all these substances, the general clinical picture presented varies considerably. Especially has it been observed that the frequency and the intensity of the icterus are not proportionate to the hemoglobinuria. The principal effect of all is not to be sought in their action on the blood. The toxic action of the different poisons varies qualitatively and in regard to its significance.

After the administration of toluylenediamin, fatty degeneration and interstitial proliferation are found in the liver. These pathologic changes, in addition to the polycholia, probably lead to icterus. The urine is diminished in quantity and contains casts of brown granular masses and epithelial debris, hemoglobin, methemoglobin, and bile-pigment. The spleen is enlarged owing to the destruction of red blood-corpuscles taking place within this organ, the leucocytes gathering up the fragments of the erythrocytes and accumulating in the spleen. If the blood in such a case is examined at the right time, it will be found to contain the shadows and fragments of red blood-corpuscles described above, and, on centrifuging, it will be seen that the serum is tinged red by the hemoglobin in solution.

The icteric discoloration of the skin and the conjunctivæ in these intoxications does not appear until the second day or later, and is frequently modified by cyanosis and by congestion of the face and the peripheral parts of the body. After poisoning with the second group the brown color imparted to the tissues by methemoglobin (from the red blood-corpuscles and the serum) still further obscures the icteric color. We see, therefore, that the shade, the intensity, and the duration of icterus may vary greatly in these cases according to the severity of the case and the character of the poison.

The entrance of dissolved hemoglobin into the liver-cells and its subsequent elaboration into bile-pigment is readily understood, but it is not entirely clear whether, and if so how, the fragments of red blood-corpuscles can be transformed by the liver-cells. According to the view of Affanassiew, which can hardly be accepted, icterus occurs more particularly in fragmentation of red blood-corpuscles (rhestocytemia) and not at all in true hemoglobinemia.

Affanassiew was enabled, further, to produce similar symptoms of intoxication by injecting into an animal its own blood changed by heat, so that blood heated to 53° C. (127.4° F.) chiefly destroyed the red blood-corpuscles, while after using blood heated to 56° or 57° C. (130.8° or 135.6° F.) a solution of the hemoglobin in the serum was produced. In extensive burns methemoglobinuria without icterus has been observed in human subjects.

It is possible that the form of icterus occasionally seen in pernicious anemia is toxic in character and is caused by a poison having hemolytic properties.

Lactophenin is ranked among the hemolytic substances. Strauss, however, who observed icterus with colorless stools in three patients who had taken 4.0 gm. daily for from nine to twenty-one days, states that this icterus is the result of a gastro-intestinal catarrh.

In the case of some of the poisons to be spoken of below, and which are accompanied by jaundice, the cause of this symptom is attributed with more or less reason to a destruction of the red blood-corpuscles.

In many of the older reports the administration of ether, chloroform, and chloral hydrate was said to be followed by icterus. I fail to find recent statements in regard to this in the literature. No very definite reports seem to have been made of late, and I personally have made no observations in this direction.

As ether, in the same manner as the bile-acid salts, is capable of dissolving hemoglobin from red blood-corpuscles, it would not surprise us if this substance had

32

the power ascribed to it of producing icterus. Naunyn injected ether subcutaneously into rabbits (1.0 and more) and found bile-pigment in the urine in one-fourth of the cases. If the ether was injected into the small intestine, bile-pigment was constantly found in the urine, for the reason, probably, that the hemoglobin was dissolved within the portal vein and in this manner was carried directly into the liver.

Geill reports a patient of fifty-eight years who took 2.0 grams of chloral hydrate on twenty-five successive days. At the expiration of this time an exanthem due to chloral appeared, on the third day thereafter icterus developed, and on the fourth day death occurred. The liver was enlarged owing to passive congestion and was strewn with a large number of stained areas varying in size from that of a lentil to that of a pea. The cells of the liver in the center of the lobules were comparatively well preserved, but elsewhere the cells were in a state of granular degeneration, contained pigment, and had no nucleus.

The administration of carbolic acid by the mouth does not seem to be followed by icterus. The latter has only been observed in three cases where carbolic acid was injected into the umbilical region of new-born infants or was applied to an abscess in the pelvic region. It is possible that in these instances a direct action on the liver was produced by way of the portal vein.

Icterus has occasionally been seen after a course of treatment for the expulsion of a tapeworm with extract of filix mas. It seems to have been particularly frequent when oil was administered at the same time, because this promoted the absorption of the poisonous filicic acid. Grawitz assumes that in these cases a solution of the hemoglobin occurs within the liver with resulting polycholia, and possibly there is also a direct toxic effect exercised on the liver-cells themselves.

In poisoning with santonin icterus has frequently been seen. Here, too, the chief effect may be exercised on the blood, as Jaffe saw hematuria in dogs following the use of the drug and Cramer observed in one human case fever and swelling of the spleen.

We will discuss phosphorus-poisoning, which leads to icterus and a considerable swelling of the liver, in another section. In this place we will only mention that Stadelmann in his experiments observed an increased excretion of bile-pigment occurring in the same way but more slowly than after toluylenediamin-poisoning; *i. e.*, after about ten hours. In the beginning a simple irritation of the liver-cells occurs, leading to pleiochromia. Later the increase in size of the liver-cells, interstitial proliferation, and catarrh of the bile-passages constitute additional obstacles to the flow of bile. It is possible that in these cases parapedesis of bile (Minkowski, Liebermeister) plays a certain rôle.

Icterus of a very mild degree is often seen in lead colic. Usually it is attributed to catarrhal conditions of the bile-passages, but it is not impossible that in this form of intoxication tonic spasms of the bile-ducts occur or that a direct toxic effect is exercised on the hepatic parenchyma.

Freyhan mentions a form of icterus observed in workmen engaged in the manufacture of storage batteries. He considers it toxic, but in his report does not distinctly state whether he attributes it to lead intoxication or not.

Icterus frequently appears with great rapidity after snake-bite, and it is said that it occurs in cases of this intoxication having a chronic course. Its mode of origin in this condition is altogether unknown.

The icterus seen after injections of tuberculin must be included among the toxic varieties. Hoppe-Seyler has shown that this icterus is accompanied by an increase of urobilin in the feces and urine, so that we may assume that it is caused by a polycholia resulting from destruction of red blood-corpuscles (see page 493).

LITERATURE.

ARSENIURETTED HYDROGEN.

Kobert: "Intoxicationen," p. 471.
Stadelmann: "*Archiv für experimentelle Pathologie,*" vol. xvi, p. 220, 1882.
— "Der Icterus," p. 193, 1891.

PHALLIN.   HELVELLIC ACID.

Kobert: Loc. cit., pp. 60, 457.

TOLUYLENEDIAMIN.

Affanassiew: "Zeitschr. für klin. Medicin," vol. vi, p. 318, 1883.
Hunter, W.: "The Action of Toluylenediamin: A Contribution to the Pathology of
    Jaundice," "Journal of Pathology and Bacteriology," iii, 1895.
Auld, A. G.: "The Experimental Evidence of Hæmatogenous Jaundice," "Brit.
    Med. Jour.," January, 1896.
Pick: "Zur Kenntniss des Toluylenediamin-Icterus," "Wiener klin. Wochenschr.,"
    1892.
Stadelmann: "Der Icterus," p. 117, "Archiv für experimentelle Pathologie," vol.
    xiv, p. 231, 1881; vol. xvi, p. 118, 1883; vol. xxiii, p. 427, 1887.

CHLORAL HYDRATE.

Arndt: "Archiv für Psychiatrie und Nervenkrankheiten," vol. iii, p. 673, 1872.
Geill: "Vierteljahrsschr. für gerichtliche Medicin," vol. xiv, p. 274, 1897.
Pelmann: "Irrenfreund," 1871, No. 2.
Wernich: "Deutsches Archiv für klin. Medicin," xii, 1874, p. 32.

CARBOLIC ACID.

Geill, Chr.: "Vierteljahrsschr. für gerichtliche Medicin," vol. xiv, 1897, p. 282.

ETHER.

Naunyn: "Reichert und Bois-Reymond's Archiv," 1868, p. 438.
Kappeler: "Anaesthetica" in Billroth-Lücke "Deutsche Chirurgie," part 20, pp. 57
    and 60, 1880.

PHOSPHORUS.

Stadelmann: "Archiv für experimentelle Pathologie," vol. xxiv, p. 270, 1888.
— "Der Icterus," p. 176, 1891.

LACTOPHENIN.

Strauss, H.: "Therapeutische Monatshefte," 1895, p. 469.
Wenzel: "Icterus nach Lactophenin," "Centralblatt für innere Medicin," xvii, 1896.
Witthauer: "Therapeutische Monatshefte," 1898, No. 2.

ANILIN.

Dehio: "Berliner klin. Wochenschr.," 1888, p. 11.

SNAKE-BITE.

Frerichs: Loc. cit., p. 167.
Kobert: Loc. cit., p. 335.

SANTONIN.

Kobert: Loc. cit., p. 633.
Cramer, H.: "Deustche med. Wochenschr.," vol. xv, 1889.

EXTRACT OF FILIX MAS.

Freyhan: "Berliner klin. Wochenschr.," 1896, p. 263.
Grawitz: "Berliner klin. Wochenschr.," 1894.

ICTERUS IN INFECTIOUS DISEASES.

Acute infectious diseases may be accompanied by other lesions causing icterus which may either have existed, possibly latent, before the infection (cirrhosis, cholelithiasis) or which may complicate the disease after it has begun to run its course (catarrhal icterus, acute yellow atrophy). Aside from these instances, we see icterus so frequently in some of the infectious diseases that we cannot consider its occurrence as an accidental complication. It is seen, moreover, more frequently in some infectious diseases than in others, so that we are forced to assume some close connection between icterus and the specific disease that it complicates. Among the diseases that are most often accompanied by icterus we may mention yellow fever, recurrent fever, Griesinger's type of bilious typhoid, pyemia, and pneumonia. In all these diseases the stools remain colored, so that the obstacle to the outflow of the bile is only a relative one, and can, as a rule, not be demonstrated at all. The appearance of icterus in these cases has been attributed to an occlusion of the smaller bile-passages by catarrhal inflammation of the ducts or catarrhal swelling of the hepatic cells. It is possible that here, too, we are dealing with pleiochromia or parapedesis of bile as a result of functional disturbances of the liver-cells.

This effect can either be exercised by the bacteria themselves or by the toxins leaborated either in the intestine or in other organs situated in parts of the body remote from the liver. Tuberculin is such a bacterial toxin, as it produces icterus even when injected in remote parts of the body. It is true, however, that in the clinical course of tuberculosis such an effect is never observed.

Recurrent fever is frequently accompanied by icterus, in some epidemics one-fourth of all the cases developing it. Griesinger observed bilious typhoid or typhus biliosus in Cairo, and characterized it as an atypical form of recurrent fever. According to the observations of Kartulis in Alexandria and of Diamantopulos in Smyrna, however, this disease is different from recurrent fever both in regard to its general course and in regard to the absence of the typical and specific spirilla. Some authors, among them Fiedler, are inclined to classify this bilious typhoid with the form of infectious icterus described by Weil.

Icterus is quite frequently seen in typhoid fever. In the first weeks of the disease it has usually been attributed to a catarrhal swelling of the bile-passages and is of subordinate importance. It is possible, at the same time, that even this initial icterus may be due to bacterial infection. In that form of icterus seen in the second half of the disease it is still more probable that the specific microbe plays a rôle, as this icterus is very much more severe and may even lead to the death of the patient.

In acute croupous pneumonia slight degrees of icterus are not infrequently seen, and in some epidemics this complication is quite common. These cases of pneumonia, designated as "bilious," seem to run a more severe course at certain times than at others, although at the same time the fact that they are complicated with icterus does not make the prognosis less favorable. On account of the gastric symptoms so pronounced in pneumonia, this icterus has been attributed to catarrhal conditions; while other authors (Gerhardt) have attempted to connect this icterus with the hemorrhagic character of the pneumonic exudate and to draw an analogy with the appearance of icterus in other forms of hemorrhagic extravasation.

In septicemia icterus is quite frequently seen. As a rule, it appears as a faint yellowish tinge, and rarely as a more intense discoloration. It is seen after septicemia following external wounds, after puerperal sepsis, after sepsis following lesions of mucous membranes, in that form arising from the endocardium, which is designated as endogenous and which, in case no distinct origin can be found during life, is called cryptogenetic septicemia. While it is true that icterus may be absent in many cases of septicemia, at the same time its appearance is a diagnostic sign of considerable value, particularly if a differential diagnosis has to be made between septicemia and certain infectious diseases.

The form of icterus occasionally seen in revaccination and called icterus epidemicus (see below) is in no way related to vaccinia itself. It must be regarded as a complication that occurs from unknown causes.

LITERATURE.

TYPHUS.

Griesinger: "Virchow's Specielle Pathologie," vol. II, 22d Ed., p. 203, 1864.
Liebermeister: "Ziemssen's Handbuch der speciellen Pathologie," vol. II, 1st and 2d Ed., p. 168, 1876.
Pal: "Wiener klin. Wochenschr.," 1894.

BILIOUS TYPHOID.

Diamantopulos: "Ueber den Typhus icterodes in Smyrna" (cited by Kartulis).
Kartulis: "Deutsche med. Wochenschr.," 1888, Nos. 4 and 5.
Karlinski: "Icterus bei Recurrens," "Fortschritte der Medicin," 1891, p. 456.
Becker: (Case following general diphtheritic infection.) "Berliner klin. Wochenschr.," 1880, p. 447.

ICTERUS EPIDEMICUS.

The appearance of icterus in many persons at the same time is well known to the laity. As such an occurrence is so striking that it could hardly be overlooked, we have descriptions of this epidemic form dating from the beginning of the eighteenth century. Hennig has collated over 86 large and small epidemics from the literature. Among these only 8 extended over large areas, and these were found particularly near the seashore. The majority of these epidemics are circumscribed in extent and attack only single families or certain communities, such as one house, barracks, prison, or boarding-house. Only 5 epidemics lasted for a considerable period of time—seven to thirteen months. In three epidemics the disease attacked children alone or at least to a great extent.

Of the epidemics recorded, 26 occurred among soldiers, 6 among soldiers and civilians, the rest among civilians alone. The epidemics that occurred among the soldiers are more reliable in regard to statistical investigations, and consequently merit particular attention. In some instances such epidemics assumed remarkable dimensions. For example, during the first year of the Civil War in the United States 10,929 cases of jaundice were observed with 40 deaths; in the Franco-Prussian war 2.4% of the men of the First Bavarian Division were afflicted from February to May. As a general rule, recently enlisted soldiers were more liable to attack than were the more seasoned men.

The course of the disease is, in general, benign. It resembles the simple, afebrile, catarrhal form of icterus, and the symptoms, aside from the yellow discoloration, are frequently very slight. In other epidemics, again, the course is similar to that form of infectious icterus known as Weil's disease. Damsch claims to have seen cataleptic rigidity, particularly in the epidemic form of icterus that occurs in children, and states that it is more frequent in this than in the sporadic form.

In only 7 of the epidemics mentioned was the disease severe and accompanied by many deaths. It appears that in pregnant women and women in the lying-in period the prognosis is grave.

The causes of epidemic icterus are manifold. Among them may be mentioned damp weather, particularly if, as in the case of soldiers, individuals are forced to wear wet clothes for a long time. The great majority of the 86 epidemics mentioned occurred in the winter and fall. Fröhlich found that in the epidemics among soldiers the spring months seemed to be the most dangerous.

The following factors may be named as further predisposing causes: errors in diet, poor or inappropriate food, a monotonous diet, bad drinking-water or the swallowing of impure river-water during bathing, and the breathing of polluted air (as in trenches containing stagnant water, from bad drains or defective foundations). In camping on moist, dirty soil several of these noxious influences may be combined.

The appearance of icterus after revaccination is very peculiar. This was observed in an epidemic that occurred in Bremen (Lurmann, Pletzer), in which over 200 workmen of a manufacturing establishment out of a total of 1500 men became afflicted with icterus in the course of four months. The limits of the incubation period were from a few days to several months. A transmission by contagion was never seen.

It is possible, therefore, to divide the predisposing factors into three groups: (1) Atmospheric, telluric, or climatic causes; (2) dietetic influences; (3) infectious causes.

It is probable that a combination of all these factors often is present, and that, for example, the first two may predispose the patient to the influence of the third. We can hardly say that infection always plays a rôle, for many of the cases present the picture of a simple catarrhal icterus that is altogether benign in character. Thus, a single company among the soldiery of a large barracks were afflicted with this simple form of icterus upon receiving a very monotonous diet, while in another company icterus appeared after these men had been ordered to take a daily bath in the river immediately after eating. In these two instances the disease disappeared as soon as the conditions mentioned were changed.

In those cases, of course, where the external conditions are such that it seems possible for bacteria to develop, it is quite probable that microbic influences play an important part in the production of icterus. Such favoring conditions are, for example, the breathing of bad air or the drinking of polluted water. The bacteria, if they enter the intestine, probably in many cases penetrate the bile-ducts and cause an inflammatory reaction leading to icterus. There is the possibility, further, that all the symptoms are produced by intoxication with the ptomains elaborated by the bacteria in the intestine and absorbed. In fact, the benign course of this icterus make the latter assumption very probable. In those cases where the breathing of polluted air seems to be the chief causative factor the intoxication theory is still more probable.

The only plausible explanation of the occurrence of icterus after revaccination is the occurrence of wound infection. It is true that the infective agency must be of a special kind, otherwise we would not see an incubation period enduring for eight months.

Damsch: "Berliner klin. Wochenschr.," 1898, p. 277.

Frölich, C.: "Ueber Icterusepidemien," "Deutsches Archiv für klin. Medicin," vol. xxiv, p. 394, 1879.

Hennig, A.: "Ueber epidem. Icterus" (literature), "Volkmann's Hefte," 1890, new series, No. 8.

Hirsch: "Historisch-geographische Pathologie," iii, p. 287, 1886.

Kelsch: "De la nature de l'ictère catarrhal," "Revue de médecine," 1886, p. 657.

Kirchner: "Deutsche militär-àrztliche Zeitschr.," p. 193, 1888.

Kramer: "Eine Epidemie von Icterus catarrhalis bei Kindern," Ugeskrift f. Lager, 1894.

Lürmann: "Eine Icterusepidemie," "Berliner klin. Wochenschr.," 1885, p. 24.

Meinert, E.: "Icterusepidemie," "Jahresbericht der Gesellschaft für Natur- und Heilkunde zu Dresden," 1890; "Schmidt's Jahrb.," vol. ccxxxi, p. 27, 1891.

Pfuhl: "Berliner klin. Wochenschr.," 1891, p. 178.

Pick, A.: "Prager med. Wochenschr.," No. 24.

Pletzer: "VII. Jahresbericht über den öffentlichen Gesundheitszustand in Bremen," 1889, p. 35.

Rankin, W.: "Brit. Med. Jour.," May 26, 1894.

Schüppel: Loc. cit., p. 16.

ICTERUS INFECTIOSUS; WEIL'S DISEASE.

(Icterus gravis.)

It has been customary to distinguish, on the one hand, favorable cases of icterus as icterus simplex and icterus catarrhalis, and, on the other hand, cases designated as icterus gravis which begin acutely, and run a severe and often fatal course lasting from several days to several weeks. Chronic icterus, even if it finally leads to death, does not properly belong under the head of icterus gravis. It is clear that a group of diseases characterized by one predominant symptom and a severe course must be a mixture of a great variety of diseases of different origin. Just as formerly fever received undue notice as the characteristic symptom of a vast number of different diseases, so now the extreme discoloration of the skin by bile may receive too exclusive attention and so lead to error.

At times pronounced changes in the hepatic parenchyma are found in some of the diseases included under icterus gravis, as in acute atrophy of the liver, in the acute terminal lesions of chronic hepatitis, in phosphorus-poisoning, in mushroom-poisoning, and in acute fatty degeneration and Winckel's disease produced by still unknown substances. At other times, again, autopsy reveals very little of note in cases of icterus gravis, and pathologic alterations in the liver might have been absent or could not be found with the incomplete methods of older investigators. We can readily, therefore, understand why older clinicians, in cases of the latter kind particularly, attempted a classification by designating all such cases as icterus gravis. Among cases of this description we can mention, for example, icterus following septicemia. Here, even in the most severe cases, no gross pathologic changes are found; and it is frequently difficult, even nowadays, to discover the place of primary infection. Bacteriologic examinations first threw some light on this subject, and we are enabled to-day to state that a great many cases of icterus gravis are of infectious origin, and that, as a rule, the bile-passages are infected. For these reasons there is a tendency to identify icterus gravis with icterus infectiosus. This is not correct, however, for the latter includes only a part of the cases of icterus gravis. Again, icterus infectiosus and infection of the bile-passages are not identical, for we see, on the one hand, cases of bacterial lesions of the bile-passages and of the liver without icterus, and, on the other hand, septicemia or infectious gastro-intestinal diseases that simulate icterus gravis without any infection of the bile-passages. We see, therefore, that for infectious icterus no definite disease-picture can be delineated and no satisfactory definition can be formulated from the fact that we are only beginning to gain an insight into the true pathogenesis of this group. The more we learn of it, the less uniform the different forms seem to be.

Clinically, icterus infectiosus is characterized by the appearance of all the symptoms of a severe infection and by icterus. In one case the one, in another case the other, of these two classes of symptoms may predominate, both in regard to intensity and in regard to the time of their appearance and their duration. In this section we will limit our discussion to those cases in which no serious lesions of the hepatic parenchyma can be found; while the latter will be described in the sections on hepatitis and acute yellow atrophy.

In our discussion of catarrhal icterus we called attention to the fact that a number of cases are seen that run their course with high fever and serious disturbances of the general health. We also mentioned the fact that it is very improbable that these grave symptoms could be due to biliary obstruction or to gastro-intestinal catarrhs alone. Cases of this character are the connecting-link between catarrhal icterus and that disease-picture that was first described by Weil in 1886 as a special form of icterus. This disease, since Weil's description, has held the attention of clinicians and has been designated as one (but not the only) type of icterus infectiosus.

Symptoms.—Weil's disease begins suddenly, without any prodromata, with fever, chills, and a rapid rise of temperature. At the same time the patient complains of vertigo, lassitude, and headache, as a result of which the sufferer soon takes to bed. Stupor early develops, and this is followed by delirium, so that the patient falls into a typhoid state much sooner than in typhoid fever. The picture resembles the latter disease more than any other infection, the tongue being coated, the spleen enlarged, and occasionally diarrhea supervening. Between the third and fifth day, rarely sooner, jaundice appears and rapidly grows intense, and at the same time the liver enlarges and becomes tender. The urine contains a moderate quantity of albumin, a few hyaline and epithelial casts, and, sometimes, a few blood-corpuscles. According to Fiedler, the swelling of the spleen and the liver are not observed in all cases, and albuminuria may be very slight and transitory.

The stools at this period are, as a rule, thin, contain bile in the beginning, and later, if the icterus be very intense, become clay-colored.

The temperature remains around 40° C. (104° F.) with fluctuations for several days. On the fourth to the eighth day of the disease the temperature drops, with remissions, and reaches normal at the end of from four to six days. At the same time the severe general symptoms disappear and the liver and spleen resume their normal size. The urine, too, becomes normal. Icterus persists for from ten to fourteen days, and then, too, gradually disappears.

In a minority of the cases (40%) a recurrence occurs some three to eight days after the final drop of the temperature to normal, manifesting itself by a rise of temperature and, as a rule, by a repetition of all the other symptoms. This recurrence is not so severe as was the primary attack.

The loss of weight that the patient suffers during the febrile period amounts to from 5 to 10 kilos (12 to 25 pounds).

In most of the cases the subject complains of violent muscular pains from the beginning of the trouble. These are chiefly localized in the muscles of the calf. During the period of stupor they are less apparent, but they persist through the febrile stage and into the stage of convalescence; in fact, they may be the last symptom to disappear. Occasionally, in the beginning of the disease, a spotted erythema is seen on the trunk, also at times there are found herpes facialis and an angina. As a result of the icterus there may be itching of the skin and a relative slowing of the pulse as compared with the temperature. Sometimes the hemorrhagic diathesis appears with hemorrhages into the skin, the conjunctivæ, and the retina, epistaxis, and blood in the urine, stools, and sputa. Parotitis, paresis of the vocal cords (Gerhardt), neuritis (Kausch), and iridocyclitis are among the rarer complications.

The duration of the febrile period, as already mentioned, is about eight to ten days; that of the apyrexia, one to eight; and that of the relapse, from five to eight days. The total duration of the disease up to complete recovery is from three to four weeks, while a feeling of weakness may persist for a much longer time.

As the termination of this disease is, as a rule, favorable, very few opportunities for postmortem study have been presented. As a result, we know very little of the anatomic changes present. Several reports of autopsies are on record, but they probably refer to cases that did not properly belong in this category. According to the reports of Wassilieff, Sumbera, and Neelsen, recent enlargement of the liver and spleen are seen, the spleen being soft and vascular. The cells of the liver are cloudy, their nuclei are increased and show mitoses. The kidneys, too, are enlarged, and in one case were seen to be filled with punctiform hemorrhages, and the renal epithelium was degenerated. In Neelsen's case there was a small-celled infiltration of the cortex of the kidneys, particularly in the region of the Malpighian bodies, the heart-muscle was in a state of fatty degeneration, and there were hemorrhages into the meninges and into the gastric and the intestinal mucosa.

Occurrence.—Weil's disease is not frequently seen. As a rule, it appears sporadically; but occasionally it affects groups of people living within circumscribed districts, and during a brief period of time, usually in hot weather. As a rule, persons in the third decade of life are afflicted. [Kissel * has recorded 96 cases in children between the ages of one and thirteen years.—Ed.] Over 90% of the cases are seen in men, while in children and in persons over fifty it is rare. It seems that butchers (Fiedler 50%, Wassilieff 20%), tanners, and laborers in sewers are particularly predisposed to the disease. In a few cases it could be shown that the use of impure drinking-water or the swallowing of contaminated river-water during bathing caused the disease. The latter was particularly apparent in different large and small epidemics that occurred quite frequently among soldiers and that had been observed and recorded long before Weil's publications appeared (Pfuhl). [Kissel states that the disease is more common in the autumn and winter than at other seasons.—Ed.]

* *Jahrb. f. Kinderheilk.*, 1898, Bd. XLVIII, p. 235.

A form of the disease has been described that is caused by drinking or unintentionally swallowing polluted water, appears in epidemics, and resembles Weil's disease in every particular with the exception of the absence of icterus. It is well to remember these cases, as they are of value in the understanding of the pathogenesis of this group of diseases.*

Nature of the Disease.—In the light of our present knowledge it is quite impossible to state whether Weil's disease is a clinical entity or not. At all events, the clinical picture presented resembles, on the one hand, severe cases of catarrhal icterus, and, on the other, febrile forms of gastrointestinal diseases that run their course without icterus and resemble an abortive form of typhoid fever. The latter are probably caused by the invasion of microbes other than the specific germ of typhoid fever.

That Weil's disease is a special form of typhoid fever produced by the entrance of the bacillus of typhoid into the bile-passages can hardly be granted. Both the occurrence of the disease and its course speak against such a theory. The French employ the name "*typhus hépatique*" for this disease (Landouzy, Mathieu), but this designation must be considered inappropriate and misleading. It is purely symptomatic.

Weil's disease resembles more the disease called bilious typhoid, or typhus biliosus, described by Griesinger in Cairo and by Kartulis in Alexandria. Fiedler is very positive in his statement that these diseases are identical.

Many investigators have attempted to find a specific bacterium in Weil's disease. Proteus flavescens, a bacillus cultivated by Jäger from the urine of living cases and from the organs of a case dead of the disease, appears to be a likely cause.

Jäger (Ulm) found the same organism in a disease of fowls, observed in a village near Ulm and characterized by icterus with enteritis. The same germ was also found in the water of the Danube in that vicinity. It is probable that the microbes had been poured into the river with the waters of a brook that flowed through the village. Some of his patients subsequently bathed in the river and probably swallowed some of the germs.

Banti succeeded in cultivating a proteus from the splenic blood of a man who was afflicted with a mild febrile icterus. This author attempts to establish certain distinctions between this germ, called by him Bacillus icterogenes capsulatus, and that of Jäger, in which the capsule is not regularly found. Banti claims a hemolytic action for his bacillus, and considers the icterus to be pleiochromic, but gives no valid arguments in support of his assumption.

Even if we should find that this parasite of Jäger really was the cause of the disease in a number of cases, we can still assume that other cases of infectious icterus are caused by other forms of parasites; in fact, I personally am very much inclined to this belief.

The micro-organisms could infect the bile-passages and could reach the liver directly from these or they could be brought to the liver from the intestine through the portal vein. In still other cases a simple intoxication with intestinal ptomains may be the cause of the trouble. All these factors must be weighed and carefully considered in every case, as general conclusions cannot be drawn from the results obtained in any one case.

In the French literature the question of the existence of an infectious icterus has been widely discussed. Landouzy, Kelch, and others assume that a bacterial infection occurs. Chauffard lays particular stress on autointoxication with intestinal putrefactive products, and even creates the word "Toxi-infection" to designate those cases where both microbian and ptomain activities are possible.

* Müller, Fr., "Die Schlammfieberepidemie in Schlesien," 1891, *Münchner med. Wochenschr.*, 1894, Nos. 40 and 41. Globig, *Deutsche militärärztliche Zeitschr.*, 1891. Possibly also Schulte, part 4 of "Veröffentlichungen aus dem Gebiete des Militär-Sanitätswesens," 1893.

As a matter of fact, many authors have included under the heading of Weil's disease several affections that do not properly belong there, such as santonin-poisoning (Cramer *), septicemia (A. Fränkel †), and acute parenchymatosis (Aufrecht ‡). Leiblinger's view,§ that Weil's disease is a form of polyarthritis rheumatica complicated by an icterus from absorption, has met with very little favor.

Chauffard is not at all justified in his statement that the recurrence of icterus and the other symptoms is characteristic of Weil's disease, although the frequency with which a relapse of the fever occurs is, it is true, quite remarkable.

It is astonishing that at the time when icterus appears, the fever and the general disturbances begin to recede. Some investigators have expressed a suspicion that the appearance of the former is responsible for the disappearance of the latter. At the same time, it is difficult to see why this should be; and it is quite probable that icterus and the other symptoms are produced at the same time, but that the former appears later than the other symptoms.

Treatment.—The treatment of Weil's disease is that of simple catarrhal icterus, on the one hand, and that of all infectious febrile diseases, on the other. The general rules and regulations that apply to the treatment of typhoid fever are proper in the treatment of this disease. Careful dietary regulations directed toward protecting and sparing the gastro-intestinal tract, evacuation and disinfection of the intestine (at least as far as this is possible), cool bathing, sponging, and the cold wet pack are symptomatically indicated. In view of the short duration of the fever, these measures are necessary for a short time only.

The administration of large quantities of water injected as enemata or even hypodermically is indicated, and has been demonstrated to be of practical value (Leick, Damsch).

LITERATURE.

Banti: "Ein Fall von infectiösem Icterus levis," "Deutsche med. Wochenschr.," 1895, Nos. 31 and 44.

Chauffard: "Revue de médecine," 1885, p. 9; Septembre, 1887.

"Deutsche militär-ärztliche Zeitschr.": Alfermann, 1892, p. 521; Hueber, 1888, p. 165; Kirchner, 1888, p. 195; Pfuhl, 1888, p. 385; Schaper, 1888, p. 202.

Fiedler, A.: "Deutsches Archiv für klin. Medicin," vol. XLII, p. 261, 1888; vol. L, p. 320, 1892 (Literature).

Freyhan, Th.: "Berliner Klinik," part 68, 1894 (Literature).

Girode: "Archives générales de médecine," 1891, I, pp. 26 and 169; 1892, I.

Goldenhorn: "Berliner klin. Wochenschr.," 1889, p 734.

Goldschmidt, F.: "Deutsches Archiv für klin. Medicin," vol. XL, p. 238, 1887.

Haas: "Prager med. Wochenschr.," 1887, Nos. 39 and 40.

Jäger: "Die Aetiologie des infectiösen fieberhaften Icterus (Weil'sche Krankheit)," "Zeitschr. für Hygiene," vol. XII, p. 525.

— "Der fieberhafte Icterus, eine Proteusinfection," "Deutsche med. Wochenschr.," 1895, Nos. 40 and 50.

Kausch, W.: "Ueber Icterus mit Neuritis," "Zeitschr. für klin. Medicin," vol. XXXII, p. 310, 1897.

Kelsch: "De la nature de l'ictère catarrhal," "Revue de médecine," 1885, p. 657.

Leick, B.: "Drei Fälle," etc., "Deutsche med. Wochenschr.," 1897, Nos. 44, 45, and 47.

* *Deutsche med. Wochenschr.*, 1889, p. 1067.

† *Deutsche med. Wochenschr.*, 1889, p. 165.

‡ *Deutsches Archiv für klin. Medicin*, 1887, vol. XL, p. 619.

§ "Ueber Resorptionsicterus im Verlauf der Polyarthritis rheumatica," *Wiener med. Wochenschr.*, 1891, No. 20.

Levi, L.: "Contribution à l'étude du foie infectieux d'une hépatite subaigue in-
    fectieuse primitive," "Archives générales de médecine," 1894, I, pp. 257 and
    444 (resembling old cirrhosis with secondary bacillary infection).
Mathieu, A.: "Typhus hépatique bénin.," "Revue de médecine," 1888.
Neelsen: "Deutsches Archiv fur klin. Medicin," vol. L, p. 285.
Munzer, E.: "Zeitschr. fur Heilkunde," 1892.
Pfuhl, A.: "Berliner klin. Wochenschr.," 1891, p. 178.
Roth: "Deutsches Archiv fur klin. Medicin," vol. XLI, p. 314, 1887.
Stirl, O. (Rosenbach): "Deutsche med. Wochenschr.," 1889, p. 738.
Wagner, E.: "Deutsches Archiv für klin. Medicin," vol. XL, 1887, p. 621.
Wassilieff, N. P.: "Ueber infectiösen Icterus" (17 cases), "Wiener Klinik," 1889,
    parts 8 and 9.
Weil, A.: "Ueber eine eigenthümliche mit Milztumor, Icterus und Nephritis einherge-
    hende acute Infectionskrankheit," "Deutsches Archiv für klin. Medicin," vol.
    XXXIX, p. 209, 1886.
Werther: "Deutsche med. Wochenschr.," 1889.
Windscheid: "Deutsches Archiv fur klin. Medicin," vol. XLV, p. 132, 1889.

CHOLANGITIS SUPPURATIVA (EXSUDATIVA, INFECTIOSA).

(Quincke.)

Purulent inflammation of the bile-passages is less frequently met with than the simple catarrhal form of inflammation. In the former the secretion contains more cells and more or less resembles pus, and the connective tissues of the walls of the bile-passages and of their surroundings show a small-celled infiltration; in the latter there is simply an increased secretion of mucus and a greater desquamation of the superficial epithelium. If the disease is of long duration, connective-tissue thickening of the walls, particularly of the larger bile-passages, is seen. As a rule, there is, in addition, obstruction to the outflow of bile, so that dilatation of the passages occurs. In this manner there is created a condition analogous to cylindric bronchiectasis. Occasionally the mucous membrane will be seen to be ulcerated in certain places, from the action of concretions or from diphtheritic or croupous inflammation. Whenever the suppurative inflammation involves the finer bile-passages, miliary accumulations of pus are formed, which are first found in the peripheral portions of the lobules. Only occasionally do these small purulent foci appear as globular collections of pus bounded by the walls of the dilated bile-passages; as a rule, they are true abscesses formed by circumscribed disintegration of the hepatic tissue. In the former case, cylindric epithelial cells from the bile-passages are seen in the pus; in the latter, we find hepatic cells in different stages of disintegration. Sometimes these small alveolar abscesses enlarge and become confluent, so that larger abscesses of irregular shape and distribution are formed. The contents of these cavities frequently shows an admixture of bile. In addition to the purulent disintegration, there is also seen at the periphery the development of connective tissue and degeneration of the hepatic cells.

Occurrence.—Purulent inflammation of the bile-passages is not very frequently met with. As a rule, it is not recognized until after the death of the patient. This form of inflammation is usually seen in subjects of advanced years and in cases where some obstacle to the normal flow of bile exists in the bile-passages. This obstacle may be either a concretion or an intestinal parasite. It is also seen as a complication and a sequel of typhoid fever, cholera, pyemia, and dysentery. Sometimes it appears without any demonstrable cause.

Etiology.—As a rule, though not necessarily always, it will be found that some microbic infection is the cause of this suppurative form of cholangitis. This fact was not recognized until recently, and we are indebted chiefly to French authors for its elucidation. Its recognition has led to an understanding in general of the importance of infections of the bile-passages. As we have seen above (page 471) microbes, as a rule, enter these passages from the intestine and travel in a direction opposed to that of the current of bile; less frequently they enter the bile-passages from the liver—*i. e.*, directly or indirectly from the systemic blood-stream. In the latter instance they produce a descending infection. In exceptional cases, finally, they may enter from the gall-bladder by penetrating the walls of this viscus from the intestine or from some neighboring focus of disease.

Microbic infection, so important in the diseases of the bile-passages, does not necessarily always produce a suppurative form of infection, but may lead to a simple catarrhal inflammation.

It is possible that occasionally the contents of the bile-passages does not resemble pus in appearance, but that at the same time (*e. g.*, in the case of Bacillus coli, according to Trantenroth) it may have a distinct feculent odor and very toxic properties, being capable of causing fever.

Sometimes the action of microbes remains altogether latent during the life of the patient, and even no anatomic changes are seen after death. As the bile-passages may present a normal appearance, cultural experiments and a microscopic examination are necessary to determine the rôle played by the bacterial invaders. By the latter procedure an increased desquamation of the epithelial lining of the bile-passages may be discovered. From the etiologic point of view, therefore, no sharp distinction can be drawn between the suppurative form of inflammation and the simplest catarrh of the biliary passages.

Bacillus coli is the most frequent cause of suppurative cholangitis, acting singly or in combination with streptococci or with Staphylococcus aureus or albus. In case the bile-passages are temporarily or incompletely occluded these microbes may penetrate beyond the obstruction and may find a suitable nidus for their development in the stagnating contents of the ducts above, from which they may even penetrate the mucous membrane, making their removal a very difficult matter.

Similar conditions favorable to a penetration of the mucous membrane by bacteria are seen in cases where the flow of bile is sluggish or where the peristaltic action of the bile-passages is reduced or the sphincters are weak. This occurs, for example, in febrile diseases of long duration in which the muscular tone of the whole body is reduced. Aside from the pathogenic germs already mentioned, a number of other bacterial species that are essentially harmless may gain an entrance and do damage only in the sense that they produce a liquefaction of tissues.

A number of cases of icterus that are in the beginning simply catarrhal or of a mild infectious type may form the starting-point for severe forms of suppurative cholangitis. This occurs if other bacteria invade the inflamed ducts or if some of the species that are already there acquire toxic properties.

When intestinal parasites, particularly ascarides, enter the biliary passages from the intestine, a suppurative cholangitis may result. This, as a rule, is probably not due to the action of these parasites themselves, but to bacteria that they carry with them.

Of all the infectious diseases, typhoid fever is most frequently complicated by a suppurative inflammation of the bile-passages. Hölscher,
among 2000 autopsies on cases of typhoid fever found evidence of this
condition in 5 cases, nearly all of which were in the stage at which the intestinal ulcers were beginning to heal, although sometimes suppuration
does not develop until the stage of convalescence. [Or even long after the
termination of the systemic infection. A sufficient number of carefully
recorded cases have been published within recent years to prove that in a
very large number of cases of typhoid fever (50%, according to Cushing)
the bile contains Bacillus typhosus, Chiari * having even found the
micro-organism in 19 out of 22 cases.—Ed.] Gilbert and Girode found
typhoid bacilli in the purulent contents of the gall-bladder and its walls
five months after convalescence from typhoid. Dupré found the bacteria
after eight months under similar conditions. [Miller † has recorded a case
of cholelithiasis in which typhoid bacilli were found in pure culture in the
gall-bladder seven years after the attack of typhoid fever, Droba ‡ has
found typhoid bacilli in the center of gall-stones seventeen years after the
primary infection, and Hunner § isolated typhoid bacilli from the bile at
operation for suppurative cholecystitis eighteen years after the attack of
typhoid fever. (For further particulars as to the rôle of the typhoid
bacillus in affections of the bile-passages see page 471.)—Ed.] Gilbert
and Dominici found the bacillus of typhoid fever and Bacillus coli
together. The bacillus of typhoid is occasionally found in the wall of the
gall-bladder without inflammation of the parts. It is not improbable
that this form of inflammation may occur by the descending route from
colonies of the typhoid bacillus that are present in the liver.

In cholera, suppurative cholangitis and cholecystitis are found still
more frequently than in typhoid fever. It seems, however, that the bacillus
of cholera is present in many cases without causing any inflammatory reaction. Girode found the bacillus in the bile fourteen times in twenty-
eight cases of cholera, but saw an inflammation of the bile-passages
extending into the finest canals in only one case.

Pneumonia, among other infectious diseases, is occasionally complicated by suppurative cholangitis. In the cases reported the pneumococcus was found within the bile-passages in combination either with pyogenic microbes or with Bacillus coli; while in some instances the latter was
found alone (Gilbert and Girode, Klemperer, Létienne). It is possible
that in pneumonia the mild form of icterus so often seen in this
disease is caused by local infection.

We may expect that the new point of view given by recent bacteriologic research in regard to the origin of these forms of suppurative cholangitis and their significance will throw light on a number of other observations. We may state now that the presence of certain infectious
germs alone is not sufficient to produce suppurative cholangitis; we must
have, in addition, either a certain virulence of the bacteria or a reduction
of the natural resisting power of the exposed tissues. The greatest
differences in this respect seem to exist in the case of the cholera bacillus,
next to this in the case of the bacillus of typhoid fever and of Bacillus coli,
while in the case of staphylococci and streptoccoci such differences are not

* *Zeitschr. f. Heilkunde*, Bd. xv, p. 199.
† *Johns Hopkins Hospital Bull.*, May, 1898.
‡ *Wien. klin. Woch.*, Nov. 16, 1899.
§ *Johns Hopkins Hospital Bull.*, August–September, 1899, p. 163.

so marked. It is important to remember that the gall-bladder in particular seems to be so frequently involved for the reason chiefly that here there are present the favoring condition of stagnation of fluids, whereas in the other portions of the bile-passages the constant stream of bile seems to effectually prevent a localization and development of bacteria.

Symptoms.—The symptoms of suppurative cholangitis are not characteristic and frequently are so indefinite that the disease is not recognized; or they may be so mild that the condition is not even suspected.

Icterus as a symptom is not so marked as are disturbances of the general health. Whenever icterus is marked, it is, as a rule, not due to cholangitis, but to some occlusion of the bile-passages that may have existed before the occurrence of the inflammation of the ducts; or it may be due to the occlusion of the bile-passages as a result of the formation of concretions.

Fever and the occurrence of enlargement of the spleen are important symptoms. As in other suppurative processes, the fever is of a remitting type with evening exacerbations, and frequently complete intermissions in the morning. Again, as in other forms of fever from absorption of purulent material, this type of fever is not necessarily maintained, but may vary in different directions. Both the number of daily maxima and minima and the time of day at which they occur may vary. The rise of temperature may be accompanied by a chill and the time of a decline by a sweat; or, again, periods of subnormal temperatures or even long afebrile periods may occur. Occasionally, the type of fever caused by the suppurative process is modified by variations in temperature induced by the impaction of gall-stones. The fever described has been called febris intermittens hepatica or febris bilioseptica, the latter designation being particularly in favor with French authors. This fever, like any other fever due to the absorption of constituents of pus, may run a similar course and cause the same subjective symptoms as the intermittent type of malarial fever; and it is even stated that a tertian and a quartan type are occasionally observed. It is not, in my opinion, demonstrated that this fever, provided careful records of temperature are made every two or three hours, resembles these malarial types of fever more than any fever from absorption of products from other suppurative foci. In both cases the fever is caused by the absorption of toxins capable of producing a febrile rise of temperature, but this does not explain the remitting type that the fever assumes. In the most serious cases microbes may even enter the blood-current.

In case other poisons capable of acting on the heart or the kidneys or of depressing the temperature are absorbed, other more or less severe general symptoms may appear. The causes of such an occurrence and the conditions under which such an absorption may take place are as unknown to us as in the case of suppurative pyelitis or of putrid bronchiectasis. The latter conditions in more ways than one resemble suppurative cholangitis and present many analogies to it. In the disease under discussion, however, the effect of biliary stasis and of the interference with the hepatic function add a specific and distinguishing factor.

In addition to icterus, which, as we have seen, is not constantly present, pain or a feeling of tension in the hepatic region often call attention to the liver as the diseased organ. In case the gall-bladder is involved, the pain as a rule is more severe. In addition to these symptoms, disturbances of the digestion, diarrhea, and vomiting are often present.

[Pick * has called attention to the absence of leucocytosis during the afebrile periods and to the diminution in the nitrogen in the urine during the days of fever. Boas † has recently called attention to a tender area in the region of the twelfth dorsal vertebra from 2 to 3 cm. from the middle line in cases of even latent inflammation of the bile-ducts.—ED.]

Some of the possible complications of suppurative cholangitis are pylephlebitis, true septicemia, endocarditis (Netter and Martha), purulent meningitis (Jossias), and, usually starting from the gall-bladder, peritonitis (Chiari).

Course.—The onset of suppurative cholangitis is, as a rule, insidious and not determinable. In case cholelithiasis exists, the symptoms of cholangitis are superadded to those of biliary stasis and of the impaction of the stone. They frequently run parallel to these symptoms, inasmuch as an increased obstruction to the flow of bile will be accompanied by an increased absorption of toxins from the pus. In cases of this kind the symptoms may vary in intensity for months, until finally the impacted stone is forced into the intestine. When this occurs, the pus that has formed finds an exit and the cholangitis may subside. The fever in these instances does not recede at once, but gradually (own observation). In the majority of cases the outflow of pus is not complete, but only partial, or occurs only at intervals. The body becomes accustomed to the absorption of toxins, so that the temperature may remain normal for a time; yet at the same time the fact that recovery is slow and incomplete soon directs attention to a focus of disease existing somewhere. If not relieved, the liver will gradually be destroyed by a process of slow purulent destruction of tissue and the patient succumb in the course of a few weeks or months. Hectic fever is always present in these cases.

In the case of infectious diseases where no obstruction of the bile-passages exists the symptoms are still more obscure. Icterus is, as a rule, absent; or if present at all, is usually slight. The fever and sometimes pain in the hepatic region are the only symptoms, and they are not characteristic. In typhoid fever these symptoms do not develop until the stage of convalescence and after the disease proper has run its course. Where the gall-bladder is particularly affected, symptoms directed to this viscus will appear (see below).

Prognosis.—The prognosis in the majority of cases is unfavorable. Where concretions exist, all the dangers of biliary stasis are present, with, in addition, the danger of multiple abscess formation. At the same time, if operative or spontaneous removal of the stone can be brought about, complete restitution to normal is possible. It seems that even ascarides can wander back into the intestine (Kartulis). [Ogilvie ‡ has reported a case in which jaundice ceased after the expulsion per anum of a round worm one-third of the length of which was stained by bile as though it had been for a time impacted in the common duct.—ED.] The typhoid form of infection seems to be the most dangerous of all, for the reason that ulceration of the gall-bladder may occur and lead to perforation and peritonitis.

Diagnosis.—In those instances where other signs point to the existence of some disease of the biliary passages, notably gall-stones, the appear-

* *Deutsches Arch. f. klin. Med.*, Bd. LXIX, Hft. 1 and 2.
† *Münch. med. Woch.*, 1902. No. 15.
‡ *British Medical Journal*, Jan. 12, 1901.

ance of a remitting type of fever and a general loss of strength will lead us to suspect cholangitis. When icterus is absent, or is so slight that it is diagnostically valueless (it might, for example, be secondary and due to pyemia), and when other local symptoms are absent, malaria might be suspected. The decision will in such a case have to be rendered from a careful study of the temperature curve. If the maximum occurs during the first half of the day, or if regular intervals, a continuous type of rise and fall, and longer periods of complete apyrexia are seen, the probability is great that the case is one of malaria; whereas the fever due to the absorption of toxins from pus usually reaches its maximum toward evening, there are more frequent rises to the highest point, and a greater irregularity in their occurrence, subnormal temperatures occur at times and the periods of apyrexia are short and not distinct. A skilled observer, in addition, will know how to interpret the absence of the plasmodium and of pigment from the blood. [The presence or absence of leucocytosis would also have great weight in differentiating the two conditions.—ED.]

If the diagnosis of fever from absorption has been made, local symptoms will have to direct attention to the bile-passages as the place of suppuration. These are, in addition to icterus, pain in the region of the liver and the gall-bladder. [And possibly the tender area described by Boas.—ED.] Certain points in the past history of the case have an important bearing on the diagnosis, such as a history of previous attacks of gall-stone colic, a recent attack of typhoid fever or of cholera.

In many respects the symptoms of suppurative cholangitis resemble those of abscess of the liver so much that it is impossible to make a differential diagnosis. In the case of the latter lesion, however, the symptoms due to involvement of the bile-ducts are not so apparent, nor is icterus or the pain in the region of the gall-bladder so marked. In the case of cholangitis fever is more apt to be absent than in the case of abscess of the liver. [Too much stress should not be placed upon the temperature in excluding a possible abscess of the liver, as in this condition the rise of temperature may be slight or even absent, while leucocytosis is frequently absent at any rate after the abscess has existed for some time.—ED.]

It is possible that later, when we shall have more experience, the determination of the species of bacteria that have infected the bile-passages may be of some diagnostic value. For the present the history of an attack of typhoid fever or of cholera alone may give us a clue. The character of the fever cannot be utilized in the determination of this point.

Netter's statement, based on some animal experiments, that Bacillus coli, in contradistinction to pyogenic microbes, causes subnormal temperatures, is certainly not universally applicable. Future investigations will have to decide whether it is at least applicable to some of the cases observed in human beings.

In the presence of symptoms pointing to cholangitis, the discovery of ascarides in the stools may reveal a possible cause.

Treatment.—One of the chief indications in the treatment of cholelithiasis is the prevention of suppurative cholangitis. The careful treatment of simple catarrhal icterus, too, has a certain prophylactic value. The importance of so-called disinfection of the intestine by drugs and milk diet, favored by French authors, is doubtful.

33

Cholangitis should be treated in the same manner as catarrhal icterus. As a general rule, the possible presence of concretions should be considered. The administration of cholagogues and the disinfection of the biliary passages is indicated on theoretic grounds, and both measures are recommended and employed. The drugs in use for this purpose are salicylic acid, salol, oleum terebinthinæ, benzonaphthol, and oleate of sodium. In cases of cholangitis due to ascarides the repeated administration of calomel and of santonin is indicated.

Kehr, of late years, has attempted to fulfil the apparently most urgent indication—that is to say, drainage of the pus that has accumulated within the bile-passages—by opening the main bile-duct and establishing permanent drainage through the skin. Sometimes opening and draining the gall-bladder is beneficial and exercises a favorable effect on the other bile-passages, particularly in those instances where the cystic duct itself is exceptionally wide and can be drained. [Terrier * has also strongly urged drainage of the biliary passages by cholecystotomy in this condition. Wilms † has reported a cure by drainage of the gall-bladder in a case of multiple abscesses due to cholangitis and cholecystitis.—Ed.]

Aubert, Pierre: "De l'endocardite ulcéreuse végétante dans les infections biliaires," Thèse de Paris, 1891.

Chauffard: Loc. cit., p. 704.

— "Etude sur les absces aréolaires du foie," "Archives de physiolog.," 1883, i, p. 263.

Dmochowski and Janowski: "Cholangitis suppurativa durch Bacterium coli," "Centralblatt für allgemeine Pathologie," 1894, No. 4.

Dominici: "Des angiocholites et cholécystites suppurées," Thèse de Paris, 1894 (fully treated, quoting largely from literature).

Dupré, E.: "Les infections biliaires," Thèse de Paris, 1891, "Archives générales de médecine," 1891, ii. p. 246.

Frerichs: Loc. cit., ii, p. 426.

Gilbert et Dominici: "Société de biologie," 1893; January and February, 1894.

Gilbert et Girode: "Société de biologie," 1890; 1891, Nos. 11 and 16; 1892.

Hólscher: "Ueber die Complicationen bei 2000 Fällen von letalem Abdominaltyphus," "Münchener med. Wochenschr.," 1891.

Jossias: "Progrès médical," 1881.

Kartulis: "Ascariden-Cholangitis," "Centralblatt für Bakteriologie," vol. i; "Bericht über den VIII. internationalen Congress für Hygiene in Budapest," 1894, vol. ii, p. 646.

Kehr: "Munchener med. Wochenschr.," 1897, No. 41.

Létienne: "De la bile dans l'état pathologique," Thèse de Paris, 1891.

— "Recherches bacteriol. sur la bile humaine," "Archives de méd. expér.," 1891, p. 761.

Naunyn: "Cholelithiasis," p. 103.

Netter et Martha: "Archives de physiolog.," 1886, p. 7.

Pick, Fr.: "Zur Kenntniss der Febris hepatica intermittens," "Congress für innere Medicin," 1897, p. 468.

Rothmund: "Endocarditis ulcerosa" (does case 10 also belong here?), Dissertation, Zurich, 1889.

Schüppel: Loc. cit., p. 36.

Sittmann: "Bakterioskopische Blutuntersuchungen" (14 cases of diseases of the liver), "Deutsches Archiv für klin. Medicin," vol. liii, p. 336, 1894.

* *Rev. de Chirurgie*, 1895, p. 966.   † *Münch. med. Woch.*, 1902, No. 13.

INFLAMMATION OF THE GALL-BLADDER.

Cholecystitis; Cystitis felleæ.

(Quincke.)

Inflammation of the gall-bladder is intimately related to inflammation of the bile-passages; as the former is probably always a complication of inflammation of the latter parts. For this reason the same etiologic factors that play a rôle in the causation of inflammations of the bile-passages can be made responsible for the same condition in the gall-bladder. Clinically, on the other hand, cholecystitis is distinguished by certain typical features, as the parts involved in this instance form a closed sac whose only exit is a narrow passage. This anatomic arrangement causes peculiarities in the development of inflammations in these parts, and also makes a cure of the affection difficult. It is for these reasons that diseases of the gall-bladder must be discussed independently. A very important element is the fact that gall-stones develop chiefly in the gall-bladder. These concretions are the most prolific cause of inflammations, since they act not so much mechanically, as was formerly assumed, but through the agency of bacteria that surround them. Many cases of gall-stone colic are not purely spastic in character, but are usually complicated by inflammatory processes in the wall of the gall-bladder and the tissues surrounding it. [For a discussion of this point see page 556.—ED.] The inflammation affects the mucous membrane, at first causing a thickening of this tissue and the secretion of an abnormal quantity of mucus in the cavity of the bladder (cholecystitis catarrhalis). This excessive secretion is soon thickened by the admixture of numerous desquamated epithelial cells, and as the walls of the cystic duct are at the same time swollen, both the viscidity of the fluid in the gall-bladder and the narrowness of the duct prevent an outflow of its contents. As a result the bladder becomes dilated. In the mean time the inflammatory process extends to the muscular wall of the bladder and to the serous membrane covering it. As it also involves the connective-tissue structures in the wall, a connective-tissue thickening of these parts results, often with peritoneal adhesions. When, later, the contents of the gall-bladder are absorbed or succeed in gaining an exit, the changes in the wall of the gall-bladder will cause a contraction of the organ, leading to a permanent reduction in its size. In addition, the gall-bladder may be distorted in shape or attached in an abnormal position, while its walls may undergo calcification.

This form of fibrinous inflammation of the gall-bladder is quite frequently seen in corset liver, where it originates from stasis of bile within the bladder caused by traction and pressure upon the cystic duct. In addition to this, gall-stones may be present and aggravate the condition. In other instances this form of inflammation extends by continuity from the serous covering of the gall-bladder in such a manner that the peritoneal investment, as a result of traumatic influences, becomes inflamed and the process extends to the internal coats of the viscus.

Purulent inflammations of the gall-bladder are less frequently met with than fibrous inflammations. The pus that is formed from the mucous lining of the gall-bladder as a rule distends the viscus, provided it was normal in size before the process began. Distention of and ulcerative processes in the gall-bladder, particularly in typhoid fever, may lead to perforation. In case suppuration follows chronic cholelithiasis, the gall-bladder is usually so thickened by previous attacks of inflammation that it is not distended by the pus, and, moreover, is less liable to perforation. At the same time a circumscribed peritonitis may result under these circumstances, or, if adhesions exist, a fistula may be formed that opens into the intestine or externally through the skin. In this manner drainage may be established, the pus evacuated, and the empyema be cured. Conditions of this kind are not infrequently found at autopsy.

The microscopic changes seen in the wall of the gall-bladder are analogous to those seen in the bile-ducts. If repeated attacks of inflammation occur and the wall becomes very much thickened, the glands of the mucous membrane disappear. In acute suppurative forms of inflammation the mucous membrane, and sometimes the whole wall, is seen to be in a state of small-celled infiltration. Occasionally, as in the case of typhoid fever, small mural abscesses may form that perforate either into the lumen of the gall-bladder or through its wall.

Symptoms.—The chief signs of inflammation of the gall-bladder are pain and enlargement. The pain may be truly inflammatory in character. In these cases it is particularly severe in acute inflammations and in involvement of the serous coat. In other instances it is caused by the distention of the wall of the gall-bladder following occlusion of the cystic duct and the filling of the bladder. The pain is increased by pressure, respiratory and general movements, and by distention and violent peristaltic movements of neighboring portions of the intestine, particularly of the duodenum and the hepatic flexure of the colon.

In cholecystitis a swelling in the region of the gall-bladder can usually be discovered by palpation and percussion. In case the gall-bladder is intact and the inflammation is recent, this swelling may be caused by an increase in the contents of the bladder and by distention. In other cases it is due to inflammatory and edematous thickening of the wall of the gall-bladder and of the neighboring peritoneal covering of the liver, abdominal parietes, and colon, or to serofibrinous masses inclosed by these inflamed parts of the peritoneum. In the first case the tumor has the same shape as the gall-bladder; in the latter, its outline is irregular and not so readily palpable, owing to the pain and the resulting tension of the abdominal muscles. The swelling may move with the liver on respiration; but frequently this respiratory motility is impaired on account of the pain, and in other instances adhesions exist and prevent it. Sometimes fecal matter accumulates in the hepatic flexure of the colon, particularly if the wall of the bowel is inflamed, and these accumulations form a mass that lies so close to the gall-bladder that it changes its outline and modifies the area of greatest pain. Owing to these possible complications, it is frequently impossible, when the disease is at its height, to diagnose more than a swelling in the right side of the abdomen, and the further course of the disease will have to reveal whether the gall-bladder, the vermiform appendix, or the colon is the seat of the trouble.

In cases of corset liver the tumor can assume a very peculiar shape from the thickening and elongation of the tongue-shaped piece of liver that is separated from the main mass of the organ by the indentation, while this piece or the thin margin of the liver situated in front of the gall-bladder may become thickened by a direct extension of the inflammatory process. As soon as the inflammation subsides this local change in the shape of the hepatic margin is corrected and normal conditions are reestablished (Riedel, compare page 394).

The intensity of this simple inflammation of the gall-bladder may vary greatly, its duration covering from one day to several weeks. Very often cystitis and pericystitis follow an attack of gall-stone colic. This is particularly true in long-drawn-out attacks; while in recent cases running an acute course the colicky seizure may be purely spastic in character.

In cases where the inflamed mucous membrane of the gall-bladder secretes pus in the place of mucus and epithelial debris, pain and swelling are particularly severe; while at the same time the fever, which may have been of a continuous type in the beginning, assumes the remitting type of an absorption fever. However, as is the case in cholangitis, this does not always occur. Pain and swelling, too, may be slight, so that, in those cases especially where purulent cholecystitis complicates some other disease, no marked change in the symptoms occurs. It may happen in this way that the condition we are discussing may not be discovered. This occurred, for example, in 11 out of 14 cases of typhoidal cholecystitis that Hagenmüller collected. In typhoid cases, in particular, it frequently happens that the small abscesses in the wall of the gall-bladder lead to perforation and fatal peritonitis (Chiari and others).

The diagnosis, therefore, of cholecystitis is in many instances as difficult or as impossible to make as is that of cholangitis. All in all, it is more easy than that of cholangitis without involvement of the gall-bladder. This is due to the more superficial position of the bladder and the typical and strictly localized symptoms that are produced by inflammations of the peritoneal covering of the organ. According to the general conditions observed and the history of the case, it is frequently an easy matter to decide what the character of the cholecystitis is and whether the bladder alone is involved or whether cholangitis coexists.

Adhesions with the abdominal parietes may be accompanied by circumscribed areas of edema of the skin. In the case of Trantenroth there was an edematous area as large as an adult hand in the hepatic region, although no peritoneal adhesions were found.

In regard to the advisability of exploratory puncture, the same arguments as in the case of simple dilatation of the gall-bladder exist, but are even more applicable than in the latter condition. [Exploratory puncture has no place in either condition at the present time. The facts learned are fewer and the danger much greater than is the case with exploratory laparotomy, while a cure is not to be expected from the former method.—ED.]

Treatment.—Both the acute and the chronic relapsing forms of cholecystitis call for rest of the inflamed parts. For this reason the patient should be instructed to remain in bed, the diet should be restricted, and opium should be administered in small doses in order to quiet the peristaltic action of the bowels. In cases where great sensitiveness to pressure exists it is advisable to apply from four to six leeches to the sore spot, applying them over as small an area as possible. An ice-bag, provided it is not too heavy, also relieves. Whenever the pain is distributed over a wider area, and where it is not so acute in character nor so violent, it is better to apply heat, either by Priessnitz bandages, or, in the more violent forms, by poultices that are kept at a constant temperature by a thermophore (Quincke). We can usually get along without hypodermic injections of morphin at the height of the disease. When the acute symptoms subside, it is well to remember that accumulations of fecal matter may occur in the hepatic flexure, and that such masses should be removed in good time either by careful enemata or by the internal administration of castor oil, a measure that may greatly ameliorate the local symptoms and favor resolution of the exudate. [The administration of an opiate is objectionable in the case of cholecystitis for the same reasons as prevail in appendicitis and it is important to bear in mind in both conditions that the relief of pain is accompanied by the danger involved in obscuring the symptoms and furnishing a false sense of security.—ED.]

If, from the local or the general symptoms, a purulent or a bacterial form of cholecystitis has been diagnosed, operative procedures must be considered. In fact, the appearance of symptoms of purulent inflammation of the gall-bladder is, as a rule, the chief indication for the surgical removal of gall-stones. If a history of previous inflammation leads us to suspect a thickening of the wall of the gall-bladder, operative interference is not so urgent. In cases, however, where the contents of the gall-bladder are very infectious, and where the bladder becomes rapidly distended, or where, as in typhoid fever, there is danger of ulceration and perforation into the peritoneal cavity, the operation should be performed as soon as possible.

Cadéac, A.: " De la cholécystite suppurée," Thèse de Paris, 1891.
Chiari: "Ueber cholecystitis typhosa," "Prager med. Wochenschr.," 1893.
Dungern: "Ueber Cholecystitis typhosa," "Munchener med. Wochenschr.," No. 26, 1897.
Ecklin, Th. (Courvoisier): "Ueber das Verhalten der Gallenblase bei dauerndem Verschluss des Ductus choledochus," Dissertation, Basel, 1896.
Fuchs: "Berliner klin. Wochenschr.," 1897, p. 647.
Gilbert et Girode: Société de biologie, 1893.
Hawkins, Fr.: "On Jaundice and on Perforation of the Gall-bladder in Typhoid Fever," "Med.-chir. Transactions," vol. LXXX, 1897.
Kleefeld (Naunyn): "Ueber die Punction der Gallenblase," etc. (diagnostic), Dissertation, Strassburg, 1894.
Mason, A. Lawrence: "Gall-bladder Infection in Typhoid Fever," "Boston Med. and Surg. Journal," vol. LXXXVI, No. 19, 1897.
Naunyn: "Deutsche med. Wochenschr.," 1891.
Quincke: "Thermophor," "Berl. klin. Wochenschr.," 1896, No. 16.
Souville, R.: "Cholécyst. scléreuse d'origine calculeuse et pericholécystite," Thèse de Paris, 1895.
Trantenroth: "Mittheilungen aus den Grenzgebieten der Medicin und Chirurgie," I, p. 703, 1896.

DILATATION OF THE GALL-BLADDER.

(Quincke.)

Dilatation of the whole system of biliary passages, either partial or throughout all its ramifications, occurs as soon as the outflow of bile from one area or the other is impeded. The longer the stasis of bile persists, the more extended the dilatation. As soon as the obstacle is removed, the dilated condition in a measure recedes; but it may persist to a varying degree. Occasionally, small ectatic protuberances are formed that are situated laterally from the main axis of the vessel.

The occurrence of dilatation of the bile-passages accompanying stasis of bile has been discussed under that heading. In case, however, the dilatation persists, the condition becomes important, for the reason that it favors infection from the intestine. During life this chronic and persisting dilatation is not recognizable, and dilatation of the gall-bladder is clinically more important. The viscus in this condition may contain (1) bile, (2) a colorless fluid, (3) pus; and in all three cases gall-stones may at the same time be present.

The gall-bladder is distended with bile in general biliary stasis or in cases where the opening of the cystic duct is occluded by a gall-stone. The obstruction may be so situated as to permit the entrance of bile into the bladder and at the same time prevent its exit. In addition to stones in the cystic duct, concretions may also be present in the bladder itself. In cases of this kind two factors are at work—viz., *first*, the direct obstruction to the outflow of the bile; *second*, a number of inflammatory processes in the bladder-wall and possibly paresis of its musculature. It is not decided to what extent such paretic conditions can lead to an enlargement of the gall-bladder without the presence of some mechanical obstruction to the flow of bile. [Kehr believes that dropsy of the gall-bladder may result from an acute infectious cholecystitis of mild grade, and that it is exceptionally due to obstruction of the cystic duct by a stone alone.—ED.]

In cases where the cystic duct is permanently occluded by a stone, cicatricial tissue, twisting, or swelling of the mucosa, the contents of the gall-bladder are absorbed and nothing remains but a colorless liquid free from all bile constituents (*hydrops cystidis felleæ*). This fluid is usually clear, resembles mucus, is viscid or may be very thin and watery. It contains mucin, squamous epithelium, and occasionally albumin from inflammatory exudation (Kleefeld). In cases of this kind the gall-bladder is usually very tense, like a cyst, and, as a rule, a little or occasionally very much larger than normal. The larger the gall-bladder, the thinner its wall; and, as a result, the glands of the mucosa are destroyed and the cylindric epithelium is replaced by squamous cells.

If the contents of the gall-bladder consist of pus (empyema), the fluid contents may be really pus or a mixture of pus and serous fluid that may be colored by bile. This fluid, as a rule, contains some albumin, occasionally mucin, cylindric and squamous epithelium and cells in a state of fatty degeneration, and also bacteria.

Symptoms.—Both the transverse and longitudinal diameters of the gall-bladder increase when the viscus becomes dilated and a swelling is formed that can often be felt during life. In slight degrees of dilatation the gall-bladder extends below the lower margin of the liver. Its outline is that of a segment of a sphere some two or three centimeters in diameter. Only when the abdominal walls are thin can the enlarged bladder be palpated. The larger the gall-bladder, the more it extends below the hepatic margin, assuming a pear-shaped outline. At the same time its motility, as compared to that of the margin of the liver, increases, particularly in a lateral direction and backward and forward. This motility is particularly apparent when the patient is lying on his side and on bimanual palpation; but the organ always quickly returns to its original position underneath the margin of the liver. With each respiratory excursion the bladder rises and falls synchronously with the margin of the liver. If the bladder becomes very much elongated, its longitudinal axis may become twisted so that the outline of the organ resembles a cucumber (Courvoisier). The fundus is turned forward and may appear to be separated from the margin of the liver by a coil of intestine that has entered between the bladder and the liver. The fundus, of course, follows all the movements of the liver. In cases of corset liver the gall-bladder may become dislocated downward and toward the median line to a considerable degree. If the gall-bladder is very much dilated,—and cases are on record where the contents of the organ amounted to over one liter,—the swelling may be confounded with echinococcus cysts, hydronephrosis, or ovarian cyst. The connection of the tumor with the liver will have to be determined in order to arrive at a decision. If the growth is the gall-bladder, it will be attached to the liver above and be situated in close contact with the abdominal wall. Ovarian cysts, on the other hand, are attached by a pedicle in the pelvis, and hydronephrosis starts from behind. Sometimes distention of the stomach with gas may be of some assistance, as this manœuver will push the gall-bladder forward and bring it in closer contact with the anterior abdominal wall.

If the abdominal walls are very thin and very much relaxed, the gall-bladder, if it is enlarged, is sometimes even visible. Palpation is less satisfactory than might be expected from the close proximity of the organ to the anterior abdominal wall. This is due to the fact that no resistance is offered behind the bladder, so that it escapes from the hand pressing on the abdomen. It is a comparatively easy matter, however, to determine whether the consistency is elastic and cystic or not, whether the walls are thickened, and whether concretions are situated within the bladder. On the other hand, it is rarely possible, even if the bladder is very much enlarged, to elicit fluctuation by bimanual palpation.

Dulness on percussion, that might be expected when the bladder is very much enlarged and distended with fluid, can only be elicited on light percussion for the reason that the fluid contents allow the impulse to be transmitted to neighboring coils of intestine so that a tympanitic sound is produced.

Dilatation of the gall-bladder rarely causes subjective symptoms. Symptoms of this character, it is true, are caused by the disease that has produced the dilatation or by inflammation that may be present at the same time. In the majority of cases the diagnosis of dilatation of the gall-bladder is difficult, and it is necessary to utilize all the symptoms of complicating conditions together with the anamnestic data of the case. These, in combination with the scanty objective symptoms presented, may lead to a satisfactory diagnosis. The same applies to the determination of the nature of the fluid contents of the bladder. Exploratory puncture has occasionally been performed for the latter purpose; but as this procedure may easily lead to peritonitis from extravasation of some of the inflammatory contents (Naunyn), many authors condemn it absolutely. If performed at all, it should be done with a thin and very long needle. [In this, as in other exploratory punctures, it would seem that aspiration of even a small quantity of fluid might tend to diminish the danger always present in intra-abdominal exploratory punctures. The simple hollow needle does not relieve tension sufficiently to render unlikely leakage into the peritoneal cavity. The removal of a larger quantity of fluid relieves tension to a greater degree and lessens this imminent risk.—ED.] Nowadays, when we have all the improved technique of modern surgery at our disposal, exploratory laparotomy must certainly be preferred. This operation is more complicated but far less dangerous; while, in addition, the opening of the gall-bladder for therapeutic purposes can follow the exploratory opening of the abdomen whenever indicated.

The prognosis and the treatment of dilatation of the gall-bladder must depend altogether on the origin of the trouble and on other circumstances. Dilatation alone would call for extirpation of the organ only in those cases where harm is being done from pressure on surrounding organs or where a rupture of the bladder is to be feared from too rapid distention. [Even in these cases drainage without extirpation is now found to be sufficient, and is a much simpler procedure.—ED.]

HEMORRHAGE INTO THE BILE-PASSAGES.
(Quincke.)

Small extravasations of blood into the mucous membrane are occasionally seen in hyperemia and inflammation, and have no significance. Larger hemorrhages into the lumen of the bile-passages and the gall-bladder, causing the bladder and the ducts to contain a bloody fluid, are rare, but may become clinically important. They are occasionally seen in passive congestion of the liver. In the cases reported no source of the hemorrhage could be found, so that it is probable that the blood oozed from the capillaries.

Quinquaud described a case of hemorrhagic cholangitis in which so large a quantity of blood was poured into the bile-ducts and into the intestine that death followed from hemorrhage. In this case the walls of the bile-passages were thickened and showed connective-tissue hyperplasia, were hyperemic and covered with ecchymotic spots, and the blood within the passages was coagulated. The patient had at different times been a sufferer from attacks of colic, although no gall-stones were found on autopsy. Cases of this character have also been reported among patients with yellow fever, in sufferers from the hemorrhagic diathesis, in carcinoma and ulceration of the gall-bladder, in contusions and abscesses of the liver, and in aneurysms of the hepatic artery that have burst into the bile-passages (see the section on this subject).

If the flow of blood into the bile-passages is very copious, the signs of acute anemia may become apparent during life. At the same time the stools will contain blood, and occasionally hematemesis will be observed. If the hemorrhage occurs very suddenly, the bile is washed out of the bile-passages, so that the blood following is pure and can coagulate. These coagulates may in their turn act as obturators and cause obstructive icterus and spasmodic contraction of the bile-ducts. It is possible, therefore, to determine that the bile-ducts are the source of blood appearing in the intestinal contents.

Treatment can only be directed against the disease that is the primary cause of the bleeding. In only one class of cases could treatment of the hemorrhage itself be successful—namely, when it would be possible to diagnose an ulcer of the gall-bladder (possibly after typhoid fever) and to remove it by surgical procedures.

Schüppel: Loc. cit., p. 62.
Quinquaud: "Les affections du foie," Paris, 1879, cited by Schüppel.

SOLUTIONS OF CONTINUITY OF THE BILE-PASSAGES.

Rupture; Perforation; Fistula.

(Quincke.)

The different possible forms of solution of continuity of the bile-passages are:

1. **Rupture** of the distended or of the normal wall of the bile-passages from pressure exercised by the contents or from without. This is seen more frequently in the gall-bladder than in the bile-passages.

2. **Perforations** from ulcerative processes. These occur more frequently from within outward than vice versâ. They, too, are more often seen in the gall-bladder than in the ducts. Perforation occurs either into the abdominal cavity directly or into some neighboring cavity after adhesions have formed between it and the gall-bladder (fistula). Diseases of the bile-passages complicated with stones or those that are inflammatory in character, owing to the presence of stones, are most frequently complicated by perforations. The direct pressure of the gall-stones may also lead to ulceration. Ulcers of a typhoidal or a carcinomatous origin are comparatively rare.

There are also so-called "primary" ulcers of uncertain origin. They have sharp margins, are circular in shape, and resemble gastric ulcers. Budd draws an analogy between the two, and infers that the ulcers seen in the bile-passages are caused by the action of the bile on the mucous membrane of the gall-bladder. Glaser has reported a case of this kind in which perforation occurred.

The diseases that may cause perforation from without into the bile-passages are usually lesions of the liver-substance itself, as abscess, echinococcus cysts, and, less frequently, purulent inflammations of the surrounding tissues, such as circumscribed accumulations of pus within the peritoneum.

Whenever perforation into some other body-cavity occurs, the bile flows into it. In case the bile flows into the intercellular tissues, these become infiltrated with bile.

Symptoms.—If the solution of continuity does not allow the bile to flow into the intestine, or if the bile cannot leave the body through some other channel, it must necessarily come in contact with deep-seated tissues. As a rule, inflammation results. Until recently this inflammation was attributed to the chemical action of the biliary constituents. Recent experiments, however, have shown that, although the bile is normally sterile, and can produce but slight inflammation, in almost all cases where marked inflammation is produced the bile is contaminated by irritating products. In these cases, therefore, the bile itself does not produce the inflammation, but certain inflammatory products of the mucous membranes, pus, or bacteria play the chief rôle. As a matter of fact, pure bile is hardly ever poured into the peritoneal cavity or into the tissues even if the trauma that causes the abnormal exit of the bile in human beings is indirect. In those cases in which the bile-passages were diseased before the perforation occurred, the bile, of course, is never sterile, so that peritonitis, either circumscribed or diffuse, is the natural result.

The symptoms of such a perforation are altogether similar to those seen in any other form of perforation, as of the stomach or the intestine, and vary, like these, in degree, intensity, and virulence according to the nature of the fluid that is poured out. That a perforation of the bile-passages has occurred can be determined only from the history of the case and from the exact location of the pain. In those cases where normal or only mildly infectious bile is poured into the peritoneal cavity (as in trauma) the symptoms of inflammation, pain, and fever are very slight. The bile that enters the peritoneal cavity forms a strictly circumscribed sac of fluid that, to judge from the large quantity of albumin that it contains, consists in large part of peritoneal exudate. In some instances this fluid may contain flakes of fibrin or may be separated from the abdominal cavity by a capsule of fibrin. Langenbuch quotes a number of cases of this kind. Many liters of exudate tinged with bile may gradually be poured into the abdominal cavity, and yet, as I have myself seen, recovery may ultimately occur. Occasionally, a mild degree of icterus of the skin and the urine is noticed, although the flow of bile from the bile-passages seems to be unimpeded. This is probably caused by the absorption of large quantities of bile from the peritoneum.

Perforations of bile into the cellular tissue always cause inflammation, which with very few exceptions leads to suppuration.

The treatment is the same as in any other form of perforation followed by peritonitis. In those cases where it is possible to determine at an early stage of the disease that the perforation occurred from the gall-bladder it may be possible to open the abdomen and to drain the peritoneal focus of inflammation through an indirect biliary fistula through the skin.

3. **Fistulæ.**—Whenever ulceration of the bile-passages leads to adhesions with one of the neighboring organs, and when ultimately, as the disease progresses, the wall of this organ is perforated, we have a direct biliary fistula. Whenever a long tortuous passage of an ulcerative character passes through connective tissue or adhesions or through a portion of the peritoneal cavity that is walled off by adhesions, we have what is called an indirect biliary fistula.

Fistulæ usually start from the gall-bladder; next in frequency from the intrahepatic bile-passages. The following varieties of fistula are described in their order of frequency:

(a) *Gastro-intestinal Biliary Fistulæ.*—As a rule, perforation occurs from the gall-bladder into the duodenum, less frequently into the transverse colon, and still less frequently into the stomach. It is usually produced by stones, not so often by carcinoma of the gall-bladder. Direct perforation into the duodenum from the ductus choledochus as the result of impaction of gall-stones may also occur. The presence of such a fistula can be suspected in all those cases in which large concretions are passed with the stools. If icterus has existed for a time and suddenly disappears, a fistula of the ductus choledochus is more probable than a fistula of the gall-bladder. In cases of this kind the chances of subsequent infection are greater. Anatomic findings have taught us that fistulæ of the gall-bladder may occasionally heal.

(b). *External Fistulæ.*—Fistulæ leading outward through the skin rarely originate from abscesses of the liver containing bile. As a rule, they start from the gall-bladder. They are frequently indirect with a long channel. The external orifice may correspond to the position of the gall-bladder, which in these cases is, as a rule, dislocated; or, on the other hand, the fistulous passage may lead along the ligamentum teres to the umbilicus or to some other even more remote portion of the abdominal wall. [Porges * has reported a case of fistula in the thigh from which gall-stones were discharged.—ED.] Formerly fistulæ of this kind occurred only as the result of spontaneous rupture of an ulcerated gall-bladder; nowadays they are often made on purpose by surgical procedures or result against the wish of the operator as the result of defective surgical methods in operations on the bile-passages. Usually bile mixed with mucus and pus or with concretions is poured from these fistulous openings. Only in rare instances do we see one of these four possible constituents poured out alone.

If bile escapes through the fistula, and if, at the same time, some obstruction to the flow of bile within the liver exists, such an exit may be very desirable. We must refer to the surgical treatment of cholelithiasis for a discussion of the various points of view that have a bearing on this question.

(c) *Perforation into the Air-passages.*—This may occur in cases of perforating hepatic abscess or in echinococcus cysts. Occasionally cholangitis may produce it. The color and the taste of the bile in the sputa are usually perceived by the patient himself. In favorable cases such a perforation may establish drainage, the pus-sac may empty itself completely, and a restitution to normal occur. [Graham † has reported 3 cases of broncho-biliary fistula, and has collected 10 recent cases in addition to the 24 collected by Courvoisier.—ED.]

(d) *The establishment of a fistulous connection between the bile-passages and the urinary bladder* is a very rare occurrence. In cases of this kind gall-stones may be voided with the urine. In one case the establishment of the fistula was favored by the anomalous persistence of a patent urachus.

(e) The occasional occurrence of a fistulous communication between the bile-passages and the blood-vessels will be discussed in the section on the diseases of the latter.

Budd: Loc. cit., p. 163.
Langenbuch: Loc. cit., pp. 362 and 346 (literature).
Schüppel: Loc. cit., pp. 147 and 64 (literature).
Riedel: "Chirurgische Behandlung der Gallensteinkrankheiten," Penzoldt u. Stintzing's "Handbuch der speciellen Therapie," vol. IV, part 6b, p. 68.
Glaser: "Jahrbuch der Hamburgischen Staatskrankenanstalten," II, 1890.

Other diseases of the bile-passages that merit discussion are neoplasms, parasites, and foreign bodies in the bile-passages. The neoplasms and the parasites are clinically so closely related to those seen in the liver that it appears to be more practical to discuss them together. Among the foreign bodies that are found in the bile-passages, or rather among the abnormalities of the contents of the bile-passages, concretions are by far the most important. These will be discussed in a separate section and their rôle in the production of a variety of diseases explained. We will only mention in this place that other substances that occlude the lumen of the bile-passages may produce symptoms similar to those of gall-stones, such as icterus and attacks of pain. Among these are echinococcus, distomata, ascarides, and blood-clots. All these are found much less frequently than gall-stones; but their presence must always

* *Wien. klin. Woch.*, 1900, No. 26.
† *Brit. Med. Jour.*, June 5, 1899, p. 1397, and *Trans. Assoc. of American Physicians*, vol. XII, p. 247.

be considered, and if possible excluded. [Membranous casts apparently formed within the gall-bladder have been found in the feces following an attack of obstructive jaundice.—ED.]

CHOLELITHIASIS.

(Hoppe-Seyler.)

HISTORICAL.

Gall-stones are seen so frequently nowadays that it is astonishing to find so little mention of this condition among the medical authors of antiquity, who are otherwise renowned for the accuracy of their observations. No data are given in the writings of antiquity that allow us to infer with certainty that the physicians of that day knew of this disease or any description that would lead us to believe that cases described were sufferers from gall-stones. In Hippocrates and in Galen, it is true, we find a few brief communications on pain in the hepatic region, on icterus as a result of constipation without fever, but these descriptions, as compared to the precise and exact communications on renal colic, convey only a very inadequate idea of hepatic colic. Nowhere, further, do we find mention of concretions in the bile-passages and in the gall-bladder. The discovery of stones in the stools is mentioned, and we are possibly justified in seeing a connection between the two. In view of the fact that the old Greek physicians were good clinical observers, and at the same time thorough students of anatomy, we are forced to the conclusion that gall-stones were less frequent in those days than they are in modern times. An explanation for this difference might be sought in the mode of life. The people of Greece ate other food than we do, and their whole régime was different. The food, moreover, was prepared in an altogether different manner than nowadays; the meals were simpler; physical exercise was an important factor during the years of adolescence, forming a large part of the curriculum of every youth, and in later years the men continued to indulge in much and varied physical exertion; the clothing, too, did not cause anything that is analogous to our corset liver.

In the middle ages medicine made very little progress. It therefore does not astonish us to find little mention of gall-stones. According to Donatus, it is true, Gentilis of Foligno in the fourteenth century is said to have found stones for the first time in the gall-bladder and the cystic duct of a corpse that he was embalming. No definite statement in regard to this discovery is made in his works. In the fourteenth and the fifteenth centuries concretions were discovered in other organs. Gall-stones were first mentioned by Antonius Benivenius, who died in 1592. He describes gall-stones that were seen in the case of a woman who had been a sufferer from pain in the abdomen. They were found both in the gall-bladder and in a sacculated cavity on the surface of the liver. He assumes that the death of this patient was caused by these stones. Cœlius Rodiginus and Lange subsequently reported similar cases. Vesalius and Fallopius, in spite of their exhaustive anatomic knowledge, say very little on concretions in the liver and the gall-bladder. Fernelius, in 1554, gives a very good description of gall-stones and of the symptoms which they produce (by some error Frerichs has dated Fernel's work 1643). The author named seems to be familiar with the fact that occlusion of the ductus choledochus leads to a swelling of the gall-bladder, a white discoloration of the feces, and the passage of dark urine, and that, in occlusion of the hepatic duct, the gall-bladder is empty. He states, further, that the concretions seen in the gall-bladder are usually black and of a low specific gravity, so that they always float on water. According to this author, they are formed from bile when this fluid cannot be evacuated, remains too long in the gall-bladder, or is not renewed. He also states that they are seen especially where an occlusion of the cystic duct exists. The symptoms of this condition are frequently so indistinct that the disease cannot be diagnosed. Colombus (who died in 1557) reports that in the liver, portal vein, kidneys, and lungs of the Jesuit General Ignatius de Loyola numerous concretions were found, and Camenicenus reports to his teacher Mattiolius, 1651, on a case in which the ductus choledochus was occluded by a stone. In this case icterus was seen, and, in addition, numerous stones were found in the dilated ramifications of the portal vein. It is probable that in this case, as well as in the case of Loyola, as Morgagni says, the intrahepatic bile-passages were confounded with the branches of the portal vein. Matteoli believed that the formation of stones occurs from the thickening of the bile and mucus as a result of an elevated bodily temperature, following in this respect the old theory of Galen, who assumes that all concretions of the body are formed in this manner. The same author makes the statement that stones in the gall-bladder are probably more common than is usually assumed, and that they frequently pass unnoticed or are confounded with intestinal concretions.

All the authors mentioned so far were under the influence of Galen's teachings. Paracelsus freed himself from all these venerable beliefs and proceeded to introduce clinical observation and chemical investigations into the study of medical phenomena. Thanks to him, a complete revolution in the views in regard to the nature of gall-stones was brought about. His doctrine of "tartarus" is based on the belief in chemical changes within the organism. In his discussion on the "tartarus disease" (1563) he mentions stones in the liver as precipitates of impure material brought about in the same way as are wine-stones from wine. "Tartarus" could also be formed from the nourishment or through destruction of the constituents of the body. He believes that the bile coagulates tartarus. In order to avoid this, gastric digestion must be regulated by the administration of amara, acids, and carbonated waters, and the diet must be regulated in such a manner that tartarus is burned and metabolism is stimulated. Paracelsus was familiar with jaundice and the attacks of colic that accompany gall-stones. As in the case of gout, also attributed to the presence of tartarus, heredity is supposed to play a certain rôle and to predispose to gall-stones.

Johann Kentmann, in 1565, in an epistle reprinted in Gessner's work ("De omnium rerum fossilium genere") describes gall-stones of different sizes and shapes, and illustrates them. He states that the more numerous they are, the more they assume an angular shape, and that on the broken surface they seem to be composed of circular structures due to their formation from bile that gradually becomes thickened. Ferrandus (1570) publishes a case of rupture of the gall-bladder caused by a large gall-stone, followed by a pouring out of the bile into the peritoneal cavity. W. Coiter (1573) describes a case in which a great accumulation of gall-stones occurred in the gall-bladder and the ductus choledochus in a woman with icterus. In this patient violent vomiting of a bilious fluid was seen. In another instance he saw a severe form of icterus get well after the passage of a gall-stone by way of the intestine. Forestus is of the opinion that gall-stones are formed in those cases where the gall-bladder is not properly emptied and the cystic duct is occluded. He attributes icterus to occlusion of this duct, and states that it runs from the gall-bladder to the intestine. He also mentions that the feces are colored white on account of the absence of bile. He also states that Arculanus of Verona (1457) was the first physician to attribute icterus to an occlusion of the bile-duct following inflammation of the intestine, and that this investigator recognized that in these conditions the orifice of the bile-duct is occluded. According to Plater (1536-1614), concretions are formed in the liver and the kidneys as a result of an earthy consistency of the serum and a separation of the mineral constituents of the latter fluid, for which reason concretions may be seen at the same time in these two organs. He reports a case in support of his view. He was in part cognizant of branched stones in the hepatic duct that are difficult to remove so that they remain in the body until the death of the animal or human being. Cardanus also knew of stones of this kind, and says that they cause incurable pain. Fabricius Hildanus (1612) describes the lamellated structure of gall-stones. He found his specimens in a count who was a sufferer from icterus, his description tallying with that of Kentmann. Van Helmont expresses the belief that concretions are formed by the action of a peculiar ferment that has the power of causing the petrifaction of all substances that come in contact with it, basing his theory on the study of renal concretions. Scultetus makes the statement that icterus is not always found in occlusion of the bile-passages. He also mentions that carcinomata of the colon, of the uterus, etc., can cause retention of bile. Huldenreich expresses similar opinions and reports a case in which stones were found in the gall-bladder and in the cystic duct in addition to calcareous masses in the mesentery. Bonet, too, is a believer in this action of retained bile, and attributes a corroding action to this excretion and believes that a case of "peri-pneumonia" that he observed was caused by its presence.

The anatomic examinations of Glisson (1654) were of fundamental importance in the further development of our knowledge of gall-stones. He described stones that had the shape of coral branches in the bile-passages of cattle, and noticed that they were formed more frequently in winter, when the animals are fed on stable forage, than in summer, when they can eat fresh herbs and are driven to pasture. He even states that old concretions can disappear when the animals begin the new régime. He also describes (chapter xxx, page 265) his own case, and delineates a good picture of an attack of hepatic colic combined with icterus, and the peculiar pain of this condition radiating into the region of the clavicle. As he was unable to demonstrate the presence of nerves in any other parts than in the hepatic capsule and in the walls of the bile-passages, he states that the pain, in the absence of nerves within the parenchyma of the liver, must originate in the bile-ducts. Wepfer (1658) utilized Gillsson's researches to draw the conclusion that the bile is formed in the liver and is poured through the bile-passages and the common duct into the intestine. He deduces from this that icterus can never occur as the result of occlusion of the cystic duct unless the ductus choledochus be occluded at the same time. In one case of hepatic colic without icterus he attributes the disease to the presence of a stone in the gall-bladder. According to this author, the pain in the precordial region, and in that of the processus ensiformis, is due to the pressure exercised by the stone on the neck of the bladder. Bartholinus (1657), quoting from Tinctorius, describes the passages of three large three-cornered stones with the stool. The latter author saw a case in which violent pain in the right side was present and a considerable quantity of blood and pus was passed. He assumed that an erosion of the ductus choledochus had occurred and that the stone had passed into the intestine in this manner. Bartholinus, on the other hand, expresses the belief that all these symptoms could have been produced by a simple dilatation of the ductus choledochus, and describes cases of this kind that he had seen. Bobrzenski ("Sepulchr. Anatomic," Lib. iii, Sect. xvi, page 281) describes the appearance of numerous gall-stones in the ducts of the liver where the gall-bladder contained no bile but was filled with gall-stones. One of these was wedged into the cystic duct. From these findings he draws the conclusion that the bile is formed in the liver and is only stored in the gall-bladder, and that icterus appears as soon as bile accumulates in the bile-passages.

At the same period we encounter the first descriptions of the formation of abscesses as the result of gall-stones. Blasius ("Sepulchr.," Lib. iii, Sect. xvii, Observ. 13) describes in a cirrhotic liver an abscess containing a black stone. Stalpart van der Wiell and Thilesius describe the evacuation of gall-stones on opening an abscess. It is unfortunate that at this time the wrong idea of Sylvius, viz., that the bile is formed in the gall-bladder and is poured into the liver by way of the cystic and hepatic ducts and later mingles with the portal blood, influenced many of the investigators that followed him, even van Swieten declaring himself a disciple. Sylvius explains the formation of gall-stones by assuming that certain acrid and acid substances enter the body and mingle with the bile and blood within the gall-bladder and cause the coagulation of the latter fluid and of the bile. He seems to have been familiar with the symptoms of biliary colic, but states that these attacks originate in the colon. He also knew the symptoms of icterus, and describes the urine in this disease and states that it is dark in color and has the power of staining paper and linen yellow. Ettmüller gives a much more lucid description of all these conditions. In his dissertation entitled "De ictero flavo, nigro et albo" ("Oper. med.," Tom. ii, page 1, Colleg. pract., Sect. 17, Cap. 4, Art. 4, page 442) he speaks of pain (*dolor compressivus*) in the precordial region, that appears in icterus and is accompanied by nausea, difficult respiration, and a reddish color of the urine. Fever is described as frequently present and in many cases pain in the right hypochondrium, which may either be readily removed or be very difficult to cure, or, lastly, may be removable, but shows a tendency to recur. In cases of the latter kind stones are said often to be found in the gall-bladder. He states that colic and icterus are also sometimes seen after child-birth, and that icterus frequently follows the attack of colic, that icterus is frequently the result of an obstruction to the flow of bile into the intestine or of insufficient secretion of bile by the liver, as is seen from the fact that icterus may occur without any obstruction in the bile-passages, following fever, the bite of wild animals, abuse of blood-letting, etc. He further says that icterus does not necessarily always follow gall-stones, and that gall-stones may be present in the bladder without causing icterus. Ettmüller bases these statements on his knowledge of the fact that the gall-bladder can be extirpated without endangering the life of the animal, and he quotes the important experiment of one of the students in Leyden, who extirpated the gall-bladder in a dog without observing any bad results. He affirms that, if the ductus choledochus is occluded, no bile is poured into the intestine, the feces turn white, the bile regurgitates into the blood, and in this manner icterus is produced. This investigator also assumes that an acid or acrid consistency of the blood leads to a thickening of the bile as it is formed in the liver or after it has reached the gall-bladder, and speaks of a "sal volatile oleosum" that, he thinks, degenerates and coagulates in the form of gall-stones. He also speaks of spasm of the bile-passages transmitted from the intestine and causing a constriction of the ductus choledochus and icterus, and intermitting, so that the color of the feces is seen to vary at different times. He claims that the chief diagnostic clue for the presence of gall-stones must be their passage per alvum. Finally, according to this author, there is no remedy for gall-stones.

Borrichius reports a case of ulceration in the region of the liver following a severe attack of pain. A number of gall-stones were passed, their derivation being correctly attributed to the gall-bladder. This investigator, and before him Plater, Schneider, and Wepfer, report the occurrence of gall-stones and concretions in the kidneys in the same individual. An interesting case is described of a woman who was a sufferer from bilateral pain and urinary difficulties. She passed a few stones with the urine, but the pain in the right side did not cease, but, on the contrary, grew worse. Suddenly this pain, too, stopped, but no stones were passed with the urine. The author here made a correct diagnosis by assuming that at the time of the pain a gall-stone attempted to leave the gall-bladder, and finally did get out, as manifested by the sudden cessation of the pain in the right side. Later, he found the gall-stone in the feces, and was, in this way, enabled to verify his diagnosis.

The discovery of glands in the walls of the gall-bladder and the bile-passages was important for the understanding of gall-stone pathology. We are indebted to Morgagni for this discovery. He draws a parallel between the occurrence of gall-stones in the liver and the appearance of concretions in the parotid gland and other glands of the body.

Sydenham ("Prax. med.," Sect. IV, Chap. VII, Par. 16) has frequently been credited with discoveries that have thrown light on the pathology of gall-stones. In reality, however, he considered gall-stone colic as an hysterical symptom, and described its occurrence in female subjects who were sufferers from other forms of hysterical seizures. He describes the symptoms of cholelithiasis at great length, mentions icterus, but says nothing whatever of gall-stones. At the same period Tyson, in the "Philosophical Transactions," for the first time mentioned a fever of a septic type with transitory icterus. According to him, it is caused by the presence of pus in the liver and of gall-stones in the gall-bladder and the bile-passages. Morton attributed pain in the gastric region to gall-stones and the dilatation of the bile-passages by obstruction to the flow of bile. Baglivi, who directed particular attention to the chemical and clinical aspects of the question, mentions that the gummy portions of the bile are combustible, and that the bile is colored green by nitric acid. He also attempted to explain the occurrence, in the same subject, of gall-stones and renal concretions. Where obstinate icterus with a tendency to recurrence existed he positively assumed the presence of gall-stones and attributed the pain of gall-stone colic to spasmodic contraction (crispatura) of the bile-passages. Bianchi attributed the pain in the hepatic region to the hepatic plexus and to the sensitiveness of the surface of the liver and of the ligamentum teres; and believed that the painful irritation of these nerve-fibers causes the contraction of the bile-ducts followed by icterus. Gall-stones, according to this investigator, are never seen within the parenchyma of the liver, but only in the bile-passages. His pupil Guidetti reported cases in which gall-stones and renal concretions were seen at the same time. He also mentions (according to Lentilius) abscesses caused by gall-stones, and subdivides gall-stones into two divisions—viz., black, hard, non-combustible, and yellowish, soft, easily combustible, and having a low melting-point. He indulges in a number of exaggerated statements, attributing a great variety of ailments to the presence of gall-stones, and expresses the belief that, whenever present, gall-stones must necessarily cause grave symptoms. His treatment of gall-stones is quite correct. He advises the employment of rhubarb, herb extracts, and alkalies. Vater (1722) attributed the fever often seen when gall-stones pass to an irritation of the nervous system following the impaction and the passage of the stone through the narrow lumen of the bile-passages, just as Hippocrates had explained the same occurrence in the case of renal concretions. Vallisnieri, at about the same time, made the discovery that gall-stones are soluble in alcohol and turpentine, and draws the deduction from this finding that turpentine is a preventive of gall-stones. He expresses himself more cautiously, however, than Durande and many others after him even to this day, for he does not state that turpentine has the power of dissolving gall-stones after they are formed, but limits himself to saying that possibly it may prevent their formation and development. He explains the occurrence of icterus by spasm of the walls of the bile-ducts, and the pain by assuming that the walls are stretched and dilated and that the rough surfaces of the stone scratch their lining membrane. He also makes the statement that the passage of a stone through the cystic duct is more painful than through the ductus choledochus, and explains this from the relative narrowness of the former channel.

The passage, finally, of a stone from the common duct into the intestine is said to be particularly painful, owing to the narrowness of the external orifice of the duct.

Friedrich Hoffmann, in his "Medicina Rationalis Systematica," carries us a step further. He attributes the formation of gall-stones to stagnation of bile, and expresses the belief that eating little and at long intervals favors their formation. This is due, he thought, to the fact that normally the stomach should be sufficiently distended to exercise a certain pressure on the liver and in this manner favor the expression of the bile from the gall-bladder. According to this author, the chief predisposing factors are age, the abuse of alcohol, especially of beer, and the female sex, particularly at the time of the menopause and immediately thereafter. He attributes the radiating pain, particularly the shoulder pain, to irritation of the phrenic nerve. Colic, he says, is particularly liable to occur at night. A violent pain in the right hypochondriac region, followed by severe icterus and the passage of gall-stones in the stools, are given as important diagnostic signs. He also stated that if the gall-stones lie quietly in the gall-bladder no pain is experienced, but as soon as the highly sensitive bile-passages are dilated pain is felt; and also that gall-stones may grow in bulk by gathering bile within the ducts. His treatment consisted in the use of almond oil, milk, warm compresses, laxatives, ferruginous and alkaline waters. Tacconi described the occurrence of an abscess of the gall-bladder followed by the evacuation of a gall-stone from the fistula that formed. In this case icterus was absent, and the author explains this phenomena by the patency of the ductus choledochus. The same writer also describes an autopsy on a case in which hydrops of the gall-bladder was found following the impaction of gall-stones in the cystic duct. In 1742 Gottfried Müller observed a perforating abscess of the gall-bladder that burrowed through the stomach and the abdominal walls. The external opening was enlarged and the stone within the gall-bladder fragmented, notwithstanding which a fistula remained that continued to excrete bile and chyme. One year later J. Petit called attention to this form of suppuration of the gall-bladder after gall-stones, and emphasized the necessity of draining the pus. He only operated, however, in cases where adhesions were present between the gall-bladder and the peritoneum (as shown by immobility of the gall-bladder and inflammation of the skin). He advised puncture, the finding of the stone with a probe, enlargement of the fistula, and extraction of the stone. He points to the analogy with concretions in the urinary bladder, and makes the statement that the formation of stones in either case is due to some obstacle to the normal outflow of the contents or to weakness of the bladder-walls. These views of Petit were generally regarded as too bold, but van Swieten defends them. The latter writer has given us a splendid description of cholelithiasis and an explanation of the progression of the stone. He states that it is caused by the gathering of bile behind the stone combined with the pressure of the diaphragm and the abdominal muscles. He also remarks that large concretions can usually effect a passage through the narrow bile-ducts owing to the elasticity of the latter. He recommended the administration of opium for colic, and advised walking and driving for the expulsion of the stone. He claims that this facilitates the progression of the stone and prevents its enlargement. Schurig, in his work entitled "Lithologia," mentions many cases of gall-stones, the abscess formation, colic, icterus, etc., without, however, describing anything new (1744).

In the second half of the eighteenth century more light is thrown on the pathology of gall-stones. The etiology and the general symptoms of the disease are elucidated by the following researches and writings: The pathologico-anatomic studies of Haller and Morgagni, the summary of all that was known on the subject up to the time of Morgagni by the latter author, the chemical examinations of Pouillettier, Fourcroy, Vicq d'Azyr, Soemmering, and others. A great deal, too, was learned by all these investigations in regard to the composition of the bile. Haller saw a great many of the possible sequels and complications of gall-stones in his numerous autopsies (peritonitis, adhesions and perforation of the gall-bladder, contraction of the gall-bladder as a result of occlusion of the cystic duct, etc.). He found that the bile is not secreted in the gall-bladder but in the liver, and that certain substances can exercise a direct chemical irritation on the gall-bladder and the ductus choledochus, causing contractions of these parts. On these grounds he assumed the presence of muscular fibers in the walls of these organs, but was unable to demonstrate their presence. Sabatier (1758) gives some very good clinical descriptions of gall-stone colic, hydrops vesicæ felleæ, and empyema of the gall-bladder as a result of occlusion of the common duct. He also mentions the occurrence of ileus following the passages of large gall-stones, of which Boucher also reported an instance. Sauvage (1760), in his "Nosologia methodica," furnishes some very clear clinical reports. Morgagni delineated a very lucid picture of the state of knowledge of that day in his celebrated work, "De sedibus et causibus morborum." After carefully sifting and collating all the literature on the subject of cholelithiasis, he reports a number of original observations, and finally arrives at important conclusions in regard to the etiology, pathology, and therapy of this class of diseases. Occlusion of the bile-passages, according to this writer, is the result of a simple contraction of the ducts, a thickening of their mucous lining, compression of the passages by swollen glands, etc. This occlusion is always followed by icterus; if the cystic duct alone is occluded, icterus is not observed. The age of the subject, sedentary habits, and other factors are mentioned as predisposing causes. He gives a detailed description of the appearance, color, form, and structure of gall-stones, and opposes the erroneous view prevalent at that time that dark stones are seen in old people and light ones in young subjects. He further gives irritation of the glands of Malpighi in the wall of the gall-bladder as another predisposing cause for gall-stone formation. Gall-stones that remain quietly within the gall-bladder are said to cause no symptoms, and the same applies to concretions within the cystic duct. He gives as the most positive diagnostic sign of gall-stones the passage of concretions in the feces, and assumes that all concretions found in the feces must have passed through the ductus cholehochus.

Pouilletier de la Salle, Galleatti (1748), J. F. Meckel (1754–1759), and Vicq d'Azyr worked out the chemical aspects of the question. The first-named investigator succeeded in isolating cholesterin for the first time; the last-named drew a distinction between gall-stones that consisted of this substance alone, others that constituted a mixture of cholesterin and the yellow bile-pigment, and others that contained the pigment alone. Fourcroy found phosphoric acid in gall-stones.

Durande, in 1782, discovered that gall-stones were soluble in turpentine, and founded a method of treatment on this fact. He used both turpentine and ether internally. Soemmering, however, in 1793, expresses doubts in regard to the efficacy of these remedies, and does not believe that they ever really reach the gall-stones. According to the latter author, gall-stones are not formed from the thickening or the decomposition of the bile, but as a result of certain excretory anomalies of the bladder-wall and the formation of acids, as tartaric and acetic acids, within the gall-bladder, these acids being said to coagulate the bile.

The surgical treatment of gall-stones was inaugurated by Sharp and Monaud (according to Gottfried Müller and Petit). Bloch, in 1774, proposed the artificial formation of adhesions in the region of the gall-bladder. Chopart and Dèsault, F. A. Walter, and Richter improved these methods. Herlin, L'Anglas, and Duchainois studied the ligation of the cystic duct, and the incision and extirpation of the gall-bladder as early as 1767.

In his work entitled "Anatomischen Museum," published in 1796, Walter gives a good description of gall-stones of various forms and furnishes very good illustrations. G. Prochaska ("Opp. min.," Pt. 2, p. 219) succeeded in differentiating the granular periphery of gall-stones from their crystalline center. Coe gives a fair picture of the etiology and the symptomatology of cholelithiasis. Pujol, in particular, in his "Mémoires sur les coliques hépatiques," describes the diseases caused by gall-stones, based to a large extent on his own experience. He attributes the pain and the thickening of the gall-bladder to this condition. Contractions of the gall-bladder are said by him to drive the stone out of the bladder into the cystic duct, where the colicky pains are produced, the pain stopping either as a result of the cessation of contractile efforts, or because the tissues adjust themselves to the dilatation, or, finally, because the stone may drop back into the gall-bladder. He also states that almond oil may form peculiar concretions in the gastro-intestinal tract that may be mistaken for gall-stones. He gives a good description of the different steps in the diagnosis, and mentions as one of the most important clinical symptoms, that the patient complains of pain in the gastric region assuming the character of very painful tension as soon as pressure is exercised in the region of the gall-bladder. Portal, in 1813, described the dilatation of the bile-ducts if the larger passages are occluded, also the possibility of perforation of a stone into the intestine, the soft character of some of the stones, their nucleus and their chalky consistency. Bramson, Hein, Buisson during the following decades occupied themselves in trying to find the origin and constitution of gall-stones. Meckel von Hemsbach was the first to emphasize in a clear manner the significance of catarrh in the formation of concretions. Andral, Trousseau, Frerichs, and others furnished valuable contributions to the clinical knowledge of cholelithiasis. Fauconneau-Dufresne, in particular, gave very detailed clinical descriptions. Charcot attempted to explain the intermittent type of fever that is seen in diseases of the bile-passages and in gall-stones. His example has stimulated French investigators, in particular, to continue investigations on this question and on cholelithiasis. As a result, we possess a clear picture of cholelithiasis, thanks chiefly to the discoveries of bacteriology. Anatomic and experimental physiologic research have thrown a brilliant light on many of the symptoms of this disease. The formation of gall-stones, too, is fairly well understood, particularly since physiologic chemistry has taught us much in regard to the nature and origin of the different biliary constituents. Naunyn especially has contributed much that is valuable to this subject.

In regard to the treatment of cholelithiasis, the greatest advance has of late years been made in the operative treatment. This is due to the discovery and introduction of aseptic methods and the application of improved methods of operating. The first attempts at surgical treatment that we have described above made a very slight impression. Kocher and Sims are really the fathers of modern gall-stone surgery, they having first attempted cholecystotomy. Langenbuch later performed cholecystectomy, Küster and Courvoisier the operation of cholecystendysis. These were followed by methods for re-establishing the flow of bile into the intestine in cases where the common duct was occluded, cholecystenterostomy, choledochotomy, etc., first taught by Winiwarter and others. The experience that these surgeons gleaned has thrown a great deal of light on the general picture of gall-stone disease and its complications. In addition to the surgeons mentioned, Riedel, Kehr, Thiriar, Lawson Tait, and others have contributed much to our knowledge on the subject.

ɛ If we look backward over the long history of cholelithiasis, we see that even in the days of remote antiquity many physicians of genius possessed correct ideas in regard to this disease. As a rule, however, these correct ideas were buried under a mass of purely speculative deductions that were enunciated by authors of renowned authority in those days. As a result of this, the kernel of truth was lost. It was not until modern chemical, anatomic, and physiologic research constructed a solid and immovable basis of facts that these old theories were established on a stable foundation.

PROPERTIES AND CLASSIFICATION OF GALL-STONES.

Guidetti, the pupil of Bianchi, distinguished two kinds of gall-stones —blackish ones, that were hard and non-combustible, and lighter ones, that melted in the flame and burned. The former, according to modern investigations, consist of bilirubin-calcium and carbonate of calcium; the latter consist of cholesterin. Gall-stones are composed of these three substances chiefly. As a rule, cholesterin and the calcium compound of bile-pigment are mixed in about equal proportions. The stones generally show a concentric arrangement similar to urinary calculi, a peculiarity to which Kentmann called attention long ago. The different layers vary in color owing to the different proportion of contained bile-pigment. Generally the nucleus is soft and the external covering hard. In addition, a radiating structure can be discerned. This was first described by Morgagni, and was attributed by Meckel to the peculiar manner in which the cholesterin that the stones contain crystallizes.

As we have stated, the chief constituents are cholesterin, bile-pigment (particularly bilirubin) in combination with calcium, and carbonate of calcium. The following substances are occasionally present in small quantities: Phosphoric acid combined with calcium and magnesium, sulphate of calcium, bile-acids, sodium, potassium, free bilirubin, silicic acid, copper, manganese, and, in some animals, occasionally zinc. A little mucus is always found. There is also a peculiar nitrogenous compound that remains undissolved if the gall-stones are treated with certain solvents. This is probably a product of the epithelial cells that are destroyed while the stone is in process of formation.

On analysis of gall-stones it will be found that the different constituents occur in varying quantities. There may be over 90% of cholesterin (v. Planta and Kekulé). In the small, dark stones, consisting chiefly of pigment and calcareous salts, and found principally in the ducts, pigment-calcium and the carbonate of lime are the principal constituents. In this variety of stone copper, manganese, and iron in combination with bilirubin are usually found. Free bile-pigment is found only in traces in concretions and probably enters into their composition from imbibition. The same applies to the small quantities of bile-acids that are sometimes found. In the bile-passages, however, Virchow found a pultaceous mixture of bilirubin crystals and cholesterin. It is stated that uric acid is occasionally found in gall-stones (Stöckhardt and Marchand). It is possible, however, that in many of these cases gall-stones were confounded with urinary calculi. In addition to the ordinary bile-pigments, bilirubin and biliverdin, a number of other pigments have been seen that were probably formed from them—viz., bilihumin, bilifuscin, biliprasin (the latter, according to Maly, being identical with biliverdin). In gall-stones examined after they have been kept for a time, it is possible that many of these substances are simply decomposition or transformation products formed by contact with the air or from putrefaction.

The color of the stones is essentially dependent on the quantity and the character of the pigment they contain. The stones that consist of cholesterin alone are the only ones that are almost pure white. If they contain a small amount of pigment, their color may be golden yellow or greenish. If they contain much pigment, it will be reddish-brown to black. The stones are never uniformly tinted throughout. The cortex, the shell, and the nucleus are always colored differently. In the shell the peculiar concentric arrangement and the striated radiating structure are seen. The surface of gall-stones is sometimes scintillating like mother-of-pearl, particularly if the shell is formed by thin layers of cholesterin that has crystallized in horizontal layers.

The consistency will also depend on the composition of the stone. The more calcium-compounds the stones contain, the harder will they be. The lighter forms of cholesterin stones can, as a rule, be easily scratched with the finger-nail, or can even be crushed between the fingers. Young concretions are generally soft. The shell, if it consists of calcareous compounds, is usually the hardest part of the stone. Occasionally it is seen to be as thin as the shell of a sparrow's egg, the contents of the stone in these cases consisting of a gruelly mass of cholesterin.

The shape of gall-stones differs according to their number and their place of origin. If several stones of medium size are present in the gall-bladder at the same time, they become faceted when still soft; from the fact that they are squeezed together when the gall-bladder contracts. It is also possible that new layers, as they form, adapt themselves to the outline of their surroundings. Octahedral, tetrahedral forms, etc., are seen if several large stones are present in the gall-bladder. The surface of the stones turned toward the mucous lining of the gall-bladder is usually rounded and rough, while the surface that is directed toward the other stones is flat and smooth. This is rarely due to grinding and polishing of one surface against the other, as it is seen that on cross-sections the individual layers are distinctly developed at the different places where compression has occurred, although of course they appear a little narrower here than at the edges. If they are colored, the stain is more intense at the narrowest point—*i. e.*, at the points of contact. This may probably be considered as proof of the assumption that the change of form is produced by compression. Large isolated stones are round or oval, and usually correspond more or less in shape to the cavity in which they have developed—*i. e.*, the gall-bladder. Nodular, raspberry-shaped concretions are occasionally met with, these being formed from the coalition of several smaller stones glued together and subsequently covered by a common layer of new deposit. If numerous small stones are present, they are usually rolled about by the contractions of the gall-bladder, so that the mass assumes a spherical shape. Leaf-shaped stones and others that are twisted and distorted in many ways may be produced by the pressure of the gall-bladder. These, however, are comparatively rare. Within the bile-passages cylindric structures may be formed, and in some instances coral-shaped stones have been found similar to those found in cattle (Glisson). Sometimes portions of the stones are dissolved in the gall-bladder, or the cholesterin may crystallize; so that the stones are broken or nicked and fragments of different size and shape are found.

The Weight of the Stones.—In former days it was considered a characteristic feature of gall-stones, and one that distinguished them from other forms of concretions, that they would float in water. As a matter of fact, only dry stones do this occasionally. Haller has called attention to the fact that this is done to air-bubbles that they contain and that become incarcerated within the cavities and cracks that are formed when the stones become desiccated. Their specific gravity varies according to their composition. If a large central cavity is present, it is lower; if they contain a large amount of calcium and are very dense and compact, it is greater. Thus, Batillat found the specific weight as high as 1.966, and Bley 1.580.

[In regard to size the concretions vary greatly. From barely perceptible grains they may attain a size which, when they reach the intestinal canal, may be sufficient to seriously interfere with peristalsis or indirectly produce complete obstruction. Among the larger stones the following are noteworthy: Richter records one weighing three ounces and five drams removed from the common duct at autopsy. Schüppel states that he has seen one measuring 7.5 cm. in length, 4 cm. in width, and 12 cm. in circumference, and refers to one (reported by Meckel) which measured 15 cm. by 6 cm. Russell reports one measuring $5\frac{3}{4}$ by $4\frac{1}{2}$ inches. Thornton removed from the common duct during life a stone 2 inches long and $3\frac{1}{2}$ inches in circumference. Frerichs says that he has seen a number of stones measuring from 2 to $2\frac{1}{2}$ inches by 1 inch. It may be roughly stated that the size of the stones as a rule varies inversely with their number.—ED.]

If all these different properties and modes of origin are taken into consideration, the following classification of gall-stones may be attempted.

To begin with, we can subdivide them into small stones that are not larger than a hazelnut, and large stones that are as large as a hazelnut and larger. Haller subdivided them into round, white, solitary, and small angular, multiple stones. Walter differentiated between concrementa striata, lamellata, and corticata. Hein, according to their composition, divided them into homogeneous and mixed stones.

Meckel von Hemsbach arranged eight classes, some of which, however, represent different stages in the development of the same class of stones: (1) Multiple jagged stones; (2) multiple warty stones (usually formed from the former by impregnation with cholesterin); (3) brown, solitary stones of round or oval shape and with layers of different color;

(4) solitary, cholesterin stones formed from the foregoing and oval in outline, produced when the process of crystallization advances as far as the periphery; (5) granular stones without any defined structure, with a nodular surface and containing much calcareous matter and pigment; (6) black, jagged stones, small and fairly hard; (7) stones with a metallic luster, loosely constructed; (8) stones consisting chiefly of carbonate of calcium, fragile, nodular, brown on the outside and white inside. The latter class is very rare, Hein having found only five concretions of this kind among 632 specimens.

Naunyn, on the ground of his careful and thorough investigations, arrived at the following more consistent classification. He distinguishes:

1. Stones consisting of cholesterin alone. These are usually perfectly spherical, pure white or yellowish, rarely colored more intensely on their surface, and smooth. On transverse section no arrangement in layers is seen, but a clearly marked, radiating, crystalline structure is found. There are only very small quantities of brown deposit, particularly near the central portions of the stone.

2. Stones consisting of cholesterin and arranged in layers. These are usually quite solid and become fissured and cracked on desiccation. The color of their surface varies, and they are faceted. On transverse section several layers are seen, of different thickness and color. Of these layers the external ones are frequently amorphous; the inner ones, particularly near the center, crystalline. Starting from this crystalline center, long streaks of crystallized material radiate toward the periphery. In addition to cholesterin, which constitutes some 90% of their bulk, they contain small quantities of bilirubin- and biliverdin-calcium, with, in addition, a considerable quantity of carbonate of calcium.

3. Ordinary gall-stones of different size, shape, and color. To this class belong the greatest number of gall-stones. They rarely grow larger than a cherry and are usually smaller. They are faceted and of a brown or white, less frequently greenish, color. When they are fresh, they are often soft and can be easily crushed; on desiccation, they grow harder and contract without forming fissures. Their shell is hard and arranged in layers; their kernel is soft and mushy and frequently contains an irregular cavity filled with a yellowish, alkaline fluid. Macroscopically no crystalline structure can be distinguished.

4. Mixed bilirubin stones. These are usually about as large as a cherry or larger. They occur singly or in numbers of two or three, and are found either in the gall-bladder or in the bile-ducts. They are arranged in concentric layers of dark or reddish-brown masses that are rarely altogether solid. The nucleus is not laminated. On drying, the outer layers contract and form cracks and fissures. The different layers readily peel off, so that sometimes different spherical layers are shed, the middle layers often being lighter in color and consisting of large crystallized masses of cholesterin. Cholesterin is also found in the external layers (even though these may appear very dark in color, they may contain as much as 25% of cholesterin). The rest of the stone consists almost exclusively of bilirubin-calcium.

5. Small stones consisting almost exclusively of bilirubin-calcium. They are not larger than a grain of sand or at most a pea, and are seen in two different forms:

(a) Solid, black-brown concretions with an irregular nodular surface, usually soft, sometimes partly compressed and conglomerated. It is probable that the larger stones originated from these smaller ones. On drying they contract considerably and disintegrate very easily.

(b) Harder stones of different forms, frequently spindle-shaped, with a smooth or a slightly nodular surface, either steel-gray or black in color, with a metallic luster that is particularly apparent when they are powdered, hard, solid, and brittle. The larger varieties show a spongy structure. These small stones of both kinds consist in great part of calcium compounds of bilirubin and its derivatives. In addition to bilirubin-calcium, which constitutes the bulk of the stones, small quantities of biliverdin-calcium and some bilihumin (up to 60%), and rarely biliprasin, are seen. Free bilirubin and cholesterin are present in small quantities only.

Naunyn mentions the following varieties as rarities:

(a) Amorphous and incompletely crystallized stones of cholesterin. They look like pearls and contain a nucleus consisting of small masses of black bilirubin-calcium or mixtures of bilirubin and cholesterin.

(b) Chalk-stones that are very hard and consist chiefly of carbonate of calcium. These are either prickled or smooth, and inclose cavities containing cholesterin, pigment-calcium, etc. In ordinary gall-stones calcium carbonate is also seen either in the shape of spheres or in columnar arrangement. As a rule, this chalky material radiates from the center of the stone toward the periphery.

(c) Concretions with inclosures, and conglomerate stones. In some stones whose shell consists of bilirubin-calcium a cholesterin stone will be found in the place of a nucleus, or, vice versâ, a stone with a cholesterin shell will contain a bilirubin stone of dark color in the place of the nucleus. Different kinds of stones are also occasionally seen conglomerated and covered with a common shell. Foreign bodies proper are rarely found within gall-stones. The following substances have been found in them: A worm of the species Anguilla (Lobstein), a piece of a Distoma hepaticum (Bouisson), a needle (Nauche), the kernel of a plum (Frerichs). Small particles of mercury have also been found in the inside of gall-stones by Frerichs, Lacarterie, and Beigel, the patients being all subjects who had been taking mercury. Recently Homans has reported gall-stones in persons who had undergone the operation of cholecystotomy for the removal of old gall-stones; here new stones had formed around the sutures of the first operation. [Kehr mentions three cases of a similar kind.—Ed.]

(d) Casts of the bile-passages. These are rarely seen in human beings. They consist chiefly of bilirubin-calcium, rarely of cholesterin (Naunyn); they are more frequently found in cattle (Glisson).

Of the different varieties of stones enumerated, the large cholesterin stones (1 and 2) and the ordinary mixed stones are principally found in the gall-bladder and in its recesses; but they are also seen in the cystic and the common ducts, usually wedged in tightly and conglomerated in masses of several stones. They are frequently adherent to the mucous membrane, or the latter may send processes into and around them. Their surface is, as a rule, rough or warty. Occasionally they are suspended in the bile and are covered with crystals. The pure form of bilirubin stones are found in the gall-bladder, and also quite frequently in the ducts of the liver.

ORIGIN OF GALL-STONES.

Following Galen's original idea, the belief was prevalent for a long time that gall-stones were formed from the coagulation of the bile. It was imagined that this occurred as a result of an increase in the temperature of the liver. Paracelsus, by teaching his doctrine of "tartarus" and of the precipitation of concretions in the body owing to certain chemical processes, is the father of the conception that disturbances of the digestion produce an acidulation of the blood, the acids formed acting on the bile and causing the formation and precipitation of concretions (Ettmüller *et al.*). Even in recent years the view has been brought forward that during fasting and on an exclusive meat diet an acidulation of the bile occurs, and that, as a result, decomposition of the alkaline carbonates takes place, followed by a precipitation of the cholesterin and bilirubin-calcium that these substances held in solution. In this manner, it was believed, gall-stone formation could occur. In the eighteenth century a more exact knowledge of the different constituents of the bile was acquired and the theory was formulated that under certain conditions the bile might contain too much of one or the other of its normal constituents, and that in this case a precipitation would occur. This view has some adherents to this day. Meckel von Hemsbach, following an idea of Morgagni, called attention to the rôle of chronic catarrhs of the mucous membranes of the gall-bladder and bile-passages, and expressed the belief that such chronic catarrhs could be made responsible for the formation of stones (stone-forming catarrh). Dramson believed that when the bile contained much calcareous matter and little alkali, pigment-calcium was precipitated and led to the deposit of cholesterin. Austin Flint's and Dujardin-Beaumetz's theory of cholesteremia following excessive nervous work and cerebral activity (?) led to the theory that gall-stones were formed as soon as abnormal quantities of cholesterin were poured into the blood. Thénard assumed that a precipitation of bile-pigment occurred as soon as the percentage of sodium salts in the bile was reduced. Frerichs, too, was inclined to see a connection between the frequent occurrence of gall-stones in old people and the increased quantity of cholesterin that the blood of the aged contains. At the same time he assumed that an excessive formation of carbonate of calcium takes place as a result of catarrhal conditions of the mucous membranes of the bile-passages. Hein assumed that gall-stones are formed around plugs of mucus that, in their turn, are the morbid product of diseased mucous membranes; and, further, that changes in the composition of the bile within the bile-passages are followed by the precipitation of bile-pigment stones, and that these reach the gall-bladder and form the nucleus for larger concretions. Finally, he believed that an excessive quantity of cholesterin is formed later as a result of alterations in the tissues of the liver itself or from a tendency to fatty deposits. Seifert believed that the epithelial cells play a certain rôle in the formation of gall-stones, for the reason that they are frequently found in the insoluble residue of dissolved gall-stones. A number of other authors attribute some importance to desiccation of bile (Fernelius, Boerhave, van Swieten, and others). It is known, however, that the bile may remain for a long time in the gall-bladder,—as, for instance, in occlusion of the cystic duct,—and that this is followed by hydrops of the gall-bladder, but not by inspissation of bile. If bile is concentrated outside of the body by evaporation, no concretions resembling gall-stones are precipitated.

The investigations of Naunyn and his pupils have, of recent years, thrown a great deal of light on the question of gall-stones. A summary of all the results obtained speaks in favor of the old view enunciated by Meckel von Hemsbach. According to this investigator, all that is needed for the formation of gall-stones is a center of crystallization. Mucus, small particles of pigment-calcium, etc., are not sufficient to cause the formation of concretions. It is found that if small particles of cholesterin, bilirubin-calcium, etc., are placed in the gall-bladder of a dog after ligation of the cystic duct, all these foreign bodies are absorbed in the course of a few months (Naunyn and Labes).

According to Naunyn, stones in the gall-bladder originate in the following manner: The bile contained in the gall-bladder always contains some desquamated epithelial cells from the mucous lining. These, as a rule, show no degenerative changes. In old people, however, and in sufferers from tuberculosis, febrile diseases, or cardiac lesions, it will be found, on autopsy, that they are in a state of fatty degeneration. This is particularly the case if gall-stones are present in the gall-bladder. Within the desquamated cells are seen large and small droplets of fat or myelin. These collections of myelin leave the cell and conglomerate to form little balls of myelin. They consist chiefly of cholesterin. In addition to soft masses, hard ones are sometimes seen, which may be crystalline. In addition, we may see a number of swollen epithelial cells which are in part disintegrated and form heaps of granular brownish debris. Other structures are seen that are apparently formed from myelin, and in which a shell of cholesterin may be seen inclosing a kernel of brown, granular material. Around these bodies new layers are formed, and in this manner the little stones continue to grow.

Another mode of origin is the following: In human bile we usually find a sediment consisting of flaky, granular, brown lumps that are composed of brownish granules and yellowish pultaceous masses. These contain cholesterin (almost 25%), and still larger quantities of bilirubin-calcium (39% in one case), fat (as much as 20%), and alkaline salts of the bile acids (as much as from 15 to 20%), albumin, and mucus. From these masses the bile-acid salts are soon eliminated and concretions form in one of the following two ways: (1) They may become covered by a hard, thin shell of bilirubin-calcium while the center remains soft. In this case a crystallization of the cholesterin occurs, the bilirubin-calcium forms granular masses; and the two constituents, in their changed form, are then deposited on the inner surface of the shell, in such a manner that in the center nothing is left but some fluid, so that when the stone dries out a cavity is found in the middle. (2) The solid parts of the gruelly mass described above may form a soft shell of crystalline cholesterin and amorphous bilirubin-calcium, again leaving nothing in the center but some fluid.

These first predecessors of future gall-stones may in some cases be poured out with the bile. In case, however, stasis of bile occurs, they undergo further changes. The contractions of the gall-bladder force out all the fluid, so that the concretions are consolidated or are pressed together into conglomerate masses forming the above-mentioned raspberry- or mulberry-shaped stones.

Within the bile-passages small stones, consisting of bilirubin-calcium, are formed and remain embedded in thickened bile. These concretions are not simply formed from inspissated bile, but they contain a number of pigments, as biliverdin, bilicyanin, etc., that can only have been formed from bilirubin by oxidation. Naunyn assumes that bacteria are the primary cause of this oxidation. As a rule, stasis of bile occurs in all these cases.

Subsequently cholesterin is deposited in layers over these minute concretions, and the same substance penetrates into and through the little stones, so that they are infiltrated with cholesterin, which later becomes crystalline.

The different layers formed in this manner may either consist of pure white cholesterin or of cholesterin mixed with bilirubin- or biliverdin-calcium. The latter mixture, of course, is colored. The layers of pure cholesterin are, as a rule, thinner than those that contain the pigments. The central cavity for a long time remains filled with fluid. Further deposits of pigment can occur only if the bile comes in contact with the stones, while cholesterin can be deposited even though no bile reaches the stones.

The most interesting feature of the further transformation of gall-stones is the recrystallization of cholesterin and the infiltration of the concretion with this substance, a phenomenon to which Meckel called attention. He was aided in his attempts to explain it by his knowledge of geologic phenomena of a similar character. In the interior of the stone the cholesterin crystallizes in a direction vertical to the layers of the shell. Only in exceptional cases do we see a crystallization in a horizontal plane. The crystals are formed from cholesterin already present in the stone, which recrystallizes, and from cholesterin that filters into the stone at a comparatively late period of its development. At first, the cholesterin crystallizes in pockets within the kernel of the stone. In many of the stones no distinct nucleus can be seen, the different layers being indistinct and the general structure crystalline. Stones are also seen in which marked differences exist between the shell and the kernel, and in which the latter may have a geodic or stalactite structure. The recrystallization of cholesterin starts from the nucleus, and the crystals shoot out toward the periphery. Cholesterin that is present in the stone at this period undergoes recrystallization, and, in addition, more cholesterin filters into the stone and, in its turn, assumes a crystalline structure. The latter occupies chiefly the fissures, cracks, and canals within the concretion. A transverse section of the stone will, as a rule, reveal these processes with great distinctness. The calcium compounds of the bile-pigments are dissolved in the mean time or are mechanically removed, so that, under certain conditions, a pure cholesterin stone may be formed from a mixed, laminated stone. A stone of this kind will have a radiating structure and will show very little of its former laminated arrangement. As the result of contraction of the peripheral parts of the stone or of expansion of the masses of cholesterin that are being deposited in the interior of the stone, cracks and fissures occur, so that the layers of the stone are pushed apart. Those parts of the different layers that contained more of the pigments naturally assume a darker color. Sometimes this tearing apart of the stones, combined with the dissolving properties of the bile, may lead to a complete destruction and solution of the gall-stone (Meckel), and in this manner a spontaneous cure of cholelithiasis may be brought about. The metamorphosis of gall-stones, in general, may be said to depend on the proportion of concretion-forming or concretion-dissolving substances that are present in the bile. We can readily appreciate that this proportion must vary considerably when we remember that all gall-stones are distinguished by layers of different substances that are imposed one upon the other without any semblance of uniformity. In hydrops of the gall-bladder we may also see a destruction of gall-stones following the change in the nature of the fluid contents of the gall-bladder. In the same manner indentations and disintegration of gall-stones may occur in the intestine. In view of all these circumstances, we must concede that Meckel was at least partly correct when he stated that the cavities so often seen in the center of gall-stones owe their origin to the solution of the central nucleus.

The most important factor in the development of gall-stones is the formation of a large amount of cholesterin in the gall-bladder. The old view that cholesterin is formed after the ingestion of large quantities of fat is untenable, Naunyn and his pupils having definitely refuted it. The theory of Bristowe, according to which cholesterin is formed from the disintegration of the epithelial cells lining the gall-bladder and the bile-ducts, seems more probable (compare page 416). The amount of calcareous matter found in the bile does not depend upon the amount of calcareous matter circulating in the tissue-fluids or ingested with the food, as it is also a product of the mucosa of the bladder and ducts. In former times it was believed that an abnormally large percentage of calcium in the serum or the drinking of large quantities of calcareous water could produce cholelithiasis.

According to Naunyn, the diseased mucous membrane excretes a large amount of calcareous matter, and this causes the formation of sediments that contain bilirubin and that play a certain rôle in the formation of gall-stones. Steinmann has demonstrated experimentally that the albuminous products of the degeneration of the bladder cells mixed with egg-albumen and calcium solutions are capable of causing the precipitation of bilirubin-calcium, a substance which in a measure favors the conglomeration of cholesterin masses. That this is its mode of action may be deduced from observations on atheromatous cysts, where we have large quantities of cholesterin but no bilirubin-calcium, and as a result we do not see the formation of concretions.

In gall-stone cases a number of glands are also seen in the wall of the gall-bladder that are not normally present. It is probable that these abnormal glands are in part responsible for the increased formation of cholesterin and of the calcium-containing mucus. They have the same type of epithelium as does the rest of the mucous membrane of the gall-bladder (Adolf Müller).

Large stones that enter the bile-ducts from the gall-bladder continue to increase within the ducts. This is due to the fact that the epithelial lining of these passages is similar to that of the gall-bladder (according to Ranvier) and also secretes cholesterin and calcium. We are forced to this conclusion, if for no other reason, because gall-stones are often found in the common duct which are so large that they could not possibly have passed the cystic duct (Friedr. Hoffmann). The occurrence of gall-stones within the bile-ducts of animals that have no gall-bladder (for example, elephants) is another argument in favor of this supposition. In the smaller bile-passages no epithelial lining is seen, and for this reason, of course, no degenerative changes and new-formation of cells like that seen in the gall-bladder and the larger bile-ducts occurs. As a result of this, then, no increased formation of cholesterin occurs in this location.

From all that has been said, we learn that a diseased condition of the mucous membrane of the gall-bladder and the bile-ducts, leading to an increased formation of cholesterin and of calcium, is the primary cause of gall-stone formation.

The question arises as to how catarrhs of this character originate. There are two possibilities: The catarrh may either be caused by certain noxious agencies that reach the mucosa by way of the blood-current, or certain poisonous principles may be present in the bile and act harmfully on the mucous lining of the bladder by direct contact. On the former assumption, many authors have postulated a connection between cholelithiasis and a great variety of diseases. Among these are: certain diseases of metabolism, such as gout, rheumatism; excessive mental exertion, arteriosclerosis, etc.; certain infectious diseases, such as tuberculosis, typhoid fever, cholera, etc.; and, finally, disturbances of nutrition, such as the taking of too much food or too little food, eating at too great intervals, etc. (Frerichs).

With regard to the second possibility—*i. e.*, the direct effect of poisonous principles contained in the bile on the mucous membrane of the gall-bladder—different theories have been formulated. Some authors believe that stasis of bile can produce the catarrh for the reason that bile is a strong protoplasmic poison. This injurious effect of the bile on the epithelium would be exaggerated if the bile should decompose, and it was assumed that this occurred regularly in stasis.

In later years the action of bacteria has been adduced as the most important factor in the causation of the catarrh under discussion. It was formerly believed that the bile possessed distinctly antiseptic properties, the idea being chiefly based upon the supposed increase of intestinal putrefaction in cases of occlusion of the biliary passages and the apparently slight tendency of the bile and its contents to cause inflammation upon contact with the peritoneum. Several authors agree in the statement that the bile is a culture-medium in which bacteria could develop abundantly but not so energetically as in bouillon (Létienne, Mieczkowski, Miyake, and others). Talma has found great variability in the supposed inhibiting action of bile on bacterial growth in different species of animals and in the same species under varying conditions. Netter, Naunyn, and others claimed that the bile of animals is normally sterile. Miyake has recently in part confirmed their results, having found micro-organisms (except in 1 out of 76 animals) only in the lower portion of the common duct. Ehret and Stolz, on the other hand, have found the bile in lower animals by no means free from micro-organisms. Gilbert, Girode, and Naunyn found the bile obtained from human cadavers sterile. Ehret and Stolz and E. Fraenkel and Krause, on the contrary, find that the bile obtained at autopsy contains micro-organisms in a large proportion of cases.

Of more significance are the bacteriologic findings in human bile obtained during life. Mieczkowski found the bile sterile in all of 15 cases from whom it had been obtained at operation for some affection other than cholelithiasis; on the other hand, in 18 out of 23 cases of cholelithiasis coming to operation the bile was found infected. The same conclusions regarding the presence of micro-organisms in the bile in cholelithiasis have been reached by other observers. Gilbert and Domenici found, by both direct and cultural examination, micro-organisms in two recently formed calculi; in two old calculi no micro-organisms were found; in one old calculus bacteria were found by staining but not on culture; and on examination of an old and a recent stone derived from one patient the former showed no micro-organisms, while the latter contained colon bacilli. Gilbert and Fournier examined 36 gall-stones, including 3 from cattle. Of these, 22 (one of which was bovine) showed no bacilli; while 9 (one of which was bovine) contained colon bacilli. In two of their cases dead bacilli were found in the calculi, the bile being sterile. Since these observations were made they have received ample confirmation. It is, therefore, definitely proved that the bile is sterile in at least a large majority of cases without calculi, that in cases of cholelithiasis the bile contains micro-organisms in those coming to operation, that in recently formed calculi micro-organisms are usually found, that in old calculi micro-organisms incapable of growth may be found while the bile shows no evidence of infection, and that in an old calculus there may be no bacteria while a more recently formed stone in the same case may contain the colon bacillus.

In order to determine the significance of the presence of bacilli in concretions Gilbert and Fournier tested the permeability of gall-stones for bacteria; gall-stones were placed in tubes of bouillon, fractionally sterilized, and then the tubes were inoculated with colon bacilli. In five days bacilli were found in the center of the calculi. The importance of this finding is offset by the discovery of bacilli in the center of calculi, the surrounding bile being sterile. It has, however, a distinct bearing upon recurring cholecystitis in cholelithiasis.

The question as to whether the infection of the bile is to be looked upon as the cause or the effect of the formation of calculi has given rise to much discussion. The micro-organisms most frequently found are the members of the colon group and Bacillus typhosus. So constantly is one of these forms present that Gilbert and Fournier divided chole-lithiasis into two groups, those due to the colon bacillus and those due to Bacillus typhosus. There is sufficient clinical evidence to prove that there is a distinct connection between typhoid fever and cholelithiasis. Chauffard found that symptoms of gall-stones were present in only 10% of a series of cases that had had typhoid fever, while 20% of cases of cholelithiasis gave a history of a previous attack of typhoid fever. Ehret and Stolz have collected from the literature 32 cases in which either at operation or at autopsy typhoidal cholecystitis was found. In 20 of these gall-stones were present. Hanot and Milan found Bacillus ty-phosus in the center of recently formed gall-stones and in the walls of the gall-bladder and bile-ducts. Since these observations abundant confirmation of the frequency of infection of the bile in typhoid fever has been obtained (50% of fatal cases, according to Cushing). There is evidently, therefore, apparently some connection between infection of the bile by typhoid bacilli and the formation of gall-stones, although this infection does not necessarily lead to the latter. The determining factor may receive its explanation in an interesting observation made by Richardson. In a case of cholecystitis he found typhoid bacilli clumped "as if a gigantic serum-reaction had taken place in the gall-bladder." Similar large clumps of typhoid bacilli in the bile were found in five out of six cases of typhoid fever. In the sixth case the blood-serum had no agglutinating power. Richardson injected 0.5 c.c. of typhoid bouillon culture clumped by the addition of typhoid serum into the gall-bladder of one rabbit, two drops of ordinary bouillon culture of typhoid bacilli into the gall-bladder of another rabbit, and used a third animal as a control. Four months later all three animals died. In the gall-bladder of the "control" animal he found a small number of rounded bodies arranged in concentric rings; in the animal injected with ordinary typhoid culture nothing was found, while in the animal injected with the clumped culture the gall-bladder was contracted about a rounded concretion.

It has been proved by many experiments that the gall-bladder can readily rid itself of micro-organisms, and in purulent cholecystitis it is known that bile and biliary pigment (Ehret and Stolz) are absent—two facts which, in addition to the absence of constant infection of the bile, may account for the escape of some cases from calculus formation after typhoid fever.

The effect of stasis of bile upon infection of that fluid is decided. After ligation of the common duct micro-organisms were found in the bile by Charcot and Gombault, by Naunyn, and by Netter. Recent observations by Ehret and Stolz and by Miyake even more definitely prove this influence.

Attempts to cause the formation of gall-stones in animals throw considerable light upon human cholelithiasis. The injection into the gall-bladder of virulent cultures produces severe cholecystitis; the injection of attenuated cultures may be followed by the formation of concretions, particularly if the flow of bile be hindered. Gilbert and Dominici injected into the gall-bladders of three dogs cultures of typhoid bacilli, and in that of one dog the bacillus of Escherich. In none of these did concretions develop. Gilbert and Fournier injected into the gall-bladder of a rabbit a culture of Bacillus typhosus attenuated by heating a bouillon culture for ten minutes at a temperature of 50° C. (122° F.). Six weeks after the injection of three drops of such an attenuated culture into the gall-bladder the rabbit was found dead. The thickened gall-bladder contained bile of a slightly yellow color and two concretions adherent to the mucous membrane. Section of these showed a central, whitish portion, from which typhoid bacilli were obtained in pure culture, and a pigmented shell. According to Miyake and others, the injection of pure or mixed cultures into the gall-bladder may be followed by cholecystitis, but is not followed by the formation of calculi if no other factors are present. Ehret and Stolz found that diminution of motility of the gall-bladder, or anything promoting the accumulation of residual bile, aids the growth of micro-organisms within the gall-bladder, while Mieczkowski found that stasis of bile increased the virulence of the bacteria present. Cushing produced true biliary concretions by injecting typhoid bacilli into the gall-bladder of rabbits when there was simultaneous restriction of motility of the gall-bladder or its ducts.

The effect of foreign bodies in the production of concretions was well illustrated by a case reported by Homans. Twenty months after a cholecystotomy for cholelithiasis pain returned, and a second operation revealed that five out of seven calculi present had developed about the remnants of two of the silk sutures remaining from the first operation. Kehr states that he has on three occasions seen a similar formation about fragments of sutures. Jacques Meyer introduced small hollow balls of ivory and of clay into the gall-bladder of dogs and failed to see any evidence of stone-formation after one year. A small amount of sediment was noticed, but no concretion even in the cavity of the balls. Small pieces of agar disappeared completely. Mignot combined the introduction of attenuated micro-organisms and sterile foreign bodies. Attenuation was obtained by diluting cultures of the micro-organisms in bile through the addition of progressively smaller quantities of bouillon or of ascitic fluid. The attenuated organisms were injected into the gall-bladder, and, after allowing a time to elapse sufficient to permit of their becoming implanted in the mucous membrane, sterile porous tampons were placed in the gall-bladder for ten or twelve days. The tampons were then withdrawn and at the same time a small sterile foreign body was introduced and fixed to the wall of the gall-bladder. After the lapse of one or two months this foreign body was found covered by a deposit of cholesterin. Foreign bodies of a size sufficient to prevent their entrance into the cystic duct, impregnated with attenuated cultures, and placed in the gall-bladder soon became covered with cholesterin. A similar proceeding with the later extraction of the foreign bodies was followed at the expiration of six months by the formation of true stratified cholesterin stones in 7 out of 19 animals. Mignot, therefore, concludes that two causes are necessary for the production of gall-stones—a weakened micro-organism and stagnation of bile.

Miyake found that the injection of pure cultures of colon bacilli obtained from a case of cholelithiasis was followed by the formation of concretions only when the caliber of the cystic duct was diminished. When there was no obstruction to the outflow of bile, simple cholecystitis resulted from either the injection of bacteria, injury to the mucous membrane, or the insertion of foreign bodies. Similar conclusions were reached by Ehret and Stolz. These authors have demonstrated the fact that the presence of foreign bodies within the gall-bladder has the same effect as does mechanical hindrance to the outflow of bile because of the layer of bile between and around these bodies, so insuring the presence of residual bile and resulting bacterial growth.

The following conclusions seem at present justified:

1. Infection of the gall-bladder by virulent micro-organisms causes acute cholecystitis without the formation of concretions, the elements necessary to their production being absent in such cases.

2. So long as complete exit of bile from the gall-bladder is possible, a cure without the formation of concretions may occur.

3. Micro-organisms of attenuated virulence only produce concretions if the complete evacuation of bile cannot occur.

4. Foreign bodies have the same effect as obstruction to the outflow of bile because of the layer of bile around, between, and within them.

5. The presence of inflammatory products or of foreign bodies purposely placed or accidentally present in the gall-bladder may cause the formation of concretions by virtue of the residual bile about them.

6. It is possible that the "clumping" of typhoid bacilli within the gall-bladder may furnish an explanation of the frequency of post-typhoidal cholelithiasis.

According to all these experiments and the anatomic findings reported, it seems probable that the stone-forming catarrh of the gall-bladder and the ducts can be attributed to microbian infection. It is, further, probable that these germs penetrate the gall-bladder during certain diseases, and that their power is increased as soon as stasis of bile occurs. As a result of catarrhal inflammation, degeneration of epithelium and desquamation of dead and dying cells occurs. At the same time the mucous membrane continues to regenerate, new glands are formed, and these in their turn furnish a mass of degenerated cellular material. This process is followed by the accumulation in the gall-bladder.or the ducts of cholesterin and pigment calcium in about equal quantities. The concretions that are formed later, therefore, are composed of equal amounts of the two ingredients, and are more or less uniform in structure. Naunyn calls attention to the fact that wherever numerous gall-stones are found they seem to be exactly alike. He draws the conclusion from this fact that cholelithiasis is, as a rule, caused by one single infection and one lesion of the walls of the gall-bladder, and that recurrences of this condition are rare. In addition to the factors enumerated, all those agencies must be considered which, by obstructing the flow of bile, prevent the evacuation of micro-organisms, concretions, etc., from the gall-bladder. These agencies will be discussed below. They may consist in certain anatomic changes in the parts or may be rendered active by an irrational mode of life, etc. As a final result of all these factors, the gall-stones continue to enlarge and to consolidate until finally the picture of a fully developed cholelithiasis is presented.

The question arises as to how the bacteria penetrate the gall-bladder. There are two possibilities: They may either gain an entrance by way of the blood-current or they may be derived from the intestine. Both experimental and anatomic evidence is overwhelmingly in favor of the latter supposition, which is made particularly apparent by the fact that Bacillus coli, the micro-organism that is most frequently seen in the gall-bladder, has its natural habitat in the intestine. It is probable that catarrhal conditions of the duodenum and ducts have something to do with this invasion, and an analogy must be sought between this condition and the invasion of the ducts in catarrhal icterus, in both instances the germs that cause the catarrh having penetrated the bile-ducts. In those cases where a partial obstruction to the flow of bile exists in the ductus choledochus, and where stasis of bile obtains, such an invasion is favored. Foreign bodies and parasites (thread-worms, flukes, etc.) may act as carriers of bacteria, and may in this manner, in addition to causing irritation and impeding the flow of bile, be the direct cause of catarrh.

Concretions form in the intrahepatic bile-passages, particularly in the course of cirrhosis of the liver. This is due to the contraction of the hepatic tissues, which causes constriction of bile-channels and impedes the flow of bile. In those cases where the flow of bile is impeded by compression of the ductus choledochus or hepaticus, or where tumors, parasites, or gall-stones occlude the bile-ducts, not only does cholangitis exist, but concretions of bilirubin-calcium are formed. These enter the gall-bladder and there form the nucleus of larger gall-stones. The different stages of this development can be clearly seen in cross-sections of the bladder and ducts.

Fernelius and Forestus were the first to point out the significance of biliary stasis in the formation of gall-stones. All modern authors concede that this is the most important predisposing factor. The flow of bile may be impeded by adhesions in the region of the porta hepatis, occlusion of the bile-ducts by parasites, etc., compression of the bile-passages by tumors of the portal lymphatic glands, the head of the pancreas, and the duodenum. Diminished contractile power of the gall-bladder may also lead to stasis, as pointed out by Petit. Charcot claims to have found in the aged atrophy of the musculature of the gall-bladder, and as a result poor evacuation of the viscus.

Constriction of the body by tight clothing may also constitute an obstruction to the flow of bile. Cruveilhier found that corset liver and gall-stones are often seen together, an association to which Heller and Marchand have especially drawn attention. Rother found evidence of corset liver in 40% of all women with gall-stones, Peters saw the same in 23%, while Schloth, in 95 cases of corset liver, found gall-stones in 15.3%. Bollinger and Riedel advocate the same view. Lacing seems to cause stasis of bile, because, in the first place, the excursions of the diaphragm during respiration are impeded so that the bile is not forced out of the bladder as well as normally; secondly, the liver becomes elongated downward, the gall-bladder becoming dislocated to the same extent, and the cystic duct, as a result, becoming twisted or bent; thirdly, the cystic duct may be compressed, especially if floating kidney of the right side exists at the same time; finally, the catarrhal conditions of the stomach and the duodenum that are engendered by lacing, as well as the compression of these parts, may readily lead to catarrh of the bile-ducts and bladder.

In women the influence of pregnancy must be considered. The uterus, when it becomes enlarged, may exercise pressure on the bile-ducts and interferes with the excursions of the diaphragm and the action of the abdominal muscles on the gall-bladder. As soon as the child is delivered this abnormal pressure may suddenly cease, and we not infrequently see symptoms of the passage of gall-stones following the improved evacuation of the gall-bladder. The general ptosis of the viscera, the stomach, intestine, kidneys, and uterus, that occurs after pregnancy, also exercises an unfavorable effect, producing traction on the large bile-passages or torsion of the ducts (Weisker, Litten, and others). The frequent relaxation of the abdominal walls is not unimportant, as it impedes the normal evacuation of the bile as the result of the action of these muscles. Schröder examined 115 bodies of women who had died during the sexual period and who had been sufferers from gall-stones. Among these, 99 had positively been pregnant at some time; in 11 only could pregnancy be definitely excluded.

All the facts enumerated, particularly the influence of pregnancy and of lacing, account for the fact that the female sex is more liable to gall-stones than the male. Attention has been called to this by nearly all authors since the day of Friedr. Hoffmann. Craz states that in nearly all the women examined postmortem in Bonn gall-stones were found. Hein found that the relative frequency of gall-stones in men as compared with women is as 2 to 3. Fiedler found gall-stones in 15% of females and in only 4% of males, Roth (Basel) in 11.7% and 4.7% (a ratio of 5 to 2), Rother (Munich) in 9.9% and 3.9%, Schröder (Strasburg) in 20.6% and 4.4%, Peters (Kiel) in 9% and 3%. [Mosher * found that in America gall-stones were present in about 10%.—ED.]

It is not impossible that the sedentary habits of most women and lack of exercise play a rôle. Such a mode of life has been considered a predisposing factor in cholelithiasis since the days of antiquity. Thus, Friedr. Hoffmann, Haller, Coe, Sömmering, Morgagni, J. P. Frank, and others state that scholars and prisoners are frequently afflicted with gallstones. A long period of convalescence with enforced rest in bed is said to predispose to gall-stones. It is possible that in the latter case stasis of bile may occur as the result of the slight movements of the diaphragm and of the abdominal muscles and from the pressure exercised on the cystic duct by the intestines. Frerichs has explained the occurrence of gall-stones in the bile-passages of cattle in winter (Glisson) by the long period of rest in the stable; while Glisson is inclined to attribute it to the change in diet. According to Bollinger, liver-flukes are the true cause. Another factor must be considered in judging of the significance of sedentary habits, and that is the possibility of catarrhal conditions of the intestine and other digestive disturbances that readily follow such a mode of life. We have no reliable statistics in regard to all these questions, and, in the very nature of the inquiry, can hardly expect to procure them.

35   * *Bull. Johns Hopkins Hosp.*, August, 1902.

[Brockbank * has drawn attention to the relative frequency of gall-stones in cases of heart disease, and especially those with mitral stenosis. Among 1347 autopsies gall-stones were found in 5.4% of cases without and in 10.9% of those with cardiac disease. Mitral stenosis was accompanied by gall-stones in a larger proportion than was any other heart lesion. He found that, on standing, bile from cases of cardiac disease showed a larger deposit of cholesterin crystals than was the case with bile obtained from cases where disease of the heart was not present. Probably the more or less sedentary life led by these patients accounts in part for the presence of gall-stones among them. Passive congestion and repeated catarrhal inflammation of the gastro-intestinal tract and its related glands may play a rôle.—Ed.]

Certain anomalies of metabolism have been credited with an important rôle in the causation of gall-stones, among them being gout, rheumatism, diabetes, obesity, arteriosclerosis, etc. French authors claim that gout, in particular, predisposes to the formation of calculi. In men, however, gout is more frequent than in women, whereas the latter are more often sufferers from cholelithiasis. The rôles of obesity and of diabetes are altogether uncertain. Beneke found arteriosclerosis and gall-stones together, and has attempted to formulate some connection between the two. As both diseases are frequently seen in old people, this connection is probably a mere coincidence. Peterssen-Borstel, moreover, failed to find any relationship between the two conditions in all the postmortem examinations he made in Kiel.

It has been claimed, further, that the taking of too much food could favor the development of cholelithiasis. This statement can be proved as little as the inverse one that poor food or deficient nourishment plays such a rôle.

The abuse of spirituous liquors (beer, etc.), too much meat, and too much fat have all been accused of causing gall-stones; but no proof for these assertions has been forthcoming. The only possible connection would be a predisposition to intestinal catarrhs that might be created by an inappropriate diet. According to Friedr. Hoffmann and Frerichs, irregular meal hours, long periods of starvation, or eating at long intervals could act unfavorably, for the reason that under these circumstances the gall-bladder is not emptied as frequently as it should be, it being known that the bile flows from the gall-bladder chiefly during the time of digestion.

The rôle of heredity, chiefly advocated by Fauconneau-Dufresne from the experience of the spa physicians in Vichy, is exceedingly doubtful. [Ehret † has reported cholelithiasis occurring in four generations. —Ed.]

The increasing frequency of gall-stones with advancing years is very striking. Friedr. Hoffmann, Morgagni, Haller, Coe, J. P. Frank, and others have emphasized this fact, and it is established by all autopsy reports. As the latter alone furnish conclusive evidence, we are justified in believing that such a connection exists. According to Peters (Kiel), only 0.62% of gall-stones were found in subjects under thirty, between thirty and forty there were 3.24%, between forty and fifty were 4.44%, between fifty and sixty were 6.98%, between sixty and seventy were 9.53%, between seventy and eighty were 13.02%, and over eighty

* *Edin. Med. Jour.*, July, 1898, p. 51.
† *Nereins-Beilage der Deutsche med. Woch.*, May, 1902, p. 143

years there were 16.36%, etc. Rother (Munich) states that the following relations between the age of the subject and the prevalence of gall-stones exist: One to thirty years, 3%; thirty-one to sixty years, 6.9%; sixty-one and over, 19.2%. Schröder (Strasburg) gives the frequency as from birth to twenty years, 2.4%; twenty-one to thirty years, 3.2%; thirty-one to forty years, 11.5%; forty-one to fifty years, 11.1%; fifty-one to sixty years, 9.9%; sixty years and over, 25.2%. We see, therefore, that a gradual increase seems to occur with the progression of years. It is true, on the other hand, that in earliest youth gall-stones are occasionally met with. Bouisson found three gall-stones in a new-born infant with narrowing of the common duct; Portal saw stones in children both in the ductus choledochus and in the bile-passages of the liver; Frerichs saw gall-stones in a girl of seven years. [John Thomson * has reported a case of gall-stones in a new-born infant. Still † has reported cases at the ages of eight and nine months and has collected twenty published cases.—Ed.] The greater tendency to cell degeneration, with a resulting increase in the formation of cholesterin, in old people may be considered a valid reason for the greater frequency of gall-stones in the aged; and the same applies to arteriosclerosis, where, as we know, the percentage of cholesterin found in the blood is markedly increased. According to Kausch, the bile of old people contains more cholesterin than does that of young subjects. Another factor, according to Charcot, is the weakness of the musculature of the gall-bladder and the bile-ducts in old people as a result of degeneration of the muscle-fibers of these parts. The action of the diaphragm and the pressure exercised by the abdominal walls are also weaker (Heidenhain). Disturbances of digestion and catarrhs of the intestine are more frequent, food is taken at longer intervals, and the production of bile is smaller—all factors that favor cholelithiasis. Finally, it must be remembered that the longer a person has lived, the more frequently has he been exposed to conditions that favor the development of the various diseases of the bile-passages that may lead to gall-stones.

In reviewing the different statistical reports, and in considering, of course, only those that are based on autopsy findings, it will be seen that gall-stones are seen more in certain localities than in others. This may in part be attributed to differences in the pathologic material, as in one location (Kiel) the majority of the autopsies were performed on children, whereas in another (Strasburg) the subjects were nearly all older people. In Kiel, according to Peterssen-Borstel, gall-stones were found in 3.95%; according to Peters, in 5%; in Munich, according to Rother, in 6%; in Dresden, according to Fiedler, in 7%; in Erlangen, according to Schloth, in 7.2%; in Basel, according to Roth, in 9 to 10%; in Vienna, according to Frank, in 10%; in Strasburg, according to Schröder, in 12%. [Mosher (*loc. cit.*) found gall-stones in 6.94% of 1655 autopsies in Baltimore. —Ed.] Naunyn is inclined to credit the differences in these statistics to the fact that the observers examined for gall-stones with more or less thoroughness. The observation that differences seem to exist in various locations in regard to the frequency with which gall-stones are seen in people of different ages speaks strongly in favor of a special tendency to the disease in these locations. The finding of gall-stones by Schröder in Strasburg in 25% of people over sixty, by Rother in Munich in only

* "Edinburgh Hospital Reports," 1898, vol. v.
† "Trans. Pathological Soc. of London," 1899.

19.2%, and by Peters in Kiel in 11.3%, for example, shows an apparent local variation in frequency.

It is, *à priori*, probable that the disease would be found with greater frequency in certain places, as has been claimed for a long time. Even in the different provinces of Germany it may be said that the mode of life is different. In addition, the influence of certain endemic diseases must be taken into consideration, causing variations in the frequency of catarrhal conditions of the gastro-intestinal tract and of the bile-passages, and in this manner indirectly leading to cholelithiasis.

PATHOLOGIC ANATOMY.

Gall-stones are often found at autopsy. In Munich (Bollinger-Rother) they were seen 66 times in 1034 autopsies (that is, in 6.3%); in Copenhagen (Poulsen) 347 times in 91,722 autopsies (that is, in 3.7%); while Conradi excluded autopsies in children and found gall-stones 87 times in 4000 autopsies (that is, in 2.4%). Halk, in 4140 autopsies in subjects over fifty, found them in 29%; Hünerhoff (Göttingen) in 4.4%; Fiedler (Dresden) in 7%, Frank (Vienna) in 10%, Schröder (Strasburg) in 12%, Roth (Basel) 9 to 10%, Schloth (Erlangen) in 4%, Peters (Kiel) in 6%. [Brockbank (*loc. cit.*) in 1347 autopsies at Edinburgh found gall-stones in 4% of males and 15% of females dying from all causes, and Mosher in this country in 6.94%.—Ed.] As a rule, the subjects during life had complained of no symptoms of gall-stones. According to Poulsen, symptoms were present in only 8% of the cases. Other authors state that in many instances·the disease runs its course without producing any symptoms, and that, notwithstanding the presence of large accumulations in the gall-bladder, no disturbances in the flow of bile, no pain, and no inflammatory phenomena become manifest. [Kehr states that only about 5% of people with gall-stones are troubled by their presence. —Ed.]

Sometimes only one large stone is found in the gall-bladder; in other cases the viscus is filled with a mass of small concretions. The bile-passages within the liver may be completely filled with these small stones. In one case Friedr. Hoffmann counted 3642, in another Otto found 7802, and Naunyn has reported 5000. As a rule, in these cases, the stones are more or less uniform; but occasionally different varieties are seen. Walter was the first to report such a finding, and Hein states that in 632 cases he found multiform stones in 28. In the great majority of cases the stones are seen in the gall-bladder alone; they are less frequently found in the large bile-ducts and the bile-passages within the liver. Conradi, for example, in 97 cases that he examined, found stones in the bladder alone in 92 cases, in the bladder and the ducts in 10 cases, and in the bile-passages alone in 5 cases. Hünerhoff in 85 cases found stones in the intrahepatic bile-passages once, in the hepatic duct twice, in the cystic duct 8 times, and in 84% in the gall-bladder. Charcot is inclined to the belief that the stones that are found in the bile-passages may be derived from the gall-bladder in cases where the ductus choledochus is occluded. In general, however, the stones found in the bile-passages consist of bilirubin-calcium, and were formed where they are found.

Within the gall-bladder the concretions are usually free and suspended in fluid, but in some instances they are adherent to the walls of the bladder or connected with it by thread-like processes. In rare cases all the stones are found within a capsule of connective tissue that is subdivided into several compartments. A conglomeration of gall-stones of this kind may perforate into the intestine as a whole and be passed in the stools. These masses must be explained by the outpouring of a fibrinous exudate between the stones, the material thus poured out later being converted into fibrous tissue. In many cases the stones are seen embedded in the walls of the gall-bladder, either inclosed in little crypts (Hedenius) or in glandular excrescences (as reported by Malpighi). Morgagni saw the formation of stones within these structures of the gallbladder wall. In these cases trabecular hypertrophy of the connective tissue and of the musculature plays a rôle. Sometimes it appears as though the stones had exercised pressure on the walls of the gall-bladder, causing ulceration of its surface, and had succeeded in penetrating in this manner. This process would be analogous to the method in which the stones perforate the wall and succeed in entering neighboring organs. The action of the stones within the gall-bladder may produce indentations and separation of certain portions of the gall-bladder. Protuberances are frequently seen in the region of the exit of the cystic duct, the "bassinet" of French authors, which may cause a change in the channel of the cystic duct so that it starts laterally from such a diverticulum. Within the cystic duct gall-stones may form cyst-like protuberances, as is also seen in the ductus choledochus, where they may be very marked (Morgagni, Cruveilhier, Frerichs and others). Within the intrahepatic bile-passages cylindric and sacculated dilatations are occasionally seen in cholelithiasis, which in rare cases may form peculiar cyst-like structures altogether separated from the duct from which they arose.

Distinct changes can usually be seen in the gall-bladder, due, as a rule, to the mechanical action of the gall-stones, to the action of bacteria that have entered the bladder, and to stasis of bile. The gall-bladder, as a rule, is distinctly enlarged, and consequently protrudes below the lower margin of the liver. [In long-standing cholelithiasis the gallbladder is apt to be small and tightly contracted about the concretions, a condition produced by inflammatory thickening of the walls.—ED.] In corset liver the gall-bladder is usually dislocated in this manner together with a tongue-shaped piece of the liver (Riedel), from the fact that a portion of the liver in close contact and connection with the gallbladder is pulled down with it. The mucous lining of the bladder shows distinct evidence of catarrh, such as degeneration, desquamation and regeneration of epithelium, round-celled infiltration in certain locations, and here and there deeper destruction of tissue consisting in ulcerations of its surface. The inflammation may in some cases extend to the serous covering of the gall-bladder and in this manner produce adhesive peritonitis and adhesions with neighboring parts, as the abdominal walls, the duodenum, the colon, the ileum, etc. As a result of the chronic irritation the wall of the gall-bladder becomes thickened; the connective-tissue part of the wall increases, glands are formed, and in rare instances cysts containing cholesterin and devoid of an epithelial lining are present (Adler). The muscularis of the bladder, too, may hypertrophy, and in this manner the inner surface assumes a trabeculated structure analogous to the conditions seen in the urinary bladder (*vessie à colonnes*) in chronic catarrh of this organ and in lithiasis of the urinary passages. Within these indentations and spaces stones may become lodged and may enlarge there (Barth and Besnier, Charcot, Bouchard, Sonville, and others). Particularly in the case of rough angular stones do we see this sclerosis of the walls of the gall-bladder, as well as in impaction of stones in the neck of the bladder and whenever very many stones are present (Durand-Fardel). Hünerhoff in 57% of his cases found changes in the walls of the gall-bladder, in 20% the fibrous form being observed. In the beginning the musculature, as a rule, is hypertrophied, but later perishes altogether in the overgrowth of connective tissue. The latter, under these circumstances, assumes the character of scar-tissue and imparts a grating feeling to the hand when cut with a knife. Sometimes it calcifies, so that a calcareous mass is found in place of the gall-bladder. In other cases the gall-bladder contracts around the stones. Here, as a rule, it is surrounded by dense adhesions in which stones or fragments of concretions may be found. Under these circumstances it may be a very difficult matter to discover the remnant of the gall-bladder. What is left of the organ generally contains a few stones and a little mucus but no bile. The inner surface of the viscus is cicatrized and is no longer covered by epithelium. When a stone occludes the lumen of the cystic duct, or when ulcerative processes produced by stones occlude the canal and the neck of the gall-bladder, thus causing an obliteration of the viscus, hydrops vesicæ may occur. The inflammation of the gall-bladder may extend to the side nearest to the liver or may even involve the latter organ by direct continuity. As a result the gall-bladder may become anchored to the liver by solid bands of adhesions or the hepatic tissues may undergo sclerosis. If pus-forming organisms penetrate the gall-bladder when it is filled with gall-stones, violent inflammation of its mucous membrane with reddening, swelling, ecchymosis, desquamation of epithelial cells, diphtheritic changes, or even necrosis of the mucosa (Jacobs, Tadéac), may be seen. The necrotic parts in these cases are colored greenish by bile-pigment. In this empyema of the gall-bladder we find that the walls of the organ are infiltrated with round cells and are brittle, so that they easily rupture, and that the serosa is often adherent to other organs by fibrinous material.

Similar changes may be produced in the larger bile-passages (the cystic, hepatic, and common ducts) whenever gall-stones are present. Diverticula are frequently seen in the cystic duct containing gall-stones, the stones seeming to be arrested here whenever the duct is twisted. The ductus choledochus, too, may be very much distended by gall-stones, and particularly near its exit do we see concretions, for the reason that this portion of the canal where it penetrates the wall of the intestine is very narrow. Gall-stones lodge less frequently in the hepatic duct, for the reason that this passage grows wider as it approaches the common duct; only in cases where the latter is filled with gall-stones do we see them in the hepatic duct. In cases of this kind the wall of the bile-ducts is inflamed or even ulcerated. In some instances, owing to ulcerative processes, the walls become very thin and perforation occurs, or, as in the walls of the gall-bladder, fibrous thickening and hypertrophy of the musculature are seen. These various inflammatory processes may extend to the serosa and cause peritoneal irritation, fibrinous exudation, and later connective-tissue adhesions with neighboring organs. As a result, particularly in the case of the cystic and the common duct, the walls of the passages may ultimately become embedded in a mass of solid cicatricial tissue, and as this contracts a considerable obstruction to the flow of bile is produced. These changes are readily transmitted to the finer biliary passages within the liver, in which case cholangitis is produced; the bile-passages become dilated, especially if stasis of bile supervenes; and as a result we see proliferation of the interstitial tissues in the liver with new-formation of bile-passages—in other words, biliary cirrhosis. These processes develop particularly in those cases where stones are present in the intrahepatic channels. These passages, if the common duct is completely occluded, may become dilated to such a degree that atrophy of the true hepatic tissue occurs. In the midst of this atrophic tissue are seen the bile-passages that sometimes attain the size of a finger (Raynaud and Sabourin), a process analogous to the changes seen in the kidneys in hydronephrosis. If the pressure that the stones exercise on the walls of the bile-passages becomes so great that perforation occurs, the stones may wander into the tissue of the liver itself. In other instances, ulcers will develop and lead to the formation of cicatrices, and ultimately to obliteration of the passages or to stenosis. In this manner a cystic cavity may be formed within the liver. If pus-forming organisms penetrate the bile-passages during the course of cholelithiasis, suppurative cholangitis is the result, with all its serious consequences; such as necrosis of the mucosa, ulceration, perforation, and the passage of gallstones into the surrounding tissues. If perforation of the large bile-passages occurs, general or circumscribed peritonitis will be the result; if perforation occurs in the intrahepatic bile-passages, abscess cavities will be formed within the liver, the latter sometimes containing one or many gall-stones.

In this manner multiple abscesses may be formed that contain staphylococci, streptococci, Bacillus coli, less frequently Bacillus typhosus, the comma bacillus, and the pneumococcus. At the same time suppurative cholangitis may be observed. As the venous blood from the gall-bladder and the bile-passages is poured into the portal vein, microorganisms may be transported into this vessel, causing pylephlebitis, inflammatory thrombosis of branches of the portal vein, and multiple abscesses. In this manner large and small abscesses consisting of numerous minute purulent foci, varying in size from that of a millet-seed to that of a hazelnut (*abscés aréolaires*), are formed and involve the branches of the hepatic veins. In addition to suppurative processes, the presence of pus-forming organisms may cause other changes, as follows: if gall-stones are present and stasis of bile occurs, the microbes may penetrate the hepatic tissues proper and cause localized areas of necrosis (*hepatitis sequestrans*, Schüppel), the same form of hepatitis being produced experimentally by the injection of pyogenic organisms and other infectious germs into the bile-passages (Dominici). These gall-stone abscesses may perforate through the liver into passages that lead out of the body, thus breaking into the abdominal walls, the intestine, through the diaphragm, into the lungs, etc., and produce purulent inflammations of surrounding tissues and organs, such as pleuritis, peritonitis, etc., in the same manner as is described in the section on abscess of the liver.

Another complication of gall-stones that is quite frequently seen is carcinomatous degeneration of the bile-passages or of the gall-bladder. This is seen particularly in old people in those locations where the irritation and the pressure exercised by the concretions have caused cicatricial constrictions and thickening. Carcinoma is caused by gall-stones and not gall-stones by carcinoma. It has been stated that the stasis of bile caused by gall-stones can be made responsible for the formation of carcinomatous growths; that this is not the case will be shown at length in the section on the tumors of the liver and the bile-passages. Here, too, the typical changes in the mucous lining of these parts will be described.

Ulcerative processes occurring in the gall-bladder are particularly important for the reason that they predispose to perforation of the walls of the viscus and the migration of gall-stones into other organs. Accidents of this character produce fistulæ and inflammations in the surrounding tissues, and complications of this kind may altogether dominate the disease-picture.

The ulcerative processes described above may lead to phlegmonous inflammation in the wall of the gall-bladder. As a rule, however, they are seen in the wall of the bladder without undermining its structure, so that a simple perforation occurs that causes no symptoms while in process of formation. All around the ulcer inflammatory processes naturally develop and adhesions form between the different layers of the peritoneum. In this manner it is brought about that the stones or jagged fragments of the concretions, when they bore through the wall of the gall-bladder, do not enter the free peritoneal cavity but are received in sacculated diverticula of the peritoneum or in connective-tissue structures. Processes of this kind are apt to develop particularly in the region of the fundus of the gall-bladder. If the fundus is situated in the usual place, it is in contact with the duodenum and the transverse colon. The fundus, therefore, can readily become adherent to these parts and the stone perforate into these divisions of the intestine. If the gall-bladder is situated more toward the median line, adhesions will form with the second part of the duodenum and the pylorus. If it is situated more externally, adhesions will form with the second part of the duodenum, the right kidney, and the first part of the transverse colon. In cases where the fundus is dislocated downward to a considerable degree, as a result of elongation of the liver (corset liver) or dilatation of the gall-bladder, adhesions may form with the jejunum. In this manner stones may perforate into the duodenum (the most frequent occurrence), the colon, the stomach, the jejunum, or the pelvis of the right kidney, without, at the same time, producing any local inflammation of the peritoneum. Adhesions with the abdominal walls may also occur in those cases where the gall-bladder is in contact with it, so that the concretions are ultimately expelled through the skin. On autopsy remnants of such fistulous passages are frequently seen, represented by connective-tissue bands and adhesions, and by protrusions and diverticula from traction in different parts of the intestine. Occasionally an open fistula is seen; but, as a rule, the lumen is occluded by cicatricial tissue. In other cases, again, a round peptic ulcer of the duodenum may be formed at the point of adhesion corresponding to the opening of the fistula (Ottiker).

Gall-stones may, further, gain an entrance into masses of connective tissue formed on the serous surface of the gall-bladder and may remain there. In this position they may constitute an irritant and produce peritonitis, the inflammation sometimes extending and ultimately leading to the formation of much cicatricial connective tissue in the region of the porta hepatis. The stones may also migrate within the peritoneal cavity and may, as a result, be encountered on autopsy in almost any part of the abdomen (Thiriar), as in the iliac fossa (Lecreux), in the female genitals, etc. In the same manner they may occasionally wander to the convex surface of the liver, to the lower surface of the diaphragm, producing inflammation and ulceration on this location, followed by pleuritis with adhesions with the lower surface of the lung, or they may penetrate the lung and be expectorated from the bronchi (Leyden, Aufrecht, Courvoisier, Graham, and others). In rare instances they may enter the urinary passages or may wander through the remnant of the urachus, and enter the urinary bladder. This occurs if by some chance they reached the region of the umbilicus.

Perforation into the free abdominal cavity is comparatively rare. As a rule, such an accident is followed by purulent peritonitis caused by the micro-organisms that usually cling to the gall-stones; whereas, if the bile were sterile, such a complication would not occur. Perforation of this kind usually follows trauma, parturition, or violent attacks of gall-stone colic. In cases where only a partial infection of localized areas of the peritoneum occurs and the pocket of pus is sacculated, the pus may burrow along the descending colon into the pelvis, perforate the rectum or the vault of the vagina, and thus be evacuated (Schabad).

Fistulæ may start from the bile-passages in the same manner as from the gall-bladder and cause ulceration of their walls. In this manner the ductus choledochus may become adherent to the duodenum, the pylorus, etc., and later become perforated, so that gall-stones that were unable to pass the opening of the duct enter the intestine or the stomach by this route. The occurrence of double common ducts or of a common duct with two orifices must be explained in this manner. Occasionally multiple fistulæ are formed, such as between the gall-bladder and the duodenum, on the one hand, and the common duct and the duodenum on the other (Ottiker).

Large concretions principally pass from the bile-passages into the intestine in this way. In old persons who have died of ileus large gall-stones are often found that constitute an obstruction within the lumen of the intestine. As a rule, the duodenum is the seat of the obstruction, less frequently the ileocecal valve or the lower portions of the intestine; in rare cases the stone has been found in the vicinity of the sphincter ani. These concretions may be the direct cause of ulceration, gangrene, and perforation of the intestine. The intestine is irritated by the presence of the stone and contracts around it; at the same time the muscles of its walls contract spasmodically, so that great pressure is exercised in the region of the stone producing the accidents named. In rare cases the stones enter the vermiform appendix and produce inflammations of this organ and of the adjacent tissues.

Gall-stones may also perforate from the bile-passages into the portal vein. They may gain an entrance into this vessel either directly from the large bile-ducts after adhesions have formed between these passages and the wall of the vein, or by a gall-stone abscess of the liver causing circumscribed suppuration at the porta hepatis, eroding the vein and allowing the perforation of a stone into it. Many cases of this kind, that have been reported particularly in the older literature, are doubtful, as it is not impossible that the different authors confounded this condition with perforation into intrahepatic bile-passages.

In cases where cholelithiasis is complicated with much inflammation of the bile-passages (cholangitis and cholecystitis) due to virulent bacteria, the latter seem to penetrate the blood-stream, even though no suppuration occurs in these parts, and infect the heart. In this way endocarditic deposits may be formed on the leaflets of the tricuspid and mitral valves (Murchison, Luys, Mathieu and Malibran, P. Aubert, Netter and Martha, and others). [Oddo * has reported a case of pericarditis complicating hepatic colic.—ED.]

SYMPTOMS AND COURSE.

In many, in fact in the majority, of the cases of concretions within the gall-bladder or the bile-passages, all symptoms are absent and the condition is only discovered at autopsy (compare page 548). In some instances, while examining a patient for some other trouble an enlargement of the gall-bladder will be discovered that rouses our suspicion in regard to the presence of cholelithiasis. In some cases large gall-stones may be passed per rectum, and this may be the first symptom to reveal their existence. As a rule, however, symptoms make their appearance as soon as the stone begins to move and attempts to enter the intestine by way of the bile-ducts. Symptoms also appear when the stones are causing inflammation and ulceration of the walls of the bile-passages, or when stasis of bile occurs, and, as a result, pus-forming microbes gain an entrance into the bile-passages and develop there, causing violent inflammatory reaction. Complicated cases of this kind may be appropriately designated as irregular cholelithiasis. Whenever the stones, on the other hand, remain in the location where they were formed,—*i. c.*, in the gall-bladder,—they usually produce no symptoms.

A number of prodromal symptoms have been described that are said to indicate the impending formation of gall-stones. These consist chiefly in certain gastric and intestinal disturbances that are probably catarrhal in character and may extend to the bile-passages and there produce the stone-forming catarrh. It is, however, a difficult matter to determine to what extent catarrhs of the stomach, the duodenum, and the bile-passages precede the actual formation of gall-stones, and what is their true significance in this respect. In many instances a careful anamnesis fails to reveal that they were ever present. The same applies to catarrhal jaundice, which is said to predispose particularly to gall-stone formation owing to the stagnation of bile and the inflammation of the mucosa of the gall-bladder and the bile-ducts that accompany it. A review of the literature on this subject fails to yield satisfactory information.

The first symptoms as a rule, therefore, do not appear until the stones are formed and fully developed.

In cases where the stones remain quiescent and do not move, the patients frequently complain of a sensation of heaviness in the hypochondriac region. This sensation changes its location with changes in the position of the body, and is particularly annoying if the patient sits or stands for a long time, especially several hours after eating—that is, toward the end of gastric digestion. In cases of this character the patients may also complain of a dull pain in the right portion of the epigastric region, radiating toward the hypogastrium, the thoracic organs, the right shoulder, or the lumbar region. At the same time the appetite may be very capricious, periods of anorexia alternating with bulimia. Slight errors of diet may be followed by nausea and vomiting of bile-colored masses. Patients of this class are apt to complain of a "weak stomach." At the same time certain nervous disturbances may be present, such as

* *Rev. de Méd.*, Sept. 10, 1893, p. 829.

great irritability, depression, and a feeling of oppression in the epigastric and precordial regions. All these symptoms may lead us to diagnose or to suspect some trouble with the stomach or heart. A number of cutaneous sensations, as itching, burning, etc., may be experienced, due to nervous irritation. Among other symptoms must be mentioned disturbances of sight, of hearing (Alison), coryza, headache *(cephale lithiasique)*, migraine, neuralgias, etc. All these symptoms may be explained by assuming that the gall-stones irritate the gall-bladder, and that certain nervous areas are reflexly irritated, that certain neurasthenic and hysteric conditions of the central nervous system are caused in this manner, and that in this way the innervation of the affected parts is disturbed. The same effect is manifested in alterations that are brought about in the composition and the secretion of the gastric juice, chiefly in regard to an increase or a decrease of the hydrochloric acid, etc. Possibly the well-known aversion to laxatives (Cyr) displayed by these patients is based on similar perversions. Such substances as rhubarb, senna, etc., are said to produce dyspeptic disturbances.

Examination of the abdomen frequently reveals that the gall-bladder is enlarged so that it can be palpated; its surface will appear nodular; in exceptional cases, when the gall-bladder contains many stones, it is possible to feel the concretions within the bladder, particularly if the viscus protrudes beyond the margin of the liver. In cases of this kind the gall-bladder will feel like a sac filled with nuts in which the different stones can be moved about. Some authors state that a peculiar rattling sound can be elicited on auscultation. This, probably, is heard in very exceptional cases only. In many instances the gall-bladder extends very far downward to the region of the crest of the ilium, and at the same time is freely movable, so that the impression is created that the swelling is a tumor of the intestine or the mesentery, or that it is a floating kidney. This will be the case particularly when the gall-bladder is covered by the colon, a contingency which is, however, rare. As a rule, it is an easy matter to determine that the tumor felt extends up to and beneath the margin of the liver, and that it is freely movable with respiration and follows the excursion of the diaphragm, provided, of course, that it is not adherent to the abdominal wall. The liver in these cases is, as a rule, distinctly enlarged, due perhaps to stasis of bile, or, in the case of women, to the effects of lacing. That portion of the liver to which the gall-bladder is attached is often elongated downward, forming a tongue-shaped extension, as described by Riedel. If the cystic duct be patent, so that the bile can enter the gall-bladder freely, it will often be found that the size of the bladder increases and decreases, following the increased or decreased secretion of bile or the closure or opening of the sphincter of the choledochus. In exceptional cases it may even be possible to evacuate the gall-bladder by pressure exercised from without, so that the organ collapses into an empty, flaccid sac (Gerhardt).

If the gall-stones are situated in the intrahepatic bile-passages they remain latent. Only in exceptional cases is it found that they cause symptoms, either by exercising direct pressure that may be painful and cause enlargement of the liver, or by producing icterus. As a rule, in these cases, the symptoms are so indefinite that their diagnostic value is slight.

If the concretions are situated in the large bile-ducts, they rarely remain quiescent, but, as a rule, begin to move, and in this way produce symptoms of violent inflammatory irritation and of icterus.

As soon as the stones begin to move severe disturbances of the general health are noticed. Such disturbances need not necessarily appear in every case; we know that occasionally gall-stones are passed with the stools without having revealed their presence to the patient by any symptom that could be interpreted to indicate the passage of concretions through the bile-ducts. In some of the cases of this kind ulcerative processes in the wall of the gall-bladder or the bile-ducts in all probability favored perforation into the intestine through fistulæ (Fiedler), a supposition made particularly probable from the large size of the stones passed in many instances. Another factor that favors the passage of large gall-stones without symptoms may be gradual dilatation of the bile-ducts following the frequent passage of concretions, so that subsequent stones can pass through without any difficulty. This would be analogous to the dilatation of the ureters after the passage of many concretions from the kidneys. In general, however, the passage of gall-stones is accompanied by violent symptoms that have been grouped under the name of hepatic or gall-stone colic. The question arises, What causes the gall-stones to enter the cystic duct from the gall-bladder and to move along the bile-ducts?

The following are some of the causes of characteristic attacks of gall-stone colic: Violent movements of the body; all kinds of succussion, such as horseback-riding, driving, dancing, jumping, etc.; stretching of the body for the purpose of reaching some object above the head; gastric and intestinal disturbances following the excessive ingestion of food or drink; and, finally, attacks of colic are often seen to follow the removal of tumors from the abdomen, the delivery of a child, the appearance of menstruation. Psychic excitement, anger, fright, and excitement of various kinds have for a long time been regarded as factors that predispose to attacks of gall-stone colic.

Of late years the action of the musculature of the gall-bladder and the bile-ducts has been made accountable for the peculiar mechanical features of the progression of gall-stones during an attack of gall-stone colic. Formerly a great deal of significance was attached to the effect of the stream of bile itself. As the pressure of the bile, however, is very slight (according to Friedländer and Barisch, Heidenhain, and others, equal to only about 200 mm. of water), this factor can hardly be credited with such a rôle. On the other hand, contraction of the wall of the gall-bladder, capable of being produced experimentally in animals by irritation of the gall-bladder, and observed in human subjects, could very readily force a gall-stone into the cystic duct. As soon as the stone reaches the duct, it is grasped by the muscular fibers, which contract around the impediment, and in this manner hold it tightly in its position. Strong peristaltic action of the musculature of the bile-passages is often caused by active peristaltic action of the duodenum communicated to the bile-ducts (compare page 421). In this manner can be explained the coincidence of attacks of gall-stone colic with certain digestive disturbances, indigestion, catarrh, etc., accompanied by an increased activity of the intestine. The same is true of many cases in which a migration of gall-stones is observed during an attack of typhoid fever or in the course of arsenical poisoning. In these latter cases the intestine is irritated, as shown by the appearance of diarrheic stools, and, as a result, there is increased peristalsis of the intestine that, as we have seen, can be communicated to the bile-ducts. If, in emergencies of this kind, the bile-passages are filled with bile (and this will usually be the case in digestive disturbances following the ingestion of too abundant or unsuitable food), the latter will have a tendency to force the stones forward in the bile-ducts, for the reason that it is itself being propelled forward by the pressure of the muscles of the gall-bladder and the duct that contract behind it. In cases where the body is violently shaken, a displacement of the stones may occur, and at the same time the stones moving to and fro within the narrow passage will exercise an irritation on the mucous lining of the ducts, and indirectly on the musculature, that will be followed by expulsive efforts. Patients under these circumstances frequently complain of a feeling of distress or of pain in the region of the gall-bladder or of the bile-ducts without at the same time developing any of the symptoms of impaction of gall-stones. The symptoms enumerated are, of course, due to the irritation exercised by the stones on the mucous lining of the bile-ducts and the gall-bladder. An irritation of this character may lead to muscular contractions of the walls of the parts, and in this way produce the same result as the other factors already mentioned.

Contraction of the abdominal muscles also has a certain significance in the expulsion of gall-stones. Such contractions followed by colic may occur after stretching movements of the body, after coughing, defecation, etc. This will be particularly the case if the gall-bladder and the bile-ducts are filled with bile, as is the case after a full meal, dinner or supper, at the time of digestion.

It is not quite easy to understand the effect that certain psychic alterations, such as emotional disturbances, sorrow, fright, etc., seem to exercise on the propulsion of gall-stones. The supposition that they influence the peristaltic action of the bile-passages in the same manner as they affect the musculature of the stomach and the intestine must be considered, especially as fibers of the vagus and the splanchnics innervate the musculature of the bile-passages and the duodenal sphincter of the common duct. Attacks of hepatic colic following nervous excitement without the presence of concretions can be best explained on the same basis. The possibility that the various emotions may exercise a cholagogue action is not probable, but cannot, at the same time, be completely ignored. Another factor that must be considered is the contraction of the abdominal muscles that occurs during laughing, crying, sobbing, etc.

It is probable that a certain nervous factor is responsible for the occurrence of gall-stone colic following menstruation. There can be no doubt that in many cases the peristaltic action of the intestine is stimulated during menstruation. It is possible that this peristalsis may occasionally be so excessive that it is transferred to the bile-ducts and the gall-bladder.

Pregnancy and abdominal tumors have a twofold effect on gall-stones, for, on the one hand, the increased abdominal pressure present in these conditions favors the formation of gall-stones, and, on the other, the pressure exercised on the gall-bladder favors the expulsion of gall-stones that are already formed. As soon as the great abdominal pressure is relieved by the delivery of the child or the removal of the tumor, the gall-stones will enter the narrower portions of the ducts, whereas previously they were located in the wider portions filled with bile. In this manner they produce symptoms of impaction by irritating the mucous lining of the ducts, producing spasmodic contractions of the walls, etc. During parturition it is not impossible that the action of the abdominal muscles favors the propulsion of gall-stones along the bile-ducts.

Riedel makes an inflammatory exudation of fluid into the gall-bladder and the bile-passages responsible for gall-stone colic. According to this investigator, the mucous membrane of these parts swells as a result of the irritation exercised by the concretions, the lumen of the passages becomes occluded, and in the parts behind the obstruction, following an extension of the inflammation, exudation is seen. All this causes the pressure within the bile-ducts to rise. It is possible that inflammatory irritation of this kind may occasionally be observed, but it can hardly be considered the exclusive cause of colic. [He distinguishes two kinds of jaundice from gall-stones—"inflammatory" and "true lithogenous icterus."—ED.] Riedel bases his views on his experience during operations. In the majority of his cases, however, old foci of inflammation of the bile-ducts and of the surrounding tissues were present. In uncomplicated gall-stone colic no inflammatory symptoms are demonstrable after the passage of the stone, as is the case after attacks of nephrolithiasis. As a rule, normal conditions are re-established almost at once after the stone has passed, so that we are hardly justified in assuming that a very strong inflammatory irritation occurs. [It is possible that the difference in the views of Riedel and, for example, Naunyn arise from the fact that Riedel has reached his conclusions from cases requiring surgical interference—in other words, cases of gall-stone colic plus inflammatory conditions.—ED.]

Numerous obstacles exist to the free propulsion of gall-stones. As soon as they leave the gall-bladder they enter the narrow cystic duct, where they can progress only with difficulty. This duct forms an angle very soon after leaving the gall-bladder, runs a tortuous course throughout, and, being attached to the neck of the gall-bladder by a mesentery, is prevented from becoming very much distended. In addition, a fold of the mucous lining runs along the whole inner surface of the duct; in a longitudinal direction, it is true, but twisted in a corkscrew manner. For all these reasons even small stones pass the duct with difficulty, and in passing cause much pain. As soon as they enter the wider channel of the common duct they can progress more rapidly toward the intestine. As soon, however, as they reach the last part of the ductus choledochus,—namely, that portion that runs through the wall of the duodenum,—they are again arrested by the sphincter-like contraction of the muscular coat of the intestine that surrounds the orifice of the duct. At times this contraction may constitute an almost insurmountable obstacle. For this reason it will often be found that the stones remain in the common duct for a long time or even permanently. For a time they may cause some disturbances, but ultimately show a tendency to become quiescent. In the latter case they produce no symptoms. If the stones are able to pass through the orifice of the common duct into the intestine, they cause most violent, spasmodic pain until they succeed in passing, when the pain stops suddenly.

Another serious obstacle to the passage of the stones is the spastic contraction of the musculature of all the bile-passages caused by the irritation of their mucous lining. Simanowski was enabled to demonstrate experimentally that the introduction of a foreign body into the ductus choledochus caused a contraction of its muscular fibers. This factor is probably less active in old people, for the reason that their musculature is atrophic. Riedel claims that another impeding cause may be the swelling of the mucous membrane around the concretion.

Very much depends on the elasticity of the walls of the ducts and the degree to which they are able to yield. This elasticity is probably considerable during life; much greater, at all events, than would appear from postmortem examination of the parts. After death it is frequently quite difficult to force even a very small concretion through the bile-passages. At the same time the natural elasticity of the bile-passage may be much hampered by adhesions with neighboring parts, the formation of cicatrices, tumors, etc., in the vicinity of the bile-ducts.

The size and the shape of the stone are, of course, very important. Very large stones—that is, stones as large as a hazelnut—probably pass the bile-ducts in exceptional cases only. In many instances stones of this character are expelled through fistulæ that develop in a latent manner (Fiedler). Rough and angular stones have a tendency to cause spasmodic contractions of the musculature, and become impacted very readily, more so than those which are round or oval. Faceted stones do not completely fill the gall-bladder, but allow some of the bile to pass. As a result they do not lead to such degrees of stasis of bile, and in consequence the *vis a tergo* is smaller. If long stones occupy a position transverse to the direction of the duct, they cannot pass. As a rule, however, a change of position is brought about, so that their longitudinal axis is pointed in the same direction as that of the cystic duct. Stones of this kind, if they are oval or cone-shaped, are particularly liable to cause gradual dilatation of the duct, by acting like a bougie. I once saw a gall-stone as large as an almond impacted within the common duct. It had almost passed into the duodenum, and was situated so that its narrowest, cone-shaped end protruded into the duodenum, while the bulk of the stone was still in the duct. The duodenal end of the duct was greatly dilated by the action of the stone. Stones that are very soft or have brittle walls may sometimes be broken by the contraction of the muscles of the walls of the duct, and in this way succeed in passing without any difficulty and much more readily than old, hard stones.

The forces that impel the concretions forward are approximately the same as those that cause the original migration of the stone and precipitate the attack of colic. The pressure of the biliary secretion is of subordinate importance in this respect, and has probably been overestimated. The pressure within the gall-bladder and the bile-ducts, however, is increased as soon as stasis of bile occurs. At the same time stasis exercises pressure on the dilated portions of the bile-ducts, ultimately acting on the constricting portion of the channel, and in this manner aiding the propulsion of the stone. As the portions of the bile-passages that are situated immediately behind the stone are congested with bile, pressure that is exercised in remote parts of the system of biliary passages is transferred as far as the stone. In this manner such agencies as contractions of the musculature of the gall-bladder and the bile-ducts, compression from tumors situated in the vicinity of the gall-bladder or of the liver in general, the action of the abdominal muscles or of respiratory movements, etc., may all help to increase the pressure behind the stone. As the fibers of the musculature of the bile-passages run in a longitudinal direction in man, a contraction of these strands must primarily cause a shortening of the bile-passages. As a rule, it will be found that the portion of the bile-duct situated behind the stone is filled with bile, while that situated in front of the stone is empty. Naunyn has determined, by a series of animal experiments, that the contraction is most violent in the portion of the duct a short distance above the obstruction. As a result, the contraction will, in a way, pull the walls of the duct backward over the stone, and at the same time the stone will move onward in the direction of least resistance, that is, away from the portion of the duct that is filled with bile; in other words, the stone will progress toward the intestine. The assumption that the pressure exercised by voluntary contraction of the abdominal muscles is often brought to bear in order to aid the expulsion of the stone is seemingly justified, especially as we know that an increase in the intra-abdominal pressure can produce a dislocation of the abdominal contents in many different directions. In the majority of instances, however, the patients do not employ this adjuvant, owing to the consequent increase of pain. In other cases, again, it can be clearly demonstrated that the patients perform violent contractile efforts during an attack of colic. The same effect is exercised by the gagging and vomiting that occur during many of the attacks, since these acts cause violent contractions of the abdominal walls which certainly aid in the propulsion of the gall-stone. At the same time the evacuation of the stomach that follows vomiting is a valuable adjuvant.

In many instances the attack of gall-stone colic proper is preceded by certain prodromal symptoms, such as pain in the region of the liver or the gall-bladder, and a distressing feeling of pressure in the same region due to swelling of the liver, to the filling of the gall-bladder, or to the incipient irritation of the mucous lining of the bile-ducts by the concretion.

The attack usually begins with violent pain. Suddenly, as a rule after midnight or during the late afternoon hours, a boring, stabbing, or tearing pain is felt, this being usually so violent that the patients become very much excited, scream, or shriek, or moan. Women describe the pain as much more violent than the pains of child-birth. The pain is frequently localized in the right hypochondriac region, in the site of the gall-bladder. In many cases it appears to be rather in the epigastrium, or it may even be felt in the left hypochondriac region, in the mamma, etc. It radiates in all directions, toward the abdomen, the chest, the back, occasionally toward the right shoulder, the extremities, less frequently toward the genitalia. If the pain is most pronounced in the back and in the right side, the suspicion may be aroused that the case is one of renal colic. If the pain is felt in the epigastrium, the possibility of gastric pain—for instance, from gastric ulcer—must be excluded. The latter may be the case where the formation of gall-stones occurs within the intrahepatic bile-passages, as in this case the pain is located in the epigastrium. If the pain appears suddenly after a meal, the suspicion of some intoxication may be aroused. Respiration, in particular inspiration, is painful, for the reason that respiratory movements, by causing movements of the diaphragm, exercise traction or pressure on the sensitive parts. As a result, respiration is, as a rule, accelerated and shallow and of a purely costal type. The patients in their efforts to avoid all pressure on the part frequently twist the body toward the right side in order to relax the abdominal muscles of the right side as much as possible, and at the same time they draw up their legs or rest the chin on the knee. On the other hand, we not infrequently see tonic rigidity of the abdominal muscles and spastic contractures, particularly on the right side, notwithstanding the great pain that these spasms produce. The pain may remit temporarily, only to be renewed with greater violence. At times a long pause may occur, particularly in case the stone has succeeded in entering the common duct. As soon, however, as the stone attempts to pass the orifice of this duct the pain reappears with great intensity. The latter pain usually ceases suddenly. The pain may also stop in case the stone drops back into the gall-bladder, or if the spastic contraction of the cystic duct ceases, or, finally, if the stone comes to rest in the common duct. In case a feeling of soreness persists after the cessation of the violent pain, and the region of the gall-bladder is still sensitive, this indicates that the stone is still within the gall-bladder or the bile-ducts, but that the contractions of the walls of these parts have ceased. During motion or during digestion, however, the pain is very liable to recur.

The pain caused by the migration of the gall-stones (compare page 456) is chiefly due to the spasmodic contraction of the musculature of the bile-passages, as was first emphasized by Baglivi. It is also in part caused by the pressure exercised on the sensitive mucous membrane; in other words, it is a true colicky pain. Simanowski was enabled to determine that in animals violent pain was experienced and a contraction of the bile-duct was observed when foreign bodies were introduced into the ductus choledochus. Riedel, as has been said, attributes the pain to inflammatory processes going on in the wall of the bile-passages, and, consequently, does not make a clear distinction between this pain and that felt in ulcerative processes and in circumscribed forms of peritonitis.

The distribution of the pain follows, in general, the distribution of the phrenic and the sympathetic nerves. The irregularity of the pulse sometimes observed may be due to an involvement of the vagus system by which an influence is exerted, by reflex action, on the heart. In some instances the pain may be due to a swelling of the liver and an irritation of the nerves in Glisson's capsule. These nerves can easily transmit the irritation to the phrenic nerve and the nerves that anastomose with it.

As a result of the violent nervous irritation the central nervous system becomes excited, as is manifested by a variety of nervous disturbances of a general character, such as spasms, hysterical seizures, etc. (the "hystero-traumatisme" of Bychofski).

In many people the passage of the stone is accompanied by no symptoms whatever or is characterized by very slight disturbances only. This may be due to the slight irritability of their mucous membranes or to weakness of the musculature of the bile-passages, as is particularly the case in old subjects. It may also be seen in those who have been sufferers from repeated attacks of gall-stone colic, for the reason that here a gradual dilatation of the bile-passages has occurred as a result of the frequent passage of stones.

Together with pain, vomiting may be present, and, as a rule, vomiting

36

in this condition is very violent. At first remnants of food are vomited, later masses of material that are tinged deeply with bile. During vomiting of this character it is even possible for gall-stones that are in the duodenum to be vomited (Petit, Fauconneau-Dufresne, and others). The vomiting of bile is an indication that the common duct is at least not altogether occluded. In rare instances stones have been known to enter the stomach through some abnormal communicating passage between the gall-bladder and that viscus, and to have been evacuated *per os* in the act of vomiting. Occurrences of the latter character, however, are certainly very rare. Notwithstanding the violent and the persistent character of the vomiting feculent masses are rarely raised; this occurs only when a large gall-stone occludes the lumen of the intestine in some place; and in the course of regular cholelithiasis a complication of this kind can never occur.

A feeling of chilliness, or even a real chill, may be complained of in the course of an attack of gall-stone colic. At the same time a rise of temperature may be observed, the thermometer indicating temperatures as high as 40° C. (104° F.). In some cases a rise of temperature may occur without any feeling of chilliness, so that there is complaint only of the sensation of heat that usually should follow chilliness. Sweating is less frequently seen. The fever, as a rule, persists for a few hours only; rarely, for several days. It may, however, reappear later during subsequent attacks. In general, it may be said that the rise of temperature follows the attacks of colic pretty closely. In case the attacks are frequently repeated a rapid rise and fall of the temperature may at times be noticed; in other words, an intermittent type of fever. This fever is strictly differentiated from that type that Charcot has called *fièvre hépatique intermittente*. The latter is an expression of the septico-pyemic action of infectious agencies that have penetrated the bile-passages, the former is characterized by the close connection that is seen to exist between it and the attacks of gall-stone colic. The type of fever described by Charcot, it is true, is quite often seen in chole-lithiasis, but it is also observed in carcinoma, compression, etc., of the bile-passages. This is due to the fact that micro-organisms can readily penetrate the bile-passages in all these conditions owing to the stasis of bile accompanying them. Under conditions of this kind bacteria can readily exercise their deleterious influence.

[Special mention should be made of the not infrequent "ball-valve" action of a stone in the ampulla of Vater. Suspicion of the existence of such a condition should be aroused by recurring attacks of pain followed by chilliness, rise of temperature, and renewed or increased jaundice. Between the periods of occlusion the health may be but little impaired, although usually infection of the bile-passages causes a mild toxemia.—ED.]

It is for the present undetermined whether micro-organisms participate at all in the production of the fever that accompanies attacks of gall-stone colic. Numerous investigators have compared this type of fever to the fever following catheterization of the urethra, so-called urethral fever. It is quite conceivable that the severe irritation of the mucous membranes may be transmitted to the central nervous system and may cause a rise of temperature. In support of this view the observation might be adduced that the temperature returns to normal immediately on the cessation of the attack. Riedel attributes the fever to a transitory inflammation of the mucous lining of the bile-passages, even in the absence of bacteria. This view seems quite tenable. An argument against it is the fact that other symptoms of inflammation are frequently absent. As bacteria have occasionally been found on puncture of the gall-bladder during an attack of gall-stone colic (Osler), and as bacteria are, in general, frequently found in the bile-passages in cholelithiasis, the possibility that they play an important part in the causation of the fever under discussion cannot be denied, even though in many instances the bacteria found were not very virulent.

For a long time icterus has been regarded as one of the most important symptoms of gall-stone colic. It is true that icterus is not always present. If it is present, however, it constitutes one of the most important diagnostic clues. As long as the origin of the bile was misunderstood and investigators believed, for instance, that it was formed in the gall-bladder, the significance of icterus as a symptom in cholelithiasis was not thoroughly appreciated nor understood. Wepfer was familiar with the fact that icterus is absent in those cases where occlusion of the neck of the bladder alone existed; and Ettmüller mentions the fundamental experiment of a medical student in Leyden who extirpated the gall-bladder of a dog without causing any disturbances in the general health of the animal. It was not until the end of the eighteenth century that the researches of Haller, Morgagni, and others definitely cleared this question. Icterus can only arise in the course of cholelithiasis if the ductus choledochus or hepaticus or large branches of these passages are occluded. If, on the other hand, the cystic duct alone is occluded in the course of uncomplicated cholelithiasis, icterus does not occur, even though the gall-bladder be filled with bile and the occlusion be complete. Wolff stated that he had seen icterus in only one-half of the cases he observed in which the existence of cholelithiasis was demonstrated by the discovery of gall-stones in the stools. Fürbringer saw icterus in only one-fourth of his cases. In cases where the stone enters the cystic duct and remains there after the irritation of the mucous lining and the spasmodic contraction of the muscularis have ceased, icterus does not occur—a statement which applies also to cases in which the stone drops back into the gall-bladder or in which it enters the ductus choledochus but does not completely occlude the passages owing to its angular form or its small size. Again, a gall-stone may succeed in migrating into the intestine without having caused occlusion of the common duct that was sufficiently complete or lasted for a sufficient period of time to produce icterus from stasis of bile. In view of these different possibilities, it cannot surprise us to encounter cases that present all the clinical features of an attack of gall-stone colic, but in which icterus is absent. In the same subject a second attack may be complicated by short and mild attacks of icterus, or, again, the subject may become afflicted with severe and protracted forms of icterus. In other instances icterus may be absent for the reason that the gall-stones succeed in entering the intestine through a fistulous opening. We are not justified, however, in assuming that the formation of a fistula has occurred whenever we find gall-stones in the intestine without the occurrence of icterus, for we know that, particularly in old chronic cases of cholelithiasis in which a great many stones have passed through the ductus choledochus at one time or another, this passage may be so dilated that gall-stones can traverse it without causing any stasis of bile; or, on the other hand, the gall-stones may be faceted, and as a result allow a certain proportion of the bile to pass through the duct. Gall-stones that occlude smaller channels within the liver may not cause icterus because of the small size of the district in which stasis occurs. Icterus will only be seen if one of the large biliary passages or a number of the smaller ducts are occluded. Attacks of gall-stone colic of this kind, that run their course without producing icterus, particularly those that occur in the region of the smaller intrahepatic channels, present the greatest diagnostic difficulties. They are frequently confounded with cardialgia, symptoms of gastric or cardiac lesions, hysterical or other nervous seizures, intestinal colic, etc.

Icterus does not appear at the beginning of the attack of gall-stone colic. As a rule, several hours, often twenty-four, elapse before it is noticed. This can readily be explained. The gall-stone, as a rule, must pass through the cystic duct before it enters the common duct, where alone it can produce stasis of bile within the liver. Besides, it is essential that the stone become impacted in the common duct, and this does not always occur at once. The same applies to gall-stones that come from the intrahepatic bile-passages. They, too, as a rule must enter the common duct before they can produce icterus. But even in those cases in which the gall-stone enters the common duct at once or was already present within this channel icterus cannot occur until a certain amount of bile has been secreted, an amount sufficient to constitute a stasis of bile. The bile-passages behind the impacted gall-stone must be filled with bile before biliary constituents can enter the blood and cause icterus. Further, some time must elapse before the bile-pigments that enter the blood can color the skin, sclera, etc., sufficiently to make the coloration visible to the eye. Icterus, moreover, is difficult to detect in artificial light; for which reason, if icterus appears at night or in the evening, it may not be recognized until the morning.

In this manner it may happen that the true nature of the disease is not recognized for a day. Sometimes we must be content to make the diagnosis *post festum*, because the irritation of the mucous membranes and the spasmodic contractions of the musculature may have subsided before icterus appears and suddenly throws light on the diagnosis. In some instances icterus is of a transitory character, in others it may persist for weeks or months. It may persist long after the attack itself has subsided, as occurs in those cases where a gall-stone becomes impacted in and occludes the common duct. In cases of this character we see the development of hepatic intoxication (cholemia) which will be described below. In addition, we see intense coloration of the skin and mucous membranes, while in the icterus that accompanies ordinary attacks of gall-stone colic the coloration of the skin and mucous membranes is only slight.

At the same time bile-pigment is found in the urine. As a rule, the quantities excreted are very small, so that the urine is colored only slightly reddish-yellow. Bilirubin appears in the urine before it is deposited in the tissues, and, on the other hand, disappears more rapidly from the urine than from the skin, mucous membranes, etc. Consequently the absorption of urobilin can in many instances be demonstrated from an analysis of the urine before icterus appears, and, on the other hand, no bile-pigment may be discovered in the urine even though it is noticed that the skin and mucous membranes are stained.

Corresponding to the removal of the obturator, the urine becomes very dark-red owing to the excretion of large quantities of urobilin. This is due to the fact that as soon as the obstacle to the flow of bile is removed there occurs a sudden outpouring of a large quantity of bile that was arrested behind the gall-stone. In the intestine the bile-pigment is converted into urobilin and is voided as such in part by the urine. Urobilin can be recognized in the urine by spectroscopic methods and by the fluorescence seen on the addition of ammonia and a little chlorid of zinc. At the same time, it is not impossible that a part of the urobilin may be formed within the bile-passages, as sometimes bacteria enter them and inaugurate different processes of reduction, in this manner causing the reduction of bilirubin to urobilin. The consensus of opinion nowadays condemns the theory that the exclusive excretion of urobilin without the presence of any bilirubin in the urine is due to so-called hepatic insufficiency (*insuffisance hépatique*, Gubler); that is, a deficient formation of bilirubin in the liver; nor is it believed that the yellow color of the various icteric tissues is due to the presence of urobilin (compare page 445).

The obstruction to the flow of bile into the intestine and the consequent absence of bile from the intestine is manifested, further, by the passage of whitish or grayish stools containing very little converted bile-pigment or none at all. In this manner it is often possible to determine that occlusion of bile has occurred even after several days have elapsed. Even in the complete absence of icterus, the periodic passage of stools without bile-staining may lead us to suspect cholelithiasis, even though no attacks of gall-stone colic were at any time complained of. On the other hand, icterus of the skin and the mucous membranes may exist and attacks of gall-stone colic may occur, yet the stools retain their color. This may happen, in the first place, if the obstruction to the flow of bile through the ducts is almost but not quite complete, a small quantity of bile being able to pass, but the greater part being retained within the ducts; in other words, the quantity entering the intestine not corresponding to the quantity that is secreted. In cases of this kind the contents of the intestine may still be decidedly colored by bile-pigment. In the second place, complete decoloration of the stools may not be seen in cholelithiasis when even large parts of the system of bile-passages within the liver are obstructed with stasis of bile in these areas, causing some bile-pigment to enter the blood, provided that, at the same time, a small quantity of bile can flow into the intestine through those channels that are not occluded. The stools appear very dark and contain a great deal of urobilin whenever the obstruction of the cystic, hepatic, or common ducts is suddenly removed, so that large quantities of retained bile are poured into the intestine at once.

Enlargement of the liver and of the gall-bladder are also related to the stasis of bile. The older authors were familiar with this phenomenon, and Charcot has called attention to the fact that a swelling of these parts can be determined in almost every case of gall-stone colic if the patients are only examined with sufficient care. Particularly in cases of complete occlusion of the common duct do we find the bile-passages greatly dilated; the gall-bladder, too, enlarges considerably, provided, of course, that it is not contracted as a result of previous inflammations or that the duct that leads from it is not occluded. [More emphasis must be placed upon the absence of enlargement of the gall-bladder in long-standing cholelithiasis (Courvoisier's law). In primary attacks with but little thickening from previous catarrhal processes the gall-bladder may be distensible, but absence of gall-bladder tumor points strongly to cholelithiasis as compared to other causes of biliary obstruction in chronic jaundice.—Ed.] As a result of the rapid enlargement of the liver its capsule is distended and severe pain results. At the same time, a distinct contraction of the abdominal muscles will be noticed, particularly of the right rectus. Owing to this muscular rigidity and contraction, it is often a difficult matter to satisfactorily perform percussion and palpation of the liver, and to determine whether the organ is enlarged or not. In many instances, however, the enlargement of the liver is so great that it can be readily detected and the gall-bladder may be felt at the margin of the rectus muscle as a round, tense, elastic, tender swelling. In very rare cases it may even be possible to determine a swelling or a shrinkage of this tumor following the retention or the liberation of bile when the cystic duct is alternately occluded and patent. Different factors may lead to this: new stones may cause occlusion of the cystic duct after the first one has passed, or the original stone may change its location so that in one position it occludes the duct and in another permits the bile to pass. Again, an increase or a decrease in the degree of spasmodic contracture of the musculature of the duct or the secretion of inflammatory exudates into the duct may all lead to alternate occlusion and patency of the channel. In cases in which the cystic duct alone is occluded, the gall-bladder alone may be enlarged; in cases, on the other hand, in which the common duct is occluded both the liver and the gall-bladder are liable to swell. As soon as the gall-stones have passed, the swelling is reduced very rapidly and the tenderness ceases. In cases, of course, that are complicated—where, for instance, a severe degree of cholangitis or of cholecystitis exists—the swelling of the organ and the pain will persist for a longer time. In complications of this kind a tumor of the spleen may also be observed, although this complication is rare and is invariably absent in ordinary cholelithiasis.

The effect of the attack of gall-stone colic on the digestive tract is manifested by a loss of appetite, that may persist after the attack itself has subsided, and by constipation. In some cases, particularly if the patient vomits a great deal, severe thirst may be complained of.

The demonstration of the presence of gall-stones in the stools is, of course, of paramount importance in determining the cause of an attack of colic. It is true that many cases occur in which no stone can be found in the feces even though cholelithiasis has existed for a long time. Many authors (for instance, Wolff) claim to have found gall-stones in every case that they examined; others claim that they have not found them in the majority of cases. A great deal will depend, in the first place, on the method of examination that is employed. If the stools are not examined with the greatest care, and if the examinations are not performed for several consecutive days, they may be readily overlooked. At a time when the belief was prevalent that gall-stones always float on water it was customary to stir up the feces with water and then to examine only those portions that rose to the surface. By this method, of course, it is a very easy matter not to find the gall-stones. The method described was originated by Prout. It is necessary to dilute the feces with much water and then to filter the mixture through a hair-sieve, the insoluble solid particles remaining on the sieve, where they can be examined.

One should persist in these examinations for days, as the concretions may remain in the intestine for a varying length of time. Even if all these precautions are taken, the stones are not always discovered. There are several possible explanations for the absence of gall-stones in the stools after the termination of an attack of gall-stone colic. Among these are:

1. Dropping back of the stone into the gall-bladder (Charcot), probably not a frequent occurrence.

2. Cessation of the contractions of the musculature of the bile-duct or cessation of the irritability of its mucous lining. If this occurs, the stone will remain quietly in one place.

3. Entrance of the gall-stone into the wide, common duct.

4. Disintegration and dissolution of the stone in the intestine.

Naunyn in particular has emphasized the latter possibility. He administered several gall-stones of the size of peas by the mouth, but despite the most diligent search did not succeed in recovering all of them from the feces. Only those that had a solid shell of cholesterin retained their original shape and size, those that consisted of bilirubin-chalk and the ordinary laminated forms of gall-stones seeming to be readily disintegrated. It has also been known for a long time that gall-stones leaving the body per rectum show a variety of indentations and fissures. For all these reasons, the occasional absence of gall-stones in the feces following an attack of gall-stone colic is not surprising after all, and we are not justified in drawing the conclusion from their absence that a large proportion of gall-stone attacks, so called, are not due to the passage of gall-stones. The theory advanced by Riedel that such attacks are simply the mani-. festation of inflammations of the gall-bladder and of the bile-passages, that appear and disappear suddenly, seems hardly tenable.

It is true that a great variety of different things that are found in the stools are occasionally taken for gall-stones. Thus, the hard masses found in pears and all those hard particles that are found around the kernel of different kinds of fruit may be mistaken for concretions. All these substances are insoluble in acids and alkalies, in ether, alcohol, etc. If oil is administered by mouth, soft masses of various kinds are often seen in the stools. They consist of soaps (the salts of oleic acid). In case it is doubtful what kind of concretions are present, it is well to examine for cholesterin. For this purpose the concretions are powdered and treated either with a mixture of ether and alcohol or with chloroform, the solution being then evaporated. If cholesterin be present, it will crystallize in characteristic needles that give the typical reaction with iodin and sulphuric acid. The solution in chloroform also gives a characteristic color-reaction with concentrated sulphuric acid, etc. If the concretions seem to consist of the calcium compound of bilirubin, the latter substance may be detected by Gmelin's reaction.

We have already mentioned that gall-stones that can pass through the common duct are rarely larger than a hazelnut. Quite frequently very large numbers, possibly hundreds, of smaller stones are passed in the feces. As a rule, they are faceted and are all approximately of the same size. They are either passed in several small batches or pass all at once. In this manner it may occur that conglomerates of many stones, held together by ordinary intestinal contents, are discovered in the feces. It may also occur that a large quantity of material resembling sand, consisting principally of bilirubin-calcium, is passed with the stools.

If all the stones are passed after an attack, a recurrence is rarely seen, from the fact that the formation of gall-stones rarely occurs again—in other words, the passage of all the stones frequently constitutes a cure of the disease.

The principal sequels of an attack of gall-stone colic aside from the complications that may arise as the result of violent inflammatory processes, etc., consist in a feeling of weakness, loss of appetite, defective nutrition, disturbed sleep, etc. In general, however, sufferers from cholelithiasis feel fairly well after the attack is over. Only in those cases where the stones do not succeed in entering the intestine, or where a more violent irritation of the mucous lining of the bile-passages exists, or where, finally, infectious agencies gain an entrance into the ducts or the bladder, a swelling of the gall-bladder or of the liver and a general feeling of distress and of pain may be present. Death rarely occurs at the height of the attack; when it does occur, it follows after the patient has shown alarming symptoms of increasing weakness, an irregular and weak heart-beat, etc. It is often impossible on postmortem examination to find a definite cause for the fatal issue. [Chauffard* has reported a case of sudden death after the disappearance of the pain, and attributed by him to toxemia.—Ed.]

Finally, a peculiar accident that has been reported several times may be mentioned in this place. It has happened that the mucous membrane of the bile-ducts ruptured, that the stone, as a result, perforated the wall of the duct, and, together with a certain quantity of bile, entered the peritoneal cavity. In cases where the mucous lining of the bile-ducts is intact, an accident of this character can probably never happen. It might be possible, however, that long-continued pressure exercised by the gall-stone might weaken the wall to such an extent that it finally yields. If the bile—as, for instance, in long-standing uncomplicated cholelithiasis—contains no virulent bacteria, the peritonitis that results from an accident of this kind need not necessarily be fatal. A serous fluid tinged with bile will accumulate in the peritoneal cavity in these cases. If the fluid be evacuated, or if the opening made by the perforation be closed by operation, complete recovery may ensue. If, on the other hand, virulent colon bacilli, pyogenic cocci, etc., gain an entrance into the abdominal cavity, the course of the disease is naturally quite different (see below).

If we summarize the symptoms of the general disease-picture and the course of an attack of gall-stone colic, the following can be stated:

In the beginning certain vague symptoms described above may exist pointing to the existence of gall-stones; or, on the other hand, there may be no premonitory symptoms whatever and the attack set in suddenly and unexpectedly. As a rule, the first symptom is a violent pain in the right hypochondriac region and the epigastrium. The patients, as a rule, go to bed at once. They bend the body toward the right side in order to relieve their distress. The region of the gall-bladder is usually painful to pressure, while the liver may be enlarged and its margin may be palpable. Vomiting now sets in; there is a complete loss of appetite; in many cases a chill and a rise of temperature; occasionally, irregular action of the heart. Frequently, icterus appears after the lapse of a certain time. The pain usually stops after a few hours, but may recur again as violently as before. A condition of this kind may persist for

* *Gaz. des Hôp.*, 1899.

days. Then, suddenly, all pain stops and the patient, aside from a slight feeling of lassitude as a result of the suffering undergone, may otherwise be none the worse for the attack. In general, the stools are not colorless until after the attack is over. The concretions, too, are naturally found after the attack.

Abortive attacks of gall-stone colic may precede the typical seizure. They consist in attacks of mild headache, pain in the epigastric and hypochondriac regions, loss of appetite, a tendency to vomiting, certain nervous symptoms, as excitement and peculiar undefined sensations in various parts of the body; occasionally, too, slight degrees of icterus are seen with temporary decoloration of the feces, a slight degree of swelling of the liver, and tenderness over the region of the gall-bladder and the liver. Attacks of this kind are apt to occur if the gall-stones are small or if the mucous lining of the bile-ducts or of the gall-bladder is only slightly irritated or possibly is normally less irritable. Finally, they may occur in subjects whose bile-passages are dilated and relaxed.

COMPLICATIONS.

Irregular Cholelithiasis.—Uncomplicated *regular* cholelithiasis presents many varying symptoms, the difficulties of diagnosis are considerable, and the disease may assume a very grave character. If this is the case in the regular form of the disease, so called, how much more must all these difficulties be emphasized in those cases that are irregular in their course owing to the occurrence of various complications! Complications may consist in infection of the bile-passages by virulent pathogenic bacteria followed by cholecystitis and cholangitis or by the formation of abscesses of the liver. In the regular form of cholelithiasis, we frequently encounter bacteria in the bile-ducts and the gall-bladder, but, as a rule, they are harmless or not very virulent forms and only produce slight symptoms of irritation and of inflammation wherever they happen to be located. Other serious and dangerous complications may occur if the stones become impacted. Among these are, for instance, ulcerations, cicatricial constrictions or strictures, formation of pockets, and separation of parts of the ducts. Permanent occlusion of the bile-passages may be brought about, leading to renewed stasis of bile and the formation of more concretions. This is seen particularly in cases where the ductus choledochus is occluded; and is then often followed by the formation of new concretions in the hepatic duct and its main branches by stasis of bile, changes in the smaller intrahepatic ducts, and, finally, of the interstitial tissues of the liver itself (cirrhosis). The retention of bile within the liver following occlusion of the common duct is, further, particularly dangerous in view of the grave form of icterus that it may cause. Finally, very serious complications may arise in cases where gall-stones attempt to penetrate the walls of the gall-bladder or of the bile-ducts and cause inflammation of surrounding parts. This inflammation of the neighboring tissues may be purulent in character, but, as a rule, leads to the formation of solid masses of connective tissue. After this, fistulæ are easily formed, so that the gall-stones can wander into other organs and there cause serious disturbances.

Occlusion of the cystic duct by a gall-stone or cicatricial contraction of the walls of this duct and obliteration of its lumen is not generally followed by any very serious consequences. The gall-bladder in cases of this kind is reduced in size. At first its contents are reabsorbed; then the bladder contracts around any gall-stones that it may still contain, forming a mass resembling cicatricial tissue. This is often seen during laparotomies for gall-stones. It may happen that the gall-bladder cannot be felt, or that it may be difficult to find even after opening the abdomen during a laparotomy. It is often particularly difficult to find the gall-bladder under these circumstances, for the reason that inflammatory processes occasionally develop around the organ, so that it becomes embedded in a mass of connective tissue. In other cases, again, in which occlusion of the cystic duct occurs, the gall-bladder may be felt as a tumor protruding beyond the margin of the liver. In such an event it is generally filled, tense and elastic at the same time; and in some instances fluctuation can be elicited. In the latter case we can assume that hydrops of the gall-bladder (*hydrops vesicæ felleæ*) has occurred. Hydrops as well as contraction of the gall-bladder may develop without causing any symptoms, the patients experiencing no abnormal sensations. In the case of hydrops of the gall-bladder, they occasionally complain of a sensation of weight in the right hypochondriac region. In cases where the gall-bladder is contracted and small, stones or fragments of concretions may attempt to perforate the walls of the bladder, causing circumscribed peritonitis to develop. Attacks of this complication resemble in general outlines any attack of gall-stone colic; but they do not run so typical a course, not beginning and ending so suddenly. Icterus is always absent in this localized form of peritonitis except in those instances where adhesions form in the region of the hepatic or the common duct and later contract and occlude these ducts. Vomiting, loss of appetite, and pain may all be present, as in an attack of gall-stone colic. In case pyogenic germs enter the gall-bladder, hydrops of the organ may be followed by symptoms of inflammation, peritonitic irritation, etc.

Whenever the ductus choledochus is occluded, a variety of serious complications may occur. Permanent icterus with all its dangerous consequences may often be seen as a sequel of this condition. Icterus, as a rule, appears after several attacks of gall-stones have occurred and have passed off; and it is rare to see it immediately after the first attack or without the appearance of any symptoms of colic. After it has once appeared icterus may persist for many months. In case the bile cannot escape, the disease-picture of hepatic intoxication (cholemia) appears, which is characterized by a tendency to hemorrhages, digestive disturbances, a weak heart action, finally coma, etc. The bile usually, however, succeeds in forcing an exit into the intestine or some other organ. This may result from expulsion of the stone from the duct or from the formation of a fistulous communication between the bile-passages and the intestine or with the exterior through the skin. The latter exit is created by ulcerative processes followed by adhesions and perforation. Finally, the accumulated bile may be liberated by one of the many possible operative measures that we have at our disposal.

In cases where the bile is completely prevented from entering the intestine, we see the skin and mucous membranes turn an intense yellow or greenish-yellow, the coloration gradually and progressively increasing in intensity. At an early stage of the disease the patients are liable to complain of an itching of the skin; and this symptom may be present in cases where cholelithiasis exists and gall-stone attacks have occurred without the development of icterus, so that it must be considered in many instances independent of the presence or absence of icterus, and must be attributed to nervous disturbances. It probably ranks with the other purely nervous symptoms seen in the course of most cases of chole- lithiasis. In icterus the stools are permanently decolorized. In cases, on the other hand, where the common duct is not permanently occluded, but where the flow of bile from the bile-passages into the intestine is periodically arrested, so that the bile alternately enters the intestine or is excluded from it, the stools are alternately colored and uncolored and show varying percentages of urobilin, etc. At this stage the appear- ance of furuncles is often noted. The frequency of the heart-beat is reduced and the pulse is slow. Hemorrhages from the skin and the mucous membranes occur very easily, so that in many cases operations are complicated by severe and almost uncontrollable hemorrhages from the cut tissues. The passage of bile into the *intestine* is not neces- sary to cause an arrest of all these symptoms. All that is needed is that the stasis of bile and the resulting absorption are stopped. In this way is explained why the passage of the bile through a cutaneous fistula is usually followed by a comparative amelioration of the symptoms enumerated. In prolonged cases it may happen that the icteric dis- coloration grows less intense after a time from the fact that the liver- cells perish in part as a result of the continued stasis of bile; or if they do not perish, they are at least seriously impaired in the exercise of their functions; consequently the production of bile is reduced or arrested altogether. The liver in these cases may enlarge considerably as a result of the distention of many of the bile-passages due to stasis of bile. It may even happen that the parenchyma of the liver may disappear be- tween the dilated passages or be present only in remnants (Raynaud and Sabourin). In case the tissue of the liver happened to be cirrhotic before, so that it was contracted, swelling of the liver as described above can, of course, not occur. If the cystic duct is patent, the gall-bladder appears in the shape of a round, tensely distended tumor at the lower margin of the liver. In many instances, however, the lumen of the cystic duct is also occluded by gall-stones, or the gall-bladder may already be contracted as described above, or both conditions may exist; in which case, of course, no tumor of the gall-bladder can be formed. The swelling of the liver does not cause serious disturbances in the area of the portal vein for the reason that no compression of the branches of this vessel occurs within the liver, and what little occlusion and obliteration of the blood-vessel occurs is not sufficient to cause symptoms of portal stasis. In this way it happens that the spleen is not enlarged and that ascites is absent; if, on the other hand, the cirrhotic changes within the liver assume greater dimensions, or if wide-spread cholangitis exists, some of the symptoms of portal stasis may appear. The common duct may become excessively dilated behind the gall-stone, forming a cylindric or sacculated tube that may be dilated to such a degree as to contain as much as a liter of fluid. The same may occur in the case of the cystic or the hepatic ducts, so that the dilated portions of these ducts may readily be mistaken for the gall-bladder. Very frequently the discovery is made on the operating table that the gall-bladder is small, atrophied, and contracted, and that the swelling that was taken for the gall-bladder was nothing more nor less than one of the dilated bile-ducts filled and distended with retained fluid. Permanent occlusion of the common duct may also be brought about in cholelithiasis by pressure exercised on it by the gall-bladder itself, when it is permanently dilated to a great degree following the complete occlusion of the cystic duct by large gall-stones. The latter are then usually found either in the cystic duct itself or in a diverticulum of this channel. This explains the observation that has been made several times that an operation on the gall-bladder and the cystic duct, consisting in the evacuation of the bile accumulated in the gall-bladder and the removal of the stone or stones occluding the cystic duct, was followed by the cure of chronic icterus without the removal of any stone or other obstruction from the common duct itself. At autopsy, too, occasionally nothing more is found to explain the occurrence of chronic icterus and occlusion of the common duct during life than a very much enlarged gall-bladder filled and distended with bile and compressing the ductus choledochus. It is even stated by some (Naunyn, Petit, Jakob and Cyr) that biliary stasis can be produced through pressure upon the common duct by a gall-bladder which is completely flaccid, with reduced tonus of its walls, and inability to completely empty itself.

In many cases of long-continued occlusion of the common duct incarcerated gall-stones are not the only form of obstruction, as quite frequently we see the formation of a common annular carcinoma of the walls of the duct which has probably resulted from long-continued irritation of the parts, particularly of the mucous lining of the duct. In fact some authors attribute most of the cases of chronic occlusion of the common duct in the aged to the formation of carcinoma. This hypothesis, however, goes too far, for we know of very many cases of long-continued simple obstruction of the common duct without the development of carcinoma. Simple carcinomata of the common duct and carcinomata of the head of the pancreas may also lead to chronic stasis of bile and to severe icterus. In these cases the gall-bladder will be found to be enlarged; in cholelithiasis, on the other hand, it is usually contracted and no longer permeable for bile.

With regard to the duration of icterus in complete obstruction of the common duct, it may be stated that this condition can last several months, in rarer instances over a year, and that it can then eventually disappear if the gall-stone is passed or removed in some other way. Occasionally the stone escapes through a fistula, so that the orifice of the common duct may remain occluded. If no passage of bile occurs, death usually takes place after a few months,—as a rule, between the sixth and the twelfth month,—with all the symptoms of cholemia.

The entrance of pathogenic microbes, notably of the pus-forming species, into the bile-passages in cholelithiasis is very important in view of its bearing on the subsequent course of the disease. As we have repeatedly emphasized, stasis of bile seems to favor the development of these germs and seems to predispose to the subsequent development of severe forms of cholangitis and of cholecystitis. In exploratory punctures during operations for gall-stones and at postmortems, the following bacteria have at different times been found in the bile-passages: Bacillus coli, the bacillus of typhoid and the bacillus of cholera, pneumococci, and, finally, in combination with many other species, streptococci and staphylococci. All these germs have been found both in the gall-bladder and in the bile-ducts. Virulent colon bacilli are found, and can be cultivated from the contents of the gall-bladder and the bile-ducts

(Netter and Martha, Naunyn, Levy, Dominici, and others). Dupré, Fauraytier, and many later authors have found Bacillus typhosus alone in suppurative cholangitis, etc.; and occasionally this micro-organism has been associated with Bacillus coli. Pneumococci and the spirilla of cholera are less frequently found (Girode). Pyogenic germs have frequently been found alone or in association with bacteria of the above species. Cholelithiasis plays a very important rôle in the causation of cholangitis. Dominici states that in 65% of the cases of cholangitis observed by him attacks of gall-stones had preceded the disease or gall-stones were present when the disease developed. [The rôle of gall-stones in insuring the retention of residual bile, as explained by Ehret and Stolz (see above), has a marked bearing in this connection, especially as regards the operative removal of gall-stones in order to avoid the danger of infective and dangerous inflammation of the gall-bladder and its ducts. —ED.]

It is true that in cases of typhoid fever, cholera, or pneumonia, where a severe attack of inflammation of the bile-passages is caused by the specific germ of the disease, all symptoms of this complication may be absent. The symptoms of the primary disease are so violent, and the symptoms of involvement of other organs dominate the disease-picture so completely, that the disturbances in the liver and its appendages are comparatively insignificant and are overlooked. Thus, Hagenmüller found that out of eighteen cases of typhoid fever in which cholecystitis typhosa was found after death, symptoms of this condition were present in only eleven of the cases during life. Infection with colon bacilli may cause suppuration and still run a purely latent course, so that we may be very much surprised to find pus in the gall-bladder and the bile-passages postmortem.

The course of infectious cholangitis seems to be most acute in cases of invasion by Bacillus coli, particularly if the bacilli are very virulent. In infections with streptococci and with staphylococci the course of the disease is apt to be more chronic. In infections with Bacillus coli, purulent inflammation of the peritoneum is most frequently seen; in infection with pus cocci, on the other hand, abscess formation in the liver is more often encountered. The picture of insidious and slowly developing septicopyemia is also frequently seen. Bacillus coli may, however, also lead to the formation of hepatic abscesses, which, as a rule, develop from the bile-passages. To these symptoms of cholangitis are frequently added the symptoms of endocarditis (Netter and Martha, Mathieu, Malabran, and others). In some cases ulcerative endocarditis may develop. In other words, a general septicopyemia may arise in which the local symptoms in the liver are of such subordinate importance, and are so much relegated to the background, that the primary source of the general septicopyemic involvement is not discovered until an autopsy is performed and the disease of the bile-passages is discovered.

In many cases the occurrence of cholangitis is manifested as follows: After the patient has undergone one or several attacks of gall-stone colic, a tendency to slight febrile disturbances, an icteric color, a dull pain in the region of the liver, and other symptoms are observed, all pointing to the possible presence of some infectious process in the affected parts. An intermittent type of fever is frequently seen. Charcot was the first to describe this and to call attention to a possible connection between these febrile disturbances and septic processes; he designated this fever "*fièvre intermittente hépatique*" (compare page 511). If a temperature curve of this kind is seen in the course of cholangitis, it signifies that micro-organisms or their toxins have entered the blood from the bile-passages; although it is not necessary that suppurative processes should occur in the bile-passages themselves, for it seems possible for pyogenic germs to pass through the bile-passages into the blood without infecting the former. Pathogenic germs have, in fact, at different times been found in the blood. The attacks of fever are liable to appear toward evening or during the night with chills, cyanosis, etc. The temperature may rise as high as 40° C. (104° F.). The feeling of chilliness may last for a short time only or it may continue for a long time, even lasting for two or three hours. Following this, a feeling of heat is complained of and the pulse grows tense and rapid. Finally, profuse sweating occurs, and the temperature drops back to normal. Following an attack of this kind, comes a period of apyrexia of varying duration, before the next attack begins. It will be seen that depending on the length of the period of apyrexia, all types of intermittent fever may be simulated: viz., quotidian, tertian, quartan. The sequence of the different attacks is not, however, as regular as in malaria. It must also be emphasized that in cases where the inflammatory processes in the bile-passages increase, or where they extend to the surrounding tissues, the type of fever may change and assume the characteristic course of a remittent or of a continuous fever. When the fever runs a course like this, the patient usually dies; whereas the intermittent type of fever seems to be less dangerous. In many of the more severe cases it may be found that the fever is remittent from the very beginning. In other cases, again, particularly in old subjects and in cases where the hepatic cells are very much altered, all fever may be absent; in fact, the temperature may be subnormal during the whole course of the attack. Migration of the gall-stones seems to favor the occurrence of fever. This is probably due to the slight injury which they always inflict on the mucous membrane lining the bile-passages, in this way throwing the doors open for the entrance of germs or of their virulent products into the blood. This is the reason why the fever we are discussing follows attacks of gall-stone colic. The intermittent type of this fever has been explained as follows: owing to the fluctuations in the quantity of bile secreted and the fluctuations of pressure to which the secretion is exposed during the contraction and relaxation of the walls of the bile-passages, the quantity of pathogenic material that can be absorbed varies, so that at different times different quantities of the latter products or of virulent germs themselves enter the blood and the tissues.

In the urine we find, in addition to bile-pigment and urobilin, albumin and indoxyl. It has even been stated that tyrosin and leucin are occasionally encountered in the urine. Regnard claims that in biliary fever a decrease of the excretion of urea occurs; but all other investigators (Brouardel, Lecorché, Talamon, and others) have reported that in the case of this fever, as in all other forms of febrile infection, the excretion of urea is increased.

In some instances the gall-bladder can be felt, palpation being, as a rule, easy if the organ is filled. The region of the gall-bladder is frequently sensitive to pressure. Sometimes it will be found that pericholecystitis has developed, a diffuse swelling will be felt around the gall-bladder, and, later, fluctuation may even be elicited in the center of this swelling. Death usually results in cases of this character from acute peritonitis. In other instances it may happen that the cystic duct is occluded by a gall-stone or that its lumen is completely obliterated by cicatricial contractions, etc. In this event, the biliary constituents within the gall-bladder are gradually absorbed and the fluid contents is converted into a thin, sanious, or serous liquid. At the same time the gall-bladder continues to increase in size and becomes very much distended, its walls growing thicker, and, finally, hydrops of the gall-bladder developing. The fluid contained within the gall-bladder at the end of this process is sterile, for the reason that all micro-organisms that may have been present have perished. Before the establishment of this stationary condition, however, various influences, as traumata, digestive disorders, intercurrent infections, etc., may cause a revival of the infectious germs present in the gall-bladder or may cause the entrance of new micro-organisms into the viscus, and in this manner produce ulcerative processes, by which the danger of circumscribed or of diffuse peritonitis is made imminent. Gall-stone fistulæ may also be formed as a sequel of such an attack of cholecystitis.

A further complication of cholelithiasis is hepatic abscess. The formation of purulent collections in the liver may follow an attack of cholangitis, disease of the small branches of the portal vein, or infection of the bile-passages or the parenchyma from pus in the gall-bladder. If this complication occurs, the disease-picture becomes complicated; and the lesion exercises a considerable influence on the course of the disease. In the majority of cases of hepatic abscess a definite diagnosis of the condition cannot be made. This is particularly the case if multiple abscesses develop. In the latter instance the general symptoms of grave septicopyemia completely dominate the disease-picture. As a rule, furthermore, death occurs before the formation of the abscess can be discovered. The suspicion of abscess of the liver may be entertained if a pyemic type of fever develops, characterized by the alternate appearance of intermittent and of remittent temperature curves, and if at the same time symptoms of inflammation of the surface of the liver are observed, particularly if the diaphragm or the right pleural cavity is involved. The general loss of strength, the rise in temperature, and the swelling of the spleen seem to be greater in abscess than in simple cholangitis, while the fever is, as a rule, more intermittent than remittent in character. In the intermittent form the temperature may run very high and may suddenly drop to subnormal. Occasionally, the formation of an abscess is manifested by symptoms of circumscribed peritonitis. In other instances the complicating pleuritis, that may be either purulent or serous, may so dominate the picture that the primary cause and seat of the trouble are overlooked. Owing to adhesions that may form between the peritoneal covering of the hepatic abscess and many different organs or tissues, the abscess may perforate through the skin, the diaphragm, the intestine, etc., and in this manner the pus may be poured into the pleural cavity, the lungs, the bronchi, etc., and be evacuated in this manner. It may also happen that the pus enters the peritoneal cavity, an accident which is, of course, followed by most dire results.

The diagnosis of abscess is established in case a protuberance develops somewhere on the surface of the liver, sensitive to pressure, particularly painful during the period of the chill (Naunyn, Osler), and later developing fluctuation. On opening a cavity of this kind not only pus and bile, but also gall-stones, are evacuated. It is possible, at the same time, that many of the described abscesses of the liver that contained gall-stones, and were evacuated by spontaneous rupture or on operative interference, were nothing else than empyemata of the gall-bladder. It is a very difficult matter, and it may, in fact, be impossible, to make a differential diagnosis between abscess and a softened carcinoma, etc., in case the latter lesion develops in the course of cholelithiasis.

Ulceration of the bile-passages may develop insidiously and in a latent manner, so that fistulæ, adhesions, etc., may develop without causing any symptoms. Ulcers of this kind, however, generally lead to formidable complications. In many instances they may cause hemorrhages by eroding branches of the hepatic artery or even that artery itself, and permitting the occurrence of a hemorrhagé into the bile-passages or the formation of spurious aneurysms, etc. It may also happen that some of the vessels of the stomach or the intestine are eroded and opened by gall-stone ulcerations, so causing profuse hemorrhages leading to increasing anemia, collapse, and death. Hemorrhage into the abdominal cavity has also been observed from time to time. Aufrecht reports a case of this kind in which a gall-stone penetrated the parenchyma of the liver from the gall-bladder and caused so violent a hemorrhage into the cavity it had formed that the blood, aside from pouring through the bile-ducts into the intestine, ruptured the wall of the sac and poured into the abdominal cavity. Following hemorrhages into the bile-passages, the intestine, or the stomach, blood is found in an altered form in the stools or in the vomitus. The diagnosis is very difficult, particularly if no symptoms previously pointed to the existence of cholelithiasis. As a rule, the diagnosis of hemorrhage from a gastric or duodenal ulcer is made. Even on autopsy it may be a difficult matter to completely explain the connection existing between the presence of blood in the stomach and intestine and the presence of gall-stones. Aside from hemorrhages of this kind bleeding into the stomach and the intestine is occasionally seen following severe forms of icterus, particularly that following occlusion of the common duct. The origin of these hemorrhages must be explained from a weakening of the vessel walls as a result of hepatic intoxication; *i. e.*, of the circulation in the blood of deleterious substances absorbed from the liver. Thrombosis of the portal vein as a result of compression by a gall-stone in the ductus choledochus is rarely seen, consequently stasis in the blood-vessels of the wall of the stomach and hemorrhage from this source are not often encountered. The same applies to hemorrhages of this character from the walls of the intestine. In discussing abscess formation following cholelithiasis, we called attention to the possibility of pylephlebitis and its sequel, multiple hepatic abscesses. It may even happen that gall-stones perforate into the portal vein, an occurrence indicated by a series of older reports and the descriptions of Deway, Murchison, and Roth. If this occurs, the picture of occlusion and inflammation of the portal vein develops, and, in addition, we see ascites, swelling of the spleen, passive congestion in the stomach and intestine, and at the same time pyemia.

One of the most important complications of cholelithiasis is the formation of fistulous tracts between the gall-bladder and the bile-passages, on the one hand, and the intestinal tract, on the other. We have at different times mentioned such fistulæ.

Concretions occasionally enter the stomach, although this accident must be considered comparatively rare. We are not justified in concluding that such a perforation has occurred merely because gall-stones are found in the vomitus, for we know that violent retching and vomiting may occasionally allow bile to flow backward into the stomach and to appear in the vomitus, and the same applies to small gall-stones during an attack of gall-stone colic. In the case of larger stones this cannot occur so readily, as these concretions can pass the pyloric orifice of the stomach only with difficulty. In case larger gall-stones are vomited the formation of a fistula must be considered. It has been definitely determined by anatomic examination that a fistulous connection between the bile-passages and the stomach occasionally occurs (Cruveilhier, Oppolzer, Frerichs, Murchison, Jeaffreson, and others). As a rule, the evacuation of gall-stones by vomiting is preceded by attacks of violent pain in the region of the stomach, and violent and persistent vomiting of bile, food, etc. Sometimes several stones are vomited at the same time, or the vomiting of gall-stones recurs several times in the course of the disease.

Fistulæ are most frequently formed between the gall-bladder or the common duct and the duodenum. There can be no doubt that our statistics in regard to the frequency of this occurrence are much too low. In many instances the fistula is mistaken for the dilated orifice of the common duct in old cases of cholelithiasis examined postmortem. The gall-bladder, the common duct, and the duodenum are situated in such close proximity to each other that the formation of fistulous connections between any two of these parts can proceed so insidiously and so quietly that the patient is not aware of it. In this manner the passage through the intestine of gall-stones that are larger than a hazelnut must be explained. This, as we know, may occur without the development of any inflammatory or peritonitic symptoms. Hemorrhages of varying degree of intensity probably occur during the passage of so large a concretion; but, as a rule, they are overlooked unless the stools are examined carefully for the appearance of blood.

If symptoms are present at all, they consist in pain, the formation of an exudate in the region of the gall-bladder, etc., so that a doughy, soft swelling is developed around the gall-bladder and can be felt in the region of that organ; in addition, vomiting may occur and both bile and blood may be raised. Icterus rarely appears in these cases. On the other hand, it may happen that icterus that has existed for some time prior to the development of the above symptoms may disappear because, of course, the bile that was pent up behind the occlusion can pass as soon as the gall-stone has dropped into the duodenum. Finally, the stone is passed per rectum. It may be, as we have already stated, that the appearance of the stone in the stools is the only symptom noticed. In rare instances, finally, when the stone is very large and angular, occlusion of the lumen of the intestine and ileus may result.

Among 384 cases of formation of internal and external gall-stone fistulæ (of these, 200 were internal) that Courvoisier collected in the literature, 108 were duodenal fistulæ; and of these, 15 started from the common duct and 93 from the gall-bladder. According to the results obtained from an examination of the autopsy material investigated by Roth, Schröder, and Schloth, gall-bladder fistulæ were found in 19 cases, and choledochus-duodenal fistulæ in 5 cases (Naunyn). Cour-

37

voisier mentions gastric fistulæ only twelve times, and found only one case among the postmortem examinations chronicled above.

On account of the great motility of the small intestine, it rarely happens that a gall-stone perforates its walls. In the case of the colon it is different, and fistulæ into that viscus are quite frequently seen. As a rule, they start from the gall-bladder, as the fundus of this organ is in close proximity to the transverse colon. Adhesions are very liable to form between the gall-bladder and the transverse colon, and later perforation can easily occur. This process is, as a rule, more favorable to the patient than the formation of a fistulous connection between the gall-bladder and the duodenum, for the reason that even large gall-stones can pass through the colon without any difficulty, and in this way be evacuated with the feces without threatening to occlude the lumen of the intestine at any time during their transit. In cases of this kind the general symptoms of the formation of a fistulous connection are quite insignificant, and the passage of the gall-stone through the fistula remains altogether unnoticed. Courvoisier found 50 cases of colonic fistula in his collection; while Roth, Schröder, and Schloth, in their autopsy material, found 16 cases. Combinations of cutaneous or colonic fistulæ with duodenal fistulæ have also been described. In cases where a fistula through the skin and one into the intestine existed, it might even be possible for some of the intestinal contents to pass out through the skin. If the fistula into the colon is very wide, fecal matter might enter the gall-bladder or the bile-passages, producing a very serious infection. It is hardly probable that an accident of this kind will happen frequently, for the reason that the fistula closes very rapidly after the gall-stone has passed.

Fistulæ formed between different bile-passages are of subordinate clinical importance.

In the course of their wanderings through the abdominal cavity, it may also happen that gall-stones enter the urinary bladder. In cases of this kind the symptoms of urinary calculi in the bladder are produced, and the gall-stones can be crushed or removed just as are ordinary urinary stones. If concretions of this kind are carefully examined, they will be found to contain the calcium compound of bilirubin and cholesterin, these constituents, of course, distinguishing them from renal or urinary stones. Güterbock has described cases of this character: I have also, on one occasion, examined a stone, removed by Bier from the urinary bladder, which consisted almost exclusively of cholesterin and was arranged in characteristic layers, with, in addition, a radiating structure. As a rule, all symptoms of inflammation of the peritoneum are absent. It may also happen that small stones, not larger than a bean, perforate the pelvis of the kidney and pass along the ureters, reaching the bladder in this way. Murchison assumes that this happened in two cases that he reports. In one of his cases some 200 small stones were gradually passed through the urinary bladder. Under these circumstances the concretions may produce the symptoms of urinary colic, particularly if they become lodged somewhere in the ureters. In one or two cases they have been known to occlude the lumen of the urethra so that the operation of urethrotomy had to be performed in order to remove the obstruction.

J. P. Frank describes the very unique case of a gall-stone passed from the gall-bladder through some adhesive tissue that had formed between that viscus and the uterus, and voided from the vagina during labor.

• If gall-stones wander to the convex surface of the liver, they may become encapsulated in a subphrenic abscess and remain there. Under certain circumstances, however, they may perforate the diaphragm and lead to the development of empyema, pyopneumothorax, or to perforation and evacuation of the pus into the lungs or the bronchi.

In many cases the lung is already adherent to the diaphragm, owing to previous attacks of inflammation of the diaphragmatic pleura. In cases of this character a perforation into the tissues of the lung may occur without the formation of any fluid exudate in the pleural cavity. Within the lung, the symptoms of an abscess may develop and quantities of pus and bile may be expectorated for a long time. It may happen that the left pleural cavity is entered from the left lobe of the liver (Cayley). It has even been observed that in one case gall-stones entered the mediastinum (Simons), or the pericardial cavity (Legg), or that they wandered from the mediastinum into one of the main bronchi. Symptoms of subphrenic abscess, of suppurative pleuritis, of pyopneumothorax, as is seen in thoracic fistulæ, may all exist for a long time and still their connection with gall-stones remain obscure and undiscovered. The expectoration of bile-tinged sputum first calls attention to this possibility. The latter symptom is, however, still more frequently seen in echinococcus or in abscesses of the liver that break through into the lungs or pleural cavity. The diagnosis, therefore, will have to be supported by a history of gall-stone colic, with the passage of gall-stones at some time in the past. In case perforation into the lungs occurs, the gall-stones themselves are rarely expectorated; although this did happen in a case reported by Vissering.

Perforation of the abdominal walls by gall-stones has always played an important rôle in our studies of gall-stones and the pathology of cholelithiasis. This accident does not occur as frequently as we might be led to believe from the statements made in the literature. Courvoisier, among 384 cases of gall-stone fistula reported in the literature, found 184 in which the fistula had perforated the external abdominal wall. Duodenal fistulæ are, however, more frequent than would appear from statistics. This is due to the fact that they are frequently not discovered, whereas fistulæ that penetrate the skin necessarily cannot be overlooked.

In the production of fistulæ through the abdominal walls and the skin adhesions first form between the gall-bladder and the layers of the parietal peritoneum, then the peritoneum and the abdominal wall are perforated, the inflammatory symptoms arising incident to this process being, as a rule, very slight. In other cases the gall-bladder may be very much distended as a result of some violent inflammation, forms adhesions with the peritoneum and the abdominal walls, and the pus that it contains finally burrows through the muscular walls of the abdomen and the skin and is either spontaneously evacuated or removed by operative interference. As a rule, the presence of an abscess of the liver is suspected. When the swelling is opened, pus and sometimes bile are evacuated; after a time it may happen that concretions appear, and then only is the diagnosis in many cases cleared. The fistula is often situated in the region of the fundus of the gall-bladder. Occasionally, the inflammatory process follows the course of the suspensory ligament, so that the direction of the fistula is downward, in which case the abscess will open in the region of the umbilicus. It may even occur that gall-stones are evacuated to the left of the median line near the pubes, or in the region of the clitoris. Stones as large as a hen's egg may be passed through these abnormal channels and hundreds of individual stones may be passed in the course of time.

As a rule, it is not possible to follow the development of the different stages of the processes described. This can be done only in those exceptional cases where the symptoms of a perforation of the gall-bladder appear first, followed immediately by symptoms of abscess formation in the peritoneal cavity, as was present in a case described by Reichardt. The first symptom observed is, generally, a tender swelling in the place where the abscess is developing. The swelling increases in size and occasionally gall-stones can be felt in it. In general, however, all that can be determined is that an abscess is forming and that the site of the swelling is growing redder and is gradually protruding more and more above the level of the abdomen. Slowly the reddened and edematous skin becomes thinner; and finally, unless an incision is made into the abscess, the pus will break through the skin. In cases where the cystic duct is occluded, only pus and mucus are evacuated; whereas if the lumen of the cystic duct is patent, bile is passed with the pus. Gall-stones, as a rule, do not appear in the spontaneous opening of the abscess until later. If the abscess is incised, the gall-stones are generally evacuated with the rest of the contents of the abscess cavity. They may, on the other hand, remain in the gall-bladder or in the fistulous passage and not come away spontaneously, so that it becomes necessary to follow the course of the fistula and to remove the stones by a special operation. It may also occur that the rupture of the abscess follows an empyema of the gall-bladder. This may be the sequel of an attack of suppurative cholangitis which, in its turn, was caused by the occlusion of the common duct by a gall-stone. In a case of this kind, of course, no gall-stones are found in the pus. Icterus following an accident of this character will be relieved as soon as the fistulous opening is established.

The fistulous channels are frequently very long and tortuous, and sometimes diverticula are formed along their course that may be filled with mucus, pus, or bile, or may occasionally contain a gall-stone. The walls of these passages are often thickened by deposits of fibrinous material. Even though the lumen of such a fistula appears very narrow on postmortem examination, this does not exclude the possibility that at some time there had passed through it a gall-stone larger than the opening appears to be. This is explainable from the fact that cicatricial contractions and partial obliteration of the lumen frequently follow the passage of the concretion. Sometimes a fistula may close and the superficial opening heal, only to be broken open again at some later time to allow the passage of another gall-stone. It may also happen that a gall-stone becomes impacted in a fistulous channel, completely occluding it. If this occurs and other gall-stones attempt to pass, abscesses may form in other places in the vicinity of the gall-bladder. Patients often lose all the bile through a fistula of this kind, particularly if the common duct is occluded by a gall-stone; but it may even occur if the ductus choledochus is patent. In certain cases there has been reported a loss of 250 gm. (9 ounces), in some cases as much as 500 gm. to 600 gm. (17.50 to 21 ounces), or even a quart, of bile daily. Generally, this fluid is not pure bile; but contains also watery transudates, pus, mucus, etc.

Many investigators have attributed the marasmus that often follows such a flow of fluid to the loss of bile and the deficient elaboration of the chyme which they claim follows the absence of bile from the intestine. This view is rendered untenable by the existence of many cases in which the loss of bile through a fistula was well borne for many years without any disturbance of the general nutrition. It is more probable that the marasmus is caused by the continuous formation and evacuation of pus usually observed in these cases.

Gall-stones that enter the gastro-intestinal tract in one of the different ways described may cause a variety of disturbances chiefly brought about by occlusion of the lumen of the intestine. It may happen that occlusion of the pylorus occurs. The pylorus may be compressed from without in case a large stone is passing through the common duct and is attempting to perforate into the stomach or the duodenum; or, again, an ulcer may be discovered in the pylorus within which is seen a concretion that comes from the gall-bladder. Cicatricial contraction may cause traction on the pylorus and narrow this passage, or, finally, inflammatory swelling around a gall-stone may lead to traction or compression of the pylorus. [Fibrous bands of adhesion stretching from the gall-bladder to other structures may compress the duodenum or cause kinking long after the gall-stones have escaped.—ED.] The natural result of all these conditions will be obstruction to the exit of the stomach-contents, with dilatation of the organ and fermentation and decomposition of the food that it contains. In cases of this kind cicatricial narrowing of the pylorus as a result of gastric ulcer is usually diagnosed; or if the gall-stone is felt in the region of the pylorus or the swelling caused by its presence is palpated, the diagnosis of carcinoma of the pylorus is made. Occasionally the gall-stone is subsequently passed in the stools or vomited, and in this manner the passage opened. Leichtenstern reports a case of dilatation of the stomach that persisted until on one occasion, during lavage of the stomach, the lumen of the stomach-tube was occluded by numerous gall-stones; after this the patient recovered.

Sabatier, Boucher, and others have described a dangerous form of ileus following the impaction of a gall-stone, their reports dating from the eighteenth century. An accident of this character is particularly liable to happen in cases where the gall-stone perforates the walls of the duodenum and enters this part of the intestine. When the fistula opens into the colon, occlusion of the lumen of the intestine is less apt to occur on account of the greater width of the canal. If the gall-stone becomes impacted in the duodenum, the same symptoms as those observed in stenosis of the pylorus may appear, such as regurgitation of bile into the stomach, dilatation of the stomach, and obstinate vomiting of food. More frequently, however, the gall-stone lodges somewhere in the lower portions of the small intestine, in the jejunum or the ileum, producing violent colicky pains with vomiting of food and, later, of bile-stained and feculent masses. Gradually the symptoms of ileus may increase, with the development of peritonitic inflammation in the region of the obstruction, followed, finally, by the death of the patient. Occasionally the obturator may be dislodged and the opening re-established. This has been known to occur during the manipulations incident to palpation. In cases of this kind the gall-stone slides along and the patients themselves may describe a sensation as though something were moving in the intestine. It may, however, happen that the gall-stone becomes impacted a second time either at the ileocecal valve or in the rectum. Obstruction in the region of the cecum and the lower part of the ileum is particularly to be dreaded, notably in the portion of the intestine situated immediately above Bauhin's valve, as stones seem to lodge there with greater frequency than in other parts of the intestine. This may happen even if the stones are not very large. If a stone becomes lodged in the region of this valve, it may act as a ball-valve; in other words, the lumen of the intestine may be alternately occluded and patent; as a result the symptoms of ileus alternate with the symptoms of patency of the intestine. In the first instance we know that the gall-stone has become impacted within the valve, completely occluding the passage; in the second, we must infer that the stone has again become dislodged by antiperistaltic movements, by concussion of the body, or some change of position. It appears that this change in the symptoms occurs more frequently in cases where the occlusion of the intestine is due to gall-stones than in cases where it is due to other causes. Le Gros Clark reports a case in which the symptoms of ileus disappeared completely for three weeks, so that the patient's intestinal functions were normal; but at the end of this time the symptoms of ileus suddenly reappeared and caused the death of the patient. Gall-stones situated in the large intestine may also occasionally act as ball-valves in the sense that they only allow the passage of pultaceous, soft stools. Such a condition is, however, compatible with many months of life. If the occlusion of the intestine is due to gall-stones, it appears that the passage of flatus is less impeded than in other forms of occlusion of the bowels; probably from the fact that closure by gall-stones is not quite hermetic (Maclagan, Naunyn). This may also explain the frequent absence of meteorism in the form of ileus under discussion.

Gall-stones that become impacted in the intestine are usually as large as a pigeon's or a hen's egg; occasionally they are smaller. Occlusion of the intestine by conglomerations of small stones, held together by solid masses of intestinal contents, has also occasionally been observed (Puyroyer). Similar conglomerates are occasionally formed by masses of raisin-pips or plum-kernels. On the other hand, very large gall-stones have been seen to pass from the anus without having caused any symptoms of ileus or any other intestinal disturbance. The latter may be even 4 by 9 cm. (1½ by 3½ in.) in diameter (Blackburne).

If gall-stones are impacted in the ileocecal region, they may simulate typhlitis; and the diagnosis can in these cases be definitely established only by an operation (Th. Kölliker). It may even happen, in rare instances, that small gall-stones enter the vermiform appendix and produce appendicitis.

In former days a great deal of significance was attached to the growth of gall-stones within the intestine. It has been found, however, that no enlargement ever occurs; if anything, the gall-stones decrease in size within the intestinal canal and disintegrate if they remain there for a long time. In rare instances, they may form the nucleus of large coproliths.

It is, as a rule, impossible to determine the exact location of a gall-stone in the intestine. If the patient vomits large masses of material tinged with bile and not mixed with feces, the diagnosis of occlusion of the duodenum is very probable. In cases of occlusion of the colon it is frequently possible to feel the concretion per rectum.

Even after the occlusion of the intestine has been remedied, attacks of ileus may recur at any time as long as the gall-stone is still within the intestinal canal. After the stone has been voided a series of sequels may remain, affecting principally the mucous membrane of the intestine and manifesting themselves by diarrhea, etc.

The fatal issue is usually precipitated by exhaustion and collapse of the patient. Many authors emphasize the frequency with which peritonitis is seen following ileus from occlusion by gall-stones, and have stated that this complication is the result of perforation and inflammation of the mucous membrane of the intestine so often seen in cases where hard concretions are present. To this possibility of perforation they attribute the fatal issue from peritonitis occasionally seen after the occluding gall-stones have been removed. Other authors (Kirmisson and Rochard) state that peritonitis is very rare in ileus from gall-stones. According to the last-named authors, death occurs in 50 to 70% of the cases; according to Courvoisier, in 44%; according to Schüller, in 56%. The disease, therefore, is a very serious one. The duration of the disease varies, and may fluctuate from one to twenty-eight days. Kirmisson and Rochard found that the cases that terminated in recovery lasted, on an average, eight days; those that terminated fatally, ten days.

As old women seem to be particularly predisposed to cholelithiasis, ileus from gall-stones is very frequently seen in such subjects. In case, therefore, an old woman is afflicted with ileus, we are always justified in suspecting that it may be caused by a gall-stone. Kirmisson and Rochard found that among 105 cases, 70 occurred in female subjects and only 35 in males. Among 127 cases observed by Schüller, 34 occurred in men.

Robson mentions among possible additional causes for ileus following cholelithiasis local peritonitis in the region of the gall-bladder, volvulus as a result of a violent attack of gall-stone colic, stenosis of the intestine following adhesions due in their turn to local peritonitis. All these factors are certainly less important than direct occlusion of the intestine by a gall-stone.

Cirrhosis of the liver is not infrequently seen in cholelithiasis. Dodonæus, Forestus, and others, stated that the liver may appear indurated in cases of cholelithiasis. During the century just past, Gubler, Virchow, and Liebermeister, in particular, have more exhaustively described cases of this character. The last-named author sees a connection between the concretions and the proliferation of connective tissue and the atrophy of liver-tissue observed in his case with intrahepatic ducts filled with stones. Hanot has written a treatise on the connection between gall-stones and cirrhosis of the liver. Meyer and Legg observed that ligation of the common duct in cats and rabbits is followed by a proliferation of interstitial tissue. Charcot and Gombault arrived at the same conclusion as the result of their experiments, but attributed the proliferation of tissue to the action of the stasis of bile. Thomson, also, observed biliary cirrhosis in congenital obliteration of the large bile-passages. In case, therefore, stasis of bile occurs in cholelithiasis this may be the cause of cirrhosis (see the section on cirrhosis). In many cases of this kind, however, where proliferation of connective tissue occurs, as in the case of Liebermeister, icterus may be very slight or completely absent. In these cases it must be assumed that the proliferation of connective tissue in the periportal region (a proliferation that may extend into the region of the periphery of the acini) is a direct continuation of the chronic inflammatory processes prevailing in the bile-passages, and caused by micro-organisms and by the mechanical injury to which the mucous lining of the walls of the bile-channels is subjected. In cirrhosis of the liver following gall-stones the organ is, as a rule, hard, usually smooth, and easily palpated. A tumor of the spleen is present, but is not characteristic, as this complication may be seen as a result of cholangitis in any case of cholelithiasis. Ascites is rarely present and is only seen toward the end of the disease. Icterus may be absent or may be present in a mild form only, except in cases that are caused by general stasis of bile. Even after the gall-stones have been evacuated, the liver preserves its hard consistency and remains enlarged, owing to the fact that cirrhosis, after it has once formed, cannot retrogress to any great extent. If the process is very far advanced, it may happen that icterus persists even after the flow of bile from the gall-bladder has been re-established. Frequently severe degrees of cholangitis develop in the widened channels of a liver of this kind, and consequently we see the development of multiple abscesses (Leichtenstern, Braubach).

We have, in several places, mentioned the occasional occurrence of carcinoma of the gall-bladder and of the bile-passages as one of the possible complications of cholelithiasis. We will give a detailed description of the disease-picture of carcinoma of the liver in the section entitled "Cancer of the Liver and the Bile-passages." In this place we will limit ourselves to a discussion of a few of the salient features of this condition. If the carcinoma develops in the gall-bladder, and if this organ is enlarged and filled with gall-stones, a painful, nodular, gradually enlarging tumor can often be felt. This tumor, in the course of its development, may involve the cystic, the hepatic, and the common ducts, and in this manner compress these passages and cause biliary stasis. In many other cases the development of the carcinoma is so slight that it is hardly perceptible; or the tumor may grow exclusively on that side of the gall-bladder directed toward the liver, and in this way evade detection. In cases of this character the carcinomatous involvement of the gall-bladder may be completely overlooked and no diagnosis made other than carcinoma of the liver. The carcinomatous involvement of the whole organ may be the result of metastatic, secondary infection from the gall-bladder or of extension of the growth in the gall-bladder by direct continuity of tissue. Those annular forms of carcinoma that develop around a gall-stone in the duct often cause such serious disturbances at an early stage of their development that death may result from cholemia before the presence of a tumor can be diagnosed. This effect is, of course, due to the complete occlusion of the duct and the consequent impeded flow of bile. It may happen, therefore, that the presence of such a carcinoma is not discovered until after the death of the patient, and even then a microscopic examination of the tissues may be necessary before the presence of neoplastic tissue is discovered. We may assume, therefore, that a good many cases of carcinoma of the gall-bladder remain unrecognized, and it is probable that the disease is more frequent than we are led to believe from our statistics. Tumor of the spleen is, as a rule, absent. Ascites may be present, and at the same time other transudates as a result of the existing cachexia; or, finally, a carcinoma of the peritoneum may be present and cause ascites. Other important symptoms are progressive loss of strength, the cachectic appearance of the patient, the formation of secondary carcinomata in the liver, the peritoneum, etc. Only very rarely will an exploratory puncture of the gall-bladder reveal the presence of carcinoma by demonstrating small particles of carcinomatous tissue in the aspirated fluid. As a rule, if carcinoma exists the aspirated fluid will consist of a mixture of an albuminous exudate and blood. If, in the case of old subjects, an obstinate and persistent occlusion of the common duct is observed, and if at the same time the patient grows cachectic, the probability that a carcinoma is present is great. In doubtful cases an exploratory laparotomy may be attempted, and will furnish information that is of fundamental importance for prognosis and treatment.

Chronic peritonitic lesions are liable to develop principally in the region of the porta hepatis and of the gall-bladder, these locations seeming to be particular points of predilection in cholelithiasis. These lesions may lead to the formation of adhesions and to the development of connective-tissue strands. The adhesions may, in the first place, cause all the disturbances that we have described, such as compression of the bileducts with all its results; and, in addition, they may exercise traction on certain parts of the intestine, and in this manner hinder their free movement, cause stasis of their contents, digestive disturbances of various kinds, and particularly violent attacks of pain that usually assume the character of attacks of intestinal colic. An examination of the abdomen, as a rule, furnishes very little information, for the reason that the adhesive strands are not palpable. It is often possible to localize the pain and the other disturbances within a circumscribed area in the vicinity of the region of the fundus of the gall-bladder, this applying particularly to the tenderness and the spontaneous pain. If such a localization can be made, this may be considered a diagnostic clue of some significance. The suspicion will often be aroused that we are dealing with an ulcer or a carcinoma of this region until some serious disturbance arises that calls for a laparotomy, and the diagnosis is made in this way. Loosening of the adhesions is usually followed by a complete restoration to health; but unfortunately, as a rule, new adhesions form.

It is also possible for a diffuse form of perihepatitis to develop after inflammation of the gall-bladder or of the intrahepatic bile-passages, particularly of those that are situated immediately beneath the capsule of the liver (Leichtenstern, Raynaud and Sabourin). If this occurs, the first symptom to be noticed will be a distinct respiratory friction sound; which, later, may be heard over a large area. The liver, as a rule, is very sensitive to pressure. Singultus may occur as a result of irritation of the diaphragm. Gerhardt states that he has heard the respiratory friction sound described above in the region of the gallbladder following transitory attacks of gall-stone colic. The perihepatitis under discussion ultimately must lead to a thickening and later to a contraction of Glisson's capsule and of the peritoneum covering the surface of the liver; and, in addition, strands of connective tissue may extend from the surface of the organ into the interior, and in this manner cause atrophy of the liver (Poulin).

Many authors consider diabetes mellitus one of the possible sequels of cholelithiasis, for the reason that these investigators have found sugar in the urine at different times following attacks of gall-stone colic. Naunyn has submitted these views to sharp criticism and has demonstrated that a clear and positive connection cannot be proved to exist in the present state of our knowledge between the two conditions. Most of the cases were probably diabetics in whom the existence of cholelithiasis had not been discovered because it ran its course without causing any symptoms or without causing any disturbances of the general health of the patient. Owing to the severe nervous commotion incident to an attack of gall-stone colic, it is possible that the excretion of sugar in cases of this kind became increased, and that after the subsidence of the attack the excretion of sugar was again reduced or disappeared altogether.   In addition, it must be remembered that many factors that may lead to cholelithiasis may also cause diabetes, particularly the so-called fatty form of the disease.   If cirrhosis of the liver is present at the same time, it may be that an alimentary form of glycosuria plays a certain rôle. [Exner * found sugar in all but one of 40 patients with cholelithiasis, the glycosuria disappearing in from three to four weeks after operation. Zinn † found, on the other hand, that glycosuria was present in only 2 out of 89 cases; Kausch ‡ found it in only one out of 85 cases; while Strauss § failed to produce glycosuria by feeding three cases of chole-lithiasis with 100 gm. of glucose.—Ed.]

If the disease is of long duration and the strength of the body is severely taxed, and particularly if chronic and persistent icterus is present, emaciation, cachexia, and anemia are seen.   It has even been stated that the latter may assume the character of a pernicious form of anemia. It is probable that some of the retained biliary constituents exercise a deleterious effect on the blood-corpuscles.

Finally, disturbances in the sphere of the nervous system must not be underestimated.   They are caused mainly by the long-continued character of the disease, the frequent attacks of intense pain, the dis-turbance of sleep and of the power to move about freely, and other causes.   In this manner, hysteria, neurasthenia, melancholia, or, on the other hand, states of excitement may be produced.   Both the laity and physicians since the days of antiquity have known that such nervous disturbances may develop and play an important rôle in the course of diseases of the liver.

[Opie has recently been able to demonstrate the close etiologic con-nection between cholelithiasis and certain cases of hemorrhagic pan-creatitis.   In the instance observed by him at autopsy a small concre-tion blocked the orifice of the common duct and the pancreatic duc-showed distinct evidence of the entrance of bile into its lumen.—Ed.]

PROGNOSIS.

As cholelithiasis generally runs its course without disturbance, and only rarely causes complicating inflammation of the bile-passages and of the tissues surrounding them, the prognosis, as a rule, is favorable. Gall-stones, at the same time, always constitute a danger for the patient, as they may at any time begin to migrate and produce inflammatory and ulcerative processes which, in their turn, cause a variety of diseases. These appear at times when they are least expected, and may suddenly attack the patient and endanger his life.   All this must be taken into con-

* *Deutsche med. Woch.*, Aug., 1898, 4p. 491.
† *Centralbl. f. innere Med.*, Sept. 24, 1898.
‡ *Deutsche med. Woch.*, Feb. 16, 1899.
§ *Berlin. klin. Woch.*, Dec. 19, 1898.

sideration when making a prognosis, and even though the stones be perfectly quiescent, the prognosis in regard to some of the lesions complicating cholelithiasis must be guarded. In cases where icterus appears, or where colic and great swelling of the liver or of the gall-bladder are present, or symptoms appear that indicate that the gall-stone is moving, the prognosis becomes unfavorable. Even under these circumstances, however, it need not necessarily be altogether bad.

If a violent form of intermittent or of remittent fever appears, or if a gall-stone becomes impacted within the common duct and causes permanent obstruction to the escape of bile, the prognosis is bad. The same can be said if signs of circumscribed peritonitis appear, or if empyema of the gall-bladder, suppurative cholangitis, or abscess of the liver complicate the disease. The prognosis is particularly bad if sudden perforation into the peritoneal cavity occurs, and if, following this rupture, larger or smaller quantities of the contents of the bile-passages or of the gall-bladder are poured into the abdomen, the contents of the bile-passages being, as a rule, changed and abnormal, and therefore dangerous. The prognosis is also very bad if a gall-stone or gall-stones become impacted in the intestine and cause ileus, or, finally, if the presence of a carcinoma can be diagnosed from the appearance of long-continued icterus, great loss of strength, ascites, etc.

DIAGNOSIS.

The diagnosis of cholelithiasis can be made from all the symptoms discussed above in all their essential features.

If the gall-stones remain quiescent, the diagnosis may often be very difficult. In many instances an examination of the region of the liver and the gall-bladder will lead to the discovery of a tumor of the gall-bladder in which the gall-stones can be distinctly felt. This can, however, rarely be done, and it is still more difficult to elicit the sensation of crepitation described by older authors. In many cases the walls of the gall-bladder are so thick that the gall-stones cannot possibly be felt through them. Nodular tumors of the gall-bladder may, moreover, be due to carcinoma of the viscus. In the case of the latter lesion, however, the further course of the disease, and the discovery of metastases, will clear the diagnosis. Schwartz describes the following differences between a tumor of the kidney and an enlarged gall-bladder: A tumor of the gall-bladder can be depressed or pushed into the abdomen, but immediately returns to its original position; a tumor of the kidney, on the other hand, that extends into the region of the liver, will remain in the position into which it is pressed until it is pushed forward again by the hand of the physician. Gerard-Marchand calls attention to the fact that tumors of the gall-bladder cannot be pushed upward.

Puncture of the gall-bladder and palpation of the contained gall-stones is quite dangerous, although this procedure has been recommended by Harley and others. As we can never know, however, whether the contents of the gall-bladder are septic or not, it is dangerous to puncture the gall-bladder, as some of its contents may exude through the opening and, if it should be infectious, cause peritonitis.

Gall-stones cannot be demonstrated by the Röntgen rays for the reason that they are permeable for these rays owing to the cholesterin and relatively large proportion of organic matter which they always contain, as well as to the obscuring shadow of the liver.

In the majority of cases an attack of gall-stone colic will be the first positive sign that reveals the presence of gall-stones. The diffuse pain and the other vague and varying sensations complained of, the feeling of pressure in the region of the gall-bladder, etc., are all of subordinate importance in the diagnosis of the disease.

It is also possible to misinterpret the significance of the attack of colic and to confound it with intestinal colic, cardialgia, nervous hepatic colic, etc. Whereas, however, in the case of peptic ulcer the pain is liable to occur after eating, the pain in gall-stone colic usually appears toward midnight; that is, some time after a meal, and particularly after some error of diet of which the patient has been guilty. In other instances, again, it is true, the attack of gall-stone colic may occur very soon after eating, and the pain may even be felt in the median line, in the epigastric region, so that the similarity to a case of gastric ulcer is indeed very great. The pain will be in this location if the gall-stone is impacted near the orifice of the common duct. Violent retching and vomiting are more frequently seen in gall-stone colic than in the other condition. In intestinal colic the pain is usually located in the right hypochondriac region and is not quite so violent; and, as a rule, it disappears as soon as belching, the passage of flatus, or defecation occurs. Lead colic is a disease that causes very violent symptoms, and the pain is located in a region so similar to that in cholelithiasis that the two may often be confounded. The former is seen particularly in men, whereas the latter occurs more frequently in women. Certain occupations, the handling of lead by the patient, a blue line on the gums, the absence of pain and swelling of the liver and of icterus, will all speak in favor of lead colic. The pain of renal colic is situated more in the lumbar region, while that of gall-stone colic very rarely radiates into this region. The former usually radiates along the course of the ureter into the bladder and the genitals, while this rarely happens in gall-stone colic. An attack of peritonitis, particularly if it is localized in the right hypochondriac region and is circumscribed, may cause diagnostic difficulties. Collapse, changes in the pulse-beat, and sensitiveness to pressure may be observed in both conditions. As a rule, the pain on pressure, the frequency and the smallness of the pulse, and the collapse are more pronounced in peritonitis. At the same time, cases of inflammation of the peritoneum may occur in which all these symptoms are indistinct and only present to a slight degree, and, on the other hand, all these symptoms may be present in an aggravated form in attacks of gall-stone colic. The type of breathing, it is true, is almost always purely costal in peritonitis, while in gall-stone colic a distinct movement of the diaphragm will generally be seen. Further, large quantities of indoxyl are, as a rule, voided in the urine during an attack of peritonitis; this does not occur in simple uncomplicated cholelithiasis. It is often possible to make a differential diagnosis between cholelithiasis and an attack of perityphlitis extending upward along the right side of the abdominal cavity (as a result of dislocation of the appendix) by the aid of this indoxyl reaction of the urine.

[Mention must be made of the possibility of an attack of gall-stone colic being erroneously looked upon as "gout of the stomach." The latter is extremely rare, and the diagnosis should never be positively made except by exclusion and from the simultaneous retrocession of more characteristic distant uratic manifestations.—ED.]

Icterus is without doubt of the greatest importance in the recognition of cholelithiasis. It is true that this valuable sign is often absent in cases where the gall-stones are situated in the cystic duct or in the intrahepatic bile-passages, or where they pass through the common duct very rapidly. The change in the intensity of icterus is of particular importance in the diagnosis of gall-stones. In the catarrhal form of icterus, in that form of icterus that is the result of compression of the bile-ducts from tumors or some external obstruction, icterus may persist for weeks and months without fluctuations in its intensity. This may, of course, also occur if the ductus choledochus is completely occluded for a long time by gall-stones. This, however, rarely occurs in simple cholelithiasis; it is possibly more frequent if carcinoma complicates the disease. Icterus usually appears during the course of an attack of gall-stone colic and soon disappears again. As a rule, this icterus is not very severe, but it has a tendency to recur, and, even if it persists for a long time, considerable fluctuations in its intensity are apt to occur. At the same time colored and acholic stools are alternately evacuated. It is not at all necessary that icterus of the skin should exist.

What can be found out in regard to the localization of the gall-stones —that is, whether they are located in the gall-bladder, the cystic duct, the common duct, etc.—has been described in the section on symptomatology; and the same statements apply to the diagnosis of ulceration, the formation of fistulæ, the entrance of gall-stones into the intestine, etc.

From a therapeutic point of view, it is, in addition, important to determine whether pyogenic organisms have penetrated the bile-passages; in other words, it is important to determine the presence or absence of suppurative cholangitis and cholecystitis.

The chief symptom of these conditions is the appearance of an intermittent or remittent type of fever of long duration. At the same time a tumor of the spleen may be noticed, while septicopyemic metastases in other organs and symptoms of infectious endocarditis point toward the diagnosis. Empyema of the gall-bladder produces swelling of and pain in the organ. Sometimes it is possible to aspirate a purulent fluid. Puncture of the gall-bladder, however, is severely condemned by the majority of physicians, and particularly by surgeons, for the reason that great danger of peritonitis exists in case some of the contents of the gall-bladder should enter the abdominal cavity. Even if all possible precautions are taken,—if, for instance, very thin needles are employed, etc.,—a circumscribed form of peritonitis will almost invariably be produced. Naunyn—who, by the way, is a strong advocate of exploratory puncture of the gall-bladder for diagnostic purposes—makes this statement himself. In cases where the walls of the gall-bladder are very thin and are under pressure from the tension of the fluid they inclose, it will be well to be exceptionally careful. After the little operation, an ice-bag should be applied to the region of the gall-bladder and the patient kept in bed for at least eight hours. If the fluid that is aspirated is dark brown or yellowish in color and contains some of the bile-constituents but no micro-organisms, then we are dealing with a simple ectasy of the gall-bladder; if a colorless or slightly colored fluid containing mucus or squamous epithelium but no bile constituents is aspirated, and if this fluid is watery or viscid, then we have hydrops of the gall-bladder; again, if the fluid aspirated is colorless or slightly bile-stained and contains albumin, desquamated cylindric and squamous epithelium, micro-organisms, in particular Bacillus coli, we are dealing with cholecystitis seropurulenta; finally, if the fluid is purulent and contains no bile whatever, the case is one of empyema of the gall-bladder (Kleefeld).

The formation of abscesses of the liver, which are as a rule multiple, frequently cannot be recognized. In many instances the abscesses are in a location where they cannot be palpated; circumscribed pain, fluctuation, etc., may be absent; while exploratory puncture for diagnostic purposes is as dangerous here as in empyema of the gall-bladder. (For details see the section on abscess of the liver.) The existence of this lesion can be suspected if the symptoms of suppurative cholangitis persist for a very long time in cholelithiasis, if the liver is painful, if symptoms of pyemia appear, and if purulent inflammation of neighboring parts can be recognized.

In all cases of cholelithiasis the most positive criterion for the presence of gall-stones is the discovery of concretions in the stools. While some authors—as, for instance, Wolff—claim to have found them in all cases, still there are instances in which they cannot be discovered in spite of the most careful and diligent search. They may be retained within the gall-bladder or the bile-passages and there cause attacks of colic from time to time; they may also become disintegrated in the intestine or may be retained within the bowels for a long time even without producing any of the symptoms of occlusion or of ileus. For all these reasons it is often necessary to search the stools for days before they are found. It is not well to employ the old method of Prout, which consists in diluting the stools with water, in stirring them and then limiting the examination to the particles that float on top; but the stools, after dilution with water, should be filtered through a fine sieve and the residue washed out repeatedly with water; it is not advisable during this manipulation to crush the stools, for the reason that the more recently formed stones are often very soft and may be crushed beyond recognition. If the stools are analyzed as above, it will often be possible to detect the presence of very small and quite soft stones. Gall-stones may readily be confounded with all sorts of pips and kernels from berries, pears, etc.; in addition, small hardened masses of fecal matter, and concretions of calcium- and magnesia-soaps, that are found after an abundant ingestion of fat, may lead to confusion. If the masses found are carefully examined for cholesterin, bile-pigment, and the characteristic structure of gall-stones, mistakes of this kind are not liable to happen.

[The "ball-valve" stone in the common duct at times gives rise to difficulties in diagnosis. The recurrence of attacks of pain, followed by fever and increasing icterus, make a picture easily recognized if the condition is borne in mind.—ED.]

PROPHYLAXIS.

In order to prevent the formation of gall-stones the following measures, recommended in our discussion on the etiology of gall-stones, should be employed:

1. Stasis of bile should be prevented.

2. All factors that may lead to an infection of the bile-passages, and in this manner to a stone-forming catarrh, should be strenuously avoided.

If sufficient care is taken that the clothing in the region of the liver and the gall-bladder is not too tight, congestion of these parts is not so liable to occur. In subjects, therefore, whose bones are slender and delicately constructed, who are thin with a poorly developed muscular system and no adipose layer, tight corsets should be forbidden; and they should be instructed never to wear tight skirt-bands nor to attach their clothing by tight bands nor to wear tight apron-bands, belts, etc. Women who are constructed in this way should be told to wear loose clothing and corsets that are made like jackets and are suspended by shoulder-straps and that permit the other clothing, shirts, underwear, etc., to be buttoned on' (see page 395). If the clothing is arranged in this way, its weight will be brought to bear on the shoulders and not on the epigastric and hypochondriac regions. It is also well to advise people predisposed to gall-stones and of the peculiar build described above to loosen their clothing after eating; *i. e.*, as soon as the flow of bile begins.

Physical exercise also counteracts the stasis of bile. Walking, gymnastic exercises, fencing, horseback-riding, etc., are efficient preventives. Bathing, too, may exercise a favorable effect, particularly with swimming. In the case of those who cannot or will not persevere in these exercises, it may be well to advise massage of the body or medico-mechanical exercises. Energetic physical exercise influences the flow of bile not only directly and mechanically, but also indirectly by increasing the peristaltic action of the bowels and the evacuation of the contents of the intestine.

Constipation must be relieved as much as possible by the administration of laxatives, particularly of Glauber's and Epsom salts. In the same way a course in one of the bathing resorts, such as Carlsbad, Marienbad, Kissingen, etc., may act in a prophylactic manner.

Fr. Hoffmann has sounded a warning against eating at too long intervals. Frerichs has also emphasized this, for the reason that under these conditions the bile is retained too long in the bile-passages and the gall-bladder. A diet that is too uniform and that contains too much fatty food is also to be avoided. A régime of this kind seems to predispose to catarrh of the stomach and intestine, and this may readily extend to the bile-ducts.

Particular care should be taken to avoid all infections of the intestine, so obviating the development of a stone-forming catarrh of the bile-passages. It is, of course, a difficult matter to guard against these infections, because a small quantity of spoiled food or any of the pathogenic germs may induce infectious processes of different kinds. As accidents of this kind are most apt to occur if the diet is too uniform or if too much food is eaten, so that the digestion is overtaxed in one or in several directions, it will be best to advise a moderate mode of life and the taking of a mixed and not too abundant diet. The general rules and regulations formulated in the paragraphs on diet in the section on treatment may be followed to advantage. A close observance of these rules will do much toward an avoidance of gall-stone formation.

TREATMENT.

The treatment of gall-stones will depend greatly on the presence or absence of complications; *i. e.*, whether the object desired is simply to remove gall-stones that may be present, and thus do away with the symptoms caused by their presence, or whether the disease is complicated by cholecystitis and cholangitis and it is desired to cure or relieve these conditions.

In the former, the regular form of gall-stone disease, dietetic measures, the drinking of certain waters, etc., and treatment with drugs must be chiefly considered. In rare cases only will it be necessary to consider the advisability of surgical measures from the beginning.

In the dietetics of cholelithiasis the views of different authorities are in part diametrically opposed. This is explainable from the different views entertained by different authors in regard to the formation of gall-stones, the genesis of cholesterin, the importance of intestinal catarrhs, etc., some of these views being necessarily quite incorrect.

Some, as Bouchard, J. Kraus, and others, debar all fatty food, for the reason that they believe that such a diet increases the formation of cholesterin. They base their view on certain investigations that seemed to show that the administration of large quantities of fatty food causes an increase in the quantity of cholesterin. Naunyn and Thomas oppose and combat this idea. According to Jankau, the introduction of cholesterin itself into the organism does not increase the amount of cholesterin formed. The amount of cholesterin is dependent on the degree of catarrh present in the bile-passages.

On the other hand, the administration of large quantities of fat, as recommended by Dujardin-Beaumetz, is not indicated, as the cholagogue action which he claims for fat is only slightly manifested; in fact, could not be determined at all in several investigations that were undertaken for this purpose.

It seems well in the case of gall-stones to avoid the ingestion of too much fat, for the reason that such a diet seems to predispose particularly to disturbances of the gastric digestion, and may in this manner lead to the formation of intestinal catarrhs which, in their turn, may extend to the bile-passages. For the same reason the patients should be advised to avoid all excesses of whatever kind, including excessive eating and drinking, the abuse of alcohol, of spices, etc. These restrictions will be particularly indicated in all those cases in which disturbances of gastric or intestinal digestion, such as catarrhal conditions, already exist. In all cases of this character it will be well, therefore, to advise a very light and readily digestible diet, corresponding to the abnormal digestive conditions indicated. The most suitable diet seems to be a mixed one containing plenty of proteid, not too scanty or uniform, so that an abundant quantity of bile-acids is produced, and so that the flow of bile may be stimulated and maintained. It is a good plan to advise frequent meals only three hours apart during the course of the day. It seems superfluous to advise eating something in the middle of the night as long as the patient will surely eat a breakfast soon after rising. It is also well to advise the ingestion of an abundant amount of fluid, for while an abundant or an excessive amount of water does not stimulate the flow of bile or increase it, at the same time too little water is known to cause thickening of the bile, and in this manner possibly indirectly constitute an impediment to its flow.

Bramson has argued particularly against the use of water containing much calcareous material, as he believes that this will lead to an increased excretion of chalky matter through the bile. Hankau, however, has demonstrated that the ingestion of water containing much lime does not lead to an increased excretion of this substance in the bile, and that the amount of calcium excreted in the bile is independent of the amount ingested at any given time.

In order to promote an unobstructed flow of bile, it is necessary to instruct the patient to wear loose clothing—a point already discussed in the section on the prophylaxis of gall-stone formation. For this reason women should be advised to wear loose, soft, and wide corsets attached by shoulder-straps; to these the skirts, etc., should be attached by buttons, and all tight belts, skirt-bands, or other supports constricting the waist should be discarded. After eating, particular care should be taken that the patient rests quietly and that the clothing is loosened.

Exercise favors the flow of bile, and for this reason patients who are lazy and fat should be induced to take regular physical exercise. Walking is a very good form of exercise; and, particularly in the case of women, long walks should be advised. Domestic duties, housework of all kinds, do not furnish sufficient exercise of the right kind, since patients in doing housework sit down or stand a great deal more than they realize. Other forms of exercise are also good, as, for instance, horseback-riding, riding a bicycle, rowing, swimming, mountain-climbing, gymnastic exercise, medico-mechanical exercises, etc. In the course of such exercises it may happen that a gall-stone becomes dislodged and begins to wander, so that an attack of colic is produced in this manner. This may happen during horseback-riding, jumping, dancing, etc. In case the gall-stone passes through the ducts and is evacuated, such an accident will of course in its ultimate consequences be of use to the patient. On the other hand, it may of course happen that gall-stones become lodged in the cystic or the common duct and remain firmly impacted. In a case of this kind all the unfortunate results of such an occurrence may be witnessed—inflammatory processes may be set up in the vicinity of the stone, icterus may occur, or perforation of the duct with all its sequels may take place. It may also happen that rapid or sudden motions of the body may cause an impacted gall-stone to perforate the walls of the duct in cases where the latter had become attenuated, an occurrence from which serious damage may result. In uncomplicated cases of cholelithiasis the latter emergency will be exceedingly rare. In cases where the presence of ulcerative processes or of other complications is suspected, the patient should be warned against indulging in too violent exercise, and should be particularly advised against performing sudden movements that cause a succussion of the body. Among these may be mentioned horseback-riding, jumping, dancing, or such acts as riding in a wagon with bad springs over defective roads.

Massage of the body acts favorably in the same sense as exercise of other kinds. In cases where the sluggishness of the bowels can be relieved by massage, the effect is especially good, as an increased peristaltic action of the bowels is induced, and this is, as a rule, transferred to the bile-ducts, by which the musculature of the bile-passages is stimulated to increased action and the stagnation of bile counteracted and corrected. Direct massage of the gall-bladder rarely leads to an evacuation of gall-stones, although some cases are on record in which, following repeated palpation and manipulation of the gall-bladder, gall-stones were induced to move, entered the bile-ducts, and were finally evacuated. Van Swieten long ago recommended tapping the gall-bladder with the fingers in the treatment of gall-stones. The employment of electricity,

38

either in the form of the galvanic or of the faradic current, has been advised by some authors, but is of doubtful value.

For a great many years one of the aims in the treatment of chole-lithiasis has been to promote the solution of gall-stones within the bile-passages after they had formed there. All attempts in this direction have, however, so far been altogether unsuccessful. It may at times occur that a solution of gall-stones takes place. Naunyn has demonstrated this by introducing gall-stones into the gall-bladder of dogs. Normally disintegration and fragmentation of gall-stones is, moreover, quite frequently observed. The bile is a good solvent for cholesterin, but not to such a degree for stones that contain a considerable portion of calcium. The alkaline salts of the bile-acids in particular seem to exercise this effect (Schiff and others). As gall-stones are soluble in alkaline fluids, alkalies were recommended for the treatment of gall-stones (Fr. Hoff-mann) even as early as the eighteenth century. Since that time their value in the treatment of gall-stones has become established. They are employed especially in the form of different mineral waters, as the waters of Carlsbad, Vichy, Ems, Bertrich, and many others. Warm saline waters have also been recommended for this purpose, as the waters of Wiesbaden, Soden, Nauheim, and others. Some benefit is unquestion-ably derived from the use of these waters. From all experimental in-vestigations, however, it seems more than doubtful whether these waters in any way influence the alkalinity of the bile and in this manner dis-solve gall-stones. Their cholagogue action is also doubtful and has not been experimentally demonstrated. Many authors attribute a beneficial effect to the large quantities of water that are swallowed in the course of such a line of treatment (Leichtenstern), and express the belief that the ingestion of all this fluid promotes the flow of bile and causes an increased excretion. Animal experiments, however, do not show that such an effect on the bile is exercised by excessive drinking of water. It is probable that the effect of large quantities of water on the stomach and the intestine is the chief factor and acts favorably on the bile-passages. Catarrhal conditions of these organs are ameliorated by this procedure and indirectly act on similar catarrhal conditions that may be present in the bile-ducts or the gall-bladder. The waters of those springs that contain Glauber salts act favorably on the bowels, promote regular evacuations, and in this manner the peristaltic action of the bowel musculature is stimulated, and this stimulus is transmitted to the musculature of the bile-ducts, causing increased peristalsis in these parts and aiding the passage of the gall-stone. Consequently the drink-ing of these waters is often followed by the passage of gall-stones. The use of bitter waters—a course of treatment in Marienbad and other places—often leads to the same result. The change in the mode of life of the patients during the time they are taking the course of treatment plays a most important rôle, the regulation of physical exercise, the moderation and regulation of the diet, and other features explaining to a great extent the beneficial effects of the waters of Carlsbad, Vichy, and of other places. This also explains why certain patients who could be benefited as much if they remained at home, lived sensibly, and took Carlsbad waters, bicarbonate of sodium, Glauber salts, or rhubarb, never really notice any benefit until they go to the different watering-places and take the waters there. It appears to these patients that all their complaints are much relieved as soon as they arrive at these places, and, in fact, the treatment they undergo is often followed by the passage of gall-stones, etc.

The different herb extracts that were formerly so popular (Hoffmann and others) probably act in a similar manner, the administration of these infusions having been based on Glisson's observation that in cattle gall-stones seem to disappear in summer as soon as the animals begin to eat green herbs and grass.

The administration of fats, particularly of olive oil, has also been recommended in order to promote the dissolution of gall-stones. It is doubtful, however, whether fats really enter the bile, although Virchow and Thoma have made statements to this effect. At all events, they cannot possibly exercise any effect on gall-stones that consist largely of chalky material.

Durande, in 1782, recommended a remedy that created a great deal of interest. It consisted of equal parts of ether and turpentine. According to this author, twenty to thirty drops of the remedy should be taken three to four times daily. In many cases the bad taste of this remedy makes it difficult to take (Pujol, J. P. Frank, and others), for which reason Durande modified his prescription and ordered a mixture of three parts of ether with one part of turpentine. Later Soemmering and others used ether alone mixed with the yolk of an egg. Of late years the remedy has again been recommended by Lewaschew, who bases his recommendation on the experiments of Botkin and on his own experience. It is true that ether and turpentine are excreted in part by the bile, but in so small a quantity that they cannot possibly exercise a solvent effect. Vallisnieri recognized this quite correctly long before Durande recommended the remedy, and discovered the fact that gall-stones are soluble in turpentine, but refrained from advising the internal use of the remedy for the solution of gall-stones for the reason stated. Some authors (Frerichs) have attributed the favorable effect sometimes exercised by Durande's remedy in cases of gall-stones to the calming effect of the ether; while others state that peristalsis is stimulated or that efforts at vomiting are induced that help to expel the stone. It is known that ipecacuanha and tartar emetic have been employed for the same purpose. Duparcque has seen beneficial effects follow the administration of a mixture of ether and castor oil.

Chloroform belongs to the same class of remedies. This drug was recommended by Corlieu, Bouchut, Gobley, and others. As a rule, it is administered in the dose of 5 or 6 drops in water or of 1 gm. in 150 of water, a tablespoonful being given at a time; or it may be given in capsules of 0.1 gm. Many physicians recommend the drug highly; others claim to have seen no benefit from its employment. It does not seem to possess any anodyne properties and cannot stop the pain of an attack of colic. If ether or chloroform is inhaled during the attack, according to Murchison, the effect is, of course, different.

The oil treatment even to this day plays a prominent rôle in the treatment of gall-stones. This method is of American origin, was first introduced by Kennedy, and later advocated warmly by Chauffard in France and Rosenberg in Germany. [Lindley Scott * found no difference in the solvent action of petroleum or almond and olive oil. A quarter of the weight of calculi was lost in twelve hours, a half of their weight in twenty-four hours, and all but the nucleus was dissolved in thirty-six

* *Brit. Med. Jour.*, Sept. 25, 1887, p. 798.

hours.—Ed.] It is erroneous to attribute a cholagogue action to oil, as has been done by several writers. Rosenberg recommends the administration of 180 to 200 gm. of olive oil with 0.5 of menthol, 20 to 30 gm. of cognac, and the yolks of two eggs to be taken in one or in several doses. Senator has recommended the use of lipanin instead of olive oil, Blum advises the oleate of sodium. [Clemm * also employs the latter remedy in doses of 0.75 gm., and Artault † has claimed a prophylactic effect from the taking of 8 to 16 minims of olive oil before breakfast for ten days in each month.—Ed.] It is probably best to swallow the disagreeable remedy at one dose instead of distributing it in tablespoonful doses over the whole day, although the latter plan has many advocates. Friedr. Hoffmann, it may be mentioned, recommended almond oil for the treatment of gall-stones in the eighteenth century; cottonseed oil, too, has been recommended. It is true that after the administration of these different oils gall-stones often pass. The best explanation for this is that the remedy, like many other drugs, acts as an emetic or a laxative, and in this manner promotes the emptying of the bile-passages. There can be no question in regard to the utility of castor oil, and this drug has often been employed with great advantage. Another factor must be remembered in judging of the value of all these oils in promoting the passages of gall-stones, and that is the possibility of their forming concretions of saponified oleic acid in the intestine. These masses, when they appear in the stools, may very well simulate small gall-stones (Chauffard, Dupré, Rosenberg, Prentiss, Fürbringer, and others). Pujol long ago described masses of this kind formed from almond oil. Undigested particles of food, pieces of pear, etc., may also lead to errors.

Enemata of 400 to 500 c.c. (13 to 17 fluidounces) of oil at 30° C. (86°·F.), at first recommended by Blum, may act favorably by regulating the action of the bowels. They should be given at first daily, later at longer intervals.

Glycerin administered with Vichy in daily doses of 15 to 20 gm. seems to be without value. This treatment was first recommended by Ferraud.

The attempt has frequently been made to introduce calomel into the therapeutics of cholelithiasis, as has been done lately by Sacharjin.

Very often the physician is called while the patient is suffering from an attack of gall-stones, and it is his first duty to alleviate the suffering. He must also attempt to cut short the attack by promoting the passage of the stone, and, finally, avoid many of the complications, like ulceration, inflammation of the surrounding tissues, etc., that might follow impaction of the stone.

Opium or morphin has for a long time been recommended to stop the pain (van Swieten, Coe, J. P. Frank, and others). These drugs not only relieve the great pain, but also help to relax the spasm of the muscles of the bile-ducts. Pujol, it is true, warns against this procedure because he fears that the gall-stone will remain where it is, and in this manner "the wolf be locked up in the sheepfold"; but as it is known that the spasmodic contractions of the muscles of the walls of the bile-ducts are, if anything, an obstacle to the free passage of the gall-stone, an arrest of these contractions can only be of use. The administration of narcotics is therefore indicated, and is of value in promoting the passage of a gall-stone. At first a hypodermic injection of from 0.01 to 0.02 of the hydrochlorate of morphin is given, or 20 drops of the tincture

* *Wien. med. Woch.*, 1902, No. 16.   † *La Med. Moderne*, 1901, p. 392.

of opium are administered by mouth, followed in from two to four hours by another 5 to 10 drops, the dose to be repeated every two to four hours.

Belladonna has further been recommended for its antispasmodic action (Trousseau, Frerichs, Murchison, Stricker, and others). It does seem as if this drug were capable of relieving the spasmodic contraction of the muscles and in this manner of promoting the evacuation of the gall-stone. It is best administered as the extract of belladonna in powders of 0.02 to 0.03 or dissolved in aqua amygdala amara (1.0 to 10.0), 5 to 10 drops every two hours. It is well in giving belladonna to watch the patient carefully, for the reason that excessive doses may produce symptoms of poisoning, while doses that are too small exercise no effect whatever.

Antinervines, as antipyrin, phenacetin, preparations of salicylic acid, etc., sometimes stop the violent pain. Inhalations of chloroform should be administered only in cases with exceptional excitement. Chloral hydrate and other narcotics of this class as a rule are without effect. In case they do not put the patient to sleep, they are apt to produce great excitement, and later unconsciousness.

Warm applications in the form of cataplasms, of dry or wet cloths, of poultices kept warm by means of a thermophor applied over the region of the liver are recommended, and seem in fact to be able to relieve much of the distress; but if inflammatory processes are going on in the region of the gall-bladder, they are frequently not so well borne. In cases of this kind leeches or applications of cold by an ice-bag placed over the painful region will often relieve. If the patient is very sensitive to pressure, the ice-bag can be suspended over the painful spot, barely touching it without exercising any pressure (Bricheteau). In plethoric subjects, following the procedure of older physicians, blood-letting is often beneficial and may relieve the spasms. Drinking warm fluids, different herb-infusions, etc., occasionally does good.

If it is possible to place the patient in a warm bath of about 40° C. (104° F.), the pain and the spasm will usually be relieved, and many patients are comforted if kept for a long time in a warm bath. Hysterical seizures, too, are best aborted and treated by immersing patients in a warm bath or by pouring cold water over them.

It is advisable at the same time to procure a good evacuation of the bowels during the attack of gall-stone colic. This is best accomplished by the administration of castor oil, Epsom salts, artificial Carlsbad salts, etc. As, however, all these laxatives are vomited in many cases, it is imperative to employ enemata. Large quantities of cold or of hot water applied in this way act very beneficially, as do also 1 to 2 liters of chamomile tea, or, if the stools are very hard, 200 to 300 gm. of olive oil injected into the rectum. If the patients are very weak and if the pulse is small and rapid, wine, champagne, and similar stimulants must be administered. Here camphor injected hypodermically in doses of from 0.1 to 0.2 in oil is often very useful.

In cases, finally, where all internal medication is without avail, and where despite all the remedial measures employed attacks of gall-stone colic recur, and where the strength of the patient is being undermined, his nervous system shattered, and he is rendered incapable of attending to his affairs, surgical interference should be advised. In the present state of our knowledge of surgical technique and experience such an operation is indicated, and the patient may thus for all time get rid of his gall-stones.

At the same time it must be remembered that each attack of gall-stone colic may be the last one, and that a permanent cure of the condition may occur even after many severe and grave attacks of gall-stone colic. In some cases, too, operations have been performed at a time when the last gall-stone had been evacuated and passed through the common duct. It must also be remembered, on the other hand, that in cases where impaction of gall-stones occurs repeatedly the danger of cholangitis and ulceration with all its consequences exists, and that a number of local changes may develop insidiously that complicate a subsequent operation—I refer to adhesions, stenoses, narrowing of the bile-passages, etc. [The danger of acute hemorrhagic pancreatitis is an additional reason for operative interference.—Ed.]

Operative interference should be advised at once if signs of suppurative cholangitis, of cholecystitis, or of incipient peritonitis appear.

It is true that even in these cases recovery may occur without operative interference; but the prospect of a cure and the general outlook are much better if the bile-passages are opened as soon as possible and a fistulous opening is created. This operation will be described below. Under circumstances of this kind the hepatic and the common duct have been drained through a fistula with good results; while in some instances it has been necessary to open the common ducts and to flush the channel thoroughly through a bent metal tube (Kehr).

In case the operation, notwithstanding the presence of cholelithiasis, is not permitted by the patient, it will be necessary to attempt to allay the inflammation by hot or cold applications in the shape of warm compresses, the ice-bag, etc.; at the same time the bowels must be regulated and the feces regularly evacuated by the use of enemata, laxatives, etc., in the manner indicated above. Antibacterial remedies have also been recommended, such as salicylic acid and the preparations of this drug (such as salol), oil of turpentine, quinin, etc. The most rational method of administering salicylic acid appears to be in the form of the salicylate of sodium (four to six times daily in doses of 1.0). According to Naunyn, the cholagogue action of this preparation can in this way be utilized, in addition to its antibacterial powers. If we succeed, by the application of all these measures, in allaying the inflammation, and if the gall-stone is passed through the common duct or through a fistula, a Carlsbad cure or a course of some other waters should be advised, by which we may help remove the last traces of the inflammation and prevent a recurrence of attacks of gall-stone colic.

In cases where the common duct is occluded by a gall-stone, great danger arises to the patient from stasis of bile, and an operation becomes imperative.

If icterus has persisted for a long time, and a tendency to hemorrhage exists as a result, the operation will be fraught with considerable danger. Death from bleeding may occur very rapidly even if all the blood-vessels are carefully ligated and if all hemorrhage is stopped by careful packing and tamponage. It is, therefore, advisable not to wait too long before operating in cases that are complicated by severe grades of icterus. At the same time a great many operations for gall-stones are on record which terminated favorably despite the presence of icterus and the resulting tendency to hemorrhage, so that, if no other prospect of relief or of cure exists, the operation should by all means be advised.

As soon as peritonitic symptoms appear with any degree of severity this should, too, be considered an indication for operation.

The operative treatment of cholelithiasis has only been generally employed during the last fifteen years; and, as a result of the constant improvement in the technique of operating and the introduction of aseptic and antiseptic methods, the results obtained have grown more and more favorable.

Petit, the first surgeon to attempt opening of the gall-bladder for inflammation following cholelithiasis, limited the operation to cases in which he was positive that adhesions had formed between the gall-bladder and the walls of the abdomen. Even under these conditions a majority of the clinicians of the end of the eighteenth and the beginning of the nineteenth century condemned it. Sharp, Morand, and Haller supported Petit in his views during this time, and Herlin, l'Anglas, and Duchainois attempted to demonstrate their feasibility by experimentally extirpating the gall-bladder from animals without detriment. Bloch went even further than Petit and advised the artificial creation of adhesions between the gall-bladder and the abdominal walls as a step preliminary to the operation of incision. Richter, Sebastian, Graves, Fauconneau-Dufresne, and others made similar suggestions. Thudichum, in 1859, advised sewing the gall-bladder to the abdominal walls as a preliminary step, and opening the viscus after six days. In 1867 Bobbs performed a cholecystotomy, having mistaken the tumor of the gall-bladder for a cyst of the ovary. In 1878 Kocher performed a successful operation for empyema of the gall-bladder, and at the same period Sims operated on a case of cholelithiasis according to the method of Thudichum, with an unfavorable result. After this time Keen, Lawson Tait, Rosenbach, and Ransohoff performed numerous operations for gall-stones. In 1882 Langenbuch was the first to perform extirpation of the gall-bladder (cystectomy), and Winiwarter performed the first cholecystenterostomy in a case in which the common duct was occluded. Following these operations, Kuster recommended the ideal operation of cystotomy: viz., cystendesis (Courvoisier). This consisted in opening the gall-bladder, evacuating its contents, closing it again, and replacing it in the abdominal cavity. Of late years the bile-ducts themselves, in cases where the gall-stones were situated within these passages, were incised directly (cysticotomy and choledochotomy). The last operation was usually undertaken from the front of the body; in some instances from the lumbar region. Finally, an operation has been performed several times that consists in making an artificial fistula between the ductus choledochus and the intestine—choledochoduodenostomy and choledochoenterostomy, both of which operations are indicated whenever the common duct is occluded.

This is not the place to describe the different operations and to go into the detail of their technique. All these descriptions will be found in the works of Riedel, Kehr, and others, and, above all, in the book on this subject written by Langenbuch.

The operation is rarely performed in a typical manner, particularly in complicated cases. The presence or absence of gall-stones, the existence or non-existence of adhesions, are all complications that can only be discovered after the abdomen has been opened, and the surgeon will have to be largely governed by what he finds. In many instances the case will appear to be a simple one and the operation will appear easy, but as soon as the abdomen is opened unsuspected difficulties may be discovered that necessitate a complete change of plan.

Cystotomy is the operation that is most frequently performed. If several large gall-stones are present in the gall-bladder without any inflammatory symptoms and without any evidence of irritation of the surrounding tissues, and if, finally, gall-stones are absent from the bile-ducts, the ideal form of cystotomy, *i. e.*, cystendesis, may be performed.

The gall-bladder is opened and its contents evacuated; the organ is then thoroughly flushed and cleansed. If it is found that the bile can flow through the cystic duct,—in other words, if this channel is patent,— and if no gall-stones can be found in the other ducts, the gall-bladder is closed by suturing and replaced in the abdomen. It must be remembered that whereas new gall-stones rarely form (as, for instance, around silk sutures, Homans), it may nevertheless happen that small concretions are left in the gall-bladder and that inflammatory symptoms may appear later as a result of infection of the gall-bladder. All these sequels and complications may endanger the replaced gall-bladder and may lead to peritonitis; if this occurs, the abdomen and the gall-bladder must be reopened.

Cystotomy performed in the ordinary manner protects against all these dangers, but has the disagreeable feature that it leaves the patient with a bothersome biliary fistula that may call for a tedious after-operation in those cases where spontaneous closure does not occur. In performing the operation the gall-bladder is found, pulled as far as possible toward the abdominal wall, and attached to it by stitching. If the gall-bladder contains pus and there seems to be danger of the inflammation spreading to the peritoneum, it is best to open the gall-bladder at once and to evacuate its contents, the gall-stones that the organ may contain being removed with forceps and spoon-shaped instruments. In the case of old subjects, the attempt should be made to open the gall-bladder at once and to remove the gall-stones, as this does away with the necessity of a second operation (single cystotomy).

Cystotomy in two stages is indicated in cases where the gall-bladder is contracted and is situated so deep down in the abdomen that it cannot readily be approximated to the abdominal walls. All adhesions that may exist are loosened and the place marked (by a thread) where it is purposed, later, to make the incision. A cavity is formed by parts of the mesentery (that is pulled up for this purpose), the parietal peritoneum, the liver, etc., and filled with tampons. At the expiration of from twelve to twenty-four hours the tampons are removed, the gall-bladder is opened, evacuated, etc.

Following this operation a fistula remains; through the new channel are poured changed contents of the gall-bladder, gall-stones, and later, in case the cystic duct is patent, bile. If the common duct is occluded all the bile is poured out through the fistula. In cases of this character it is frequently necessary to perform secondary operations (choledochotomy, enterostomy). As a rule, the fistula closes spontaneously, particularly if the flow of bile into the intestine is not impeded.

Cholecystectomy as well as the ideal operation of cystotomy prevent the formation of a fistula; at the same time this operation may be more readily followed by disagreeable complications. The absence of the gall-bladder is of subordinate significance. Although it has been claimed that the continuous flow of bile into the intestine and the deficient retention of this excretion can produce certain digestive disturbances, such as emaciation, diarrhea, etc. (Oddi), all these troubles are soon relieved and in a measure compensated by a vicarious dilatation of the common duct. In those cases, however, where gall-stones are situated in the cystic, the common, or the hepatic duct, and are not discovered during the operation, it is quite possible that these concretions may cause much trouble, as they cannot be reached so easily as if a fistula had been formed, a fact constituting an objection to the operation. Besides, the gall-bladder may be adherent to the liver and other adjacent tissues, and the extirpation of the organ may be very difficult under these circumstances. If empyema is present, it can, further, very well happen that the neighboring tissues become infected when it is attempted to loosen the gall-bladder from its surroundings. On the other hand, it must be emphasized that in cases where the wall of the gall-bladder is diseased but the bile-passages are intact extirpation of the organ is followed by splendid results (see Langenbuch and others).

If gall-stones are present in the cystic duct, the attempt can be made to reach them from the incised gall-bladder, as they can often be reached under these circumstances by spoon-shaped instruments, by forceps, etc.; or the attempt may be made to reach them with the fingers and to enucleate them from their surroundings with the finger-nails; or, finally, it may be tried to crush them from without and to push the fragments back into the gall-bladder. If all these measures fail, the attempt must be made to find the exact location of the stone in the duct and to incise the walls immediately over the stone. This is often a very difficult procedure owing to the hidden location of the stone, and it may be impossible to extract it in this manner. Too great pressure must be avoided in attempting to crush the stone through the walls of the duct, for the reason that the mucous lining of the cystic duct may be bruised, and this may be followed by serious complications.

If the gall-stones are situated in the common duct, the attempt should also be made to reach them through the gall-bladder, to crush them (Langenbuch, Kehr, Credé), and to push the fragments back into the gall-bladder. This may succeed, particularly if the common and the cystic ducts are dilated, as is often seen in cases of this character. If all these measures fail, the attempt must be made to create a fistula through the abdominal walls and to allow it to remain open, or to make some connection between the gall-bladder and the intestine (Winiwarter). The latter procedures will be particularly indicated in cases where the general condition of the patient, severe degrees of icterus, etc., make it impossible to perform more radical operations, and where, at the same time, the outflow of bile must be established. In the last-named operation the danger of infection of the gall-bladder from the intestine always exists (Dujardin-Beaumetz), and in cases where the fistula was made between the gall-bladder and the colon fecal fistulæ have been known to occur (Chavasse). If icterus is very severe, it is best to wait until it is less intense as a result of the outpouring of bile through the external fistula, and then, after the tissues have recovered somewhat, the more serious operation may be attempted.

Of late years the attempt has, finally, been made to incise the common duct and to remove gall-stones in this way (Heusner, Küster, Courvoisier, Riedel, and others). After removal of the stone the wall was closed by sutures. In many cases it is a very difficult matter to feel the stones through the wall of the duct, and it may even happen that they are confounded with enlarged lymph-glands. Those gall-stones that become impacted in the posterior parts of the ductus choledochus, behind the duodenum, are especially difficult to feel, and often cannot be found. Some operators have opened the common duct through an incision made from the lumbar region (Tuffier, Poirier) and have removed the gall-stone through this channel. Others, again, have made an anastomosis between the common duct and the small intestine (Sprengel) or the duodenum (Terrier, Körte, Kocher). By means of these operations the most natural method of cure is imitated, as even without operative interference fistulæ are often formed between the gall-bladder or ducts and the small intestine, and the gall-stone passed in this way.

It is usually possible to push gall-stones that are situated in the trunk of the hepatic duct into the common duct. If the gall-stones are situated in the intrahepatic bile-ducts, they can be reached only with considerable difficulty. If they can be felt at all, the attempt should be made to slowly work them down into the trunk of the hepatic duct. Instruments pushed into the hepatic duct for the purpose of grasping and removing gall-stones situated within the hepatic channels, as a rule, produce an opposite effect to the one desired, inasmuch as they only push the concretions further into the intrahepatic ducts instead of grasping them and pulling them out. Occasionally gall-stones within the liver have been found and removed in the course of an operation for abscess of the liver.

Numerous attempts have been made, besides those enumerated, to remove gall-stones by other methods. Thus, a number of investigators have in vain tried to dissolve the concretions within the channels by injections of warm water (Taylor, Baudouin), oil (Brockbank), ether (Dujardin-Beaumetz), and other substances.

The treatment of ileus from gall-stone impaction deserves particular discussion. If opium is indicated in any form of occlusion of the intestine, it certainly is indicated here. In the form of ileus under discussion the occlusion of the intestine is not necessarily due to the gall-stone proper, but may be due to the spasmodic contractions of the musculature of the intestine around the stone. Consequently the administration of sufficiently large doses of opium (tinctura opii 20 gtt. and 5 to 10 gtt. every hour thereafter) will very often relieve the ileus. High enemata will be of additional value. If the gall-stone can be reached from the rectum directly, the attempt should be made to grasp it and to extract it. In all other cases a laparotomy must be performed, the exact location of the gall-stone determined, the intestine incised, and the stone removed through the incision. This operation has been performed a number of times (Korte and others). In many cases, unfortunately, it is impossible to determine that the occlusion of the intestine is due to gall-stone impaction, as no symptom of cholelithiasis may have preceded the attack of ileus; and, in addition, it may be impossible to find the location of the gall-stone during laparotomy. According to Kirmisson and Rochard, the operation of laparotomy was only successful in 20% of the cases; whereas of 80 cases that were not operated upon, 29 recovered and 51 died. Naunyn states that as many as 50% recovered after internal, non-operative treatment alone   The best plan, therefore, will be to inaugurate a course of treatment with opium at first. If at the expiration of two days no relief is apparent, and ulceration, perforation, and peritonitis threaten, a laparotomy should be performed.

The treatment of abscess, cirrhosis of the liver, and carcinoma hepatis following gall-stones will be discussed in the different sections on these diseases.

LITERATURE.

OLDER LITERATURE.*

Andral: "Clinique médicale," tome II, Paris, 1839.
Bartholini, Th.: "Histor. anatomic. var. Centur. III et IV," p. 335, Hafniæ, 1657.
Bianchi: "Histor. hepatica," Turin, 1716.
Blasius, G.: "Observat. medic. var. Amstelodami," 1677.
Bobrzenski in Bonet: "Sepulchret. anatomic.," Lib. III, Sect. XVI, p. 281, Lugduni, 1700.
Boerhaave: "Aphorismi de cognosc. et cur. morbis," Lugduni Batav., 1737.
Coe: "Abhandlung von den Gallensteinen," from the English, Leipzig, 1783.
Coiter, V.: "Extern. et intern. principal. human. corpor. part. tabul. . . . Norimbergæ, 1573.
Craz, H.: "De vesicæ felleæ et duct. bil. morbis," Dissertat. inaugur. Bonnæ, 1830.
Dodonaei, R.: "Medicinal. observat. exempla var. Hardervici," 1621.
Donatus, Marcellus: "De medica historia mirabili," Venetiis, 1588.
Ettmüller, M.: "Opera medica," tomus II, pars 1, p. 442, Francofurti ad Mœnum, 1708.
Fabricii, Hildani: "Observat. et curat. chirurg. centur.," Basileæ, 1606.
Fernelius: "Universa medicina. . . . Trajecti ad Rhenum," p. 141, 1656.
Forestus, P.: "Observat. et curat. medicin. et chirurg. op. omn.," observat. XIV, XV, XXI, Francofurti, 1660.
Frank, J. P.: "De cur. homin. morbis," tom. V, p. 172, Florentiæ, 1832.
Glissonii, F.: "Anatom. hepat.," p. 38 et 265, Londini, 1654.
Haller, Alb. de: "Mém. sur la nature sensible et irrit. des part. du corps animal.," tome I, p. 280, Lausanne, 1756–1760.
— "Opuscul. patholog.," p. 70, Lausannæ, 1755.
v. Helmont: "Ortus medicinæ," Amstelodami, 1648.
Hoffmann: "Medicinæ rational. systematica," 1733.
Kentmann bei Gesner: "De omni rerum fossilium genere," p. 6, Tiguri, 1565.
Morgagni, J. B.: "De sedibus et causis morbor.," Lib. III, Epistola 37, p. 127, Lugduni Batav., 1767.
Müller, Godofred: "Act. phys. med. anat.," tomus VI, observat. 69, 1742.
Paracelsus ab Hohenheim, Th. B.: "De origine morb. e tartaro," tomus I, Strassburg, 1616.
— "Von den tartarischen Krankheiten," p. 282.
Portal, A.: "Sur la nature et le traitement des maladies du foie," Paris, 1813.
Prochaska, G.: "Opera minora," Pars. I, II, Viennæ, 1800.
Pujol, A.: "Oeuvres de médecine pratique," tome IV; "Mém. sur la colique hépat.," Paris, 1823.
Schurig, M.: "Lithologia," p. 172, Dresden-Leipzig, 1744.
Scultet, J.: "Armament. chirurgiæ," p. 300, Amsterdami, 1672.
Soemmering: "De concrem. biliariis," 1793.
van Swieten, G.: "Comment. in H. Boerhaave Aphorismos" § 950, Wirceburgi, 1787–1788.
Sydenham, Th.: "Praxis medic.," p. 259, Lipsiæ, 1695.
Tacconi: "De raris quibusdam hepatis aliorumque visc. affect. observat.," Bononiæ, 1740.
Walter, J. G. und F. A.: "Anatomisches Museum," 1. und 2. Theil, Berlin, 1796.
Walter, J. G.: "Observat. anatomicæ," Berolini, 1775.
Wepfer, J. J.: "Histor. apoplectic . . . auctuarium," p. 389, Amstelædami, 1710.
— "Histor. cicut. aquatic.," cap. X, p. 225, Lugduni Batav., 1733.

COLLECTIVE WORKS.

Bouïsson: "De la bile," Montpellier, 1843.
Brockbank, E. M.: "On Gall-stones," London, 1896.
Budd, G.: "Krankheiten der Leber," translated by Henoch, Berlin, 1846.
Charcot: "Leçons sur les maladies du foie," Paris, 1877.
Chauffard: "Traité de médecine," vol. III, Paris, 1893.

* The older literature is given in full by Muleur, "Essai historique sur l'affection calculeuse du foie," Thèse de Paris, 1884.

Courvoisier: "Casuistisch-statistische Beiträge zur Pathologie und Chirurgie der Gallenwege," Leipzig. 1890.

Cyr: "Traité de l'affect. calculeuse du foie," Paris. 1884.

Dupré, F., in "Manuel de médecine" by Debove and Achard. vol. vi. Paris, 1895.

Fauconneau-Dufresne: "Traité de l'affect. calculeuse du foie," Paris. 1851.

Frerichs: "Klinik der Leberkrankheiten," vol. ii, 1861.

Harley. G.: "Diseases of the Liver." German by Kraus und Rothe, Leipzig, 1883.

Kehr, H.: "Die chirurgische Behandlung der Gallensteinkrankheite," Berlin, 1896.

Kraus: "Pathologie und Therapie der Gallensteinkrankheit," Berlin, 1891.

Langenbuch: "Chirurgie der Leber und Gallenblase," Stuttgart, 1897; "Deutsche Chirurgie." chap. 45, part 2.

Leichtenstern: in Penzoldt und Stintzing's "Handbuch der speciellen Therapie," part vi b, p. 28 *et seq.*

Murchison: "Clinical Lectures on Diseases of the Liver." London, 1877.

Naunyn. B.: "Klinik der Cholelithiasis," Leipzig. 1892.

Riedel. B.: "Chirurgische Behandlung der Gallensteinkrankheit" in Penzoldt and Stintzing's "Handbuch der speciellen Therapie," part vi b, p. 68.

Schüppel: in Ziemssen's "Handbuch der speciellen Pathologie und Therapie," vol. viii. 1, 1880.

Thudichum: "Treatise on Gall-stones," London. 1863.

Waring. H. J.: "Diseases of the Liver," Edinburgh and London, 1897.

SPECIAL WORKS.

1. PATHOLOGY.*

Adler: "Deutsche med. Wochenschr." No. 3. 1892.

Alison: "Contribution au diagnostic de la lithiase biliare," "Archives générales de médecine." p. 141, August. 1887.

Aubert. P.: "D'endocardite ulcéreuse végétante dans les infect. biliaires," Thèse de Paris. 1891.

Aufrecht: "Austritt von Gallensteinen aus der Gallenblase," "Deutsches Archiv für klin. Medicin," vol. xliii, p. 295. 1888.

Bohnstadt. F.: "Die Differentialdiagnose zwischen dem durch Gallensteine und dem durch Tumor bedingten Verschluss des Choledochus," Dissertation, Halle, 1893.

Bouchard: "Du mode de formation des ulcérations calculeuses de la vessie bil.," "Archives générales de médecine," p. 187. August. 1880.

Brissaud et Sabourin: "Deux cas d'atrophie du lobe gauche du foie," "Archives de physiologie." 3d series. vol. iii. p. 345, 1884.

Brockbank: "Edinburgh Med. Jour.," July, 1898. p. 51; "Manchester Med. Chron.," Dec., 1896.

Buxbaum: "Münchener med. Wochenschr.," p. 1368, 1897.

Bychoffski: "Contrib. à l'étude de l'hystéro-traumatisme," Thèse de Paris, 1893.

Cabot: "Medical News," Nov. 30, 1901, p. 844.

Cadéac: "Contrib. à l'étude de la cholécystite suppurée." Thèse de Paris, 1891.

Cahen: "Ein seltener Fall von Gallensteinen," "Deutsche med. Wochenschr.," No. 41. 1896.

Camac: "Am. Jour. Med. Sc.." March. 1899.

Chauffard. A.: "Valeur clinique de l'infection comme cause de lithiase bil.," "Revue de médecine." No. 2, 1897; "Gaz. des Hôp.," 1899, No. 16.

Chiari: "Zeit. f. Heilk.," Bd. xv, p. 199.

Cushing: "Johns Hopkins Hosp. Bull.." Aug.–Sept., 1899. p. 166; ibid., May, 1898.

Cyr. J.: "Causes d'erreur dans le diagnostic de l'affection calculeuse du foie," "Archives générales de médecine." p. 165. February. 1890.

Da Costa: "Amer. Jour. Med. Sc.." Aug., 1899. p. 138.

Dauriac: "Les infect. biliaires dans la fièvre typhoide." Thèse de Paris, 1897.

Dominici. S. A.: "Des angiocholites et cholécystites suppurées," Thèse de Paris, 1894.

Droba: "Wien. klin. Woch.." Nov. 16. 1899.

* The newer works only are mentioned here. For the very large number of cases we refer to the Index-Catalogue of the Library of the Surgeon-General's Office. U. S. Army. under article "Gall-stones." The collective works of Naunyn, Langenbuch, Courvoisier, Schüppel, etc., also contain many references to literature.

v. Dungern: "Ueber Cholecystitis typhosa," "Münchener med. Wochenschr.," p. 699, 1897.

Ehret: *Abstract* in "Vereins-Beilage des Deutsches med. Wochenschr.," May 8, 1902, p. 143.

Ehret and Stolz: "Mittheil. a. d. Greuzgebeit. d. Med. u. d. Chir.," 1901, Bd. vii, p. 373; "Berlin. klin. Woch.," Jan. 6, 1902, p. 13.

Exner: "Deutsche med. Woch.," 1898, No. 31, p. 491; ibid., March 16, 1899, p. 173.

Fraenkel, E., and P. Krause: "Zeitschr. f. Hyg. u. Infectionsk.," Bd. xxxii.

Fuchs: "Ein Fall von acuter Cholecystitis und Cholangitis mit Perforation der Gallenblase," "Berliner klin. Wochenschr.," p. 646, 1897.

Fürbringer: "Verhandlungen der Congresses fur innere Medicin," Leipzig, 1892.

Gerhardt, C.: "Zur physikalischen Diagnostik der Gallensteinkolik," "Deutsche med. Wochenschr.," p. 975, 1893.

Gilbert: "Arch. gén. de méd.," 1898, p. 258.

Gilbert and Dominici: "Compt. rend. de la Soc. de Biol.," June 16, 1894.

Gilbert et Fournier: "Du rôle des microbes dans la genèse des calculs bil.," "Gazette hebdomad. de méd. et de chirurg.," No. 13, 1896.

— Société de biologie Paris, October 30, 1897.

Griffon: "Calculs enclavés dans l'ampoule de Vater," "Presse médicale," No. 85, 1896; from the "Chirurgisches Centralblatt," No. 13, 1897.

Homans: "Lancet," July 31, 1897; "Johns Hopkins Hosp. Bull.," Aug.–Sept., 1899.

Hölzl: "Darmverschluss durch Gallensteine," "Deutsche med. Wochenschr.," No. 17, 1896.

Hünerhoff, H.: "Ueber Perforation der Gallenblase infolge von Ciholelthiasis," Dissertation, Göttingen, 1892.

Hunner: "Johns Hopkins Hosp. Bull.," Aug.–Sept., 1899.

Imhofer: "Prager med. Woch.," 1898, Nos. 15 and 16.

Jacobs: "Zur Kenntniss der Cholecystitis calculosa," Dissertation, München, 1890.

Janowski: "Veränderungen in der Gallenblase bei Vorhandensein von Gallensteinin," "Ziegler's Beiträge zur pathologischen Anatomie," vol. x, 1891.

Kausch: "Deutsche med. Woch.," March 16, 1899.

Kirmisson, E., and Rochard, E.: "De l'occlusion intestinale par calculs biliaires et de son traitement," "Archives générales de médecine," February and March, p. 148, 1892.

Kleefeld: "Ueber die bei Punction, Operation und Section der Gallenblase constatirten pathologischen Veränderungen des Inhaltes derselben und die daraus resultirenden diagnostischen Momente," Dissertation, Strassburg, 1894.

Kölliker, Th.: "Centralblatt. für Chirurgie," p. 1113, 1897.

Létienne: "Note sur un cas de lithiase bil.," "Archives générales de médecine," p. 734, December, 1891.

Meckel v. Hemsbach: "Mikrogeologie," Berlin, 1856.

Meczkowski: "Mittheil. a. d. Greuzgebeit. d. Med. u. d. Chir.," 1900, Bd. vi, p. 307.

Meyer, J.: "Experimentelle Beiträge zur Frage der Gallensteinbildung," "Virchow's Archiv," vol. cxxxvi, p. 651, 1894.

Mignot: "Arch. gén. de méd.," 1898, p. 129.

Miller: "Johns Hopkins Hosp. Bull.," May, 1898.

Mixter: "Boston Med. and Surg. Jour.," May 25, 1899.

Miyaki: "Mittheil. a. d. Greuzgebiet. d. Med. u. d. Chir.," 1900, Bd. vi, p. 479.

Müller, A.: "Zur pathologischen Bedeutung der Drüsen in der menschlichen Gallenblase," Dissertation, Kiel, 1895.

Naunyn: "Verhandlungen des Congresses für innere Medecin," Leipzig, 1892; "Mittheil. a. d. Greuzgebeit. u. d. Chir.," 1899, Bd. iv, pp. 1 and 602.

Netter et Martha: "De l'endocardite végétante dans les affect, des voies biliaires," "Archives de physiolog., norm. et patholog.," p. 7, 1886.

Nickel: "Zur Casuistik der durch Cholelithiasis bedingten Pericystitis vesicæ felleæ," Dissertation, Marburg, 1886.

Niemer: "Ueber einen Fall von Gallensteinen in den Lebergallengängen," Kiel, 1894.

Oddi: "Effeti dell' estirpazione della cisti fell," from the "Centralblatt. für Chirurgie," No. 8, 1889.

Opie: "Amer. Jour. Med. Sc.," Jan., 1901, p. 27.

Osler: from "Münchener med. Wochenschr.," p. 1125, 1897; "Trans. Association of American Physicians," 1897, vol. xii.

Ottiker: "Ueber Gallenfisteln," Dissertation, Erlangen, 1886.

Peters, H.: "Gallenstein-Statistik," Dissertation, Kiel, 1890.

Peterssen-Borstel: "Ueber Gallensteinbildung in ihrer Beziehung zu Krebs und chronischer Endarteriitis," Dissertation, Kiel, 1883.

Porges: "Wien. klin. Woch.," 1900, No. 26.

Pratt: "Am. Jour. Med. Sc.," Nov., 1901, p. 584.

Raynaud et Sabourin: "Note zur un cas d'énorme dilatation des voies biliares," "Archives de physiolog., normale et patholog.," No. 31, 1879.

Richardson: "Jour. Boston Soc. of Med. Sc.," Jan., 1899.

Riedel: "Ueber den zungenformigen Fortsatz der Leber," "Berliner klin. Wochenschr.," 577, 1888; "Mittheil. a. d. Greuzgebiet. Med. u. d. Chir.," 1898, Bd. iii, p. 168; ibid., 1899, Bd. iv, p. 565.

Robson, Mayo: Lecture on "Diseases of the Gallbladder," "Lancet," June 5, 1897.

— "Varieties of Intestinal Obstructions depending on Gallstones," "Medic.-chir. Transact.," vol. lxxxvii; "Edinburgh Med. Jour.," September, 1899; "Allbutt's System of Medicine."

Rother: "Zur Aetiologie und Statistik der Gallensteine," Dissertation, München, 1883.

Schabad: "Ein Fall von Gallensteinen mit Ruptur der Gallenblase," "Petersburger med. Wochenschr.," No. 3, 1896.

Schloth: "Ueber Gallensteinbildung," Dissertation, Wurzburg, 1887.

Schmitz, R.: "Intermittirendes Fieber bei Gallensteinen," "Berliner klin. Wochenschr.," p. 915, 1891.

Schüller: "Gallensteine als Ursache von Darmobstruction," Dissertation, Strassburg, 1891.

Schwartz: "Discuss. sur la lithiase de la vessie bil.," "Bull. et mém. de la société de chir. de Paris," vol. xxii, p. 245.

Simanowski, N. P.: "Zur Frage über die Gallensteinkolik," "Zeitschr. für klin. Medicin," vol. v, 501, 1882.

Sonville, P.: "Cholécystite scléreuse d'origine calcul. et pericholécystite," Thèse de Paris, 1895.

Still: "Trans. Path. Soc. of London," 1899.

Thomson: "Edinburgh Hospital Reports," 1898.

Vissering: "Ein Fall von Thorax-Gallenfistel mit Entleerung eines Gallensteines per vias naturales und nicht tödtlichem Ausgang," "Münchener med. Wochenschr.," p. 567, 1896.

Weltz: "Ueber Divertikel der Gallenblase," Dissertation, Kiel, 1894.

Wunschheim: "Prag. med. Woch.," 1898, Nos. 2 and 3.

Zinn: "Centralbl. f. innere Med.," Sept. 24, 1898.

2. THERAPY.*

(Newer Works.)

Beck: "When shall we Operate for Cholelithiasis?" "New York Med. Journal," May 8, 1897.

Braun: "Die operative Behandlung der Steine im Ductus choledochus," Dissertation, Göttingen, 1896.

Chauffard et Dupré: "Note sur le trait. de la lithiase bil.," "Gazette hebdomad.," p. 677, 1888.

Fenger: "Stones in the Common Duct and their Surgical Treatment," "American Med. Jour.," February, 1896.

Franke: "Beiträge zur Chirurgie der Gallenwege," Festschrift zur 69. Versammlung der Naturforscher und Aerzte, Braunschweig, 1897.

Kehr: "Ueber Behandlung der calculösen Cholangitis durch directe Drainage des Ductus hepaticus," "Münchener med. Wochenschr.," No. 41, 1897.

Köhler, A.: "Beiträge zur Casuistik der Operationen an der Gallenblase," "Deutsche Zeitschrift für Chirurgie," vol. xxxix, p. 549, 1894.

Kümmell: "Die ideale extraperitoneale Operation der Gallensteine," "Deutsche med. Wochenschr.," p. 578, 1897.

Lange: "Die chirurgischen Gesichtspunkte der Gallensteinerkrankungen," "New Yorker med. Wochenschr.," January, 1897.

Lejars: "Contrib. à l'étude des indic. de la cholécystotomie," "Revue de chirurg.," No. 9, 1896.

* Leichtenstern, in Penzoldt und Stintzing's "Handbuch der speciellen Therapie" (Internal Therapy). Langenbuch, "Chirurgie der Leber und Gallenblase," part 2, complete list of literature.

Lewaschew: "Ueber die therapeutische Bedeutung des Durande'schen Mittels bei der Gallensteinkrankheit," "Virchow's Archiv," vol. CI, p. 430.

Loos: "Ueber den Durchbruch des Ductus choledochus ins Duodenum," Dissertation, Kiel, 1890.

Martig, W.: "Zur Chirurgie der Gallenwege," Dissertation, Basel, 1893.

Prentiss: "Med. News," May 12, 1888.

Rosenberg: "Behandlung der Cholelithiasis," "Berliner klin. Wochenschr.," No. 48, 1889.

— "Demonstration von Gallensteinen, die nach Oelbehandlung abgegangen sind," "Berliner klin. Wochenschr.," p. 314, 1891.

Roth, Th.: "Zur Chirurgie der Gallenwege," "Archiv für klin. Chirurgie,' vol. XXII, p. 87, 1885.

Sacharjin: "Berliner klin. Wochenschr.," p. 604, 1891 (Calomel).

Schröder, A.: "Ueber die Behandlung in den Gallengängen sitzender Steine," Dissertation, Kiel, 1895.

Sendler: "Zur pathologie und Chirurgie der Gallenblase und der Leber," "Deutsche Zeitschrift für Chirurgie," vol. XL, p. 366, 1895.

— "Beiträge zur Chirurgie der Gallenwege," "Deutsche Zeitschr. für Chirurgie," vol. XXVI, p. 383, 1887.

Staub: "Divertikelbildung der Gallenblase; Cystotomie mit partieller Resection der Blasenwand," "Correspondenzblatt für Schweizer Aerzte," p. 1, 1896.

Terrier: "Sur un cas de gastrocystentérostomie," "Bulletin de la société chir.," vol. XXII, p. 565, Paris, 1897.

Trantenroth: "Acute infectiöse Cholangitis und Cholecystitis infolge von Gallensteinen; Heilung durch Operation," "Mittheilungen aus den Grenzgebieten der Medicin und Chirurgie," vol. I, p. 703.

Weber: "Klinische Betrachtung der Gallensteinkrankheit vom Standpunkte der inneren Medicin," "New Yorker med. Wochenschr.," January, 1897.

White, Sinclair: "Lancet," April 17, 1897, p. 1095.

Witzel: "Beiträge zur Chirurgie der Bauchorgane," "Deutsche Zeitschr. für Chirurgie," p. 159, 1884 (literature).

DISEASES OF THE LIVER.

HYPEREMIA OF THE LIVER.

(Quincke.)

THE liver, owing to the enormous development and capacity of its capillary system, is one of the most vascular organs of the body. If it is inspected during laparotomy or vivisection, it will be found that it presents an altogether different appearance from the organ as it is seen after death, and it is surprising to note the degree of turgescence of the liver during life and to observe how deeply it is colored. The walls of the capillaries are very thin and the parenchyma is very delicate; as a result the quantity of blood that the liver contains varies very much at different times.

Many observations, chiefly clinical, seem to indicate that at the time of greatest functional activity,—that is, at at the time of digestion,—and also under certain pathologic conditions, the quantity of blood contained within the liver increases. The blood-supply in the case of the liver, as in most other organs, is regulated by changes in the lumen of the afferent vessels. This is apparent from the fact that both the hepatic artery and the portal vein have a number of smooth muscular fibers within their walls. Some facts even point to the possibility that the capillaries of the liver are capable of spontaneously changing their caliber.

The venous system of vessels within the liver is subject to many fluctuations from the fact that the hepatic veins enter directly into the lower vena cava, and as this vessel is influenced greatly by the changes in intrathoracic pressure caused by the respiratory movements and the movements of the heart, it can be readily understood why the pressure in the hepatic veins is constantly changing. Aside from the fluctuations mentioned, that must occur constantly even during complete rest of the body, it must be remembered that all movements of the body and a variety of other causes influence the blood-pressure in the vena cava. This in its turn causes the blood to flow more rapidly or more slowly from the hepatic veins into the vena cava. When the pressure in the caval system is increased, the flow of blood from the hepatic veins is slower and the pressure within the liver is increased. The liver during this time must be able to hold and does hold quite large quantities of blood. As a matter of fact, the liver acts in this respect like a sponge, and is capable of absorbing and retaining much blood without detriment.

These fluctuations in the volume of blood contained within the liver are, as a rule, impossible to detect by palpation. Heitler,* however, claims that he can determine an increase of volume in the case of the liver as well as in the case of the spleen by careful percussion. He claims that he finds differences in the area of percussion dulness both in an upward and a downward direction of more than 3 cm. (!), and states that these fluctuations can occur within the course of two minutes or even a shorter time.

Of the two possible causes of pathologic plethora of the hepatic vessels, that which is due to passive stasis is more frequent, more important, more readily understood, and more easily controlled than the one due to active stasis. This condition of passive hyperemia is, as a rule, caused by some obstruction to the outflow of venous blood.

The external pressure on the liver is of some significance in bringing about fluctuations in the volume of blood contained within the organ. Tension of the abdominal walls in the presence of an abundant quantity of intra-abdominal fat will counteract great fluctuations, whereas flaccid abdominal walls and the presence of small quantities of fat in the mesentery, etc., possibly as a result of emaciation, will favor fluctuations. For the same reason the left lobe of the liver is probably subject to greater fluctuations than the right one; so that all the symptoms of hyperemia or stasis in the liver are clinically more apparent in the left lobe than in the right, from the fact not only that that part of the organ is more accessible to our methods of examination, but also that the changes are really more pronounced. This may also account for the observation that in atrophic and in hypertrophic cirrhosis of the liver the left lobe seems to reveal more pronounced changes, in the sense that it is more contracted in the former disease and more enlarged in the latter.

PASSIVE CONGESTION.

Etiology.—The most frequent cause of obstruction to the outflow of blood from the veins of the liver is insufficiency of the activity of the heart. This may be due either to some primary disease of the cardiac muscle or to some valvular disease with secondary involvement of the myocardium. Those cardiac lesions in which the right heart in particular

* Heitler, "Die Schwankungen der normalen Leber- und Milzdämpfung," *Wiener med. Wochenschr.*, 1892, No. 24.

is insufficient are especially adapted to cause stasis in the veins of the liver. Among these may be mentioned the final stages of mitral or pulmonary valvular disease or the sequels of tricuspid lesions. Following the course of these diseases and developing slowly, passive congestion of the liver develops in the course of many years. The acute forms of myocarditis following infectious diseases rarely cause the development of clinically recognizable passive congestion of the liver. This only occurs if, for instance, as in children, the organ is very elastic (therefore this condition is occasionally seen after diphtheria), or if slight degrees of stasis existed in a latent form for some time. In the new-born acute passive hyperemia of the stasis may follow a difficult delivery or atelectasis of the lungs.

Certain diseases of the lungs, such as emphysema, contraction of lung tissue, chronic and acute bronchitis, pleural adhesions of large dimensions, act in the same manner as do diseases of the right heart. At times several of these conditions are present at the same time. They decrease the area of the pulmonary circulation and reduce the respiratory excursions, so that they finally lead to insufficiency of the right side of the heart. Scolioses and kyphoses of the spinal column, if they are sufficiently pronounced, may act in the same manner, as may intrathoracic tumors and large exudates into the pleural cavity [and pericardial synechiæ.—ED.]. It happens sometimes, though comparatively rarely, that the inferior vena cava alone is compressed by all these lesions in that short part of its course that runs between the liver and the right auricle. Finally, cicatricial or thrombotic narrowing of the veins of the liver itself may lead to hyperemia from stasis. This may also occur in some circumscribed district within the liver, as in the neighborhood of tumors, etc.

Local hyperemia from stasis may also be seen if a lobe of the liver is separated from the main body of the organ by lacing. In this instance the veins running through the furrow between the lobe and the main body of the liver are compressed and cause stasis in the lobe, so that induration and enlargement are produced therein. General hyperemia of a mild degree may often be seen in a corset liver, particularly in those cases where the patient has a high waist or where the compression is diffuse in the lower part of the thorax so that the vena cava is compressed between the liver and the spinal column.

Anatomy.—If the flow of blood from the liver is impeded, the first result will be an engorgement and a dilatation of the hepatic veins. Following this, engorgement will occur in all the venous radicles situated behind the obstruction, so that in cases where stasis persists the organ will gradually enlarge. The dilatation of the hepatic veins then becomes permanent and is transmitted to the central venules of the lobules and to the surrounding capillaries. At the same time the trabeculæ of hepatic tissue situated between the dilated vessels are compressed and narrowed by the pressure, and finally undergo atrophic changes. For these reasons it will often be found that the lobules of the liver are colored dark red in the center, whereas the peripheral parts are much lighter in color owing to the many intact cells that these parts still contain (cyanotic or chronic red atrophy). In many instances it will be seen that those cells that remain in the central areas of the lobules are filled with brown pigment, whereas those cells that are nearer the periphery contain globules of fat. In cases of this character the brownish-yellow portal zone is clearly dif-

39

ferentiated from the center of the lobule, a peculiar picture to which the name "nutmeg liver" has been applied. The designation is hardly a happy one, because the majority of physicians are probably not familiar with this object of comparison taken from the kitchen.

After death the capillaries are in part emptied and the central portions of the lobules, as a result, often appear retracted on postmortem examination. This retraction may be apparent on the surface of the lobule or in transverse sections through it. The further the atrophic changes of the cells near the periphery have progressed, the more distinct will this retraction appear. In this manner it may happen that the surface and sections through the lobules appear finely granular. The individual granulations, however, are much smaller than in true cirrhosis —*i. e.*, they correspond in diameter and extent to exactly one lobule, whereas in cirrhosis several lobules constitute one granule. On section the whole liver in this condition appears flaccid and tough, and if the organ has been allowed to lie for some time, so that much blood has oozed out, the liver will appear very little enlarged or even smaller than normal. This may be noticed even if a very short time before, during the life of the patient, the enlargement of the liver and the tension of the capsule were apparent as a result of the great engorgement with blood.

As a rule, these changes of color and consistency are not evenly distributed throughout the whole organ, but nutmeg spots alternate with very red, flaccid, and completely retracted areas. Within the latter the liver-cells will be seen to be still more atrophied, so that nothing remains but a few scanty remnants of a brownish pigment. The surface of the liver in these cases presents a nodular, wavy appearance, which also is presented by the surface of sections through the organ. Similar changes, based chiefly on the unequal amount of stasis that exists in different parts of the organ, are also, for instance, seen in the lungs, and must be attributed to peculiarities in the ramification and the angles of division of the blood-vessels that supply the diseased areas.

The serous covering of the liver in cases of stasis from hyperemia is, as a rule, cloudy and often thickened. As the trabeculæ of hepatic tissue disappear the walls of the capillaries become more and more approximated, until finally they come in contact with each other. The material situated between the lumina of the different capillaries consists of the thickened walls of the capillaries and of strands of connective tissue that are either homogeneous or striated. This connective tissue sometimes can be traced as far as the thickened sheath of the branches of the hepatic veins. It occasionally shows small-celled infiltration.

Within the connective tissue new-formed bile-channels are sometimes seen. These either originate from epithelial proliferation or are made evident from atrophy of trabeculæ of liver-cells.

In addition to intralobular new-formation of connective tissue, that is seen principally in the center of the lobules, connective-tissue proliferation may occasionally be observed in the interlobular spaces in the vicinity of the branches of the radicles of the portal vein. Liebermeister appears to have encountered this condition more frequently than other authors. He distinguishes a circumscribed form that appears in streaks and a wide-spread form that appears over larger surfaces. This proliferation is followed by retraction, and in this manner adds to the atrophic changes that occur in the hepatic tissues. The whole picture resembles

PLATE III.

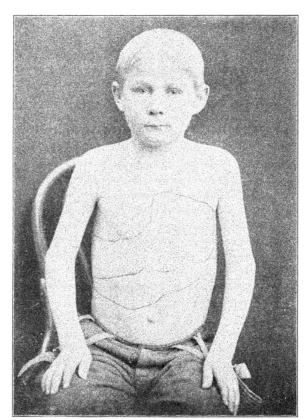

HEPATIC ENLARGEMENT DUE TO CONGESTION SECONDARY TO CARDIAC
DISEASE. OUTLINE OF CARDIAC AND HEPATIC DULNESS.

that of the ordinary form of cirrhosis, with the difference, however, that in this form the distribution of the cirrhotic areas is not uniform, but very irregular.

Under conditions of this kind the granular appearance of the surface of the liver and of sections grows still more pronounced, and the outlines of the lobules of the liver seem more circumscribed and distinct from the fact that those parts of the lobules that are really central on first sight present the outline of the interlobular reticulum.

Symptoms.—Owing to the fact that this disease of the liver develops very slowly, the first stages of engorgement of the organ with blood produce no symptoms and are not recognized until after the death of the patient.

If the enlargement of the liver has attained a certain degree, the condition can be discovered by palpation and percussion. The surface of the organ feels hard, tense, and smooth, the margin rounded and extending as far down as the umbilicus or even further. The liver is sensitive to pressure. In cases of tricuspid insufficiency it may even be possible to feel systolic pulsations over the liver as a result of regurgitation of the blood into the veins. If the condition persists for a long time, the liver gradually grows smaller as a result of atrophy of the parenchyma, increase of the connective tissue, and a reduction in the quantity of blood following the general cachexia that soon supervenes. Under these circumstances the liver does not feel so tense.

Immediately following paracentesis of the abdomen for the removal of ascitic fluid, the surface of the liver may feel nodular from the fact that the blood streams into the liver as soon as the pressure within the abdomen is relieved, and owing to the structural changes that have occurred within the organ, all parts of the surface are not evenly distended with blood, and hence the irregularity of its surface (E. Wagner).*

Occasionally the enlargement of the liver may be apparent to the eye from the protrusion of the hypochondriac region.

The subjective signs of passive hyperemia of the liver vary. They are proportionate to the rapidity with which the condition develops more than to the degree of development. It may happen that very considerable degrees of swelling cause no symptoms whatever provided the enlargement has developed gradually, whereas slight degrees of swelling in the beginning of stasis may cause a very disagreeable feeling of fulness in the epigastric region and may cause the patient to complain of the pressure of his clothing. This is particularly noticeable after eating, owing to the filling of the stomach and the hyperemia of the liver during the period of digestion. At times evidence of passive congestion is noticed in the portal system, and is usually shown by dyspeptic and gastric disturbances and by swelling of the hemorrhoidal veins.

A very mild form of icterus is quite frequently seen. As a rule, it is so slight that it is altogether overlooked on superficial examination and is manifested only by the passage in the urine of a minute quantity of urobilin. Bile-pigment itself is not necessarily found in the urine. The most probable explanation of this icterus is that it is due to absorption of bile following compression of some of the bile-channels within the liver by dilated capillaries. Grawitz † is inclined to attribute it to polycholia, for the reason that he found free hemoglobin in the blood in many cases of

* *Deutsches Archiv für klin. Medicin*, 1884, vol. xxxiv, p. 536.
† *Deutsches Archiv für klin. Medicin*, vol. liv, p. 61.

heart-lesions, and claims that this hemoglobin originates from the disintegration of red blood-corpuscles that are no longer as resistant as normal. The appearance of icterus is not universal, and its degree is variable and in no way dependent on the degree of hyperemia and stasis. According to Thierfelder, it is less frequently seen in cases where the hyperemia of the liver is caused by certain diseases of the lungs than when it is caused by diseases of the heart. I cannot indorse this view. The combination of cyanosis and of icterus often seen in cases of this character leads to a peculiar greenish coloration of the skin.

In addition to passive hyperemia of the liver, a number of the other complications of the primary disease of the heart or lungs are noticed. Thus, serous exudates, edema, diminution of the flow of urine, disturbances of respiration, etc., may all complicate the lesion of the liver. It is very noticeable, however, that the affection of the liver seems to occupy a peculiarly independent position among all the possible sequels of cardiac and pulmonary diseases. The other complications do not appear with any degree of regularity, so that at one time the one, at another time the other, is more apparent. The hyperemia of the liver, on the other hand, seems to be constantly present, and when it is once fully developed it seems to persist until the death of the patient, varying of course in intensity from time to time. In fact, the swelling of the liver may be the only symptom outside of the affected organs themselves. It is possible that in the first-named group of cases the function of the liver is to act as a safety-valve by absorbing like a sponge all the blood that the heart cannot master; in this way congestion of other organs is avoided and they do not become so hyperemic.

There are a number of other peculiarities in connection with this condition that merit particular mention. They refer to the swelling of the spleen and the origin of the ascitic fluid that is usually exuded. As a rule, cirrhosis of the liver is followed by enlargement of the spleen. In the case of passive hyperemia of the liver, however, the spleen in only indurated but not enlarged, although in both conditions the flow of blood from the spleen is impeded. It is possible that the time at which the stasis develops can be made responsible for this peculiarity, or that in cirrhosis the frequent recurrence of hyperemia of the organ during digestion plays a certain rôle.

Ascites is, as a rule, a symptom of subordinate significance in the general disease-picture of cardiac dropsy, and generally develops at a late stage of the disease, and then only to a slight degree. Ascites, moreover, stands in no relation, in regard to its intensity, to the degree of swelling of the liver that may be present. In some diseases of the heart, however, we see the development of ascites at so early a period of the disease that the suspicion of disease of the peritoneum is created. This is particularly the case when, as so often happens, all evidence of edema of the lower extremities is absent or is present only to a very slight degree. Continued observation, however, will reveal the cardiac origin of the trouble, and the comparatively favorable course that the abdominal lesion takes will soon exclude peritoneal disease. Ascites of this kind may not be accompanied by a very high degree of swelling of the liver from hyperemia or stasis. In some cases, it is true, cirrhosis of the liver from stasis proper or the induration of the organ from proliferation of connective tissue, or, in other instances, parenchymatous swelling of the liver, may play a certain rôle in the causation of ascites, but there are a number of cases on record in which isolated ascites of cardiac origin existed for a long time and finally disappeared after repeated tapping and withdrawal of the accumulated fluid. It is probable that in these instances the safety-valve action of the liver was insufficient, so that the congestion of the abdominal organs became so great that transudation of fluid occurred into the abdominal cavity or that exudative peritonitis developed. We must assume that the different vascular areas of the body are independent in a manner and that it will depend on their individual state or on individual peculiarities whether congestion, hyperemia, exudation, etc., will occur in the course of cardiac stasis in this or that part of the body.

The liver, already enlarged from passive congestion, may in the course of a few days become still larger; whereas in the case of a healthy liver, acute attacks of cardiac insufficiency cause no distinct enlargement of the organ. In other words, if the liver enlarges rapidly as a result of cardiac insufficiency, we must assume that the condition of stasis was chronic, but that the liver was comparatively small before the acute attack, and that the condition of chronic stasis had in all probability existed for some time but had evaded detection. In the case of children this does not quite hold true, since here an enormous swelling of the liver may be noticed in the course of a few days during an attack of diphtheria. The swelling is caused partly by parenchymatous swelling, partly by hyperemia of the organ from stasis, the latter condition being the result of cardiac weakness combined with disease of the bronchi. We can conclude, therefore, that the liver in children is more elastic than in adults, or that it is rendered so by the acute disease.

Diagnosis.—The most important point in the differential diagnosis of hyperemia of the liver from other lesions of the organ that are accompanied by enlargement is that a hyperemic liver constantly changes in volume, whereas in all the other diseases the volume of the liver remains uniformly large. In passive hyperemia this change is still more apparent than in simple congestion, because the capacity of the dilated blood-vessels within the liver is permanently increased in the former state. Much will depend on the power of the heart to hold the blood accumulating in it and to propel it onward. The character of the cardiac lesion, therefore, will determine whether a decrease in the swelling will occur, and to what degree the size of the swollen organ may decrease; i. e., whether the swelling persists for days, weeks, or months, or whether it disappears rapidly or slowly. In cases where the liver is very much enlarged a decrease in the size of the organ and an increase in the quantity of urine voided may be considered the first signs of improvement of the condition of the heart; on the other hand, hyperemic swelling of the liver and the consequent sensation of pressure may be one of the first indications that a cardiac lesion exists. As the distress incident to the swelling of the liver is usually increased after eating, the diagnosis of gastric trouble is frequently made.

Passive congestion of the liver is also an important symptom in other diseases of the liver, and constitutes a frequent complication. It is found in the different forms of cirrhosis and in fatty degeneration of the liver, because alcohol, the chief factor in the causation of these two diseases, affects the heart at the same time. I believe that this enlargement is frequently overlooked, and that the decrease in the size of the organ that occurs in the later stages as a result of the decrease in the volume of blood is attributed to atrophy of the liver.

Treatment.—The treatment of passive congestion of the liver from stasis must be directed primarily against the cause of the condition—viz., the cardiac insufficiency. In cases, too, in which the primary trouble is situated in the lungs, it is, as a rule, easier to direct treatment against the complicating cardiac weakness than against the lesion of the lungs. The heart should be protected from excessive work, and later should be strengthened by systematic exercise. The quantity of fluid taken should be reduced; and such drugs as digitalis, camphor, strophanthus, etc., should be given with diuretics like calomel, squill, theobromin, and potassium salts. If venous plethora is very great, blood-letting may be indicated in many cases, the favorable effects of this procedure being at once demonstrated by a marked decrease in the swelling of the liver.

The diet should be restricted, and in this manner the flow of blood to the intestine decreased, the radicles of the portal vein in this way being also freed from an excess of blood. As spontaneous hemorrhoidal bleeding is known to relieve congestion of the liver, it seems a good plan to produce such hemorrhage artificially, and for this purpose it was formerly customary to apply leeches to the region of the anus.

A course of salines, either Glauber salts or some of the saline waters, is also a valuable adjuvant in the treatment of the condition under discussion, particularly in the initial stages. Abstinence from irritating food and from alcohol is also indicated, and should be insisted upon for long periods of time. The good results obtained from these measures show conclusively what an important rôle active congestion and other disturbances of the parenchyma of the liver play in the causation and the aggravation of stasis.. All the measures discussed will be particularly effective in cases in which the stasis is due to pure hyperemia.

If the pain in the region of the liver is very severe, the same measures should be applied as in perihepatitis, such as the ice-bag, leeches, or warm compresses.

If ascites is very great, paracentesis acts both as a palliative and curative form of treatment. It acts by lessening the impediment to the circulation of the blood within the abdominal cavity, and in this manner encouraging the absorption of the transudate that has formed. It is in these cases particularly that a cure has actually been known to occur after repeated tapping and removal of the ascitic fluid.

ACTIVE HYPEREMIA OF THE LIVER; CONGESTION OF THE LIVER.

We include under this heading all those forms of engorgement of the liver with blood that are not caused by the presence of some obstruction to the flow of blood from the liver. In the case of other organs than the liver it is, as a rule, a very difficult matter to find an adequate explanation for the different hyperemic states that are occasionally noticed, nearly all the interpretations offered being purely hypothetical. In the case of the liver this is particularly true when one comes to venturing explanations on the origin of hyperemia of this organ. In the first place, no correct or even approximate estimation of the quantity of blood contained in the organ during life can be obtained from postmortem findings. Further, the blood-supply of the liver is exceedingly complicated and intricate, inasmuch as blood flows into the organ from two different directions and from two sets of vessels—the hepatic artery and the portal vein. It is impossible for us to determine to what extent the one or the other set of vessels participates in the excessive determination of blood to the liver.

We know that very peculiar conditions may exist in this respect, as the investigations of Gad demonstrate.

Gad allowed warm salt solutions, of the strength of 0.5 per cent., to flow through the liver while it was still warm, immediately after removal from the body of the animal. If the salt solution was allowed to flow into the portal opening alone, he found that more fluid percolated through the liver than if he allowed the stream to enter both the portal vein and the hepatic artery. It appears, therefore, as though the current flowing through the portal vein was impeded in its course by the current flowing through the hepatic artery. This may possibly be explained from the pressure exercised by the small branches of the hepatic artery on the small branches of the portal vein which run in their immediate vicinity. Possibly, too, the two currents oppose each other within the capillary network where they meet.

Our knowledge of hyperemia of the liver, from the very nature of the question, is based as much on general conclusions, traditions, and theoretic considerations as on exact anatomic investigations; in fact, it may be said that we know a great deal less from the latter source than from the former. While it is true, therefore, that many of our conclusions are not grounded on a substantial basis of established facts, we are not justified in completely ignoring them for that reason. They require, of course, careful and critical reviewing before we permit ourselves to constitute them the starting-point for further considerations. It is possible that many of these congestive states are due to changes in the innervation of the blood-vessels of the liver (both of the portal vein and of the hepatic artery); in other instances it is quite possible that such changes in normal innervation or changes in the parenchyma of the liver itself cause abnormal narrowing or dilatation of the lumen of the capillaries.

As a rule, probably, states of congestion are accompanied by an increased flow of blood through the liver; or, again, certain external conditions may be responsible for the change in the quantity of blood contained within the liver and the amount of blood that flows through the organ in a given time. Whenever the abdominal cavity is overfilled (by food, feces, gas, deposits of fat), the current of blood passing through the liver is impeded by the pressure exercised on the organ; at the same time the afferent part of the capillary area may be engorged. In case, on the other hand, the abdominal walls are relaxed and flaccid it may very well occur that an atonic condition of the blood-vessels results, and that they consequently become dilated.

The respiratory movements are an important factor in the regulation of the flow of blood through the liver; and they are of more significance for the flow of blood than for the quantity of blood contained in the organ at a given time. We know from observations on peripheral parts of the body and from experiments on the artificial passage of currents of blood through different isolated organs that a change of position and passive movements are capable of exercising a great influence on the capillary blood-stream as regards the rapidity of its flow. In the case of the liver the movements of the diaphragm act in this way, and, in addition, deep inspirations cause an increased suction of blood from the hepatic veins into the right heart. Any impediments to normal respiratory movements must necessarily, therefore, cause a slowing of the flow of blood through the liver. From this there results an accumulation of blood in the portal and hepatic capillaries.

Changes in the constitution of the blood ("thickening") may also possibly play a rôle.

Etiology.—Among possible causes of congestion of the liver must be mentioned increase and prolongation of the normal hyperemia during digestion as a result of too copious or too frequent meals. This overfeeding is particularly injurious in still another way if it is combined with a sedentary mode of life and lack of sufficient exercise, for under these circumstances obesity may frequently be seen to develop, followed by the usual difficulty in breathing and in the general power of locomotion. These two factors, in their turn, again impede the flow of blood through the liver.

The quality of the ingesta has much to do with digestive hyperemia. Alcohol, especially, causes high degrees of digestive hyperemia, aside from the hyperemia caused by food taken at the same time (v. Kahlden). Strong spices and coffee seem to act in a similar manner. It is also possible that certain toxins developing as a result of putrefactive changes in the intestine, particularly in gourmands, lead to disturbances of digestion and hyperemia of the liver (Dujardin-Beaumetz's stercoremia) (Bouchard).

Under all the conditions indicated above, other abnormal states besides hyperemia soon develop. Hyperemia is only the first stage, so to speak, of such changes in the parenchyma of the liver as enlargement of the organ, albuminous or fatty infiltration of the hepatic cells, and, later, proliferation of the interstitial connective tissues. Overfeeding and alcoholism act on the liver in the manner described and at the same time exercise their deleterious effects on other organs of the body, particularly the stomach and the heart, and also on the general constitution of the patient. It may be said, therefore, that the congestion of the liver is merely a more or less conspicuous part of a general disease-picture that may be called abdominal plethora, general plethora, or general obesity, which in its later stages is, as a rule, complicated by gout, gravel, and glycosuria.

If the affection of the heart is the most conspicuous symptom, passive congestion of the liver may develop, and in this way be combined with hyperemia of the organ; or it may even take the place of the latter condition.

Digestive disturbances and toxic agencies are by far the most important factors in the production of this hyperemia of the liver; all other possible causes are far less important. We may also mention contusions of the region of the liver and the effect of tropical climates.

In the tropics hyperemia of the liver, and a number of diseases of the liver that develop from this condition, are frequently seen (abscess, fatty liver, cirrhosis), particularly in the case of Europeans, a fact that has been falsely attributed to the effect of the great heat. An elevation of the temperature alone has nothing whatever to do with it, the real cause being the digestive disturbances that develop at the same time in these climates, and certain miasmatic infections, particularly malaria and dysentery, and probably others of which we are ignorant. A tropical climate is deleterious only in the sense that alcohol and irritating or abundant food can exercise a bad effect in quantities that would not be harmful in a more temperate climate where general metabolism is more active.

Domestic infectious diseases, such as typhoid fever, the acute exanthemata, and others, can produce the same changes in the liver (hyperemia and parenchymatous swelling of the organ), just as do the tropical miasms. Scurvy, too, according to the older observations on this disease, is capable of producing the same hepatic disturbances. In diabetes mellitus, a disease in which, *a priori*, a considerable involvement of the liver should be expected, hyperemia of the organ has, as a matter of fact, rarely been observed.

During menstruation we see changes in the liver corresponding to those seen in many other organs. These may consist in transitory affections of the organ that accompany menstruation *per se*, or they may be caused by sudden interruption of normal menstruation by cold, psychic disturbances, etc. These vicarious forms of hyperemia are transitory in character, but may appear for a long time during the climacteric. It is stated that the cessation of hemorrhoidal bleedings that once occurred habitually can be followed by disturbances of the above kind in the liver. Permanent disturbances, however, never develop from the stoppage of such habitual bleeding. It appears that the effect of the stoppage is exercised on the digestive organs or other parts of the body, the latter becoming congested if the plethora is not relieved by a hemorrhage, and becoming disordered, and thus in their turn helping to produce disorder of the liver.

Other possible causes of hyperemia of the liver that have been described are disturbances of the innervation of the organ in the course of hysteria, psychic excitement, terror or fright, and excessive mental effort (Monneret).

Local lesions of the liver, such as neoplasms, parasites, etc., cause an engorgement of the surrounding tissues with blood that may be due either to hyperemia or to congestion.

Symptoms.—The symptoms of congestion of the liver, owing to the different possible causes of this condition, are rarely manifested in a pure and uncomplicated form. As in the case of passive congestion, they consist chiefly in a sensation of pressure and fulness in the right hypochondriac and epigastric regions that may be so intense as to amount to actual pain, and may be increased by movement, by breathing, and on occupying a position on the side. At the same time percussion and palpation will reveal an enlargement of the liver, tenderness, and an increase in the consistency of the organ. All these disturbances are particularly apparent at the time of the greatest digestive activity, and are, as a rule, combined with other disturbances of digestion, such as pressure in the region of the stomach, flatulence, heartburn, and congestive oppression in the head.

In forms of hyperemia of the liver that are not of digestive origin all the symptoms are, in general, aggravated at the time of the greatest digestive activity, particularly after the ingestion of irritating food. This effect is more manifest in this form of hyperemia than in that which is dependent on lesions or disorders of the heart. In the latter no periodicity can be noticed, in the former a periodic aggravation seems in many instances to take place after eating. The general disease is, however, as a rule, so complicated that it is impossible to decide in each individual case whether the hyperemia is mechanical or congestive in character.

In the course of the disease, particularly if it is due to habitual congestion, icterus often appears, either following an exacerbation of the digestive disturbances or, again, without any increase in the dyspeptic symptoms. It is probably due to stasis in the bile-capillaries or to catarrhal changes in the common duct. This form of icterus may be very severe in the menstrual form of hyperemia of the liver.

Diagnosis.—In the discussion of the causes of congestion of the liver we have seen that this condition, in case it attains pathologic significance, rarely constitutes a transitory state lasting only several days or weeks. As a rule, the condition becomes permanent, and frequently becomes aggravated, so that it may in this way predispose to more serious and deep-seated diseases of the liver. It is for this reason that the symptoms are of great diagnostic significance, even though they are not very marked and are not at once apparent to the physician or to the patient. In all cases of abdominal plethora these symptoms should be particularly looked for, and if they are discovered in this or similar states, it is the duty of the physician to institute a course of treatment directed toward their removal even against the wishes of the patient. In this manner it is often possible to avoid very serious diseases. It will frequently happen that some involvement of the parenchyma of the liver is present at the time the symptoms of congestion are first discovered; but, as a rule, it is impossible to determine this at once, and the decision will have to be rendered later from the subsequent course of the disease. A valuable criterion for the seriousness of the involvement is the size of the liver; the less the organ is enlarged and the more rapidly the swelling subsides, the less danger, we may say, is there of extensive parenchymatous involvement, and the less complicated is the hyperemia.

The prognosis, of course, is dependent on the presence or absence of other conditions, and on the power of the patient to abstain from injurious indulgences, as alcohol, or to withdraw from dangerous surroundings (malaria); in other words, it is, in many instances, dependent on the calling and the character of the patient.

Treatment.—The treatment of hyperemia of the liver is essentially dependent upon the cause of the trouble. In many of the infectious diseases the treatment of the hepatic complication coincides exactly with the treatment of the primary disease. In cases of hyperemia from miasmatic infection in the tropics, temporary or permanent change of climate is essential; and in the cases due to menstrual or vicarious congestion a regulation of the disordered functions is indicated. It may even be necessary to induce bleeding by artificial means. Traumatic hyperemia calls for absolute rest, and the local application of cold in the form of an ice-bag, or leeches. If the pain is very severe, the hypodermic administration of morphin or some other form of opium to arrest the peristaltic action of the bowels is necessary. Those forms of congestion that are not due to trauma are rarely so violent as to require antiphlogistic medication. Our chief remedy is a regulation of the diet. This applies not only to the majority of cases in which the involvement of the liver is due to digestive or toxic causes, but also to all other forms, for the reason that a reduction of the congestion of the liver during digestion will protect the organ from the effects of other irritants, such as malaria, trauma, etc.

In the acute forms of hyperemia and in the acute exacerbations of chronic hyperemia the functional activity of the liver should be reduced as much as possible by limiting the amount of food taken, the diet being restricted to thin soups, water, and weak tea. The general health of the patient will have to be studied and these restrictions carried on only as long as nutrition remains fairly good, the state of the liver alone not constituting a proper guide. It if becomes necessary to give a more plentiful and a more stimulating diet, the amount should be regulated by the actual demands of the body; but all overfeeding and the ingestion of all irritating food should be avoided. Aside from the qualitative composition of the food, the latter condition can be fulfilled by causing the patient to drink much water. The greatest difficulty will be encountered in those accustomed to an abundant diet, and it is precisely in these cases that such restrictions are especially necessary; in general, although not always, such subjects will be found to be plethoric. All alcoholic beverages, irritating spices, as mustard, pepper, etc., should be completely eliminated from the diet, and the amount of salt and condiments is to be restricted. Coffee and roasted foods are to be condemned. These measures alone, combined with simplicity of food, will lead to a reduction of the amount eaten. A mixed diet is to be preferred to a monotonous one, for the reason that we must take care not to stimulate the formation of urea alone, on the one hand, or the storing of fats and glycogen, on the other. These indications are, in general, fulfilled if the patient is restricted to a milk diet or to one consisting principally of soups, vegetables, and fruits. In many instances the choice of foods will have to be governed to a large extent by the state of the stomach and bowels and by the general constitution of the patient. In fat subjects amylaceous foods will have to be restricted; in emaciated or reduced subjects fat and proteids are necessary and can be furnished by a non-stimulating diet.

The moderate employment of cathartics has for a long time been recognized as very useful in congestion of the liver. According to the experience of Thierfelder, gourmandizing is less harmful if the bowels are frequently and thoroughly evacuated than if the reverse is the case. It is difficult to decide whether the incomplete assimilation of the food ingested that may be said to follow frequent purging is best explained on this ground. Such an interpretation is the first to present itself; at the same time, it is quite probable that the removal of putrefactive products, and the influence that is exercised by the increased peristalsis on the blood-current in the portal vein are still more important. The dietetic regulations formulated above are alone capable of increasing the peristalsis of the bowels and producing free evacuations, particularly by the fruits and vegetables prescribed. Saline remedies, rhubarb, cascara, senna, and aloes are all useful. The last-named irritating drugs should be used carefully and sparingly, and certainly not for a long time, owing to the effect they exercise on the intestinal tract. I should hardly say, however, that it is best not to use them at all because they might irritate the liver, although the latter recommendation has been made by several authors (Cantani).

The administration of saline, alkaline, and alkaline-saline mineral waters plays an important rôle in the treatment of congestion of the liver and of the general disturbances of health associated with this condition. In choosing one or the other of these waters the general constitution of the patient and, in particular, the condition of the gastro-intestinal tract must be considered. Cold Glauber-salts waters (as Marienbad, Franzensbad, Elster, and Tarasp) are indicated in cases of overfeeding, abdominal plethora, and constipation. Cold saline waters, on the other hand, should be recommended where plethora is less pronounced, and in all those cases where bathing is valuable for the treatment of complicating affections of the heart. Waters of the latter class are found in Kissingen, Homburg, Nauheim, Pyrmont, and Soden. Warm waters (such as those of Carlsbad, Vichy, Aix-la-Chapelle, and Wiesbaden) are indicated in those cases in which parenchymatous changes of the liver are already present, or at least seem to be impending. Carlsbad and Vichy waters are more effective in the latter respect than the saline waters of Wiesbaden, Aix-la-Chapelle, and Baden-Baden. Bitter waters are less adapted for regular courses of treatment than of frequent use over a long time.

Enemata are also useful in treating the obstinate constipation that so often complicates this disease. It is possible that they act on the blood directly, by causing a larger absorption of water, and that, as a result, the blood is, so to say, diluted. This applies particularly to injections of warm water, if they are frequently employed, or to the administration per rectum of aromatic infusions, such as those of chamomile, valerian, etc. The old "visceral enemata of Kämpf"* possibly fulfilled this indication.

The French school of clinicians recommends such intestinal disinfectants as bismuth, naphthalin, naphthol, salol, resorcin, etc.

Acute congestion of the liver accompanied by pain calls for rest; chronic or frequently repeated attacks of hyperemia, on the other hand, call for exercise. Physical exertion in the latter cases acts beneficially by stimulating and increasing the rapidity of the blood-stream and the general circulation, as well as by promoting deeper respiratory excursions. In this manner an auto-massage of the liver is obtained which is unquestionably more effective than the external form of massage of the organ recommended by Durand-Fardel. It is probable that this external method acts indirectly through the agency of the intestine.

Pain is rarely so severe in congestion of the liver as to call for active interference. In the acute forms in which perihepatitic irritation may occur antiphlogistics are indicated; in the chronic forms warm compresses, or rarely narcotics. The latter class of drugs is particularly bad in this disease for the reason that they arrest the necessary peristaltic action of the bowels; for this reason opium and morphin should be given very sparingly.

LITERATURE.

Bamberger: Loc. cit., p. 489.

Brieger: "Beitrage zur Lehre von der fibrösen Hepatitis," "Virchow's Archiv," 1879, vol. LXXV, p. 99.

Dujardin-Beaumetz: "Des congestions du foie," "Bulletin der thérapie," 1892, vol. LXXIII; "Jahresbericht," II, p. 190.

Durand-Fardel: "Du massage du foie dans l'engorgement hépatique simple," "Bulletin de thérapie," March 30, 1881; "Jahresbericht," II, p. 186.

Frerichs: Loc. cit., I, 374.

Gad, J.: "Studien über Beziehungen des Blutstroms in der Pfortader zum Blutstrom in der Leberarterie," Dissertation, Berlin, 1873.

Hirsch: "Historisch-geographische Pathologie," 1886, p. 267.

Liebermeister: "Beitrage zur pathologischen Anatomie und Klinik der Leberkrankheiten," Tübingen, 1864, pp. 77–135.

— "Specielle Pathologie," v, p. 228.

Monneret, E.: "De la congestion non inflammatoire du foie," "Archives générales de médecine," 1861, I, p. 545.

Naunyn: (Lecture) "Berliner klin. Wochenschr.," 1886, No. 37.

Potain: "Le foie cardiaque et la cirrhose hypertrophique," "Gazette des hôpitaux," 1892, No. 53.

Senator, H.: "Ueber menstruelle Gelbsucht," "Berliner klin. Wochenschr.," 1872, No. 51, p. 615.

Thierfelder: Loc. cit., p. 60.

* Herba Centaurii minoris, Rhizom. Graminis, Rad. Saponariae, Rad. Taraxaci āā 8.0, heated with 300 c.c. of water. To be used as a clyster.

HEMORRHAGE INTO THE LIVER.

(Quincke.)

Hemorrhage into the liver is rare for the reason that there is little room for bleeding in the tissues around the blood-vessels. Hemorrhages when they do occur are seen either in small foci distributed throughout the liver parenchyma or beneath the serous covering or as a diffuse hemorrhagic infiltration of the liver-tissue. They originate from direct or indirect trauma, by wounding or crushing of the parts, and may follow either a simple solution of continuity or an actual destruction of tissue. In the new-born hemorrhages usually originate from acute passive congestion of the liver following difficult or retarded labor. In cases of chronic congestion of the liver hemorrhages are less frequently seen, for the reason that the tissues of the liver in this condition are so tough.

Hemorrhage is, further, occasionally seen in very acute cases of congestion of the organ, in tropical malaria, in mussel-poisoning, in sclerema neonatorum, in chronic experimental phosphorus-poisoning in rabbits (Aufrecht), and in carcinomatous nodule formation. Hemorrhagic infarcts, following the occlusion of small branches of the portal vein, are a rare occurrence (Dreschfeld, Woolridge). Hemorrhages resembling infarcts are sometimes seen in recurrent fever and in severe forms of puerperal infection. [Thromboses and hemorrhages in the liver (Schmorl) have recently grown to constitute an important part of the pathology of puerperal eclampsia.—ED.]

If an aneurysm of the hepatic artery bursts, larger hemorrhages may occur. It is doubtful whether circumscribed lesions of the walls of the portal system of blood-vessels within the liver can lead to similar accidents because of the low pressure therein. It is possible that a number of obscure cases that Frerichs found mentioned in the older literature and discussed were hemorrhages due to disease of some of the larger blood-vessels of the liver.

Symptoms.—Hemorrhage into the tissues of the liver might possibly be suspected in case the symptoms of hyperemia of the liver (pain in the hepatic region and enlargement of the organ), already present, are suddenly aggravated. If the hemorrhage involves the serous covering of the liver as a direct result of the solution of continuity or as a secondary effect of the bleeding, blood will be poured into the abdominal cavity. An accident of this character can sometimes be recognized from the sudden appearance of an area of dulness on percussion, together with definite peritonitic symptoms and a fall of the general blood-pressure. The life of the patient, of course, is greatly endangered by this accident. The symptoms of perforation of a hemorrhagic focus into the bile-channels or hemorrhage directly into these passages have already been discussed (see page 521).

It may occur that liver-cells, either individually or in groups, may pass through the hepatic veins from a traumatic hemorrhagic focus in the liver and enter the general circulation; they may cause embolic occlusion of pulmonary capillaries, or, in case the foramen ovale be patent, may even cause embolic occlusion of some of the capillaries of the greater circulation in the brain, the kidneys, etc. The formation of such *liver-cell emboli* is probably favored by all those conditions of the hepatic parenchyma that are accompanied by a loosening of the connection between the different hepatic cells. Such states are, for example, fatty degeneration of the liver and other parenchymatous changes. Emboli of this character are not necessarily of traumatic origin, but may occasionally be seen in necrotic lesions of different cause, such as puerperal eclampsia, scarlatina, and diphtheria. Jürgens and Klebs assume that hepatic cells carried to the different locations enumerated can proliferate where they happen to be lodged, but Lubarsch contradicts this, and states that they may remain intact for a period of about three weeks, but that, at the end of this time, they are dissolved and disappear, the only damage they are capable of doing being to cause local thromboses.

The diseases that lead to the formation of liver-cell emboli are all very severe, so that no symptoms are known that can be definitely attributed to this particular accident.

Dreschfeld: "Hämorrhagische Infarcte," "Verhandlungen des X. internationalen Congresses," 1890; "Berichte," 1891, II, p. 195.
Frerichs: Loc. cit., I, 395.
Lubarsch, O.: "Zur Lehre von der Parenchymzellenembolie," "Fortschritte der Medicin," 1893, Nos. 20 and 21.
Meyer, Arthur: "Ueber Leberzellenembolie," Dissertation, Kiel, 1888.
Thierfelder: Loc. cit., p. 73.
Wooldridge, L. C.: "On Hemorrhagic Infarction of the Liver," "Transactions of the Patholog. Society of London," 1888, vol. XXXIX, 421.

PERIHEPATITIS.

(Quincke.)

Inflammation of the peritoneal covering of the liver is always secondary, and is seen either as the result of some general peritonitic involvement or as a sequel of a variety of diseases of the liver. The latter form is particularly frequent and of great clinical importance and interest. If the perihepatitis is acute, it may be classified in accordance with its results as serous, fibrinous, or purulent. In chronic inflammation the subserous tissues are also involved or may be exclusively affected. In the latter instance we see a thickening of the serosa and the formation of connective-tissue adhesions with neighboring parts; occasionally, too, the process extends into the liver so as to involve the interstitial connective-tissue structures of the organ. The process may either extend into the liver from the surface of the organ or from the porta hepatis, following the course of Glisson's capsule.

In general, the process follows no typical course, and the inflammation is irregularly distributed and varies in intensity with the primary disease of the liver. It occasionally happens that the whole capsule of the organ is inflamed so that the exudate forms a sort of capsule around the liver. In the more pronounced cases of the latter kind the serous membrane may be several millimeters thick and be of a milk-white color. In such cases the liver will be compressed by this covering and will be deformed, and the margins of the organ will be rounded ("Zuckerguss-Leber," or "icing-liver"). When we see other deformities, such as corset liver, lobulated liver, etc., in combination with perihepatitis, we can assume, in general, that the deformities of the organ are essentially the result of the direct pressure from without or of some disease of the liver itself.

Etiology.—In all cases of diffuse peritonitis the covering of the liver is usually more or less involved. The mechanical influences that cause perihepatitis are, as a rule, of long duration and of moderate degree, as, for instance, the pressure exercised by corsets or narrow waist-bands. Less frequently acute mechanical influences can be made responsible for the occurrence of perihepatitis. In general, the former agencies produce permanent deformities of the liver at the same time.

Among the diseases of the liver itself, those that involve the paren-chyma of the organ do not lead to perihepatitis as frequently as do those that involve the interstitial connective tissues, such as abscess, cirrhosis, syphiloma, alveolar echinococcus, carcinoma, etc. The character of the primary disease will, as a rule, determine the character of the inflamma-tion of the serous membrane.

Perihepatitis, either purulent, serous, or adhesive, frequently origi-nates from the gall-bladder. The disease may also start from some of the organs adjacent to the liver, such as a pleuritis of the right side by exten-sion through the diaphragm. A simple gastric ulcer may cause peri-hepatitis, particularly on the lower surface of the liver and on the anterior margin; in this case the inflammation is generally of the adhesive kind, and it may happen that the ulcerative process in the stomach wall extends to the substance of the liver by means of adhesions between the two organs.

Symptoms.—In acute cases of perihepatitis pain is a prominent symp-tom. It may either be circumscribed or be felt throughout the whole hepatic region. From the distribution of the pain clues may sometimes be obtained in regard to the localization and the extent of the perihepatitic process. The pain is accentuated by pressure from without and by differ-ent movements, for which reason the pressure of the clothing is disagreeable to the patients and they avoid lying on the right side; at the same time and for the same reason, respiration may be slightly impeded. The pain, as in all forms of serous inflammations, is, as a rule, severe and lancinating. Palpation and percussion of the liver are, therefore, often rendered very difficult. At times a friction-sound may be heard and a fremitus may be felt over the area of perihepatitis, generally syn-chronously with respiration.

In addition, all the symptoms of the primary disease will be observed, whether this be in the liver itself or in some other organ. Peri-hepatitis rarely causes vomiting or a considerable rise of temperature. Icterus is sometimes seen in this condition, but it is doubtful what causes it. Some authors are inclined to attribute it to the reduced rhythmic movements of the liver following the impediment in the normal respira-tory excursion; but whether this theory is correct or not cannot very well be determined.

Chronic perihepatitis may run its course without causing any symp-toms whatever, and may not be noticed by the patient until ultimately the symptoms caused by adhesions with neighboring organs or thickening of the serosa of the liver appear. Adhesions between the diaphragm and the abdominal walls, if they are sufficiently developed, may hinder the respiratory motility of the lower margin of the liver, and the condition may be readily recognized in this manner.

Chronic perihepatitis may extend to the connective-tissue structures within the liver and in this way produce a true hepatic cirrhosis with its clinical manifestations (Roller, Frerichs, *loc. cit.*, II, p. 92).

In rare instances chronic inflammatory perihepatitis may cause a metamorphosis of the inflamed peritoneal covering of the liver into tough contracted connective tissue, so that the liver is inclosed in a sort of capsule. As the covering contracts, pressure is exercised on the organ and the circulation of the blood is impeded in the same way as in true cirrhosis of the organ; consequently, a disease-picture that is very similar to the latter condition may be seen, characterized, in particular, by the occurrence of ascites and the remarkable reduction in the size of the liver. The spleen, in this condition, is not generally enlarged, for the reason that this organ cannot expand owing to the callous thickening of its capsule. Cases of this kind have been occasionally described in the older literature* and have recently been studied more carefully by Curschmann, Rumpf, Pick, and Hübler, and have been called "Zuckergussleber" (*perihepatitis chronica hyperplastica*) by these authors. They are differentiated from cirrhosis by their longer course (six, even as much as fifteen years), during which the condition may become quiescent at times, or, on the other hand, an almost incredible number of paracenteses may have to be performed (as many as 301 in one case).

The capsule may be from five to ten millimeters thick, and naturally compresses the liver considerably. As a rule, the capsule consists of thick fibrous tissue. The size of the liver may be reduced to one-half. If the capsule is cut, the tissue of the liver bulges above the surface of the section. It is not changed in its microscopic structures and reveals no proliferation of connective tissue.

The exact cause for this peculiar form of thickening of the capsule is not at all clear. In the case of Hübler frequent and very violent attacks of gall-stone colic occurred and possibly constituted an irritant predisposing to inflammation. In other cases, again, the first remote cause of the trouble seems to have been an attack of pericarditis occurring long before the development of the capsule formation and which at the time of its occurrence caused obliteration of the pericardial sac. Pick mentions the latter possibility and calls the condition pericarditic pseudo-cirrhosis of the liver.

As a matter of fact, one or several of the following conditions are found at autopsy in cases of this kind, in addition, of course, to the thickening of the capsule of the liver: peritonitis, with fibrous exudates in the upper part of the abdominal cavity, in the region of the capsule of the spleen and of the parietal peritoneum, obliteration of the pericardium, and the formation of fibrous tissue in this region, and cirrhosis of the liver.

It appears, therefore, that occasionally fibrinous perihepatitis originates from extension of an inflammation of the pericardium or of the pleura. It seems possible too, that cirrhosis of the liver from stasis resulting from cardiac insufficiency plays a part in impeding the flow of blood through the portal system of vessels. Another factor that may be made responsible for the appearance of ascites is fibrinous peritonitis, a lesion which may itself lead to the formation of an exudate or, at all events, may constitute a serious obstacle to the absorption of ascitic fluid by the parietal peritoneum.

It is also possible that stasis of lymph can help produce ascites, from the fact that pericarditic or pleuritic exudates, by narrowing the intrathoracic space, compress lymph-channels situated within the thorax.

In a certain sense that form of circumscribed exudative peritonitis that occurs between the liver and the diaphragm (subphrenic abscess), and is characterized by the collection of pus in that region, must be counted among the manifestations of perihepatitis. This peritonitis may originate from a gastric or a duodenal ulcer or from echinococcus of the liver. Clinically, the disease simulates pyopneumothorax, or less often an enlargement of the liver. (This condition is discussed in detail in another volume.)

The pathologic significance, therefore, of perihepatitis and the prognosis of the disease may vary as much and be as closely dependent on the nature of the primary trouble as is, for example, pleuritis. Another analogy may be drawn between the two diseases from the fact that in

* Budd, "Diseases of the Liver," p. 495. Bamberger, "Krankheiten des chylo-poietischen Systems," 2d edition, p. 495.

both the appearance of an inflammation of the serous membrane signalizes, for the first time, a diseased condition of the organ it is covering—in the case of perihepatitis the lungs, in the case of pleuritis the liver. With the discovery of these lesions, a more careful diagnosis can be made and an intelligent prophylaxis instituted.

Diagnosis.—The pain of perihepatitis may be differentiated from pain originating within the liver by certain peculiarities. The former is of a more lancinating character and is increased by pressure, the latter (as in abscess of the liver) is more diffuse, indefinite, and radiates particularly into the region of the right shoulder-blade. It is true that this differentiation cannot always be made with absolute certainty, and it is even possible that the symptoms enumerated as characteristic of a hepatic pain are in reality due to the presence of circumscribed perihepatitis on the convex surface of the organ.

The liver may be tender on pressure in other conditions besides perihepatitis, as in acute swelling with a rapid increase in the size of the organ (acute hyperemia, phosphorus-poisoning), in cases in which the volume of the liver decreases rapidly (acute atrophy), and, finally, sometimes in gall-stone colic. In the latter disease, it is true, the pain is, as a rule, more violent, and the tenderness, while it may extend to regions outside the area of the liver proper, is still by far most pronounced immediately over the region of the gall-bladder. In concrete cases, at the same time, a reasonable doubt may exist in the mind of the diagnostician whether the pain is attributable to the tension of the walls of the gall-bladder or to inflammations in and around the liver. If the pain is due to some inflammatory process, it is usually of longer duration, and, finally, as a rule, becomes strictly localized in one place or the other.

Treatment.—Acute perihepatitis is often accompanied by such severe paroxysms of pain that the latter must be treated *per se.* In the most violent attacks leeches and the ice-bag may be applied; in the less severe, warm Priessnitz compresses or cataplasms, with rest and, possibly, the administration of narcotics. If the pain persists, vesication, or painting the painful places with iodin may be tried. In many cases it will be impossible to treat the primary disease until the pain has been alleviated and the acute attack has subsided. Treatment of the primary disease, of course, constitutes the best prophylaxis against the recurrence of attacks.

LITERATURE.

Bamberger: Loc. cit., p. 495.
Curschmann: "Zur Diagnostik der mit Ascites verbundenen Erkrankungen der Leber und des Peritoneums," "Deutsche med. Wochenschr.," 1884, p. 564.
Frerichs: Loc. cit., ii, p. 4.
Hübler: "Fall von chronischer Perihepatitis hyperplastica," "Berliner klin. Wochenschr.," 1897, p. 1118.
Longuet: "Du frottement perihépatique," "L'Union méd.," 1886, Nos. 85 and 86.
Pick, Fr.: "Pericarditische Pseudolebercirrhose," "Zeitschr. für klin. Medicin," 1896, vol. xxix, p. 388.
Roller: "Cholelithiasis als Ursache von Cirrhosis hepatis," "Berliner klin. Wochenschr.," 1879, p. 625.
Rumpf, H. (Bostroem): "Ueber die Zuckergussleber," "Deutsches Archiv für klin. Medicin," 1895, vol. lv, p. 272.
Siegert, F.: "Ueber die Zuckergussleber und die pericarditische Pseudolebercirrhose," "Virchow's Archiv," 1898, vol. cliii, p. 251.
Thierfelder: Loc. cit., p. 75.
v. Wunschheim: "Prager med. Wochenschr.," 1893, No. 15.
    Illustration in "Rumpel's Atlas," D, part 1. 2.
    40

ACUTE HEPATITIS.

(Quincke.)

Among the acute inflammatory diseases of the liver the suppurative forms are best understood, and their origin is most comprehensible. These are always, possibly with exceedingly rare exceptions, caused by micro-organisms. As a result, the same symptoms are produced as in any form of suppuration in other parts of the body. The symptoms that are attributable to the particular involvement of the liver are merely dependent on the topographic position of the organ, and have nothing whatever to do with its specific function. Of course, the flow of bile is often impeded, and this symptom may, in a sense, be designated a specific sign of involvement of the liver.

The diseases of the liver that are designated diffuse acute inflammations of the organ are more important, for the reason that they are intimately connected with the specific function of the organ and involve principally the glandular parenchyma.

We can subdivide acute hepatitis into acute parenchymatous hepatitis, acute atrophy of the liver, and acute interstitial hepatitis.

ACUTE PARENCHYMATOUS HEPATITIS.

Anatomy ; Etiology.—Parenchymatous cloudy swelling of the liver is frequently found in certain infectious diseases, particularly in septicemia, puerperal fever, typhoid fever, recurrent fever, pneumonia, and erysipelas. The substance of the organ, in these cases, appears to be more cloudy than usual and less transparent, the organ looking "as though it had been boiled." On microscopic examination, it will be seen that the hepatic cells are cloudy, as a rule contain fine granulations and, if the disease is of longer duration, coarser refractive granules. The latter consist of albumin, and in the later stages of the disease of fat. Sometimes the hepatic cells are slightly swollen, so that the liver appears anemic and enlarged, with rounded margins. The milder degrees of this cloudy swelling, it appears, do not occur during the life of the patient, but must be considered a postmortem coagulative change; it is more pronounced in the cases under discussion, however, than in normal subjects. In particularly severe cases, of sepsis, for instance, the intimacy of the hepatic cells with the interstitial tissues of the liver and their connections with one another are considerably loosened, so that the trabeculæ of hepatic cells are more or less dislocated (disassociated, Browicz). The outline of the hepatic cells becomes indistinct, necrotic changes occur within them, and both the nuclei and the protoplasm lose their normal staining properties. Similar changes are seen in malaria, but in this disease, as well as in sepsis, circumscribed areas of necrosis may appear; it may also happen that in malaria and in some of the other infectious diseases a diffuse or localized collection of embryonal cells occurs which later become organized into connective tissue. In many of these infectious diseases, particularly in malaria, sepsis, and typhoid, the specific pathogenic organisms may be found within the hepatic capillaries. As a rule, however, the latter are not present in sufficient numbers to warrant the suspicion that they cause by a purely local action the necrotic changes described. In the production of all these lesions certain chemical poisons undoubtedly play a rôle, and such poisons may be generated in remote parts of the body.

This view is strengthened by our knowledge of the fact that some of the known chemical poisons are capable of producing similar parenchymatous swelling and cloudiness of the hepatic cells. Such poisons are, for instance, phosphorus, chloroform (E. Fraenkel, Bandler), chloral (Geill), and some of the mushroom poisons, as *Amanita phalloïdes*. Lupinosis in animals and acute fatty degeneration from unknown causes in adults and in children are other similar conditions. Alcohol, too, must be mentioned. This drug, however, can only act deleteriously in one large dose provided the liver has been previously damaged by the habitual abuse of spirits. In all the cases enumerated the cloudiness of the liver-cells is accompanied by fatty degeneration, and, in the case of alcohol and of phosphorus, with fatty infiltration. If the poisons act for a long time, interstitial proliferation may supervene.

In the majority of the cases both of poisoning and of infection other organs are, as a rule, involved, and frequently to a higher degree than the liver. This may account for the fact that in the general picture of these infections and intoxications symptoms attributable to disease of the liver are frequently absent. With the exception of phosphorus-poisoning, in which the liver is infiltrated with fat and consequently very much swollen, the liver is, in general, not much enlarged. Consequently, the degree of parenchymatous change cannot be determined from the degree of enlargement, but must be deduced from the severity of the general symptoms pointing to this condition.

Liebermeister has attempted to attribute the parenchymatous clouding of the liver (and of other tissues) to the febrile rise of temperature in different infections. This explanation is not correct, for we learn from our observations on human subjects that the changes in the tissues are in nowise proportionate to the height of the fever or its duration. Animal experiments show that artificial elevation of the temperature (in the heat-box, Litten) produces a fatty degeneration of the glandular cells, but no parenchymatous degeneration. More recent experiments by Ziegler and Wernhowsky show that cloudiness, vacuolation, and fatty degeneration of the hepatic cells and a loosening of their connection can occur, but do not, as a rule, take place until the overheating of the animal has been carried on for many days.

Those cases in which the hepatic symptoms are very conspicuous, or in which we obtain the disease-picture of an acute hepatitis, are rare indeed. This form is most frequently encountered in the tropics. It is impossible, in many instances, to differentiate it from the congestive hyperemia of the liver so often seen in this climate; in fact, a gradual transition can be observed from simple changes in the vascularity of the liver and changes in the parenchyma that follow eating and are due to digestive engorgement of the organ, to active congestion, and, later, to acute parenchymatous hepatitis.

Malaria and dysentery are unquestionably the chief causes for this acute hepatitis of the tropics. Apart from these two diseases, however, the development of hepatitis may be seen in Europeans that migrate to warm climates (see page 453). This is particularly the case in young people during the first year or so, and at all ages until they have become accustomed to the change of climate and before they have learned to moderate their diet and to refrain from eating as much as they did at home, particularly if they persist in indulging in a liberal animal diet or continue to abuse alcohol. The liver in these cases is enlarged and very vascular, soft, and filled with grayish, more or less softened foci that exude serum from their cut surfaces. The immediate vicinity of these foci is more vascular and usually harder than the foci themselves. Later the foci turn yellowish, dull, and finally atrophic from degeneration of the cells and absorption of the debris (Cayley). It is probable that this form of hepatitis owes its origin to the action of intestinal ptomains that find a suitable nidus for their action in the liver when it is in a stage of chronic congestion, and which act as irritants. According to Kartulis, pathogenic microbes have been seen in a liver of this character without at the same time having caused the formation of abscesses. In Mexico, hepatitis of this kind is more frequently seen in summer than in the other seasons of the year (Mejia).

These acute forms of hepatitis are not found in the tropics alone. Kartulis has described their occurrence, for instance, in Alexandria. In Europe they are probably very rare. Talma claims that he has observed such cases in Utrecht, and several years ago described seven cases of this character. He quotes the rather scanty and vague statements of older authors. Talma is inclined to seek the primary cause of the trouble in the intestine, and believes that the liver is secondarily affected either through the blood-vessels and the portal blood or through the lymphatics.

Symptoms.—In the cases described by Talma the disease usually begins with vomiting, followed by diarrhea, a moderate degree of fever, and, after a few days, pain in the region of the liver. The liver is enlarged, its consistency increased, and it is tender on pressure. The organ is greatly swollen and on its surface nodular prominences can be felt that may be as large as a hen's egg. As a rule, icterus is present, but the feces are rarely discolored. The spleen is enlarged and readily palpable. Nothing abnormal can be discovered in the thoracic organs. The sensorium is free. The urine contains no albumin.

In the course of the second week all the symptoms seem to recede, the liver and the spleen decrease in size, and complete recovery may occur at the expiration of from eight to fourteen days. Talma saw a fatal issue in only one case, on the ninth day.

In Alexandria the course that these cases pursue is similar, and also favorable, the average duration being from two to three weeks.

The following etiologic factors have been mentioned in the production of the tropical form of acute hepatitis: catching cold, overfatigue, insolation, errors of diet, alcoholic excesses, and attacks of malaria. The disease here is more violent, frequently begins with a chill, the temperature rises higher, and all the symptoms are more pronounced and more grave. The liver may be so much enlarged that it extends 7 to 8 inches below the costal margin. The organ may be enlarged in certain circumscribed districts only; for instance, toward the ribs on its anterior surface or upward toward the diaphragm. At the same time local pain, a feeling of pressure under the costal margin, difficulty in breathing, and pain in the region of the shoulder may be present. Icterus, as a rule, is mild.

In malarial hepatitis the picture of acute malaria is complicated by certain hepatic symptoms. The liver and the spleen generally swell at the time of the fever paroxysms. Kartulis discovered plasmodia, but no bacteria, in the blood removed from the liver by aspiration.

In the form of hepatitis seen in the tropics the final outcome of the disease is favorable in those cases that are afflicted for the first time, and in which the liver was perfectly healthy before the onset of the disease. An attack of acute tropical hepatitis, however, predisposes to subsequent attacks that run a less favorable course. In case the general nutrition of the patient is not good, abscesses are liable to form, or the liver may remain permanently enlarged, and possibly atrophic cirrhosis may develop later. In Mexico the first attack generally leads to abscess-formation, and a cure of the disease is seen in exceptional cases only (Mejia).

Termination; Prognosis.—The prognosis of the primary form of parenchymatous hepatitis is favorable in temperate climates. In tropical climates the prognosis is dependent on the primary cause of the trouble and on the willingness or the ability of the patient to change his mode of life and to live in a manner suited to the exigencies of the climate. The probability of subsequent attacks grows with each recurrence of the disease, and at the same time the probability of a complete restitution to a normal condition diminishes.

Frequent recurrences of the disease lead to hypertrophy of the liver, then to chronic inflammation, and finally to cirrhosis. In malaria localized atrophic foci develop in the liver, and, in addition, nodular hyperplasias that resemble adenomata. If the disease takes this form, it is called by French authors *hépatite nodulaire* (Sabourin, Kelsch and Kiener).

In intoxications and infections the unfavorable issue may in some instances be determined by the disorders of metabolism that follow the derangement of the liver incident to parenchymatous hepatitis. In cases of this character acute atrophy of the liver may in rare instances result. This disease will be discussed in the following section.

Treatment.—In general, the patients remain in bed without being told; but complete rest is an essential part of the treatment. In the beginning of the disease purgation by calomel or salts is to be recommended, while emetics—as, for instance, ipecacuanha—are less indicated. In the subsequent course of the disease a mild laxative treatment and "disinfection of the intestine" are useful (see page 464). In the beginning the diet should be greatly restricted and remain simple and non-irritating throughout the whole course of the disease, milk and gruel soups being particularly advisable. Cayley advises the administration of chlorid of ammonium at the height of the disease in the daily dose of from 4 to 6 gm. Later he recommends tartar emetic and nitrate of potash, aqua regia with gentian, and daily doses of from 0.1 to 0.3 of euonymin with a little rhubarb. The latter prescription is intended to relieve the feeling of pressure in the side. Violent pain should be relieved by blood-letting and by the application of compresses to the hepatic region. The diet should remain non-irritating for a long time after convalescence and the use of alcohol should be eschewed. In hepatitis from malaria quinin should be administered in addition to the other remedies enumerated; as a rule, the size of the liver will decrease in a few days after the exhibition of quinin.

If attacks of tropical hepatitis recur very frequently, the patient should be advised to move to another climate.

LITERATURE.

Aufrecht: "Die acute Parenchymatose," "Deutsches Archiv für klin. Medicin," vol. XL, p. 620, case 2.

— "Die diffuse Leberentzündung nach Phosphor," "Deutsches Archiv für klin. Medicin," 1878, vol. XXIII, p. 331.

Browicz: "Dissociation der Leberläppchen," "Virchow's Archiv," 1897, vol. CXLVIII, p. 424.

Cayley, H.: "Tropical Affections of the Liver," VIII. Congress für Hygiene und Demographie in Budapest, 1894; "Berichte," vol. II, p. 695.

Dock: "Malarial Liver," "Amer. Jour. of the Med. Sci.," April, 1834.

Erdmann, L. (Bessarabien): "Virchow's Archiv," 1868, vol. XLIII, p. 291.

Frerichs: Loc. cit., II, p. 9.

Girode: "Quelques faits d'ictère infectieux," "Archives générales de médecine," 1891, I, pp. 26 and 167.

— "Infections avec ictère," "Archives générales de médecine," 1892, I, pp. 412 and 555 (mostly pyemias and septicemias with icterus).

Hirsch: "Historisch-geographische Pathologie," 1886, III, p. 267.

Kartulis: "Ueber verschiedene Leberkrankheiten in Aegypten," VIII. Congress für Hygiene und Demographie in Budapest, 1894, vol. II, pp. 643–657.

Kelsch et Kiener: "Archives de physiolog. norm. et pathol.," 1878, 1879.

— "Maladies des pays chands," Paris, 1889.

Mejia (Mexico): "L'hépatite parenchymateuse aiguë circonscrite," "Verhandlungen des X. internationalen Congresses," 1890, part v, p. 26.

Monneret: "De la congestion non-inflammatoire du foie," "Archives générales," 1861, I, p. 545.

Runge: "Krankheiten der Neugeborenen," p. 162: "Acute Fettdegeneration."

Sabourin: "Archives de physiolog. norm. et patholog.," 1880, 1884.

Talma: "Hepatitis parenchymatosa benigna," "Weekbl. v. het. Neederl. Tijdschr. vor. Geneesk.," 1891, No. 20; "Berliner klin. Wochenschr.," 1891, p. 1111.

Ziegler (u. Werhowsky): "Ueber die Wirkung der erhöbten Eigenwärme auf das Blut und die Gewebe," "Verhandlungen des Congresses für innere Medicin." 1895, p. 345.

AFTER THE USE OF CHLORAL.

Geill, Ch.: "Vierteljahresschr. für gerichtliche Medicin," 1897, vol. XIV, p. 274.

Gellhorn: "Allgemeine Zeitschr. für Psychiatrie," 1872, vol. XXVIII, p. 625; 1873, vol. XXIX, p. 428.

Ogston: "Edinburgh Med. Jour.," October, 1878, p. 289.

EFFECTS OF CHLOROFORM.

Bandler, V.: "Mittheilungen aus den Grenzgebeiten der Medicin und Chirurgie," 1896, I, p. 303.

Fränkel, E.: "Virchow's Archiv," 1892, vols. CXXVII, CXXIX.

Compare also the literature of acute atrophy of the liver, page 647, of fatty liver, and of malarial liver.

ACUTE ATROPHY OF THE LIVER.

(Icterus gravis ; Ictère typhoide.)

(Quincke.)

Acute atrophy of the liver is in the majority of cases a sequel to diffuse parenchymatous hepatitis; at the same time the disease is clinically and anatomically so clearly characterized that it merits particular discussion and deserves to be ranked as a distinct clinical entity, especially since Rokitansky, in 1842, determined and established the anatomic characteristics of this condition.

Occurrence.—Acute atrophy of the liver is a very rare disease. It is seen more frequently in women than in men (proportion 8 to 5); and about one-half of those that are afflicted, particularly among women, are from twenty to thirty years of age. About one-half to one-third of all women afflicted are in the fourth month or in later stages of pregnancy. The lying-in period seems also to predispose to the disease, although it is less frequently encountered at this time than at earlier periods of pregnancy.

Acute atrophy of the liver has also been observed in children; but it is rare. Fr. Merkel has collated 18 and R. Schmidt 16 cases that occurred from the first days of life to the tenth year. [A casual examination of the literature since 1896 adds five new cases, with a considerable number between the ages of ten and fifteen years, probably as a result of the attention drawn to the subject by the article of Merkel and the monograph of Schmidt.—ED.]

Etiology.—Very little is known in regard to the causes of acute atrophy of the liver. Older statements in regard to "fright, anger, abuse of alcohol," are very unsatisfactory. As the preliminary stages of the disease resemble catarrhal icterus, we must assume either that some particular cause existed for the development of this icterus into acute atrophy or that in the course of the ordinary catarrhal form of icterus there entered into the disease some new factor that led to atrophy. Some of the cases observed (Meder, Case III) occurred during an epidemic of icterus, all the other cases of which were benign, a fact that furnishes no clue in either direction.

Acute atrophy of the liver has been known to follow certain infectious diseases: for instance, osteomyelitis (Meder), diphtheria of the stomach (Cahn), erysipelas (Huntermann), sepsis (Drinkler, Babes), typhoid (Dorfler), recurrent fever, and syphilis (twenty cases, Meder). It is possible that in these cases the ordinary form of parenchymatous degeneration of the liver that is so frequently seen in infectious diseases attained a particularly severe degree and terminated in an exceptional manner.

In the secondary stage of syphilis, particularly in the beginning, acute atrophy of the liver has occasionally been seen following the attack of icterus that is so often seen at this time (Engel-Reymers, Senator, and others; altogether, in twenty cases). Aufrecht observed acute atrophy of the liver in sclerodermia neonatorum.

Poisons, too, may lead to acute atrophy of the liver. This has been positively demonstrated in the case of phosphorus when death does not ensue soon after the ingestion of the poison, but when the patient survives for some time, several weeks or more (Mannkopf, Litten, Hedderich). It is said that acute alcoholic poisoning (Oppolzer, Laudet) and the abuse of spirits in general lead to this condition. Sausage-poisoning (Wolf) and mushroom-poisoning (Hecker) have also been made responsible for acute atrophy of the liver. Bandler has recently described a case in which acute atrophy followed within three days after chloroform narcosis in a beer-drinker, causing the death of the patient. Bandler assumes that the chloroform was retained in the liver in large quantities and that it was there combined with the lecithin and the cholesterin normally present in the organ. He also quotes three similar cases mentioned by Bastianelli.*

It is quite probable that intoxication by ptomains occurs in many cases where the function of the intestine is deranged, and that in certain of the infectious diseases bacterial toxins play an important rôle.

Kobert † advances the theory that an intoxication by phosphoretted hydrogen may occasionally occur. This gas, he assumes, is generated in the intestine from the phosphates by the action of bacteria. He believes that the hydrogen compound of phosphorus acts in the same way as phosphorus itself.

Many attempts have been made to discover certain bacteria that could be made responsible for the occurrence of acute atrophy of the liver (Klebs, Eppinger, Hanot, and others). Thus, Babes found streptococci in

* Perhaps Bamberger's case also belongs here (" Krankheit. des Chylopoietischen Systems," 2 Aufl., S. 532).
† Kobert, " Intoxicationen," p. 416.

four cases, Strobe and v. Kahlden found in the capillaries of the liver Bacterium coli, which had been transported through the portal vein. While it is possible that bacteria have a certain significance in the isolated cases mentioned, their importance in many other instances is exceedingly doubtful (Vincent, Rangleret and Mahen); in still other cases no bacteria whatever were found, or, if they were found, could not be cultivated (Kahlder, Bloedau, Rosenheim, Gabbi, Phedran and Macallum, Sittmann).

As a rule, acute atrophy is seen in otherwise healthy livers. Occasionally, however, this condition seems to be a complication or a sequel of other diseases of the organ, particularly of cirrhosis, stasis of bile, and fatty degeneration of the liver.

General Clinical Description.—The disease usually begins, like any other form of catarrhal icterus, with symptoms of an acute gastric catarrh; following these, icterus develops in the course of a few days or, less frequently, weeks. This first, so-called prodromal stage of the disease lasts for several days or weeks, in every way resembles catarrhal icterus, and may be so mild that it is taken for one of the very slight attacks of catarrhal icterus that permit the patient to be about. Suddenly, less often gradually, the second stage of the disease develops, with stupor, delirium, restlessness, and even mania. As a rule, vomiting and convulsions are seen at the same time. Coma increases, and in the course of a few days death occurs. Recovery is very rare.

With the onset of the second stage the volume of the liver decreases, there is usually pain in the region of the liver, the spleen becomes enlarged, bloody vomiting supervenes; and epistaxis, bloody stools, hematuria, bleeding from the genitals, or ecchymoses in the skin are all seen. The urine usually contains bile-pigment and albumin, with, as a rule, some leucin, tyrosin, and other products of abnormal catabolism. Temperature is normal or subnormal, occasionally elevated toward the end.

Anatomy.—The liver is reduced in size and flaccid. Its weight may be reduced one-half or even more, the left lobe, in particular, being smaller than normal. The organ is flattened, folded on itself, and situated nearer to the spinal column. The capsule is usually wrinkled.

In many cases the color of the hepatic substance is a dirty yellow. The tissue is very soft and the outlines of the lobules indistinct. Microscopically it will be seen that the contours of the hepatic cells are also indistinct, and that the latter are in different stages of granular and fatty degeneration and are stained with bile. They are least degenerated near the center of the lobules. In the peripheral parts of the lobules they are to be seen in all stages of granular degeneration, and the columns of liver-cells are indistinct.

In other, apparently more numerous cases, a red hepatic substance is seen in addition to the yellow tissue described. This may be present in small foci or may constitute the bulk of the degenerated tissue, so that the yellow foci seem to be embedded within the red substance. The former in these cases form nodules as large as a grain of oatmeal or may reach the size of a hazelnut. As a rule, they protrude above the level of the cut surface. The red substance is tough, its cut surface is smooth, and the outlines of the lobules cannot be recognized. On microscopic examination it will be found that liver-cells are absent and that all that is left of the hepatic tissue is a homogeneous or striated mass of connective tissue inclosing detritus of different kinds. This red substance constitutes an advanced stage of degeneration. Occasionally it will be seen that the center of a lobule is colored yellow and is surrounded by a ring of the red tissue that constitutes the periphery of the lobule. According to Meder and Marchand, the degeneration of the liver-cells does not always occur in the same manner. Sometimes finely granular degeneration is seen as a result of necrosis; in other cases, fatty degeneration. These changes are always most intense at the periphery of the acini. At the same time, the epithelial cells of some of the interlobular bile-passages perish. In the beginning the blood-capillaries are intact, although they may become very brittle; but later these also perish. As soon as the columns of liver-cells in the peripheral parts of the lobules perish, the bile-capillaries, too, of course, disappear; and it is possible that the interference with the current of bile in these parts is the cause of icterus.

It may happen that so much of the yellow substance perishes that finally the whole liver presents the picture of the higher degree of degeneration and is flaccid and red throughout.

In the beginning of the disease a certain red discoloration of the cut surface of the liver may be due to hyperemia, and constitute nothing more than the preliminary stage in the formation of the yellow substance. The latter, as we have seen, is nothing more than the conglomerate of cells that have undergone swelling and clouding. According to this view, Frerichs designates the red parts of the liver as those that are least degenerated, whereas the yellow parts are those that are most atrophic. Klebs, on the other hand, in opposition to this view, considers the red substance alone as the real product of atrophy, whereas the yellow is, according to him, the expression of beginning regeneration. It may be conceded that in the yellow parts, owing to the smaller number of cells that have perished, regeneration seems to occur more actively than in the red parts.

According to Perls and v. Starck, chemical analysis of the liver-substance shows that the fat in this form of degeneration is formed from the proteid of the liver-cells. These investigators found an increase of the fat and a reduction in the quantity of dry residue that was free from fat. At the same time the water remains the same as normal or is slightly increased. In phosphorus-poisoning, on the other hand, complicated with fatty infiltration of the liver, fat takes the place of much water.

	WATER.	FAT.	DRY RESIDUE CONTAINING NO FAT.
Normal liver	76.1	3.0	20.9
Acute atrophy { (Perls)	87.6	8.7	9.7
(Perls)	76.9	7.6	15.5
(v. Starck).................	80.5	4.2	15.3
Phosphorus-poisoning (v. Starck).............	60.0	29.8	10.0
Acute fatty degeneration (v. Starck)..........	64.0	25.0	11.0

[This question as to the production of the fat from protein must still be considered an unsettled one. There has been a large amount of work upon it recently; and, as far as experimental results are concerned, the chief of these, which were obtained by Rosenfeld, A. E. Taylor, and several of the Pflüger school, indicate that the fat in fatty degeneration of the liver is not produced from protein. The subject has recently been ably reviewed by A. E. Taylor.*—ED.]

*Am. Jour. Med. Sciences, May, 1899

A remarkable finding in this disease is the excretion of crystals of tyrosin which are visible both microscopically and macroscopically, especially if the liver is allowed to lie for some time.

In addition to the degeneration of the hepatic cells, an increase of the interstitial tissues of the liver is occasionally seen. In part this increase is undoubtedly only apparent and relative, and its appearance is due to the fact that so many of the cells have perished; in part, changes of this character that are reported were longstanding; sometimes, however, recent proliferation of connective tissue may be seen with small-celled infiltration (Riess, Meder) that may occur diffusely or in foci throughout the interlobular connective tissues.

The interlobular bile-passages show progressive tissue changes in the form of an increase of the cubical epithelium lining them. These changes are more frequently seen than those described in the connective tissue of the liver. The cells penetrate the meshes of the collapsed tissue, and in this manner form new trabeculæ of liver-cells. Increase in the size of these cells and general proliferation of the cells of the liver that remain intact may also lead to regeneration of the liver tissue. These processes may be observed within the first week after the occurrence of atrophy, and may, in fact, lead to a real cure of the disease. The new liver-cells are then not arranged in the usual typical manner, and as a result the new-formed bile-channels are very long and tortuous. In a case described by Marchand, examined half a year after the onset of the disease, regeneration had not occurred in a uniform manner, but nodules of hyperplastic tissue about as large as lentils or peas were distributed all through the red substance of the liver. The yellow substance, in this case, consisted of broad tubes of cells; the red, of narrow ones. [The formation of new glandular cells from the epithelial cells lining newly formed bile-channels was clearly seen in a case described by Aly Bey Ibrahim*; the regenerative process taking place exclusively in the red areas.—Ed.]

Changes are seen in other organs besides the liver. General icterus, granular clouding, and fatty infiltration of the kidney epithelium and of the muscular fibers of the heart, sometimes, too, of the muscles of the extremities, are seen. The epithelial cells and the glandular cells of the stomach, and the bronchial and pulmonary epithelium, as well as the epithelium of the intestinal villi, may also show these changes. The spleen, as a rule, is considerably increased in size and is soft. In the intestine a catarrhal condition of the mucous membrane may be seen and the follicular and mesenteric glands may be somewhat swollen. In the majority of cases ecchymoses will be seen in the serous membranes, the external skin, the mucosa of the stomach and of the urinary passages, the connective-tissue structures of the body-cavities and of the extremities. The blood is generally thin. No definite changes are found in the brain.

Symptoms.—In the prodromal stage of the disease nothing characteristic whatever is seen. Icterus usually appears a few days after the onset of the gastric symptoms, and as a rule becomes quite intense, the stools being clay-colored or colorless, and complete stasis of bile supervening. With the onset of the second stage icterus increases. In exceptional cases icterus does not appear until severe symptoms develop, or even after this period. Occasionally the degree of icterus, like the color of the feces, fluctuates during the course of the disease, and icterus may even be completely absent, if the course of the trouble is very rapid.

* *Münch. med. Woch.*, May 21, 1901.

The liver is generally enlarged during the prodromal stage, owing either to stasis of bile or swelling of the cells. Clinically, however, this condition can rarely be recognized, and the same condition is present in ordinary catarrhal icterus. In phosphorus-poisoning a considerable degree of swelling may be noticed from the very beginning, but may even in this condition be completely absent (Hedderich).

Soon after the appearance of cerebral symptoms, rarely before, a decrease in the size of the organ may be noticed. The liver dulness may completely disappear, not alone because of the decrease in the size of the organ, but also because of its flaccidity. The liver becomes folded and drops back so that it may even be impossible to palpate it. At the same time the hepatic region is very sensitive, and this tenderness may extend into the epigastric region and other parts of the abdomen.

If the reduction of the volume of the liver leads merely to a flattening of the organ, the liver may still show the same area of percussion dulness, but the sound will be less dull and more tympanitic. This always occurs if the liver is attached to the anterior abdominal walls by adhesions (C. Gerhardt).

Leube, in a case that ran a very slow course, noticed that the hepatic region was so doughy that the pressure of the fingers left a distinct pit in the epigastric region.

With the cerebral symptoms vomiting occurs. The vomitus is slimy, sometimes bile-tinged, and toward the end bloody. Constipation is usually present and the appetite is lost. The spleen is enlarged in about two-thirds of the cases.

In the great majority of the cases hemorrhages are observed, most frequently as hematemesis and hemorrhagic ecchymosis of the skin. The vomitus is generally reddish or like coffee-grounds, large quantities of blood being rarely vomited. The stools may occasionally be bloody. Hemorrhages from the nasal mucosa, the mucous membranes of the mouth, or the urinary passages are rare. In pregnant women and in women during the lying-in period uterine hemorrhages are seen.

Litten observed retinal hemorrhage, and in one case irregular grayish-white spots caused by fatty degeneration of the elements of the retina with the formation of small granular spheres and of small sheaths of tyrosin crystals.

Fever is often present during the initial catarrhal icterus, but later the temperature is, as a rule, normal. The same applies to the second stage of the disease, although here it may become subnormal. Sometimes the temperature remains subnormal until death, while in other cases a rise of temperature occurs during the last two days or so and may attain very high degrees (42.6° C.—108.68° F.).

The action of the heart is normal or slow in the prodromal stage and in the beginning of the second stage. As the general condition of the patient grows worse, the cardiac action becomes more rapid and weaker, the heart-sounds being softer and duller and occasionally accompanied by a systolic murmur.

The urine is, as a rule, slightly decreased and, owing to the presence of icterus, contains some bile-pigment and generally small quantities of albumin and a few casts with fatty epithelium. The most important urinary constituents are a number of products of perverted metabolism, such as leucin, tyrosin, sarcolactic acid, oxymandelic acid ($C_8H_8O_4$), peptone,*

* It seems hardly necessary to call attention to the fact that peptone is believed at the present time never to appear in the urine. That substance which has been called peptone is in all probability always one of the various albumoses of the system.—Ed.

and albumose. In concentrated urine a deposit of tyrosin occurs spontaneously in the form of delicate needles or small bundles of needles.

Owing to the destruction of hepatic parenchyma and the wide-spread degeneration of the organ, an increased excretion of nitrogen is to be expected. As the disease runs such a peculiar course, and as the termination is so rapid, no very careful metabolic studies have so far been made. Von Noorden, in one case, found the nitrogen excretion to be 10.14 gm. in twenty-four hours one day before the death of the patient, this being much more than would correspond to simple fasting. P. F. Richter found an average excretion of nitrogen of 9.8 gm. during the last three days of life, with about 3.5 gm. ingested.

[Albu has reported * observations made upon a case studied by him that went on to recovery. The nitrogen output was a great deal larger than the amount ingested, but the urea nitrogen formed from 75 % to 85 % of the total quantity. This he considers strong evidence against the formation of urea in the liver from ammonia salts.—ED.]

The character of the nitrogen compounds found in the urine is particularly changed in this disease (Frerichs, Riess and Schultzen). In advanced cases the excretion of urea is diminished, sometimes reduced to nothing. In some of the cases, especially those that ultimately recover, an abundant quantity of uric acid is excreted.

The ammonia of the urine is sometimes, though not always, increased. It is for the present impossible to determine whether this is due to the formation of sarcolactic acid, discovered by Schultzen and Riess, and the flooding of the blood with acid products of proteid catabolism, or whether the increase of ammonia is due to inefficiency of the liver. In other words, whether we are dealing with a protective process or with a perverted or inhibited function.

Leucin and tyrosin were first discovered in this disease by Frerichs, and are among the most frequent findings in the urine of cases of acute atrophy of the liver. At the same time they are not always found and are not characteristic of the disease. The largest daily quantity of tyrosin found in the urine was 1.5 gm. The xanthin bodies are increased in many cases and on certain days (Röhmann and P. F. Richter), but there is no regularity in regard to the time at which this increase occurs. The same can be said of uric acid.

Carbaminic acid has never been found, although its presence might have been postulated from the animal experiments that Naunyn has reported on extirpation of the liver in dogs.

Albumoses have at times been found; but they are not constantly present, and when present are found in small quantities only (Thomson, v. Noorden). Schultzen and Riess speak of an as yet undefined "peptone-like" body which is found in considerable quantity.

Albumin is present only in small quantities, and as compared to the massive degeneration of renal epithelium, in smaller quantities than would be expected. Sugar is never present.

Von Jaksch reports alimentary glycosuria (16 gm. excretion and 100 gm. ingestion) in a case that recovered.

Besides sarcolactic acid, other acids have been found in different cases, such as oxymandelic acid (Riess and Schultzen), that was regarded as oxyhydroparacumaric acid, and inosinic acid (Boese).

* *Deutsche med. Woch.*, April 4, 1901.

ACUTE ATROPHY OF THE LIVER.	NITROGEN.			
	In Urea.	In NH₃.	In Uric Acid.	Residue.
Rosenheim	81.1%	4.7%	14.2%	
Münzer	52.4%	37%	10.59%	
v. Noorden	71%	18%	1.2%	9.7%
				In Alloxuric Bodies.
P. F. Richter*:				
Case 1: 1st to 12th day	81.2%	8.45%	3.1%	4.6%
13th to 14th day	67.5%	13%	4.3%	6.25%
Case 2	79.6%	8.5%	—	5.5%
PHOSPHORUS-POISONING.				
A. Fraenkel	43.9%	—	—	—
A. Huber	85.6%	—	—	—
v. Noorden-Badt:				
Case 1	69.9%	7.8%	3.1%	19.2%
Case 2	67.5%	25.8%	2.6%	4.1%
Normal	84–87%	2–5%	1–3%	7–10%

This table shows in what form 100 parts of the excreted nitrogen appeared in the urine in a number of cases; it will be seen that great differences exist. We will explain below why phosphorus-poisoning is included in this table.

At first sight the apparent irregularity of the urinary findings and the inconstancy of this or that abnormal excretion in acute atrophy of the liver are astonishing to the observer. The explanation of this phenomenon, however, is readily found in the differences that exist in regard to the degree of the hepatic involvement; in addition, the other organs participate to varying degrees in disturbing normal catabolism; and, finally, the rapidity with which the disease progresses must have something to do with the character of the excretions.

In the second stage of the disease nervous symptoms are particularly conspicuous. Occasionally, in the course of one single day the temperament of the patient seems to change, restlessness, insomnia, and headache appearing, to which may be added, without any premonition whatever, serious disturbances of the sensorium, stupor combined with delirium, jactitation, rapid talking, screaming, apprehension, etc., these symptoms sometimes being so aggravated that the picture of acute mania is presented.

In about a third of the cases in adults, and in nearly every case in children, convulsions occur, appearing either as regular spasms of certain muscular groups, or as general muscular spasms, or general clonic convulsions.

The pupils are generally dilated and react poorly to light. Numerous nervous symptoms in the digestive system appear. The vomiting already mentioned is, in all probability, of central origin. Sometimes the more serious nervous disturbances are ushered in by an attack of vomiting; sometimes a feeling of thirst is complained of, or ischuria, constipation, meteorism, and perspiration are present. The breathing is snoring, and occasionally irregular.

* The average figures are calculated.

All these nervous symptoms are very inconstant both as to duration and severity. They may disappear for a time and the patient may regain consciousness (particularly after child-birth), but they generally reappear. Irritative and paralytic symptoms occur simultaneously and may be observed together.

Duration ; Prognosis.—The duration of the disease fluctuates from a few days to several months. According to the figures of Thierfelder, 50 % of all cases terminate fatally between the fifth and fourteenth day; 30 % between the third and the fifth week. Death rarely occurs before the fifth day; but it may do so in pregnant women. The second characteristic stage of the disease is, as a rule, of short duration, lasting from one and a half to three days. It rarely lasts longer than a week. In the protracted cases the cerebral symptoms are less violent and all irritative symptoms are less severe. The second stage is of long duration in those cases that run a favorable course.

Certain cases that run a course of many week or months are in truth originally acute, and are only slow in recovering; others, again, run what must be called a subacute course. Leube and Wirsing report such a case (minimum size of the liver at the end of the eighth week, increase in size after three weeks, recovery after eight months).

The prognosis of acute atrophy of the liver is in the great majority of cases fatal, and is more unfavorable the sooner after the onset of the disease cerebral symptoms appear. In the case of pregnant women the prognosis is particularly unfavorable, the case being here complicated by the shock and the hemorrhage of child-birth.

In former days the possibility of recovery from acute atrophy of the liver was denied, and all cases that did recover were considered diagnostic errors. There is no reason why the damage should not be arrested prior to the complete destruction of the liver. We are justified in entertaining this view because we know that even in those cases that terminate fatally regenerative changes can be observed during the first and second week. [We have already mentioned the fact that Albu has recently reported a case * which resulted in recovery. The patient was a man, thirty-six years old. Three weeks before his illness he had experienced great emotional excitement, followed by persistent icterus. He became stupid, had fever, but no tenderness or pain. The liver dulness was only two finger's-breadths in width, and later, as delirium came on, the dulness disappeared altogether. Large amounts of leucin and tyrosin were obtained from the urine. Gradual improvement, with gradual broadening of the area of liver dulness, occurred, until absolute recovery took place. Dobie † has also reported a case of recovery.—ED.] Anatomic studies teach us this, as do also experimental studies carried on by Ponfick for the purpose of elucidating this very subject. In a case of Marchand's examined postmortem, regeneration had occurred in the form of nodular hyperplasia. In the case of Bauer the patient died from miliary tuberculosis three months after her attack of acute atrophy, and the presence of regenerative changes in the liver could be verified at the autopsy. In addition to these instances, Wirsing has collated 16 older cases from the literature, and of late years Hedderich, Senator, and von Jaksch have described other cases. [Ibrahim's case, previously mentioned as having shown

* *Deutsche med. Woch.*, April 4, 1901.
† *Brit. Med. Jour.*, Nov. 12, 1898.

marked regenerative attempts, died between the tenth and eleventh weeks after the onset.—ED.]

It is to be expected that the clinical picture and the course of those cases that recover are different in many respects from cases that terminate fatally; and, while it is true that some of the older cases must be considered doubtful from a diagnostic point of view, we are still justified in assuming that in those instances where the liver decreased in size and remained small for a long time, and where tyrosin and leucin were found in the urine (Wirsing, Senator), the diagnosis was established with sufficient certainty.

The following case, described by E. Wagner, is peculiar both in regard to symptoms and course and in regard to the anatomic findings. The author calls it a case of acute red atrophy of the liver. A young girl of twenty-one had for four weeks vague general symptoms, for a week violent abdominal pain, and after a few days ascites. There was no icterus or albuminuria. There was edema of the lower half of the body. She died quietly three weeks after the appearance of ascites. The liver was somewhat smaller than normal (1500 gm.), tough and vascular. On the surface of the organ there were adhesions and a number of nodules of the size of a pea. The portal vein was thickened from the hilus to the smallest peripheral branches The cut surface of the organ showed irregular whitish streaks. The acini were reddish-brown, smaller than normal, and contained liver-cells in their outer third or fourth, these being somewhat more granular than normal. In the central portions of the acini nothing was present but connective tissue and red blood-corpuscles that were found lying within the columns of degenerated liver-cells. Interlobular connective tissue is present only in the vicinity of the portal branches, and somewhat increased in these localities. Wagner does not favor the diagnosis of pylephlebitis with secondary atrophy of the liver, but considers the latter as the primary condition. At all events, the presence of ascites points to a considerable obstruction to the flow of blood through the portal capillaries.

Nature.—Acute atrophy of the liver occupies a peculiar position among the diseases of this organ from the rapidity of its development and the degree of change present in typical cases. The position of this disease is anomalous not only for the liver but for every other organ of the body from a general pathologico-anatomic point of view. It is variously considered as a peculiar form of acute diffuse inflammation that runs a particularly rapid course, or, again, as a retrogressive form of metamorphosis, or as a wide-spread necrosis of the cellular elements of the liver-cells. If the anatomic findings alone are considered, the initial stages of acute atrophy are most similar to parenchymatous swelling and inflammation of the liver (Busse, for example, describes a case of the disease with enlargement of the organ). Interstitial proliferation, it is true, is not a constant finding, but is in many cases present at an early stage of the disease.

The nature of the noxious agent and the manner and the rapidity with which it exercises its effect on the liver may account for the differences in the reaction. We have analogous conditions elsewhere, and it is readily understood why the acute effect of a large quantity of the poison, whatever it may be, will cause a complete destruction of the glandular parenchyma before reactive processes can develop. We will include these forms of the disease under the general heading of inflammation in the broader sense, and will refrain from looking for anything else in the whole process than an inflammation which differs from the ordinary forms of inflammation only in a quantitative sense.

How can we explain the wide-spread changes seen in other organs, such as the heart, the kidneys, etc.? Are they the result of the disease of the liver, or are they caused by the effect of the same noxious agent that affects the liver? I am inclined to the latter belief, for the reason that changes in the other organs are sometimes seen when the disease of the liver is very little developed. The lesions in the other organs closely resemble those seen in acute phosphorus-poisoning and in so-called "acute fatty degeneration." The latter disease is anatomically identical with phosphorus-poisoning and is seen sometimes after mushroom-poisoning (by *Amanita phalloïdes,* Schärer-Sahli), and frequently originates from unknown causes. All these conditions cause the fatty clouding and the parenchymatous degeneration of numerous glandular and muscular cells in common, as well as fatty infiltration of many of the epithelial cells and of the capillaries and a hemorrhagic tendency. At the same time, it is true, certain differences can be found. In poisoning and in "acute fatty degeneration," the fatty degeneration and the hemorrhages are in general more wide-spread, the accumulation of fat in the liver, in particular, sometimes assuming such dimensions that the organ swells greatly; and we must assume that an infiltration of fat from other parts of the body occurs (compare the experiments of Rosenfeld on page 410). Severe cases of acute phosphorus-poisoning die at this early stage of the disease. At this time the liver is enlarged and the general disease-picture is in some respects different from that of acute atrophy of the liver, the same disorders of metabolism not being found and some of the other symptoms not being identical. On the other hand, there are certain cases on record that finally lead to the genuine clinical and anatomic picture of acute atrophy of the liver. Hedderich has collated 33 such cases. In the majority of these cases atrophy began at the beginning of the second week, sometimes earlier; in three of the cases it was present from the very beginning of the disease; in only one-half of the cases was atrophy preceded by enlargement of the liver lasting about one week. Death occurred in the second week, generally within twenty-four hours after the beginning of atrophic changes. In three cases recovery from phosphorus-atrophy of the liver ensued.

These facts teach us that the symptoms and the anatomic changes, particularly in the case of the liver, may vary greatly even in so simple a form of intoxication as that by phosphorus. The factors that determine these differences are, in the first place, the absolute quantity of poison taken, then the rapidity with which it is absorbed, and finally the formation or non-formation of certain compounds of phosphorus in the intestine. Other factors to be considered are the possibility of the absorption of other substances at the same time and the general condition of the liver and of the system at the time of the poisoning.

We can draw certain conclusions from these considerations in regard to acute atrophy of the liver. First, a purely chemical poison (alone or aided by certain concomitant factors) can produce acute atrophy of the liver; and this poison does not act on the liver alone, but also affects other organs, so that the general disease-picture of acute atrophy of the liver cannot be deduced from the hepatic changes alone, but must be evolved from the lesions known to exist in other organs as well. It appears that certain other poisons, such as chloroform, alcohol, and chloral, may occasionally act in the same manner as phosphorus, since all of these can lead to parenchymatous hepatitis with acute degeneration. As acute atrophy of the liver is frequently ushered in by certain gastro-intestinal disturbances, we are possibly justified in assuming that there may at times be generated in the intestine certain organic poisons which exercise on the liver parenchyma an effect similar to that produced by the poisons enumerated above. We must think in particular of bacterial toxins and of ptomains, and possibly, also, of the higher derivatives of the albumin ingested, such as the albumoses, some of which are known to possess highly toxic properties.

In the second place, the relationship between phosphorus-poisoning and acute atrophy of the liver throws some light on those cases of acute fatty degeneration that have been seen to follow mushroom-poisoning or that were caused by unknown agencies. The same noxious principles may cause these cases; and possibly several poisons may act at the same time and cause a more intense form of poisoning (?), so that they produce acute swelling of the liver and infiltration of the organ with fat to such a degree that death ensues very soon. In less intense forms of poisoning, on the other hand, or owing to other causes, the primary swelling of the liver is not produced, and, as is sometimes seen in the case of phosphorus, atrophy alone is present from the very beginning.

From all that we know in regard to acute atrophy of the liver we can conclude that we are not dealing with a uniform clinical entity, but that a variety of noxious agencies may affect the liver and at the same time some of the other organs as well. This factor and the varying intensity of the poisoning explain the different forms of the disease and the different ana-atomic findings. All the forms have in common the great disturbance in general health naturally following in the path of wide-spread destruction of liver parenchyma, and present a most pronounced picture of so-called "hepatargy" (see page 458) and of the autointoxication that is the result of this perversion. In view of the manifold functions of the liver in general metabolism, these changes are necessarily varied in quality and in severity, and we can readily understand why the urinary constituents are different from those excreted normally both in quantity and character, and also that they show certain peculiarities not constant and not typical of the disease. This is also due to the fact that the number of liver-cells that have perished may vary, and that, in addition, the function of the surviving cells may be impaired in different ways. In other words, we cannot draw any conclusions in regard to the nature of the functional disturbances that existed during life from the size of the organ after death. In addition, the lesions of the heart and the kidneys necessarily lead to certain disturbances of the circulation and of the excretion of urine, so that the latter is no index alone of purely metabolic perversions within the organism, for the reason that the excretion of some of the most strikingly abnormal products may be prevented. As an example of this, the discovery of tyrosin in the blood (Schultzen and Riess), the liver, and the retina may be mentioned.

The most conspicuous disturbances are the perversions in nitrogen metabolism, the decreased excretion of urea, the increased excretion of ammonia, and the appearance in the urine of such intermediary bodies as leucin and tyrosin. The increased excretion of nitrogen can be explained from the death of so many liver-cells, and at the same time the increased catabolism of the nuclei of these cells may explain the increase of uric acid and of the alloxuric bodies. Disturbances in carbohydrate metabolism are, as a rule, not perceptible, because the amount of food ingested is so much reduced.

The absence of the "detoxicating" function of the liver may also

41

become apparent in acute atrophy, so that ptomains formed in the intestine are allowed to enter the general circulation and there exercise their deleterious effects.

As in other toxic conditions (uremia, diabetes), the general symptoms of intoxication are not constant, and vary according to the nature and the composition of the complicated poisons concerned.

As the etiology of acute atrophy was so obscure and the symptoms of the disease are so violent, it can be readily understood why the disease was considered an infection, particularly as at the time of its discovery the trend of medical thought was in that direction. We have learned, however, from our discussion that it is to be considered an *intoxication*, in which chemical damage to the liver as well as other organs is the essential feature. The most frequent poison appears to consist of certain substances that are formed within the intestinal canal and are absorbed and act on the liver; in other words, we are dealing with a form of bacterial dyspepsia or of intestinal autointoxication. In cases in which acute atrophy of the liver follows osteomyelitis, erysipelas, or some other infectious disease, the bacterial toxins possibly are formed in some other organ and are carried to the liver by the blood.

In a minority of the cases the liver may be damaged by the local action of certain bacteria. The latter may enter the liver either in the blood or through the bile-passages. The cases of Babes, Ströbe, and v. Kahlden furnish examples of the former kind. Here masses of streptococci or of Bacterium coli were found in the capillaries of the portal vein, so that the suspicion is justified that these organisms produced their toxins in these localities and acted deleteriously on the neighboring hepatic cells.

The assumption that bacteria can invade the liver through the bile-passages is supported by our knowledge of certain cases of infectious icterus in which this has been known to occur. This is the most probable explanation, particularly of those forms of acute atrophy of the liver that begin with catarrhal icterus. The anatomic findings in many of the cases, the irregular distribution of the different foci throughout the organ, the variety in the changes of the parenchyma seen in different localities (resembling bronchopneumonia), all point to the bile-passages as the point of entrance.

Finally, I would like to call attention to another possibility that has so far never been mentioned. When we consider that the ducts of the liver and of the pancreas enter the intestine through a common opening, it might well be possible, in case this opening becomes occluded, for some of the pancreatic secretion to enter the liver and there to digest the liver-cells; this would be particularly the case in those parts of the organ where trypsin penetrates as far as the capillaries. Whether this hypothesis is a correct one can be determined only by experiments performed in this direction; as a single observer will rarely have occasion to study clinically many cases of this character, I will content myself with formulating this hypothesis. [This theory receives some support from the analogous result upon the pancreas from the entrance of bile into the duct of Wirsung as discovered by Opie. Our views concerning the nature of acute yellow atrophy, as well as of phosphorus-poisoning, must be largely influenced by the recent work on autolysis of the liver. Salkowski's original work upon the latter question has lately been repeatedly confirmed, and was very strikingly extended by M. Jacoby,[*] who demonstrated very definitely

[*] *Zeitsch. f. physiol. Chemie*, Bd. xxx.

that the liver after death, under aseptic conditions, shows very marked proteolytic digestive action. He also showed that in acute phosphorus-poisoning this proteolysis is very largely increased. He considers that this definitely confirms the idea that phosphorus-poisoning is closely related to ferment action, and is, indeed, apparently in large part, really increased ferment action; although what the actual cause of the increase is cannot as yet be definitely stated.

A. E. Taylor * has recently studied elaborately a case of acute yellow atrophy from this standpoint. He found large amounts of leucin and asparaginic acid in the liver, but, strangely enough, hexon bases were apparently absent. Still it has become increasingly probable that the chief process in acute yellow atrophy may be a pathologically active and rapid autodigestion, although if this be true it cannot yet be stated what the cause of the increase in the autolytic process in the liver is due to. It seems likely that it is set in motion at times by bacterial, at times by enterogenous or other metabolic toxic substances.—Ed.]

A review of all the factors enumerated leads us to the conclusion that acute atrophy of the liver may not only be due to a great variety of causes, but that the pathologic processes that ultimately lead to atrophy may be different in themselves. This will also explain why the course of the disease may be so varying and still lead to the same final condition.

We are stimulated, therefore, particularly in those cases that recover, to direct our attention, for the sake of study, to those diseases from which it originated or to which it is related. Among these may be named: parenchymatous hepatitis, catarrhal icterus, particularly those cases that may be classified separately as infectious icterus, and, finally, those infectious diseases that are accompanied by parenchymatous changes in the liver and serious cerebral disturbances or icterus. It is probable that in many of these diseases cases will be found in which the liver shows changes similar to those found in acute atrophy, and that would have led to the development of this disease had the patient lived longer. The development of atrophy occurs only in the great minority of cases—namely, in those cases where the disturbance of the hepatic function continues for a long time or where certain concomitant features are apparent. In the majority of cases, however, death occurs before the development of atrophy, or before the damaged parenchyma undergoes regeneration. It is possible that even under these circumstances some of the liver-cells perish, but the number of cells that are destroyed is not great enough to cause a decrease in the size of the organ or to cause intoxication. It is probable that the surviving cells engage in compensatory activity. At the same time there are to be noticed in all the conditions enumerated a number of cases which ultimately run a favorable course, but which for a time develop such serious symptoms that they resemble the syndrome of acute atrophy of the liver. These are probably abortive cases.

We will attempt to explain the symptoms and the course of the disease by the theoretic views developed. It seems hardly probable that the serious anatomic changes seen postmortem and the atrophic process leading to them began only when symptoms of the disease assumed so grave a character. Particularly in those cases that run a less acute course, and in which there is a prodromal stage of from eight to fourteen days, atrophy unquestionably must have begun during this time. At

* *Zeitsch. f. physiol. Chemie.* Bd. xxxiv.

this period, however, compensation was sufficiently active to prevent the most serious symptoms, as compensation does not fail until atrophy and disturbance of function have reached a certain degree. At this time the severe symptoms appear so suddenly that they seem to be caused by some acutely acting agency; whereas in reality they have been preparing for a long time. The conditions observed here are the same as in other forms of autointoxication, such as uremia and diabetic coma; in all of which it is the last drop that causes the cup to overflow.

The decrease in the size of the liver that appears at the time of the development of cerebral symptoms is usually explained by the assumption that at this time a large portion of the degenerated parenchyma is absorbed. Hirschberg assumes that a decrease in the quantity of blood flowing into the liver may also be in part responsible for the decrease in size, and that the liver looks so very small because after death the volume of blood is still less.

Icterus is probably caused in several different ways in this condition. In the beginning of the disease, when the stools are clay-colored, we must assume that some occlusion of the larger bile-passages exists. In the atrophic stage of the disease we believe that the interlobular passages are occluded by desquamated epithelial cells or that the passages are collapsed or twisted in the same manner as the intralobular channels. This is due to a destruction of parenchyma that robs them of support and direction. The central cells of the lobules are better preserved and still contain bile-pigment, and this has been adduced as an argument in favor of the above explanation. It is true that the larger bile-passages contain a colorless fluid devoid of all pigment; at the same time, it is possible that diapedesis of bile (Minkowski) occurs—in other words, that the damaged liver-cells allow the bile to flow both into the bile-ducts and into the blood-channels. This is a theory which has, of course, not been proved.

The old theories that explained the cerebral symptoms on the ground of inanition or the absorption of bile-products possess historic interest only. There can be no doubt that these symptoms are the result of intoxication by products of perverted metabolism; but no one, as is the case in uremia, has so far succeeded in demonstrating any one substance that can be made accountable for these symptoms. The intoxication following inhibition of the hepatic function must be considered as a very complicated one, and the toxic agent is a mixture of poisons of varying composition.

It is impossible to decide whether leucin and tyrosin belong to these toxic substances. Panum * and Billroth † injected large quantities of these bodies into the blood of certain animals without producing any damage and without the appearance of nervous symptoms. At the same time, this does not exclude the possibility that in acute atrophy of the liver these substances exercise a deleterious effect, for the reason that in normal animals they are possibly rendered harmless by the liver, whereas in the disease under discussion the liver has lost this power. The same reasoning applies to sarcolactic acid and other bodies, which the liver can no longer oxidize.

As tyrosin is one of the aromatic group, and as these bodies are otherwise produced only by bacteria, the suspicion has been created that the tyrosin found in acute atrophy owes its origin to the same source. The statement has been made that it is generated either by bacteria in the liver or by putrefactive organisms in the intestine. It has, however, never been demonstrated that this is the only source of

* Schmidt's "Jahrbücher der gesammten Medicin," 1858, vol. ci, p. 215.
† Langenbeck's "Archiv," vol. vi, p. 396.

tyrosin in the body, and it is not excluded that metabolic processes play an important rôle in its formation.

The hemorrhages in this disease, as in other similar conditions, can best be explained from the general disturbance of nutrition. It is possible that fatty degeneration of the vessel-walls has some influence. In the intestinal area a possible adjuvant is stasis in the portal system due to collapse of intrahepatic capillaries. The swelling of the spleen can be explained on the same basis.

Diagnosis.—As acute atrophy of the liver is relatively rare in those diseases in which it could occur, it would be a very interesting and useful task to examine all the cases in which this complication threatens as soon as possible. Unfortunately this is not always possible; at the same time, particularly severe disturbances of the general health or the occurrence of certain unusual symptoms should arouse our suspicion as to the possibility of atrophy. Possibly quantitative analyses of the urine would enable us to detect the condition in its prodromal stages. In a practical sense, the first available symptoms are the nervous disorders, which sometimes are mild and hardly noticeable, while in other cases they appear so rapidly as to take us by surprise.

The decrease in the size of the liver is usually not noticed until the following day, rarely before. It may be well to mention again that tympanites or coils of intestine situated between the liver and the abdominal wall may simulate a decrease in the size of the organ, and that, on the other hand, atrophy may not be discovered in case adhesions fix the liver in certain positions or if the organ is enlarged or very resistant from the presence of other older disease, such as cirrhosis.

The determination of perversions of metabolism by urinalysis is of great diagnostic importance. The presence of tyrosin and leucin is easy to discover because these bodies are either precipitated spontaneously or crystallize as soon as the urine is concentrated. On the other hand, it is true that these bodies are not always found in acute atrophy, and that, as a rule, they do not appear until late in the disease.

Typical cases of atrophy can usually be diagnosed as soon as the symptoms of the second stage appear; but the diagnosis may be difficult if the cases are seen for the first time after the patient has relapsed into stupor, unless a history of the case can be elicited, or if the patient is a sufferer from some chronic disease of the liver.

Severe cerebral symptoms as well as icterus may be due to a variety of causes. If the two appear together there is created a very striking picture to which the term *icterus gravis* has been applied. This name explains nothing whatever; but it has a certain value as a descriptive term because there are, in fact, a number of cases whose course, origin, and pathologic anatomy remain unexplainable. The term, at the same time, includes a great variety of known pathologic conditions (sepsis, puerperal fever, pneumonia, yellow fever, recurrent fever, Griesinger's bilious typhoid, peritonitis, chronic alcoholism), which can appear as icterus gravis in the same manner as in the case of icterus infectiosus, phosphorus-poisoning, or acute atrophy of the liver. Since we have learned to isolate the last-named disease from this group, it is not practicable to follow the example of Dupré and to reserve the name icterus gravis for this condition alone.

Mossé distinguishes: (1) Ictère typhoide ou grave primitif (ictère grave proper); (2) ictères graves secondaires (insuffisance hepatique), (3) ictères aggravés. This division, captivating as it may seem on first sight, is neither correct nor practical, for many cases of acute atrophy would have to be ranked with the cases of ictère aggravés of the third category, and, besides, many of the cases that Mossé designates as ictères graves primitifs would certainly not be cases of acute atrophy.

Boix formulates the following division, not limiting icterus gravis to acute atrophy, but extending it to other diseases:

		TEMPERATURE.
Specific and primary	{ Phosphorus	Subnormal.
	{ Yellow fever	Febrile.
Non-specific and always secondary	/ Due to staphylococcus \	
	" streptococcus	
	" pneumococcus }	Febrile.
	" proteus, etc. /	
	" Bacillus coli	Subnormal.

It may be a difficult matter to differentiate acute atrophy of the liver from some of the other conditions enumerated above; but, as a rule, it can be done. Symptoms in favor of the diagnosis of acute atrophy are the intensity of the icterus, the small size of the hepatic dulness, the absence of fever in the majority of cases, and the serious cerebral symptoms that are changeable, and in which symptoms of irritation alternate with symptoms of paralysis, and, further, the appearance of leucin and tyrosin in the urine. Although, as we have stated, phosphorus-poisoning may ultimately lead to acute atrophy of the liver, the differential diagnosis between the two conditions will sometimes have to be made in cases that are acutely seized and are seen for the first time after severe icterus has developed. This is particularly necessary if no definite information in regard to the swallowing of phosphorus can be obtained. For these cases the following points in the differential diagnosis may be given. As in the case of many other diseases, they are not altogether reliable in cases that run an atypical course.

ACUTE ATROPHY OF THE LIVER.	ACUTE PHOSPHORUS-POISONING.
Preceded by an extended period of illness (one to two weeks) and icterus.	Gastritis immediately after poisoning, icterus on the third day following a pause of two days.
Icterus as a rule more intense and older.	Icterus recent, less dark.
Liver sensitive, reduced in size.	Liver sensitive after the beginning of the third day and enlarged.
Cerebral symptoms appear suddenly (combination of excitement and depression), appearing one or two days before the end.	Cerebral symptoms corresponding to general prostration, more of a depressive type, appearing toward the end.
In the urine:	In the urine:
Oxymandelic acid.	Much sarcolactic acid.
Leucin.	
Much tyrosin.	

(In both, peptone, sarcolactic acid, tyrosin.)

Hemorrhages smaller, fewer.	Hemorrhages large, wide-spread.
Duration several weeks.	Duration shorter, less than a week

Treatment.—In the prodromal stage of the disease something may possibly be expected from treatment. As danger of infection of the bile-passages and of "intestinal mycosis" is present in every case of catarrhal icterus, every such case is threatened with acute atrophy of the liver. This should be remembered whenever threatening symptoms or abnormal signs of any kind develop in the course of icterus, particularly if the disease is present in women and, above all, in pregnant women. In cases of this sort the patient should not be allowed to be out of bed, the diet should be very plain and moderate, and care should be taken that the bowels are regularly evacuated. Asepsis of the intestinal tract is a great desideratum, and may be attempted by the administration of small doses of calomel, bismuth, salol, naphthalin, etc., frequently repeated. At the same time, enemata and laxatives should be administered from time to time to insure evacuation. The latter remedies cause increased diuresis, and special drugs should be given to encourage copious urination, as the poisons are to a great extent removed from the body by this channel.

In the second stage the same principles hold good, and in those cases that have terminated favorably it appears that a good share in this happy result must be attributed to the administration of purges, notably calomel. In this stage the treatment must be essentially symptomatic. For the restlessness, bromid of sodium, lukewarm baths (narcotics are not so good); for the vomiting, ice pills, cocain, extract of nux vomica, small doses of morphin; for coma and collapse, stimulants.

In cases where no fluid is absorbed from the stomach and the rectum, subcutaneous infusions of physiologic salt solution should be attempted.

Where phosphorus-poisoning cannot be altogether excluded, drastic purges and antidotal treatment with old oil of turpentine are indicated. Traces of phosphorus, according to my own observation, may still be present in the intestine on the fourth day of the poisoning.

LITERATURE.

Babes: "Ueber die durch Streptococceninvasion bedingte acute Lebererkrankung," "Virchow's Archiv," vol. cxxxvi, p. 1.

Bamberger: Loc. cit., p. 527.

Bauer (recovered case): "Verhandlungen des Congresses für innere Medicin," 1893, p. 185.

Bloedau: "Ueber acute gelbe Leberatrophie," Dissertation, Würzburg, 1887.

Boix, E.: "Nature et pathogénie de l'ictère grave," "Archives générales de médecine," 1896, ii, p. 77, 202 (literature).

Buss: "Beginnende acute Leberatrophie," "Berliner klin. Wochenschr.," 1889, p. 975.

Favre und Pfyffer: "Weitere Mittheilungen über die Genese der acuten gelben Leberatrophie," "Virchow's Archiv," vol. cxxxix, p. 189.

Frerichs: Loc. cit., i, p. 204.

Gabbi: "Sperimentale," 1892, iii, p. 232.

Gerhardt, C.: "Verkleinerung der Leber bei gleichbleibender Dämpfung," "Zeitschr. für klin. Medicin," 1892, vol. xxi, p. 374.

Hanot: "Contribution à la pathogénie de l'ictère grave," "Bericht des VIII. internationalen Congresses für Hygiene in Budapest," 1894, vol. ii, p. 623.

— "De l'ictère grave hypothermique," "Archives générales de médecine," August, 1893.

v. Haren-Noman: "Ein Fall von acuter Leberatrophie," "Virchow's Archiv," 1883, vol. xci, p. 334.

Hirschberg: "Drei Fälle von acuter gelber Leberatrophie," Dissertation, Dorpat, 1886.

v. Jaksch (recovered case): "Alimentary Glycosuria," "Prager med. Wochenschr.," May, 1895.

v. Kahlden: "Ueber acute parenchymatöse Leberatrophie und Lebercirrhose," "Münchener med. Wochenschr.," 1897, No. 40.

Kahler: "Prager med. Wochenschr," 1885, Nos. 22 and 23.

Klebs: "Handbuch der pathologischen Anatomie," i, p. 417.

Lewitsky und Brodowsky: "Ein Fall von acuter Leberatrophie," "Virchow's Archiv," 1877, vol. lxx, p. 421.

Litten: "Augenveränderungen bei acuter Leberatrophie," "Zeitschr. für klin. Medicin," 1882, vol. v, p. 58.

Marchand, F.: " Ueber Ausgang der acuten Leberatrophie in multiple knotige Hyperplasie," " Ziegler's Beiträge," 1895, vol. xvii, p. 206.
Meder, E.: " Ueber acute Leberatrophie mit besonderer Berücksichtigung der Regeneration" (literature), " Ziegler's Beiträge," 1895. vol. xvii, p. 143.
Nepveu et Bourdillon: " Bactérie dans l'ictère grave," " Gazette méd. de Paris," 1892, No. 41.
v. Noorden: " Pathologie des Stoffwechsels," p. 290.
Perls: " Zur Unterscheidung zwischen Fettinfiltration und fettiger Degeneration," " Centralblatt für die med. Wissenschaft," 1873, No. 51; " Allgemeine Pathologie," 1877, p. 171.
Phedran and Macallum: " The Lancet," February, 1894.
Podwyssotzky: " Petersburger Wochenschr.," 1888; " Centralblatt für die med. Wissenschaft," 1889, p. 173.
Ranglaret et Mahen: " Recherches sur un microbe nouveau de l'ictère grave," " Gazette hebdomad.," 1893, No. 32
Richter, P. F.: " Stoffwechseluntersuchungen bei acuter Leberatrophie," " Berliner klin. Wochenschr.," 1896, p. 453.
Riess: " Eulenburg's encyklopädische Jahrbücher," 1897, i, 177.
— " Charité-Annalen," 1864, vol. xii, p. 141.
Rosenheim: " Zeitschr. für klin. Medicin," 1889, vol. xv, p. 441.
Schultzen, O., und Riess, L.: " Acute Phosphorvergiftung und acute Leberatrophie," " Charité-Annalen," 1869, vol. xv.
v. Starck: " Deutsches Archiv für klin. Medicin," 1884, vol. xxxv, p. 481.
Stroebe: " Zur Kenntniss der acuten Leberatrophie mit besonderer Berücksichtigung der Spatstadien," " Ziegler's Beitrage," vol. xxi, p. 379.
Thierfelder: Loc. cit., p. 215.
Wagner, E.: " Die acute rothe Atrophie der Leber," " Deutsches Archiv für klin. Medicin," 1884, vol. xxxiv, p. 524.
Wirsing, E.: " Acute parenchymatöse Leberatrophie mit günstigem Ausgang," Dissertation, Würzburg, 1892. " Verhandlungen der physikalisch-med. Gesellschaft zu Würzburg," 1892, vol. xxvi.
Zenker: " Zur pathologischen Anatomie der acuten Leberatrophie," " Deutsches Archiv für klin. Medicin," 1872, vol. x, p. 167.
        Illustrations in the works of Zenker, Riess, Marchand.

CASES IN CHILDHOOD.

Ashby: " British Med. Journal," November, 1882.
Aufrecht: " Acute Leberatrophie bei Sclerema neonatorum," " Centralblatt für innere Medicin," 1896, No. 11.
Cavafy: " The Lancet," July 17, 1897.
Lanz: " Wiener klin. Wochenschr.," 1896, No. 39.
Merkel, Fr.: " Münchener med. Wochenschr.," 1894, p. 89.
Schmidt, R.: " Ein Fall von acuter parenchymatöser Leberatrophie," etc. (collection of 16 cases of new-born up to 10 years), Dissertation, Kiel, 1897.

FOLLOWING SYPHILIS.

Engel-Reimers: " Jahrbücher der Hamburger Krankenhäuser," 1889, i (three cases). " Monatshefte für Dermatologie," 1892, vol. xv, p. 476.
Goldscheider und Moxter: " Fortschritte der Medecin," 1897, vol. xv, Nos. 14 and 15.
Naunyn, Fleischhauer: " Congress für innere Medicin," 1893.
Neumann: " Syphilis," Nothnagel's Encylcopedia, vol. xxiii, p. 411 (literature list pp. 412 and 413, Remarks).
Senator: " Congress für innere Medicin," 1893, p. 180 (two cases).
— " Charité-Annalen," 1893, p. 322.
Talamon: " Médecine moderne," February, 1897; " Centralblatt für Dermatologie," i, p. 25.

AS TO VARIOUS OTHER DISEASES.

Bandler, V.: " Ueber den Einfluss der Chloroform- und Aethernarkose auf die Leber," " Mittheilungen aus den Grenzgebieten der Medicin und Chirurgie," 1896, i, p. 303.
Cahn: " Acute Leberatrophie nach Diphtherie des Magens," " Deutsches Archiv für klin. Medicin," 1884, vol. xxxiv, p. 113.
Dinckler, M.: " Ueber Bindegewebs- und Gallengangsneubildung in der Leber bei

chronischer Phosphorvergiftung und acuter Leberatrophie," Dissertation, Halle, 1887.

Dörfler: "Acute Leberatrophie nach Typhus," "Münchener med. Wochenschr.," 1889, p. 878.

Hecker: "Acute Leberatrophie nach Pilzvergiftung," "Monatsschr. für Geburtskunde," vol. xxi, p. 210.

Hedderich: "Acute Leberatrophie bei Phosphorvergiftung" (literature), "Münchener med. Wochenschr.," 1895, p. 93.

Hüntemann: "Acute Leberatrophie nach Erysipel," Dissertation, Würzburg, 1882.

Schärer und Sahli: "Vergiftung mit Amanita phalloides," "Correspondenzblatt für Schweizer Aerzte," 1885, No. 19, p. 464.

Wolf: "Acute Leberatrophie nach Wurstvergiftung," "Memorabilien," 1876, No. 3; Virchow-Hirsch's "Jahresbericht," ii, 216.

ACUTE INTERSTITIAL HEPATITIS.

(Quincke.)

Small-celled infiltration and proliferation of connective tissue have at different times been described as occurring in parenchymatous hepatitis and in acute atrophy of the liver (Riess and others).* This condition is found particularly in those cases that are examined postmortem after the disease had lasted for a long time; and also in cases of phosphorus-poisoning.

Sometimes the hyperplasia of connective tissue is more conspicuous than the parenchymatous changes, or the latter may be completely absent. Such cases have been called "acute cirrhosis," the condition being called acute from the appearance of the new tissue and the short duration of the pathologic process. Both these criteria are, however, very uncertain and misleading; we shall see, for instance, in the case of chronic hepatitis, that a condition of this kind may be present in a latent form for a long time and cause no symptoms until the disease has advanced to a complicated stage. Many of the cases with an acute course are unquestionably old cases of interstitial hepatitis (ordinary cirrhoses) that have become complicated by fresh proliferation of connective tissue with an increase of the cellular elements and cell infiltration, or by parenchymatous changes that finally lead to acute atrophy.

An example of the former combination is a case reported by Eichhorst, that terminated fatally within two weeks; of the latter are the cases reported by Clarke † and Richter.‡

In a few cases it is possible, however, that we are dealing with a true acute interstitial proliferation leading, secondarily, to atrophy of hepatic cells (Obrzut) or appearing simultaneously with parenchymatous changes (Debove, Polqèure, Blocq, and Gillet).

It is not possible to estimate the duration of the process from the anatomic findings. It is true that we know, from the experiments of Hochhaus with cold applications, that small-celled infiltration may occur in the course of from two to three days, but at the same time other observations teach us that this condition may persist for months without leading to further changes.

Since in chronic cirrhosis recent increase of connective tissue is found principally in the interstitial tissues between the lobules, or even in the interior of these parts, we cannot attach any particular significance to the appearance of the one or the other form of distribution.

* See Meder's arrangement. p. 182.   † *British Med. Journal*, 1890, i, p. 1000.
‡ Richter, "Schmidt's Jahrbücher," 1858, vol. xcviii, p. 181.

The same causes are given for interstitial hepatitis as for the parenchymatous forms—chemical irritants coming from food-stuffs and condiments, intestinal ptomains, and bacterial toxins. Whenever bacteria lodge in the capillaries of the portal vein, small-celled infiltration may take place around them. This is particularly so in the case of tubercle bacilli, in which case so many single foci develop that an increase in the size of the liver may be brought about. To a slighter degree staphylococci, typhoid bacilli, and the malarial parasite can exercise the same effect. All these germs, as well as syphilis, may cause acute proliferations, which, however, persist for a long time.

In one case reported by Dreschfeld interstitial proliferation was complicated by thrombosis of small branches of the portal vein with hemorrhagic infarcts.

Symptoms.—The symptoms of acute interstitial hepatitis resemble those of the parenchymatous form and of acute atrophy. Possibly icterus in these cases is a little more pronounced in the beginning, and the onset and the course are not so acute. The duration of the disease is several weeks, occasionally several months. One group of the cases (malarial and syphilitic) becomes chronic and leads to the ordinary picture of cirrhosis. Those cases in which a considerable degree of degeneration of liver-cells occurs (Blocq and Gillet) have been called *cirrhoses graisseuses;* but other authors have used this designation for a disease of altogether different origin (compare page 732).

In typical cases the picture of parenchymatous and of interstitial hepatitis is widely different; there are, however, a number of cases that constitute intermediary forms in which the sequence of events, and consequently the classification, becomes doubtful. The same statements apply to these diseases of the liver as to the same conditions in the kidney. In the latter organ the attempt to distinguish strictly between interstitial and parenchymatous nephritis, as we know, fails in many instances. The differentiation of the clinical picture of these diseases in both the liver and the kidneys is still more difficult. This cannot surprise us when we remember how similar are the primary causes of the two diseases in the case of both organs. The symptoms, therefore, are exceedingly similar, with this distinction—that the course of those cases where interstitial changes predominate is less violent.

Blocq et Gillet: "Des cirrhoses graisseuses considérées comme hépatites infectieuses," "Archives générales de médecine," 1888, ii, pp. 60 and 181.
Carrington: "Transactions of the Patholog. Society," 1885, vol. xxxvi, pp. 221–224; "Jahresbericht," ii, p. 201.
Debove: "De la cirrhose aiguë du foie," "Gazette hebdomad.," 1887, No. 30; "Jahresbericht," ii, p 278.
Dock: "American Journal of the Med. Sciences," April, 1894.
Dreschfeld: "Ueber eine seltene Form von Hepatitis interstitialis mit hämorrhagischen Infarcten," "Verhandlungen des X. internationalen Congresses," 1890; "Berichte," 1891, ii, p. 195.
Eichhorst: "Ueber acute Lebercirrhose," "Virchow's Archiv," 1897, vol. cxlviii, p. 339.
Gastou: "Le foie infectieux" (illustrated), literature, Thèse de Paris, 1893.
Obrzut: "Chronische gelbe Leberatrophie oder acute Cirrhose?" "Wiener med. Jahrbücher," 1886, New Series, i, p. 463.
Polguère: "Cas d'hépatite graisseuse primitive," "Gazette méd. de Paris," 1887; "Jahresbericht," ii, p. 278.

ABSCESS OF THE LIVER.

(Hoppe-Seyler.)

ETIOLOGY.

The chief cause of abscess of the liver is the entrance of pus-forming micro-organisms (bacteria, amebæ) into the parenchyma of the liver. The paths that these organisms travel are various, and from this fact, and because of the differences in species and virulence of the different germs, the varieties of the clinical course and the localization and distribution of the purulent foci must be explained.

The following germs have been found in abscesses: streptococci (Kirmisson, Pantaloni, Kruse, Zancarol, and others), Bacillus coli (Ewald, Pantaloni, Achard, and others), Fraenkel's pneumococcus (Hermes), bacilli resembling typhoid germs, Bacillus pyocyaneus, actinomycosis, etc. Kruse, Kartulis, and others have found amebæ, and Grimm has found flagellated organisms. Experimentally, abscess can in many instances be produced by the injection of these germs.

As carriers of these infective organisms we may have foreign bodies, such as fish-bones, parasites (ascaris), etc.; such bodies have often been found in abscesses of the liver.

A distinction has always been made between primary and secondary abscesses of the liver. Among the former are those that are caused by injuries and by the extension of ulcerative processes from neighboring organs, as from the gall-bladder and the bile-passages. In the secondary forms infection occurs through the blood-stream. In many instances this differentiation is not possible. Sometimes the liver is ruptured without contusion or laceration of the overlying parts. If the abscess develops under these conditions, we must assume that infection occurred through the blood, and that germs contained in the blood-stream found a suitable nidus in the wounded hepatic tissue. On the other hand, primary traumatic abscesses may follow gunshot or stab wounds in case bacteria enter the wound through the channel so created.

Gastric ulcers, particularly peptic ones, may extend to the liver after adhesions have formed between the two organs, and may lead to suppuration. An extension from an intestinal or peritoneal purulent focus is not so often encountered.

Ulcers of the gall-bladder and of the bile-passages may perforate the mucosa and produce suppuration in the hepatic parenchyma in all cases in which pyogenic germs are present. In this manner abscesses are formed between the wall of the bile-passages on the one hand and the hepatic tissue on the other, or abscesses may be formed that are situated within liver tissue but communicate with a bile-passage filled with pus. In these foci there are often found gall-stones or parasites which ultimately lead to occlusion of bile-ducts and inflammatory irritation, so that the development of the bacteria in the retained bile is favored and the organisms can easily penetrate the injured mucosa. In addition, the retained bile exercises a deleterious effect on the parenchyma of the liver, so that, in combination with the action of the bacteria, necrosis and disintegration of the tissues (*hepatitis sequestrans*) are produced. This condition can be experimentally produced by the injection into the bile-passages of certain bacteria, such as staphylococci, streptococci, pneumococci, bacillus of typhoid and cholera, Proteus vulgaris, etc. In the course of a suppurative cholangitis the walls of the interlobular bile-passages may become softened and inflamed, this process extending to the surrounding tissues (suppurative pericholangitis) and leading to purulent disintegration of neighboring parts of the hepatic parenchyma. In this manner there originate some of the confluent multiple abscesses of the liver called *abscès aréolaires* by Charcot.

In the majority of cases the pyogenic organisms penetrate the liver by way of the blood-channels (secondary abscess of the liver). This may occur by the following three channels: (1) through branches of the hepatic artery; (2) through branches of the portal vein; (3) through the radicles of the hepatic vein.

Infectious germs gain an entrance into the hepatic artery in general pyemia, in ulcerative endocarditis (endocarditis ulcerosa), in suppuration and gangrene of the lungs, and in purulent and putrid bronchitis (bronchiectasis). In connection with these processes numerous metastatic purulent foci are formed in the liver, following the transportation of infected emboli and bacteria from the heart or other sources. In infected wounds combined with septicopyemia, abscess of the liver occurs in 15% of the cases, according to the statistics of Bärensprung in the Berlin Pathologic Institute. This form was seen more frequently in former days before the introduction of asepsis and antisepsis. It plays a subordinate rôle clinically, for the reason that in pyemia the disease in general is so violent that the abscesses are not discovered, particularly as they develop slowly and at a late stage of the disease. Death as a result occurs before typical symptoms point to an involvement of the liver. Abscess of the liver is, therefore, in these cases generally found unexpectedly after the death of the patient.

If the liver, on the other hand, is infected through the portal vein, there generally appear very distinct clinical symptoms which allow us to diagnose purulent hepatitis. Abscess of the liver originates most frequently in this manner.

Morgagni long ago called attention to the possible connection between abscess of the liver and disease of the portal system. Dance and Cruveilhier elaborated this idea upon the discovery that operations on the rectum and operations for hernia at times led to abscess of the liver. Experimentally this was corroborated later by injecting mercury into the radicles of the portal vein, an operation that was followed by the formation of abscess of the liver containing globules of mercury. Ulcerations of the intestine in particular favor the entrance of pathogenic organisms into the portal vein. Dysenteric ulcers are the principal cause for this accident. In the beginning of the nineteenth century certain authors saw a connection between dysentery and abscess of the liver, and since the writings of Budd this view has found many adherents. It is even stated that dysentery is one of the most prolific causes for that form of abscess of the liver so frequently seen in the tropics. Cheyne, Abercrombie, and Annesley in the first half of the nineteenth century found abscesses in dysentery, but they could not decide whether dysentery was the result or the cause of the abscess of the liver. Budd believed that dysentery was the cause of the abscesses even in those cases where the latter appeared before the former. He assumed, in these cases, that dysentery was present for some time, but had not been discovered. He opposed the view of Annesley, who claimed that the purulent secretion of an abscess of the liver was so irritating as to cause dysentery, and strengthened his argument by demonstrating that the dysenteric process left the duodenum and the jejunum free. In later years the views of Budd have been sharply antagonized. Fayrer, Sachs, and others attributed tropical abscesses to certain climatic influences (heat, deficient oxygenation, etc.) and to an irrational mode of life. They designated those abscesses that appeared in the course of dysentery or that followed trauma as septico-pyemic forms. Statistics collated since those days all speak in favor of Budd's views. Kelsch and Kiener, for instance, found dysentery in 260 cases among 314 cases of abscess; that is, in 75%. Zancarol states that 59% of his cases had dysentery. Waring, in 300 cases of abscess, found dysentery in only 27%. According to Murchison, 51 cases in which intestinal scars were present were seen among 204 cases of abscess of the liver; that is, in about one-fourth of the cases. While, therefore, dysentery is not found in all the cases of abscess of the liver, and is not the only etiologic factor, it certainly plays an important rôle in the causation of this disease. The fact that there are seen a great many cases of hepatic abscess in which no symptoms of dysentery preceded the disease, and the knowledge that many autopsies are performed in tropical hepatic abscess in which no traces of dysentery are discoverable, does not militate against this statement. In India, Algiers, and the south of Russia it is generally accepted to-day that dysentery is etiologically related to abscess of the liver (Magulies). If it is argued that there are certain regions, such as Cayenne, in which dysentery is very frequent, but where abscess of the liver is very rare, this argument does not invalidate the position taken. In our discussion on the rôle of dysentery we will show that dysentery alone cannot produce abscess of the liver, but that certain other factors are brought into play, particularly the mode of life, and that damage to the liver in other directions creates the necessary predisposition to abscess. The argument, too, that in the dysentery of temperate zones abscess of the liver is not frequent is not valid, for, in the first place, this form is different from the tropical form, and may even be due to another causative factor; in the second place, climatic influences do not exercise their deleterious effects under these conditions; and, in the third place, a number of cases are on record in which abscess of the liver did follow dysentery in subjects that had never lived in other than a temperate climate (France, England).

The fact that thrombi have been of rare occurrence in the portal vein in cases of abscess of the liver following dysentery is not a forcible argument against the existence of a connection between dysentery and hepatic abscess, since other diseases are known in which pyogenic organisms are carried through the veins without causing thrombosis. Even though a tropical abscess is found in the liver, and if ulcers and cicatrices are not present in the intestine, it is still possible that the specific virus of dysentery may have caused the abscess; for it may have penetrated through some slight abrasion of the intestinal mucosa, that healed later without leaving any trace. Unfortunately, the etiology of dysentery is not quite clear. Certain amebæ (as Amœba coli felis—Quincke), Bacillus coli, streptococci, etc., have all been credited with the causation of dysentery; it has also been held that the disease is due to the combined action of different germs. All the germs enumerated have been found at various times in abscesses of the liver. Amebæ have been found in hepatic abscesses by Osler, Kruse, Kartulis, and others, and are looked upon especially by Kartulis as the cause of the dysentery. [Osler has recently reported five cases of hepatic abscess of amebic origin. In all, the symptoms were obscure and latent. Osler calls especial attention to the absence of leucocytosis in three of these cases. In one case there was no ulceration of the intestine, though the history admitted the possibility of dysentery months previously.—ED.] Kruse found amebæ in every case that was preceded by dysentery or in which dysentery was present at the time. Other pathogenic bacteria were also frequently found, though there are many cases on record in which amebæ alone were present (Kartulis, Kruse and Pasquale). Kartulis believes that amebæ are of themselves capable of producing suppuration. Other authors assume that the amebæ act as carriers of bacteria, as do the distoma, the ascarides, etc., and that, owing to these bacteria, suppuration is produced. It must be remembered that although abscesses containing only amebæ seem to demonstrate that these organisms alone can cause suppuration, the possibility cannot be excluded that other bacteria were present but perished in the fluid. In the tropics certain forms of abscess are seen the pus of which is sterile and incapable of producing suppuration in the pleura and the peritoneum in case perforation occurs into these cavities (Tuffier, Peyrot, Windsor, and others). This seems to be due to the fact that the medium upon which the bacteria have developed gradually becomes exhausted and insufficient for their support. In certain cases, however, bacteria could be cultivated from the pus (Achard); in such cases we can neither assume that the medium was exhausted nor that a complete destruction of the germs had been accomplished by some toxic substance in the pus. It is possible in any event that the bacteria are not very virulent, and an argument in favor of this supposition is supplied by the fact that serious complications are absent in the case of many of these abscesses. Thus, although amebæ play an important part in dysentery, and in the abscesses that occur in this disease, this does not exclude the possibility that occasionally other germs (streptococci [Zancarol], staphylococci, colon bacilli) may cause an abscess in the course of an attack of dysentery without any action on the part of the amebæ themselves. All of the germs named are constantly present in intestinal ulcers, and may penetrate the connective tissues and thus reach the liver even before the amebæ. [Through the portal vein.—ED.] It is also possible to discover amebæ deep down in the layers of the intestinal wall, at the bottom of the ulcers, so that it seems very probable that they also may enter the intestinal veins.

[In the light of the recent work of Shiga in Japan, Kruse in Germany, and Flexner in the Philippines and in America, there is now no question that at least a large percentage of all cases of dysentery are directly due to the influence of a specific bacillus, of the typhoid group of organisms, but differing in many respects from the typhoid bacillus. The cases in which this bacillus has been isolated have been almost invariably of the acute variety, a class in which hepatic abscess is a rare occurrence. Nearly all of the typically chronic cases have appeared to be due to Amœba coli. Notwithstanding this seeming exclusion of the dysentery bacillus from the number of organisms that cause hepatic abscess, it seems likely that cases will be found that will give unmistakable evidence of the presence of this organism, in the same manner that the typhoid, and many other bacilli and cocci, have been found to be causal factors. The lesions of the form of dysentery due to the specific bacillus differ somewhat from those that are seen in amebic dysentery, but they none the less consist of typical serpiginous ulcers, and offer a seemingly ready source of infection for the portal circulation, and through the latter for involvement of the liver parenchyma.—ED.]

It would be a very prejudiced view that assumed that all abscesses occurring in the tropics or after return from the tropics are attributable to dysentery. The appearance of so-called idiopathic abscesses in the complete absence of a history or of symptoms of dysentery may well be attributed to the entrance of bacteria that perforate the intestinal wall through lesions other than those of dysentery. [J. Alison Scott has recently reported a case of hepatic abscess in which there was no antecedent history of dysentery. Evacuation took place suddenly into the right pleural sac, with signs of acute hemorrhagic pleurisy and the development and subsequent disappearance of pyopneumothorax. The pleural fluid was brownish-red, with a heavy flocculent brownish sediment containing fatty leucocytes, resembling liver-cells, also bile-pigment and fat crystals. A culture from this fluid proved sterile. There was present a very old lesion in the colon. Amebæ were not found in the pleural fluid, but were later demonstrated by Flexner in the scrapings from the abscess wall.—ED.] The fact that climatic and other injurious influences also render the liver a suitable nidus for the development of the different germs greatly favors such an invasion. In such cases Kruse has found only bacteria, and no amebæ; in all cases that were preceded by dysentery, however, amebæ were invariably present in the hepatic abscess.

We have repeatedly intimated that in order to explain the occurrence of tropical abscess of the liver in isolated localities and among such various classes of people we must assume that other factors are at work reducing the natural powers of resistance of the liver, and thus favoring the origin of abscess.

[Robinson's paper upon tropical abscess of the liver covers thoroughly the course and behavior of this condition in the Philippines and Cuba. He states that in the First Reserve Hospital of Manila there were in one year 2251 cases of diarrhea and 1391 of pronounced dysentery, following in the main in the course of the rainy season. Manson (quoted) reports 3680 autopsies made on dysenteric patients in various tropical countries. Of these 21 % showed abscess of the liver. In 96 dysentery autopsies made at the above station in Manila in 1899, abscess of the liver was present in over 12 %. This forms the average percentage for Europeans in tropical countries. The part played by the amœba coli has not yet been determined. It was always present in the stools, but only in five of these cases in the abscess, and most of these were cases of long standing.—ED.]

In Egypt, India, and in certain other localities the female sex is rarely involved, notwithstanding the fact that women are frequent sufferers from dysentery. Sachs found only 6 cases in women among 113 cases of abscess of the liver, Rouis only 8 among 258 cases, and Waring only 9 among 300 cases. The latter two series are of less value than those of Sachs, however, for the reason that they are obtained from localities with an overwhelmingly military population.

Europeans are more liable to develop abscess than the natives. Negroes, Fellahs, Hindoos, etc., are rarely afflicted with abscess, although they are frequent sufferers from dysentery.

Fayrer states that from 1888 to 1892, out of 1000 men in the Indian army 0.97 % to 1.24 % of the European soldiers and 0.03 % to 0.1 % of the native soldiers died of abscess of the liver; of the Europeans, 0.45 % to 0.81 %, and of the natives 0.85 % to 1.11 % died of dysentery. Cayley corroborates these figures. Among the European troops in India from 1880 to 1889, 26.8 % of abscess occurred among every 1000 men, with 1.34 % of deaths; in the preceding decade the proportion was still worse. Of the native Indian troops, only 0.05 % were afflicted during this period and only 0.03 % died (Davidson).

Nearly all authors attempt to explain this striking fact by the assumption that the use of alcohol predisposes especially to suppurative hepatitis. Those soldiers who were abstainers were afflicted far less frequently than those who were not. In the French possessions in India, for the same reason, diseases of the liver are less frequent than in the English ones, owing to the simpler mode of life of the inhabitants. Europeans, particularly the English, were in the habit some years ago, and are still to-day, of indulging in large quantities of alcoholic beverages, spices, coffee, tea, etc., and of living luxuriously; the natives, on the other hand, particularly the Mohammedans, are very frugal in their habits. It is generally recognized that alcohol, spices, improper diet, etc., exercise an unfavorable effect upon the liver (compare page 454). It is also probable that food that is too abundant, or nourishment that is too rich in proteids and in fat, undergoes abnormal changes in the intestine, which result in the formation of toxic products. These enter the portal vein and reach the liver, where they are capable of exercising a deleterious effect. It is also possible that in the tropics the bacteria that inhabit the intestine are of a different nature from those found in more temperate zones, and that the products of metabolism are, as a result, so different as to exert a distinct influence upon the parenchyma of the liver. It is remarkable how few cases of alcoholic cirrhosis of the liver are seen in tropical and subtropical climates, as compared with the many cases of liver abscess. Even if, moreover, by the mode of life and the influence of the climate the parenchyma of the liver is so predisposed to the development of suppurative processes, we are not justified in stating, as is sometimes done, that the climate, the nourishment, imperfect metabolism in the lungs, an improper diet, hyperemia of the liver, etc., are the only causes for the formation of abscess of the liver.

It appears that **sudden changes of temperature,** traveling from a cold to a warm climate and vice versa, exert an important influence upon the development of abscess of the liver. A blow, or some other injury in the region of the liver, seems also to predispose to the disease; this seems quite plausible in the light of all that has been said above.

When we consider all the etiologic factors enumerated, we can readily understand why the female sex, which is less given to excesses in alcohol, and the Mohammedan natives, who lead a frugal life, are attacked relatively less frequently. As soon as the natives or the women begin to indulge in alcoholic excesses, they also fall ready victims to the disease. The fact that the Antilles and Cheyenne do not seem to have as many cases of abscess of the liver, notwithstanding the presence of much dysentery, may be accounted for by the equable character of the climate.

It appears that no direct connection can be traced between the disease under discussion and malaria, although for a long time a relationship was claimed between the two. It is, however, easy to understand that an attack of malaria may inflict such damage to the parenchyma of the liver that it becomes a favorable soil for the lodgment and development of bacteria, amebæ, etc.

In colder climates, as we have already stated, abscess of the liver is seen as a sequel of dysentery in relatively few cases. **Typhlitis** and **perityphlitis** are the two chief diseases that seem to produce abscesses of the liver with or without thrombosis of a branch of the portal vein. Together with the abscess following gall-stones, this is the most frequent form of the disease encountered in our part of the world. The explanation is simple, inasmuch as inflammations and ulcerations are relatively most frequent in this particular part of the intestine. Körte believes that the suppurative process travels through the retrocecal tissues to the liver, and deduces this view from the fact that the portal vein shows no evidence of inflammation. It is much more plausible, however, to assume that the process is similar to the formation of metastases elsewhere, and that the infected particles travel very rapidly through the blood of the portal vein without being arrested and that they do not become lodged until they reach the narrower channels of the liver. Abscess of the liver is quite frequently seen in otherwise benign forms of typhlitis.

Einhorn, in 100 autopsies on cases of inflammation of the vermiform appendix, saw 6 cases in which infection of the portal vein and the liver had occurred; Langfeld, among 112 cases, saw pylephlebitis in 4 and abscess of the liver in 2 cases. Reginald Fitz saw pylephlebitis and infection of the liver in 11 cases out of 257 cases of appendicitis. In actinomycosis of the liver, too, the primary focus of the trouble will in general have to be sought in the region of the cecum and appendix (Barth, Langhans, Lubarsch, Partsch, Ranson, Samter, Schartau, Uzkow, Vassiliew).

Many case reports in regard to the etiologic rôle of appendicitis have been published. It may happen that the appendicitis is cured, and is causing no symptoms of any kind, when an abscess of the liver develops as the result of the primary condition. [Dale has recently reported a case of multiple abscesses of the liver following latent appendicitis.—Ed.]

Gastric ulcers, either peptic or carcinomatous, may also, apart from direct extension, in rarer instances, render possible the transference of infectious germs into the portal vein, and in this manner cause the formation of abscess (Andral and others). Duodenal ulcers may result in the same misfortune (Reinhold, Romberg, and others). Simple catarrhal, typhoid, or tubercular ulcers (Andral) rarely lead to this complication. In the case of a tubercular condition this is probably due to the fact that there is present a tendency to obliteration of the blood-vessels, which acts as a hindrance to the transference of infectious germs to the liver (Chauffard). Actinomycotic foci of the liver may originate from ulcers of the small intestine (Zemann, Vassiliew), or of the colon (Bargum and Heller, Hoeffner, Kimla, Lüning and Hanau, Ullmann, Uzkow), or of the rectum (Samter). Ulcers of the rectum, degenerating carcinomata, hemorrhoids, and purulent inflammation of the same tract, when operated upon may easily lead to the formation of abscess of the liver, as has been known for a long time (Morgagni, Cruveilhier, Dance, Arnaud, et al.).

Inflammatory processes **in the bile-passages** may also occasionally lead to a more or less pronounced inflammation of the portal vein and to the formation of hepatic abscess, since the blood-vessels of these passages enter the portal vein. In this manner infectious material may be carried from ulcers of these ducts into the parenchyma of the liver (Geigel). Gall-stones situated in the cystic or the common duct may also cause compression of the portal vein, so that inflammatory processes may extend to the latter vessel, causing thrombosis and phlebitis followed by suppurative processes in the liver (Klesser). In the new-born, infectious germs sometimes penetrate the portal vein through the umbilical vein in cases of infection of the umbilicus; these, entering the liver, cause abscess. Inflammation of the splenic vein in cases of abscess of the spleen, abscess of the pancreas, and purulent pancreatitis, may all rarely produce abscess of the liver. Owing to the anastomoses existing between the pelvic veins, inflammations of the uterus may occasionally be the starting-point for the entrance of infectious organisms into the portal system and the liver (Handford, Roughton). In pyemia infectious thrombi may form in abnormal conditions of the veins of the pelvis or the mesentery (varicose, etc.), and from these the liver may again be infected via the portal vein (Virchow). Finally, circumscribed peritonitic exudates (*i. e.*, between the pancreas and the liver, Beveridge) may cause pylephlebitis and abscess of the liver.

Any form of pylephlebitis may lead to abscess of the liver. Thus we sometimes see the disease after injuries of the portal vein followed by infection of the vessel, as, for instance, in a case in which a fishbone penetrated the vessel from the intestine (Winge).

Inflammations of the liver starting from the roots of the hepatic vein have often been observed, and are characterized by the development of microscopically determinable changes around the vena centralis of each infected lobule. The process extends to neighboring parts, and, generally, a number of small abscesses are formed that later become confluent. This variety is not easy to explain. As a rule, it is assumed that infectious germs penetrate the hepatic vein from some primary focus in one of the lower extremities, the uterus, the adnexa, or neighboring parts. The infectious agent probably first enters the vena cava inferior, and as soon as a retrograde flow of blood occurs (following stasis or forced respiratory movements) it is forced into the hepatic veins and its branches.

· That this can and does occur has been demonstrated by Heller, who noted the formation of a metastasis in a branch of the hepatic vein from a carcinoma of the abdominal lymph-glands; he also proved the occurrence experimentally. Infection may also enter the hepatic veins from the superior cava, providing even a minute quantity of the blood from the superior cava that pours into the right auricle is forced by the contraction of the right ventricle into the inferior cava (Diemer has demonstrated this in the rabbit). In this way it may be carried into and infect the hepatic veins. Ever since the days of Hippocrates a connection has been formulated between injuries of the head and abscess of the liver. Ambroise Paré encouraged this belief; Morgagni, on the other hand, discredited it. To-day we have less faith in a connection of this kind, and it is more than probable that in the days before antiseptic treatment of scalp wounds was inaugurated injuries about the head led to general pyemia more frequently than they do to-day, and that as a result the liver was more frequently involved. Langenbuch has thoroughly discussed this question, one particularly interesting to surgeons, and has shown that there is no apparent connection between abscess of the liver and injuries of the head.

It would appear that infection of the liver by way of the hepatic veins occurs primarily in the presence of some weakness of the heart, so that stasis of venous blood occurs. Thierfelder, in a case of purulent throm-

42

bosis of the subclavian vein, noted multiple miliary abscesses of the liver that originated from the center of the acini and were due to infection of the organ by pus germs via the right auricle and the hepatic vein.

The bile-passages exert in many respects the same influence as the blood-vessels. Such germs as streptococci, staphylococci, Bacillus coli, Proteus vulgaris, and other bacteria, may penetrate deep into the tissues of the liver through the fine divisions of the veins in the interlobular tissue, and lead to the formation of abscess (Chauffard, Gouget, and others).

Abscesses may originate in the bile-passages in three different ways:

1. By direct extension to the hepatic tissues from ulcers due to gall-stones (compare page 651).

2. By extension of a purulent cholangitis or pericholangitis to the interlobular tissues and the subsequent formation of tiny multiple abscesses.

3. By the entrance of pathogenic germs into the blood-vessels of the mucosa, and thence into the portal vein (compare page 657).

Suppurative processes are rarely noted in the liver as the result of infection via the lymph-channels. In cases of perihepatitis an abscess may occasionally develop beneath the surface, but clinically such an occurrence assumes little, if any, importance.

Finally, the echinococcus may appear as the cause of hepatic abscess; in such cases the cysts become purulent as a result of secondary infection following trauma or inflammation of the bile-passages. This subject is discussed in detail under Echinococcus of the Liver.

With regard to the frequency of the various forms of non-tropical abscess of the liver, the following statistics may be given. Bärensprung observed 108 cases (among 7326 autopsies), of which 11 followed ulceration of the bile-passages, and 18 followed ulceration in the territory of the portal vein. The latter included 8 cases of affection of the cecum and appendix, 5 of carcinoma ventriculi, 1 of carcinoma of the pancreas, 3 of carcinoma of the uterus or the vagina, 4 followed gangrene of the lung or abscess of the lung, and 55 followed injuries of other parts of the body.

Luda (unpublished communication) in the Pathologic Institute of Kiel found only 29 abscesses of the liver among 10,089 autopsies (0.28 %). Of these, more than half were due to pyemia (55 %), and 31 % were due to disease of the portal system.

[Oddo cites nine recent cases of traumatic abscess of the liver in children. The symptoms in some cases appeared at once, in others only after a latent period. The liver abscess seemed sometimes to be affected primarily by the trauma, and occasionally it seemed to be secondary to injury of some other portion of the abdomen. Four of these cases died.—Ed.]

A summary of the principal etiologic factors leads us to conclude that life in the tropics is the most frequent cause of hepatic abscess, and that an attack of dysentery or an improper mode of living is usually the antecedent condition. Typhlitis and perityphlitis, and then cholelithiasis, together with the suppurative processes that accompany this condition, must then be considered. Direct injuries in the region of the liver are less frequent causal factors, as are also the entrance of foreign bodies, ulceration of the gastro-intestinal tract, purulent infection of echinococcus cysts. General pyemia of varying origin is finally to be looked upon as one of the most frequent causes. This form of abscess of the liver is of subordinate clinical interest.

PATHOLOGIC ANATOMY.

The anatomic picture presented by the liver in purulent hepatitis varies decidedly, not only with reference to the stage of the disease, but especially with regard to the nature of the infectious agent, the virulence of the germ, and its mode of entry. In this manner the differences can be explained that are seen on examining the liver in a case of tropical abscess and in one of general pyemia. The differences are by no means so pronounced between some cases of multiple tropical abscess, on the other hand, and certain abscesses that are seen in temperate climates following infection via the portal vein from an intestinal ulceration, pus accumulation in the peritoneal cavity, the mesentery, etc. This is particularly apparent if the reports on the different forms of tropical abscess are compared, and is readily explainable when we remember that tropical abscesses owe their origin to the entrance of infectious material through the portal vein. Consequently no sharp distinction can be drawn between acute multiple tropical abscesses and those that occur in colder climates as the result of infection through the portal vein. In the case of traumatic pyemic abscess, abscess from gall-stone infection, and chronic tropical abscess, such a distinction is possible.

Little need be said in regard to traumatic abscess. The condition is either one of an injury of the abdominal or even the thoracic wall, accompanied by trauma of the liver, as the result of which the parenchyma undergoes a process of disintegration and of suppuration; or the substance of the liver may be ruptured within the organ itself and this accident be followed by inflammation. In the affected portion of the organ we find actual destruction of tissue, the formation of pus, hyperemia, later the formation of a pyogenic membrane and the encapsulation of the abscess within a connective-tissue covering. Microscopically, we can see the leucocytes passing from the wound into the interlobular tissues, and making their way between the columns of hepatic cells. Sooner or later the liver-cells undergo coagulation necrosis and degenerate into fat and detritus. In this manner the process extends to the center of the acinus, ultimately destroying even this portion (Koster). The result is the formation of an irregular cavity containing sero-purulent masses, disintegrated liver-cells, fat-droplets, leucocytes, etc. The wall of the cavity in the beginning is formed by the parenchyma of the liver; later by a distinct pyogenic membrane. In case the abscess is formed near the surface of the liver, perihepatitis will as a rule be observed.

If abscess of the liver is caused by infection through the hepatic artery or the portal vein, the enlarged organ is riddled with many diminutive abscesses, so that its surface often appears mottled by prominent, soft, yellowish spots corresponding to the pus foci. On transverse section the liver appears hyperemic and cloudy; numerous abscesses, varying in size from that of a millet-seed to that of an apple, are seen in different stages of softening and disintegration. If of long standing, they pour out a purulent fluid mixed with particles of disintegrated tissue. The pus may be either serous, creamy, bloody, or bile-tinged. Occasionally it is very offensive, and particularly if the abscess has had its origin in intestinal ulcers, or from gangrenous cavities in the vicinity. The abscesses are often of a bright yellow color from the presence of bile-pigment, which is known to have particular staining affinities for necrotic tissue. Occasionally a dark green zone will be seen around the abscess, owing to the action of bacteria and their products on the surrounding liver-tissues and to discoloration by the hemosiderin contained in the liver-cells. In many instances the formation of pus does not occur, nor is there any destruction of tissue; instead we see numerous dark spots on the cut surface of the organ; this is particularly the case where the infection has originated in the intestine, and especially when the subject has succumbed very rapidly to the disease.

On microscopic examination an accumulation of bacteria will be seen in the dilated capillaries between the liver-cells in the vicinity of the abscess, and, in addition, numerous leucocytes in the interlobular tissue. If infection has occurred through the portal vein, the leucocytes will be seen particularly around the branches of this vessel. Leucocytes also accumulate around the vena centralis, and in dense plugs fill the spaces between the columns of liver-cells. Later changes take place in the liver-cells, their nuclei stain poorly, the protoplasm undergoes granular degeneration, and coagulation necrosis gradually occurs. Ultimately nothing remains but undefined masses and fat-globules, which, together with the leucocytes and the bacteria, form the essential contents of the abscess-cavity. Abscesses that originate from the bile-passages may, apart from such as are due to gall-stones which have ruptured the bladder-wall, entered the liver-tissue, and caused suppuration (these abscesses have been described in detail in the section on cholangitis), be caused by pericholangitis. In the latter case the abscesses resemble those that are caused by infection through the blood. In the beginning numerous miliary abscesses form around the bile-passages. These may vary in size from that of a millet-seed to that of a grain of hemp; at the same time the walls of the bile-passages become infiltrated with round cells, as is also the case in their immediate vicinity. This area of infiltration soon assumes the character of a purulent focus and invades the parenchyma of the liver and the branches of the portal vein, destroying liver-cells and causing a pylephlebitis. Peritonitic inflammation often begins on the surface of the liver. Such a picture is seen particularly in cases in which stasis exists in the bile-ducts.

Chauffard distinguishes a particular form of abscess that he calls *abscès aréolaire.* He believes that these are always caused by infection from the bile-passages. Multilocular abscesses of this kind were observed even before his day as the result of inflammation of the vena hepatica, and especially following disease of the portal vein. Quite often they occurred in connection with disease of the vermiform appendix. These abscesses are characterized by their resemblance to infarcts. On the surface of the liver there may be seen a circular area, somewhat raised above the surface of the organ, and of a different color from the rest of the liver. If this portion is incised, it is seen to constitute the base of a wedge-shaped lesion the apex of which is directed toward the center of the liver. On transverse section the abscess presents the appearance of a spongy mass filled with numerous pus cavities that communicate with one another. These cavities originate from the confluence of the many acini that have undergone purulent degeneration; they form multiple round abscesses that are in contact with each other, gradually unite, become confluent, form a hive-like structure, and usually contain a large cavity in the center. In older cases the mass is surrounded by a pyogenic membrane that may become converted into a connective-tissue capsule. In portions more recently affected, near the edge of the abscess, changes are seen in the lobules, also round-cell infiltration in the interlobular tissues around the branches of the portal vein, and cholangitis or pericholangitis is present; in some cases thrombosis of the central vein and necrosis and destruction of the surrounding parts are observed. This form of multilocular abscess seems to owe its origin to the infection of some one of the larger blood-vessels or bile-passages. Bacillus coli, streptococci, and staphylococci have all been found in the pus.

Actinomycotic foci may appear in any part of the liver either singly or in multiple form. Sometimes they penetrate from without by extension of a peritonitic abscess or of a phlegmon in the posterior abdominal wall. These foci present the characteristic structure of actinomycotic eruptions, *i. e.*, exuberant granulation tissue, covered with a pus that contains the characteristic radiating fungi. Older foci may have a fan-shaped structure. Perforation through the diaphragm into the pleura or the lungs may occur, and often metastases are present in the lungs, the brain, etc., at the same time.

Tropical abscesses usually run a more chronic course, and are, as a rule, surrounded by a firm capsule. Usually they are single and leave the rest of the fiver intact.

Rouis has collected the statistics obtained from 756 autopsies on this disease, and has found the abscess located as follows: in 53 cases it was near the upper surface, in 39 in the anterior portion, in 46 in the inferior, in 47 on the right border, in 36 on the posterior surface, and in 67 cases in the interior of the liver. We learn from this that the abscess is in many cases situated, for instance, in the upper portion of the organ, or in other parts where it is not accessible to palpation. The right lobe seems to be a place of predilection. According to Rouis, the abscess was found 154 times in the right lobe, 33 times in the left lobe, and 9 times in the lobus Spigelii. The abscesses may even occupy an entire lobe, and the latter may constitute one large abscess-cavity. [Manson's report of 3680 autopsies has already been referred to. He found that 21 % of all dysentery patients had abscess of the liver. The right lobe was most often affected, in one series of 13 cases, only two presenting an abscess of the left lobe. Sometimes patches of necrosis were present, but no pus. Had the patient lived these also would probably have formed abscesses.—ED.] In 75 % of the cases quoted by Rouis the abscess was single. A good idea of the size of these abscess cavities may be obtained from the amount of pus contained, varying from 20 to 4500 c.c. Corresponding to the amount of pus, the liver is enlarged to a greater or lesser degree. In 101 autopsies it was found that the liver was enlarged in 70 cases, normal in 28, and decreased in size in 3 instances.

In those forms of tropical abscess that run an acute course the tissues rapidly undergo extensive softening, with round-cell infiltration of the lobules and the surrounding area, as well as coagulation necrosis of the liver-cells, as is the case with other metastatic abscesses. Sometimes death occurs before a true abscess has formed. In the early stages and before the appearance of true suppuration, the liver is very hyperemic, deep red on transverse section, and soft (Davidson). In the tissue grayish-white spots are visible that exude a serous fluid on section. Later on, the parenchyma becomes brittle, grayish-yellow, exudes droplets of pus on the cut surface, and shows microscopically a marked round-cell infiltration and fatty degeneration.

If the abscess forms more slowly, more characteristic pus-formation occurs. The wall of the abscess consists of the liver parenchyma, and is later lined by a pyogenic membrane; this is a layer of young connective tissue that soon becomes covered with fibrin, leucocytes, bacteria, amebæ, etc. From this wall there extend into the interior of the cavity processes consisting of more or less altered liver-tissue covered with the membrane. This abscess-wall may subsequently become so much thickened as to assume the consistency of cartilage and in it proliferation of the bile-passages may occur. The surrounding parenchyma is usually more or less hyperemic, and the liver-cells are sometimes atrophic and spindle-shaped. In other cases the abscess consists of a perfectly dry mass of leucocytes. Abscesses of this kind offer the most favorable opportunity for a spontaneous cure by contraction and cicatrization. On the other hand, the fluid from a young abscess contains leucocytes, necrotic liver-cells, fat-droplets, amebæ, and bacteria. If an abscess of this kind is incised, or if spontaneous evacuation of the pus occurs externally, a cure usually results with the formation of a firm cicatrix, the site of which is marked by a depression in the tissues; sometimes calcification occurs. Occasionally, calcareous cicatrices of this kind have been found in the liver that have pointed to the existence of an abscess at some time. It has also been observed that tiny new abscesses may form in the walls of an old one, even after all the pus has been evacuated.

Kelsch and Kiener draw a distinction between the foregoing and fibrous abscesses. The latter, even when they are small, are invested with a firm capsule of connective tissue. This capsule consists of fibrillar connective tissue containing spindle cells, while around it is a zone of granulation tissue with round papillæ, and around this again there is a layer of flat cells, filled with fat-globules; these cells are the transformed round cells which furnish the contents of the abscess. According to the writers, a nodule of connective tissue is formed which breaks down in its center, and thus creates the picture as described. These abscesses may be single or multiple; occasionally they resemble a degenerating gumma.

The tissues surrounding an abscess may become necrotic or even gangrenous, particularly after the abscess has been opened. As a rule, the arteries in the walls of the abscess are obliterated and appear as fibrous cords; the branches of the hepatic veins are especially liable to occlusion by thromboses. Often the latter undergo suppuration and form small abscesses that later communicate with the cavity of the main abscess. Usually the bile-passages remain patulous and the blood-vessels, with the exception of those in the immediate vicinity of the abscess, as a rule, show no changes. In rare instances only have abscesses been found that have broken into the branches of the hepatic vein, and in the same manner perforation into the bile-ducts may occur.

Peritonitis and perihepatitis with the formation of adhesions to the parietal peritoneum are seldom seen in tropical abscesses, even though the abscess may be situated near the surface of the organ. In cases in which perforation of the liver capsule threatens, however, adhesive inflammation of the serosa usually develops. For this reason an abscess is rarely seen opening into the abdominal cavity; such an accident probably never occurs except as the result of trauma. It is much more likely that perforation will occur into the peritoneal cavity at some point from which the capsule has been previously removed; thus a pus collection forms in the abdomen which may rupture again externally, into the bowel, etc. Perforation into the right lung has been described very frequently. This may happen if adhesions form with the diaphragm, and if the inflammation extends through the diaphragm to the right pleura. Inflammatory adhesion of the pleura with the base of the lung occurs, then more or less extensive infiltration of the involved portions of the lung. If the pus then burrows through the diaphragm, it may empty directly into the lung, or into a bronchus. In this way an abscess of the lung may be formed. Often, however, the evacuation of pus may be so complete that entire healing occurs. It may also happen that a subphrenic abscess develops, and leads to purulent pleuritis, the empyema finally perforating the lung. Cases are also described in which empyema has occurred without perforation of the diaphragm; in such instances pus-producing organisms have penetrated the diaphragm and caused the inflammation in the pleural cavity. There is found in such cases merely a thin membrane in the place of the diaphragm, between the abscess and the empyema. Serous pleurisy may also originate in this manner.

Perforation into the pericardium is rare, and usually results in early death, so that no characteristic changes are to be seen in this membrane.

It may also happen that adhesions form with the abdominal wall, and that the abscess perforates these parts, evacuating itself through the skin. In these cases fistulous passages of greater or less length are present, and lead from the inguinal, the axillary, or other regions of the body to the abscess.

On rare occasions perforation into the colon, the duodenum, the stomach, the bile-passages, or the inferior vena cava, is seen postmortem. It may also happen that an abscess, in case it is situated in close proximity to the right kidney, may form adhesions with this organ; the pus may then perforate the renal parenchyma and be evacuated through the pelvis of the kidney.

The abscess may discharge itself into other parts of the body, and can easily make its way into the circulation and thus give rise to metastatic foci in the brain, the spleen, etc.

COURSE.

The course and the general symptom-complex of abscess of the liver vary decidedly according to the origin of the disease and the nature of the infectious agency. We may differentiate acute, subacute, and chronic abscesses. It is, however, hardly possible to draw sharp distinctions, for the reason that an abscess that may have been latent for a time can suddenly become active, owing to some intercurrent disease, trauma, etc. In this manner a serious condition may be produced that will present all the symptoms of acute abscess. On the other hand, an acute suppuration may gradually become encapsulated, and in this way be converted into a chronic abscess.

Traumatic abscess is really a surgical condition. At times, however, the traumatic origin of the abscess is so remote that it can be established only with difficulty, and the impression is then created that the abscess owes its origin to some internal cause.

An **open wound** may extend through the skin and fascia to the liver, and through suppuration this may become still more extensive, until it involves the parenchyma of the liver. Under such conditions the pus will contain particles of liver tissue and some bile; by scraping the base of the pus-cavity liver-cells will be obtained. Under such circumstances a large abscess-cavity may be formed and the same picture be present as in suppurative processes of the liver following contusion or internal tearing.

In certain cases of contusion of the liver (a fall, crushing, or a blow in the region of the organ) the symptom-complex of hepatic abscess may develop in the absence of a penetrating wound.

Statistics show that abscess is not a frequent sequel of such traumata. Dudly analyzed 28,034 autopsies in Zürich and failed to find a single case of traumatic abscess of the liver. Christianson had the same experience in another series of 2450 autopsies. In America it seems to be more common; Dabney found 12 cases due to trauma among 110 abscesses. Thierfelder found only 11 cases in the literature of thirty years, and Langenbuch failed to find more than 39 cases in the whole literature. [Attention has already been called to Oddo's series of nine cases of traumatic abscess in children, all of which ended fatally.—Ed.]

The great majority of cases of injury of the liver go on to healing without suppuration, unless the patient dies in consequence of profuse loss of blood.

If an abscess forms, we see an enlargement of the liver, pain in the region of that organ, signs of peritonitic irritation, icterus as a result of the compression of bile-passages, etc. These symptoms, however, are not pathognomonic of abscess of the liver. The diagnosis cannot be made until the symptoms that are indicative of all the forms of abscess of the liver appear: viz., fever, pain in the right shoulder, a fluctuating tumor, etc. The subsequent course of the traumatic abscess resembles that of the other forms. It usually appears singly. The resemblance between the pictures of traumatic and non-traumatic abscesses can readily be understood, since both owe their origin to infection, from some outside source, such as the bowel, or the outside air, and the trauma is only a predisposing factor.

In cases of general septicopyemia or of ulcerative endocarditis the presence of an abscess is, as a rule, not discovered. Other symptoms are so prominent that those about the liver are obscured; the disturbances of the heart, the circulation, the inflammatory processes that develop in serous cavities, the symptoms of involvement of the central nervous system, etc., dominate the scene. If pain is present in the region of the liver, it is usually attributed to some other cause, for the reason that no fluctuating abscess of the organ develops, since death ensues too early in the course of the necrosis and destruction of the liver. The type of fever is dependent upon the nature of the general infection. Pain in the shoulder is often attributed to an involvement of the joint. In very rare instances it is possible to feel fluctuating spots or prominent areas on the surface of the liver or to find places that seem painful on pressure. In some instances, however, in the course of pyemia, pain appears at localized points over the liver, the organ seems enlarged, without exhibiting the hardness of an enlargement from stasis, and here and there peritonitic friction sounds may be heard. As a rule, however, no diagnosis can be made during life, and the hepatic abscess is first found at the postmortem examination.

The diagnosis of those abscesses that develop slowly and are due to **infection from the intestine** is generally much simpler. This is particularly the case in tropical abscesses. On the other hand, it may also happen that the development of the abscess is altogether latent, and the patient may have an abscess of the liver containing as much as two liters of pus and not become aware of the fact until some intercurrent affection, trauma, etc., causes the condition to be recognized.

In many of these abscesses the clinical development can be studied. The symptoms of some intestinal trouble, dysentery, typhlitis, perityphlitis, may precede the abscess-formation or exist simultaneously. The first symptoms that point to an involvement of the liver are pain in the region of the organ, and hepatic enlargement, as well as a dull feeling of discomfort or pressure in these parts. Pain is felt particularly in the right hypochondriac region. The liver dulness is increased, and sometimes more in an upward direction than downward, if the suppurative process is developing in the upper part of the liver; in this event the characteristic outline of the organ is revealed with the upper margin bent convexly upward. The appetite becomes poor, often nausea and vomiting are present, the stools become thin, and often the patient is constipated. Pain is often noted in the right shoulder. Icterus is rare. A continuous or a remittent type of fever develops. The pleura may be irritated at an early stage of the disease, and as a result a dry cough may appear. The patient always appears to be very sick, usually lying on the back or turned a little to the right, with the legs flexed.

This inflammatory stage, which is usually supposed to last a week in tropical abscess, may terminate favorably in cure of the disease. This is stated to be the case particularly in the tropical form of hepatitis. We must assume that in these cases the process is arrested before the development of true suppuration, and that the inflammatory products are reabsorbed. It is a difficult matter to prove that this takes place, though we are justified in assuming that it can occur from analogous conditions observed in other organs.

The symptoms of suppuration soon appear; the pain becomes more localized in the affected part, and in most cases active shoulder pain develops. The temperature curve is decidedly that of a septic condition, rising to a high point with chills, and falling again with a sweat; in general, however, the attacks of pyrexia are not so severe as in pyemia. Loss of appetite and intestinal disturbances are present, as well as vomiting, if pressure is exercised over the stomach or intestine. Respiration is more and more impeded by the abscess and the consequent swelling of the liver. If the abscess is situated so that it can be palpated, distinct fluctuation will, as a rule, be felt. Neighboring organs are next involved; peritonitis, usually localized in character, inflammation of the pleura, more rarely of the pericardium, and pneumonic infiltration of the right lower lobe, may all appear. Perforation may also occur, either through the lungs into a bronchus (in which case pus may be expectorated for months), or externally through the abdominal walls, or into the intestine; in the latter case pus will be found in the stools. Perforation may also occur more rarely into the peritoneal cavity, the pericardium, the right kidney, the inferior vena cava, etc.

If the abscess becomes indolent in consequence of encapsulation, as is the case quite frequently in the tropical form, the liver remains enlarged and a feeling of oppression or of pain persists in the hepatic region. The patient emaciates more and more, the skin turns yellowish-gray, the strength gradually fails, and a cure can be brought about only by operative interference, or by spontaneous rupture of the sac and evacuation of the pus through the lung, the intestine, etc. Resorption or calcification occurs only in very rare instances.

The duration of the disease varies from three weeks to six months. If the walls of the abscess are very dense, it may persist for years. In these cases some intercurrent disease or trauma may cause rupture of the abscess into the peritoneum and death.

Actinomycotic abscesses usually develop very slowly, and with very slight inflammatory symptoms; or all symptoms of a metastasis in the liver may be absent if the process develops in the interior of the organ. In general the symptoms are the same as in the case of any abscess that owes its origin to infection of the portal system from the intestine with organisms of slight virulence. Later in the disease metastases may develop in the lungs or general pyemia may supervene (Beari).

Now that we have given this brief description of the course of a condition which, as we have said, may vary decidedly under different circumstances, we will discuss individual symptoms and explain their significance.

SYMPTOMS.

General Symptoms.—A sufferer from abscess of the liver always appears to be a very sick person, even in the absence of marked symptoms of suppuration or of inflammation, and even though fever and local symptoms are lacking. This is the reason why errors in diagnosis are so frequently made in a condition in which little or nothing seems to point to the liver as the seat of the trouble, and the patients are often considered sufferers from phthisis, carcinoma, malarial cachexia, etc. The great psychic depression that is generally present is also misleading.

The color of the skin is usually a grayish-yellow, the sclera are yellowish, but icterus is, in general, absent, for the reason that no compression of bile-passages occurs; if present at all, it may be looked for in the first stage of the disease. If icterus is very pronounced, the suspicion is aroused that the condition is complicated by some such disease as cholelithiasis, that leads to stasis of bile. As a rule, the tension within the abscess is not sufficiently strong to cause symptoms of pressure on surrounding parts; it rarely develops in the region of the porta. The color of the skin recalls that of cirrhosis. In subjects suffering from septicopyemia, or from very acute forms of abscess, this color is, of course, not seen. After the abscess is cured this color disappears from the skin, which very slowly resumes its normal tint.

Owing to the destruction of much of the parenchyma of an organ that is so important in all the processes of life, and that plays such a large rôle in the regulation of the composition of the blood, **anemia** is frequently quite pronounced.

Fever is almost always present, at least for a time; in the beginning it is usually continuous or remittent, until the development of suppuration. It may be absent in the period preceding suppuration or may be of an intermittent, and sometimes an altogether irregular type. During the period of suppuration chills occur, followed by sudden rises of temperature, and then a rapid fall, with the breaking-out of a severe sweat. This has been denominated septic fever, and is not characteristic of abscess of the liver. The rise of temperature usually occurs toward evening, and the fall with sweating during the night, so that the sleep of the patient is often disturbed by dreams, etc. The intermittent type of fever may resemble the hectic type of tuberculosis, or the type of malarial fever, and consequently lead to confusion with these two diseases. It is, however, distinguished from malarial fever by its more irregular character and, in addition, by remaining uninfluenced by the administration of quinin. It may happen that this fever, after having persisted for some time, suddenly ceases, owing possibly to an arrest of the suppurative process; at the same time it may rise again in these cases and usher in the perforation by the pus, and death from exhaustion. The **pulse** during the fever is rapid, tense, and later is small. The **sensorium** is in many cases clear until death, notwithstanding the pyrexia. Sometimes, however, typhoid symptoms develop: stupor, restlessness, delirium, etc., that may lead on to the death of the patient. Abscesses have been reported in which all fever was absent; this seems to be particularly the case in those forms that are surrounded by a dense capsule and in which the symptoms of cachexia, etc., are prominent, and in which pain, inflammation, and swelling are slight. On the other hand, local symptoms may be altogether absent, though the fever-curve points to the presence of some pus-focus that is not discovered until after death.

[Leucocytosis, if present, may prove a valuable differential sign, and especially if the observer is fortunate enough to have begun a series of examinations at the beginning of pus formation. If a leucocytosis then forms, there will be a distinct gradual increase in the total numerical count. Osler has, as already noted, reported a series of cases in which there was no evidence of a leucocytosis, and in many cases it is undoubtedly absent. In his, as in nearly all reported cases, no differential count of the leucocytes was made.—ED.]

The prominent symptoms relate directly to the involvement of the liver, and particularly the **pain in the liver region.** In the beginning there is a feeling of weight and oppression, generally in the right hypochondriac region, but occasionally extending to the epigastrium, or the region of the left lobe. This feeling sometimes slowly, sometimes suddenly, merges into positive pain radiating into different areas of the body, according to the location of the abscess. It may be dull or crushing, but can also be cutting, stabbing, tearing, or boring. Its intensity varies greatly in different cases; it may be exceedingly severe or very mild. Much will depend on the location of the lesion. If the abscess is situated deep down in the organ, no pain may be felt until the abscess reaches the capsule, which has a rich nerve-supply. If the abscess develops near the periphery, pain is an early symptom, owing to the irritation of the integument of the liver. Movements of the body, respiration, a recumbent position on the left side, all cause an aggravation of this pain, in the latter case because the inflamed suspensory ligaments of the organ are put on the stretch. Pressure on the liver and even percussion increase the pain. A throbbing, pulsating, pain is rarely complained of. As a rule, the pain is not continuous, but varies in intensity; there may even be periods in which all pain is absent; these alternate with periods of excessive distress, as is readily explainable from the irregular progress of the suppurative process. In this manner a remitting or intermitting type of pain-accession may occur, similar to the course of the fever. Later, and especially if the abscess becomes encapsulated by fibrous membrane, all pain may disappear; if trauma supervenes and the process again becomes acute, the pain returns.

Pain in the shoulder has for a long time been considered a particularly characteristic symptom of abscess of the liver. This pain is generally felt in the region of the right shoulder, in the cucullaris muscle, the scapula, the upper arm, more rarely in the left shoulder, or on both sides. Its origin may be traced to the distribution of the branches of the right phrenic that extend to the capsule of the liver. If the capsule is inflamed, the branches of this nerve are irritated, and the stimulus is transmitted to the fourth cervical, which anastomoses with the phrenic. As the fourth cervical nerve sends sensory branches to the shoulder, the pain is transmitted to this portion of the body (compare page 456). In isolated cases atrophy of the deltoid has been seen (Rouis), pointing to a neuritic process. That the pain is less frequently felt in the left shoulder is readily explained from the relatively rare involvement of the left lobe of the liver, and from the fact that this lobe is supplied by a very small branch from the phrenic. In 17 % of the cases Rouis found this symptom pronounced; Sachs, among 36 cases, found it twenty-five times. As a rule, the pain appears synchronously with the beginning of suppuration, more rarely before or after; it also appears simultaneously with the pain in the liver, seldom after, and very rarely before. The pain may either be very slight or most severe; it may be that of oppression or may seem as though the shoulders were being torn apart.

Swelling of the liver is usually an early symptom. The liver is, as a rule, fairly soft in the beginning, but the enlargement can be clearly felt, and if the degree of swelling is considerable, can be seen to cause bulging of the right hypochondrium. The ribs protrude, and the intercostal spaces disappear or become enlarged. Sometimes a distinct bulging corresponding to the liver can be seen underneath the costal arch in the epigastric region. Usually the appearance is disguised by the contractions of the abdominal muscles, particularly of the right rectus. The margin of the liver, if it can be grasped, appears rounded. The superficial abdominal veins over the liver are often dilated. Percussion furnishes definite information. It is stated that the dulness extends more in an upward direction than downward, and this is considered characteristic. As a rule, however, the boundary between the liver and the lung is not regular, but is indented so that the upper boundary forms a convexity instead of the normal concave line. Frerichs has described this phenomenon as a semicircular protrusion of the lung-liver boundary. In abscess this line is not so angular as in echinococcus disease, and the decline on either side of the greatest concavity is more gradual in the case of hepatic abscess. The concavity can be determined between the parasternal and the mammillary lines or in the axillary region or even more posteriorly. Enlargement of the liver in an upward direction is especially apt to occur in case adhesions exist with the anterior abdominal wall or with the costal arch, so that the organ is prevented from enlarging downward. In large abscesses of the liver containing several liters of pus the dulness may extend upward as far as the apex of the right lung and downward as far as the crest of the ilium. The right lobe may also push the left far to one side, so that a distinct enlargement occurs toward the left. At the upper margin of the liver dulness respiratory excursion of the lower edge of the liver is generally absent or at best very slight. This impaired excursive power of the lungs is in part explainable by the pain that is caused by the slightest respiratory efforts. Sometimes symptoms of compression may be elicited at the margins of the lung.

Circumscribed bulging is produced if an abscess develops on the anterior surface of the liver or if a large abscess situated posteriorly or deep down in the organ grows to such a size as to press the liver forward as the result of the resistance offered by the ribs, the spinal column, etc., to the posterior surface of the liver. Such protuberances are most often found underneath the right costal arch, or they may be below this line, or in the epigastrium. If the abscess is near the surface of the liver, distinct nodules may be felt or even seen; and if suppuration is far advanced, it may even be possible to elicit fluctuation. Even a circumscribed edema of the abdominal wall is sometimes seen over the abscess. The patients are usually found lying on the back in order to decrease the tension of the liver capsule caused by traction or pressure. Some•observers state that the patients usually flex the right leg in order to decrease the tension of the abdominal walls; also that they turn a little to the right with the same object in view. Others, as Pel, claim that this position causes the ribs to press against the liver, and that consequently these patients never occupy it. Pel, Sachs, and others attach no importance to the tension of the right rectus (a symptom which Twining mentions as characteristic), for the reason that this symptom is seen in other conditions, as gall-stone colic, intestinal colic, etc.

Disturbances of the digestive tract are frequently associated with abscess of the liver. As already mentioned, dysentery may be one of the causes of the disease, and this condition may either persist after the abscess has formed, or it may become chronic, so that diarrhea and constipation are alternately present. Symptoms of typhlitis, gastric ulcer, etc., may also complicate the condition. Obstinate loss of appetite, sometimes alternating with a sensation of hunger, vomiting, a coated tongue, etc., may, however, be ascribed to the influence of the abscess itself. If the liver is very much enlarged, the ingestion of food may be disagreeable, owing to the pressure exercised on the liver as soon as the stomach becomes distended. There may be quite obstinate vomiting of mucus or of bile-tinged masses. This symptom, according to Maclean, is seen particularly in those cases in which the abscess develops on the concave surface of the liver, and presses upon the stomach and intestines. It is possible that the fever and the absorption of septic material into the blood are concerned in these digestive disorders; disturbances of the bile secretion are probably of less active importance in this respect.

Ascites may appear as the result of the general cachexia, together with anasarca, hydrothorax, etc.; or it may be the result of direct compression of the portal vein by the abscess itself. Circumscribed peritonitis and perihepatitis follow superficial abscesses, and often manifest their presence by friction sounds on breathing; in rare instances inflammatory sero-fibrinous exudates form within the peritoneal cavity.

In pyemia of the liver the **spleen** naturally is enlarged; in the more chronic forms of tropical abscess, however, this is said not to be the case unless malaria has preceded the abscess. Amyloid degeneration of the organ may occasionally be the result of chronic suppurative processes, and in this way lead to a dense tumefaction of the spleen.

Owing to the facility with which inflammations that involve organs beneath the diaphragm may extend to the pleura and lungs, respiratory disturbances are often noted in abscess of the liver. The right pleura and lung are involved with especial frequency. At an early stage a dry cough may develop, as the result of irritation of the diaphragmatic pleura; or a purely nervous cough may be complained of, as the result of the peripheral irritation of certain nerve-fibers in the liver which act reflexly on the central nervous system. This has been described by many authors. Active excitation of the pleura is followed by serous pleurisy, a condition manifested by dulness, reduced breath sounds, etc. Pleuritic friction sounds are not frequently heard. This is probably due to the fact that the fibrinous exudate occurs chiefly in the diaphragmatic pleura, and in a locality removed almost beyond our range of observation. Empyemata may appear as the result of microbic invasion, and for this to occur it is not necessary that the diaphragm be perforated; the same physical signs are seen in this condition as in serous effusions. Exploratory puncture will best reveal the nature of the inflammation. Dulness on percussion, with reduction or absence of the normal breath sounds, is most likely to occur if the liver enlarges upward to such a degree as to compress the lung. This compression may be so considerable as to cause a tympanitic percussion dulness and weak breathing over the right apex. Loud crepitant râles are heard on inspiration at the same time at the lower margin of the lung. As a result of the upward pressure of the diaphragm, dyspnea becomes more or less evident, particularly upon violent effort, exercise, etc. This symptom may appear even in slight cases of hepatic suppuration, owing, even in such conditions, to impairment of the movements of the diaphragm, (1) because of the enlargement of the liver; (2) owing to the pain that is caused by the pressure of the diaphragm upon the surface of the liver; and to the friction between the liver and the abdominal parietes during respiration, particularly when perihepatitis is present; and, finally, to pleuritic inflammation; (3) because of adhesions between the liver and the abdominal walls.

Pneumonia may also occur, particularly in the right lower lobe, by direct extension of the inflammation from the diaphragmatic pleura to the lung.

The outcome of these processes, as we shall show more in detail below, may be a perforation into a bronchus and the evacuation of the abscess by this channel; healing of the abscess cavity may follow. Kelsch and Kiener describe certain forms of pneumonia which, as in the case of malarial processes in the liver, are occasionally seen in abscess of the liver, and involve both the right and left lungs; such pneumonias are probably due to infection of the lungs through the circulation.

The **circulatory apparatus** exhibits the changes seen ordinarily in pyemia: emboli and consequent abscess formation in the lungs and other organs, endocarditis, etc. If the suppuration persists for a long time, symptoms of myocarditis develop, dilatation, irregular and weak heart action, and anemic murmurs. At the same time edema of the dependent regions of the body, the feet, the lumbar region, etc., develops. Abscesses in the left lobe of the liver displace the heart upward; in abscess of the right side the heart is much less frequently pushed to the left. The pericardium is very occasionally involved by direct infection through the diaphragm from an abscess in the left lobe, and a serous or purulent pericarditis may develop. Perforation of the abscess itself into the pericardium is exceedingly rare.

In a few cases aneurysmal dilatation of the branches of the hepatic artery in the walls of the abscess cavity has been noted. If these rupture, a severe and usually fatal hemorrhage is the result. The blood pours into the cavity and, if this already communicates with some outside part, or if it ruptures as a result of the increased pressure, the blood passes out from it; in one case, reported by Irvine, it ran into the intestine, so that blood was vomited, and enormous quantities were evacuated in the stools.

No characteristic changes are to be observed in the urine in abscess of the liver. Bile is seldom present. The urine is often colored red from urobilin, and in case there are fever and sweating, urates are deposited in quantity.

Parks states that a decrease in the quantity of urea passed is characteristic of the beginning of suppuration; other investigators deny this. Lecorché and Talamon found an increase of urea during the stage of inflammation, also an increase of the uric acid and of phosphoric acid, and a decrease of all those substances as soon as the abscess had formed. Kelsch, however, was not able to corroborate these statements. In these investigations much may be learned from careful determination of the nitrogen supply, and these studies are not always carried out with sufficient care. It is possible that in large abscesses with much destruction of liver tissue a decrease in the output of urea may be noticed. This decrease may, however, also be due to deficient assimilation, and a reduction in the amount of food owing to digestive disturbances. On the other hand, an increase may be due to increased proteid catabolism as a result of the destruction of tissue, or as a direct result of the fever, etc.

Disturbances of the **central nervous system** may be the result of the fever, of the cachexia, or of exhaustion. Delirium, insomnia, stupor, etc., are occasionally observed, and in rare instances these conditions may be due to the formation of secondary abscesses in the brain.

Perforation of hepatic abscess.—Descriptions of the different methods of perforation through the skin, or into internal organs, occasionally in several directions at the same time, are to be found scattered in numerous reports throughout the literature; particularly in English writings. The works of Rouis, Murchison, Thierfelder, Davidson, Langenbuch, and others give detailed accounts of this occurrence, and, particularly as they are of special interest from their surgical aspect only, it will be impossible at this time to enter into a discussion of all the symptoms.

Perforation through the skin usually occurs in such a manner that adhesions first form between the liver and the parietal peritoneum; the fibrous tissue thus formed is perforated and the pus burrows through either the soft tissues of the abdominal wall, the lower intercostal spaces on the right side, or the tissues of the lumbar region, until it finally reaches and ruptures the skin surface. At the point of perforation a doughy swelling is noticed, which gradually extends, bulges, and the skin becomes edematous. The parts become red, and present the feeling of a hernia-sac; on pressure a dull feeling of oppression is felt in the hepatic region. Soon a softer portion of the swelling becomes apparent, surrounded by more solid tissue, and often distinct fluctuation is present. If an incision or puncture is made, vesicles form on the surface, the skin ruptures, and necrotic portions of the skin are cast off, the contents of the abscess evacuating through the opening. The fluid is often tinged with blood, and resembles a fat emulsion; frequently it contains pieces of necrotic liver tissue and shreds of connective tissue. Sometimes the fluid is viscid and stringy, at other times creamy or purulent. In cases of actinomycosis it contains the typical granules that represent aggregations of the fungi. Occasionally necrotic portions of the soft parts, particles of muscle, pieces of rib, etc., are extruded through a considerable opening. The pus is often malodorous, as, for instance, in cases of infection following an attack of typhlitis or some lesion caused by the colon bacillus. The opening of the abscess does not always correspond to the exact location of the latter, and it is possible that a long fistulous passage may lead to it. Abscesses have been known to perforate in the neighborhood of the spinal column, on the inner surface of the thigh, in the inguinal region, etc.; they may even perforate in the region of the umbilicus if the fistula follows the course of the suspensory ligament.

The pus is often evacuated by means of a fistula formation through the lung, especially the right, and by the discharge of the pus through the bronchus. Cases of this kind that have recovered have been reported since the last century, and the literature is full of such instances. As a rule, the occurrence is not preceded by symptoms on the part of the pleura; the evacuation of pus is preceded by the expectoration of bright red (bloody) sputum (Budd, Köllner, and Schlossberger), though only very slight pneumonic symptoms appear. The latter consist of dulness over several of the intercostal spaces, crepitation, and possibly bronchial breathing. Suddenly the patient is seized with a coughing spell, and a large quantity of pus is raised by coughing; this is usually more or less bloody, sometimes bright red, and occasionally brown in color. Often it is partly seropurulent and sometimes contains shreds of liver and lung tissue. It may also contain bile, and subsequently, following the evacuation of the pus, bile may be coughed up and expectorated for a considerable time. The quantity expectorated is often very large, sometimes as much as one liter in a few hours. Feltham states that in one case 500 c.c. of pus were expectorated daily. This may continue for several weeks, and has been known to last even for the space of a year and a half (Pel). In the majority of cases the expectoration of pus gradually stops, the pulmonary symptoms subside, and the patient recovers. In other cases the abscess does not heal, owing to the formation of adhesions or to the stiffness of the capsule, so that the abscess cavity cannot close; or, again, infection of the lung may have occurred with the formation of abscesses of that organ. These may continue to spread until they may involve the greater portion of the lower lobe. This condition is recognized by symptoms of cavity formation in the affected portion. In all such instances the cough and the expectoration continue, the fever remains high, hemorrhages occur from time to time, the patient grows cachectic, and ultimately dies. Thierfelder's statistics show the frequency of perforation into the lungs. In 170 cases perforation occurred into the bronchi 74 times, into the right pleura 26 times, the intestine 32 times, the abdominal cavity 23 times, the stomach 13 times, the pericardium 4 times. According to a table by Cyr, perforation into the lungs was the most frequent accident among 563 cases of spontaneous evacuation of pus.

If perforation occurs into the pleura, empyema results. Sometimes the opening through the diaphragm is very small, so that empyema develops slowly with increasing dulness and diminution of the breath sounds over the lower part of the right lung. Purulent pleuritis occurs more frequently in this manner than by infection through the diaphragm, without perforation. The pus often forces the liver downward (in case it is not adherent), compresses the lung, and pushes the heart to the left. Dyspnea increases gradually. The pus may now be expectorated through a bronchus after penetrating the lung, or it may burrow through the chest-wall and be evacuated externally. Occasionally pyopneumothorax is seen (Northrup). Only rarely does perforation occur into the left pleura.

If an abscess of the left lobe perforates into the **pericardium,** severe pain is felt in the cardiac area as well as a sense of oppression and dyspnea. Collapse and death occur in a short time, and prior to the development of symptoms of pericarditis, except a marked increase in the heart dulness. Graves, in one case in which a communication existed between the pericardium and the stomach, heard a metallic sound with each heart-beat from the presence of air or of gas in the pericardium.

Abscesses of the liver are emptied not rarely into the **intestinal tract,** and with particular frequency into the stomach, the duodenum, and the colon. If the abscess is situated on the lower surface of the liver, it is very liable to perforate in this manner. If perforation occurs into the stomach, a large quantity of blood-tinged fetid pus is suddenly vomited, and a portion may be passed in the stools. More rarely vomiting does not occur at all, and all of the pus passes per rectum. In the same manner, when perforation occurs into the duodenum, usually through adhesions or through the bile-ducts, a portion of the pus is vomited, though the greater part is intimately mixed with the intestinal contents and is passed in the feces. Under these circumstances it is often difficult to recognize the pus in the stools. There is a sudden collapse of the hepatic tumor, often with the feeling that something has ruptured within the body; copious diarrheic stools then supervene. If this occurs, we are justified in assuming that the pus has perforated into the intestine, although it is impossible in the event of a recovery to state into what part of the intestine the perforation has occurred. If the abscess perforates into the colon, the contents appear in the stools almost unchanged, distinctly purulent, serous, of a brick-red color, and containing small particles of gangrenous tissue. If the opening remains patulous, some of the gastric or intestinal contents, especially gas, may enter the cavity in the liver and there cause a tympanitic percussion note, splashing, etc.

Perforation into the **free peritoneal cav**ity is rare. It is said to occur especially after trauma in cases in which the abscess is not adherent to its surroundings, or in which the adhesions have been torn (Davidson). The result is the appearance of a free exudate in the abdomen, accompanied by violent pain, collapse, weakness and rapidity of the pulse-beat—in short, all the symptoms of a diffuse peritonitis, to which the patient succumbs in a short time.

More frequently we see **a sacculated form** of peritonitic exudate in cases in which the perforation takes place slowly. Subphrenic abscesses may develop in this way, and cause a bulging of the diaphragm upward; later, perforation occurs into the pleura and the lungs. Or an abscess may be formed in the mesentery which is subsequently evacuated into the colon or through the abdominal wall. Abscesses may also develop between the coils of intestine in the posterior abdominal wall, and either be evacuated into neighboring organs, or burrow through the inguinal canal into the scrotum, etc.

It may also happen that the abscess perforates into the **portal vein,** resulting in an acute pylephlebitis. The symptoms are so obscure that a certain diagnosis cannot be made. If the pus enters the **inferior vena cava,** the right heart and the pulmonary artery are filled with purulent fluid. The result will be rapid death with symptoms of asphyxia, as in all forms of embolism of the pulmonary artery.

Very rarely perforation occurs into the **right kidney,** and into the pelvis of the kidney; cases of this kind have been reported by Huet, Annesley, Naumann, Roughton, and Hashimoto. The urine contains pure pus, and possibly blood and liver-cells, and is brown-red in color. After a time the urine may become clear and the condition pass on to recovery.

The frequency with which the different possible forms of evacuation of an abscess of the liver occur may be learned from the following figures collated by Cyr from all the cases discovered by him in the literature: Of 563 abscesses, 311 (55 %) found no opening whatsoever; 83 (14.9 %)

43

were operated; 59 (10.5 %) perforated into the lung; 39 (7 %) into the abdomen; 31 (5.5 %) into the pleura; 13 (2.3 %) into the colon; 8 (1.4 %) into the stomach or the duodenum; 4 (0.7 %) into the bile-passages; 3 into the vena cava; 2 into the kidney; 2 through the abdominal walls; 1 into the pericardium. Thierfelder quotes similar figures (see page 672).

If several abscesses are present, they may either become confluent and be evacuated together, or each one may make its own passageway. It has also occurred that one abscess has burrowed in various directions; *e. g.*, into the pleura and the lungs (Eames, Peacock), pleura and abdomen (Haspel), pleura and pericardium (Legg), pericardium and colon (Marroin), bronchi and intestine (Janeway, Depesselche, Webb), stomach and abdominal wall (Budd, Krieg, and Goodwin), duodenum and peritoneal cavity (Juhel-Rénoy), colon and abdominal walls (Domenichetti), colon and duodenum (Bristowe), etc.   .

Amyloid degeneration of the liver may complicate the condition if hepatic abscess persists for a long time, and also cause changes in the kidneys, spleen, and intestine, that will be discussed in the proper section. The appearance of septicemia is particularly alarming; this condition may be present if pus or pus-producing organisms enter the hepatic circulation. In cases of tropical abscess the lesions of dysentery or its traces can often be seen in the bowel. Finally the symptoms of malaria may occasionally complicate those of abscess of the liver: viz., dense tumefaction of the spleen and liver, fever, etc.

PROGNOSIS.

The prognosis in abscess of the liver is always uncertain with regard to recovery. Pyemic abscesses are probably always fatal. Traumatic abscesses, and those that follow acute infection through the portal vein, are also, as a rule, unfavorable in their outlook. Only such abscesses as occur singly, and contain no very virulent germs, go on to recovery after evacuation of the pus by operation or perforation externally. Such a recovery occurs quite frequently in abscesses following gall-stones. Tropical abscesses seem to offer the most favorable prognosis, for the reason that their contents seem to be less toxic, and may even be sterile. The more chronic forms of this type of abscess frequently perforate the intestine, the skin, and especially through the lungs, and are cured in this way. In cases of perforation into the lungs the prognosis appears to be by no means a bad one; Ughetti, for example, met with only 14 % of fatalities after this accident. If the abscess is incised or aspirated in the case of these subacute and chronic suppurations of the liver at an early stage, the prognosis becomes still better. In rare cases only do we see absorption of the pus, and cicatricial obliteration of the abscess-cavity. It may happen that an abscess that has been successfully aspirated recurs after many years (fourteen years in a case of Rebryend), and it becomes necessary to evacuate the pus a second time. In making the prognosis the following features must be considered: whether septic or pyemic symptoms are present; whether the pleura, the lungs, the pericardium, the peritoneum, etc., are involved; and whether amyloid degeneration or other intercurrent diseases are present, reducing the vital forces of the patient. These factors, if present, render the prognosis very doubtful.

DIAGNOSIS.

The difficulty of the diagnosis of abscess of the liver has already been emphasized. The older authors have called attention to this, and consider it a rare event indeed if the diagnosis is made at all.

Multiple abscesses, such as follow septicopyemic conditions, acute cholangitis, or pylephlebitis, are generally not recognized *intra vitam.* They can only be suspected if the region of the liver is acutely painful, and particularly if the painful area is circumscribed.

Solitary abscesses, on the other hand, following life in the tropics, or dependent upon gall-stones, perityphlitis, and traumata, can be diagnosed. The chief symptoms of these conditions have been enumerated above, the most important diagnostic signs being pain in the region of the liver, enlargement of the organ in an upward direction, pain in the shoulder, septic fever, circumscribed bulging, and, eventually, fluctuation over the liver. In pyemia a tumor of the spleen is usually present; its absence in the last-named forms of abscess is said to constitute a point in the differential diagnosis between this condition and malaria in cases where intermittent fever is present. If the abscess develops in the superior portion of the liver, the condition may be mistaken for pleuritis or pneumonia. The convex outline of the dulness, the pronounced bulging (circumscribed, as a rule) of the lower costal area, the absence of a distinct hepatic enlargement downward, usually indicate the presence of an abscess. Exploratory puncture may render important aid in the final decision. It may, of course, happen that both a pleuritic effusion and a hepatic abscess are present; in such an event the diagnosis, of course, becomes very difficult. [The Röntgen rays have in certain favorable cases given valuable aid in differentiating between localized conditions, and extensive effusions. F. H. Williams, in an excellent series of studies has shown that certain pathologic processes result in products which appear as dark areas when reproduced upon the negative. Purulent fluids are included in this class, owing to their great density, and these, by obstructing the passage of the rays, throw a shadow upon the otherwise clear area. Williams has demonstrated distinctly in this way the extent and locality of an empyema, and a number of observers have demonstrated the presence of abscesses in the lung. The procedure is of less value in the case of a localized collection of pus in the liver, owing to the density of the organ itself, but may at times be of signal service. The position of the liver in the body, requiring the passage of the rays through its longest diameter, also offers a hindrance to the success of this method.—ED.] The differential diagnosis from **subphrenic abscess** is also a difficult one, though, as a whole, the history of the case will lend material aid. Softened **carcinomatous nodules** of the liver have been mistaken for abscess. As a rule, however, the course of malignant disease is without marked fever, and usually evidence of carcinomatous growths will be discovered in other portions of the liver and of the body. It may, of course, happen that infection of the liver occurs from some carcinomatous ulceration of the intestine, and that in a case of this kind the patients are very cachectic, but do not develop any fever.

Suppurations posterior to the liver, as, for instance, **paranephritic abscess,** have simulated abscess of the liver, and the diagnosis has only been assured upon the passage of pus in the urine, or of uriniferous pus from the incision.

Abscesses of the left **lobe** may be mistaken for carcinoma ventriculi, particularly if inflammatory symptoms are absent, and gastric symptoms are prominent. The age of the patient, the history, and a careful examination of the stomach-contents will render the diagnosis clear. Abscesses of the liver have also been taken for **aneurysm of the aorta,** owing to the fact that the pulsations of the aorta are transmitted to the abscess; the pulsation will, however, be found to occur in one direction, usually from behind forward, and is not expansile in character.

Empyema of the gall-bladder is often mistaken for liver abscess; the situation of the pus-sac and its contour offer the most certain protection against error in this regard.

Echinococcus cysts develop more slowly and without any inflammatory symptoms; they are hard, tense, and elastic; they do not show distinct fluctuation, and are characterized by a thrill on percussion. Exploratory puncture will decide the question as to their nature. The tumor present in **hydronephrosis and pyonephro**sis is not palpably movable with respiration; it is situated behind the colon, and may decrease in size coincidently with the passage of large quantities of pus or of urine.

Cysts and inflammations of the pancreas may also simulate suppuration of the liver. The stomach should in such cases be distended with carbonic acid gas or with air, and it will then be found that the tumor is situated behind the stomach; the outline of the pancreatic tumor is, moreover, elongated and situated transversely across the epigastrium.

The seat of the abscess may sometimes be determined upon the following considerations: if the convex surface is involved, the liver is enlarged in an upward direction, there is pain in the shoulder, dyspnea, and bulging of the right hypochondrium. If the tumor is in the interior of the organ, no characteristic signs are present and there is only general enlargement and pain. If the tumor is on the under surface of the liver, pressure is exercised upon the stomach and the intestine, and, as a result, distress after eating, nausea and vomiting, etc., occur; icterus may also appear.

After perforation the purulent collections formed by lodgment of the pus in different localities may lead to confusion with psoas abscess; or they may appear at the inguinal ring and create the impression that a cold abscess of the spinal column exists; it is necessary, therefore, to examine both the vertebræ and the liver carefully. Perforation by a hepatic abscess into the lung may rouse suspicion of perforating empyema; the anamnesis and a careful examination of the liver should, however, clear the diagnosis.

Exploratory puncture is of paramount importance in rendering judgment upon the presence or absence of an abscess of the liver, its location, the character of its contents, and of the micro-organisms causing it. Especially in the case of tropical abscess, in which the contents of the cavity are usually non-virulent, puncture is a harmless procedure, even if frequently repeated.

The operation is performed as follows: Puncture is made in the suspected area with a fine needle or with the fine trocar of the apparatus of Potain or Dieulafoy. The skin is first disinfected, the air evacuated from the apparatus, and the sterile needle inserted; the cock of the apparatus is opened as soon as the needle enters the soft parts; this is done in order that pus may be aspirated as soon as it is reached; and in order that it may not pass alongside of the needle. If pus is found, the needle should be removed and a note should be made of the distance to which the needle penetrated; the cock should be kept open so that aspiration is continuous. Sometimes the cannula becomes occluded, and in this case the puncture must be repeated. Occasionally a Pravaz needle is employed, but it is less suitable for the purpose because the point of the needle is likely to make large excursions that may tear the abscess-wall. Sometimes, however, no other instrument can be obtained; if, therefore, this syringe is used, the needle should be pushed into the soft parts and the plunger pulled out when the point of the needle enters. The respiratory movements should be followed as soon as the needle enters the liver, it being possible in this way to aspirate the pus without doing any harm. The small wound should be closed with cotton, iodoform collodion, a suitable plaster, etc.

Sometimes it becomes necessary to perform puncture in different places before pus is obtained.

Peritonitic irritation is rarely seen after this trifling procedure, and it has repeatedly been found on autopsy that the puncture did no harm. As the walls of the abscess are not so tense and rigid as in echinococcus, the small opening closes rapidly and does not permit any of the fluid to ooze out. The needle may also be inserted through the lower portions of the thorax, without fear of harmful results.

In contradistinction to an empyema of the pleura, the pus of a subphrenic abscess shows an increase of pressure during inspiration and a decrease during expiration, so that more pus flows out during inspiration than during expiration; in purulent pleuritis the reverse is the case.

A careful study of the aspirated pus will reveal the presence or absence of micro-organisms, etc.

It should be noticed whether particles of liver tissue, echinococcus hooklets, actinomycosis granules, etc., are present; the odor of the fluid should also be determined to see whether it is fetid or pure. At the same time the exploratory puncture gives a certain direction to subsequent surgical procedures, as we shall see below.

PROPHYLAXIS.

In order to prevent the formation of liver abscess, such diseases should be guarded against as may lead to the entrance of infectious material into the liver, and especially dysentery and typhlitis. If such diseases are present, everything should be done to promote as rapid a cure as possible. Care should also be taken that the liver, particularly in hot climates, is not abused, so that there may be no predisposition to the formation of abscess.

The treatment of tropical dysentery, both by dietetic and medicinal measures, should, therefore, be begun at once; people living in regions in which dysentery is prevalent should take exceptional care not to acquire the disease. Suitable internal treatment of typhlitis from the very beginning, the careful treatment of recurrences, and, if necessary, prompt surgical procedures for the relief of disease of the appendix are all powerful preventives against abscess of the liver.

People living in the tropics should observe every care in avoiding the abuse of spirits, condiments, and indigestible food, as all these factors reduce the resisting powers of the liver.

These precautions will be particularly necessary if disease of the intestines is already present or has been present; this applies as well to inflammations of the bowels in our own climate. If some injury of the liver has been sustained, the condition of the bowels and general dietetic measures should be considered in addition to surgical procedures, in order to prevent the entrance of infectious germs into the diseased liver-substance.

TREATMENT.

Abscesses of the liver are rarely presented for treatment in the stage of inflammation preceding the formation of pus. As a rule, there is already a distinct accumulation of pus in the organs and the problem is to remove the pus as soon and as completely as possible. Conse-quently the treatment is almost exclusively surgical. Some abscesses cannot be treated at all. Such are pyemic abscesses, and the smaller pus foci that are seen in certain intestinal diseases, or that follow chol-angitis with or without cholelithiasis. They are not recognized, and, even though suspected, may be so numerous or so small that they baffle all attempts at treatment.

If a patient presents himself for treatment **at a time prior to the development of the abscess, but when evidence of a circumscribed inflammation of the liver** is **already present,** antiphlogistic measures should be employed. The patient should remain in bed, a light and digestible diet (milk, gruel, meal- or milk-soups) should be given, and all spirituous liquors avoided. An **ice-bag** should be placed over the liver and leeches (as many as 12) may be applied over the affected region; these may also be placed around the anus in order to relieve the engorge-ment of the portal system. Blood-letting, formerly a favorite measure, is useless even in robust individuals; in anemic subjects it may do harm. [Remlinger has reported four cases of apparently acute hepatitis, with symptoms strongly indicating the presence of abscess of the liver, in four cases of dysentery. Exploratory puncture gave exit to a quantity of blood, but no pus was found. In all four cases the local blood-letting was followed by immediate relief and subsequent continued improve-ment in the hepatic symptoms.—ED.] The application of vesicants to the abdomen has also been recommended; it is better, however, not to employ this measure in view of a subsequent operation. Tincture of iodin docs no harm if the case is a protracted one. Internally, laxatives should be given, and particularly calomel (1 gm. divided into three or four doses); vegetable purges may then be used, such as rhubarb, senna, castor oil, etc., in order to insure copious stools. The long-continued use of calomel is, however, bad (Rouis), because this treatment weakens the patient, particularly if poisoning occurs, rendering him less fit to undergo a subsequent operation. Emetics, such as ipecac, tartar emetic, sal ammonia, etc., are useless, and are not employed as much as formerly.

In some cases a change of climate does good; in others the develop-ment of an abscess is observed as soon as the patient returns from a pro-longed sojourn in the tropics.

Formerly considerable time was wasted with these preliminary meas-ures. To-day the most important point is considered to be the earliest possible discovery of the abscess by exploratory puncture, and, as soon as its position is determined, immediate evacuation. This marks a great advance in treatment, as formerly an operation was not undertaken until rupture externally was threatened; multiple incisions were then made and a cure often followed. At the present time, owing to the danger known to exist of perforation into other organs, sepsis, etc., such delay is not tolerated.

It will be, of course, impossible to describe all the different operations, or to outline the measures that have to be adopted to suit the location of the abscess, the complications, etc. A detailed description of all these matters will be found in Langenbuch's hand-book, and in other text-books of surgery.

Aspiration by means of the trocar comes first into consideration. It consists in evacuating the pus through a hollow needle or a trocar or with one of the instruments designated for the purpose by Potain or Dieulafoy. The procedure is the same as that described as exploratory puncture, except that now the attempt is made to evacuate the pus as completely as possible. In this manner complete cures have been brought about (Cameron, Dieulafoy, and others). Sometimes puncture must be repeated; in one case it was performed twenty-four times before the patient was cured. Certain cases at least demand incision and drainage. Tropical abscesses, owing to the non-virulent character of the pus, are particularly adapted to treatment by aspiration; the metastatic forms of abscess of our climate, on the other hand, do not act favorably under such treatment. As the result in the latter cases is, therefore, always doubtful, the method will probably never be extensively employed; and, particularly in those cases that can be treated in a hospital with all aseptic precautions, incision is much to be preferred. On the other hand, puncture has the advantage of being so simple of execution that it can be performed in private practice; moreover, it gives the physician a convenient means of evacuating an abscess, even in the upper part of the liver, by puncturing through the pleural space and the diaphragm without necessitating a major operation.

Puncture combined with drainage is also a valuable form of treatment. This operation is performed with a thick trocar, the cannula being retained in the wound until adhesions have formed or until a fistula has developed; it is then replaced by a rubber tube.

That form of the operation is to be condemned which directs the immediate withdrawal of the cannula after tapping, and neglects drainage precautions. Pus may enter the peritoneum through the large wound in the liver, particularly if the abscess was large and had extended nearly to the abdominal walls, and, as a result, suppurative peritonitis may develop.

If the cannula is allowed to remain, the liver tissue closes around it, and a fibrinous exudate, and later adhesions, form as a result of the irritating influence of the instrument; in this manner the wound is inclosed and separated from the peritoneal cavity. If the trocar pierces the pleura, the same process may occur there; the soft tissues, muscles, skin, etc., tightly grasp the cannula at the same time. In this manner a wound-fistula develops through which the pus can flow without danger to the patient.

The operation is performed as follows: The skin is incised (2 to 4 cm.) over the point under which the abscess has been found to lie by exploratory puncture, and a trocar, about as thick as the little finger, is rapidly plunged through the incision into the abscess. The pus is allowed to flow out and the cannula retained in place; an aseptic dressing is then applied to absorb the pus that continues to flow through the cannula. It is not so advisable to introduce a rubber drain at once through the cannula, since this has to be removed frequently, and this manipulation prevents so thorough an occlusion of the canal from the abdominal cavity; as a result the danger of peritonitis is greater. The cannula is attached to the skin by a few stitches, this being best accomplished by boring a few holes in the instrument to allow the threads to pass. At the expiration of two or three days the cannula becomes loosened, and can now be removed and replaced by a suitable drainage-tube. It may sometimes be a good plan, particularly in hot climates, to irrigate the abscess cavity with a 2 % or 3 % boric acid solution in order to prevent decomposition of its contents. At the same time the intestine is quieted by opium, and a light diet administered. If the pus is very thick, or if it contains shreds of necrotic tissue, gall-stones, etc., that cannot pass the cannula or the drainage-tube, the opening may be dilated by sponge tents or by the insertion of drainage-tubes of different sizes.

The operation as described has been performed with success in the tropics, and also in our climate, by Renvers, Israël, Garré, and others. It has the advantage of being easy of execution even under unfavorable external circumstances; it is particularly useful, therefore, for the same reasons as the capillary puncture in the case of tropical abscess, and under all circumstances where the patient cannot have the benefit of hospital treatment. Physicians in the colonies employ it largely, and among them Cameron, Cambay, Jiminez, Ramirez, de Castro, and others. In Alexandria 50 % of the cases of liver abscess that were operated in this way terminated fatally, and of those that were not operated 71 % succumbed to the disease.

[Manson recommends a modification of this form of treatment that has given eminent satisfaction in his hands. James Cantlee has also reported a series of cases successfully treated by Manson's method as follows: A trocar and cannula are first introduced. Then a large tube stretched upon a metal rod is passed through the cannula, and by means of this siphon drainage is applied. Of four cases, all operated within the past twelve months, three recovered and one died, the fourth case being moribund when operated. The chief danger is hemorrhage from the vena cava. These four cases completed a series of 28, all operated by this method, of which 24 recovered.—Ed.]

Cauterization Methods.—In order to open an abscess through a sufficiently large opening, without at the same time running the risk of entering the peritoneum as a result of deficient adhesions, a number of methods have been employed by which the different parts of the abdominal wall are successively perforated by cauterization until finally the peritoneum is reached, and this is also opened by some caustic application. In this manner adhesions are formed, as a result of the fibrinous inflammation caused by the caustic; and only when these have developed is the abscess incised.

For this purpose Récamier employed caustic potash, Demarquay "Vienna caustic paste" (equal parts of caustic potash and quicklime). The same author used the chlorid of zinc paste of Cauquoin (chlorid of zinc with flour or starch, kneaded into a dough and cut into small strips). Finsen employed the Vienna preparation for the skin, and the zinc preparation for the deeper parts. The abscess may then be allowed either to open by itself, or, if the adhesions are sufficiently solid, an incision may be made or a trocar inserted.

It is probably best, in order to abbreviate the treatment, to incise the skin and muscles first and then to apply the zinc paste to the wound with tampons of iodoform gauze. After a few days the necrotic shreds of muscle tissue are removed, more paste is applied, and this treatment continued until the formation of adhesions has surely taken place. This usually requires fourteen days. The abscess may then be carefully incised, slowly evacuated, and drainage established.

This method is tedious (requiring at least two weeks), painful, and uncertain, and is seldom employed; in its stead the method of single or double incision has been introduced.

The **method of double incision** has much in common with the caustic method; it was introduced by Graves. An incision is made down to the peritoneum, and the wound is closed with tampons for a week or longer; the abscess is then incised. The application of the tampons causes inflammation of the parts and the formation of peritoneal adhesions, so that the incision can be performed without danger. The method is safe, but requires delay, and as there is always meanwhile the danger of perforation of the abscess into other organs, it is not a practical procedure.

The method of Récamiers and Bégins, which consists in incising the peritoneum directly and in tamponing the wound, is dangerous, and was particularly so in the days before aseptic surgery. At the present time, with all proper precautions, it may be allowable.

Owing to the greater certainty of a successful issue the following operation of single incision is the best if carried out under strict aseptic methods:

In the beginning of the eighteenth century Horner opened the abdomen, stitched the liver to the abdominal wall, punctured the abscess, inserted a cannula, left it in place for fifty-four hours, and, finally, replaced it by a drainage-tube. His method, which is generally employed to-day, could not recommend itself in his time owing to deficient facilities for cleanliness and antisepsis. His method was first employed in echinococcus disease; later Sänger employed it in abscess, stitching the abscess-wall to the abdominal muscles and later making his incision and evacuating the pus. Tait first performed puncture, evacuated the pus, and then stitched the abscess-wall fast. Ransohoff performed the operation with the thermocautery instead of with the knife. Some operators, among others Defontaine, allow the aspirating needle to remain in place and use it as a guide for subsequent incision. The liver is exposed, and the pus removed with the aspirator through the needle; the liver is then attached, and the abscess opened by incision, and drained. It seems a good plan to allow the needle to remain in place, particularly in deep-seated abscesses; in superficial abscesses it seems better to remove it before the operation in order to prevent the entrance of pus into the peritoneal cavity following movements of the patient. The incision into the skin should be from 8 to 10 cm. long. It will be well to aspirate the pus before making this incision, because the liver after evacuation changes its form and its position relative to the wound. It is best, therefore, to attach the organ after evacuation in order to avoid too great a tension on the stitches. It is also recommended to resect a semilunar piece of the abdominal wall in case the wound does not gape sufficiently, also to apply a ring of sutures through the capsule of the liver, the muscles and the fascia of the abdominal wall, and to incise the wall of the abscess between two forceps by a cut of 6 to 8 cm. The margins of the liver incision, after all bleeding has stopped, are sutured to the abdominal wound. It is useless to curette the abscess-cavity, and harm may be done. Thick drainage-tubes should be placed in the wound and the cavity washed out with a 2 % solution of boric acid. [Thompson found amebæ in the pus of a case of a liver abscess, and as long as boric acid solution was used to wash out the cavity living amebæ could be found in the discharge. A solution of quinin was then substituted (1 : 1000), and from that time, and during the next few days, only dead amebæ were to be found, and later none at all.—ED.]

This method gives good results if it is carefully performed, and seems to be safer than the rapid method of Stromeyer-Little:

This operator inserts a knife directly into the abscess, beside the aspirating needle, irrespective of the presence or absence of adhesions. With a broad incision, while the liver is being pressed against the abdominal wall, he severs the wall of the abscess, the peritoneum, the abdominal walls, and sometimes an intercostal space. He then washes out and drains the abscess-cavity. This method attracted much attention, particularly in England and France. Langenbuch has criticized it and has called attention to its many defects. If adhesions are present, the result may, of course, be good; and even if this is not the case, a cure may result if the liver is close to the abdominal wall, and if the pus is sterile. Oftentimes, however, the hepatic and the abdominal openings do not coincide after the pus is evacuated, and, as a result, pus enters the peritoneum, and a fatal peritonitis results. It is also possible to injure the gall-bladder, the large blood-vessels, the intestine, the mesentery, etc. For all these reasons this method should be condemned as dangerous, and the method of incising the abscess only after the formation of adhesions, recommended in its stead.

If the abscess is situated under the costal cartilages on the right side, it is possible, according to Lannelongue, to resect the latter over an area that does not communicate with the pleural cavity. It may even be possible to push the pleural sac upward a little, to suture the peritoneum, and then to incise the abscess.

In case it becomes necessary to enter the right axillary region and to penetrate to the abscess through the pleural space, the ribs should be resected, the leaves of the pleura united by tamponing or by stitching, the diaphragm incised, and the abscess (which is usually adherent to the diaphragm) opened. If no adhesions are present, the diaphragm must be stitched to the abscess-wall; it may also be practical to attach the former to the skin in order to insure perfect closure.

Bichon's suggestion, to evacuate the pus into the colon through an artificial fistula into that part of the intestine, appears dangerous, in that it is very possible that this might lead to the entrance of intestinal contents into the abscess-cavity.

If the abscess perforates the pleura, the empyema must be evacuated as soon as possible by thoracentesis and resection of ribs, and drained in order to prevent further perforation into the lungs. If the lung is already perforated, it will still be necessary to evacuate the pleural cavity through an external incision.

If the lung is perforated owing to adhesions with the diaphragm, it will be well to promote expectoration by the exhibition of expectorants, as senega, apomorphin, etc.; preferably, however, by inhalations of turpentine and of similar preparations, also by the internal administration of these drugs and of preparations of creosote, etc. In this manner, too, the further development of suppurative processes in the lungs and bronchi may be in a measure impeded. Life at a high altitude or at the seashore is to be advised. If an abscess of the lungs has developed, pneumotomy may have to be performed; the thorax over the affected portion should be made more elastic by extensive resection of the ribs and the abscess caused to shrink in this manner.

In case the pus is poured into the abdominal cavity, laparotomy must be performed at once and the pus removed; this does not often happen. As a rule, it occurs after some trauma, and even though the operation is performed at once it is often too late. If the contents of the abscess are sterile or not very virulent, the operation may be successful; it is even stated that in cases of this kind the administration of opium and the use of cold applications have led to a cure without operative measures.

If the abscess spontaneously perforates the abdominal walls, thorough evacuation of the pus should be promoted, and, if necessary, by enlarging the opening, by inserting drainage-tubes, etc.

If the pus is poured into the intestine, no treatment is called for, unless peritonitic symptoms appear at the same time. In the event of some of the intestinal contents entering the abscess-cavity and causing gangrenous inflammation, the abscess must at once be opened externally and thoroughly drained.

Perforation into the pelvis of the kidney is rare, and calls for no special treatment.

Frequently an operation and a complete evacuation of the pus are not all that is required. Fistulous openings may persist, and continue to suppurate; or the patient may become anemic, or his nutrition remains poor. It is well, therefore, to advise these patients to seek a better climate; to send them to sanatoria in tropical climates, in the mountains, to the seashore, or to send them home. In our climate [Germany] it will be best to send them to the seashore, into the mountains, or to advise a mild course of alkaline-saline waters, or of some thermal springs.

LITERATURE.

GENERAL ARTICLES.

Bamberger: "Krankheiten des chylopoëtischen Systems," "Virchow's Handbuch der speciellen Pathologie und Therapie," Erlangen, 1847.

Budd: "Krankheiten der Leber," p. 50, Berlin, 1846.

Davidson, A.: "Hygiene and Diseases of Warm Climates," Edinburgh and London, 1893.

Des Portes Pouppé: "Histoire des maladies de S. Dominique," tome II, Paris, 1770.

Frerichs: "Klinik der Leberkrankheiten," 1861, vol. II, p. 96.

Gasser: "Abscès du foie," in "Manuel de médecine" von Debove und Achard, vol. VI, p. 188, Paris, 1895.

Kelsch et Kiener: "Traité des maladies des pays chauds," Paris, 1889.

Langenbuch: "Chirurgie der Leber und der Gallenwege," vol. I, p. 199, Stuttgart, 1894.

Madelung: "Chirurgische Behandlung der Leberkrankheiten," in "Handbuch der speciellen Therapie," von Penzoldt und Stintzing, Bd. IV, Theil 2, p. 198.

Pruner: "Die Krankheiten des Orients," Erlangen, 1847.

Rouis: "Recherches sur les suppurations endémiques du foie," Paris, 1860.

Scheube: "Die Krankheiten der warmen Länder," Jena, 1896.

Thierfelder: "Suppurative Leberentzündung (Leberabscess)," Ziemssen's "Handbuch der speciellen Pathologie und Therapie," Bd. VIII, 1. Hälfte, 1. Abth., p. 78.

HEPATIC ABSCESS.

Aubert, Th.: "Etude sur les abscès aréolaires du foie," Thèse de Paris, 1891.

Bärensprung, C.: "Der Leberabscess nach Kopfverletzungen," "Archiv für klin. Chirurgie," 1875, vol. XVIII, p. 557.

Bajon: "Abhandlung von Krankheiten auf der Insel Cayenne" . . . Erfurt, 1781.

Bettelheim: "Beitrag zur Casuistik der Leberkrankheiten," "Deutsches Archiv für klin. Medicin," 1891, vol. XLVIII.

Blank: "On the Causes of Hepatic Abscess," "The Lancet," February 20, 1886.

Carl: "Ueber Hepatitis sequestrans," "Deutsche med. Wochenschr.," 1880, Nos. 19 and 20.

Cayley: "Tropical Affections of the Liver," "Verhandlungen des VIII. Congresses für Hygiene und Demographie in Budapest," 1896, vol. II, p. 695.

Chauffard: "Etude sur les abscès aréolaires du foie," "Archives de physiologie," 1883, p. 263.

Christiansen: "Zwei Fälle von Leberabscess mit Durchbruch ins Pericard," "Norsk. Magazin for Läger," 1890, p. 211, nach "Virchow-Hirsch's Jahresbericht," II, p. 259.

Dudly: "Ueber Leberabscess," "Deutsches Archiv für klin. Medicin," 1893, vol. L, p. 317.

Ewald: "Leberabscess nach Dysenterie," "Deutsche med. Wochenschr.," 1897, p. 67.

Fayrer: "Liver Abscess and Dysentery," "The Lancet," May 14, 1881.

Flexner: "Perfor. of the Infer. Vena Cava in Amœbic Abscess of the Liver," "American Journal of the Med. Sciences," May, 1897.

Funke: "Zwei Fälle von Leberabscess," Dissertation, Würzburg, 1893.
Geigel: "Ueber Hepatitis suppurativa," "Sitzungsberichte der physikalisch-med.,"
    "Gesellschaft zu Würzburg," 1889, p. 35.
de Gennes et Kirmisson: "Note sur deux cas d'abscès volumineux du foie,"
    "Archives genéralés de médecine," 1886, tome CLVIII, p. 288.
Gouget: "Injections hépatiques expériment. par le Proteus vulgaris," "Archives de
    médecine experiment.," 1· Serie, tome IX, p. 708.
Grimm: "Ueber einen Leberabscess . . . · mit Protozoen," "Archiv für klin.
    Chirurgie," 1894, vol. XLVIII, p. 478.
Hashimoto: "Zwei Fälle von Leberabscess," in "Archiv für klin. Chirurgie," 1885,
    vol. XXXII, p. 38.
Hengesbach: "Ueber Leberabscess," Dissertation, Berlin, 1894.
Hermes: "Casuistischer Beitrag zur Chirurgie der Leber," "Deutsche Zeitschr. für
    Chirurgie," 1895, vol. XLI, p. 458.
Kartulis: "Ueber tropische Leberabscesse und ihr Verhalten zur Dysenterie," "Vir-
    chow's Archiv," 1889, vol. CXVIII, p 97.
— "Ueber verschiedene Leberkrankheiten in Aegypten," "Verhandlungen des VIII.
    Congresses für Hygiene und Demographie in Budapest," 1896, vol. II, p. 643.
Kiener et Kelsch: "Affections paludéennes du foie," "Archives de physiologie,"
    1879, p. 398.
Klesser: "Ein Fall von Hepatitis suppurativa," Würzburg, 1887.
Klose: "Ein Fall von primärem Leberabscess bei einem Neugeborenen," Disserta-
    tion, Würzburg, 1893.
Köllner und Schlossberger: "Beitrag zur Casuistik der Leberabscesse," "Deutsches
    Archiv für klin. Medicin," 1883, vol. XXXII, p. 605.
Koster: "Untersuchung über Entzündung und Eiterung in der Leber," "Central-
    blatt für die med. Wissenschaft," 1868, p. 17.
Kruse und Pasquale: "Eine Expedition nach Aegypten," "Deutsche med. Wochen-
    schr.," 1893, p. 354.
Laveran: "Contrib. à l'anat. des abscès du foie," "Archives de physiologie," 1879,
    p. 654.
Leyden: "Fall von multiplem Abscess infolge von Gallensteinen," "Charité-Anna-
    len," 1886, p. 167.
Mejía: "L'hépatite parenchym. aigué circonscrite," "Verhandlungen des X. inter-
    nationalen med. Congresses," Berlin, 1890, vol. II, p. 126.
Menzzer: "Fall von Leberabscess infolge von eitriger Pylephlebitis," Dissertation,
    Erlangen, 1889.
Mosler: "Ueber traumatischen Doppelabscess der Leber " " Zeitschr. für klin. Medi-
    cin," 1883, vol. VI, p. 173.
Northrup: "Abscess of the Liver," "New York Med. Record," February 2, 1884,
    vol. XXV.
Pel: "Ueber die Diagnose der Leberabscesse," "Berliner klin. Wochenschr.," 1890,
    p. 765.
Rajgrodski: "Zur Casuistik der Leberabscesse," Dissertation, Jena, 1879.
Ransohoff: "Beitrag zur Chirurgie der Leber," "Berliner klin. Wochenschr.," 1882,
    p. 600.
Rassow: "Zur Aetiologie der Leberabscesse," Dissertation, Greifswald, 1895.
Rebreyend: "Sur un cas de récidive à longue échéance d'un abscès du foie," " Ar-
    chives générales de médecine," 1897, p. 226.
Reinhold: "Fälle von Leberabscess nach veralteter, völlig latent verlaufener Peri-
    typhlitis," "Münchener med. Wochenschr.," 1887, Nos. 34 and 35.
Renvers: "Beitrag zur Behandlung der Leberabscesse," "Berliner klin. Wochen-
    schr.," 1890, p. 165.
Roughton: "A Case of Hep. Abscess," "The Lancet," August 22, 1891.
Sachs: "Ueber die Hepatitis der heissen Länder," "Archiv für klin. Chirurgie,"
    1876, vol. XIX, p. 235.
Schinke: "Zur Casuistik der Leberkrankheiten," Dissertation, Greifswald, 1887.
Singer: "Zur Casuistik und Symptomatologie der Leberabscesse," "Prager med.
    Wochenschr.," 1884, No. 29–32.
Sym: "Case of Double Hep. Abscess," "Edinburgh Med. Journal," 1887, p. 879.
Ughetti: "Contrib. allo studio della epatite suppur.," "Riv. clinica," 1884, No. 12,
    p. 1057.
Vosswinkel: "Vorstellung von zwei geheilten Fällen von Leberabscess," "Berliner
    klin. Wochenschr.," 1895, p. 419.
Wettergren: "Hygiea," 1880, p. 37, Nach "Virchow-Hirsch's Jahresbericht," vol.
    II, p. 197.

Whittaker: "Traumatic Abscess of the Liver," "New York Med Record," 1880, vol. xvii, p. 587.

Windsor: "A Brief Account of Tropical Abscess of Liver," "The Lancet," December 4, 1897, p. 1447.

Zancarol: "Dysent. tropicale et abscès du foie," "Verhandlungen des VIII. Congresses für Hygiene und Demographie in Budapest," 1896, vol. ii, p. 759.

Robinson: "Hepat. Abscess," "Jour. Am. Med. Assoc.," May 11, 1901.

Scott, J. A.: "Hepat. Abscess," "Proc. Path. Soc. Phila.," Nov., 1901.

Dale: "Abscess," "Jour. Am. Med. Assoc.," Mar. 23, 1901, p 835.

Glenard: "Bull. d. l. Soc. de Med. de Paris," April 25, 1901.

Oddo: "Revue des Mal. Enf.," Paris, Jan. and Feb., 1901.

Osler: "Med. News." April 12, 1902.

Willson: "American Medicine," Mar. 29, 1902.

Cantlee: "Brit Med. Jour.," Sept. 14, 1901.

Remlinger: "Rev. de Med.," Aug. 10, 1900.

Thompson: "Phila. Med. News," Feb. 3, 1894.

Berndt: "Deut. Zeitschr. f. Chir.," vol. xl, 1894, p. 163.

Moncorvo: "Rev. mes. des Mal. de l'Enf.," 1899, xvii, p. 544.

CHRONIC INFLAMMATION OF THE LIVER.

(Quincke.)

When speaking of chronic inflammation of the liver, chronic interstitial hepatitis is usually implied. If the word interstitial were intended to signify merely a particular kind of chronic inflammation of the liver, then the chronic parenchymatous form must needs also be discussed. This, however, is never done, for reasons that we will explain below. It would appear that the word interstitial is merely an explanatory addendum, and that every form of chronic hepatitis is necessarily interstitial. This is, however, by no means the case. In certain of the diseases that we will discuss (phosphorus- and alcohol-liver) we know that the parenchymatous cells of the liver are involved, and in some cases to a great extent; in other diseases we have every reason to assume that the same thing is true. In the latter class it is often difficult to prove that the liver-cells are primarily involved, for their appearance even in a normal liver is so variable, microscopically, and it is so difficult to determine the presence of disturbances of the hepatic cells during life, that such a task is almost hopeless. We see, therefore, that mild initial changes in the parenchyma can readily evade detection; whereas even the slightest abnormalities in the interstitial tissues are at once perceived, for the reason that this tissue is normally so scanty.

Although in certain cases the changes in the interstitial tissues are primary, yet we know that they may also be secondary to primary changes in the liver-cells. Different investigators fail to agree with regard to the primary or secondary origin of the condition.

The same difficulty is experienced in chronic inflammations of other organs, as in tabes, neuritis, and nephritis. A study of the latter disease will throw some light on the processes that occur in the liver. For a long time the various authors attempted to distinguish between interstitial and parenchymatous nephritis, and to formulate certain anatomic types for the one or the other lesion. To-day we have learned to recognize that this distinction cannot be carried through, and that often parenchymatous and interstitial changes are seen simultaneously, and may develop from one another. We know also that the same influences (alcohol, scarlatina) can produce either or both forms of nephritis, and we can imagine that the quantity of poison present, the rapidity of its action, and its joint action with other harmful influences determine the cause of the various forms, as well as the course of the disease. In the case of the liver, too, we know that the same poisons—alcohol or phosphorus—may produce either parenchymatous (fatty infiltration, as a rule) or interstitial changes, and that the two forms are related to one another; we see, therefore, that a differentiation of the two diseases is not justifiable either from a histologic or an etiologic point of view.

In describing the pathologic anatomy of these diseases, the interstitial changes will be emphasized, for the reason that they are more conspicuous and because they are more lasting; our present knowledge indicates that, as a result, chronic hepatitis generally appears to be of the interstitial form.

A complete description of the interstitial changes is, however, not possible, since the relation between the anatomic conditions and the clinical phenomena has not only been the subject of much investigation, but consequently of much discussion during recent decades. Laennec's cirrhosis, the atrophic stage of alcohol liver, was for a long time the only form of interstitial hepatitis known, and it was in regard to this disease that the discussion first began. All forms of interstitial hepatitis that were observed later were compared with this form; some authors simply identified all forms with this form of cirrhosis, others attempted to base certain clinical differences on the anatomic and etiologic differences that had been found. So far, however, there has been only partial success in this altogether warranted endeavor.

In order to understand the present status of our knowledge on this subject it will be best to describe the manner in which the different possible causative factors can produce interstitial changes in the liver. Such changes are seen:

1. In **chronic stasis and hyperemia** of the liver, particularly in the central portions of the lobules. In this location the proliferated connective-tissue structures of the vessel-sheaths extend into the acini, following the direction of the dilated and thickened capillaries and passing between the atrophic columns of liver-cells. The tissue is usually homogeneous or fibrous, and consists in part of metamorphosed capillaries (Brieger); less often there is a cellular infiltration. In describing congestion of the liver due to stasis we mentioned the fact that occasionally proliferation of connective tissue occurs in the interlobular spaces between the branches of the portal vein (Liebermeister). This proliferation may occur in streaks or over a large surface, so that the lobules become constricted and atrophic, and the occlusion of numerous branches of the portal vein may lead to general disturbances of the circulation in the liver, and to ascites.

2. **Stasis of bile** from occlusion of the bile-passages. Many experiments have shown that stasis of bile may lead to the formation of foci of necrotic liver-cells, and to a proliferation of interstitial tissue which remains after the cells are destroyed; these experiments were made chiefly in rabbits and guinea-pigs. The proliferation begins in the interlobular spaces and penetrates the interior of the lobule from the periphery. The course of the whole process may not extend over more than a few weeks (compare page 428).

The results of these animal-experiments were applied to human subjects by Charcot and his pupils, and in this way a distinct anatomic and clinical picture called biliary cirrhosis was constructed, which was considered identical with "hypertrophic cirrhosis of the liver"; this view, as I will show, is untenable for several reasons. In other animals—for example, the dog and the cat—these changes are completely absent or very slight; here, however, a thickening of the walls of the gall-bladder and of the bile-passages is seen.

In man the consequences of biliary congestion resemble more frequently those seen in dogs than those observed in guinea-pigs. Cases of the latter kind do occur, however, and have been described by Janowski. Two weeks after the occurrence of stasis of bile (from a gall-stone) this author found yellow foci of necrotic liver-cells in the marginal zone of the lobules. These are reabsorbed; at the same time, a small round-celled infiltration is seen in their vicinity, and, later, cicatricial formations occur. At the same time the epithelium of the bile-passages desquamates, the walls of the ducts become infiltrated, there is a formation of new connective tissue, and a proliferation of bile-passages, as in the liver of guinea-pigs. A certain number of the new bile-passages originate from metamorphosed columns of liver-cells.

The proliferation of connective tissue and the atrophy of the liver-cells may attain as marked a degree as that seen in atrophic cirrhosis; so that it may lead to congestion of the portal system. No characteristic anatomic difference can be found between cirrhosis due to biliary stasis and other forms of cirrhosis (Litten, Mangelsdorff, Janowski). The proliferation of the bile-ducts, which Charcot's pupils consider so characteristic, is by no means specific; on the contrary, the same picture is seen not only in every form of interstitial hepatic inflammation, but in acute atrophy as well. (Brieger has seen it in hepatic congestion.)

Stasis of bile, therefore, while it is certainly to be included among the causes of interstitial cirrhosis of the liver, is not an important factor, because in man it rarely leads to this condition and (perhaps only in the presence of other influences, such as infection of the bile-passages), because in cases in which it does produce such changes the picture is dominated by the symptoms of biliary stasis.

3. Botkin and Solowieff have claimed to have demonstrated by experiment, as well as on anatomic grounds, that stasis in the portal system can lead to interstitial hepatitis; this, however, has never been proved. Simple occlusion of the portal vein or of some of its branches leads to complete or partial atrophy of the liver (vide thrombosis of the portal vein). Inflammation is seen only when the obstruction is not a purely mechanical one, but contains toxins or micro-organisms that enter the liver at the same time. This may easily occur if the main trunk or some of the branches of the portal vein become inflamed. Activity on the part of the different noxious agents is favored by a slowing of the blood-current. Only in this sense may we say that many cases of interstitial hepatitis start from the capillaries of the portal vein. [An instructive case has been described by E. Mihel in which, in a nutmeg liver, such a marked deposit of calcareous salts occurred around the central veins as undoubtedly to cause both a mechanical pressure upon the vessels, and at the same time to act as an irritating foreign body in the parenchyma of the liver. The process was so marked that the liver grated on section.—ED.]

4. Duplaix * has observed interstitial proliferation of the hepatic connective tissue in arteriosclerosis and in cases of thickening of the smaller vessels that so often accompanies this condition. He also saw enlargement of the interlobular spaces and foci of embryonal cells within them. He compares these changes with similar but much more marked processes which are seen in the heart, the kidneys, and the spleen, and finds that they occur particularly after malaria, lead intoxication, gout, rheumatism, alcohol-poisoning, etc. The lesions of the liver are too insignificant in these cases to produce any clinical symptoms

5. Chronic inflammation of the liver may be caused by **chemical poisons.** Alcohol and phosphorus produce fatty infiltration in man, and the former is also capable of causing the condition which we call cirrhosis of the liver. Experiments have demonstrated the latter fact. In the case of phosphorus-poisoning they show that the drug may produce not only the ordinary picture of phosphorus liver but that a subacute or chronic intoxication, albuminous and fatty clouding of the hepatic cells (Aufrecht, Ackermann), a degeneration of the protoplasm and of the nuclei (Krönig, Ziegler, and Obolensky), and, finally, a proliferation of the connective tissue, may occur. The degeneration of hepatic cells occurs diffusely throughout the acini, but the proliferation of connective tissues is at first only interacinous. Gradually the latter process extends until it leads up to the typical picture of cirrhosis (rabbits, Wegner). During this process the usual granular atrophy, also a smooth induration, occur, and even the lobulated form of liver may be produced. These facts are of great importance in the understanding of chronic inflammation of the liver, even though chronic phosphorus-poisoning has as yet never been observed in the human being, since they show that a poison may cause isolated foci of disease, either slight or of excessive degree. Aufrecht's observations appear to refute Krönig's belief that the changes seen simply represent a filling-out of the spaces that were occupied by the destroyed parenchyma; since the former has observed proliferation of connective tissue in cases in which the cells were not yet necrotic, but were only slightly changed in appearance. It is impossible to state whether the diseased cells or the poison caused the connective-tissue changes; this question is of purely theoretic interest, and probably cannot be answered. Even if the proliferation of the cells does not coincide exactly with the changes in the liver-cells, this fact does not disprove the etiologic rôle of the latter, since they may very well exercise an influence on the nutrition of remote tissues.

Basing his conclusions upon more recent experiments with artificial chronic phosphorus-poisoning in rabbits, Aufrecht arrives at the conclusion that vacuolar degeneration of cells and nuclear changes occur only in the periphery of the lobules. Some of the cells perish altogether, others merely become atrophic. The peripheral portion of the lobules where this occurs suggests the formation of young interlobular connective tissue, whereas in reality this new formation does not occur.

Experiments with alcohol do not give such pregnant results as with phosphorus. Certain writers have found only a severe degree of hyperemia in spite of intoxication lasting for several months (v. Kahlden); also fatty infiltration of the liver-cells (and of the stellate cells) (Ruge, Strassmann, Affanassiew, v. Kahlden) without nuclear or cellular degene-

* "Contribution à l'étude de la sclerose," "Archives gen. de. med.," 1885, i, p. 166. Also see Eichhorst's "Handbuch der spec. Pathologie," 1890, ii, pp. 391–398.

ration. Lafitte saw in a rabbit, atrophy of the hepatic cells and dilatation of the capillaries, also many punctiform hemorrhages; Affanassiew, on the other hand, noted collections of round cells around the bile-ducts, Strauss and Blocq and Pupier made the same observation in the peripheral parts of the acini. Contraction and shrinking of the tissues were never observed.

In any event it may be said that alcohol acts less energetically upon the liver of animals than phosphorus, but that its first effect, as in the case of phosphorus, is exercised on the cells of the parenchyma. The alcohol may itself be changed; it does not enter the bile, for Weintraud failed to find it there after acute poisoning. The fact that conditions analogous to the alcoholic liver of the human being have not been produced may well be accounted for by the fact that the artificial influence has not been sufficiently long-continued, and that the single doses administered were relatively too large. We can very well imagine that small doses of a certain poison frequently administered may produce purely functional changes in the cells that would ultimately lead to a proliferation of connective tissue.

Mertens, it appears, has succeeded in administering alcohol in sufficiently small doses by allowing rabbits to live in an atmosphere saturated with the fumes of alcohol. Some died at the end of a few months, some at the end of a year or longer. In the former animals the liver was brownish-green, there was profuse ascites, and the liver-cells were much altered; in the latter the liver was enlarged, pale, hard, and the liver-cells only slightly altered, though occasionally degenerated. In all the cases of sufficiently long exposure the development of connective tissue was seen in the portal spaces extending to the hepatic veins.

Other poisons that act similarly to phosphorus, both experimentally and actually, are arsenic, antimony, and, according to Langowoi,[*] cantharides.

According to H. Mertens, chloroform acts very energetically; if injections of $\frac{1}{8}$ to $\frac{1}{5}$ cm. were made every three to five days, the liver, at the expiraton of several weeks or months, was found to be harder, paler, and more nodular than usual, and the surface was seen to be granular; the different incisures were more clearly marked than usual. The liver-cells are affected first; they grow cloudy, fatty, become vacuolated, and atrophy. Strands of connective tissue develop, inclosing bile-channels; these start from the portal spaces and extend to the hepatic veins. Boix [†] produced atrophic cirrhosis in rabbits by administering small doses of butyric acid (three months), and of acetic acid (thirty-five days); the changes seen were not so pronounced in the case of lactic and valerianic acid.

6. Chronic inflammation may occur around localized foci of disease and foreign bodies in the liver.

Welch [‡] saw numerous foci of this kind around small particles of coal in a human liver. Neisser [§] injected carbolic acid solution into the liver parenchyma of animals and saw the development of aseptic foci of inflammation with round- and giant-cells. Connective-tissue proliferation is also seen in the vicinity of tumors of the most various kinds, and if there are many individual tumors the connective-tissue changes may be wide-spread. It is possible that certain chemical agencies play a rôle here in addition to the pressure of the growth. The extension of chronic inflammatory processes from neighboring organs acts in the same manner as does a gastric ulcer that extends to the

[*] "Fortschritte der Medicin," 1884, p. 437.
[†] Boix, "Le foie des dyspeptiques," etc., Thèse de Paris, 1894.
[‡] Welch, "Cirrhosis hepatis anthracotica," "Johns Hopkins Hosp. Rep.," 1891.
[§] Neisser, quoted by Mangelsdorf, p. 561.

44

liver, or a chronic inflammation of the peritoneal covering (either diffuse, tubercular, or simple, or circumscribed, as after lacing). The connective-tissue increase occurs in the interlobular spaces and involves only the vicinity of the inflammatory foci; occasionally it becomes diffuse and spreads to other parts of the organ.

The same applies to the parasites that are so often seen in the liver of animals. In the liver of rabbits the presence of psorospermia or of cysticercus may cause this process to assume extensive proportions. In the dog Distomum campanulatum, which has its habitat in the bile-passages, may, according to Zwaardemaker,* cause a thickening of the walls of the larger and finer ducts (without icterus); and in other places circumscribed granulations, or even a connective-tissue development that starts from the portal branches or the branches of the hepatic veins and enters the acini at this point, causing destruction of liver-cells from pressure. In this manner a certain form of cirrhosis is produced that is not uniform, but none the less diffuse; it ultimately leads to ascites from stasis.

In human beings Echinococcus alveolaris acts in a similar manner; also bacteria that lodge in the liver after entering the organ through the blood. In miliary tuberculosis of the liver especially, this form of proliferation assumes high degrees; in typhoid fever the development is scanty and the foci are, as a rule, very small.

M. Wolff † injected saprophytic germs (putrefying blood in Pasteur's fluid) subcutaneously into guinea-pigs, and observed the development of localized cheesy abscesses and inflammatory foci in the lungs, the kidneys, and the liver; these foci in the course of a few months led to a diffuse small-cell infiltration, and to the formation of fibrous connective tissue, a picture that greatly resembled human cirrhosis. It is probable that in this case wide-spread bacterial embolization occurred, although the fact could not be determined owing to the imperfect methods of examination of that day.

Krawkow introduced Staphylococcus aureus, Bacillus choleræ, pyocyaneus, and saprophytic bacteria into the muscles and the stomach of birds for long periods of time; he observed the development of an atrophic, and more rarely of a hypertrophic form of cirrhosis of the liver.

Malarial disease of the liver is probably analogous to bacterial hepatitis, and to that form due to the presence of a foreign body. It is possible that the mechanical occlusion of the blood-vessels by the profuse pigment may play a rôle in the former disease.

In some of the inflammatory processes described here the liver-cells sustain the first injury; in others the interstitial tissues are first affected. Nothing definite is known in regard to the origin of the small cells that are seen in these lesions; it is even uncertain whether they immigrate from the blood-vessels or whether they are a product of the proliferation of the connective tissue itself, though the latter is probably true in most instances.

The appearance on section, as well as that of the surface of the liver, is usually little changed, and frequently the condition is only discovered on microscopic examination. The initial stages may, on the other hand, be manifested, as in other organs, by an increase in the consistency of the liver or in the toughness of the tissues. In more pronounced cases these changes are so apparent that we may actually speak of hardening of the liver.

In addition to interlobular and intralobular proliferation of connective

* Zwaardemaker, "Cirrhosis parasitaria," *Virchow's Archiv*, 1890, vol. cxx, p. 197.

† Wolff, "Ueber entzunde. Veränderung. inner. Organe nach experimentel erzeugten subcutanen Käseherden," *Virchow's Archiv*, 1876, vol. lxvii, p. 234.

tissue, some authors speak of biliary, venous, portal, and bivenous proliferation, or cirrhosis. Different meanings are attached to these terms. Some merely indicate the starting-point of the process (periphery or center of the lobule); others, again, wish to show that the proliferation starts from the walls of the channels designated, or is due to some irritation starting from these channels. It must be remembered that the use of the terms in the second sense is often based on assumptions that have not been proved to be correct.

One peculiarity of all processes that are accompanied by connective-tissue proliferation is the development of many tortuous channels, and of ramified or reticulated canals of a different size; these are lined with epithelium of the flat or the cylindric variety. Undoubtedly these canals are in some way related to the finest bile-ducts, and may be injected from the latter vessels (Ackermann). They are not, however, as was formerly believed, found only in stasis of bile, but may be formed in the course of all interstitial proliferative processes. In cases in which much of the parenchyma has perished these canals may be the remnants of normal bile-channels that have been dislocated and approximated to one another by the displacement of the liver-tissues. In part (according to Aufrecht, exclusively) these originate from the columns of liver-cells that have become converted into channels and are metamorphosed into flattened epithelium. Thirdly, they may be due to a true new-formation by branching and bulging of older channels. It will depend on the nature of the process which of these three procedures is the most concerned in the formation of new channels.

We will now discuss the forms of interstitial hepatic inflammation that are seen in man; the description of the anatomic changes will for practical reasons be combined with that of the clinical aspects of the disease.

LITERATURE.

EXPERIMENTAL ALCOHOLIC CIRRHOSIS.

Ruge, P.: "Wirkung des Alkohols auf den thierischen Organismus," "Virchow's Archiv," 1870, vol. XLIX, p. 252.

Dujardin-Beaumetz et Audigé: "Recherches expérimentales sur l'alcoolisme chronique" (in swine), "Comptes-rendus de l'Académie des sciences," 1883, tome XCVI, p. 1557.

Straus et Blocq: "Etude expér. sur la cirrhose alcoolique du foie," "Archives de physiolog. normale et patholog.," 1887, p. 408 (rabbits).

Pupier, Z.: "Action des boissons dites spiritueuses sur le foie," "Archives de physiolog. normale et patholog.," 1888, p. 417.

Strassmann, F.: "Experimentelle Untersuchungen zur Lehre vom chronischen Alkoholismus," "Vierteljahrsschr. für gerichtliche Medicin," 1888, vol. XLIX, p. 232.

Affanassiew: "Zur Pathologie des acuten und chronischen Alkoholismus," Ziegler's "Beiträge zur pathologischen Anatomie," 1890, vol. VIII, p. 443.

v. Kahlden: "Experimentelle Untersuchungen über die Wirkung des Alkohols auf Leber und Nieren," Ziegler's "Beiträge zur pathologischen Anatomie," 1891, vol. IX, p. 348.

Lafitte: "L'intoxication alcoolique expérimentale et la cirrhose de Laënnec," Dissertation, Paris, 1892.

Mertens, H. (Gent): "Lésions anatomiques du foie du lapin au cours de l'intoxication chronique par le chloroforme et par l'alcool," "Archives de pharmacodynamie," Gand et Paris, 1895, tome II, fasc. 2; Jahresbericht I, p. 214.

PHOSPHORUS LIVER.

Ackermann: "Die Histogenese und Histologie der Lebercirrhose," "Virchow's Archiv," vol. CXV, p. 216.

Aufrecht: "Die diffuse Leberentzündung nach Phosphor," "Deutsches Archiv für klin. Medicin," 1879, vol. xxiii, p. 331.
— "Experimentelle Lebercirrhose nach Phosphor," "Deutsches Archiv für klin. Medicin," 1897, vol. lviii, p. 302.
Krönig: "Die Genese der chronischen interstitiellen Phosphorhepatitis," "Virchow's Archiv," vol: cx, p. 502.
Wegner: "Der Einfluss der Phosphors auf den Organismus," "Virchow's Archiv," 1872, vol. lv, p. 11.
Wyss, O.: "Beiträge zur Anatomie der Leber bei Phosphorvergiftung," "Virchow's Archiv," 1865, vol. xxxiii, p. 432.
Zeigler und Obolenski: "Experimentelle Untersuchungen über die Wirkung des Phosphors und Arsens auf Leber und Nieren," Ziegler's "Beiträge zur pathologischen Anatomie," 1883, vol. ii, p. 293.

CIRRHOSIS OF THE LIVER; CHRONIC INTERSTITIAL HEPATITIS.

(Laennec's or Atrophic Cirrhosis; Granular Atrophy.)

Of the different forms of chronic inflammation of the liver, and of the different stages of this disease, that one which leads to a reduction in the size of the organ, and granular change in the parenchyma, although it was not described for the first time by Laennec, is named after him for the reason that he first called the disease cirrhosis. His reason for so doing was the fact that he observed a peculiar yellow color in the granular tissue. This is not a constant finding, and is, at best, one of subordinate importance; Laennec, moreover, considered the yellow granulations to be neoplasms, whereas in reality they are deformed portions of the liver-tissue inclosed by connective tissue.

The name "granular atrophy" is in the majority of cases suitable to the last stages; but it must be remembered that not only in many cases does the organ remain perfectly smooth, but that, on the other hand, granular changes are seen in other conditions, as, for instance, congested liver due to stasis.

Occurrence.—Atrophic cirrhosis of the liver is seen principally in men of middle age, owing to its usual origin through the abuse of alcohol; only one-half to one-third as many women are afflicted with the disease as is the case with men. In children the condition is still more rare, sometimes being caused by alcohol, and in the new-born by congenital lues (see page 743).

The frequency of the disease varies according to the cause in different regions.

G. Förster found the disease in 31 (1 %) cases among 3200 autopsies at the Berlin Pathologic Institute, in subjects between thirty and ninety years.

In Kiel, the initial stages of alcoholic cirrhosis are among the conditions most frequently seen on the autopsy table. H. Lange found hepatic cirrhosis (in autopsies on subjects over fifteen) 43 times in 1835 men (2.34 %), in 1296 women 13 times (1 %). "Induration" (diffuse hyperplasia of the connective tissue) occurred in men 49 times (2.67 %) and in women 8 times (0.7 %). In one-half of the cases of both varieties of interstitial nephritis alcoholism was determined. In 16 cases of the first, and in 17 cases of the second category, chronic hyperemia from stasis seemed to be the cause. Of the 56 cases of true cirrhosis, 8 were of high degree, 32 of medium grade, and 16 were in the incipient stages, or were mild in character.

Etiology.—The chief cause of cirrhosis of the liver is continued indulgence in alcoholic liquors. The fact that we fail to find more cases of the disease, in spite of the wide-spread abuse of alcohol, does not signify that this abuse cannot cause the disease, but that, as Rosenstein says, other concomitant features must be present in this as in so many other diseases.

Dickinson * found 22 cases of cirrhosis among 149 men whose occupation was concerned in some way with the handling of alcoholic beverages; among 149 men whose occupation did not involve constant association with alcoholic liquors he found the disease 8 times.

Charcot mentions cases of alcoholic cirrhosis in children (loc. cit.), Demme also describes such cases.

[R. Abrahams † has reported a case of alcoholic cirrhosis occurring in a baby of sixteen months, and Hermann Biggs ‡ one noted in a boy of thirteen years. The latter had taken whisky in small quantities over a period of two and one-half years. His liver weighed 1430 grams.—ED.]

The habitual abuse of wine and beer may also produce cirrhosis, although not so frequently as the abuse of distilled liquors; to this I can testify from my own observations. We can only form conjectures in regard to the exact manner in which alcohol acts. According to Weintraud,§ alcohol could not be found in the bile after experimental acute poisoning; and yet it is very probable that it is carried to the liver in the portal vein, the fact that the pathologic processes began in the periphery of the lobules speaking in favor of this view. The fact that no one has so far succeeded [vide editorial note following.—ED.] in producing experimental cirrhosis in animals by the administration of alcohol simply shows that the duration of the intoxication and the method of introducing the alcohol are not sufficiently similar to the conditions actually existing; it appears that in order to cause cirrhosis alcohol must be given continuously every day and in frequently repeated doses.

[Rosenfeld ‖ has carried out a series of experiments with reference to the influence of alcohol upon the liver. After reviewing the work already done upon this subject he states that he fed twice daily through a stomach-tube, to dogs that had been starved for six or seven days, 3.5 to 4 c.c. of 90 % alcohol in large quantities of water. The animals became intoxicated. The poisoning was continued as long as practicable and the animals were then killed before spontaneous death took place. The conclusions arrived at from the autopsies were that doses of 3.5 to 4 c.c. of alcohol per kilo of body-weight, when given more than four times daily, result in the deposition in the liver of more than 22 % fat. The amount in an unpoisoned animal was about 1 %. The livers of these animals were poor in glycogen, and in this way gave evidence that alcohol not only exerts an influence upon the albuminous portions of the cells, but also upon the carbohydrate retaining function. It was noted that the animals that were given a few large doses recovered if the alcohol were stopped. When smaller doses were given constantly, poisoning invariably resulted. Rosenfeld declines, however, to accept the results in animals as explaining all the observations in man.

Ramond ** has, however, produced typical alcoholic cirrhosis in animals by feeding with alcohol in combination with various toxic substances. His conclusions were that as a result of toxemia alone the liver degenerates but does not become sclerotic. He injected (1) alcohol; (2) toxins of bacillus coli; (3) other cultures of pathogenic micro-organisms, and (4) alcohol and the toxins together. The animals from (1) gave a picture of fatty degeneration after four months' feeding, but·no sclerosis; (2) after seven months gave no result, if small;

* Med. Chir. Trans., 1873, p. 27; cited by Charcot, p. 220.
† R. Abrahams, Pediatrics, Mar. 1, 1900.
‡ Biggs, N. Y. Med. Record, Sept. 3, 1890.   § Quoted by Stadelmann, page 105.
‖ Rosenfeld, Centralbl. f. inn. Med., Oct. 20, 1900.
** Ramond, La Presse Méd., April 21, 1897

when larger animals were used, fatty degeneration was noted, but no sclerosis. (3) Gave no result except septicemia. (4) After ten months gave atrophy of the hepatic cells, with a granular and pigmentary degeneration, and at certain points fibrous tracts were in the process of formation. These fibrous areas almost completely encircled one or more lobules.

Marckwald * has also carried out a series of experiments on the same line as the foregoing, but with small doses of antipyrin used subcutaneously, instead of alcohol. The frogs died of malnutrition and dropsy. The liver-cells (and kidneys) showed degeneration but no regenerative processes. In small, continued doses, the drug produced hepatic cirrhosis as a reactive process against the destructive process in the parenchyma. Injection of large doses led to acute destruction of hepatic tissue.—ED.]

We can only suggest, in the following general way, the different factors that lead to cirrhosis in individual cases: concentration of the alcohol, drinking on an empty stomach or a full stomach, taking it in one or in many doses in the day, irritation of the liver by excess of food, and individual predisposition.

The other possible ingredients of alcoholic beverages are also of importance in this connection. These are in part fermentative products, in part artificial additions, and vary with the nature of the drink, its manufacture, etc. Among them may be mentioned amyl alcohol, and other alcohols with a higher boiling-point than ordinary ethyl alcohol; also the aldehyds, and the natural and manufactured aromatic substances.

According to Allison,† sedentary habits predispose to the disease He found that in field-workers alcoholic cirrhosis was present in the proportion of 1 : 85; among city dwellers who led a sedentary life, 1 : 25; among city dwellers who indulged in much exercise, 1 : 42.

[A considerable number of undoubted cases of congenital hepatic cirrhosis have been reported in the literature. In some of these there has been discovered a syphilitic taint in the family history, and in many an antecedent history of alcoholism. In certain other cases neither condition has seemed to be present in the parents and the hepatic disease has remained unexplained. Among the most important cases are those reported by Rolleston and Hayne ("Brit. Med. Jour.," Mar. 30, 1901; no family history of syphilis), who note 59 other cases as on record; H. Neumann ("Berlin. klin. Woch.," Bd. xxx, p. 445; syphilitic family history); Parker, Dunbar and Fisher ("Lancet," Sept. 24, 1901; several cases); F. X. Walls ("Pediatrics," Mar. 15, 1902). There are many others.—ED.]

Syphilis ranks next in importance to alcohol. Not only does this disease lead to the formation of circumscribed or multiple foci of inflammation around gummata, that later are converted into connective tissue, but it also produces a diffuse form of interstitial hepatitis that is analogous to alcoholic cirrhosis. This form is found most frequently in children with congenital lues, not so often in adults. In the former it assumes the form of smooth cirrhosis, the so-called "Feuerstein" liver.

Where **malaria** is endemic, it frequently leads to cirrhosis of the liver; here, too, the duration of the primary disease and other concomitant circumstances exert their influence; in southern Italy, for instance, malarial cirrhosis is very frequent; in other parts of the world (Baltimore ‡), and the tropics,§ it is comparatively rare.

* Marckwald, *Münch. med. Woch.*, April 26, 1901.
† *Archiv. Gen. de Med.*, 1888, ii, p. 294.
‡ Osler, *Practice of Medicine*, p. 440.   § Hirsch, *Pathologie*, iii, p. 286.

Other possible, though not yet established, and in any event less frequent causes are: cholera, typhoid, and other infectious diseases (Botkin *), scarlatina (Osler) [Duckworth † has also reported a similar case.—ED.], gout, rachitis (Dickinson‡). The interstitial changes in the liver that occur in the course of these diseases appear clinically, as a rule, insignificant; this is also true of the more extensive forms of interstitial proliferation that are seen in miliary tuberculosis of the liver (see section on this disease and the complication of cirrhosis with peritoneal tuberculosis).

Chronic perihepatitis occasionally seems to extend to the interlobular tissues and in this manner to produce a pathologic picture similar to cirrhosis ₰; in other cases there is simply a capsular compression of the organ, and in this way indirectly the same result is accomplished (see "Zuckergussleber").

Talma, ‖ in particular, has emphasized the possibility of the development of hepatitis from peritonitis; this author, however, furnishes no positive proof of such an occurrence, simply assuming that the "causes" of the primary disease can be directly transferred to the peritoneal covering of the organ or can affect the liver through the lymph-channels.

It is said that other substances besides alcohol may be absorbed from the intestine and produce cirrhosis; among these are mentioned certain condiments (Curry, Budd), drastics (Cantani **), and lead.†† In view of the great prevalence of chronic alcoholism, the action of the poison can hardly ever be excluded, and it would appear likely that the other irritants named only aid in the production of cirrhosis.

Many of the French authors include diabetes among the causes of cirrhosis; in Germany we are inclined to regard the connection of the two diseases as a matter of chance, or, if anything, we reverse the order of cause and effect. Hanot claims that diabetic cirrhosis starts from the central venules "owing to the excessive quantity of sugar that passes through these channels" (! ?); Saundby ‡‡ claims to have seen moderate degrees of interstitial hepatitis in many (!) cases of diabetes.

Grawitz,§§ from an isolated observation, suspects the extended use of extractum filicis maris of a possible influence in the causation of cirrhosis.

Welch ‖‖ describes a case which he calls cirrhosis anthracotica, in which the liver was filled with a number of circumscribed round, oval, or elongated foci of sclerotic tissue that were colored black by deposits of carbon. Lancereaux *** has observed similar cases in copper smelters.

Sometimes several factors act together; for instance, malaria and whisky, syphilis and whisky, etc.

[Longridge ††† and others have called attention to a *focal necrosis* that is found in the hepatic substance in many toxemias. Heretofore these foci of necrotic tissue have been looked upon as lymphatic nodules, commonly found in typhoid fever, eclampsia, etc. Longridge also suggests that these foci by coalescing may produce the anatomic picture of acute yellow atrophy. He gives an elaborate histologic description of the necrotic areas. It appears at least possible that such conditions as

* Botkin, also Laure and Honorat, *Revue mens. de l'Enf.*, 1887; Siredey, *Rev. de Med.*, VI, 1886; Bourdillon, *Assoc. franç. p. l'avanc. des sci.*, 1891.
  † Duckworth "The Sequels of Disease," *Lancet*, April 4, 1896, p. 907.
  ‡ *Med. chir. Transactions*, LII, p. 359; *Schmidt's Jahrb*, Bd. CLIV, p. 284.
  § Frerich, "Leberkrankheiten," II, p. 92. Bassi, *Rev. clinica*, 1889.
  ‖ Talma, *Zeitschr. f. klin. Med.*, 1896, Bd. XXVII, p. 14.
  ** *Il Morgagni*, Luglio, 1890.
  †† Especially noted by French observers: Lafitte, *Thèse de Paris*, 1892, p. 71. Potain, *La Semaine Med.*, 1888, p. 230.
  ‡‡ Saundby, *The Lancet*, 1890, II, p. 383.   §§ *Berlin. klin. Woch.*, 1894, p. 1173.
  ‖‖ *Johns Hopkins Hosp. Bulletin*, 1891, No. 11; Yearly Report, II, p. 194.
  *** Lancereaux, *Union Mèdicale*, 1886.
  ††† Longridge, *Brit. Med. Jour.*, Sept. 21, 1901.

that noted by Welch, and many other conditions of localized and focal sclerosis, may be the result of just such an antecedent process as this focal necrosis, which, instead of going on to full degeneration, has passed on to cicatricial contraction and healing. In this process we may also have another source of chronic interstitial hepatitis.—Ed.]

There are a number of cases in which none of the causes mentioned can be made responsible. We must conclude, therefore, that other causes that are unknown to us may cause the disease; it seems probable that these are certain poisons that are absorbed from the intestine, particularly toxins of bacterial origin (Bouchard). Micro-organisms may lodge in the liver, and start the inflammatory process.

[Weaver * inoculated guinea-pigs with a bacillus, apparently of the colon group, obtained from the body of another guinea-pig dying from apparently natural conditions. In guinea-pigs inoculated subcutaneously and intraperitoneally with this bacillus there were found in one or two animals evidences of beginning fibrous change in the liver, and in one animal there was not only marked growth of connective tissue, but some bile-duct proliferation.

Adami † reported the finding in a certain number of cases of atrophic cirrhosis of the liver a minute micro-organism in the liver and abdominal lymphatic glands which closely resembled the organism found in infective cirrhosis of the liver in cattle. The same organism was also found in certain cases of hypertrophic cirrhosis. ·It is described as very minute, difficult to stain, and appearing as a small diplococcus which when grown in broth tended to assume a distinctly bacillary form. In a later communication in the same journal Adami reports the finding of this same poorly stained organism in the liver-cells within twenty-four hours after the injection of colon bacilli or of growths of this minute diplobacillus into the ear vein of rabbits. While Adami at first believed that in this finding he had an explanation of the occurrence of cirrhosis of the liver in the human being, he later modified his views after finding that there could be almost always found in non-cirrhotic livers the same organism, although in smaller number than in those with distinct sclerotic change. In a later communication ‡ he still further emphasized the view that this supposedly new variety of micro-organism was simply a changed form of colon bacillus. While the original apparent importance of the finding has been somewhat diminished by Adami's further researches, his discovery is by no means without interest, although it cannot at the present time be determined whether the excess in the numbers of this bacillus has any etiologic relation to the anatomic change in the liver. The finding of the diplococcus form of the colon bacillus in cirrhosis of the liver has, however, a considerable bearing upon the bactericidal function of this organ. In marked cases of cirrhosis of the liver this form of the colon bacillus is found in larger number and possesses greater staining capacity than in the normal organ. In addition to this, Adami found that on injecting into the ear vein of rabbits either colon bacilli (the ordinary form) or cultures of the diplococcus formerly described by him, these organisms were found in large numbers in the liver-cells, while the bile of the animal remained sterile. The two

---

* "Contributions to the Science of Medicine"; Dedicated to Professor Welch, 1900, p. 297.
† *Montreal Med. Jour.*, July, 1898, p. 485.
‡ "Trans. Assoc. Amer. Phys.," 1899, vol. xiv, p. 300.

facts taken together certainly point to a marked bactericidal function possessed by the hepatic cells.—ED.]

Many of the French authors also speak of the cirrhosis of dyspeptics.*

Alcoholism is so wide-spread, however, that it will be necessary to analyze carefully each individual case before accepting dyspepsia as the only cause of the disease. It is possible that morbid products of digestion act deleteriously in combination with alcohol, or that the alcohol promotes the formation of these morbid products.

[Reference should also be made to *malignant growths* as a cause of hepatic cirrhosis. W. W. Ford,† among others, reports a case of sarcoma of the liver, in which the liver showed a marked cirrhotic change. No cause was evident other than the malignant growth. A number of cases of the same condition (cirrhosis) associated with cancer of the liver were reported and discussed in a symposium before the Pathologic Society of London.‡ In a number of these cases, also, there was no cause evident other than the carcinomatous change.—ED.]

As in all other diseases, **individual predisposition** is an important factor.

Sometimes several brothers and sisters are afflicted (Staples,§ "children of a drunkard"). In a case of this kind that came under my own observation both brothers were drinkers. [Hasenclever ‖ reports three cases of hypertrophic cirrhosis of the liver of the type described by Hanot, in three children of the same family, probably the subjects of congenital syphilis.—ED.]

General Outline of the Disease.—The first stages of a chronic inflammation of the liver which ultimately lead to cirrhosis produce no symptoms for a number of years. In a small number of cases the signs of active hyperemia are found during this period, with a feeling of pressure in the right hypochondrium, tenderness and enlargement of the liver, sometimes gastric disturbances, fever, and icterus. These symptoms seem to appear in attacks of short duration; they are vague, and by no means characteristic. As a rule, the shrinking and contraction of the tissues are well advanced by the time typical symptoms appear. These are seen in the organs in the area of the portal system, and affect the general health; they include disturbance of the appetite and of the digestion, a feeling of pressure in the epigastrium, and bloating from ascites. As ascites often replaces a previously fat abdomen the general emaciation is often not perceived by the patient; the skin grows grayish in color, finally light yellow; the liver will now be found decreased in size, and the spleen enlarged.

In alcoholic cirrhosis the effects of the general intoxication are often seen in other organs besides the liver: viz., the heart and the kidneys. When this is not the case, the cachexia gradually increases and certain mechanical disturbances of respiration, circulation, and digestion follow the further development of ascites. As a rule, the patient succumbs to these disorders within a few months after the appearance of the first serious symptoms; in other cases hematemesis, intestinal hemorrhage, violent diarrhea, or an acute organic disease brings on a fatal termination at a still earlier period.

Pathologic Anatomy.—A cirrhotic liver is, as a rule, decidedly

* Boix, Thèse de Paris, 1894.   † *Amer. Jour. Med. Sci.*, Oct., 1900. p. 413.
‡ "Transactions," *Lancet*, Jan. 19, 1901.   § Staples, *Lancet*, May, 1886.
‖ *Berliner klin. Woch.*, Nov. 7, 1898.

smaller than normal; this is particularly true of the left lobe. The surface presents round protuberances that are as large as a millet-seed or a pea; these are usually covered by a thickened layer of serosa, and consequently do not show their peculiar color so well on the surface of the organ as on cross-section, when they vary in color from light yellow to greenish-yellow and brown. They are separated from one another by a reticulum of whitish or reddish-gray connective tissue, the meshes and the single strands of which vary greatly in size. From these meshes single granules protrude. On microscopic examination it will be found that each granule corresponds to one or several hepatic lobules. The size of these lobules is markedly reduced and their typical structure changed as a result of the arrangement of the vessels. In some livers the lobules will be found to be of about equal size, in others of different sizes (monolobular and multilobular cirrhosis). Occasionally single lobules appear to be subdivided; they are sometimes outlined clearly against the connective tissue, and again their boundaries are indistinct. The hepatic cells under these conditions may be infiltrated either with fat, with bile-pigment, or some other brownish pigment; some show no changes except that they vary in size. Certain of the capillaries of the lobules are dilated.

The connective tissue is principally fibrous, though in places a great many cells are seen and are to be traced here and there between the columns of liver-cells.

According to Frerichs, and of late Hohenemser,* elastic fibers are always present in this connective tissue (demonstrable by orcein). The more advanced the constriction, the more conspicuous these fibers. They may, in fact, constitute the greater portion of the connective tissue. It is probable that they originate from the sheaths of the smaller arteries and portal branches.

[Flexner † has published some very thorough studies in regard to the nature and distribution of the new tissue formation in cirrhosis of the liver. He concludes that (1) in all forms of cirrhosis the white fibrous tissue is increased. (2) Along with this new tissue there is formed elastic tissue which is derived from preexisting elastic fibers in the blood-vessels and hepatic cells. (3) Both forms of tissue may in all kinds of cirrhosis penetrate into the lobules. This penetration takes place along the line of the capillary walls and follows the architecture of the reticulum. The chief distinction between the histology of atrophic and hypertrophic cirrhosis depends on the degree of extralobular growth, and the freedom with which the lobules are invaded. In the hypertrophic form there would appear to be less interlobular growth and an earlier and finer intralobular growth. (4) Alterations in the reticulum *per se* seem to constitute a hypertrophy rather than a hyperplasia of fibers.—ED.]

Within the connective tissue we see numerous tortuous bile-ducts, arranged in a ramifying network; their lumen varies markedly in size, and the cells lining them are either cuboid, or flat, or resemble liver-cells. Their connection with the bile-passages can be demonstrated by injection; they constitute in part efferent channels of liver lobules that have perished, and in part represent genuine new-formations.

The blood-vessels that are formed in the new tissue are numerous, patulous, thin-walled, and resemble erectile tissue. By injection it can be shown that they belong to the system of the hepatic artery, and are

* *Virchow's Archiv*, 1895, Bd. CXL, p. 193.
† *Univ. of Penna. Med. Mag.*, Nov., 1900.

not related, or but distantly related, to the portal system.* The inter-lobular branches of the portal vein show a thickening of their walls, and occasionally endophlebitis obliterans.

Rather less frequently than the granular liver is occasionally seen the atrophic cirrhotic liver with a smooth or almost smooth surface. The capsule of the organ is thickened, and has a reddish-gray color with a tinge of yellow. Although differing macroscopically from the granular form on the outside, this variety will be found to show the same micro-scopic changes; the difference consists simply in a more uniform prolifera-tion of the connective tissue, so that the lobules or groups of lobules are not isolated. There are all intermediate stages between these two forms, from the smooth and finely granular to the coarsely granular liver with the irregular surface.

This atrophy of the liver with proliferation of connective tissue is the final stage in a process of many years' duration. Not only in its initial stages, but even in more advanced periods, the process produces only very slight disturbances, so that the anatomy of the early stages can only be studied in individuals who have died of some other disease. I agree, however, with Leichtenstern in saying that the opportunity to study this stage frequently occurs, and especially in Kiel. The inter-lobular connective-tissue changes may be overlooked macroscopically, and the only manifestation of their presence may be hardness of the organ; they are often determined for the first time by the microscope.

The connective-tissue proliferation is first seen in the region of the portal branches either in regular distribution or particularly developed in certain interstices, so that later on either whole lobules or groups of lobules are inclosed within the strands of connective tissue (*monolobular and multilobular cirrhosis*). This form of cirrhosis is called *venous* by French authors, on account of its origin in the venous branches of the portal vein (in contradistinction to biliary). According to Sabourin, the proliferation often starts simultaneously from the portal and the central venules; such forms are called *bivenous cirrhoses*. In this form also proliferation may occur into the lobule and cause a splitting of the latter in such a manner that the different nodules often consist of portions of one lobule. In rare cases Sabourin claims that the central veins of the lobules may, even in cases of alcoholic origin, be the only starting-point of the cirrhotic process; there is then often combined with the latter a fatty degeneration of the liver.

According to Aufrecht, no increase of connective tissue occurs in atrophic cir-rhosis; he claims that the disease is primarily one of the liver-cells; and that these undergo atrophic changes, and are converted into narrow spindles that contain no nuclei. [*Vide* foregoing editorial note quoting Flexner's studies.—ED.]

I am not inclined to believe that the proliferation of connective tissue *per se* causes an increase in the size of the liver, because of the physiologic fluctuation in the size of the organ, and because of the influence, par-ticularly in drunkards, which fatty infiltration and hyperemia (active and passive) exert upon its volume. These very factors help greatly to determine the size and the color of the organ also in the later stages of the disease.

Owing to the progressive proliferation of connective tissue in the vicinity of the interlobular portal branches, the blood-supply of the lobules is interfered with; at the same time, these structures are con-stricted by the contracting tissues. In this manner atrophy of the cells and partial obliteration of the capillaries are brought about. The dis-appearance of the cells is often preceded by changes in their protoplasm, especially by fatty degeneration; these changes are in part passive

* Frerichs, Atlas ii, Taf. iii.

(necrobiotic), in part active, produced directly by the action of the morbid agency.

Partial regeneration of the liver tissues, it appears, may occur in spite of and alongside of all these changes. This is most pronounced in the adenomatous nodules that are often seen in cirrhotic livers. These are as large as lentils or hazelnuts, yellowish-gray in color, and consist of liver-cells. The cells are arranged in columns, as in the lobules; with this difference, however, that the rows are broader, and the individual cells are unequal in size. Some are very large, with enormous, multiple nuclei. These adenomata resemble active neoplasms; and are sharply outlined against the surrounding tissues; they are often very numerous, and have a tendency to fatty degeneration. They are not found in cirrhosis of the liver alone, but occur so frequently that a relationship between the two conditions must be assumed. They are probably the expression of some tendency to regeneration. The large hypertrophic nodules that are occasionally seen within the liver tissues in cirrhosis probably belong to the same class (Sabourin, Kelsch, Kiener, Pennato).

As a result of the destruction of so many of the capillaries of the lobules, the total lumen of the blood-vessels within the organ is reduced, and we see, as a result, the effects of portal stasis; the great overdevelopment of the capillaries of the hepatic artery cannot compensate this defect. At the same time the contracting connective tissue may occlude some of the larger branches of the portal vein, or capillaries may be occluded here and there by the pressure of swollen neighboring liver-cells. The portal vein itself is dilated as far up as its bifurcation and the starting-point of its first branches; its walls are thickened by an overgrowth of endothelial tissue as a result of endophlebitis and periphlebitis. We will discuss the effect of these changes when speaking of the general symptoms of cirrhosis. They first become evident, in many instances, at a late stage of the disease, so that granular atrophy of the liver may be found incidentally during an autopsy on a case that has died of some altogether independent condition.

Symptomatology.—*Prodromal Symptoms.*—The initial stage of chronic hepatitis usually runs its course without causing any symptoms; when they do appear, they are, as a rule, the manifestation of some accompanying disease, as, for instance, gastro-intestinal catarrh in drunkards, evidenced by loss of appetite, symptoms of pressure in the stomach-region, diarrhea, etc. The feeling of fulness in the epigastrium and the right hypochondrium is increased particularly after eating, in cases in which the liver is enlarged, or in which there is general adiposity of the abdomen, as a result of fatty infiltration. Occasional brief attacks of pain in the liver are due to transient digestive hyperemia. These may even be accompanied by fever, swelling, and pain that may persist for several days.

Liver.—In subjects that are later afflicted with cirrhosis, the liver will often be found enlarged for years before. As we have said, this is not so much due to the connective-tissue hyperplasia as to other circumstances, such as fatty infiltration, fluxionary or stasis hyperemia. The enlarged organ is more resistant than normal and more readily palpable, also more sensitive.

The enlargement in these cases is not characteristic of the disease and not different from other forms. Borelli * claims that the upper boundary is forced upward partly as the result of meteorism, and partly owing to paresis of the diaphragm following perihepatitis.

* *Verhandlungen der phys. med. Gesellsch. z. Würzburg*, Neue Folge, Bd. VIII, 1875, p. 87.

A decrease in the size of the organ is more difficult to determine than an enlargement. The proof of the former is the disappearance of the lower boundary into the cupola of the diaphragm. This is no positive criterion, for meteorism may produce the same effect; emphysema of the lungs may also aid in decreasing the area of dulness of the whole organ; on the other hand, adhesions may prevent the movement of the lower margin upward. Early atrophy of the left lobe is important and significant; if this occurs, the presence of the left lobe in the epigastrium can no longer be determined. As a rule, the study of the size of the organ is performed by percussion, and it may happen that in cirrhosis there is no hepatic dulness whatsoever in the mammillary line. Palpation, for reasons mentioned, is often impossible in cirrhosis; in certain other cases the nodules can be distinctly felt and the margin distinctly palpated.

If perihepatitis exists, friction sounds can be felt and heard. At the same time, there may be local tenderness, while the other subjective symptoms in the hepatic region have disappeared; particularly during the period of contraction.

Icterus is not a typical symptom of atrophic cirrhosis. In many cases it is altogether absent, in others present to a slight degree; conspicuous jaundice is rare, and usually points to some complication in the bile-passages.

The results of the disease of the liver are: (1) Disturbances in the circulation of the portal system; (2) reduced functional activity of the atrophying gland; (3) secondary results of these two disturbances.

The **circulatory disturbances** are the most conspicuous. As compression of the portal capillaries takes place, stasis of blood results throughout the portal area, and leads to congestion of the spleen and the intestinal tract. This may be favored by the absence of valves in the portal veins. The most conspicuous, though at the same time one of the latest symptoms, is ascites. Hyperemia from stasis of the gastric and intestinal mucosa is seen at a much earlier stage and produces functional disorders of these organs; even in the absence of alcoholism, lack of appetite, oppression after eating, etc., may occur. Sometimes diarrhea relieves the congested capillaries, or atony exists with constipation or meteorism. Venous hyperemia seems to lead to a reduction of the normal secretions as well as to a lessening of the peristaltic activity, and absorbing power of the intestine.

Fr. Müller, even in the presence of ascites, failed to find the absorption of the ingesta reduced; fat resorption, too, was normal, so that sufficient bile entered the intestine; if diarrhea was present, and as a result water absorption was reduced, the assimilative power was also diminished.

Other authors, however, disagree with this statement; Fawitzky (discussion of the older literature) finds that nitrogenous material is poorly absorbed (in one case 13.8 % of the ingested nitrogen in the stools); Münzer, on the other hand, calls attention to the relatively small amount of urinary nitrogen (61 %); it seems, therefore, that in serious cases 26.9 % of nitrogen is retained (!?). Münzer regained only 58 % of the nitrogen from the urine.

Hemorrhoidal tendencies should be increased by stasis in the portal system, but are not very troublesome in this disease.

Portal stasis produces induration and swelling of the **spleen.** The former or latter condition may predominate; if the first is present, however, the second cannot fully develop. According to Frerichs and H.

* *Verhandlungen des Congresses für. inn. Med.*, 1887, p. 408.

Lange, enlargement of the spleen is seen in one-half of the cases; according to Bamberger, in nine-tenths.

It seems doubtful whether the enlargement of the spleen is due to stasis alone; for the spleen in the congestion of cardiac disease has a different appearance, is more solid, is darker, and not so large as in cirrhosis. In the latter disease swelling of the spleen appears very early, before other symptoms of stasis, and a hyperplastic condition of the pulp followed by a connective-tissue increase are noted (Oestreich). It appears, therefore, that active processes occur also in the spleen and vary with the primary cause of the disease. In malaria and syphilis the direct influence is known. It is also probable that in different subjects the spleen may show variations in its elasticity, so that it responds to congestion in a varying manner.

Bouchard and Leudet* have reported systolic blowing over the spleen similar to the placental murmur.

Ascites is one of the late symptoms of the disease, although the serous lining of the intestine probably is congested very early in the disease, and may cause an increased exudation of fluid into the peritoneal cavity. This exudate is, however, reabsorbed by the lymphatics of the diaphragm and the parietal peritoneum, which are independent of the portal system†; for this reason ascites appears only when the exudate is so massive that these channels grow insufficient.

As a rule, the liver is contracted at the time of the appearance of ascites, but this is not always the case; it is sometimes enlarged. This may be due to complications (stasis, fatty infiltration), or enlarged liver-cells may exercise pressure upon the portal capillaries.

Slight degrees of ascites cause no trouble; occasionally the physician will be surprised to find a considerable degree of ascites, and particularly in patients who have habitually a large, obese abdomen.

Less often ascites appears suddenly after some injury, as a cold in the abdomen (Potain).‡ The fluid is freely movable, the intestine pressed against the spinal column, and, as a result, a tympanitic sound is only perceptible on deep percussion.

The fluid is generally of a clear yellow color, specific gravity **1012 to 1014**, and contains albumin 0.6 % to 1.2 %. Bile-pigment and sugar are rare; sometimes a little blood will be found as a result of the congestion. Sometimes the latter condition will cause a subacute peritonitis, that may be hemorrhagic in type; in such cases the fluid is heavier, coagulates more readily, contains more albumin, and possibly some blood.

[Barjon and Henry§ regard hemorrhagic pleural and peritoneal effusions as rare occurrences in hepatic cirrhosis. They report four cases that have come under their observation. Two cases presented both hemorrhagic pleurisy and ascites.—ED.]

As in the case of other forms of ascites, edema of the lower extremities and a reduction of the urinary excretion follow the compression of the veins of the lower half of the body. In severe degrees the diaphragm is pressed upward, and respiration and heart action are impeded. If

*Revue de méd., 1890. p. 868.
† Quincke, "Ascites," Deutsches Archiv für klin. Med., 1882, Bd. xxx.
‡ Semaine Méd., 1888, p. 9.   § Lyon Médicale, June 19, 1890.

PLATE IV.

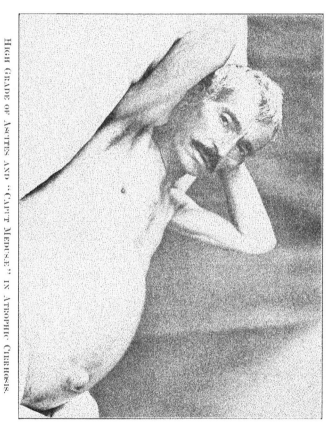

HIGH GRADE OF ASCITES AND "CAPUT MEDUSÆ" IN ATROPHIC CIRRHOSIS.

نزن
ن

ascites develops during the course of uncomplicated (!) cirrhosis, it rarely disappears.

MacDonald * reports two such cases in which ascites disappeared after 31 and 60 punctures respectively; Casati † performed puncture 111 times. [Cheadle, in his Lumleian lectures (1900), mentions a case that lived eight years from the onset of the cirrhosis with ascites. He was tapped 19 times, the last time eight years before death. Another case was still living twelve years after first coming under observation. The last tapping was done two years before the report was made.—ED.]

If stasis is very severe, the capillaries of the stomach and intestine may burst and cause vomiting of blood and the passage of blood in the stools; it may be that occasionally a gastric ulcer will develop from hemorrhagic erosion of the gastric mucosa.

As a result of the increase of pressure in the portal system, the **collateral veins** are enlarged, *e. g.*, the hemorrhoidal vein ‡ leading to the hypogastric vein; the inferior esophageal veins that anastomose, on the one hand, with the vena corona ventriculi, and, on the other, with the vena azygos; also the vessels running in the ligamentum hepatis, and in the perihepatic tissue (these are newly formed vessels). The latter form a direct connection between the liver and the diaphragm. Within the ligamentum teres a vein of some 1 to 6 mm. in diameter establishes a connection between the portal system and the veins of the abdominal wall; a part of the portal blood escapes through this channel and empties itself into the upper epigastric veins. As a result the subcutaneous vessels of the abdominal wall in the vicinity of the navel are dilated and can be distinctly seen; at the same time the skin becomes slightly edematous.

The shape and the caliber of these dilatations vary greatly; in rare cases only is the fantastic name *caput medusæ* justified. The radiating group of blood-vessels around the umbilicus must not be confounded with the network of dilated vessels that connect the superior and inferior epigastric veins, and that are seen in every form of ascites (even though not of portal origin), and that constitute collaterals of the compressed inferior cava.

Some authors consider the vein in the ligamentum teres as a rudiment of the umbilical vein (Bamberger,§ Hoffman,‖ Baumgarten**; others regard it as a paraumbilical vein entering into it, or as an accessory portal vein.

It can be shown by compression that the blood flows from the navel in the umbilical garland of vessels; sometimes a murmur can be felt and heard in these vessels (Bamberger,†† *loc. cit.*, page 519). Von Jacksch ‡‡ heard and felt a buzzing sound between the umbilicus and the xyphoid process, which, as the autopsy showed, probably originated in the dilated vena coronaria ventriculi.

Leyden observed that the ductus Arantii had remained patulous in one case; Drummond,§§ in another instance, saw a communication between the paraumbilical vein through an abdominal vein with the right iliac vein.

Although these veins all help divert the portal blood, they are not capable (compare an Eck fistula) of carrying off all the surplus and of reestablishing a normal vascularity, and in this manner removing the

* *Med. News*, Oct., 1889; "Jahresbericht," ii, p. 297.
† *Il raccoglitore medico*, Aug. 20, 1893.
‡ Z. B. Drummond, *Brit. Med. Jour.*, Feb., 1881; and "Jahresbericht," ii, p. 289.
§ "Krankheiten des chylopoetischen Systems," p. 520.
‖ *Correspondenzbl. f. Schweizer Aerzte*, 1872.
** *Bull. de l'Acad. de Soc. Med.*, 1859, t. xxiv, p. 943.
†† Koppel, Dissertation, Marburg, 1885.   ‡‡ Jaksch, *Prager med. Woch.*, 1895.
§§ Drummond, *Brit. Med. Jour.*, Feb. 4, 1888.

ascites.* Whenever this occurs, we must assume that the liver itself has become more passable to fluid.

Occasionally, profuse, fatal hemorrhage occurs from the dilated esophageal veins; the blood is in such cases poured into the stomach (compare page 707).

[Preble† has analyzed 60 cases of fatal *gastro-intestinal hemorrhage* in cirrhosis of the liver. He concludes that it is infrequent but not rare; that in the majority of cases the cirrhosis is atrophic, but may be hypertrophic; that in one-third of the cases the first hemorrhage is fatal, but that in the remainder the hemorrhages may continue at intervals for a long period; that esophageal varices are present in 80 %, and that in more than half of these macroscopic ruptures are present; that in certain cases fatal hemorrhage can occur without esophageal varices, and that in only 60 % of the cases with esophageal varices was the cirrhosis accompanied by typical symptoms and signs. He reports four new cases. Curschmann also notes in detail a case of fatal hematemesis in the same condition,‡ and mentions 13 fatal cases observed by him.

E. Stein § cites cases of *intestinal hemorrhage.* Mannesse,‖ Lubet-Barbon,** Ewald,†† and many others have noted cases of fatal hemorrhage from *dilated and ruptured esophageal and laryngeal veins.*—ED.]

It is stated that the congestion may be transmitted to the vena azygos and the intercostal vein, and in this manner cause right-sided hydrothorax§§ [Cheadle, Barjon and Henry, and others have called attention to the frequency of right-sided pleural effusion in hepatic cirrhosis. It rarely occurs in sufficient quantity to cause trouble. Villain‖‖ has observed 9 such cases in which the diagnosis was confirmed by puncture.—ED.]

The *urine* in cirrhosis of the liver is usually scanty, of a high specific gravity, and of a reddish color. The decrease in quantity is due to deficient absorption of fluid from the intestine and to accumulation of water in the belly during ascites. At the same time, the kidneys are compressed, and, when cachexia supervenes, the arterial pressure is lowered.

Albuminuria may be due to alcoholic nephritis, hematuria to hyperemia of the bladder (Langenbeck).*** The reddish color is in part due to urobilin; icterus is rarely so severe as to cause the appearance of bile-pigment.

G. Hoppe-Seyler ††† found an increase in the urobilin excretion to 0.24 and 0.3 in two cases of cirrhosis (instead of the normal 0.123). In some cases the increase is only apparent, owing to the decreased secretion of urine. Von Noorden's conclusion that a cirrhotic liver forms abundant quantities of bile-pigment does not appear justified to me. Changes in normal intestinal absorption and other circumstances may very well lead to an increase of the urobilin excretion.

Urea is generally reduced, ammonia increased, and sugar is sometimes present. We will discuss the significance of these findings in our paragraphs on metabolism.

* Monneret, quoted by Frerichs, "Leberkrankheiten," II, p. 40; Pel, *Neederl. Tijdschr. f. Geneesk.,* 1882; "Jahresbericht," II, p. 174.
† *Amer. Jour. Med. Sci.,* Mar., 1900, p. 263.
‡ *Deutsche med. Woch.,* April 17, 1902.
§ *Archiv. f. Verdauungskr.,* May 6, 1899.   ‖ *Gaz. hebd. de med.,* Jan., 1899.
** *Archiv. de Laryngol.,* July–Aug., 1897.
†† *Berlin. klin. Woch.,* 1892, No. 23.
§§ Piazza-Martini, *Rev. clinica,* June 30, 1892; "Jahresbericht," II, p. 195.
‖‖ *Riforma Med,* 1895.   *** *Archiv. f. klin. Chirurgie,* Bd. I, p. 41.
††† G. Hoppe-Seyler, *Virchow's Archiv,* 1890, Bd. CXXIV, p. 43.

Sometimes "peptones" [albumoses—Ed.] are found in the urine (Stadelmann, Bouchard), also leucin and tyrosin (?), sarcolactic acid (v. Noorden, Stadelmann), and abnormal amounts of volatile fatty acids (v. Jaksch).*

Respiration is greatly impeded as ascites increases; this is due to obstruction of the movements of the diaphragm, and to the deposit of fat in the abdominal walls, and the mediastinum. The heart action, also, is mechanically impeded in ascites; in addition, the heart muscle is weakened by the alcohol and the cachexia. The pulse, therefore, grows small and rapid, the breathing shallow and labored, and there is a subjective sensation of oppression.

Hypertrophy of the left ventricle, as Wagner † says, is due to narrowing of the arteries in the liver; its cause is analogous to that in contraction of the kidneys. As a matter of fact, the arteries are not reduced in size in the liver; and the condition is due to other causes, alcohol, etc.

The temperature shows no abnormal fluctuations, or at most they are insignificant; fever, if present, is due to inflammatory complications (perihepatitis); in the final stages the temperature may be subnormal.‡ [Carrington§ discusses the question of pyrexia in cirrhosis of the liver and concludes that there may be a range of temperature from 100° to 102.5° F. —Ed.]

The **general nutrition and health** of the patient are greatly impaired. Unless malaria or alcoholic catarrh of the stomach is present, the cachexia may not appear until late in the disease; *i. e.*, at the time of contraction. The patients look sallow and flabby, the general muscular and vascular tone is reduced, though, at the same time, they may be obese; soon the fat disappears, however, and an emaciation sets in that may be disguised by edema and ascites.

The emaciation may be explained in part by the deficient nourishment, and the interference with the absorption of food. At the same time, the cirrhotic changes of the liver cause certain metabolic disturbances that also play a rôle. These disturbances would be greater than they usually are in view of the great destruction of liver tissue, if the shrinkage did not occur so gradually that the organism becomes to a certain degree accustomed to it.

The chief manifestation of this perversion of metabolism is the decreased excretion of urea and the increased excretion of ammonia; this was first noticed by Hallervorden, later by Stadelmann, Favitsky, and others. It appears that the urea-forming power of the liver is still present to a surprising degree, even in advanced stages of atrophy, for large quantities of ammonia salts are, under these circumstances, converted into urea.

According to v. Noorden, the normal ammonia of the urine is 2 % to 5 %, according to Weintraud 3 % to 5 %, an average of 4.1 % of the total nitrogen. In cirrhosis as much as 10 % of the total nitrogen passes as ammonia, and the absolute quantity of ammonia in twenty-four hours may be 1.4 to 2.5 gm., according to Hallervorden. In less advanced cases this increase may be absent (Stadelmann). It is interesting from a theoretic point of view that, according to Weintraud, a person with cirrhosis is capable of transforming as large quantities of ammonia (administered as the citrate) as a healthy person, so that the proportion of ammonia-

Zeitschr. f. physiol. Chemie, Bd. x.   † *Archiv. de Heilkunde*, Bd. iii, p. 459.
‡ Janssen, *Deutsche Archiv. f. klin. Med.*, 1894, Bd. liii.
§ "Guy's Hosp. Reports," 1884.

nitrogen to total nitrogen is not increased. In the agonal period this power seems to be lost. The remnant of liver tissue, therefore, seems to retain the power of forming urea; it is even possible that death occurs as soon as this function grows insufficient. [It must be recalled, however, that recent experiments have proved conclusively that urea formation is to a large extent the function of other tissues than the liver. The muscles seem especially active in this direction.—ED.] Some facts point to the possibility that the great amount of ammonia excreted is the result of excessive acid formation (as in diabetes). Von Jaksch* found the alkalinity of the blood reduced, and discovered volatile fatty acids in the blood†; Stadelmann, v. Noorden, and Weintraud discovered sarcolactic acid in the urine of cirrhotics.

Chauffard observed a great increase in the urea excretion (40 to 50 gm. *pro die*) at the period of the initial congestion.

Sugar is occasionally voided in cirrhosis, though not as a rule. It may appear in as large quantities and as constantly as in a case observed by the author (100 gm.); as a rule, this occurs only after the ingestion of large quantities of sugar. The explanation must be sought for in the inability of the liver to store large amounts of sugar as glycogen; besides, a portion of the portal blood containing sugar does not go through the liver, but enters the systemic circulation through collateral branches.

[In cirrhosis many liver-cells retain their reserve of glycogen intact, and renew this reserve even when isolated. Cells may be separated into groups (as shown by Brault ‡) or isolated by disease, but the trabeculæ do not destroy the histochemical properties of the cells with which they come in contact, and especially is their glycogenic function retained. This glycogen integrity suggests a retention of other functional activities, and thus confirms histologic evidences of persistent hepatic capacity despite considerable cirrhosis. This explains the latent period of cirrhosis to a certain extent, and also those cases in which a respite from symptoms occurs. It also demonstrates the possibility of cure, and also of living with a functionally active though anatomically cirrhotic liver.—ED.]

French authors are inclined to attach a certain diagnostic significance to the occasional occurrence of alimentary glycosuria following a moderate ingestion of carbohydrates.

Couturier made the first statement of this kind after Cl. Bernard had produced alimentary glycosuria in a dog by gradual obliteration of the portal vein. As the normal boundary for sugar assimilation fluctuates markedly (between 100 and 250 gm.), it is not surprising to find differences in the excretion of sugar in a series of determinations made even by the same author. German authors (Frerichs, the author, Kraus and Ludwig, Bloch, v. Noorden) all arrive at negative conclusions.

In certain rare cases sugar was constantly excreted even if an ordinary diet was given; these possibly were real cases of glycosuria, or even of diabetes mellitus (Quincke, Palma). In my case 4 % to 6 % of sugar was excreted daily, although the total quantity of the urine was normal. Finally, both the sugar and the total quantity were decreased, and in the last weeks before death the sugar was no longer determinable. In another case, a drunkard who clinically showed symptoms of contracted kidney, I observed glycosuria (0.2 %); here, too, the sugar disappeared in the last weeks.

Pusinelli observed a diabetic for eight years; in the beginning the liver was enlarged, but ultimately became atrophic and cirrhotic. In this case two years before death ascites was noticed for several months, and during the persistence of this condition the sugar excretion ceased; as soon as the ascites was relieved the sugar reappeared. It is impossible to explain the connection between glycosuria and ascites in this case.

*v. Jaksch, *Zeitschr. klin. Med.*, 1888, Bd. XIII, p. 350.
†v. Jaksch, *Zeitschr. f. phys. Chemie*, 1886, Bd. x, p. 553.
‡*Presse Médicale*, May 29, 1901.

[Lefas * has studied the relations of the pancreas and the liver in cirrhosis of the latter organs, and has drawn some highly interesting conclusions. In atrophic cirrhosis of the liver he. found the pancreas increased in size, with relative atrophy of the head and body. The color was yellowish-gray, and the organ appeared somewhat waxy. Its density was increased. The cirrhotic process, he found, might affect part only, or the entire organ. When the process was intense, he found proliferation of connective tissue around the vessels, with changes in the walls of the latter, and a tendency to form fibrous plaques externally. Fatty degeneration of the organ was a frequent condition. Pigmentary degeneration was rare.—Ed.]

· The appearance of ammonia and of sugar does not indicate the entire disturbance of metabolism caused by the destruction of so much of the liver tissue; sometimes, toward the end of the disease, we see serious nervous disturbances, stupor, or delirium. These symptoms recall the picture of hepatargy following icterus from stasis and the last stages of acute atrophy; they are symptoms of an autointoxication. They appear as soon as compensation for the disturbances of metabolism fails. They may be seen in the absence of jaundice, or when very slight degrees of icterus only are present; so that they cannot be attributed to retention of bile-constituents. They must be due to other products of metabolism that are no longer utilized by the liver. It is possible that carbaminic acid, a substance closely related to ammonia, or that abnormally formed acids play an important rôle.

Hemorrhages are also to be regarded as the result of general disturbances of nutrition; they may occur in the last stages of cirrhosis (without icterus), and are seen not only in the area of stasis, but in other parts of the body; as petechiæ of the skin, the retina, the subcutaneous tissues, the surface of the nasal, pulmonary, and urinary passages, and hemorrhagic exudates into the pleural and peritoneal cavities. They are not so frequent in this condition as in hypertrophic cirrhosis. Death may result from violent epistaxis.

Certain dyscrasias may be made responsible for some of the hemorrhages in the portal area in addition to the purely mechanical factors (hemorrhages into the mucosa of the stomach and intestine and into inflammatory peritoneal exudates). At a rule, the bleeding is capillary, and in the case of the stomach it may lead to ulceration. Hematemesis in cirrhotics is usually due to rupture of esophageal veins (Litten); it appears suddenly without any premonitory gastric symptoms. In gastric ulcer such prodromata are generally present. Sometimes hemorrhage relieves by disgorging the portal system; in the majority of cases, however, it leads to the death of the patient.

Among 56 cases of cirrhosis Lange found hemorrhages 10 times (18 %) (stomach, esophagus, air-passages, and serous cavities); 37 % of these occurred in advanced cases, and not one case occurred in the beginning of the disease.

Leichtenstern mentions cases in which the clinical picture of gastric hemorrhage with severe anemia was simulated, and in which (possibly as a result of the many hemorrhages) neither ascites nor swelling of the spleen developed.

[E. Stein † reports a case of cirrhosis of the liver of which repeated

---

* *Archiv. gen. de med.*, May, 1900.
† *Arch. f. Verdauungs-krankheit.*, Bd. v, Heft 1.

hemorrhage from the bowel was the chief symptom and was the cause of death.   H. Curschmann * notes 13 fatal cases of hemorrhage from varices, from the digestive tract, etc.. Webber † reports a case with repeated epistaxis, hemorrhage from the ears, spongy and bleeding gums, and long-continued irregular temperature. Lubet-Barbon ‡ cites a case of hemorrhage from the larynx, and Ewald, Mannesse, and Müller all cases of fatality from the bleeding of esophageal varices.

Carrington ₰ has shown that the course of the disease may be alto-gether *afebrile*. The temperature may, however, rise as high as 100° to 102.5° F., though it never reaches a point that could be called hyperpy-rexia. *Increased frequency of the pulse and diminished arterial tension* have been found in cirrhosis of the liver by Gilbert and Garnier.‖   They attri-bute at least some of the lowering of pressure to portal obstruction, as they had found a corresponding decrease in blood-pressure on ligating the portal vein.—ED.]

Sometimes diseases of the interior of the eye follow cirrhosis of the liver, retinitis pigmentosa and choroiditis atrophicans **; certain authors have attempted to find anatomic analogies between these lesions and the cirrhosis of the liver.

[Hayem †† has found diminution or absence of hydrochloric acid in the gastric secretion in atrophic cirrhosis, whereas in hypertrophic cir-rhosis an excess of acid was found.—ED.]

Complications.—In many cases other organs than the liver are in-volved in the cirrhotic process because they, too, are affected by the same harmful influences (alcohol, malaria, syphilis) that act on the liver; it is for this reason that albuminuria as a result of interstitial and paren-chymatous **nephritis** is so often seen in the course of hepatic cirrhosis.

Jones‡‡ found inflammation of the kidneys 26 times among 30 cases of cirrhosis of the liver; Wallmann§§ found it 17 times among 24 cases, Price 25 times among 142 cases, G. Förster ‖‖ 10 times among 31 cases. Alcohol, syphilis, and malaria are chiefly responsible for these changes.

Alcohol may also cause chronic meningitis and pachymeningitis; also arteriosclerosis and myocarditis.   Clinically, the disturbances of the heart become very prominent, and are manifested by the development of edema and of hyperemias from stasis.

[Oestreich,*** Posselt,††† and Banti ‡‡‡ all make special reference to the cirrhosis with enlargement of the spleen.—ED.]

Complications affecting the liver itself are: fatty infiltration and hyperemia from stasis; both are caused chiefly by alcohol; both are, therefore, important because they produce an enlargement of the organ at a stage of the disease in which interstitial proliferation alone would have led to a decrease in the size of the organ.

Icterus, aside from the mildest degrees, is not one of the symptoms of atrophic liver cirrhosis *per se;* it may, however, be produced by cicatricial

* *Deutsche med. Woch.,* April 17, 1902.   † *Lancet,* April 21, 1894.
‡ *Archiv. de Laryngol.,* July–Aug., 1897.   § "Guy's Hospital Reports," 1884.
‖ *Presse Médicale,* Feb. 4, 1899.
** Litten, *Zeitschr. f. klin. Med.,* Bd. v, H. 1.   Baas, *Münch. med. Woch.,* 1894, No. 32.
†† *Bull. Medicale,* 1898, No. 26.   ‡‡ Quoted by Duplaix, p. 146.
§§ Wallmann, *Oesterr. Zeitschr. f. praktische Heilkunde,* Bd. v, No. 9.
‖‖ Forster, Dissertation, Berlin, 1868.   *** *Virchow's Archiv,* 1895.
††† *Deutsch. Archiv. f. klin. Med.,* Bd. LXII.
‡‡‡ *Beitrage zur path. Anat. u. zur allg. Pathologie,* Bd. XXIV.

compression of the finer, as well as of the larger bile-passages, and even of the ducts at the porta hepatis.

The obstruction to the portal flow in the liver, and the cicatrices that are sometimes seen at the porta, all favor the formation of thrombosis of the portal vein; and this, in its turn, increases the tendency to stasis in the whole portal area.

Abscess, amyloid degeneration, carcinoma, and adenoma may also develop in a cirrhotic liver.

In certain cases of cirrhosis there is a development of circumscribed tumor-like structures that are arranged like liver tissue and may be called adenomata; the cells of these tumors are young hepatic cells. They have been considered attempts at regeneration. The so-called *hépatite nodulaire* of French authors differs from this form, which is seen particularly in malaria-liver. The columns of liver-cells are arranged in spherical form, and the cells in the center of the nodules are large and contain one or more large nuclei (Kelsch and Kiener, Sabourin).

Finally, true multiple primary carcinoma may occur in cirrhosis. It seems to develop from isolated aggregations of liver-cells (encapsulated, so to speak, within connective tissue), or from the epithelium of the finer bile-passages. Carcinoma may also develop from an adenoma.*

The rare occurrence of glycosuria as a complication has already been mentioned.

The peritoneum is often chronically inflamed and thickened. This factor may aid the development of ascites or may lead to contraction and shortening of the mesentery.

According to Gratia,† a slowly progressing, retracting peritonitis leads to a thickening of the walls of the intestines and to shortening of the intestine (small intestine, 5.8 m. instead of 8 m., the large intestine 1.5 m. instead of 1.83 m., on an average). In this manner it is claimed that absorption is interfered with. Botazzi,‡ too, found thickening and shortening of the intestine; he attributes it to some primary disease of the blood-vessels.

Sometimes the peritonitis is hemorrhagic in character with the development of bloody adhesive strands of fibrin and the exudation of bloody ascitic fluid. **Tuberculosis of the peritoneum** is found with astonishing frequency in combination with cirrhosis of the liver. Aside from those rare and doubtful cases in which tuberculosis is the primary disease, and in which, possibly, the cirrhosis of the liver is caused by tuberculosis, and in this way causes secondary peritonitis, the cirrhosis is generally the primary and the more chronic disease, whereas the peritoneal tuberculosis is secondary and more recent. Brieger assumed that the reverse was the case in the instances studied by him; such a sequence is, however, probably exceptional. Although often not recognizable clinically, older tubercular foci will, as a rule, be found in the lungs, the intestine, etc., postmortem.

The relative frequency with which the two diseases are seen together proves that certain factors must favor the development of the peritoneal involvement. It is probable that the exudate forms a favorable nidus for the development of the bacteria that may enter it, though if we judge from the analogy with other organs the venous hyperemic condition of the intestine should, if anything, be a protection against

* Naunyn, *Reichert u. du Bois-Reymond's Archiv*, 1866, p. 725. Fetzer, Dissertation, Tübingen, 1868. Wulff, Dissertation, Tübingen, 1876. Rohwedder, Dissertation, Kiel, 1888.

† *Journal méd. de Bruxelles*, 1890, No. 5.

‡ *Archivio per le sci. med.*, vol. XIII, 1894, No. 3.

the invasion of tubercle bacilli. In some of the cases that I have personally observed (autopsy by Heller) the tubercular process was limited to the peritoneum, so that an invasion of bacilli probably occurred through the uninjured (possibly edematous) mucosa of the intestine.

It is very difficult to make a differential diagnosis between cirrhosis of the liver and tuberculosis of the intestine, and, as a result, the true condition of affairs frequently remains unrecognized during the life of the patient. There are, however, certain diagnostic clues that may be obtained in the course of the disease, even apart from the presence of involvement of the organs. The moderate exudation, after running a chronic course and remaining altogether hidden, suddenly becomes excessive; at the same time the abdomen often becomes painful, and fever sets in. It becomes necessary to aspirate repeatedly; and the fluid aspirated will often be found to be hemorrhagic or, at least, to contain more cells than the fluid of ordinary stasis ascites. Death occurs within a few months, after a rapid and progressive loss of strength.

Duration; Termination; Prognosis.—Owing to the mild character of the initial disturbances, it is often impossible to recognize the beginning of the disease; there are many cases of contraction of the liver on record that have been found postmortem and caused no symptoms whatever during the life of the patient. It is only possible, therefore, to form a conjecture as to the probable duration of the disease; the majority of cases run a course of many (ten and more) years.

As the disease is the result of alcohol and other poisons, it is probable that remissions or even a total arrest of the process may occur if abuse of these substances is stopped. It is, of course, hardly possible to prove this, because fatty infiltration of the liver and hyperemia from stasis develop from the same intoxications, and are diseases characterized by great fluctuations in the size of the liver.

In a case quoted by Hardt,[*] that presented all the features of Laennec's cirrhosis, both anatomically and clinically, the liver was enlarged up to the death of the patient; this was due to the mass of connective tissue that had developed; the parenchyma at the same time was essentially intact.

In cases in which cirrhosis can be positively diagnosed, the disease is, as a rule, in an advanced stage, and death may be expected within a few months.

I do not believe that cirrhosis can run an acute course and terminate in a few months; the nature of the process makes this improbable. Stricker,[†] Lenhartz,[‡] and others [§] describe cases of this kind; the former claims to have observed the transformation of an enlarged liver into a contracted one within a period of six weeks. In all cases of this kind I should be very much inclined to the belief that the case was one of fatty infiltration or of hyperemia from stasis, and that these conditions disappeared and caused the reduction in the size of the organ. In the cases described by Hanot that terminated fatally in from 2 to 6 months, the cirrhosis seems to have been complicated by a subacute parenchymatous hepatitis with disintegration of the parenchyma.

[*] " Hypertrophische Form der portalen Lebercirrhose," Tübingen, 1894.
[†] Stricker, *Charité-Annalen*, 1874, p. 324.
[‡] *Verhandlungen des Cong. f. inn. Med.*, 1892, p. 125.
[§] Cornillon and Scheven, quoted by Mangelsdorff, *Deutsch. Archiv f. klin. Med.*, 1882, Bd. xxxi, p. 519.

The outcome of a case of cirrhosis with distinct reduction in the size of the liver is death from general malnutrition, heart failure, edema of the lungs, or some intercurrent acute disease; more rarely from hepatargia.

The prognosis of the atrophic stage is unfavorable. In the earlier stages, which can never be positively recognized, the prognosis is not so bad, provided we can remove the causal condition (malaria, syphilis), or bring to an end the chronic intoxication with alcohol.

In those cases, too, in which ascites is already present, but in which the liver, though hardened, is not reduced in size, the swelling of the liver may sometimes recede and the ascites disappear. In these cases improvement may last for many years. Such a result probably depends upon the removal of stasis hyperemia (by strengthening the heart), or of the parenchymatous swelling or fatty infiltration of the liver.

The assertion that the development of a collateral circulation in the veins that anastomose with the portal system can aid in reducing ascites does not appear to me to be very probable. It is true, however, that a most pronounced ascites may disappear in cases in which peritonitis (often difficult to recognize) has existed in addition to the stasis. [For a discussion of operative treatment see below under Treatment.—ED.]

Diagnosis.—For the reasons mentioned an early diagnosis of chronic hepatitis would be very desirable. As the symptoms are so indefinite, a great deal of importance must needs be attached to general considerations, to the etiology, and to apparently insignificant liver-symptoms. Further, in making the diagnosis of such diseases as fatty infiltration of the liver, hyperemia, and perihepatitis, it will be well to remember that these conditions may be complicated with interstitial hepatitis. A tumor of the spleen that cannot be explained, but which appears in the very first stages of the disease, is of real diagnostic importance; in the later stages, when this lesion is combined with a small liver, it is still more suggestive. If ascites is present, it will be a difficult matter to recognize the presence of cirrhosis, owing to the uncertainty of palpation under these circumstances. All kinds of peritoneal diseases will have to be excluded, chiefly tuberculosis and carcinoma of the peritoneum. It is advisable, therefore, to look for these diseases in other organs (the lungs, the intestine, the testicles, the tubes, the stomach). Diseases of the peritoneum, if they develop acutely, are usually painful, tuberculosis usually is accompanied by fever, and is characterized by nodules and strands that can be felt through the abdominal walls and through Douglas' pouch. Sometimes the diagnosis can be aided by palpation following immediately upon the removal of the ascitic fluid; a particularly important point is the presence of a thick strand of omentum running transversely across the abdomen. It will also be well to remember that cirrhosis and peritoneal tuberculosis may occur together. It is only in rare cases that it is possible to palpate the nodular surface of the liver, even after tapping.

Definite information may be obtained by an analysis of the ascitic fluid. In simple cirrhosis it contains very few cells, and its specific gravity is not above 1014. In peritoneal disease the specific gravity is frequently higher, there is often more albumin, and numerous epithelial or carcinomatous cells are found in the sediment precipitated by centrifuging.

Chronic pylephlebitis and contracting perihepatitis may lead to the same pathologic picture as cirrhosis; the liver, moreover, may be small and symptoms of stasis may be present in these conditions. The differential diagnosis must be made from a study of the etiology and the course of the disease. [Colpi has reported a case * in which pylephlebitis was present in a typical case of hepatic cirrhosis, and as a complicating rather than a causal condition.—Ed.] The latter is, as a rule, more rapid in occlusion of the portal vein than in cirrhosis; in chronic perihepatitis (Zuckergussleber) it is much slower, sometimes lasting for years with intermissions. Sometimes pain in the beginning of the disease will point to the inflammatory character of the trouble, or, again, the whole disease may appear to start from an attack of pericarditis (see perihepatitis and cirrhosis from stasis). [J. B. Herrick † has written an instructive account of a case under his observation in which the condition was regarded as an instance of Pick's "pericarditic pseudocirrhosis of the liver." The clinical picture was one of relatively slight edema of the lower extremities, enlarged liver, and rather obscure cardiac symptoms. Three similar cases described in 1896 by Pick showed on the autopsy table an adhesive obliterative pericarditis, adhesive pleuritis, and changes in the liver described as the nutmeg type, cirrhosis and a coarsely granular liver. From his studies he concludes that this symptom-complex resembling true cirrhosis was caused by a pericarditis that induced circulatory disturbances in the liver, leading to fibrous connective-tissue change. In this way portal stasis and ascites resulted. He emphasizes the importance of inquiring into the history and the symptoms for the presence of pericardio-mediastinitis.—Ed.]

Treatment.—Prophylaxis would be the ideal therapy in alcoholic cirrhosis if it were possible to carry it out. Cases in which dyspeptic symptoms appear with disagreeable sensations in the epigastric region and the right hypochondrium are particularly suited for an intelligent prophylaxis, and should be advised, accordingly. This also applies to cases in which transitory enlargement of the liver and increase in its consistency point to an irritable state. There can be no doubt that a withdrawal, or at least a decided reduction in the quantity of alcohol ingested will arrest the progress of the disease. It is likewise important to avoid other exciting factors, such as excessive eating, irritating food, condiments, etc.

A simple diet will alone prevent overnourishment, and if good care is taken to treat all catarrhal conditions of the stomach and the intestine, the formation of irritating and poisonous decomposition products can to a large degree be prevented. Milk, buttermilk, gruel, fruits, and vegetables are all advantageous; but the selection of the diet should be different in each individual case, and be governed by the state of the intestinal tract, and of the general nutrition, since the liver is never the only damaged organ. In some instances a milk diet may be useful; the French and Italians are strong advocates of this plan.

In the initial stages, particularly if plethora exists, the use of laxatives (salines, rhubarb, aloes), certain waters containing alkaline Glauber salts (Karlsbad, Marienbad, Tarasp) or saline waters (Kissingen, Homburg, Wiesbaden), is indicated. The actual success at-

*La Riforma Medica, 1900, 84–89.
† Chicago Med. Recorder, p. 15, 1902.

tained by a course of these different waters suggests a direct influence on the liver.

The same can be said of iodid of potash and of mercury, drugs that should be employed in cases that are not complicated by gastric or intestinal catarrh, also in cases of uncertain origin, and not only in those of syphilitic origin.

In cases in which pain and acute swelling are noted in the beginning, perihepatitis is often the cause of these symptoms. Rest, the use of laxatives, and a restricted diet, are the chief remedies; in addition, local blood-letting and warm compresses may be employed.

As a rule, chronic inflammation of the liver is seen for the first time in the more advanced stages; in these cases the diet (suited to the individual) is the most important factor in the treatment. The principles enunciated above cannot always be enforced owing to the individual appetite, tastes, habits, or the state of the patient's nutrition; sometimes it remains necessary to give a little alcohol, and to allow a certain variety of food. The treatment is, therefore, essentially symptomatic, and is concerned with the regulation of disorders of digestion (constipation, dyspepsia, diarrhea), and with the ascites.

For the dyspepsia alkalies, bitter tonics, rhubarb and hydrochloric acid, are to be given; for the constipation the milder class of laxatives and enemata; for the diarrhea astringents and disinfectants (bismuth, salol, naphthalin, creosote). It is well not to stop the diarrhea in all cases, and in fact only when it interferes with general nutrition. The diarrhea may even act beneficially by relieving the engorgement of the intestinal capillaries, and in this way removing ascites. The same effect may be produced, provided the strength of the patient will permit it, by the use of purgatives; these drugs should be given in doses sufficiently large to insure from one to four liquid stools during the forenoon.

Sometimes an increased diuresis will promote the absorption of ascitic fluid; this can be brought about by such drugs as potassium salts, squills, diuretic infusions, theobromin, resina copaibæ (1.5 pro die, for from eight to fourteen days), calomel (0.1 to 0.2 t. i. d. for three days, then a pause). [Apocynum cannabinum has been used recently by a number of observers with great success. It slows and steadies the cardiac action, increases blood-pressure, stimulates the kidneys (probably by dilating their arterioles), and seems to have a tonic effect on the general capillary system, thus lessening the transudation of serum. Lloyd's tincture is generally used in doses of 2 or 3 minims (0.12 to 0.18 cc.) every three or four hours. The drug is not, however, free from dangerous qualities.—ED.]

Sasaki administered for months cream of tartar in doses that insured a stool two or three times a day (dose 10 to 20 gm. pro die); Schwass praises the action of digitalis; Klemperer has recently advised the administration of urea in doses of 10 to 20 gm. pro die for from two to three weeks.

The difference in the effect of certain drugs in the course of ascites can best be explained by the fact that ascites is not always due to compression of the portal venules alone, but may also be due to parenchymatous swelling of the liver, chronic peritonitis, and cardiac insufficiency. Thus digitalis may act beneficially in some cases; and in others the reduction of the fluid may be spontaneous and create a false impression in regard to the beneficial effect of a certain drug that happened to be adminstered during this time. Diaphoresis will probably be contraindicated in many cases because of the reduced strength of the patient.

Whenever the ascitic fluid exerts enough pressure upward upon the diaphragm to interfere with respiration and circulation the ascites should be removed by abdominal puncture.

The evacuation of the fluid acts beneficially in other ways than by relieving the pressure. The ingestion of larger amounts of food is made possible, the stools are passed with less difficulty, and diuresis is improved, owing to the removal of excessive work from the kidneys. Perhaps owing to the lessened tension of the peritoneum there will be a more thorough absorption of the fluid exuded from the intestinal serosa. These advantages, in many cases, are so considerable that puncture is followed by a prolonged improvement in the condition of the patient. In other cases the fluid accumulates rapidly and calls for repeated tapping. This procedure has among its drawbacks the loss of considerable nutritive material, and at the same time the danger that the sudden diminution of the intra-abdominal pressure may exert an irritant influence upon the peritoneum. The significance of these disadvantages and their effect on each case varies with the ordinary capacity for food and the condition of the peritoneum. In each individual case, therefore, the advantages and the disadvantages of repeated puncture should be carefully weighed, and the physician must be governed accordingly. It is manifestly impossible to predict what effect puncture will have on a patient, and it is often necessary to perform the operation once or twice before deciding as to its benefits or disadvantages.

The operation should not be performed very early in the course of the disease (Murchison* advises differently), and its first indication should be difficulty of breathing, and signs of interference with the circulation, or with nutrition. On the other hand, it is not well to wait very long. Of course, nothing can be said in regard to the amount of fluid that should be present before paracentesis is demanded, as this factor will depend upon the tension of the abdominal walls.

Talma has proposed stitching the mesentery to the abdominal wall, and in this way causing an artificial collateral path for the blood in the portal system, allowing it to flow by this channel directly into the systemic circulation. Lens performed this operation, but the results are not sufficiently definite as yet to allow us to render judgment on the value of the procedure.

[Since Talma first suggested epiplopexy as an operative cure for cirrhosis of the liver, many cases have been treated in this way, and a fair opportunity has been afforded to judge of the value of the measure.

Neumann,† in a case of cirrhosis of the liver 'with ascites, opened the abdomen, curetted the parietal peritoneum and omentum, and stitched these two together. After many months distinct dilatation of the vessels of the abdominal wall around the navel had formed and the ascites had not returned.

Rolleston and Turner ‡ operated on two cases of ascites from cirrhosis of the liver. In one of these improvement occurred and the ascites had not returned for three and a half months.

Scherweneky § has reported a successful case; Herman Kümmell ‖

* Duncan, *Brit. Med. Jour.*, June 4, 1887.
† *Deutsche med. Woch.*, 1899, No. 26.   ‡ *Lancet*, Dec. 16, 1899.
§ *Medicinkoie Obosvenie*, Mar. 1, 1901.   ‖ *Deutsche med. Woch.*, April 3, 1902.

seven cases, of which two died of exhaustion (two some time after the operation) and three recovered, but the ascites remained as before. Grisson operated upon a patient with a high grade of ascites, who showed such improvement as to be able to work actively for two years before death supervened. J. B. Roberts* reports two immediately fatal cases. C. H. Frazier † reports a cure. Geo. E. Brewer ‡ reports 5 cases, of which 4 were fatal. Of 60 cases from the literature, however, he found 38 which recovered. Baldwin § reports 3 cases, of which one recovered completely and two died. In one of the latter cases the patient lived three months, and ascites did not reappear. Drummond and Morison ‖ also reported a cure.

A résumé of the modern status of the operation in hepatic cirrhosis may be found in an article by Packard and LeConte,** with the report of two fatal cases. They collect twenty-two recent cases, which they analyze as follows:

Immediate death	22.7 %
Ultimate death	13.6 "
Unimproved	13.6 "
Improved	9.1 "
Recovered	40.9 "

Many of these cases were complicated by serious independent conditions, and in some the operation certainly was performed in a faulty manner. Excluding such cases the table would read:

Immediate death	7.1 %
Ultimate death	7.1 "
Unimproved	7.1 "
Improved	14.3 "
Recovered	64.3 "

Contrasting the worst and best aspects of the operation, they conclude that the percentage of recoveries must lie somewhere between 41 % and 64%. Montgomery†† adds sixteen cases to the above list of twenty-two. The whole question is one of a preference between almost certain fatality in the case of expectant and symptomatic treatment, and 40 % to 60 % of recoveries under operative measures. When cases of hepatic cirrhosis become bedridden, and the case is evidently hopeless unless some extreme and radical intervention is made, the only hope is in operation. Unfortunately, the operation has been neglected until too late and until the reactionary powers of the patient are gone. The results, on the whole, have been encouraging, and even as a *dernier ressort* the operation has not proved as much of a failure as the less active medical treatment. —Ed.]

LITERATURE.

Aufrecht: Article on "Lebercirrhose," in Eulenburg's "Realencyklopädie der gesammten Heilkunde."
Bamberger: "Krankheiten des chylopoetischen Systems," 2. Aufl., 1864, pp. 510–526.
v. Birch-Hirschfeld: "Leberkrankheiten," in Gerhardt's "Handbuch der Kinderkrankheiten," 1880, Bd. IV, Abth. 2, p. 743.

* *Phila. Med. Jour.*, Jan. 26, 1901.   † *Amer. Jour. Med. Sci.*, Dec., 1900.
‡ *Med. News*, Feb. 8, 1902.   § *Jour. Am. Med. Assoc.*, July 26, 1902.
‖ *Brit. Med. Jour.*, Oct. 19, 1896.   ** *Amer. Jour. Med. Sci.*, March, 1901.
†† *Med. Chronicle*, April, 1902.

Budd: "Diseases of the Liver," pp. 105–132, London, 1845.
Carswell: "Illustr. of the Elementary Forms of Diseases," Fasc. 10, Pl. 2, London, 1838.
Charcot: "Leçons sur les maladies du foie," etc., 1877.
Chauffard: "Maladies du foie," in Charcot, Bouchard et Brissaud's "Traité de médecine," 1892, III, p. 822.
Cruveilhier: "Anat.-patholog.," Livr. 12, Pl. 1.
Frerichs: "Leberkrankheiten," 1861, Bd. II, p. 19.
Laennec: "Traité de l'auscultation médiate," 4. éd., tome II, p. 501.
Leichtenstern: "Behandlung der Krankheiten der Leber," in Penzoldt-Stintzing's "Handbuch der speciellen Therapie," Bd. IV, p. 138.
Thierfelder: "Leberkrankheiten," in Ziemssen's "Handbuch der speciellen Pathologie und Therapie," Bd. VIII, 1, p. 148, 1880.

Botkin: "Krankengeschichte eines Falles von Pfortaderthrombose," "Virchow's Archiv," Bd. XXX, p. 449.
Brieger, L.: "Zur Lehre von der fibrösen Hepatitis," "Virchow's Archiv," 1879, Bd. LXXV.
Bristowe: "Observations on the Cure or Subsidence of Ascites due to Hepatic Disease," "Brit. Med. Jour.," April 23, 1892, p. 847.
Dieulafoy: "Les cirrhoses du foie (nimmt Uebergangsformen an zwischen der hypertrophischen und atrophischen Cirrhose)," "Gazette des hôpitaux," 1881, 20, 39, 40, 41, 43.
Dujardin-Beaumetz: "Dés Cirrhoses," "Bulletin de thérapie," Nov., 1892.
Förster, G.: "Die Lebercirrhose nach pathologisch-anatomischen Erfahrungen" (31 cases), Dissertation, Berlin, 1868.
Goodhart: "A Case of Cirrhosis of the Liver probably Originating in Phlebitis," "Pathological Transactions," 1890, vol. XI; "Jahresbericht," II, p. 257.
Hanot: "Cirrhose sans ascite," "Archives générales de médecine," Nov., 1886.
Janowski: "Beitrag zur pathologischen Anatomie der biliären Lebercirrhose," in Ziegler's "Beiträge zur pathologischen Anatomie," 1893, p. 79.
Kabanoff: "Quelques donné es sur la question de l'étiologie des cirrhoses du foie," "Archives générales de médecine," Feb., 1894.
Küssner, B.: "Ueber Lebercirrhose," Volkmann's "Sammlung klinischer Vorträge," 1877, No. 141.
Lange, H.: "Ein Beitrag zur Statistik und pathologischen Anatomie der interstitiellen Hepatitis" (205 cases), Dissertation, Kiel, 1888.
Liebermeister, C.: "Beitrag zur pathologischen Anatomie und Klinik der Leberkrankheiten," Tübingen, 1864.
Litten: "Klinischer Beitrag zur biliären Form der Lebercirrhose," "Charité-Annalen," 1880.
Mangelsdorff: "Deutsches Archiv für klin. Medicin," Bd. XXXI, p. 522.
Oestreich, R.: "Die Milzschwellung bei Lebercirrhose," "Virchow's Archiv," 1895, Bd. CXLII, p. 285.
Potiquet: "De l'albuminurie dans la cirrhose atrophique," Thèse de Paris, 1888.
Price: "Remarks on the Pathology of Cirrhosis" (142 cases), "Guy's Hospital Reports," 1884, vol. XXVII.
Rosenstein: "Ueber chronische Leberentzündung," "XI. Congress für innere Medicin," 1892, p. 65, und "Berliner klin. Wochenschr.," 1892, Nos. 23–26.
Saundby: "Remarks on the Variety of Hep. Cirrhosis," "Brit. Med. Jour.," Dec. 27, 1890.
Simmonds: "Ueber chronische, interstitielle Erkrankungen der Leber," "Deutsches Archiv für klin. Medicin," 1880, Bd. XXVII.
Solowieff: "Veränderungen in der Leber unter dem Einfluss künstlicher Pfortader verstopfung," "Virchow's Archiv," Bd. LXII, p. 195.
Stadelmann: "XI. Congress für innere Medicin," 1892, p. 90.
Steinmetz: "Beitrag zur Lehre von der Lebercirrhose" (35 cases), Dissertation, Göttingen, 1894.
White, H.: "The Cause and Progression of Ascites due to Alcoholic Cirrhosis, to Perihepatitis and to Chronic Peritonitis," "Guy's Hospital Reports," 1893, vol. XXXIV.

Occurrence of Cirrhosis in Children.

Taylor, F.: "Transactions of the Pathological Society," 1881.
Demme: "XXII. Jahresbericht des Berner Kinderspitals," Bern, 1885.

Hébrard: Thèse de Lyon, 1886.
v. Kahlden: "Münchener med. Wochenschr.," 1886.
Howard, P.: "American Journal of the Med. Sciences," Oct., 1887.
Laure et Honorat: "Revue mensuelle de l'enfance," Mar. and April, 1887.
Henoch: "Charité-Annalen," 1888, p. 636.
Biggs, H.: "Med. Record," Aug., 1890.
Target: "Med. Record," 1890; "Transactions of the Pathological Society."
Ormerod: "St. Bartholomew's Hospital Report," 1890; Lafitte: "L'intoxication alcoolique expér. et la cirrhose de Laennec," Thèse de Paris, 1892 (cites 9 cases between 9 and 15 years of age).
Clarke: "British Med. Journal," June 30, 1894.
Hall, J. G.: "British Med. Journal," 1893, vol. xxviii.

HEMORRHAGES.

Hirsch, M.: "Ueber Blutungen bei Lebercirrhose" (with references to literature), Dissertation, Berlin, 1891.
Lange, H.: "Ein Beitrag zur Statistik und pathologischen Anatomie der institiellen Hepatitis," Dissertation, Kiel, 1888.
Gaillard: "Hémorrh. pulmonaires et pleurales dans la cirrhose du foie," "L'Union méd.," 1880, Nos. 155, 156.
v. d. Porten: "Venenerweiterungen bei Lebercirrhose," "Deutsche med. Wochenschr.," 1884, No. 40, p. 652.

HEMORRHAGE FROM THE ESOPHAGUS AND HEMATEMESIS.

Litten: "Verhandlungen des X. internationalen medicinischen Congresses," 1890, Abth. v, p. 212; "Virchow's Archiv," 1880, Bd. lxxx, p. 279.
Notthaft: "Münchener med. Wochenschr.," 1895, No. 15.
Wilson and Ratcliffe: "British Med. Journal," December 27, 1890.
Reitmann: "Wiener klin. Wochenschr.," 1890, No. 20-22.
Schilling: "Aerztliches Intelligenzblatt," 1883, No. 36.
Völkel, G.: Inaugural-Dissertation, Halle, 1891.
Ehrhardt: "Des hémorrh. gastro-intest. profuses dans la cirrhose," Thèse de Paris, 1891.
Garland: "Boston Med. and Surgical Journal," 1896, No. 12; "Jahrsberichte," ii, p. 199.

EPISTAXIS.

Verneuil: "Bulletin de l'académie de médecine," 1894, No. 22.
Zarnack: "Beitrag zur Casuistik der Blutungen bei Lebercirrhose" (7 cases), Dissertation, Kiel, 1894.
Garnier: "Gazette hebdomadaire," 1887, No. 10.
Bogie: "Med. Times," July 15, 1881.

METABOLISM IN CIRRHOSIS OF THE LIVER.

v. Noorden: "Lehrbuch der Pathologie des Stoffwechsels," p. 283.
Hallervorden: "Ueber Ausscheidung von NH_3 im Urin bei pathologischen Zuständen," "Archiv für experimentelle Pathologie," 1880, Bd. xii, p. 274.
Stadelmann: "Ueber Stoffwechsel anomalien bei einzelnen Lebererkrankungen," "Deutsches Archiv für klin. Medicin," 1883, Bd. xxxiii, p. 526.
Fawitzky, A. P.: "Ueber den Stoffumsatz bei Lebercirrhose," etc., "Deutsches Archiv für klin. Medicin," 1889, Bd. xlv, p. 429.
Stadelmann: "Ueber chronische Leberentzündung," "Verhandlungen des Congresses für innere Medicin," 1892, p. 108.
Aillo e Solaro: "Il Morgagni," 1893, Nos. 1 and 2; "Jahresbericht," ii, p. 273.
Weintraud: "Untersuchungen über den Stickstoffumsatz bei der Lebercirrhose," "Archiv für experimentelle Pathologie," 1893, Bd. xxxi, p. 30.
Münzer and Winterberg: "Die harnstoffbildende Function der Leber," "Archiv für experimentelle Pathologie," Bd. xxxiii, p. 164.

CIRRHOSIS OF THE LIVER AND TUBERCULOSIS OF THE PERITONEUM.

Brieger: Loc. cit.
Brodowski: "Gazeta lekarska," 1881, No. 13; Virchow-Hirsch's "Jahresbericht," ii, p. 189.

Moroux: "Des Rapports de la cirrhose du foie et la peritonite tuberculeuse" (13 cases), Thèse de Paris, 1883.
Weigert, C.: "Die Wege des Tuberkelgiftes zu den serösen Häuten," "Deutsche med. Wochenschr.," 1883, No. 472.
Wagner, E.: "Beitrag zur Pathologie und pathologischen Anatomie der Leber" (10 cases), "Deutsches Archiv für klin. Medicin," 1884, Bd. xxxiv, p. 520.
Lauth: "Etude sur la cirrhose tuberculeuse," Thèse de Paris, 1888, p. 38.

GLYCOSURIA AND CIRRHOSIS OF THE LIVER.

v. Noorden: Loc. cit., pp. 289 and 391 (with references to literature).
Couturier: "De la glycosurie dans les cas d'obstruction totale ou partielle de la veine porte," Thèse de Paris, 1875.
Quincke, H.: "Symptomatische Glykosurie," "Berliner klin. Wochenschr.," 1876, No. 38.
Roger, G. H.: "Contrib. à l'ét. des glycosuries d'origine hépatique," "Revue de médecine," 1886, tome vi, p. 935.
Kraus, Fr., and Ludwig, H.: "Klinischer Beitrag zur alimeatären Glykosurie," "Wiener klin. Wochenschr.," 1891, Nos. 46 and 48.
Bloch, G.: "Ueber alimentare Glykosurie," "Zeitschr. für klin. Medicin," 1893, Bd. xxii, p. 531.
Casati, C.: "Ueber alimentäre Glykosurie," "Il raccoglitore medico," Aug., 1893; "Jahresbericht," ii, p. 273.
Palma, P.: "Zwei Fälle von Diabetes mellitus und Lebercirrhose," "Berliner klin. Wochenschr.," 1893, p. 815.
Pusinelli: "Ueber die Beziehungen zwischen Lebercirrhose und Diabetes," "Berliner klin. Wochenschr.," 1896, p. 739.

TREATMENT.

Lanceraux: "Bulletin de l'académie de médecine," 1887, No. 35.
Deshayes: "Gazette hebdomad.," 1888, No. 34 (milk diet and potassium iodid).
Boccanera: "Il Morgagni," 1888, Luglio (Milchdiät).
Elhöt, G. R.: "New York Med. Record," May 26, 1888 (strophanthus).
Millard: "Trois cas de guérison de cirrhose alcoolique," "Gazette hebdomad.," 1888, No. 52.
Schwass: "Berliner klin. Wochenschr.," 1888, p. 762 (calomel and digitalis).
Gilbert: "De la curabilité et du traitement des cirrhoses alcooliques," "Gazette hebdomad.," April 10, 1890.
Sacharjin: "Klinische Abhandlungen," Berlin, 1890 (calomel).
Frémont: "L'Union medicale," 1892, No. 70 (Vichywasser).
Kramm, H.: "Zur Therapie der Lebercirrhose" (Gerhardt's clinic, sweat-baths used in every stage of cirrhosis of the liver), Dissertation, Berlin, 1892.
Lens: "Hechting van het omentum majus aon den buikwand bi cirrh. hep. Weekbl. van het.," "Neederland. Tijdschr. f. Geneesk.," 1892, i, No. 20; "Jahresbericht," ii, p. 197.
Sasaki, M.: "Ueber die Behandlung des Ascites bei Lebercirrhose und Lebersyphilis mit Cremor tartari in grösseren Dosen," "Berliner klin. Wochenschr.," 1892, No. 47.
Casati, C.: "Il raccoglitore medico," Aug., 1893 (111 tappings).
Palma: "Therapeutische Monatshefte," Mar., 1893 (calomel).
Klemperer: "Berliner klin. Wochenschr.," 1896, p. 6 (urea).

HYPERTROPHIC CIRRHOSIS OF THE LIVER.

Anatomy.—In hypertrophic cirrhosis the appearance of the liver differs greatly from that of Laennec's cirrhosis. The organ is greatly enlarged throughout the whole course of the disease and may attain a weight of from 2200 to 4000 gm. The general outline of the liver is preserved, though the left lobe is sometimes a little more enlarged than the right, and the surface of the organ is granular. The individual nodules on the surface do not differ in size, as in atrophic cirrhosis, and are, as a rule, somewhat larger (the size of a lentil or a pea). The serosa is usually thickened and adherent to the surrounding parts.

• The liver is hard, and at the same time elastic; its surface is mottled, but icteric throughout, playing from yellow to green. On transverse section the lobules will be seen to be separated by broad, grayish or reddish-gray bands of connective tissue. The large bile-passages are completely patulous.

On microscopic examination it will be found that the connective tissue consists of fine fibrils and scanty elastic fibers; these are not so numerous nor so coarse as in the other form of cirrhosis. Between these fibers are seen nests of young cells. The connective tissue stains readily with carmin; it is found not only in the interlobular spaces, but penetrates the lobules, and runs between the columns of hepatic cells within the lobules. In the beginning it is said that this development of connective tissue starts from small centers situated within the lobules; Charcot for this reason has called the process "insular." Notwithstanding the increase in connective tissue, the amount of hepatic parenchyma is not reduced. The trabecular structure of the lobules is well preserved, and the appearance of the individual cell is normal. Some of the cells may even be enlarged and contain nuclei with mitotic figures (Prus); Aufrecht states that all the liver-cells are enlarged and multinuclear. Only a few of the lobules, the bile-passages leading from which are occluded by bile pigment, show a disarrangement of the lobular structure by the invasion of strands of connective tissue; in these cases the lobules atrophy and become pigmented.

Within the connective tissue the walls of the interlobular bile-passages are seen to be twice or three times as thick as normal, owing to the development of connective tissue containing many cells. The lumen of these channels may be patulous, or it may be occluded by desquamated epithelia or flakes of pigment. In addition, the connective tissue contains numerous tortuous bile-passages like those described above, and, according to the statements of all authors, in much greater numbers than in the atrophic form of cirrhosis. In some places these channels are dilated and form reticula that resemble angiomata in structure; or they may become dilated and form cysts containing bile-tinged fluid or mucus (Sabourin). French authors designate these structures as *pseudo-canalicules biliaires*, and claim that they are formed from the columns of liver-cells by a metamorphosis of the normal liver-cells into small indifferent cuboid cells; according to Hanot (I fail to see a great difference between the two views), the intercellular bile-capillaries simply become dilated. Certainly a definite proportion of these cells is formed from the division and budding of preformed bile-passages.

The blood-vessels of the portal system and the hepatic artery take no part whatever in the pathologic process; even the smaller branches remain patulous and their walls do not become thickened. This can be readily shown by artificial injection. Only in the later stages does it appear possible for the connective-tissue proliferation to involve the vessel-walls.

In 1857 Todd, in a clinical lecture, emphasized briefly the difference between atrophic and hypertrophic cirrhosis, and called particular attention to the predominance of icterus and the insignificance of ascites in the latter disease. Until the beginning of the seventies these statements remained unnoticed. At that time French authors began to study the disease; and among them Ollivier, Hayem, Charcot and Gombault, Hanot, and Sabourin. They described the anatomic and clinical differences in contrast with those of atrophic cirrhosis. The French school (which has been in the habit of designating hypertrophic cirrhosis as Hanot's disease) consider periangiocholitis of the interlobular bile-passages as the primary factor, and believe that the connective-tissue proliferation extends from this point to the lobules of the liver.

So far no explanation has been given for the slight effect exercised by this development of connective tissue upon the parenchyma of the organ; sometimes the latter may even appear to increase in volume. Thus the main difference between the atrophic and hypertrophic forms of cirrhosis of the liver is the preservation of the parenchyma in the latter. In the last stages of the disease and when death is impending, fatty and parenchymatous degeneration of the liver-cells is seen.

General Clinical Picture.—The affection begins with dyspeptic outbreaks, that occur at considerable intervals, and are always accompanied by icterus, and a painful enlargement of the liver. At first, during the intervals these symptoms all disappear, but later in the disease the liver remains enlarged, and the icterus persists; the swelling of the liver may attain a very considerable degree, and there is also an enlargement of the spleen. Ascites is absent. General emaciation sets in, with a tendency to hemorrhages from various sources. Death occurs after several years, as the result of general exhaustion and complicating conditions; sometimes with cerebral symptoms.

Etiology.—Hypertrophic cirrhosis is a rather rare condition, much more rare than the atrophic form. It is seen chiefly in men (according to Schachmann, 22 times in 26 cases), and particularly among comparatively young men between twenty and thirty; it is sometimes seen in children.

[Among a considerable number of cases reported Mirinesca [*] has studied one of hypertrophic cirrhosis with chronic icterus in a boy of fourteen years; and Gilbert and Fournier [†] seven cases in infants. J. T. Bruigier [‡] has observed a case of acute hypertrophic cirrhosis in a boy of seven years, and Pierre Roy [§] one in a child in whom death occurred after exploratory laparotomy. F. W. Jollye[||] has reported two cases in children of the same family.—ED.]

The causes of the condition are not thoroughly understood; according to some authors, alcohol has no influence in its production; according to others (P. Ollivier, observation by myself), it has. Malaria and syphilis are doubtful causes, and the same may be said of typhoid and cholera (Hayem).

If, as it appears, alcoholism is indeed one of the predisposing causes of hypertrophic cirrhosis, there must be other unknown causes that assist in producing a type of disease that is clinically and anatomically so different from the usual and more frequent form of atrophic cirrhosis. The location seems to have something to do with its occurrence, and the fact that so many more cases are described in France can hardly be attributed to the fact that Hanot first clearly defined the disease and in this way called the attention of French physicians to the lesion. It must also in part be actually due to the more frequent appearance of this condition in France than, for instance, in Germany. This observation might be adduced as an argument favoring the parasitic nature

---

[*] *Rev. des Mal. de l'Enfance*, Oct., 1894.   [†] Ibid., July, 1895.
[‡] *Phila. Med. Jour.*, vol. v, No. 22, 1900.   [§] *Soc. de Pœdiatrie*, Dec. 10, 1901.
[||] *Brit. Med. Jour.*, April 23, 1892.

of the disease; it might be a primary infection of the bile-passages either by bacteria or by protozoa.

Vincenzo succeeded in cultivating cocci and bacilli from a hypertrophic-cirrhotic liver. A guinea-pig was injected and died in forty-five days; on autopsy interstitial sclerotic hepatitis was found.

[We have already (vide Atrophic Cirrhosis) called attention to numerous bacteriologic studies of the liver along clinical and experimental lines. There would seem, however, to be no direct constant causal connection between either form of cirrhosis and any specific micro-organism. The toxins produced by bacteria seem able to cause cirrhotic processes, not only in the liver but in the lungs, spleen, kidneys, etc., but alcohol can accomplish this with equal facility. It seems necessary to confess that at the present date we do not know the exact etiologic process followed in either the atrophic or hypertrophic form, and still less in the latter than the former.—ED.]

Symptoms.—The digestive disturbances that usher in the disease are very indefinite and by no means characteristic. There is loss of appetite, vomiting in the morning, a feeling of pressure in the epigastrium, and particularly in the right hypochondrium. Icterus soon appears, and with it the liver enlarges and becomes painful; the other symptoms increase in severity until the icterus disappears, when they also disappear. The liver may remain slightly enlarged. Such light attacks of icterus with febrile dyspepsia recur at intervals of many months, and sometimes of years; each attack is more severe than the preceding one, and lasts a little longer; at the same time the enlargement of the liver increases. Finally icterus becomes permanent, although fluctuating periodically in intensity, and at the same time the general disease-picture grows more pronounced. The discoloration of the skin is moderate, sulphur yellow, and rarely has the greenish tint that characterizes complete stasis of bile; enough bile always enters the intestine to give the stools their normal color. As a rule, the latter are pultaceous, and if anything only a little lighter than normal.

The liver at the height of the disease is so much enlarged that it causes the right costal arch to bulge out and changes the form of the thorax. It protrudes below the margin of the thorax and may extend downward as far as the crest of the ilium. The organ is hard, its margin dull, the surface smooth, and appears to be irregular only here and there, owing to the constrictions caused by strands of connective tissue. The liver is sensitive to pressure and, in addition, there is a dull sensation of pain or of distress in the whole hepatic region. The swelling of the organ increases by stages; at the same time the icterus grows more intense and the pain more severe. The size of the organ persists until the death of the patient; occasionally the malnutrition becomes so marked that the liver shrinks a little.

The spleen becomes enlarged in the same manner as the liver, the organ protruding below the costal arch. It is painful owing to perisplenitis. In atrophic cirrhosis the cause of the swelling of the spleen was in part, at least, stasis; in hypertrophic cirrhosis the genesis of this enlargement is obscure. All symptoms of stasis are absent in this form, there is no ascites, and the collateral veins of the portal system are not enlarged. In those rare cases in which a slight exudate is poured into the abdominal cavity, the condition is usually due to a complicating peritonitis.

46

The loss of appetite that is so conspicuous a symptom in the beginning of the disease gives way to a normal appetite in the later stages, or even to bulimia. Notwithstanding this fact, the general nutrition of the patients remains low, they emaciate and feel miserable, and the enlargement of the liver is particularly conspicuous as the patients grow thinner.

The quantity and the concentration of the urine fluctuate with the condition of the digestion; as a rule, it contains bile-pigment. As soon as a slight improvement occurs marked polyuria sets in.

[Minute traces of bile-acid and bile-pigment can be detected by means of flowers of sulphur. A very scanty amount is powdered upon the surface of the urine and will at once begin to fall to the bottom if the slightest traces of bile are present (Hay's test). Otherwise the sulphur floats upon the surface of the liquid. We have had a number of opportunities of proving the value of this test.—ED.]

According to Chauffard, the abundant ingestion of carbohydrates is followed by glycosuria, but not so readily in this form of cirrhosis as in the atrophic form. [Lefas has shown that in hypertrophic cirrhosis there is no increase in the size of the pancreas (vide atrophic cirrhosis in contrast), but that its density is markedly increased. The interlobular connective tissue, especially around the excretory ducts, is increased, and there is also a certain amount of intralobular sclerosis. The sclerotic tissue seems to take its origin from the excretory ducts, and consists largely of round cells. The islands of Langerhans are numerous, and filled with a large number of cells.—ED.] Chauffard also claims that urobilin is not found so frequently (? Q.); both of these facts are interpreted to signify a slighter interference with the liver function than is true in the atrophic form.

Myocarditis, with disturbance of the heart action, takes rank as the most important complication, after peritonitis. Occasionally accidental (?) systolic murmurs are heard, particularly at the apex; the number of red blood-corpuscles is said to be reduced (Rosenstein), and the number of leucocytes increased to from 9000 to 20,000 per cubic millimeter (Hanot, Hayem). Disease of the kidneys and albuminuria are less frequently encountered than in the contracting form of cirrhosis. Gilbert and Fournier describe a thickening of the epiphysis of the lower arm and the leg in children, and claim that this lesion is due to the action of a toxin that is characteristic of this disease. As the disease progresses, the hemorrhagic diathesis develops; epistaxis, hemorrhages into the skin, the gums, or into the intestinal tract are seen; these hemorrhages are, however, not so conspicuous as in atrophic cirrhosis.

The **course** of the disease is slow, with many ups and downs; the duration, after icterus has become permanent, is on an average four to five years, and sometimes ten to twelve. The patients can, therefore, follow their calling for a long period. From time to time, and often as a result of dietary indiscretions that cannot always be determined, the above-mentioned attacks of icterus and digestive disturbances set in. Toward the end of the disease icterus becomes more severe, the hemorrhages recur with greater frequency. At the same time, a remittent type of fever may appear and death occur from general weakness, from some intercurrent complication, or from hepatargia or hepatic intoxication. In the latter case a slight decrease in the size of the liver may be noticed. In children * physical development is impeded, and the swelling of the spleen becomes particularly conspicuous. The terminal phalanges of the fingers and toes occasionally show drumstick enlargement, and

* Gilbert and Fournier, *Soc. de biologie*, June 1, 1895.

sometimes the same changes are seen in the articular ends of the long bones of the lower extremity.

The **diagnosis** cannot be made in the beginning of the disease; it resembles catarrhal icterus, which also shows a tendency to recurrence. If the enlargement of the liver persists, the diagnosis of cirrhosis becomes a probability. The uniform enlargement excludes neoplasms to a certain extent, but may be due to cirrhosis with fatty infiltration, to venous hyperemia, or to chronic biliary stasis. In cases of this kind the decision must be based upon the constant increase in the size of the liver, and upon the persistence of icterus without loss of color on the part of the stools. In other words, the diagnosis must depend essentially upon the course of the disease; the most significant symptoms are the early swelling of the spleen, and the absence of ascites.

[A point of much interest in relation to the disturbance of general health in hypertrophic cirrhosis, and one that may possibly prove to be of some diagnostic value in various diseases of the liver, is that recently recorded by v. Jaksch.* This investigator found that the amido-acid nitrogen excreted in the urine in two cases of hypertrophic cirrhosis constituted a very abnormally large part of the total urinary nitrogen. This is not a wholly unexpected result, since such large amounts of leucin and tyrosin, and perhaps other amido-acids, are excreted in acute yellow atrophy and phosphorus-poisoning. The increase in the amido-acid nitrogen of the urine was naturally not confined to hypertrophic cirrhosis; it was found in typhoid fever and diabetes insipidus also, but not in some other conditions of importance, as, for instance, nephritis.—ED.]

The **prognosis** is unfavorable, and a cure of the fully developed disease has never been known to occur. A slow course is, however, a relatively favorable one. It seems on its face probable that the initial stages may be arrested and recovery sometimes take place, though this has so far never been determined by exact observation.

Treatment.—In the beginning the treatment is that of gastric and intestinal catarrh, of catarrhal icterus, and of congestion of the liver. In the intervals a non-irritating diet and complete abstinence from alcohol are especially indicated. It is doubtful, however, whether good results can be expected from any treatment after the disease is once fully developed. The reports of good results have been recorded in cases in which cirrhotic fatty liver, etc., was not excluded.

Iodid of potash and calomel are recommended in this disease; they are to be given in small doses (0.06, six times a day, Sacharjin) over a long period.

It is possible that even in the advanced stages a purely symptomatic treatment, by helping to avoid exacerbations and too many attacks, may do some good.

Ackermann: "Virchow's Archiv," 1880, Bd. LXXX, p. 396.
Carrington: "Observ. on the Occurrence of Fever with Cirrhosis," "Guy's Hospital Reports," 1884, vol. XXVII.
Charcot: "Maladies du foie," 1877, p. 206.
Charcot et Gombault: "Archives de physiologie," 1876.
Duckworth: "British Med. Journal," January, 1892.
Freyhan: "Virchow's Archiv," 1892, Bd. CXXVIII, p. 20; "Berliner klin. Wochenschr.," 1893, p. 746.
Gilbert et Fournier: "La cirrhose hyp. chez l'enfant," "Revue mens. d. Mal. de l'Enfance," 1895, tome XIII, p. 309.

* *Zeitsch. f. klin. Med.*, Bd. XLVII, Hefte 1 u. 2

Goluboff, N.: "Zeitschr. für klin. Medicin," 1893, Bd. xxiv, pp. 353–373.
Hanot: "Et. sur une forme de cirrhose hyp. du foie," Thèse de Paris, 1876.
— "Des différentes formes de cirrhose du foie," "Archives générales de médecine," 1877, tome ii, p. 444.
— "Cirrhose hyp. avec ictère chron.," "Archives générales de médecine," 1879, tome i, p. 87.
— et Schachmann: "Archives de physiologie," 1887, tome i, p. 1.
Hayem: "Archives de physiologie," 1874.
Litten: "Charité-Annalen," 1880.
Mangelsdorff: "Deutsches Archiv fur klin. Medicin," 1882, Bd. xxxi, pp. 522–603.
Olivier: "Mém. p. servir à l'histoire de la cirrhose hyp.," "L'Union médicale," 1871, Nos. 68, 71, 75.
Rosenstein, Stadelmann: "Verhandlungen des XI. Congresses für innere Medicin," 1892, pp. 65 and 90.
Senator, H.: "Ueber atrophische und hypertrophische Lebercirrhose," "Berliner klin. Wochenschr.," 1893, No. 51.
Todd: "Abstract of a Clinical Lecture on the Chronic Contraction of the Liver," "Med. Times and Gazette," December 5, 1857, p. 571.
Thue: "Norsk Magazin," 1892, p. 795.
Vincenzo: "Lo Sperimentale," Sept., 1889; "Jahresbericht," ii, p. 298.

Calomel in the Treatment of Hypertrophic Cirrhosis of the Liver.

Nothnagel: "Internationale klin. Rundschau," 1889, Nos. 49 and 50.
Sacharjin: "Klinische Abhandlungen," Berlin, 1890.
Sior: "Berliner klin. Wochenschr.," 1892, No. 52.

In the preceding sections the pathologic pictures of atrophic and of hypertrophic cirrhosis have been delineated according to current views on this subject. The atrophic form has been known for a great many years, and the later stages are fully understood; what doubt exists relates to the initial stages. The hypertrophic form, however, has been known for only twenty years or so, and has only recently become generally recognized, chiefly through the studies of French authors. A certain amount of confusion has arisen from the endeavor of Charcot and Gombault to connect the lesions of the liver that are the result of simple stasis of bile with the disease that Hanot has described. Moreover, the fact that Hanot's cirrhosis is not seen so frequently elsewhere as in France prevented many from recognizing the disease as a clinical entity. There can be no doubt, however, that the disease called *cirrhose hypertrophique avec ictère* is clinically and anatomically different from atrophic cirrhosis. At the same time, both have in common the development of connective tissue that for a long time was considered characteristic only of the atrophic form of the disease.

In order to clear up some of the doubtful points the tables appended below have been constructed (see page 725), and the points in the differential diagnosis have been contrasted. Every attempt at classification, however, is weak when considered from a pathologic standpoint; there is a tendency to consider only the extremes, and by neglecting transition-forms to overemphasize extreme cases and to emphasize in an improper manner their peculiarities, with a total neglect of the transitional forms. Outside of France the contrast and the identity of the two diseases has not been so fully recognized; even in France, Dieulafoy, by formulating the picture of mixed cirrhosis, has attempted to do full justice to the actual facts of the case.

Eichhorst * has recently described such a mixed case; there was a great development of connective tissue that was in part multilobular, containing few cells; in

* Eichhorst, *Virchow's Archiv*, 1897, Bd. cxlviii, p. 339.

part monolobular, containing many round-cells. The liver-cells themselves were unchanged and neither icterus nor ascites was present.

There is a disease among New Foundlanders that can be included in this category of mixed cirrhoses. These people eat large quantities of mussels (5 to 10 kg. in a day) and a certain disease of the liver seems to be the result. It begins as hypertrophic cirrhosis with icterus, and finally leads to atrophy with terminal hemorrhages.* It is possible that mytilitoxin (a poison isolated by Brieger) plays a certain rôle in this connection.

[Jakowleff † reports an interesting case of mixed cirrhosis, as does also Ullmann.‡ The latter ran a fatal acute course. At the present time the mixed form of cirrhosis is not looked upon as a rare occurrence.—Ed.]

ANATOMY.

ATROPHIC CIRRHOSIS.	HYPERTROPHIC CIRRHOSIS.
Liver somewhat enlarged (?) in the beginning; later contracted.	Liver permanently much enlarged.
Connective-tissue proliferation begins between the lobules extralobular, interlobular, penetrates the lobules only in the later stages.	Connective-tissue proliferation enters the lobules from the very beginning, is both extralobular and intralobular.
It surrounds the lobules in an annular or capsular arrangement.	It is "insular," and starts from certain points within the lobules.
The nodules, inclosed by connective tissue, are multilobular, rarely monolobular.	The nodules are monolobular.
The *boundary* between glandular and connective tissue *is distinct.*	Boundary *is not distinct.*
The connective tissue is more tough, cicatricial, contractile.	The connective tissue is more delicate, retains its nuclei for a longer time; resembles that of elephantiasis.
The connective-tissue proliferation starts: from interlobular branches of the portal vein (Hanot) (*venous cirrhosis*); from the interlobular branches of the portal vein and the central venules (*bivenous cirrhosis*) (Sabourin); from the capillaries of the hepatic artery (Ackermann).	from interlobular bile-channels (periangiocholitis) "biliary cirrhosis"—more correctly, cholangic cirrhosis (Q.);
"New-formed bile-channels" within the connective tissue are always present;	more abundant;
The capillaries of the liver lobules cannot be well injected or cannot be injected at all from the portal vein;	can be well injected from the portal vein.
Liver-cells involved early in the disease, show fatty degeneration; gradually disappear.	Liver-cells remain intact for a long time.

CLINICAL SYMPTOMS.

ATROPHIC CIRRHOSIS.	HYPERTROPHIC CIRRHOSIS.	MIXED CIRRHOSIS. (Secondary Contracted Liver.)
Liver smaller than normal, usually granular.	enlarged permanently, of great size, granulation indistinct.	permanently enlarged (contraction only manifested by symptoms of stasis in the portal system).
Icterus absent or slight.	very distinct from beginning to end.	absent or slight.

* Segers, *Semaine Med.*, 1891, p. 448.   † *Deutsche med. Woch.*, Nov. 18, 1894.
‡ *Munch. med. Woch.*, Mar. 26, 1901.

CLINICAL SYMPTOMS.—(*Continued.*)

ATROPHIC CIRRHOSIS.	HYPERTROPHIC CIRRHOSIS.	MIXED CIRRHOSIS. (Secondary Contracted Liver.)
Ascites		
considerable.	absent. (Sometimes appears toward the end, but is slight.)	develops gradually, not considerable.
Spleen		
usually enlarged.	always much enlarged.	enlarged.
Hemorrhages		
hemorrhagic diathesis, chiefly in stomach and intestine.	hemorrhages seen also in other locations.	
Onset		
imperceptible.	repeated gastric attacks.	
Duration		
at most, 2 or 3 years.	5 or 10 years.	3 or 4 years.
Death		
usually from hemorrhages in the portal area.	from complications or from hepatargia.	
Complications		
contracted kidney, relatively often peritoneal tuberculosis.	very rare.	
Occurrence		
usually *after* the fortieth year.	usually *before* the fortieth year.	
Alcohol		
a very frequent cause.	not generally recognized as a frequent cause.	

If those cases of cirrhotic liver are excluded that develop in a latent manner, and that are not seen until the stage of atrophy with ascites, we shall find that a great many cases are left that show considerable variations in their course and in the anatomic changes that are found after death. The chronic process is seen not only in the interstitial tissues, but also in the parenchyma, and may attain different degrees of severity. In many cases other organs than the liver will be found to be involved; these, in their turn, exert a certain influence on the liver and on the general health of the patient. For all these reasons the so-called mixed forms of cirrhosis of the liver vary greatly, both anatomically and clinically; they have the negative characteristic in common, however, that they are examples neither of Laennec's atrophic cirrhosis, nor of typical Hanot's hypertrophic cirrhosis. It should also be remembered that the latter is not the only form of hepatic disease that can cause enlargement of the liver; fatty infiltration, hyperemia from stasis, possibly, also, certain processes of regeneration, may all cause an enlargement of the liver, though the atrophic form of cirrhosis may be present (see case of Hardt, for instance, on page 710).

Thus it is seen that any and every classification of the different cirrhoses is somewhat forced; the only value of the different subdivisions consists in a certain clearness obtained and a general diagrammatic summary of the most important etiologic and anatomic points in the different forms.

With this object in view the following classification of Chauffard may be given; it is both anatomic and etiologic:

CIRRHOSES.

I. Vascular:

(a) toxic
{ 1. from ingested poisons,
{ 2. from autochthonous poisons;

(b) infectious
{ 1. direct microbic infection,
{ 2. hematogenous infection { local,
{ extra hepatic;

(c) dystrophic.
{ 1. from arteriosclerosis,
{ 2. from venous stasis,
{ 3. (from portal phlebitis should be added).

II. Biliary:

(a) from retention of bile;
(b) from radicular angiocholitis

III. Capsular:

(a) from chronic localized perihepatitis;
(b) from chronic general perihepatitis.

Simmonds (and Heller) distinguish three groups, and divide them according to anatomic peculiarities:

1. *Cirrhosis:* interlobular proliferation, early inclosure of lobules and groups of lobules; boundaries between connective tissue and liver-cells indistinct;

2. *Induration:* interlobular proliferation without tendency to constriction (this form often follows malaria owing to the stasis of blood and of bile);

3. *Diffuse fibrous hepatitis:* uniform interlobular and intralobular proliferation of connective tissue (hereditary syphilitic liver).

Even these groups occasionally originate from the same cause and may develop from one another.

It may be well to discuss certain distinct groups of cirrhotic diseases of the liver that can be differentiated clinically, anatomically, and etiologically. These forms of "special cirrhosis" are not altogether different from one another nor are they altogether different from the two principal types described. The differentiation is given for other reasons, and is, to a large extent, evolved from our ignorance of the true significance of the different groups. The groups are: (1) Cirrhosis from stasis of bile; (2) cirrhosis from stasis of blood; (3) tuberculous interstitial hepatitis; (4) *cirrhose graisseuse;* (5) *hepatitis interstitialis flaccida;* (6) malaria liver; (7) pigmentary cirrhosis of diabetes; (8) syphilitic hepatitis.

1. CIRRHOSIS FROM STASIS OF BILE.

Cirrhosis biliaris.

The French distinguish two forms of biliary cirrhosis: the one, *cirrhose biliare hypertrophique* (Hanot), caused by disease of the small bile-passages, and a *cirrhose biliare calculeuse* accompanied by sclerotic thickening of the large bile-ducts. This classification is not justified, however, and is confusing for several reasons; above all, because the word "*biliare*" in the one case is used to designate the bile as the disease-producing agent, and in the other to designate the anatomic significance of the bile-passages in the pathologic picture.

In "hypertrophic" cirrhosis, in any event, the walls of the bile-passages are thickened. In case the disease really starts from these canals, as the French seem to believe, this form should be called cirrhosis of the bile-passages, *cirrhosis cholangica*. Cirrhosis biliaris is that form of cirrhosis that originates from stasis of bile; the fact that this stasis leads to thickening of the walls of the bile-passages is unimportant; the chief and most important factor is the action of the bile itself upon the substance of the liver. Cirrhosis is produced by this chemical irritation.

Icterus, which is common to both forms of cirrhosis, establishes merely a semiotic relation between them, but does not bring them into pathogenetic relation, owing to the fact that the origin of icterus is different in each case. The atrophic form may also occasionally be accompanied by icterus.

We have already described the anatomic changes that are brought about in the liver by the action of the bile (see pages 428, 686). Rabbits and guinea-pigs do not bear experimental stasis well, dogs and cats bear it comparatively well; in man it is borne fairly well, as in the second group of animals, though there are individual differences in susceptibility.

The parenchymatous cells in the marginal zones of the liver undergo focalized necrosis and are separated by connective tissue; in the finer bile-passages epithelial desquamation and cellular infiltration are seen. In the larger bile-passages a thickening of the walls can also be noted, but the disease does not, as the French claim, start from these ducts; the primary focus must be sought within the numerous affected areas of liver-cells that can only be recognized microscopically.

The most frequent cause for persistent stasis of bile is occlusion of the efferent ducts by gall-stones; it is not, however, the only cause; narrowing of ducts by carcinomata or by cicatrices may also lead to chronic stasis and to connective-tissue hyperplasia, as I have myself been able to demonstrate. The French designation of *cirrhose biliaire calculeuse* is therefore not the proper one.

An important point in occlusion of bile-passages and stasis in chole-lithiasis is the fact that occlusion varies in degree and is frequently not complete, so that infection of the ducts by intestinal bacteria is rendered possible. The frequent presence of suppurative complicating processes demonstrates the frequency of this occurrence. Interstitial proliferation may be favored by the presence of bacteria; at the same time interstitial change may and does occur independently of the action of germs, as has been demonstrated by a number of careful animal experiments.

In the majority of cases the interstitial proliferation remains without influence upon the clinical course of the disease. The condition is recognized on microscopic examination of the liver, but the atrophy of the parenchyma due to the influence of the bile is much more important. The clinical picture is that of chronic cholemia and hepatargia; toward the end there is an exaggeration of the auto-intoxication. It cannot be shown that the interstitial proliferation exercises any influence on the course of the disease.

In exceptionl cases only, that last from two to three years, granulation of the interstitial tissue is seen, and sometimes, in rare cases, a reduction in the size of the liver. In such cases the picture of atrophic cirrhosis with ascites and swelling of the spleen develops, modified however, by severe icterus and complete decoloration of the feces (Litten, Janowski).

The microscopic appearance of the liver in a case of this kind differs in no respect from that of ordinary contracted liver. We see the same fibrous strands of connective tissue compressing the acini and separating them into single acini or into groups. Within the new tissue are the "newly formed bile-ducts" the interlobular branches of the portal vein have thickened walls and are not permeable (Litten).

The essential difference lies in the appearance of icterus at the earliest stage of the disease; as a rule, some symptoms of gall-stones will be elicited from the history.

According to v. Fragstein, icterus may disappear as soon as the stone has passed; the diagnosis in the case described by him is, however, not a clear one.

In cases in which the liver remains enlarged gall-stone cirrhosis to a certain extent resembles "hypertrophic cirrhosis." In the former condition, however, the development of icterus is much more rapid, sometimes sudden, and the duration of the disease is shorter (two or three years, as against five and more in the hypertrophic form). Icterus is, as a rule, more intense in gall-stone cirrhosis, the stools are devoid of color, and ascites is present. The liver, too, is only moderately enlarged and decreases in size during the course of the disease; the reverse is the case in hypertrophic cirrhosis.

Treatment, apart from that which is purely symptomatic, should be directed against the stasis of bile. As soon as we are convinced of the formation of connective tissue and of the development of atrophic changes in the liver following chronic stasis of bile, we should attempt a prophylaxis of these lesions by operative measures. The calculi should be removed, if possible; if not, a fistula should be made from the gall-bladder through the skin or into the intestine.

Brissaud, E., et Sabourin,Ch.: "Deux cas d'atrophie du lobe gauche du foie d'origine biliaire," "Archives de physiologie," 1884, tome i, pp. 345, 444.
v. Fragstein: "Cholelithiasis als Ursache von Cirrhosis hepatis," "Berliner klin. Wochenschr.," 1877, pp. 209, 229, 264.
Janowski: "Beitrag zur pathologischen Anatomie der biliären Lebercirrhose," Ziegler's "Beiträge zur pathologischen Anatomie," 1892, Bd. ii, p. 344.
Liebermeister: "Beitrag, etc., Leberkrankheiten," 1864, p. 135.
Litten: "Ueber die biliäre Form der Lebercirrhose und den diagnostischen Werth des Icterus," "Charité-Annalen," 1880, p. 173.
Mangelsdorff, J.: "Ueber biliare Lebercirrhose" (numerous references to literature) "Deutsches Archiv für klin. Medicin," 1882, Bd. xxxi, p. 522.
Raynaud et Sabourin: "Un cas de dilatation énorme des voies biliares," etc., "Archives de physiologie," 1879, p. 37.
Simmonds, M.: "Ueber chronische interstitielle Erkrankungen der Leber," "Deutsches Archiv für klin. Medicin," 1880, Bd. xxvii, p. 73.
Smith, Hingleton, R.: "Case of Acute Biliary Cirrhosis Clinically Simulating Acute Yellow Atrophy of the Liver," "British Med. Journal," Jan. 19, 1884.

2. CIRRHOSIS FROM STASIS OF BLOOD.

Cirrhose cardiaque.

In discussing hyperemia of the liver from stasis we have already called attention to the fact that the proliferation of connective tissue that occurs in the vicinity of the hepatic veins and the central veins of the lobules may occasionally involve the interlobular spaces, and in this manner lead to a constricting cirrhosis with narrowing of the portal circulation. From these lesions the picture of atrophic cirrhosis with ascites from stasis may develop; this may either be added to the general picture of cardiac insufficiency or it may overshadow this condition completely.

According to Sabourin, a similar form of cirrhosis from stasis of blood can be caused by alcohol. It may start from the hepatic veins; it is said to appear in combination with fatty liver.

We wish to again emphasize the fact that in cirrhosis of other organs than that under discussion, particularly the cirrhosis from alcoholism, the heart may be damaged at the same time as the liver, and in this way the microscopic picture of connective-tissue hyperplasia be modified, and a swelling, followed by a reduction in the size of the liver, be produced during the life of the patient.

Liebermeister: "Beitrag zur pathologischen Anatomie und Klinik der Leberkrank-
    heiten," Tübingen, 1864.
Curschmann: "Zur Diagnostik der mit Ascites verbundenen Erkrankungen der
    Leber und des Peritoneums," "Deutsche med. Wochenschr.," 1884, p. 564.
Rumpf, H. (Giessen): "Ueber die Zuckergussleber," "Deutsches Archiv für klin.
    Medicin," 1895, Bd. LV, p. 272.
Pick, Fr.: "Pericarditische Pseudolebercirrhose," "Zeitschr. für klin. Medicin,"
    1896, Bd. XXIX, p. 385.

3. TUBERCULAR INTERSTITIAL HEPATITIS AND TUBERCULOSIS OF THE LIVER IN GENERAL.

Secondary tuberculosis of the liver is a very common condition. It is always seen in general tuberculosis, the organ probably becoming infected through the blood of the hepatic artery. The foci are situated within the lobules, are very small, and are often recognizable by means of the microscope only. In chronic tuberculosis, particularly of the intestine, the liver is often involved; here infection occurs *via* the portal vein.

Occasionally no inflammation is to be seen around these little foci; sometimes punctiform hemorrhagic spots are seen. If the process continues for some time, small nodules are formed by interstitial infiltration and the development of connective tissue. If the primary foci are very numerous, a form of cirrhosis is produced that resembles diffuse hepatitis, and which, according to its origin from single foci, should be called "insular" (after the French type). At the same time the disease is "diffuse," as it is not limited to the interlobular spaces, but also involves the lobules.

New formation of bile-passages also occurs in this form of interstitial hepatitis. There is less tendency to contractions than in ordinary cirrhosis, for the reason that death ensues before high degrees of contraction can develop.

It is clear from the frequency of tuberculosis that a liver which is cirrhotic from some other cause than tuberculosis may be infected secondarily in very many cases; thus tuberculosis of the liver combined with cirrhosis may be found under these circumstances.

Cheesy nodules of the size of a pea or a hazelnut are frequently seen, though not as often as miliary tubercles; the former start from the interlobular tissues in the form of a periangiocholitis (Simmonds) and lead to the formation of small cavities containing a grumous, bile-tinged substance. It is possible that in these cases infection starts from the bile-passages, or from the lymph-vessels, whereas, in general, infection occurs through the blood.

v. Lauth calls particular attention to the fatty infiltration of the liver-cells in the peripheral parts of the lobules. This condition is so frequently seen that its connection with tuberculosis is doubtful, and is probably a result of the general phthisical dyscrasia (toxins). This is especially probable as Lauth does not make a clear differentiation between real tuberculosis of the liver and the fatty liver of a tubercular case. According to Pilliet, coagulation necrosis of the liver-cells is seen in addition to fatty degeneration.

In cases in which the liver and the peritoneum are both found to be tubercular, the suspicion is justified that they have both become infected from some other organ; in rare instances the tubercular process may involve the liver of the peritoneum.

Tuberculosis of the liver has been thoroughly studied in animals, both experimentally and in chance observations. The histologic picture of spontaneous tuberculosis varies with the species; that of experimental tuberculosis according to the method of inoculation and the dose. In general, inoculation-tuberculosis runs a more acute course and produces diffuse interstitial inflammation, and, in the case of the guinea-pig, circumscribed necrosis of the liver parenchyma.

Symptoms.—Clinically, tuberculosis of the liver is unimportant. In cases of serious involvement of the liver the function of the organ, and even the general metabolism, may be perverted; but the symptoms of liver infection cannot be distinguished and differentiated from the general pathologic picture. In some instances the appearance of icterus may point to an involvement of the liver (A. Fränkel).

It is said that occasionally a painless form of ascites develops (E. Wagner). In children with acute miliary tuberculosis Wagner saw enlargement of the liver and sensitiveness to pressure, and considers these symptoms of value in the diagnosis of tuberculosis of the liver and of general tuberculosis.

Whether tuberculosis of the liver is really capable of producing cirrhosis, with contraction and subsequent symptoms of stasis, is doubtful, although Hanot and his school claim that this can occur. In the majority of the cases of this kind there was probably a cirrhosis of some other origin with secondary tubercular infection.

Hanot and Gilbert, in addition to latent tuberculosis, distinguish the following forms:

1. *Acute:* Fatty hypertrophic tubercular hepatitis.
2. *Subacute:*
   (*a*) Fatty tuberculous hepatitis which is atrophic (or without hypertrophy).
   (*b*) Nodular parenchymatous tubercular hepatitis.
3. *Chronic:*
   (*a*) Tuberculous cirrhosis,
   (*b*) Fatty tuberculous liver.

In the latter form the tubercles of the liver may be completely absent.

TUBERCULOSIS OF THE LIVER.

Arnold: "Ueber Lebertuberculose," "Virchow's Archiv," 1880, Bd. LXXXII, p. 377.
Brieger, L.: "Beitrag zur Lehre von der fibrösen Hepatitis," "Virchow's Archiv," 1879, Bd. LXXV, p. 85.
Fränkel, A.: "Klinische Mittheilungen über Lebertuberculose," "Zeitschr. für klin. Medicin," 1882, Bd. V, p. 107.
Hanot et Gilbert: "Sur les formes de la tuberculose hépatique," "Archives générales de médecine," 1889, tome II, pp. 513–521.
Lauth, E.: "Essai sur la cirrhose tub.," Thèse de Paris, 1888.
MacPhedran et Caven: "Diff. tub. hepatitis," "American Med. Journal," May, 1893; "Jahresbericht," II, p. 273.
Pilliet: "Cirrh. tub. et la tub. diffuse dans le foie," "Progres médicale," 1892, No. 3; "Jahresbericht," II, p. 193.
— "Cirrhose nécrotique hypertrophique," "Mercredi méd." 1892, No. 4; "Jahresbericht," II, p. 195.

— "Et. sur la tub. expér. et spontanée du foie," Thèse de Paris, 1891.
Wagner, E.: "Die acute miliare Tuberculose der Leber," "Deutsches Archiv für klin. Medicin," 1884, Bd. xxxiv, p. 534.

TUBERCULOSIS OF THE GALL-PASSAGES.
Simmonds: "Deutsches Archiv für klin. Medicin," 1880, Bd. xxvii, p. 452.
Tublet, L.: "Thèse de Paris, 1872.
Sabourin: "Archives de physiologie normale et pathologique," 1883.

4. CIRRHOSIS ADIPOSA; CIRRHOSE GRAISSEUSE.

French authors, and first Hutinel and Sabourin, have distinguished a form of cirrhosis of the liver in which there is interstitial proliferation and fatty infiltration of the liver-cells; this disease they called cirrhose graisseuse (*cirrhose avec stéatose*). The liver is enlarged, and for this reason there is distinguished *cirrhose graisseuse atrophique* and *hyper-trophique*. It is found in alcoholics, and in tuberculous cases, some-times in combination with tuberculosis even of the liver itself. Some claim that the fat is present as a result of infiltration; others that it is the result of fatty degeneration.

It appears to me that to emphasize this form of the disease is con-fusing. In the majority of cases we are dealing with cirrhosis and fatty infiltration, in which the latter condition appears first or in rare cases only after the cirrhosis. Alcoholism may produce both processes; phthisis of the lung may lead to fatty liver; tuberculosis of the liver to interstitial proliferation, and (according to Lauth) to fatty infiltration.

Hanot, Hérard, Dalché, and Debove, have described cases that are altogether different, in which the cirrhosis of the liver was far advanced. Subsequently fatty degeneration of the cells occurred and, as a result, a diminution in the size of the organ. Death occurred in from four to six months; these were cases, therefore, of chronic interstitial hepatitis followed by subacute parenchymatous inflammation and death from atrophy.

Blocq and Gillet, finally, include under the category of cirrhoses graisseuses certain cases that run a still shorter course of five or six weeks, which they attribute to infection. These cases must be regarded as acute parenchymatous and interstitial hepatitis. [Eichhorst * cites a case in which the patient died in two days from the onset of the evident disease. At the autopsy an old multilobular hepatic cirrhosis was found, to which had lately been added a monolobular condition, with an enormous increase of small bile-ducts. The hepatic lymph-glands, and also the parotid gland were enlarged and inflamed. The case appears to have been one of acute autoinfection in which the low type glandular structures (parotid) were more seriously affected than the higher (liver). No jaundice was present.—ED.]

Hutinel: "Et sur quelques cas de cirrhose avec stéatose du foie," "France médicale," 1881.
Sabourin: "Sur une variété de cirrhose hypertr. du foie," "Archives de physiologie normale et pathologique," 1882, p. 584.
Hanot, V.: "Sur la cirrhose atrophique à marche rapide," "Archives générales de médecine," 1882, i, p. 641; ii, p. 33, und 1883, tome cl, p. 33.
Dalcbé et Lebreton: "Cirrhose atrophique à marche rapide," "Gazette médicale de Paris," 1883, No. 26.

* *Virchow's Archiv*, Bd. cxlviii, H. 12, 1898.

Hayem et Girandeau: "Contrib. à l'étude de la cirrhose hyp. gr.," "Gazette heb-
domad.," 1883, No. 9.
Hérard: "Cirrhose hypertr. graisseuse à marche subaigue," "Gazette des hôpitaux,"
1884, No. 67; "Jahresbericht," ii, p. 201.
Bellanger, G.: "Etude sur la cirrhose graisseuse," Thèse de Paris, 1884.
Gilson, H.: "De la cirrhose alcoolique graisseuse," Thèse de Paris, 1884.
For further discussion and references to literature see Lauth, Thèse de Paris,
1888, p. 15.)
Debove: "De la cirrhose aiguë do foie," "Gazette hebdomad.," 1887, No. 30;
"Jahresbericht," ii, p. 278.
Blocq et Gillet: "Des cirrhoses graisseuses considérés comme hépatites infectieuses,"
"Archives générales de médecine," 1888, tome ii, p. 60–181.
Carpentier: "Cirrhose hépatique," "Presse médicale belge," 1888; "Jahresbericht,"
ii, p. 286.

5. HEPATITIS INTERSTITIALIS FLACCIDA.

Italian authors have described certain cases under the above name in which proliferation of the interstitial tissue occurred and the liver decreased in size, at the same time becoming soft, flaccid, and tough. It is very questionable whether this striking condition of the liver is always produced by the same causes.

In the case of Ughetti, a sulphur-worker of seventeen suddenly developed fever and a swelling of the liver two months before death; the abdomen was en-larged, the liver small; there was ascites, and swelling of the spleen. Death occurred in stupor. The liver was reduced one-third; yellowish mottled; there were red and brown portions and the whole organ was softer than normal. The surface was granular. Microscopically vascular connective tissue was seen, young and containing many nuclei; this isolated the liver-cells into lobules of various sizes, and even forced its way into the lobules. The hepatic cells were degenerated and contained fat and bile-pigment. The spleen was eight times larger than normal. Alcohol and malaria could be excluded.

This case is differentiated from ordinary cirrhosis by the subacute course and the character of the connective tissue. The latter is embryonal, as in still another case described by Mazzotti in a young woman. It is stated, however, that in the latter case and in the case reported by Galvagni the clinical picture of cirrhosis was present; in the last case the liver was particularly reduced in size (870 g.) and pale yellow in color; the acini were rounded or oval instead of polygonal. It is possible that in these cases an exceptionally wide-spread degeneration of parenchyma occurred.

Galvagni, E.: "Sopra un caso singolarissimo di epatite interstitiale flaccida," "Riv.
clin. di Bologna," Nov., 1880.
Ughetti: "Archivio medico italiano," 1882, i, p. 444.
Mazzotti: "Riv. clin. di Bologna," 1883, No. 6.

6. MALARIAL LIVER.

In the type of malaria noted in Germany the liver does not seem to be markedly involved, and anatomic changes are hardly to be dis-covered in the organ. Formerly when malaria was more severe than it appears to be nowadays, and occurred more frequently, such lesions of the liver were occasionally seen. The formation of pigment in the blood and its deposition in the various organs, particularly the liver, were recognized and closely studied fifty years ago by Frerichs. The severe forms of malaria are to-day found only in Mediterranean countries and in the tropics. French and Italian physicians have, as a couse-quence, contributed most largely to our knowledge of these diseases.

Acute malaria leads to the formation of pigment within the plas-modia, and the more severe the infection, the more pigment is formed.

It is dark-brown in color and is called melanin. This pigment circulates in the blood, and within the leucocytes in the spleen and in the liver capillaries, also in the brain and the kidneys. In the liver it is found in leucocytes that are situated at the peripheral parts of the capillary lumen, and here it often leads to the formation of capillary thromboses or of large flakes of pigment. In addition, Kelsch and Kiener have described a rust-colored pigment occurring in granules or in little heaps, that are found in the center and at the margin of the lobules. If much of this pigment is present, the liver assumes a brown color that is perceptible to the naked eye; and if melanin is present at the same time, a dirty-grayish color.

The older granules of this pigment give microchemic tests for iron, turning a blackish-green upon the addition of ammonium sulphid; the malaria pigment, melanin, on the other hand, is colored orange by ammonium sulphid and later is decolorized. Sometimes the nuclei of the capillaries are increased in number, and the beginning of hypertrophy of the liver can be seen. In severe, acute cases the liver is very vascular, and the excretion of bile-pigment abundant.

Dock observed a dark green color of the liver in a fatal case of malaria of seven days' duration. There were present microscopic foci of interstitial inflammation and (separated from these) necrotic foci in which the protoplasm was cloudy and the nuclei could not be stained. In the interacinous capillaries granules of pigment were seen. Barker, too, has pictured necrotic foci of this kind.

The clinical manifestations of involvement of the liver in malaria are icterus of mild degree, bile-tinged vomit, and diarrhea, painful swelling of the liver, and a dark color of the urine.

In certain forms of tropical malaria, particularly in the form of blackwater fever seen in Kamerun, the urine contains dissolved blood-corpuscles and hemoglobin during the attack; icterus is also present.

[There is considerable discussion at the present time as to the origin of the pigment in blackwater fever. Karamitsao * and others believe that the process is entirely the result of the malarial poison. Koch, on the other hand, holds that blackwater fever is nothing more or less than a malarial infection to which quinin intoxication has been superadded. Sambon † believes that the blackwater fever and the quinin have no connection as cause and effect, but that coincidence is alone responsible. It would appear that Koch's theory of quinin-poisoning was gaining ground, and that the pigment deposit is the result of the injurious action of quinin rather than of the malarial toxin.—ED.]

The **changes of the liver in chronic malaria** are more pronounced and more conspicuous. The liver is not only hyperemic, but also enlarged, owing to an increase in the bulk of the parenchyma. The weight of the organ may be from 2000 to 3000 gm.; perihepatitis is often seen. Microscopically it will be found that the columns of liver-cells are increased to twice their normal thickness, and that the cells are enlarged and cloudy with large nuclei and mitoses. In the periphery of the lobules are seen granules giving the iron reaction; in the capillaries, masses of leucocytes and large polymorphous cells are seen containing brown iron pigment that probably comes from the spleen; the periportal tissues, too, are swollen, nucleated, and contain pigment.

This initial stage may develop in different ways as follows:

* *Wien. med. Woch.*, Nov. 3, 1900.   † *Practitioner*, Mar., 1901.

It may **retrogress** and lead to ischemic atrophy. In these cases the liver is small (700 to 1300 gm.), solid, the cut surface is smooth, light brown, or gray; the liver-cells are small and filled with pigment, their nuclei do not stain well; the tissues are dry and contain little blood; the bile is scanty and light in color; there is only a slight thickening of the connective tissue, the latter is also true with regard to the capillaries. melanotic pigment may sometimes be found in the spleen. It is difficult to inject the capillaries through the portal vein.

In another class of cases Kelsch and Kieners *hépatite parenchymateuse nodulaire* is seen; here the liver is enlarged (to 4000 gm.), soft, and covered with little nodules that are visible on the surface and on cross-sections. The latter may be as large as a millet-seed or even as large as a pea; and are distinguished by their whitish, golden-yellow color or by a greenish tint, and are very conspicuous objects against the red background of the parenchyma. Within these nodules the columns of liver-cells will be found to be thickened to four times their normal size; the cells are cloudy with a large nucleus or with three or four nuclei; the proliferation of the cells displaces the peripheral trabeculæ and flattens them out. The center of each one of these nodules corresponds to an interlobular space and the branches of the hepatic vein are found in their periphery; in other words, the normal arrangement of the lobule appears to be inverted.

Many leucocytes are also found in the capillaries and in the nodules; there is thickening of the walls of the smaller bile-passages, stasis of bile, and yellow coloration of the cells, and the formation of microscopic concretions. If several of the nodules unite, peculiar structures may be formed that look like concrements; in these colloid or fatty degeneration may occur or they may assume the character of neoplasms; *i. e.*, of true adenomata.

Thirdly, **interstitial hepatitis** may develop from the initial stage of hyperemic-parenchymatous swelling of the liver, which, starting from the interlobular spaces, assumes the ordinary type of cirrhosis. As in this type of the disease, certain areas of the liver are surrounded by connective-tissue strands and become isolated; these "granules" cover the surface of the organ, are visible to the naked eye on the surface on cross-section, and may be of varying size.

These three forms of development, simple atrophy, nodular hypertrophy, and cirrhosis, may be seen side by side in the same organ, and in this manner very peculiar pictures are created. The volume of the organ may be reduced, normal, or it may be greater than usual. It is possible to differentiate the hyperplastic nodules from the granules of hypertrophic cirrhosis by the appearance of their nuclei; in the former the nuclei are sometimes larger, sometimes smaller, than normal, are irregularly distributed, and are often multiple in the single cell. In cirrhosis the hyperplastic nodules frequently undergo degeneration and atrophy.

The causes for these various forms of development of malaria-liver are not understood. The presence of iron pigment in the liver has nothing to do with it, since cases are seen in which there are great accumulations of pigment and still no parenchymatous changes or connective-tissue hyperplasia are observed. On the other hand, nodular hyperplasia of the liver and cirrhosis are often seen in the absence of pigment. It appears, therefore, that the accumulation of pigment in the liver and the spleen is not a necessary sequel of malarial intoxication, and that the pigment is only deposited under stated conditions after it is liberated from the blood-corpuscles. Further, the serious lesions of the liver seem to be caused by some other agent, either by the direct action of the plasmodia, by certain poisons, or by pigment emboli.

The iron of the liver is often found increased to such a degree that its presence can be detected by chemical methods; this occurs in a variety of chronic diseases, and is most pronounced in pernicious anemia, a condition that is probably due to some miasmatic or toxic influence acting upon the blood. When I described this condition, siderosis, for the first time, particular attention was called to the fact that the iron reaction with ammonium sulphid is frequently not found in the rust-colored particles within the liver, but whether present or not it is always obtained with the colorless portions of the liver-cells. The colorless constituent that gives this reaction may be in solution or granular. In the only case of malaria liver that I have ever examined the iron reaction was present in the periphery of the lobules, and seemed to be given particularly by very fine intracellular granules, though these cells did not contain any brown granules. Deposition of iron seems to occur here, as in other places, independently of pigmentation. Examination of siderotic livers of other origin than malaria shows that the presence of iron of itself does not necessarily imply the development of interstitial hepatitis.

According to Kelsch and Kiener, whose description I have followed in the main, malaria liver is characterized by the frequent presence of the iron reaction and the nodular form of hyperplasia. In Southern Italy, I am informed by Professor Ughetti (in Cantania), no appreciable difference is seen between the anatomic and histologic features of malarial cirrhosis and those of the ordinary cirrhosis of alcoholism. It is possible that the unfavorable conditions of life in Sicily and a poor diet are responsible for the fact that no material is furnished for storing iron in the liver, and that consequently all the inflammatory changes are retrogressive. There seems to be no doubt that among these people the cirrhosis is produced by malaria *per se*, whereas among the European population of Algiers alcohol certainly also plays a definite rôle.

[P. Bielfield * has made an interesting study of the contents of the liver-cells of healthy persons with especial reference to the presence of iron. He makes the assertion, as the result of his experiments, that former failures to find iron have been due to faulty methods. By using Smith's method (removing the gall-bladder, and then cutting the liver into small pieces, by means of glass, scraping with a horn spatula, mixing with salt solution—7 : 1000—and straining through clean linen) he obtained a filtrate of liver-cells and salt solution. This is placed in a cylinder of 10 liters capacity filled to the brim, and set aside in a cool place for twelve hours. The liver-cells by this time subside. The salt solution is changed repeatedly until spectroscopic bands of hemoglobin fail to appear. The fluid is then decanted and the remainder centrifugated. The liver-cells he then dries and divides into two parts, one of which he uses for the determination of the quantity of NaCl, and the other for the determination of the iron. The latter portion is washed with hot water, filtered, and incinerated. The ash is dissolved in HCl, the latter evaporated, the residue treated with H_2SO_4, and a piece of zinc added to reduce the iron ; its amount of which is determined by titration with a standard solution of permanganate. Bielfield concludes: (1) There is considerable variation in the amount of iron present in the hepatic cells during health. (2) The average amount

* *Russk. Arch. Patholog. klin. med. Bact.*, March, 1901.

of iron present in a healthy liver is about 0.19 %. (3) There is more iron in the liver of the male than the female. (4) The amount of iron in the hepatic cells increases with age. (5) The amount is less between the ages of twenty and twenty-five.—ED.]

Symptoms.—When only parenchymatous hepatitis and nodular hyperplasia are present, the symptoms are limited to the appearance of slight degrees of icterus and a feeling of pain or of heaviness in the right hypochondrium. At times there are attacks of congestion of the liver with polycholia. The liver is slightly enlarged.

In typical cirrhosis ascites develops, the spleen is enlarged and painful from perisplenitis, the skin is sallow or icteroid. Loss of strength progresses rapidly as the combined result of the malarial cachexia and the disease of the liver.

In the less frequent form of ischemic atrophy the liver is small, there is much ascites, and the fluid returns rapidly after aspiration.

Frerichs: "Leberkrankheiten," Bd. I, p. 325; Atlas, Taf. IX–XI.
Chauffard: "Mal. du foie," loc. cit., p. 886.
Auscher: "Manuel de méd. de Debove et Achard," tome VI, p. 119.
Kelsch et Kiener: "Des affections paludéennes du foie," "Archives de physiologie," 1878, tome X, p. 571, 1879.
— "Maladies des pays chauds," Paris, 1889, pp. 420, 547, 684, Table V, VI.
Véron: "Cirrhoses pseudo-alcooliques," "Archives générales de médecine," Sept., 1884, p. 308.
Pampoukis: "Bulletin de la société anatomique de Paris," June, 1889.
Barker, L. F.: "Johns Hopkins' Hospital Report," vol. V, 1895.
Bordori: "Lo Sperimentale," 1891, No. 21.
Cantani, A.: "Il Morgagni," Luglio, 1890.
Dock: "American Journal of the Medical Sciences," April, 1894.
Jacobson, O.: "Malaria und Diabetes," Dissertation, Kiel, 1896.
de Renzi: "Riforma medica," 1890.
Rubino, A.: "Giorn. internaz. di science mediche," Napoli, 1884.
Ughetti, G. B.: "Archivo medico Italiano," Dec., 1882, 1883.
— "Giorn. internaz. di science mediche," Napoli, 1883.

7. PIGMENTARY CIRRHOSIS OF DIABETICS.

Cirrhosis of the liver may occur in combination with diabetes. Their simultaneous appearance seems to be rare in Germany, more frequent in France and England. This fact of itself suggests that particular conditions must be held responsible for the occurrence, and I assume that coincidence plays an important rôle, rather than that there is any more serious connection between the two conditions. As often as the attempt has been made to discover a relation between the two diseases, there have been some authors that have called the one, and some the other, the primary disease (compare page 706).

In some of the cases sclerosis of the pancreas may have been the cause of diabetes; at least this condition has been found accompanying pigmentation in a number of cases of *diabète bronzé* (Achard).

Hanot and Chauffard, in 1882, described a special disease-picture under the name of *cirrhose pigmentaire hypertrophique* in diabetes mellitus; they stated that it was characterized by great pigmentation of a cirrhotic liver and by melanodermia. Other similar cases with slight variations have been described since then, particularly by French authors. Trousseau, it appears, described a case of the kind in his day (*loc. cit.*).

. 47

[Condon,* in reporting a case with autopsy, mentions three theories relating to the nature of the condition: (1) That it is a distinct pathologic entity—advanced by Marie, Hanot, and other French writers. (2) That the primary condition is a diabetes mellitus, and that the poisons of the diabetes are responsible for the hemachromotosis, cirrhosis of the liver, pancreas, etc.—supported by Letulle. (3) That hemachromotosis is the primary condition, and that the deposition of pigment causes the hypertrophic cirrhosis of the liver and pancreas; the diabetes resulting only when the pancreatitis reaches a certain stage. This view is advanced by Opie.—Ed.]

The cases are, as a rule, afflicted with diabetes of medium degree, but are at the same time very cachectic; they may be alcoholics or tuberculous cases. The disease often sets in with disturbances of the appetite, diarrhea alternating with constipation, and other gastric disturbances. There is a feeling of pressure in the epigastrium, great polydypsia, polyphagia, and progressive cachexia. Later ascites appears, with edema of the legs, and a recession of the diabetic symptoms; the liver is usually enlarged.

With the onset of diabetes the skin usually turns a uniformly dirty brown color, and hence the name *diabète bronzé*. The mucous membranes are not colored. It is said that this melanodermia is different from that of Addison's disease, argyria, and carcinomatous cachexia; the tint is said to approach a sooty shade (bistre), and resembles chronic arsenic-poisoning more than any other condition. The discoloration of the skin may be of many different degrees of color, and may even be completely absent. The disease lasts for nine months to one year, and at the end of this time the patients die of cachexia, usually in coma.

[Anschutz † has published a comprehensive review of the subject of cirrhosis with pigmentation, as has also Futcher ‡ at a still more recent date. Both point to the fact that pigmentation occurs rather with the hypertrophic form, and almost never with the atrophic cirrhosis of Laennec. Futcher notes a case occurring in the Johns Hopkins Hospital, which he claims is the fifth to be reported in this country (America), two having been noted previously by Opie (1899), and Adami and Abbott (1889–1900), and two by Osler in 1899. Nearly all recent writers look upon the condition as one in which the diabetes is secondary or even a coincident condition, the diabetic symptoms usually appearing only within a year of the termination of the case. Nearly all cases have been observed in males. The liver shows at autopsy enlargement and the general picture of a pigmentary cirrhosis. The hepatic cells and the connective tissue show a brownish pigment containing iron; this has also been found in the cardiac muscle-fibers and in the lymph-glands. —Ed.]

The liver is generally larger than normal, heavier, and more solid; it may weigh 2000 gm. or more; in one case, however, the typical picture of an atrophic cirrhosis was seen. The color of the organ is rusty, the pancreas, the abdominal and the salivary glands, and the spleen are solid and colored brown in the same manner as the heart-muscle; in some of the cases a slate-like discoloration is seen in certain areas over the parietal peritoneum, and on the serosa of the stomach and intestine. The cirrhosis may be seen microscopically to be portal or bivenous.

* *Medicine*, Dec., 1900.   † *Deutsch. Arch. f. klin. med.*, Bd. LXII, 1899.
‡ *Jour. Amer. Med. Assoc.*, Sept. 28, 1901.

PLATE V.

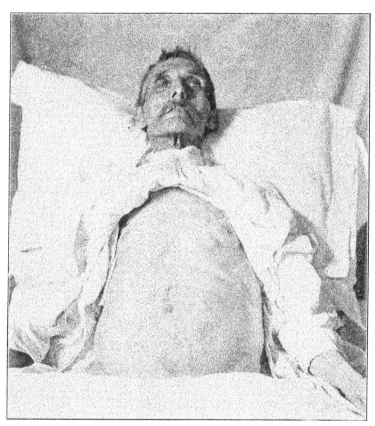

PIGMENTARY CIRRHOSIS OF THE LIVER WITH DIABETES. MARKED HEPATIC ENLARGEMENT AND ASCITES, WITH BRONZED SKIN (DIABÈTE BRONZÉ).

The pigment is most abundant in the periphery of the lobules, in the liver-cells surrounding the nucleus, and often covering the latter; it is, as a rule, finely granular. Dutournier and others have designated this condition as "pigmentary necrobiosis"; this name can hardly be reconciled, however, with the usual enlargement of the liver. Pigment is also found in the endothelia of the capillaries and in a coarser form in the connective tissue, the migrating cells, the fixed cells, Kupfer's stellate cells, and in the glandular cells of the pancreas, the salivary glands, the cells of the spleen, and of the abdominal lymph-glands, the fibers of the heart-muscle, and the smooth muscle-fibers of the vessel walls.

The first observers did not analyze the pigment; later ones (Gilbert Pottier, Auscher, and Lapicque) demonstrated the presence of iron with ammonium sulphid (greenish-black color). Auscher and Lapicque claim that colloid ferric-hydroxid is present; the blackish pigment of the peritoneum and the intestinal serosa is a different substance, showing no iron reaction, and being decolorized by reducing agents. The color is brought back by oxygen; the pigment is soluble in alkalies.

According to all these findings, there can be no doubt that the brownish pigment or the brownish masses are derivatives of hemoglobin; *i. e.*, of destroyed red blood-corpuscles. Different authors have assumed that this destruction occurs in a variety of organs, including the liver; others claim that the red corpuscles are destroyed in the liver alone, and that pigment is carried from there to the other organs.

According to my opinion, the pathologic picture as formulated is not justified, particularly as it is based on so small a number of isolated observations. The iron pigment has been examined only in cirrhotic livers, whereas in reality it is found in a great many diseases of the liver other than cirrhosis. [Attention has already been directed to the statement of Bielfield that iron is to be found in quantity in normal liver-cells.—ED.]

Many years ago I described this finding and called it siderosis of the liver (and of other organs), and showed that not only can pigmented portions of the liver parenchyma but colorless portions as well give the iron reactions. In the more pronounced cases, it is true, the substances that react are colored brown or blackish and are present in such abundant quantities that the color of the whole organ is changed. This deposit of iron may be present in the liver-cells without causing any histologic changes, and may be present in large quantities, as, for instance, in pernicious anemia. Even in cases in which there accumulate large quantities of coarse granules and cells the latter obstruct the capillaries of the liver and form circumscribed foci; cirrhotic changes are never produced by the accumulation of iron *per se*.

Diabetes mellitus is one of the diseases that is sometimes accompanied by the accumulation of iron in the liver. It was a case of diabetes in which I saw and described siderosis for the first time both in the liver, and in other organs (1877). In this case, it is true, the interstitial tissues were slightly increased, but not to such a degree that it could be called cirrhosis. I have since then seen the accumulation of small quantities of iron in diabetic livers in several cases, and without a trace of cirrhosis. This condition, it may be stated, was present only in the minority of the cases of diabetes that were examined. [Teleky *
reports two cases of men, fifty and fifty-one years of age, in

* *Wien. klin. Woch.*, 1902, No. 29.

both of whom the first pathologic symptoms were those of glycosuria. In both cases antidiabetic diet failed to cause the disappearance of the sugar from the urine. In both also, after a few weeks, marked icterus appeared, the sugar disappearing from the urine at once, and permanently, notwithstanding a diet that was finally constituted almost entirely of fats and carbohydrates. The assimilation of the ingested fats was very limited. The icterus persisted until death took place. In both cases the autopsy showed marked changes in the pancreas, and an almost normal condition of all the other organs. The cause of the icterus appeared to be a narrowing of the ductus choledochus, dependent upon pathologic changes in the pancreas. In the second case cholecystenterostomy was performed with one of the coils of the jejunum, and the point of anastomosis sutured to the mesocolon. Death followed on the fourth day after the operation.—ED.]

Siderosis appears, therefore, to be a fairly frequent occurrence in diabetics. The same accumulation is, of course, seen if the case happens to be afflicted with a **cirrhotic liver**; it appears that these cirrhotic livers have interested French authors more than the non-cirrhotic ones.

Siderosis is of frequent occurrence in *pernicious anemia.* Quite recently, and for the first time, I saw cirrhosis in combination; the patient, age 52, was cachectic and icteric when he was admitted and had some gastric disturbances; the first diagnosis was carcinoma ventriculi with secondary carcinoma of the liver. From the blood-picture and the absence of all changes in the liver, pernicious anemia was diagnosed later on. The patient died cachectic and without ascites. At autopsy the liver was found to be slightly decreased in size, cirrhotic, and brown. The microscopic picture was that of diabetic pigment-cirrhosis. The iron reaction very pronounced; it was present also in the spleen (that had remained small owing to thickening of its capsule), and in the convoluted tubules of the kidney. The cirrhosis was apparently of long duration prior to the development of pernicious anemia (instead of diabetes). The only symptom of the cirrhosis was a moderate icterus.

Marchand has described a case of siderosis with hepatic cirrhosis in a tubercular case.

Very striking is the frequency with which French investigators have found the complication of diabetes with cirrhosis. It is possible that in France an unusual number of the diabetics are constant drinkers, and that the deposit of iron produced by diabetes occurs more readily in a liver that is cirrhotic, and persists in such an organ after the deposit has once occurred.

It appears that the cases described as *diabète bronzé* are similar to the disease hemochromatosis v. Recklinghausen has described; further communications in regard to the latter disease must be awaited.

The discoloration of the skin—which, by the way, is not constantly present—remains unexplained; it is not stated that the pigment found in these cases contains iron, nor is it probable that it does. It is quite probable that the cases reported were simply cachectic, and that particular attention was directed to the color of the skin owing to the pigmentary anomalies observed in the internal organs. It is also possible that an icterus levissimus modified the cachectic color of the skin.

[A case of bronzed diabetes mellitus with cirrhosis of the liver and pancreas and hemochromatosis has been reported by Condon.* Gilbert, Casteigne, and Lereboullet † look upon the diabetes as the result and not the cause of cirrhosis, and believe that it is due to a hyper-function of the liver-cells—"hyperhepitization." Their views are based on two

* *Medicine,* Dec., 1900.   † *Gaz. Hebd. de Méd. et de Chir.,* 1900, No. 39.

observations: The hyperactivity of the liver they believe to be shown by the parallel appearance and increase of glycosuria and azoturia. Osler * has reported two cases of hypertrophic cirrhosis of the liver with hemachromatosis without glycosuria.

Opie † gives a full account of a case of hemochromatosis without glycosuria. He draws attention to the two kinds of pigment—hemosiderin, containing iron, and hemofuscin, not containing iron. The absence of pigmentation from the skin in some cases is also noted. He says, as does Anschutz, that no case of hemochromatosis or of bronzed diabetes has been observed in the female. He believes that the hemosiderin must be derived more or less directly from the hemoglobin, and draws attention to the iron-containing liver of pernicious anemia. He speaks of the fact that the deposition of iron-containing pigment in the liver and other organs has been experimentally produced by the injection of toluylenediamin in animals through destruction of the red blood-cells, but that the pigmentation is never such as is seen in hemochromatosis. Opie believes that the diabetes seen in some of these cases is secondary to the hemochromatosis. He believes that the diabetic condition is of pancreatic origin and appears when the pancreatitis has reached a sufficient intensity. In Opie's own case intercurrent typhoid fever killed the patient before the chronic interstitial pancreatitis had reached a degree sufficient to produce glycosuria. He arrives at the following conclusions: (1) There exists a distinct morbid entity—hemochromatosis—characterized by the wide-spread deposition of an iron-containing pigment in certain cells and an associated formation of iron-free pigments in a variety of localities in which pigment is found in moderate amount under physiologic conditions. (2) With the pigment accumulation there is degeneration and death of the containing cells and consequent interstitial inflammation, notably of the liver and pancreas, which become the seat of inflammatory changes accompanied by hypertrophy of the organ. (3) When chronic interstitial pancreatitis has reached a certain grade of intensity diabetes ensues and is the terminal event in the disease.

In further studies of the relation of pancreatic disease to diabetes Opie and others have found that disease of the islands of Langerhans, certain collections of round cells differing from the pancreatic cells proper, plays a most important rôle in the development of diabetes. When these islands are spared, diabetes does not occur.—ED.]

Chauffard groups diabetic cirrhosis and malaria cirrhosis as *cirrhoses pigmentaires.* The above discussion will show that the author cannot indorse such a classification. The presence of pigment has nothing to do with the cirrhosis; it can be seen in the absence of cirrhosis, and, on the other hand, cirrhosis may occur without pigmentation.

A typical pigment is, moreover, seen only in malaria; and iron-containing pigments are found more frequently in other diseases than in cirrhosis. [We have already noted a number of cases in which typical iron pigment was present sufficient to show that at the present time this statement cannot be considered as generally accepted. Hemosiderin undoubtedly occurs in most of these cases as the prominent pigment.—ED.] (Compare the paragraph on "siderosis of the liver" and "pigment liver.")

* *Brit. Med. Jour.*, Dec. 9, 1889.
† *Trans. Assoc. Am. Phys.*, 1899, vol. xiv; p. 253.

Auscher: in Debove and Achard's, "Manuel de médecine," vi, p. 105.
— et Lapicque: "Recherches sur le pigment du diabète bronzé," Société de biologie, May 25, 1895.
— — "Accumulation d'hydrate ferrique dans l'organisme animal," "Archives de physiologie," April, 1896.
Achard, E. A.: "Contribution à l'étude des cirrhoses pigmentaires," etc., Thèse de Paris, 1895.
Barth: "Bulletin de la société d'Anatomie," 1888, p. 500
Brault et Gaillard: "Sur un cas de cirrhose hypertroph. pigmentaire dans le diabète sucré," "Archives générales de médecine," 1888, tome CLXI, p. 38.
Buss, W.: "Diabetes mellitus, Lebercirrhose, Hämochromatose," Dissertation, Göttingen, 1894.
Chauffard: in Charcot, "Traité de médecine," iii, p. 891.
Dutournier, A.: "Contribution à l'étude du diabète bronzé," Thèse de Paris, 1895.
Hanot et Chauffard: "Cirrhose hypertroph. pigmentaire dans le diabète sucré," "Revue de médecine," 1882, p. 385.
— et Schachmann: "Cirrhose pigmentaire dans le diabète sucré," "Archives de physiologie normale et pathologique," 1886, tome XVIII, p. 50.
Kretz: "Hämosiderin-Pigmentirung der Leber und Lebercirrhose," "Beiträge zur klin. Medicin und Therapie," No. 15, Wien, 1896.
Marchand: "Siderotisch-cirrhotische Leber bei Phthisis," "Berliner klin. Wochenschr.," 1882, p. 406.
Minkowski: "Störungen der Leberfunction," Lubarsch und Ostertag's "Ergebnisse der allgemeinen Pathologie," 1897, p. 721.
Quincke, H.: "Ueber Siderosis," Festschrift zum Andenken an Albrecht v. Haller, Bern, 1877. "Deutsches Achiv für klin. Medicin," Bd. xxv und xxvii, 1880.
v. Recklinghausen: "Ueber Hämochromatose," "Bericht der Naturforscher-Versammlung zu Heidelberg," 1889, p. 324.
Saundby: "British Med. Journal," 1890; "The Lancet," ii, p. 381.
Trousseau: "Clinique médicale," 4. éd., ii, p. 780

8. SYPHILITIC HEPATITIS.

The interstitial changes produced in the liver by syphilis differ as to location, nature, and extent; in many cases their genetic relationship is not recognized until late in the disease. The formation of connective tissue containing many cells is common to all syphilitic processes in the liver; this tissue consists of round and spindle cells, and is either converted into cicatricial tissue, or it may undergo fatty degeneration and be absorbed. We will discuss separately the lesions seen in adults after acquired syphilis, and those that occur in the hereditary form of the disease.

In *adults* acquired syphilis may appear in the diffuse or the circumscribed form, the former being identical with the ordinary interstitial hepatitis that we have described under the caption cirrhosis. The interstitial proliferation is chiefly interacinous, but seems to penetrate between the columns of liver-cells more frequently than in alcoholic cirrhosis; just as in the latter, it may lead to contraction, and cannot be distinguished from it; in fact, the two diseases are occasionally seen together.

The circumscribed form of syphilis of the liver is more clearly characterized and probably occurs with greater frequency; it is called the **gummatous hepatitis or** syphiloma. In this condition a few, or perhaps very many, single foci are seen, varying in size from that of a millet-seed to a walnut. They are reddish-gray to white in color, radiating in structure, and are of an irregular form, more or less differentiated from the surrounding liver tissue. In their centers are seen yellowish-white cheesy or dry masses that form irregular figures on transverse section, and by this appearance recall the centers of cheesy, tubercular nodules;

at the same time they differ from the latter in that they are much more solid. These foci are found principally on the surface of the liver, and particularly near the suspensory ligament. If seen in the interior of the organ, they follow the periportal connective tissues, Glisson's capsule (*peripylephlebitis syphilitica,* Schüppel). The more recent proliferations consist of round and spindle cells, embedded in a homogeneous matrix; they are reddish-gray in color; the cheesy portions are yellow and inclose globules of fat.

In addition to these gummatous nodules, there are often seen true cicatrices that start from the surface of the organ and penetrate the liver as deep furrows. It is probable that these scars originate from the first-named foci in such a manner that a portion of the cellular tissue is converted into connective tissue, and another portion undergoes fatty degeneration and is absorbed. In some cases only a few of these scars are seen, and these may or may not inclose cheesy portions. Again, the form of the liver may be considerably changed by these scars; there may be appendices to the organ consisting of pieces of the liver paren-chyma that have become separated from the main part of the organ; these may be as large as nuts or apples, or the whole liver may appear to be made up of such fragments. The round shape of these lobes can only be explained by the great elasticity of the liver tissue; it is possible also that a process of vicarious hyperplasia has something to do with their formation.

In gummatous hepatitis the capsule is always thickened and adherent. The adhesions vary in extent and character and may reach beyond the area of the scars proper, and in this way they are usually developed to a greater extent than in any other form of liver disease.

Miliary syphilomata are less frequently seen and produce less striking deformities than the form described. The large foci are not present in great numbers, whereas the miliary areas are seen in enormous numbers and are disseminated all through the liver like tubercles, or neoplasms.

Occasionally gummatous, deforming hepatitis is combined with the diffuse interstitial form; sometimes the normal liver tissue between the cicatrices undergoes fatty or amyloid degeneration; or, again, there may be disease of the bile-passages, with the formation of concretions.

In **hereditary** syphilis the reverse is the case. The circumscribed form is rare, and the diffuse form frequent. The condition is found as early as the sixth month of fetal life or even in the new-born. It may also develop in the first weeks or months of life, and in the latter case appears in the form of hypertrophic induration of the connective tissue. The liver is enlarged and heavy (according to Birch-Hirschfeld, 6 % instead of only 4.6 % of the body-weight). Its color varies from a grayish-red to dirty brown ("Feuerstein," Gubler), and in mild cases is brownish or mottled. At the same time the liver-substance is hard ("like sole-leather," Trousseau), contains little blood, and the outlines of the lobules are indistinct. According to Hutinel and Hudelo, the microscopic picture is that of hyperemia with dilatation of capillaries, accumulation of leucocytes, and proliferation of the endothelium of the capillaries. Round cells are seen later in the broadened interstices of the lobules, which are inclosed in new-formed fibrous tissue. These cells are also seen in the interior of the lobules between the capillary walls and the columns of liver-cells. They are, finally, also seen in the walls of the blood-vessels, extending as far as the intima. In the course of time, connective tissue takes the place of the round-cell infiltration. In the beginning the hepatic cells show nuclear mitoses; later their form changes, their protoplasm becomes transparent, and they disappear.

Although the connective-tissue proliferation is in general diffuse, it may, in certain places, be circumscribed and focalized.

As a rule, the liver of a new-born child will be found enlarged if it is afflicted with indurative syphilis; this is due to the fact that the children do not live long; in the further course of the disease smooth atrophy or granular atrophy of the organ may develop. If hereditary syphilis leads to the formation of gummatous nodules, these usually assume the form of miliary nodules, that are disseminated throughout the liver in large numbers.

[Obendorfer * has reported the case of a child who died of hereditary syphilis when about sixteen months old. The liver showed a marked and characteristic hypertrophic cirrhosis with much destruction of hepatic tissue and a replacement by connective tissue. The arteries were normal in part, and in part almost obliterated by hyperplasia of the intima. The adventitia also showed round-cell infiltration in places. The veins were even more extensively involved than the arteries, their walls being full of newly forming connective tissue. The biliary channels showed proliferation, and were surrounded by newly formed connective tissue. In the areas of connective tissue many nodules with central caseation were seen surrounded by nuclear remnants and round cells. The normal and pathologic tissues were distinctly demarcated, and over the diseased areas the capsule was thickened. The lesions, contrary to the usual diffuse process, were localized to the anterior surface, and its lower portion. Usually the lesions are most marked at the transverse fissure, but in this case the tissues in the neighborhood were free from the process.—ED.]

The lesions of syphilis of the liver greatly resemble the lesions of the same disease in other organs, as the meninges, the testicles, the heart-muscle, the bones. Proliferation of the connective tissue occurs and occupies an intermediate position between new formation and chronic inflammation. The newly formed tissue shows a tendency, on the one hand, to degeneration, and to the formation of molecular fatty detritus that may be absorbed; and, on the other, to the formation of cicatricial tissue.

In the newly born syphilis produces a number of other pronounced lesions in different portions of the body; as, for instance, tumor of the spleen, cicatrices of the placenta, general atrophy, etc. In the adult the hepatic lesion may be the only manifestation of the disease.

Occurrence.—Syphilitic hepatitis appears in the tertiary stage of the disease, and at approximately the same time as gummata in the meninges, the bones, the mucous membranes, etc.; in general, therefore, it is noted a number of years after infection. As the development of the different lesions of lues fluctuates greatly in regard to time, it may be that the lesion under discussion may occasionally develop earlier in the disease. Key † and Biermer have reported cases in which the interval between infection and the development of hepatitis was only six and nine months; these cases, however, are not above criticism.

In acquired syphilis the liver is one of the most frequently affected

* *Centralbl. f. allg. Path. u. path. Anat.*, Mar. 15, 1900.
† Schmidt's "Jahrbücher," Bd. CLXI, p. 142.

organs; in hereditary syphilis, possibly after the lungs, the liver certainly is the most frequently involved organ. The disease may begin during fetal life and is seen in the prematurely born, in the still-born, and in children that die at the age of a few weeks or months.

The frequency of the disease may be learned from statistics that Hofmeister and Feige have gathered from autopsies performed from 1873 to 1885, and from 1886 to 1895, in the pathologic Institute of Kiel. Among nurslings under six months, 123 and 189 were syphilitic; a record of 20.1 % and 16.5 %. Of these syphilitic children, 48 and 123 (39 % and 65 %) showed evidence of interstitial hepatitis. The lungs were frequently involved at the same time; less frequently, the bones and the skin.

Symptoms.—In the adult the circumscribed form of syphilis of the liver rarely produces any conspicuous symptoms, and is usually found by chance at the autopsy. As the serosa is frequently involved, pain in the liver region may be felt, or there may be friction sounds present.

Fresh gummata may be felt as nodules on the margin or on the convex surface of the organ; the cicatricial deformities are more frequently felt. Pieces of the liver as large as a hazelnut or an apple may become separated from the main body of the organ by scar tissue and may give the impression of independent tumors, or may lead to confusion with floating kidney. These separated parts remain in a stationary condition for a long time, or at least are little changed; gummata proper, on the other hand, often undergo retrogressive changes. Oppolzer and Bochdalek * mistook such softened gummata for cured liver carcinomata.

The perihepatic adhesions frequently anchor the liver to the anterior abdominal wall and interfere with the respiratory motility of the organ.

Notwithstanding all these lesions, the general health may remain unimpaired, provided the healthy portion of the organ continues to functionate properly; if disturbances occur, they usually originate from the portal vein, and occasionally from the bile-passages.

If there is compression of the portal vein, and the picture of stasis of this system appears with ascites, the disease may resemble cirrhosis, particularly as a swelling of the spleen may develop both as a result of stasis and of amyloid degeneration, or of syphilitic hyperplasia. Icterus from compression of bile-passages is less frequently seen, and still less frequently a congestion of the liver from occlusion of the hepatic veins.

In some cases the course of the disease is fatal, as in cirrhosis. If antisyphilitic treatment is instituted at the right time, all the symptoms may recede. Sometimes recurrences and exacerbations occur, and this, very protracted and varying course of the disease may aid in differentiating the condition from alcoholic cirrhosis.

Diffuse syphilitic hepatitis in adults may, in fact, at the beginning, lead to an enlargement of the liver more frequently than alcoholic intoxication. The onset has appeared to me to be somewhat more sudden, and the course of the disease more rapid than in the latter condition.

If syphilitic hepatitis is present in the new-born, the children show signs of bad health within a short time after birth; they are emaciated, flabby, and do not thrive. The abdomen protrudes, the liver can be palpated as a large, smooth, and hard tumor, and, in addition, ascites is present or soon develops. The spleen is usually enlarged to several times its normal volume and can be readily palpated. Icterus is not a constant symptom, and if present varies in intensity. Children afflicted

* *Prager Vierteljahrsschr.*, 1845, Bd. ii, p. 59.

in this manner die in spite of all treatment, usually with diarrhea, cachexia, or peritonitis. Lesser degrees of hepatitis, that cause no symptoms in the beginning, are compatible with longer life, and develop into those cases that show all the characteristics of Laennec's cirrhosis in the later years of childhood, without revealing any clue to their origin.

Many of these cases of late syphilitic hepatitis run an atypical or irregular clinical course, but are characterized anatomically by the uneven distribution of intralobular connective tissue.▸ Occasionally miliary, cheesy foci, or amyloid areas will be seen in these cases.

The older the child in which hepatitis develops, the more difficult will it be to determine whether the case is one of retarded hereditary syphilis or of acquired infection. Barthélémy has collated some 30 cases of this kind; showing that they occur most commonly between the sixth and thirteenth years, but may be seen as late as the twentieth (a case of Ebermaier) year. The mildest cases are not very characteristic, and have been termed congestive cases (Barthélémy). They show some dyspeptic and intestinal disturbances and an enlargement and sensitiveness of the liver. In more pronounced cases the liver is large and hard and there is ascites, and a collateral venous network on the abdomen. There is also a tumor of the spleen; in rare instances the liver is small or deformed. Icterus is rare.

Sometimes acute parenchymatous hepatitis may develop in an organ that is affected with such an hereditary cirrhosis. If this occurs, the picture of icterus gravis and of acute atrophy appears, and death ensues in a short time; the same complication is occasionally seen in hypertrophic cirrhosis. A case from the Kiel clinic, described by Thielen, belongs to this category.

Diagnosis.—In the new-born the diagnosis of syphilitic hepatitis is comparatively easy, because the organ can be readily palpated and no other disease has to be considered. The diagnosis of hereditary syphilis is not so simple in the later years of childhood because this disease produces only vague symptoms; sometimes it is necessary to await the results of antisyphilitic treatment before rendering a decision.

In the adult the diagnosis will have to be made between syphilitic hepatitis, and carcinoma, or alcoholic cirrhosis. It is an easy matter to confound gummata with cancer nodules; both are capable of retrogressive changes. In the case of gumma, however, this process is, as a rule, more complete, whereas carcinomatous nodules soften in the center only and form central delle; at the same time new nodules may appear.

Separated portions of the liver may simulate neoplasms; they are distinguished by their smooth surface, their spherical shape, tense consistency, constant size, and by the lack of pain. A large palpable tumor of the spleen and albuminuria speak in favor of hepatitis syphilitica. Cachexia is not so severe as in cancer.

In contradistinction to ordinary cirrhosis, gummatous hepatitis has larger nodules, of varying size, a larger tumor of the spleen, and, in general, less constant symptoms. Even ascites may disappear, and there may be long periods of comparative well-being. If these changes in the condition of the patient can be traced back for a period of years, this speaks in favor of gummatous hepatitis.

Perihepatitic adhesions are, in a measure, characteristic of syphilis of the liver, and especially if they are wide-spread and to be noted in many places. Similar symptoms may, it is true, be caused by gall-stones, as pain, fever, etc., so that the diagnosis must be made between these two diseases.*

The anamnesis is of subordinate value for the diagnosis, because other diseases of the liver may be present, even in the presence of a history of luetic infection; objective symptoms in other organs are more important, as, gummata or scars of the skin, of the mucous membranes, or of the bones.

It must be remembered, finally, that even ordinary lacing may cause the separation of a ball-shaped piece of the liver from the lower margin, that may resemble similar masses of syphilitic origin. The lobe produced by lacing is, however, always single or indentated by the incisure of the gall-bladder, and is always situated in the mammillary line, and at the lower margin of the right lobe of the liver.

Treatment.—As in other organs, provided an early diagnosis is made, antisyphilitic therapy will lead to the disappearance of the gummatous process. Treatment directed primarily with reference to other organs may, it appears, cause cicatrization and the formation of scar tissue in the liver that is seen by chance only postmortem. Specific treatment may only act symptomatically and temporarily; in many cases, particularly those in which the diagnosis is positive, no success is obtained by the treatment because the process is already arrested and the cicatrices cannot be influenced by iodin or mercury any more actively than upon the skin or the pharyngeal mucosa.

Even if the diagnosis is not positive, antisyphilitic medication is justifiable. As in the case of involvement of other organs, the diagnosis can sometimes be made only from the positive or negative results of specific treatment.

If there is painful gummatous perihepatitis, sodium or iodid potassium should be given. The same drugs are employed in diagnostic treatment or in cases in which mercury, for one reason or another, cannot be given. More permanent results and a prophylaxis against further complications are obtained by a thorough course of mercury lasting over a period of six to eight weeks. Inunction is probably the best method from a practical point of view, although theoretically the internal administration of calomel seems indicated, because the drug is necessarily absorbed in the intestine and carried directly to the liver. The dose should be 0.05 twice daily in the beginning, increasing gradually to 0.4 or 0.6 per day.

In addition to specific treatment, some of the complications and symptoms call for attention, and are provided for by the measures advocated for this purpose in the section on Cirrhosis and Perihepatitis.

Barthélémy, M.: "Syphilis héréd. tardive. Lésions du foie," (Mit Literaturangaben), "Archives générales de médecine," 1884, tome CLIII, pp. 513, 674.
Biermer: "Ueber Syphilis der Leber und Milz," "Schweizerische Zeitschr. für Heilkunde," 1862, I, p. 119, 2 Tafeln.
Bristowe: "Observ. on the Cure and Subsidence of Ascites due to Hepatic Diseases," "British Med. Journal," April 23, 1892, p. 847.
Dalton, N.: "Infiltrating Growth in Liver and Suprarenal Capsule," "Transactions of the Pathological Society," 1885, vol. XXXVI.
Dittrich: "Prager Vierteljahrsschr.," 1849, Jahrgang 6, I, pp. 1–33.
Ebermaier, A.: "Ein Fall von Syphilis hereditaria tarda," Dissertation, Kiel, 1888.
Feige, E.: "Ueber die Todesursachen der Säuglinge bis zum sechsten Lebensmonate, Dissertation, Kiel, 1896.

* Compare, Riedel, *Archiv f. klin. Chir.,* 1894, Bd. XLIX, p. 206.

Gubler: "Gazette médicale de Paris," 1852, p. 262; "Memoire de la société de biologie," 1852.

Haas, G.: "Beitrag zur Lehre von der diffusen congenitalen Lebersyphilis," Dissertation, Kiel, 1891.

Hochsinger, C.: "Eine neue Theorie der congenital-syphilitischen Frühaffecte," "Wiener med. Wochenschr.," 1897, No. 25–27.

Homeister, F.: "Ueber die Todesursachen der Säuglinge bis zum sechsten Lebensmonate," Dissertation, Kiel, 1886.

Hutinel et Hudelo: "Etudes sur les lésions syph. du foie chez les foetus et les nouveaunés," "Archives de médecine expérimentale," 1890, p. 509.

Cedac: "Cirrhose hépatique d'origine syphilitique," etc., "Progrès médicale," No. 22.

Thielen, A.: "Ueber Lebercirrhose bei Kindern durch congenitale Syphilis," Dissertation, Kiel, 1894.

Wronka, L.: "Beitrag zur Kenntniss der angeborenen Leberkrankheiten," Dissertation, Breslau, 1872.

Bäumler: "Syphilis," in Ziemssen's "Handbuch der speciellen Pathologie," 1886, Bd. iii, 1, pp. 187–193.

Neumann, J.: "Syphilis," in Nothnagel's "Specieller Pathologie und Therapie," 1896, Bd. xxiii, pp. 407–435.

Thierfelder: Loc. cit., p. 198.

Frerichs: Loc. cit., Bd. ii, pp. 69 and 152; Abbildungen, pp. 73, 80, 163, und Atlas, Heft 2, Taf. iv und v.

Budd: Loc. cit., p. 328.

NEOPLASMS.

(Hoppe-Seyler.)

FIBROMATA.

Fibromata are benign tumors consisting of dense connective tissue, and are quite frequently found in the liver. As a rule, however, they are so small that they cause no symptoms during life, and are only found at the postmortem examination. On section they appear as small yellowish-white solid nodules embedded in the liver tissue. They vary in size from that of a pinhead to a pea.

If multiple fibroneuromata develop in the body, they may form upon the branches of the sympathetic nerve within the liver.[*] They rarely cause any disturbance.

Chiari [†] reports a large fibroma which was situated in the under surface of the right lobe of the liver to the right of the gall-bladder, and was 7.5 cm. long and 4.5 cm. wide. The growth was found at the autopsy, and it is not stated whether it caused any disturbance during life.

The majority of fibromata are not dangerous, and their presence interferes in no way with the health of the patient. The following case, however, observed by Quincke, in Bern, shows that if the tumor is large and unfortunately situated it may even endanger life:

The case was that of a boy, two and a half years old, who was received in the Inselspital on June 19, 1873. In the fall of 1872 icterus had appeared, and in the beginning of 1873 enlargement and tumor formation had been noted in the middle of the abdomen. Fever was present on admission, the patient showed marked icterus, the stools were discolored, the right lobe of the liver was greatly enlarged, extending from the sixth rib to the crest of the ilium. The left lobe could not be palpated distinctly. The liver was hard, and protruded distinctly; the gall-bladder could be felt, and consisted of a spherical, tensely distended swelling, about as large as a pigeon's egg, and fluctuating. At the same time a splenic tumor was

* Ziegler, "Lehrbuch der path. Anat.," Bd. ii, p. 599.

† Chiari, *Wien. med. Wochenschr.*, 1877, p. 16; Langenbuch, loc. cit., Bd. ii, p. 16.

felt, there was bile-pigment in the urine, itching of the skin, and slowing of the pulse. Ascites was not present. The temperature was elevated toward evening (38° to 39° C.), in the morning it was normal. The liver was punctured several times, but nothing except blood and liver-cells was aspirated. The condition remained unchanged for several months. In October the patient contracted whooping-cough; and then became so emaciated that the liver could be palpated without any difficulty. The size of the organ was unchanged. The gall-bladder was very prominent, and assumed the shape of a conical cylindric body, whose diameter was 3.5 cm., the axis running in an antero-posterior direction. The fundus was soft, the deeper parts hard and uneven. To the right of the gall-bladder a nodular, round tumor was felt, on the lower surface of the liver. The symptoms as described remained stationary for months, a slight attack of bronchitis being the only additional feature. The icterus persisted. In April, 1874, a swelling of the parotid and of the lymph-glands of the neck occurred, hemorrhages from the nose and the mouth appeared, and on the 19th of April, 1874, the patient succumbed to the disease.

At autopsy (Langhans) nothing abnormal was found about the heart. The lower lobe of the right lung was hepatized, there was general icterus, and slight congestion of the kidneys. The spleen was swollen and hard; the follicles numerous, and somewhat opaque; the pulp was brownish-red.

The liver was 24 cm. long, 6 cm. wide, and 3.5 cm. thick; tough (though not inflexible), icteroid, and showed no clouding. The left lobe was very small. On the under surface a round tumor about as large as a hen's egg was found. Its color was reddish, and its consistency hard. The tumor merged directly into liver tissue, and was found to be a fibroma. The gall-bladder was very much distended, and contained a gelatinous, clear, transparent fluid. The common duct was not patulous.

In addition, there was swelling of the parotid and of the lymph-glands of the neck and mesentery.

In this case the tumor, owing to its size and its position, probably led to compression of the bile-passages and complete exclusion of the bile from the intestine, so that death occurred from hepatargia (cholemia).

In similar cases, should they be observed in future, the tumor might be removed by operation, and a cure of the disease be reached in this manner. This has been done successfully in the case of sarcomatous tumors. It is necessary, of course, that the diagnosis should be made early, and possibly with the aid of exploratory laparotomy.

ANGIOMATA.

(Cavernoma. Telangiectasis.)

Angiomata of the liver are, as a rule, clinically insignificant, and are found most often at the postmortem examination. In rare instances, however, large tumors develop, consisting of cavernous tissue, and produce certain disturbances in a mechanical way; *i. e.*, by limiting the interabdominal space, and by exercising pressure on neighboring organs.

v. Eiselsberg reports a tumor of this kind weighing 470 gm., and situated at the margin of the right lobe. Rosenthal observed a fibrous angioma of the lobus Spigelii, and succeeded in removing it.

Birch-Hirschfeld reports an angioma of the liver that was partially extirpated by Hagedorn. It was as large as a pregnant uterus, and completely filled the abdomen.

The majority of angiomata do not protrude above the surface of the liver. They are usually found in old people, and more frequently in men than in women. They develop by taking the place of the liver tissue, and consequently do not produce any symptoms of compression. In the vicinity of a recent angioma fatty degeneration or brownish atrophy of liver-cells can sometimes be seen near the margin of the tumor.

[Schmieden* reports his study of 32 cases of hepatic cavernomas, and of 13 livers that presented appearances of angioma-formation. He discusses the various theories of causation,—primary proliferation of the connective tissue, congestion, primary atrophy of the liver-cells, obstruction to the flow of bile, hemorrhage, etc.,—and states that none of these theories is tenable. He believes that cavernomata of the liver should be ascribed to a local transposition or constriction, or segmentation of tissue, or a defect in the arrangement of the liver tissue. Evidences of the latter he claims are to be detected in the newborn. In short, they correspond to aberrant "rests," and take on tumor formation through secondary changes and alterations. They are distinct from cavernous angiomata of the organs, or of the skin, which are true blood-vessel tumors. He suggests as a better name than angioma "nævus cavernosus hepatis." These growths may occur at any age and have been noted in the embryo; they show little tendency to a sudden increase in size.—Ed.]

In general the tumors are wedge-shaped, with their bases at the surface of the liver, underneath the capsule. They resemble infarcts in this respect. They appear as circumscribed reddish or black spots on the surface of the organ; these may be as large as a pinhead or a nut, and on superficial inspection look like hemorrhages. On transverse section they present the appearance of spongy tissue, consisting of numerous vascular spaces intercommunicating with one another, and separated by septa of connective tissue. (Virchow found some smooth muscle-fibers.) Sometimes the septa are thickened; and in such cases we speak of a fibrous angioma (Böttcher). Occasionally the tumors are inclosed in a dense capsule, though, as a rule, they are not so sharply separated from the parenchyma. If the blood-vessels that lead to these angiomata become occluded, cystic metamorphosis may occur with exudation of serous fluid into the cavity. Occasionally dark pigment is deposited in the septa and in the neighboring liver tissue constituting the so-called melanotic angioma (Hanot and Gilbert). Quite frequently angiomata are found co-existing in the kidney, just as cysts are found in these organs together with cysts in the liver.

The cavernous tumors have usually a distinct connection with the branches of the portal vein; at the same time it is possible to inject them from the hepatic artery, as branches of this vessel supply the septa. Some authors (Birch-Hirschfeld, Hanot and Gilbert) believe that they originate in ectases of capillaries, combined with atrophy of the columns of liver-cells. Other authors believe that they are the result of senile marasmus, and that they represent circumscribed atrophy of liver-cells, and secondary ectasy of capillaries (Ziegler). Still others, like Virchow, claim that they develop from dilated branches of the portal vein, secondary to a primary inflammatory proliferation of connective tissue. Lilienfeld, working under Ribbert, arrives at the conclusion that they are formed from the interacinous vessels; in the beginning, from branches of the portal vein alone that become dilated to cavernous spaces and later in the disease the smaller vessels that originate from these spaces participate in the process; finally, the capillaries of the acini are also involved. In this manner inflammatory processes take place in the interacinous tissues around the vessels, so that their elasticity is reduced, and they become dilated as a consequence. The liver-cells atrophy, and are frequently found very narrow in the immediate vicinity of the cavernous tissue. An abnormal number

* *Virchow's Archiv*, CLXI, 373, 1900.

of leucocytes is found in the blood of these cavernomata; free liver-cells are also seen. Ribbert has lately arrived at a conclusion that is similar to that of Virchow and Rindfleisch—namely, that newly formed connective tissue penetrates the liver substance, and that this tissue is later filled with vascular spaces. He believes that the first cause of a cavernoma consists in a small independent area inserted atypically into the liver-tissue, where the process develops independently.

Virchow's view that a chronic inflammatory process plays a rôle in the formation of multiple angiomata appears to be the most plausible one; at the same time, it is possible that dilatation of capillaries together with secondary atrophy of liver-cells may produce the tumor, while, at the same time, in other cases the degeneration and atrophy of the liver-cells may be primary. Beneke, for instance, describes a case in which capillary ectasis developed in a wedge-shaped area of the liver, combined with atrophy of liver-cells. In the apex of this cone-shaped district was found an obstructed bile-duct (as a result of a tubercular process), and Beneke draws the following conclusion: At first there was obliteration of the bile-duct, then stasis of bile, followed by degeneration and atrophy of the liver-cells, and ultimately dilatation of capillaries.

Congenital angiomata must be distinguished from this acquired form. Steffen describes a solitary tumor of this kind that was as large as an apple. Chervinsky saw a large number of cavernomata in the enlarged liver of a child of seven months; these growths made the surface of the liver nodular. They resemble the cases of v. Eiselsberg and Rosenthal that were described above, and appeared to be genuine tumors and not the result of interacinous inflammation. Pilliet thinks that they are fetal inclusions of mesenchyma similar to the vascular nevi of the skin and fissural angiomata.

The **diagnosis** of cavernoma can probably only be made during life by an exploratory incision in those cases in which a large tumor is present causing distress, and calling for an operation. In all other cases the presence of cavernomata will remain unrecognized.

The **prognosis** is favorable.

Treatment of the condition is unnecessary in the ordinary form of multiple angioma, as these forms are harmless. In the case of large solitary tumors the advisability of resection must be considered. This operation is very bloody, but usually successful.

Beneke: "Zur Genese der Leberangiome," "Virchow's Archiv," Bd. cxix, p. 54.
Birch-Hirschfeld: "Lehrbuch der pathologischen Anatomie," Bd. ii, p. 615.
Böttcher: "Virchow's Archiv," Bd. xxviii, p. 421.
Chervinsky: "Archives de physiologie normale et pathologique," 1885, tome ii, p. 553.
v. Eiselsberg: "Wiener klin. Wochenschr.," 1893, No. 1.
Frerichs: "Klinik der Leberkrankheiten," Bd. ii, p. 210.
Hanot et Gilbert: "Etudes sur les mal. du foie," 1888, p. 314.
Journiac: "Archives de physiologie normale et pathologique," 1879, p. 58.
Langhans: "Virchow's Archiv," Bd. lxxv, p. 273.
Lilienfeld: "Ueber die Entstehung der Cavernome in der Leber," Dissertation, Bonn, 1889.
Pilliet: "Verhandlungen der Pariser anatomischen Gesellschaft," July 3, 1891.
Ribbert: "Ueber Bau, Wachsthum und Genese der Angiome," "Virchow's Archiv," Bd. cli, p. 381.
Steffen: "Jahrbuch für Kinderheilkunde," 1883, Bd. xix, p. 348.
Virchow: "Virchow's Archiv," Bd. vi, p. 527.

CYSTS.

(Cystoma, Cystadenoma, Cystic Liver.)

Cavities filled with fluid may originate in the liver in different ways. The most important examples of this nature are echinococcus cysts; these we will discuss in another place. The bile-ducts may become occluded by tumors, scars, parasites, etc., or gall-stones, so that the bile and the mucous secretion of the bile-duct epithelium is retained; cavities may be formed in this way that may be single, or may ramify in different directions through the tissues of the liver. Dilatation of the gall-bladder by stasis, the so-called hydrops of the gall-bladder, may also be seen; or tumors may soften and form fluctuating swellings. Of all these conditions we will speak in other sections.

We limit our discussion at present to those cavities that are filled with fluid, and to such as originate in the liver independently of any of the above-mentioned causes. Among these we must distinguish two classes—namely, first, simple (usually solitary) cysts that represent, in the main, malformations; and, secondly, multiple cysts, disseminated throughout the liver, and in this way causing more or less serious damage (cystic liver, cystadenoma, cystic degeneration of the liver). The former type is usually observed at birth, or perhaps at the postmortem examination. Cystic liver, on the other hand, is a pathologic process intimately related to tumor formation in the liver, and forming a distinct transition toward those neoplasms which we usually designate as adenomata, and which in many instances are malign. Some authors believe that the formation of multiple cysts in the liver may also be congenital, and it is possible that this is occasionally the case; it is, however, striking that so many cases of cysts that develop later in life show some proliferation and the same histologic structure as the congenital type. Cystic degeneration in the liver is often accompanied by the same process in the kidneys, the ovaries, the broad ligaments, or in other organs of the body. Cystic liver is a condition that progresses rapidly, and causes serious disturbance in a short time; this statement does not, however, apply to the first category of cases.

Simple cysts of the liver of the first class often show in a most pronounced manner that they originate in malformations; this applies, for instance, to the hepatic cysts described by Witzel, Sänger and Klopp.

These growths were so large that they obstructed the delivery of the child.

In the case described by Sänger and Kloop a pedunculated cyst was observed in the liver, in addition to a marked ascites. The cyst contained a third of a liter of a cloudy, dark, yellow, slimy fluid, containing mucin, bile-pigment, albumin, squamous and cuboid epithelial cells. It was surrounded by a capsule of connective tissue, in which were found clumps of liver tissue inlaid with flattened cells. In another case liver tissue was found embedded in the wall of the cyst. The two authors consider the first cyst as an accessory liver with an accessory gall-bladder; the second case appeared to present an accessory liver with a cyst of an accessory bile-duct. In addition, a number of cysts were found in the vicinity of the stomach and intestine that also contained liver tissue in their wall, and which were considered accessory livers developing from Meckel's diverticulum. Other authors (Morgagni, Wagner, Gruber) have also described accessory livers. Occasionally the gall-bladder may be divided into two parts, situated next to or behind one another (Ahlfeld and others). In the monster described the spleen was also divided into numerous single spleens; there was also a transposition of the viscera, hemicephalus, etc.

In Witzel's case three liters of fluid were evacuated from the cavity before birth could take place. The cyst occupied both the left and the right lobe of the liver, and communicated with the common duct, which ended in a culdesac in the region of the duodenum; this, too, was a monster, with transposed viscera. The kidneys were filled with numerous cysts.

A number of other cases have been described in which cysts were found in the vicinity of the suspensory ligament, and which caused no disturbance during the life of the patient.

Friedreich describes a cyst that was as large as a hazelnut, and was connected with the liver by loose connective tissue; ciliated epithelium were noted on top of a layer of round embryonal cells. The fluid contents were viscid, yellowish-gray, and slimy. Eberth describes a similar case. We owe the most careful description of cysts of this kind to von Recklinghausen, who notes a cyst of the size of a hazelnut containing a thick pasty mass, with granules of albumin and mucin; the epithelium was long and ciliated, and was placed upon an embryonal layer of cells. In those cases in which the cells were not so long the second layer and the cilia were lost. This cyst communicated with a mucous gland in the hepatic wall, which was dilated and cavernous, and apparently manufactured the contents of the cyst. In addition, numerous canals were found in the wall, which Friedreich considered as lymph-spaces. Von Recklinghausen, however, believed them to be bile-passages, vasa aberrantia, and observed hyaline metamorphosis of their epithelium. He attributes the formation of these subserous mucous cysts to an isolation of bile-passages, and believes that mucus, formed by the glands situated in the walls of these bile-passages, is retained within these canals. Waring has described two similar cases of cysts in the lower margin of the liver, and has made drawings of them. Virchow has described structures of this kind containing mucus or colloid, and situated near the surface of the liver; one of these was situated in the suspensory ligament. Virchow is inclined to the belief that it was formed by the isolation of vasa aberrantia. It can very well be understood why these cysts contained no bile, as such passages are not connected with secreting liver tissue. The ciliated character of the epithelium lining these cysts need not surprise us, for we know that the form and the size of the epithelial cells vary with the conditions of nutrition, in the same manner as in ovarian cysts, cysts of the glands of Bartholini, etc. Von Recklinghausen considers the cyst formation to be the result of a myxadenitis, in combination with isolation of bile-passages.

Zahn, on the other hand, considers cysts containing ciliated epithelium to be fetal growths of organs that have nothing to do with the liver; he bases this conclusion upon the fact that in all cases observed by him he found the cysts always in the same location—namely, the vicinity of the suspensory ligament between the peritoneum and the membrana propria of the liver. He believes that they are the remnants of some organ that is present in the embryonal stage and disappears subsequently. Another case, reported by Girode and published by Hanot and Gilbert, belongs to this class. This was a cavity lined with ciliated epithelium and situated in the vicinity of the suspensory ligament. The growth was found by chance at the autopsy.

We are probably justified in including certain cysts of the liver, treated surgically, among these congenital structures. These cysts were very large, but were similarly situated. No general cystic degeneration of the liver or the kidneys appeared to be present.

As these cases recovered after the operation this question could not be decided.

A case reported by Winkler must be included in this category. He describes it as a cystoma of the ovary, but found later that it was connected with the lower margin of the liver; not, however, until he had evacuated some eight liters of a yellow, brownish-red fluid, alkaline in reaction, of a specific gravity of 1014, and containing much albumin and mucin, a little bile-pigment, much cholesterin, and colloid round structures that were about as large as a leucocyte. The wall of this cyst contained no epithelium, but consisted exclusively of connective tissue. After the operation a bile-tinged, and later a mucopurulent fluid, continued to ooze from the wound. It is possible that this was a congenital cyst that later became inflamed so that an abundant secretion occurred into the cavity, or that it was a mucous cyst which had originated in a vas aberrans as a result of inflammation of the mucous membrane and occlusion of the duct. v. Recklinghausen describes a cyst of this kind in a case which he reports.

48

The other category of cysts of the liver—namely, **multiple cysto-mata,** or cystic liver, cystic degeneration, etc.—has an intimate connection with the bile-passages. These cases, and others that were less carefully investigated, presented tumors that were probably mucous cysts developing from vasa aberrantia or bile-passages that did not end within the liver tissue, but ended blindly in the region of the suspensory ligament. In the cases now to be discussed the intrahepatic bile-passages developed into cysts, probably in a manner analogous to the development of cysts from urinary tubules within the kidneys. Older authors (Rokitansky) believed that these cysts developed from blood-vessels or lymph-channels; more recent investigators, however, have demonstrated that they develop from bile-passages, and particularly from ducts formed during certain pathologic conditions. They are related to adenomata; and the cystadenomata form a connecting-link. These cysts show a tendency to rupture into blood-vessels in the same way as do bile-duct adenomata (v. Hippel).

As a sharp differentiation cannot be made, we will describe cyst adenomata and the so-called cystic degeneration as one and the same condition. Cysts hold their place among the tumor formations of the liver. Coexisting cirrhosis has frequently been observed and some authors have even expressed their belief that the cirrhotic process has a decided influence upon the development of the cysts. Thus, Sabourin states that they develop from the new bile-passages that are seen in interlobular cirrhosis, that these canals become dilated, and form a cavernous network (*angiome biliaire*); that they then develop further, become confluent, and in this way form a cyst inclosing several biliary cavities. Juhel-Rénoy, in his case, observed new-formation of bile-passages in the condensed interacinous connective tissue, and in these canals signs of cholangitis and pericholangitis; further, dilatation and the formation of cysts; all these conditions he ascribes originally to the occlusion of these bile-passages. Rolleston and Kanthack describe dilatation of bile-passages in the newborn in cases complicated with portal cirrhosis. On the other hand, cases have been described in which cirrhotic lesions were absent, or present only to a very slight degree, so that it can hardly be assumed that cirrhosis is concerned etiologically in the formation of these cysts. The new-formation of bile-passages which precedes the development of the cysts apparently is not only a result of proliferation of interlobular bile-passages and budding of these canals into the acini of the liver, but also a result of the metamorphosis of columns of liver-cells into canals that contain rows of cells similar to the epithelia of the bile-passages. We will describe the development of this process when discussing the genesis of adenomata and adenocarcinomata (compare page 765). Naunyn describes a case of cystadenoma which he calls a cystosarcoma, in which the transition of bile-passages into cysts is noted. This author shows how buds are formed on these passages, and how these again become dilated and increased by new cells until, finally, a cavity results that continues to enlarge. v. Hippel, Manski, and others have also described the formation of cysts from bile-passages, some of which sent dendritic ramifications into the acini (v. Kahlden). In the bile-passages of the liver cholangitis, thickening of the walls, and occlusion of the lumen by desquamated epithelium is frequently seen; the fully developed cysts have a cylindrical or cuboid epithelium, or a squamous polyhedric epithelium. In the larger cysts the epithelium is lower and flatter than in the small variety, owing to the stretching of the cyst-wall by the fluid. In the largest cysts cells may be completely absent owing to atrophy or desquamation; hemorrhage, too, may cause separation of the epithelium. Occasionally the walls are folded, and show connective-tissue processes; in other cases the walls are smooth. In the manner described cysts may be formed that contain many liters of fluid, and these may be seen side by side with cysts that are no larger than a pinhead. The contents consist of a more or less albuminous fluid containing mucin and peculiar colloid structures; further, epithelium, leucocytes, red blood-corpuscles, granular masses of albumin, crystals of hematoidin, and cholesterin. As a rule, bile-pigment is absent; traces of phosphates and chlorids are found. The color is usually watery, or yellowish-brown, or chocolate color; the latter is seen particularly in cases where hemorrhages have occurred into the cyst.

Sometimes a process of repair may be observed in these cysts, consisting of a proliferation of connective tissue in the wall, that gradually fills the cavity. The liver tissue is often atrophic and degenerated; the columns of liver-cells are flattened, and remnants are occasionally seen in the wall of the cyst. Branches of the portal vein may show cavernous dilatation. Macroscopically a liver of this kind presents a very peculiar picture; large and small cysts form dark and light protrusions on the surface and the transverse section of the organ. The interior of the liver is converted into a series of innumerable cavities varying in size from a pinhead to a child's skull; between these cavities a little of the liver substance may be seen. Some of the cysts are so large that they inclose several liters of fluid (Manski); at the same time stasis of bile or of blood may be present and give the organ a still more peculiar aspect. Occasionally the liver is hard and cirrhotic and only slightly or not at all enlarged; in the majority of cases, however, the organ is soft and very large, so that it weighs as much as 10 kg. (Dmochowski and Janowski). Stasis may be present in the portal vein and lead to ascites, swelling of the spleen, and congestive catarrh of the stomach and intestine.

Terburgh describes peculiar round, protoplasmic bodies with a radiating striated zone; and other bodies that are inclosed in a radiating striated shell, and contain granular masses and sometimes nuclei resembling the eggs of tenia. These were found in the fresh fluid aspirated from the cystic liver; the author believes it likely that psorospermia were involved in the cyst formation, particularly as in rabbits the presence of this parasite often causes the formation of large cavities in the liver filled with a thick whitish mass. He was not enabled to examine these structures carefully. Gubler found a number of spherical tumors in the liver of a man of forty-five, containing a viscid, slimy substance in which psorospermia were present. Leuckart also describes a similar case (see page 789). We expect that further investigation will throw more light upon this subject; it is necessary, however, that analyses should be made of fresh material, as Terburgh reports that he could no longer discover the structures he has described if the fluid was allowed to stand.

[Shupell called attention in December, 1900, to a case of simple retention cyst of the liver. He was led to look upon the case as one of that nature because of the histologic formation, the fact that it was full of bile, and because of the total absence of hooklets. A similar

case has recently been reported by Israel Cleaver * that again brings
up the question of origin of these cystic growths. His specimen obtained at autopsy measured 12½ inches in width, the left lobe 4 inches,
the vertical length 8 inches, and the thickness 5½ inches. A large cyst
projected above the surface measuring 7½ inches in circumference,
occupying the under surface of the right lobe, and crowding the gall-
bladder, which was itself much enlarged. There was also a second
cyst, walnut-sized, sessile, on the upper margin of the left lobe, and
four more of the size of hulled shellbarks on the surface of the same
face, but to the right of the large cyst. Sections of the portions of the
organ not involved by the cysts showed no parenchymatous change.
The gall-bladder contained 26 calculi. He refers to similar cases reported
by Roberts† and Robson.‡ No hooklets were found in the fluid from
any of the cases. The symptoms were invariably such as to lead to the
diagnosis of distended gall-bladder.—ED.]

Symptoms.—Congenital cysts, like those described by Witzel, Sänger
and Klopp, may be so large as to cause ascites, and constitute
an obstacle to the delivery of the child. If the tumor is perforated
or tears, the fetus dies. It may, however, not be so large as this, and
may remain latent during the life of the subject and be found at autopsy;
or it may continue to grow owing to some irritant influence, the origin
of which we do not understand, and later on form a large cystic tumor
that will endanger life.

Bayer reports a case in which a large, rapidly developing cyst was found, and
in which he assumes that the growth was the result of an inflammatory process in
the bile passages. It is possible, however, that this was a congenital cyst that
later became inflamed and hemorrhagic.

A cyst of this size may fill a large part of the abdomen, may push
the diaphragm upward, compress the right lung, lead to icterus from
stasis, and cause swelling of the liver and of the gall-bladder. All of
these conditions I have observed in the following case:

A girl of four years was admitted on the 19th of July, 1895; during the six weeks
preceding this date she suffered from diarrhea, loss of appetite, emaciation, and,
later, fever, icterus, and itching of the skin. A tumor was felt that was evidently
connected with the liver, fluctuated, and extended below the navel. On July 21st
Neuber performed a laparotomy, when it was found that the intestine was situated
in front of the swelling, that the liver was pushed upward, the gall-bladder filled
and resting on the tumor. Violent parenchymatous hemorrhage occurred, and for
this reason the cyst was not opened, and the wound was closed with tampons.
The child died from collapse a few hours after the operation. It was found that
the cyst contained over a liter of a mucous, clear fluid, was situated between the
kidney and under surface of the liver and the intestine, and was connected with
the liver in the region of the porta hepatis; in addition there were peritonitic adhesions
existed to neighboring organs. The cyst had compressed the bile-passages at the
hilum, principally the common duct, and for this reason there was stasis of bile in
the liver and the gall-bladder, the latter viscus containing about 100 cm. of a bile-
tinged fluid. The cystic duct was dilated, and also filled with bile. The wall of
the cyst could be divided into two layers, the inner one of which showed the structure of mucous membrane. Unfortunately a more careful microscopic examination was not undertaken.

It appears that ascites does not occur as frequently in the case of
these cysts as in general cystic degeneration, probably because the
isolated form of cyst develops near the anterior margin of the liver

---

Phila. Med. Jour., Dec. 28, 1901.   † *Annals of Surgery*, vol. XIX, p. 251.
‡ "Treat's Annual," 1895.

and increases in size toward the open abdominal cavity, and, therefore, does not compress the portal vein. Another reason may exist in the fact that in multiple cystic degeneration changes are frequently observed that are not present in the case of other cysts.

Multiple cysts of the liver are frequently unexpectedly found at autopsy, as they may produce no symptoms during life. Cystic degeneration of the liver, however, is more frequently diagnosed than the same condition in the kidneys, principally because the former organ is more accessible to palpation, and because the nodulated surface, with fluctuations here and there, is to an extent characteristic. If abundant ascites is present, this peculiarity may be masked, as the ascitic fluid will push the liver upward, and also cover its surface; if the fluid is evacuated, the change of form can usually be recognized. Sometimes exploratory puncture of a fluctuating tumor may establish a diagnosis; as, for instance, the presence of albumin and mucin, the absence of hooks, scolices, shreds of membrane, will help differentiate the cyst from echinococcus. It is necessary, however, to proceed very carefully, and with all aseptic precautions, as purulent infection of the cyst may occur. In addition to ascites, a considerable degree of edema of the lower extremity may result from compression of the inferior vena cava. Other symptoms of condensation of peri-portal connective tissue, hemorrhages, catarrh in the intestine, may be seen as in typical cirrhosis; sometimes, but not frequently, icterus develops. Changes in the kidneys are particularly important, and modify the course of the symptom-complex, particularly cystic degeneration of these organs, a condition that is so frequently seen together with cystic degeneration of the liver. The symptoms of chronic nephritis or of contracted kidney frequently complicate this form of degeneration, so that patients in whom a diagnosis of cystic degeneration of the liver was made during life, or in whom this condition was found postmortem have died of albuminuria, suppression of urine, uremia, and coma.

Prognosis.—The prognosis of solitary cysts of the liver and of cystic degeneration of the organ depends very much on the involvement of the bile-passages, the portal vein, or of other organs. If the kidneys are diseased, or if cirrhosis of the liver is present as a complication, the prognosis becomes graver.

Treatment is of little avail in multiple cyst formation, and consists exclusively in aspiration of the ascitic fluid or drainage of the lower extremities in case of compression of the vena cava. The renal condition will require the greatest amount of attention. If large solitary cysts are present, an operation may be necessary. Such growths have been successfully extirpated (Hueter), and others have been sutured to the abdominal wall and drained (Winckler).

Bayer, C.: "Ueber eine durch Operation geheilte, mannskopfgrosse Lebercyste," "Prager med. Wochenschr.," 1892, p. 637.
Chotinsky: Dissertation, Bern, 1882.
Dmochowski und Janowski: "Ein seltener Fall von totaler cystischer Entartung der Leber," "Ziegler's Beiträge," 1894, Bd. xvi, p. 102.
Frerichs: "Klinik der Leberkrankheiten," Bd. ii, p. 216.
Friedreich: "Cyste mit Flimmerepithel in der Leber," "Virchow's Archiv," Bd. xi, p. 466.
Hanot et Gilbert: "Etudes sur les mal. du foie," 1888, p. 295.
v. Hippel: "Ein Fall von multiplen Cystadenomen der Gallengänge," "Virchow's Archiv," Bd. cxxiii, p. 473.

Hueter: "Ein grosses Cystom der Leber," Dissertation, Göttingen, 1887.
Juhel-Rénoy: "Observation de dégénérescence kystique du foie et des reins," "Revue de médecine," 1881, p. 929.
v. Kahlden: "Ueber die Genese der multiplen Cystenniere und der Cystenleber," "Ziegler's Beitrage," Bd. xiii, p. 291.
Manski: "Ueber Cystadenome der Leber," Dissertation, Kiel, 1895.
North: "Case of Cystic Tumor of the Liver," "New York Med Record," Sept. 23, 1882, p. 344.
Opitz: "Ein Fall von Leber- und Nierencysten," Dissertation, Kiel, 1895.
v. Recklinghausen: "Ueber die Ranula, die Cyste der Bartholin'schen Drüse und die Flimmercyste der Leber," "Virchow's Archiv," 1884, Bd. lxxxiv, p. 473.
Rolleston und Kanthack: "Beiträge zur Pathologie der cystischen Erkrankung der Leber im Neugeborenen," "Virchow's Archiv," Bd. cxxx, p. 488.
Sabourin: "Contribution à l'ét. de la dégénérescence kystique des reins et du foie," "Archives de physiologie," 1882, tome ii, p. 63.
Sänger und Klopp: "Zur anatomischen Kenntniss der angeborenen Bauchcysten," "Archiv für Gynàkologie," 1880, Bd. xvi, p. 415.
Siegmund: "Ueber eine cystische Geschwulst der Leber," "Virchow's Archiv," 1889, Bd. cxv, p. 155.
Terburgh: "Ueber Leber- und Nierencysten," Dissertation, Freiburg, 1891.
Virchow: "Geschwülste," Bd. i, p. 256.
Waring: "Diseases of the Liver," p. 148.
Winckler: "Zur Casuistik der Lebercysten," Dissertation, Marburg, 1891.
Witzel: "Hemicephalus mit grossen Lebercysten," "Centralblatt f. Gynäkologie," 1880.
Zahn: "Ueber die mit Flimmerepithel ausgekleideten Cysten . . . der Leber," "Virchow's Archiv," Bd. cxliii, p. 170.

CARCINOMA, SARCOMA, ADENOMA.

As a rule, carcinoma and other malignant neoplasms of the liver are discussed apart from a connection with similar growths of the gall-bladder and the bile-passages. The clinical picture, however, does not admit of a strict differentiation, for the reason that a primary carcinoma of the liver may be complicated by a secondary carcinoma of the gall-bladder or bile-passages; and because, inversely, a carcinoma of the gall-bladder may make its way into liver tissue, and develop princi-pally within the liver substance. Finally, carcinomata of intrahepatic bile-passages act just as do primary growths of the liver parenchyma. For all these reasons we will discuss these different forms of neoplasms together.

Etiology.—The nature of the virus of carcinoma is so obscure that we will not discuss it. If we assume that such a virus exists, we must also admit that it must enter the liver through the blood in cases of primary carcinoma; and we will have to assume that this occurs through the portal vein, as in the case of all other diseases-producers that become localized in the liver (animal parasites, etc.). In other words, the virus must come from the intestine, pass through the venules into the portal vein, and thus be carried into the liver. Secondary carcinomata of the liver certainly originate in this manner. In cases of carcinoma of the stomach, the intestine, the rectum, and the pancreas, carcinoma-tous involvement of the liver is often seen, and may develop into a larger tumor than the original focus. Such a growth in the liver was at one time looked upon as the primary tumor with greater frequency than to-day, because the larger tumor was, as a rule, considered to be the primary one, and, moreover, the general examination of the abdomi-nal organs was often imperfect. It is also possible for metastases to develop in the liver by means of the general circulation through the hepatic artery, as, for instance, after carcinoma of the breast, and other neoplasms in remote organs. In carcinoma of the female genitals, particularly in cancer of the uterus, the infection probably enters the liver from certain portions of the body the veins of which anastomose with the portal system.

Primary carcinomata of the bile-passages and of the gall-bladder from the intestine through the ducts, may very possibly result from infection from the bowel through the ducts. Secondary growths of these parts may come from the liver, or especially from carcinomata of the lower abdominal organs.

A certain amount of importance has been attached to *heredity* in the case of carcinoma of the liver. Up to this time writers on this question have offered little that is convincing. Paget and West state that hereditary predisposition exists in 17 % of all cases; Lebert finds it in 14 %, Sibley in 11 %. Leichtenstern, who has summarized these and other statistics, finds a hereditary predisposition in 192 out of 1137 cases (17 %).

It may also happen that several individuals are afflicted with carcinoma in the same house, and all contract a carcinoma of the liver and die from this lesion (D'Arcy, Power, Scott, Langenbuch).

Carcinoma of the liver is less frequent than carcinoma of the uterus, the stomach, or the breast.

According to Leichtenstern, out of 10,007 cases of carcinoma, 31 % were of the uterus, 27 % were of gastric carcinoma, 12 % of breast carcinoma, and 6 % of liver carcinoma.

Carcinoma of the liver is particularly frequent in advanced age, after forty.

According to Leichtenstern, 7.8 % of all cases were found between twenty and thirty years, 12.9 % between thirty and forty, 53.1 % between forty and sixty, 19.3 % between sixty and seventy, and 6.9 % above seventy. In children carcinoma is rare, but does occur. Thus, it has been found in the new-born (Siebold) and in a child of six months (Bohn). Farré found a secondary carcinoma in a child of three months, and in two children of two years and a half. Wulff saw carcinoma of the liver in a child of three years, Kottmann in a child of nine years, Deschamps in a child of eleven years, and Roberts in a child of twelve years. Leichtenstern and Langenbuch have also seen carcinoma of the liver in children.

[A considerable number of cases of primary carcinoma of the liver in children have been reported within the past few years, of which the most interesting were those noted by Descroizille * and 10 cases noted by Schlesinger.† The ages ranged from four to eleven and a half years.—ED.]

The female sex is afflicted more frequently with secondary carcinoma than the male, this being due to the great tendency to primary carcinoma of the breast, the uterus, and the ovaries. Primary carcinoma of the liver is more frequent in men because male subjects are more frequently afflicted with cirrhosis, and because this disease seems to favor the development of carcinoma. It is stated that malaria and the abuse of alcohol are predisposing factors.

[This latter belief is of especial interest in view of the recent attempts to cure carcinoma by producing a malarial infection (Löffler ‡). The procedure has since been proved to be an absolute failure as regards the cure of the cancerous growth.—ED.]

* *Rev. mens. des Mall. de l'Enf.*, June, 1894.
† "Jahrbuch. f. Kinderh.," March, 1902.
‡ *Deutsche med. Woch.*, Oct. 17, 1901.

Traumata of the liver may have something to do with the formation of carcinoma, just as we sometimes see the development of neoplasms, parasites, and the lodgment of infectious material in other parts of the body following slight injury.

Chronic irritation seems to be an important factor in the etiology of carcinoma of the bile-passages and the gall-bladder; for this reason we see this form of tumor quite frequently in cholelithiasis. Courvoisier found carcinoma of the gall-bladder in 2.7 % of cases with gall-stones; Siegert found gall-stones almost without exception (95 %) in primary carcinoma of the gall-bladder; in secondary carcinoma they were rarely found (15 to 16 %). It seems natural, then, that carcinomata of this character are more frequently found in women than in men, because the former, are more frequently afflicted with gall-stones. It may be that lacing, which is made responsible for the frequency of cholelithiasis in women (Heller, Marchand, and others), exercises a pernicious effect on the gall-bladder, and thus favors the development of carcinoma.

Tiedemann has collated 79 cases of carcinoma of the gall-bladder, and found that 11.3 % were in men, 88.7 % in women, and that gall-stones were present in 79.7 %. Siegert mentions 99 cases of primary carcinoma of the gall-bladder, of which 15 % occurred in men, 82 % in women, and in two no statements are made. Musser found carcinoma of the gall-bladder in women three times more frequently than in men; Kelynack four times more frequently.

The view that carcinoma of the bile-forming organs leads to stasis of bile, and in this manner favors the development of gall-stones, seems less justifiable than that carcinoma is the result of the action of gall-stones.

The effect of gall-stones on the epithelium of the mucous membrane is to convert it into a horny flat epithelium, and as this is the same tissue as that seen in carcinoma, we may have here an argument in favor of the rôle of gall-stones in the formation of carcinoma. Willigk has stated that stasis of bile in the bile-passages may be the cause of carcinoma even in the absence of gall-stones.

In contradistinction to primary carcinoma of the liver, a condition that is often seen at an age when carcinoma elsewhere is rare [*vide* foregoing exceptions—Ed.], primary carcinoma of the gall-bladder is chiefly seen in old age. Tiedemann states that sixty is the average age for carcinoma of the gall-bladder; whereas Leichtenstern states that in primary carcinoma of the liver the average age is below forty.

Carcinoma of the gall-bladder is the most frequent of the primary carcinomata about the liver. Genuine primary carcinoma of the parenchyma of the liver is rare. Primary carcinomata of the bile-passages are very rare. Among 258 cases of carcinoma of the liver in the Berlin Pathologic Institute, Hansemann found 25 cases of primary carcinoma of the gall-bladder, 6 true primary carcinomata of the liver, 2 of which were indefinite, and 2 primary carcinomata of the large bile-ducts.

The rare cases of **primary sarcoma** of the liver that have been reported are usually seen in persons still younger than those afflicted with carcinoma; they are seen more frequently in childhood. Some observations seem to indicate that cirrhotic changes in the liver predispose to the development of this form of tumor, but this has not been proved. [Axtell reported a case of primary sarcoma of the liver in a child,* as

* *N. Y. Med. Jour.*, March 3, 1894.

did Samuel West.* The latter case was fifteen years old. Williamson †
reports 11 cases of melanotic sarcoma of the liver, in 3 of which melano-
gen was twice found in the urine. Hamburger also reports 2 cases
of melanosarcoma of the liver following sarcoma of the eye; in the urine
of these cases also melanin was found. Pepper has recently reported a
case of congenital sarcoma of the liver and suprarenal capsule.‡—Ed.]
Secondary sarcomata are also found in young persons, and may
originate from sarcomata in various parts of the body by metastasis.
This is particularly the case in melanotic sarcomata of the choroid and
of the skin. The causes of **malignant adenoma** are obscure; it seems
that cirrhosis of the liver favors their development.

Pathologic Anatomy.—Primary carcinoma of the liver: Within
the last decade it has been shown that primary carcinoma of the liver is
of rare occurrence compared with its secondary occurrence, and as
a result great care has since been taken to exclude the presence of carcinoma in other organs. The anatomic conditions were soon better
understood, and it became possible to differentiate between primary
and secondary tumors of the liver, and to-day it seems fair to draw
a conclusion from histologic examination of the liver whether the metastasis is from the stomach, the intestine, the uterus, or whether the
tumor is a primary growth of the parenchyma of the liver. The investigations of Naunyn, Waldeyer, Schüppel, and of his pupils; also those
of Weigert, Hanot and Gilbert, Hansemann, Siegenbeck van Heukelom (dissertations published from the Pathologic Institute in Kiel
by Rohwedder, Nölke, and others), as well as numerous other publications, give us a clear insight into the structure and genesis of primary
carcinoma of the liver.

Some points are not clear, and are still the subjects of controversy.
This is particularly the case in regard to adenomata of the liver, of
the kind first described by Rindfleisch and Griesinger; also of carcinomata. Occasionally adenomatous and carcinomatous growths are seen
side by side in the liver, so that the suspicion seems somewhat justified
that the one may merge into the other. Naunyn believed that there was
no difference between the two diseases, and Schüppel expressed the
opinion that nodular hyperplasia, adenoma, and carcinoma form a
chain. The adenoma, according to his view, persists for a long time,
or permanently, owing to its histologic structure as a typical new-formation of glandular epithelium. Under certain circumstances, however,—
in case, for instance, irritation sets in,—the tissues are stimulated to
increased growth, and may develop into an atypical carcinomatous
form of growth. Hanot and Gilbert, also Siegenbeck van Heukelom
(adenocarcinoma of the liver), are in favor of this view. Rindfleisch,
Simmonds, Kelsch and Kiener, Sabourin, and others, differentiate the
two diseases. Clinically no difference can be formulated between an
adenoma that is complicated by cirrhosis and a carcinoma with cirrhosis, and for this reason we will discuss them as one condition.

Primary carcinoma may appear in various forms. It may be solitary
or multiple, and with or without proliferation of interstitial connective
tissue. The parenchymatous cells of the liver and the epithelium of
the bile-passages may participate in the formation of the neoplasm.
In this manner totally different pictures are created.

* *Brit. Med. Jour.*, Oct. 25, 1902.   † *Lancet*, Dec. 2, 1900.
‡ *Amer. Jour. Med. Sci.*, Mar., 1901.

The following constitute the three principal types:

First, massive **carcinoma.** In the interior of the liver, and usually surrounded by healthy liver tissue (almond-carcinoma), there appears a round, rapidly developing tumor that later on sends metastasis into the liver parenchyma. The organ is much enlarged, with a smooth surface, or with a surface that is covered with large flat ridges in case the neoplasm penetrates far into the liver. These spots appear pale, whitish-yellow, or grayish, and are clearly differentiated from the rest of the liver tissue. Occasionally the capsule is thickened, but never adherent to the parietal peritoneum. On transverse section the differences in color are very apparent. The healthy liver tissue shows no cirrhotic induration, and the cut surface of the carcinoma no distinct softening, because there is very little tendency to degeneration of a primary carcinoma of the liver. Numerous strands of connective tissue are seen on the cut surface; these are white, in part transparent, and inclose nodules of carcinomatous tissue which are as large as a cherry, and appear softer in the center than at the periphery. The neoplasm is distinctly demarcated from the normal tissue. Metastases are found in the lymph-glands of the hilum, and less frequently in the peritoneum, the kidneys, and the lungs.

Second, **nodular carcinoma.** The appearance of the liver resembles that of secondary carcinoma. There are numerous whitish-gray or yellowish nodules throughout the liver and protruding above the surface. There is usually no depression in the center as a result of softening. The liver is not as large as in the preceding case; generally, there is wide-spread cirrhosis, and consequently a contraction and induration of the parenchyma. Sometimes one large and numerous small nodules of carcinoma are found, so that it appears as though the latter originated from the former. Transition stages between massive and nodular carcinoma are also seen.

Third, **infiltrating carcinoma.** This consists of a diffuse carcinomatous degeneration of liver parenchyma. The liver is uniformly enlarged, the capsule cloudy and frequently thickened, and occasionally adherent to other organs. The surface of the liver shows flat ridges and nodules, as large as peas or cherries. On transverse section the outline of the lobules can be seen as in cirrhosis; the nodules are, however, considerably larger than normal liver acini, and are colored whitish-yellow, or grayish. The connective tissue between them is usually reddish in color owing to its greater vascularity. The lobules will be found to be masses of carcinoma of a fibrous structure, from which a considerable quantity of carcinoma juice can be expressed (Fetzer).

Hanot and Gilbert differentiate between massive cancer, nodular cancer, and cancer with cirrhosis. The first two correspond to the two forms we have discussed above; the last corresponds to adenocarcinoma as described by Siegenbeck van Heukelom and the adenoma of the liver described by Kelsch and Kiener, Sabourin, and others.

In addition to numerous connective-tissue new-formations, a number of acinous neoplasms are seen that merge into masses of carcinoma; the liver is enlarged and cirrhotic; on transverse section numerous nodules are seen which when young appear yellowish and dry, and when old are softened and juicy; some of them are indented.

The **histologic picture** is, in many respects, more varied than the macroscopic picture. Frequently cirrhotic changes and proliferations, particularly of the portal, and sometimes of the intralobular, connective tissue are seen. Connective-tissue strands pass between the columns of liver-cells from the condensed interlobular tissue, and extend as far as the central veins, which are also surrounded by connective tissue. In other rare cases cirrhosis is absent, particularly if there is only one carcinomatous nodule. Sometimes the cirrhotic changes are so conspicuous that the carcinomatous element is not discovered. For this reason some authors (Perls, Thorel) speak of carcinomatous cirrhosis. Cirrhosis may be due to different causes in carcinoma of the liver; generally it is the result of the same agent that causes the formation of carcinoma, so that it originates at the same time. It is possible, however, that in some cases it precedes the carcinomatous change, as in drunkards and in stasis of bile following occlusion of the common duct. Such cases have been reported by Naunyn and Thorel. That cirrhosis, as Laveran assumes, is the result of carcinoma does not seem probable, although proliferation of connective tissue is occasionally seen in the vicinity of carcinoma. The origin of cancer-cells in primary carcinoma of the liver is also subject to controversy. Naunyn in his case saw the transition of bile-duct epithelium into carcinoma-cells; he saw the entrance of connective-tissue strands, between which bile-duct epithelium was placed, into the acini, and some of the newly formed rows of cells merged into rows of liver-cells. During this transition into carcinoma-cells the protoplasm becomes clear and the nucleus enlarges. It is possible that in cases of this kind a primary carcinoma of the smaller intrahepatic bile-ducts has existed that has grown into the acini of the liver, a condition similar to that seen in tubular adenomata. Naunyn was not able to arrive at the definite conclusion that liver-cells become transformed into cancer-cells; in other cases, however, this is distinctly so. Schüppel and his pupils observed that liver-cells became enlarged, that the protoplasm of several cells became confluent and inclosed the nuclei of all the cells; and that, following this, mitosis of the nuclei occurred, while the protoplasm became clear and surrounded the new nuclei. He also saw a circular arrangement of the new cells around a lumen, and in this way, by atypical proliferation of cells, the formation of alveolar carcinoma. The capillaries situated between the columns of liver-cells form the fibrous stroma of the carcinoma together with the strands of connective tissue that surround them. A portion of the columns of liver-cells becomes atrophic from pressure of the carcinomatous growth. Rohwedder, Siegenbeck van Heukelom, and others have also seen the formation of multinuclear clumps of protoplasm during the genesis of cancer; many authors have not been able to demonstrate this intermediary stage. Some observers have noted the fact that the transformation of liver-cells into cancer-cells occurs at the margin of the cancer nodule, and in the following way: From the tumor a round-cell infiltration starts and makes its way between the different columns of liver-cells. The round cells completely surrounded the liver-cells, new connective tissue is formed, and in this way the surrounded liver-cells are isolated from their acinus. These cells then become converted into cancer alveoli, there is a clearing of the protoplasm, an enlargement and mitosis of the nuclei, and consequently a formation of new cells. In this manner the acini are partly destroyed from the periphery. Thorel describes a peculiar extension of the columns of liver-cell into the condensed intralobular connective tissue; at the same time he saw a metamorphosis of the cells into cancer-cells, later isolation of these cells within connective tissue, the formation of nests and of alveoli. In many instances the liver-cells will be flat-tened, narrow, and elongated in the immediate vicinity of carcinoma nodules. These elongated cells radiate at a tangent to the periphery of the tumor; in these radiating stripes some authors, as Siegenbeck van Heukelom, have noted the metamorphosis of cells into cancer elements; other authors describe atrophy and fatty de-generation of these parts. Some of the nodules are surrounded by a solid capsule of connective and fatty tissue, and are necrotic in their center. Septa originate from the condensed connective tissue around the capillaries of the acini and from the intralobular connective tissue; these impart a peculiar fan-like shape or fibrous structure to many carcinomata that may be seen with the naked eye. We have already mentioned the fact that the color and the granular consistency of normal liver protoplasm are lost when the metamorphosis into cancer-cells occurs. Any pigment granules that may be present disappear, or congregate near the periphery of the cancer, or may even be carried off by the blood-vessels. This separation of pigment from the remaining protoplasm has been described in detail by Harris. In addition to the metamorphosis of liver-cells, proliferative processes are seen in the bile-passages, which form buds and branches, and sometimes penetrate between the columns of liver-cells of the acini. Their epithelium under-goes proliferation, and is changed from cylindric to cuboid or irregular forms. As a result of the abundant new-formation of·cells, the lumen is filled with young smooth cells, dilatation occurs in this manner, and the tubular form develops into an alveolar structure. Cystic dilatation may also be seen, and in this event the wall is covered with a cylindric or cuboid epithelium similar to that of cystadenoma (von Hippel and others). Within the cirrhotic connective tissue situated between the acini, new-formations are often seen developing from bile-passages; they usually have a trabecular structure, and consist of numerous tor-tuous bile-passages, with well-arranged symmetric cylindric epithelium. In other words, they have all the characteristics of that form of adenoma that has been described by Rindfleisch. Sometimes collections of small liver-cells are seen within the intralobular connective tissue. Heller regards these as vicarious processes of regeneration intended to com-pensate for the loss of such liver-cells as have perished by cirrhosis or tumor-formation, and he believes that they may easily be converted into carcinomatous alveoli. Hansemann finally describes certain cavernous capillary ectasies that originate from compressions of blood-vessels by contracting connective tissue. In many instances hyperplasia of the liver parenchyma has been seen, principally in the form of small nodules. Occasionally the tumor masses grow into branches of the portal vein or of the hepatic veins, and in this manner long fibrous structures are formed. In case the carcinoma is of an adenomatous structure these strands protrude from the branches of the hepatic artery and travel for a long distance in the lumen of the latter vessel or of the inferior vena cava. In the portal vein they grow against the blood-stream and lead to the formation of metastases in other parts of the liver. These metastases, in secondary carcinoma of the liver, develop from a cancerous thrombus of a small branch of the portal vein. Metastases do not occur so frequently in the lungs and other organs as the result of transportation of cancerous material from the hepatic vein. Secondary cancer of the gall-bladder is seen relatively often; the tumor may also grow into the bile-passages, and in this way form a tumor mass that extends to the large bile-ducts and involves the intrahepatic passages, thus leading to occlusion and to stasis of bile. Sometimes this condition of biliary stasis may aid in the development of cirrhosis (Claude and Gilbert). Cancerous degeneration of the lymph-vessels and metastases to the portal glands are seen very frequently, the latter in this case becoming enlarged.

A differentiation of the various forms of carcinoma of the liver, based on the shape of the tumor-cells, has been attempted by Hanot and Gilbert. The attempt is interesting anatomically, but can have no clinical significance. These investigators distinguish the ordinary form of *epitheliome alveolaire*, and subdivide it into (1) that with polymorphous and (2) with small polyhedric cells. They also designate tumors that contain giant and cylindric cells as unusual forms.

As we have mentioned above, a number of authors, as Rindfleisch, Kelsch, and Kiener, draw a sharp distinction between adenoma of the liver (adenoid) and carcinoma, notwithstanding the fact that in pronounced cancer-formation many places are seen in the liver that are constructed like trabecular adenomata. These adenomata have the appearance of tubular glands, and consist of numerous solid or hollow cylinders similar to the convoluted tubules of the kidney. These cylinders originate as the result of a metamorphosis of columns of liver-cells resulting in a lining of the former by rows of cylindric cuboid cells. The illustrations prepared by Kelsch and Kiener clearly show the transition of liver-cells into these atypical forms. Hanot and Gilbert, therefore, call this form of adenoma trabecular epithelioma, and differentiate between it and the above-mentioned alveolar cancers. They also describe a case of this kind that presented the appearance of a massive carcinoma, but in its interior showed a lobular structure. The cells within the growth were arranged in columns, as in the normal parenchyma, though with this difference, that the liver-cells had been converted into tumor-cells.

Adenomatous nodules originate within the acini and gradually enlarge at the expense of the parenchyma, which can sometimes be seen to one side, presenting the appearance of a semilunar remnant, and usually in a state of brown atrophy. At the same time there is more or less cirrhosis, particularly of the interlobular type. The adenomata usually appear as numerous icteric nodules, varying in size from a pinhead to a pea; solitary neoplasms of this kind are also seen. They resemble the adenomata of the breast, and, like these also run a more benign course than typical lobular cancers. They too, however, show a tendency to degenerative change if they persist for a long time. At first they undergo fatty degeneration, and later cheesy or colloid transformation of the central portion develops.

[W. H. Porter and W. T. Brooks have within the current year * reported a case of primary adenocarcinoma of the liver, with metastases in the choroid, lungs, spleen, and kidneys.—ED.]

Cheesy necrosis is seen when the single tubules are so close to one another that the already scanty circulation of the blood is occluded; a cheesy mass results, surrounded by the connective-tissue capsule of the tumor nodule.

* *Postgraduate*, June, 1902.

Colloid metamorphosis occurs in the neighboring cylinders in the following manner: As long as the circulation of the blood is sufficient, or even overabundant, the cells swell, and later become soft, and are converted into a shiny mass in which fat-droplets and large round cells with vacuolated nuclei are seen. In this manner cavities may be formed, filled with blood or a serous fluid or with a purulent brownish substance. These cavities are also surrounded by the connective-tissue capsule of the tumor nodule.

As the adenomata spread and disintegrate they gradually cause severe disturbances within the liver, impeding the circulation and secretion of bile, destroying liver tissue, and appearing to exercise a toxic influence on the whole body, causing cachexia, like typical carcinomata. It appears, however, that they rarely form metastases, even though they are known to proliferate into the hepatic veins and into the branches of the portal vein.

It is not at all clear why in certain cases these adenomata should become converted into typical carcinomata of an alveolar structure, and in other cases retain their tubular structure until death occurs from cirrhosis or from a destruction of liver parenchyma by direct displacement. Our knowledge, however, is very deficient in regard to the formation of cancerous tumors, and the causes of the various structure of these tumors even when found in the same organ.

We must differentiate between benign tumors and more or less malignant adenoid growths of the liver. In the benign growths the cells differ in no way from those of normal liver parenchyma.

Sometimes only a single tumor is present (Rokitansky, Klob, Hoffmann, Mahomed, Simmonds, and others).

The tumors may be congenital, and have been considered as accessory livers by Klob. They may be situated upon the surface of the organ or in its interior. Occasionally they are encapsulated, in other cases they are not. The connective-tissue stroma is frequently increased, the veins dilated; there may also be a central cyst formation so that the whole process appears as a cavernoma or a cyst of the liver. These structures do not participate in the performance of the functions of the liver, and if the latter are perverted as a result of stasis, corresponding changes will not be seen in the new-growth. Benign tumors, consisting of tubules lined with epithelium, occur in a solitary form in the liver, and have been described by Wagner, Greenish, and others; they have never, however, been studied with scientific care. We have already discussed the cystadenomata that belong to this class.

There is another form of growth which may be characterized as a multiple nodular hyperplasia; it is seen in livers that are altered pathologically, and particularly in those that are cirrhotic (see page 700). They are not encapsulated, show no proliferation of connective tissue in their interior, and must be regarded, possibly, as compensatory structures intended to assume vicariously the function of those liver-cells that have been destroyed by the primary disease. The liver-cells in these hyperplasias are enlarged, and hyperplastic rows may be in direct connection with atrophic ones. Sometimes a proliferation of the cells, less frequently a softening of the tissue, is seen (Kelsch and Kiener, Kelynack). The nodules are usually as large as hazelnuts, and can be seen with the naked eye on the surface of the liver. The organ usually is reduced in size from cirrhosis. The nodules protrude, and appear, on transverse section, as yellowish-gray or brownish structures that are in part confluent. Cases of this character have been described by Friedreich, Willigk, Birch-Hirschfeld, Simmonds, Kelynack, and others. Kelsch and Kiener have described similar hyperplasias in diseases of the liver that follows intermittent fever (*hépatite parenchymateuse nodulaire*) (see page 735). This multiple nodular form of hyperplasia shows a greater tendency to degeneration and proliferation, and, according to Schüppel (see above), it is possible that malign adenomata and carcinomata may occasionally develop from these nodules.

Secondary cancer of the liver may often be distinguished macroscopically from the primary form by the greater enlargement of the liver, the formation of nodules on its surface, a greater tendency to degenerative change, and, therefore, to the formation of depressions in the nodules. The tumors are usually light in color, whitish-grayish or greenish, and are clearly outlined, both on transverse sections, and upon the surface of the organ, from the rest of the normal liver substance. As a result of compression of blood-vessels stasis may occur here and there, and as a result reddish hyperemic portions are seen between the light carcinomatous masses. In other cases stasis of bile occurs, and an icteric color develops; the picture consequently is very varied. The cancer masses may fill the liver to such an extent that hardly a trace of normal parenchyma is visible. The organ may weigh 8 kg. and more. Sometimes degeneration of the carcinomatous tissue leads to the formation of cavities with a serous content (cystic carcinoma); hemorrhages may occur into these cavities, which may rupture and blood be poured into the peritoneal cavity. This is seen particularly in metastasis of the *fungus hæmatodes*, a great development of blood-vessels occurring in the connective tissue of the carcinoma.

In many cases of secondary carcinoma of the liver cancerous thrombi are seen in the portal vein or in its branches.

In rare cases it may happen that carcinomatous infiltration of the liver tissue occurs, particularly in many primary cancers of the liver. Schüppel describes this event in a gelatinous carcinoma that penetrated the liver from the peritoneum *via* the subserous lymph-passages, followed the lymph-channels of the vessels into the organ, and developed there. The lymph-vessels of the surface of the liver formed a gelatinous network, becoming more and more condensed, and were ultimately converted into plates. At the same time the intrahepatic lymph-channels became cancerous, pushed the parenchyma aside, continued to proliferate, and in this manner filled the entire interior of the organ without changing its form. Litten describes a similar infiltration in a secondary carcinoma of the liver, the primary seat of which was in the pancreas. Carcinomata of the gall-bladder may also grow into the liver by forming a massive growth in its interior similar to primary carcinoma. At the same time they do not change the outward shape of the organ.

The histologic findings vary according to the origin of the cancer. In general, the capillaries of the portal vein are filled with cancer masses of a characteristic structure. From these vessels proliferation takes place into the surrounding liver tissues; the liver-cells are compressed, and become atrophic. Later, colloid degeneration, fatty changes, or cheesy degeneration are seen in the central portions of the new tissue. Naunyn, Fetzer, Perls, Rindfleisch, and others have recorded a number of observations, according to which the liver-cells, and also the epithelia of the bile-passages and the endothelia of the blood-vessels, do not always atrophy, but, on the contrary, seem to proliferate and by alteration of their contents aid in the development of cancer.

In secondary carcinoma, also, cirrhotic changes are seen, as is the case in primary cancer. This may be due to the action of the cancer nodules in penetrating the branches of the portal vein, and thus acting as foreign bodies. In this manner an irritation of the surrounding tissues is produced that leads to the new-formation of connective tissue. In addition, just as occurs in ulcerative carcinoma of the stomach, intestine, etc., micro-organisms and toxic material may be carried with the cancerous masses and cause round-cell infiltration and later proliferation of connective tissue. Finally, in some cases stasis in the bile-channels must be regarded as a possible cause, particularly if the primary focus is situated in the common duct, at the orifice of this channel into the intestine or in the head of the pancreas, constituting in this manner an obstruction to the outflow of bile.

Carcinoma of the gall-bladder and of the bile-passages may be either secondary or primary. It may be secondary to carcinoma of the stomach, the intestine, and the pancreas, or it may extend from the pancreas or the duodenum by direct continuity of tissue. Less frequently it extends from the stomach to the common duct, and thence to the bile-passages in the liver and the gall-bladder. Sometimes primary cancer of the liver may send metastases to the gall-bladder or extend to the intrahepatic bile-passages and spread along their course. In this way different forms of cancer are developed, depending upon the form of the primary growth for their type.

Primary carcinoma of the gall-bladder is a more frequent occurrence than cancerous involvement of the bile-passages. As we have already stated, it usually follows cholelithiasis, and is the direct result of the irritation exercised by the concretions on the walls of the gall-bladder; a change in the structure of the wall is the first sign.

There is a marked development of fibrous tissue, hypertrophy, and later obliteration of the musculature, ulceration, and the formation of cicatrices in the mucous lining, and a loss of or transformation of the epithelial lining into layers of flat cells. At the same time, as in cholelithiasis, numerous glands of the mucosa atrophy and perish as a result of the sclerotic processes of the wall, and the proliferation of connective tissue. These glands may, on the other hand, enlarge by sending out processes, and in this manner possibly compensate the loss of destroyed glands. In other cases certain of the glands may be separated by connective tissue, and this, according to Ribbert, may cause the development of cancer. Those parts that are inclosed within connective tissue may, as in the case of ulcer of the stomach, undergo carcinomatous degeneration by a metamorphosis into cancerous tissue of the cells that constitute the glandular tubules. This leads to proliferation of the epithelium and to an obliteration of the lumen by young cells. In these cancerous alveoli mucoid degeneration of the cells is occasionally seen; the protoplasm swells and perishes and the picture of a gelatinous carcinoma is created; or, on the other hand, a scirrhus may develop with abundant proliferation of connective tissue. Sometimes large villous tumors are formed with numbers of soft cancerous alveoli; these readily undergo degeneration and form a cancerous ulcer. Owing to the transformation of the glandular epithelium into cancer-cells, and the metamorphosis of the cylindric cells of the gall-bladder wall into flattened tumor-cells, the alveoli may assume the shape of a flat-cell epithelioma—*i. e.*, with the characteristic onion-shaped configuration. Some authors have even described a metamorphosis of the cells of the gall-bladder and also of the cancer into horny cells.

In carcinoma of the gall-bladder the latter organ appears as a large nodular tumor; at times it is embedded in cancerous tissue that extends underneath the liver; in the latter instance the gall-bladder is not seen until the growth is divided. In other instances the gall-bladder is small and may be contracted around a gall-stone; from the organ cancerous tissue may extend far into the liver. As a rule, concretions will be found in the bladder; in other cases the stones will no longer be present, but their former existence be revealed by the discovery of scars and ulcerations, or there may be evidence of their passage, such as adhesions with the intestine or lesions of the cystic and common ducts. At times the cancer is limited to a small portion of the gall-bladder wall while the rest of the organ is found to be intact; at the site of the cancer a scar or some proliferation of tissue will usually be seen. A cancer of this kind, although small, may be the starting-point of a large growth of the liver. Quite frequently a diverticulum will be seen at the fundus in which are contained one or several gall-stones; this is usually separated from the rest of the organ by a dense ring. Cancer develops in this ring with great frequency.

The cancer spreads from the gall-bladder to the surrounding liver tissue and forms a tumor that appears like a primary carcinoma; atrophy of the parenchyma occurs and the tumor finally occupies a large part of the organ. Cancer of the gall-bladder also shows a tendency to travel along the lymph-channels, and in this way to infect the peritoneum; it may also travel along the lymph-channels of the cystic duct and by this path involve the common and the hepatic ducts. As a result of this malignant growth a tumor is formed in the region of the porta hepatis that compresses the bile-ducts and the portal vein and causes stasis of bile as well as congestion of the portal system.

In some cases the process extends to the smaller intrahepatic bile-passages, so that on transverse section these channels appear as cancerous rings. Starting from these new bile-passages are tubules filled with cylindric epithelium extending into the acini; these cause atrophy of the columns of liver-cells. Occlusion of bile-ducts may also result from thickening of their outer walls; the bile may in this manner be retained, so that cysts form that are lined by the epithelium of the bile-passages.

Carcinomata which develop as primary growths in the walls of the bile-passages usually start from a proliferation of the mural glands at some point at which a gall-stone causes, or has at some time caused, irritation of the mucosa; these concretions produce lesions and cicatricial tissue, and cause general irritation of the mucous membrane with proliferation of the epithelium. Such cancers may be annular (Willigk, Deetjen), or polypoid, and their malignant character may be recognized only on microscopic examination. In the center of these growths a gall-stone is sometimes found. Such a stone need not be very large in order to cause serious disturbances and death in a short time, particularly if it is situated in the common duct or in the stem of the hepatic duct, and in order to rapidly lead to retention of bile and cholemia. If it is situated in the cystic duct, the common and the hepatic ducts are soon involved, and in this way there is soon produced a complete occlusion of all the ducts with stasis of bile and all that this entails. If the cancer is situated at the orifice of the common duct (Marfan, Deetjen), it may cause very serious disturbances even if it be very small. It can be readily determined microscopically that these cancers originate from glandular epithelium; that they proliferate and send out tubules filled with epithelium into the muscularis and the subserous tissues; and that these canals continue to enlarge and in this way produce a carcinoma of alveolar construction.

Sarcoma of the liver is not seen as frequently as carcinoma. Sarcomata are also usually secondary, although it is often a difficult matter to discover the primary focus. It may be a small sarcoma of a muscle tendon, or a growth in the choroid that is no larger than a hop-seed.

For a time the existence of primary sarcoma of the liver was denied, but we have to-day a number of well-authenticated cases. The tumors are, as a rule, spindle- or round-celled sarcomata (cases of Hörup, Lancereaux, Arnold, Windrath, Waring, v. Kahlden, and others).

These growths usually start from the region of the branches of the portal vein, and generally from the walls of the smaller vessels; the latter show characteristic sarcomatous proliferation. At the same time old cirrhotic changes are seen in many cases (v. Kahlden).

Sometimes they appear clearly differentiated from the healthy liver tissue, which is compressed by the tumor and undergoes atrophic degeneration, and finally

49

disappears. Sometimes, indeed, extensions are sent off from the margin of the tumor that enter the liver tissue in such a manner that the cells of the sarcoma penetrate between the columns of liver-cells, and cause these to atrophy or separate some of the cells from their attachments. They penetrate the blood-vessels and fill the capillaries of the acini, exercise pressure on the liver-cells, and cause their disappearance. In this manner the alveolar structure can be explained; in some cases the construction of the tumor is *per se* alveolar.

In rare cases it appears that **melanosarcoma** can appear as a primary tumor; this is shown by a case of Block, in which a distinct alveolar arrangement of pigmented epithelial cells could be seen. Belin, too, has described a primary melanosarcoma of the liver. In another similar case of Frerichs only a partial pigmentation of the cells was observed. These sarcomata can grow to considerable dimensions, as shown by a case of Bramwell and Leith; here the tumor contained numerous blood-vessels and cavities with hemorrhagic contents. Occasionally, the tumors are situated altogether on the surface of the liver, or may even be pedunculated, as in a case of sarcomatous fibromyoma reported by Sklifosowsky.

Secondary sarcomata constitute especially large tumors. They may occur in two forms; either as nodular neoplasms disseminated through the whole liver or as diffuse infiltrating growths. In the infiltrating form, however, small nodules are seen, as a rule, within the sarcomatous tissue; and in the nodular form a diffuse sarcomatous infiltration of the adjacent portions of liver tissue is noted near the periphery of the tumor.

Particularly in the case of pigmented sarcomata (pigment-cancer), which are usually metastases from choroid tumors or from pigmented nevi of the skin that have undergone sarcomatous degeneration, infiltration of liver tissue occurs at the periphery. Dark masses of tumor tissue penetrate the liver; from the portal or hepatic veins extension occurs into the intra-acinous capillaries, and at the same time the liver-cells of the affected areas undergo atrophic changes and disappear. In this manner there is produced a peculiar configuration of the transverse section through the organ resembling granite. In addition to these changes (in some cases without other change), dark-pigmented nodules are seen in which the cells containing melanin are arranged in an alveolar manner. These peculiarities have given this form of tumor the name of pigment cancer.

In addition, numerous spindle-cell, round cell, and lymphosarcomata are seen, less frequently chondro-, cysto-, myxo-, and leiomyosarcomata. Osteosarcomata may also send metastases into the liver; here they are osteosarcomata without bone-formation. Lymphosarcomata of the liver consist of numerous miliary cavities filled with a serous fluid and lined by endothelium; they usually originate from the periosteum or the bone-marrow. Bizzozero, in one case saw a metastasis of a gliosarcoma.

In general it may be said that all these tumors are differentiated from the tissue in which they are embedded by their light color; particularly as the neighboring parts are usually compressed and of an icteroid color from stasis of bile, or are hyperemic. On the surface of the organ the tumor masses form large or small elevations that are rarely indented or hollowed, owing to the fact that sarcomata do not show as great a tendency to degeneration as carcinomata.

In cases of infiltrating sarcoma, as in infiltrating carcinoma, the form and size of the liver are not very much changed; the organ is often somewhat enlarged, however, and the surface is irregular from the presence of flat ridges.

In some cases it has been possible to trace the path by which sarcomatous material is carried to the liver; this may be either the portal vein or the hepatic artery; in the former instance the spleen is frequently involved at first and the material is then carried into the liver.

Symptoms and Course.—The symptoms and the course of malignant neoplasms of the liver may be very various, and will depend on the starting-point of the tumor as well as upon the individual tendencies of the growth to extension or to degenerative processes. The relations of the tumor to neighboring blood-vessels and bile-passages must also be considered, and, finally, the nature of the growth, *i. e.*, whether a carcinoma, a sarcoma, or a malignant adenoma, and whether primary or secondary. The presence or absence of cirrhotic changes in the liver, and of gall-stones, is also important.

We may say that the symptomatology of carcinoma of the liver and of similar neoplasms is composed in the main of the following features:

1. *Carcinomatous cachexia.* This is frequently the first symptom, and may remain the chief feature throughout the disease.

2. The *development of a tumor* either within or upon the liver. Sometimes we see a uniform enlargement, more frequently the formation of nodules on the surface and margin of the organ.

3. Symptoms of *compression* by the neoplasm: (*a*) of blood-vessels (portal vein and vena cava), (*b*) of bile-passages.

4. The *development of metastases* in the peritoneum, in the pleura, the lungs, etc.

5. *Cirrhosis and its consequences.* This lesion may be caused by the cancer, or it may exist before the advent of the growth.

Certain forms of cancer of the liver may remain altogether latent; especially is this true of metastases of carcinoma or sarcoma from other organs. This is likely to be the case if the growth develops in the interior of the liver or on its upper surface underneath the diaphragm. Primary carcinomata that develop in the form of massive cancers cause an increase in the size of the liver; but the presence of carcinoma may remain unrecognized for a long time. Adenomata have frequently been found in the liver postmortem without having caused any symptoms during life.

In general the **course** of a carcinoma of the liver is the following: At first disturbances of appetite and disgust for meats and fats appear; the patient begins to emaciate even if he forces himself to take sufficient nourishment; he grows pale, the skin becomes dry, fragile, wrinkled, and sallow, sometimes icteroid. He complains of pressure and a sense of fulness in the right hypochondrium; later of pain, radiating to the abdomen, the breast, the right shoulder, etc. On examination the liver will be found enlarged, sensitive to pressure, and usually nodular. Following these symptoms we usually see icterus as a result of compression of bile-passages, and ascites from compression of the portal vein or occlusion of the vessel by carcinomatous thrombi. These symptoms do not always appear, but are usually present, and particularly in primary carcinoma and sarcoma. Finally, general edema appears, and the formation of carcinomatous metastases, as, for instance, carcinomatosis of the peritoneum and the pleura. The patient finally dies of cachexia and heart failure. Sarcomata run a similar course. In adenomata and other neoplasms that are accompanied by cirrhosis, ascites appears earlier in the disease, the liver is harder, the course more protracted, and the disease, which in rapidly developing massive primary carcinomata lasts a few months, may, in these cases, persist for many years, and finally terminates in a cachectic condition.

The course and the symptomatology differ according to the nature of the tumor. We will refer to these differences in detail at a later point in the discussion.

In **secondary tumors of the** liver the duration and character of the disease will often be dependent upon the character of the primary tumor. In other instances the nature of the tumor is comparatively unimportant, and the primary tumor will be so insignificant that no light is thrown upon the condition until the autopsy is performed.

Carcinoma of the gall-bladder and of the bile-passages does not usually cause such distinct symptoms of cachexia or of digestive disorders. Often the symptoms of the condition are gradually added to those of cholelithiasis. Sometimes a characteristic tumor develops in the region of the gall-bladder. Icterus soon appears, owing to complete occlusion of the biliary passages. The tumors of the hepatic and common ducts rapidly close the lumen of the latter and cause the gall-bladder and the cystic duct to become involved early in the disease. Ascites also develops soon because the carcinomatous infiltration at the hilum of the liver usually involves the portal vein. This form of cancer usually ends with symptoms of hepatic intoxication (cholemia), particularly if it starts from the common duct. Occasionally, however, in cancers of the gall-bladder that grow into the liver tissue an altogether different symptom-complex is seen, similar to that of genuine carcinomata of the liver.

The disturbances of the **general health, of the blood,** and of the **nutrition of the bod**y, included under the name of carcinomatous cachexia, are probably due to the action of toxic substances produced by malignant tumors, such as carcinomata, sarcomata, and malignant adenomata. The symptoms have a definite relation to the size of the tumor and the rapidity of its development. The more rapidly the tumor spreads, the more deleterious the influence of the growth upon the general health. Many observations point to the formation of toxic substances in malignant growths, as, for instance, the increased toxicity of the urine (Gautier and Hilt, Moraczewski, and others), and the destruction of proteid tissue as manifested by an increased excretion of nitrogen as compared to the small amount ingested (F. Müller, Klemperer, and others). We know nothing, however, of the nature of these substances, as no one has so far succeeded in isolating them, or in determining their properties. For this reason we cannot say what rôle poisons of this kind play in the causation of carcinomatous cachexia.

There can be no doubt that in extensive carcinomatous processes, such as are usually seen when the liver is involved, the general metabolism is influenced not only by the supply of nourishment, but also by the direct effect of the neoplasm upon the proteid constituents of the organs. This is manifested by a loss in volume of the muscle tissues, and by atrophic processes in other organs containing much proteid. This occurs even when the nutritive supply is ample, the analyses of F. Muller, Klemperer, and others showing that more nitrogen is excreted than ingested. A decrease in the quantity of chlorids excreted in the urine has frequently been observed; this is due, in part at least, to the ingestion of small quantities owing to the lack of appetite; it may also be due in part to a retention of the chlorids in serous transudates, as ascites, anasarca, etc. Occasionally, in carcinoma the amount of phosphorus excreted is increased in proportion to the nitrogen. The occurrence would seem to point to nutritive disturbances in the bones.

In carcinoma of the liver Sjöquist found a distinct increase in the excretion of ammonia and of other nitrogenous substances, as compared to urea. This can be attributed to a decrease in the urea formation in the liver. According to Töpfer's analyses, the proportion of nitrogenous substances excreted is as follows: urea 65.2 % to 79.4 %; nitrogenous extracts 13 % to 23 %. In the normal subject the corresponding figures are 84.9 % to 96.2 % of urea nitrogen, and 0.6 % to 0.8 % of extractive nitrogen. If catabolism of the proteids is very great, acetone and diacetic acid, also β-oxybutyric acid, are excreted, as in certain other diseases. At the same time the alkalinity of the blood is reduced, and coma may appear, as in diabetes mellitus. v. Noorden states that in a case of carcinoma of the stomach with extensive metastases in the liver, lactic acid was found in the urine, and he attributes its presence to involvement of the liver.

Other changes in the blood condition, aside from the decreased alkalinity, are a decrease in the red blood-corpuscles and the hemoglobin. The blood becomes watery, and its specific gravity is lowered. The number of leucocytes, on the other hand, is relatively and absolutely increased. There is sometimes an increase of the blood-sugar (E. Freund), although this is not a constant occurrence, and is seen in other serious diseases.

v. Moraczewski found the phosphorus of the blood decreased in carcinoma, the conditions being similar to those present in the blood in anemia. He also found an increase of the chlorin and nitrogen.

As a result of the disturbances of nutrition and the destruction of protoplasm, as well as owing to anemia and hydremia, edema develops, with exudation of serous fluids into the body-cavities and the subcutaneous cellular tissues, particularly of the dependent portions of the body. In this manner the accumulation of fluid in the abdominal cavity may sometimes be explained, although, as a rule, it is dependent upon an extension of the cancer to the peritoneum, or an occlusion of branches of the portal vein. The color of the skin grows pale-yellowish even in the absence of icterus; the skin becomes atrophic, dry, and desquamates, owing to a deficient secretion of sweat and sebaceous material.

It is possible to raise the skin in large folds. The adipose layer disappears rapidly, and remains intact in rare cases only (Frerich, Oppolzer). The patient may become fatigued, dyspneic, and complain of palpitation; others become irritable, and cannot sleep well even though pain is absent. Their mental faculties become impaired, they slowly relapse into stupor, and die in coma.

On physical examination the chief symptoms of the disease will be discovered in the liver. With few exceptions, the organ is enlarged in part or as a whole. If the tumor develops in the interior, or on the diaphragmatic surface of the liver, it cannot be palpated; in the latter case the tumor may, however, protrude below the costal arch on deep inspiration, and in this way be detected. Occasionally a general enlargement of the liver can be determined, and presents a smooth surface of increased resistance to the touch. This occurs particularly when the tumor is situated in the interior of the organ, as is frequently the case in infiltrating carcinomata and sarcomata. In massive carcinoma the liver is usually as hard as a board. If many nodules are present the surface is rough, as, for instance, in those forms of carcinoma and adenoma that develop near the surface. In cases of this character the margin is not sharp and clean cut, but nodular, thickened, and projecting. This is seen especially in secondary tumors, but may also occur in primary carcinomata, and especially adenocarcinomata. Depressions in the nodules are rarely determinable, but sometimes the latter show a varying consistency according to the character and stage of development; thus, primary carcinomata are usually denser than secondary carcinomata. The latter, if they are of the scirrhous type, may also feel very hard; more frequently, however, they are metastases from medullary or gelatinous carcinomata, or lymphosarcomata, etc., so that they feel softer than the surrounding tissue, and may even simulate fluctuation. The latter sensation is also experienced if softening of metamorphosis into cavernous tissue occurs, or, finally, if hemorrhage occurs and leads to the formation of cavities filled with blood. As a rule, the nodules are of different size, sometimes large and constituting the primary foci, while around will be found a large number of smaller nodules. In enlargements of the liver without change of its form, as well as in that enlargement that occurs with the development of nodules, large tumors are found that extend deep into the abdomen, below the umbilicus and as far as the crest of the ilium, or even to Poupart's ligament, and very far toward the left. They may fill the greater part of the abdomen. In slight degrees of development the diaphragm is pushed upward so that on percussion the margin of the lung will be found higher than normal. The latter is particularly true in cases in which the tumor is very large, and cannot expand into the abdomen; also if ascites is present. Meteorism may occasionally cause the same picture. In one case that I observed the margin of the liver barely protruded below the costal arch in the mammillary line, while there was at the same time a large area of dulness in the lower part of the thorax on the right side, that extended very far upward. The reason for this was an adhesion between the lower margin of the organ and the parietal peritoneum. The adhesive bands consisted of connective tissue, infiltrated with the carcinomatous growth.

In secondary carcinomata very large livers are often felt, covered with many soft nodules. In massive primary carcinoma and sarcoma, and in infiltrating carcinoma and sarcoma, the liver is usually large and smooth. In those forms of carcinoma and malignant adenoma that are complicated by cirrhosis the liver is not very much enlarged, but very nodular.

Sometimes the enlargement of the liver can be seen. The right hypochondrium may bulge and protrude, and the outlines of the liver may be determined through the thin abdominal walls; occasionally the nodules even may be distinguished. On palpation (which should be carried out as described on page 390) the outline of the tumor can usually be distinguished more distinctly than by percussion, and the single nodules may be felt. At the same time the character of the pain which carcinomatous nodules often give on pressure should be noted; the peculiarities as to consistency, fluctuation, etc., should be determined. Occasionally respiratory friction sounds or grating may be heard by means of the stethoscope placed over the liver, a frequent complication of carcinoma of the liver. It is also stated by some that the nodules give this peculiar grating when they are palpated.

In **carcinoma of the gall-bladder and the bile-ducts** the liver is also generally enlarged. The surface is smooth, particularly if biliary stasis is present. The liver enlarges as a result of the dilatation of the intrahepatic bile-passages, and if the condition exists for a long time, the consistency of the organ increases, owing to the development of biliary cirrhosis. As a rule, the organ is not large, as in cancer of the liver. In the place of the gall-bladder a large, nodular, sensitive tumor is often felt protruding below the margin of the liver, particularly if gall-stones or hydrops are present. In other cases it is difficult to palpate the tumor, owing to its situation beneath the liver. If the abdominal walls are very much relaxed, however, it is usually possible to feel it. Tumors of the common and hepatic duct cannot be palpated. In case of occlusion of the former, the bile accumulates in the gall-bladder so that this viscus can be felt as a dense, elastic fluctuating mass. In addition to the tumor of the gall-bladder, metastatic nodules are frequently felt in other parts of the liver. Occasionally a large nodular or flat, ridge-like tumor starts from the gall-bladder.

In the event that ascites is present, the palpation of the tumor, whether it is a neoplasm of the liver or of the bile-passages, is difficult. Palpation, however, is possible if the patient is instructed to lie on the left side, or if the ascitic fluid is first evacuated. Sometimes it is possible to distinguish the presence of a tumor by ballottement, when only a thin layer of fluid is present.

From the beginning of the trouble, or possibly soon after, the patient complains of pain in the liver, frequently preceded by a feeling of pressure and fulness in the hepatic region. This pain may appear spasmodically or may be continuous. It radiates from the right hypochondrium or epigastrium into the chest, the abdomen, or the back. Pain in the right shoulder is also complained of. Skorna describes a case of primary cancer of the liver in which pain was present only in this location. [A case has been reported by Mackenzie * of a woman, aged twenty-four, suffering from carcinoma of the liver. One of the prominent symptoms had been **neuralgia of the right arm,** which Mackenzie attributed to the anastomotic connection between the phrenic and the fourth and fifth cervical nerves, branches from the latter of which supply the shoulder and upper arm.—ED.] Spontaneous pain, as well as pain on pressure, is observed particularly in cases in which the cancer is situated on the surface of the organ, and thus irritates the peritoneum and the nerves of the liver capsule. Tumors situated in the interior of the organ may also cause pain by irritation of the nerves that enter the liver with the arteries, or by causing rapid enlargement of the organ, and a consequent tension of the serosa. Pain of this kind may be very annoying to the patient, rob him of his sleep, and in this manner hasten the general collapse.

Symptoms of **compression** and **obstruction** may be subdivided into those that occur in the bile-passages and those that occur in the blood-vessels. **Occlusion of bile-passages** is particularly seen in carcinomata that start from the common, hepatic, or cystic ducts, or from the gall-bladder. Intrahepatic tumors may lead to this obstruction either by occluding a large number of bile-passages, by compression, or by direct growth, or by infiltrating the porta hepatis, causing cancerous degeneration of the glands of the hilum; or, finally, by compression of the large bile-ducts on the lower surface of the liver. Such a condition always results in icterus. At first there is a yellowish discoloration of the sclera, and later an icteroid discoloration of the skin and mucous membranes that lead to the black-green color of melas icterus. The urine contains bile-pigment, bile-acids, and albumin, as in other forms of icterus from stasis. If the cancer is situated in the common duct, complete occlusion of bile usually occurs. None of the bile consequently can enter the in-

* *Brit. Med. Jour.,* Feb. 2, 1901.

testine, and characteristic clay-colored, whitish or gray stools are the
result. These are frequently covered by icteroid mucus. This may also
be the case in cancerous involvement of the root of the hepatic duct. If,
on the other hand, the bile-passages are not completely compressed or
occluded, or if only one of the larger branches of the hepatic duct is closed,
icterus of the skin and mucous membranes will yet occur, and bile-
pigment will be found in the urine; but the stools will not be devoid of
color. In addition to bile-pigment, I have repeatedly found urobilin in
the urine, even if the bile was not completely excluded from the intestine.
If the occlusion is complete, large quantities of urobilin are voided.
Some carcinomata and sarcomata never produce icterus, particularly
primary massive carcinomata; at the same time, however, there may be
an abundant excretion of urobilin, which is reduced later, owing to the
cachexia, deficient nutrition, and the decrease in the formation of bile.
It seems possible that the excessive urobilinuria is due to a rapid disintegration of red blood-corpuscles. [An interesting case was seen during
the past year which presented a high degree of cachexia, deep jaundice,
emaciation, rapid loss of weight (from 120 to 96 pounds within a few
weeks), and an entire absence of bile and biliary acids from the urine.
There was constantly present, however, a marked urobilinuria. The
liver seemed normal in size, and a few days before the operation the gall-
bladder appeared to be palpable. On incision the liver was found to be
normal, while the gall-bladder contained a number of small hard calculi.
Impacted in the cystic duct was a large single stone. There was no
malignant growth evident either in the liver or in the gall-bladder, the
latter being subjected to a thorough microscopic examination. The
patient recovered from the operation, and both the jaundice and the
urobilinuria promptly abated, and soon disappeared.—ED.] Sometimes
in the intrahepatic form of tumor icterus is so slight that it is not recognized; only in the presence of a yellowish or brownish color of the skin,
and especially of the sclera, or in case bilirubin can be detected in the
newly voided urine, can stasis of bile be diagnosed. An intense form
of icterus may, on the other hand, be caused by the simultaneous presence
of gall-stones and the development of carcinoma of the liver. Such an
occurrence is by no means rare, and is seen especially in combination
with tumors of the bile-ducts.

Neoplasms that cause a complete retention of bile, particularly those
that develop in the common duct, sooner or later lead to **hepatargy,**
(cholemia), characterized by hemorrhages into the skin and mucous
membranes, epistaxis, hematemesis, bloody stools, etc. The patient
becomes exhausted and even more anemic than can be accounted for by
the deleterious action of the bile-constituents on the blood. As a result
of the damage to the liver-cells due to the biliary cirrhotic change the
secretion of bile is diminished, consequently the icteric color becomes
less intense. Death usually results, less as a consequence of the malignant cachexia than from the disturbances within the liver parenchyma.

In carcinomata situated near the orifice of the common duct, the duct of Wirsung may be occluded, and in this manner the pancreatic juice may be excluded
from the intestine. Further, there will be dilatation of the pancreatic duct and
a proliferation of the connective tissue of the pancreas. Similar conditions may
be caused by a carcinoma of the pancreas which develops in the head of the organ,
involves the papillæ, and occludes the common duct secondarily. The occlusion
of the common duct leads to defective intestinal digestion, and consequently to
deficient assimilation of fluid. In this way it will accelerate the death of the patient.

Neoplasms of the liver may involve the blood-vessels, and among them the portal vein, the inferior vena cava, the hepatic vein, and, rarely, the hepatic artery. The portal vein may either be compressed by tumors of the liver, its branches being individually involved, or the capillary system; or it may be occluded by means of the formation of a new-growth which may penetrate the walls of the vessel. Finally, carcinomatous masses may develop at the hilum of the liver and there occlude the vein. The result of all these occurrences is stasis in the portal system, evidenced by ascites, less frequently by tumor of the spleen, icterus, and hemorrhages into the intestine. Sometimes ectasies of collateral venous branches occur. Certain cirrhotic changes may also be concerned in the occlusion of the portal vein. Among these are the processes which we have already described, including such forms of cancer of the liver as adenocarcinoma, carcinomatous cirrhosis, etc. Ascites soon results from all these conditions, so that the diagnosis of simple cirrhosis may be made; particularly is this true in the case of malignant adenomata. Analogous changes in the inferior vena cava lead to stasis in the veins of the legs, anasarca, and dilatation of the subcutaneous veins of the abdomen (which act as collateral paths). The portal vein is usually involved at the same time. If occlusion or compression of the hepatic vein occurs, the stasis of blood will extend to the portal system, and there cause the symptoms enumerated above. Symptoms of stasis in the portal vein are particularly apparent in cases of carcinoma of the liver that are complicated by weakness of the heart, for in these cases the flow of blood to the heart and the lungs is insufficient.

If malignant growths make their way into the vena cava or the hepatic veins, metastases are frequently formed in the lungs and in other organs as a result. The appearance of metastases in remote parts of the body is comparatively rare in primary carcinomata of the liver, particularly in the massive forms that run an acute course. This also applies to the cases of malignant adenoma that are complicated by cirrhosis. In the nodular form of carcinoma, however, metastasis is a frequent occurrence, and secondary tumors of the liver, in particular, show a tendency to spread by way of the blood- and lymph-channels. Secondary more frequently than primary cancers of the liver are carried to other organs through the blood. Primary growths seem to have a predilection for the lymph-channels at the hilum, so that carcinomatous infiltration of portal lymph-glands or of mesenteric and retroperitoneal glands frequently occurs.

Extension of the cancer to the peritoneum occurs particularly in secondary growths; only the nodular form of primary cancer seems to bring this about. Thus ascites, which is so frequent in secondary carcinoma, may be explained, for we often see the development of small cancer nodules all over the peritoneum, or a cancerous infiltration of the mesentery. The exudate may be so abundant that aspiration becomes necessary. In the fluid will be found leucocytes and large cells whose protoplasm gives a glycogen reaction. Red blood-corpuscles are also frequently found. In fact, the whole fluid may be hemorrhagic from small hemorrhages that originate in the nodules of neoplasm. The percentage of albumin and the specific gravity of the exudate vary greatly; if the carcinomatosis and the chronic inflammation of the peritoneum are the primary causes of the exudation, or if there is congestion of the portal vein, general dropsy will complicate the condition. If icterus is present, the ascitic fluid, of course, contains bilirubin; urobilin may also be found in the effusion. If cancerous nodules upon the surface of the liver degenerate, severe hemorrhages may occur into the abdominal cavity, so that it is sometimes found filled with blood. In addition to other symptoms of exudate and the characteristic signs of adhesions between abdominal organs, etc., cancerous masses may frequently be felt in the peritoneum. They present the sensation of nodular masses, sensitive to pressure; the mesentery may be converted into a nodular strand running transversely across the upper portion of the abdomen. Peritonitic friction sounds may be heard and felt at the anterior surface of the liver provided the organ is not separated from the abdominal wall by fluid. Adhesions with other organs, particularly the intestine, are also found in carcinoma. In carcinoma of the gall-bladder the fundus may be adherent to the duodenum and lead to twisting and stenosis of the intestine, causing symptoms of gastric ectasy (Ewald). In secondary carcinoma adhesions frequently form with the diaphragm, which becomes perforated. In this way a right-sided pleurisy may develop. The inflammation may be serofibrinous or complicated by carcinomatosis. A serous exudate is formed that compresses the lung and causes dulness, dislocates the heart, produces dyspnea, etc. The most dangerous exudates are those that are caused by the perforation of a gangrenous carcinoma nodule into the pleura.

Leichtenstern has called attention to a swelling of the jugular gland that is occasionally observed. In primary carcinoma this sign is not always present. [Jarchette * details two cases of carcinoma of the liver in which an early sign was enlargement of the supraclavicular and cervical glands. He found that the enlarged inguinal gland in two cases of abdominal carcinoma did not show any metastasis, merely a sclerotic change, consisting in a substitution of connective for the adenoid tissue. He concludes (1) that enlargement of the left supraclavicular gland is an occasional sign of carcinoma of the abdomen and should always be looked for; (2) this enlargement may occur in carcinoma of other abdominal organs than the stomach; (3) its appearance may be early enough to be an aid in diagnosis; (4) the appearance of a metastasis in the supraclavicular glands is readily recognized without a microscopic examination; (5) slight enlargement of the supraclavicular and cervical glands, and increase in their consistency, are frequently observed in cancer, but are usually not due to metastasis, and are not of diagnostic importance.—Ed.]

If marked cirrhotic changes are also present in the liver parenchyma symptoms of stasis in the portal system make their appearance: ascites, tumor of the spleen, hemorrhages into the stomach and intestine, and occasionally profuse diarrheas. The liver is not much enlarged,—in fact it may be smaller than usual,—and is hard and nodular; sometimes it is possible to feel smaller nodules that correspond to the cirrhotic areas and larger areas that correspond to the carcinomatous nodules.

The symptoms presented by disease of other organs are primarily caused by the main complications of carcinoma as described above: cachexia, enlargement of the liver, stasis of the blood and biliary circulations, metastases of the neoplasm, etc. General disturbances of health, such as weakness, emaciation, and anemia, may be caused by the cachexia and by the deficient assimilation or ingestion of food, or may be the result of loss of blood.

* *Deutsch. Archiv f. klin. Med.,* Bd. LXVII.

In some cases fever is seen. This may be either remittent, intermittent, or irregular. It may be due to complicating inflammations, particularly to cholangitis; this is noticed with particular frequency in carcinomata of the bile-passages. [Hawthorne mentions * a case of carcinoma of the liver with distinct febrile reaction, and points to the fact that this sign is not therefore distinctive of impacted gall-stone, abscess, and other inflammatory conditions. A diagnosis based chiefly on the existence of fever is, he insists, always open to error.—ED.]

Achard, in a patient with fever suffering from hepatic carcinoma, found Staphylococcus albus in blood aspirated from the liver. Hanot found streptococci in a case of secondary carcinoma of the liver with cholangitis that was complicated by fever and icterus.

In some cases a long-continued fever is seen that cannot be traced to any inflammatory cause; here the rise of temperature must be due to the rapid proliferation of the tissues and the formation and absorption of large quantities of toxic material. This type of fever is frequently seen in cases of primary carcinoma that grow rapidly, and in extended metastases in the liver. Sarcomata, too, show a chronic type of fever, particularly lymphosarcomata; Ebstein has called the fever in the latter form chronic recurrent fever.

In the blood a decrease in the number of red blood-corpuscles will be seen; their number may be reduced even to 600,000. At the same time there is a corresponding decrease of the blood-pigment, of the specific gravity, and of the alkalinity. The white cells may be increased in proportion to the red cells; occasionally they are absolutely increased. Poikilocytosis is seen in the severe cases. Rarely there is a concentration and thickening of the blood owing to impoverization of the water-supply of the body following deficient ingestion or profuse diarrheas (Leichtenstern).

In the region of the heart the signs of dilatation, of exudation into the pericardium, or anemia are occasionally detected. The heart action is weak toward the end of the disease and the pulse correspondingly small, rapid, and irregular; edema may appear in the dependent parts of the body. Sometimes thromboses form in the femoral veins.

The respiration is sometimes affected by the development of a right-sided pleuritis following perforation of a carcinoma through the diaphragm or by the development of metastases in the lungs following the entrance of tumors into the hepatic vein or the inferior cava. Finally, hypostatic pneumonia and hydrothorax may occasionally develop.

The disturbances of the organs of digestion are particularly important. The appetite is lost at an early period of the disease and the secretion of gastric juice, particularly of the hydrochloric acid, is reduced. Sometimes vomiting occurs as a result of irritation of the peritoneum or as a result of irritation of the nerves of the liver ; it may also be due to traction or irritation on the pylorus by adhesions. Intestinal digestion is also disturbed, particularly if the bile cannot enter the duodenum or if an insufficient quantity of bile is formed in the liver. As a result there are decomposition of the intestinal contents, meteorism, and the passage of disagreeable gases; undigested food is passed in the stools; these contain very little bile or none at all, but much of the calcium and magnesium salts. As a rule, the patients cannot digest meats and fats as well as milk and carbohydrate foods.

* *Brit. Med. Jour.*, Mar. 16, 1901.

In the beginning the bowels are constipated, this condition perhaps being due to stasis in the portal system; later in the disease diarrhea and constipation alternate. At the same time the symptoms of a severe catarrh of the colon develop, accompanied by ulcerations of the mucosa. Death may be hastened by the profuse diarrheas that follow the development of these lesions.

The spleen in many cases is small and atrophic, especially if there is an absence of stasis in the portal system. In the forms of cancer that develop slowly the organ may be swollen, particularly if the cancer is complicated by cirrhosis of the liver. In many cases the size of the spleen remains normal. Metastases are rarely found in the organ.

In case there is ascites, or if too little water is taken, or if there are profuse diarrheas, the urine may be much reduced in quantity; only half a liter may be voided per diem. The color is dependent upon the presence or absence of bile-pigment and of urobilin; these bodies are often excreted in large quantities. Urobilin is excreted in those cases of carcinoma that develop and disintegrate rapidly or in those that are complicated with cirrhosis; bile-pigment is found whenever the bile-ducts are occluded by the tumor. The bile constituents irritate the kidneys so that a little albumin is often passed, also a few tube-casts and epithelial cells. In melanosarcoma melanin is found in the urine, coloring it dark brown; or it may be present in its leuco-combination, and may be converted into melanin by contact with oxidizing substances such as bromin-water. If decomposition in the intestine is very great, the aromatic substances of the urine are increased; in such cases indoxyl, phenol, and the ethereal sulphates in general are found in considerable quantities. The total daily excretion of nitrogen and the quantity of urea appear to be diminished.

The disturbances of the **nervous** system are caused in part by the neoplasm; pain in the region of the liver is caused directly by irritation of the nerves; pain in the shoulder is caused by radiation along the path of the phrenic and the cervical nerves. Sometimes attacks of hepatic colic are seen that may be due to the impaction of gall-stones or of tumor masses in the ducts, or to irritation of these passages by such bodies. The patient becomes irritable, there is loss of sleep, a decrease in the mental faculties and powers; later there is stupor, delirium, and possibly coma (cancer-coma or cholemia).

The **skin** is a pale yellow in simple cachexia, yellow to blackish-green in icterus. In the latter case there are scratches and small hemorrhages. As a rule, the skin is flaccid, dry, and peeling. Decubitus may develop, and toward the end edema may supervene.

According to the localization and the nature of the tumor, the pathologic picture may vary greatly. It is probably carrying subdivision too far, however, to formulate a dyspeptic, an icteric, a cachectic, even a painful form, as has been done by Hanot and Gilbert.

Prognosis.—The prognosis is absolutely unfavorable, except in those rare cases in which a neoplasm is so situated on the surface of the liver that it can be removed by an operation and the disease cured in this way (Sklifosowski, Bardeleben, and others).

In massive carcinoma, sarcoma, and those forms of nodular carcinoma that increase and develop rapidly, the course is very rapid, and leads to death within a few weeks or months. In adenocarcinomata complicated by cirrhosis the course of the disease is slower.

Diagnosis.—It is often impossible to determine the nature of the neoplasm. We will frequently have to content ourselves with establishing the presence of a tumor.

In the case of carcinomata and sarcomata which produce a large and smooth swelling of the liver, hypertrophic cirrhosis of the liver, amyloid degeneration, deep-seated echinococcus disease, or abscesses will have to be considered as well as occlusion of the common or the hepatic duct by a gall-stone, leukemia, and other conditions. The rapid loss of strength, the age of the patient, the absence of biliary stasis and such etiologic factors as alcohol, malaria or syphilis, tuberculosis, persistent suppuration, gall-stone colic, etc., will all speak in favor of tumor of the liver; the blood picture, the rapid growth of the swelling without fluctuation, or the aspiration of a characteristic fluid, will all assist in arriving at a conclusion.

In nodular carcinoma and sarcoma a primary focus is sometimes present. If no such focus can be found, echinococcus cysticus or alveolaris (particularly the latter), cystic liver, cysts of the bile-ducts following intrahepatic cholelithiasis, syphilis, abscesses, etc., must all be considered. In echinococcus the age of the patient, local conditions, fluctuation, exploratory puncture, the hardness of the tumor (echinococcus alveolaris), will enable us to make the differential diagnosis. Cystic liver is usually a chronic condition that produces few symptoms. Occasionally attacks of colic precede the formation of cysts of the bile-passages and give a clue. Syphilis of the liver is principally found in young individuals in whom a history of specific disease or some typical symptoms will aid in making the diagnosis. Abscesses can also be diagnosed from the history, and the appearance of inflammatory symptoms, and from an examination of the aspirated fluid.

It is often difficult to differentiate simple cirrhosis from cirrhosis complicated by cancer. The rapid loss of strength, the nodular character of the liver surface, and the absence of a tumor of the spleen will enable us to make this diagnosis.

Sarcomata of the liver are to a great extent secondary growths. In melanotic sarcoma the characteristic primary tumor will usually be found in the choroid or the skin; in other forms the primary tumor will be seen in other possibly more accessible parts of the body, as the muscles, bones, etc. Their malignancy is established by a rapid growth, and by the rapid loss of strength suffered by the patient. In melanotic tumors the examination of the urine will yield positive information.

Neoplasms of the gall-bladder may be confounded with stagnation of bile due to gall-stones, hydrops of the gall-bladder, and filling of the bladder with calculi. Here again the age of the patient, the symptoms of general carcinomatosis, the nodular consistency of the tumor, the extension of the growth to the liver and the bile-passages, the resulting icterus, and carcinomatosis of the peritoneum will assist in the diagnosis.

Carcinoma of the ductus choledochus and the hepatic ducts may be confounded with simple impaction of gall-stones. In this condition, however, the exclusion of the bile from the intestine is not so complete; besides the long duration of the occlusion and its persistency, the age of the patient, the presence of metastases, ascites, and cachexia all speak for cancer. The question whether or not a cancer of the pancreas is closing the orifice of the common duct is a difficult one to answer. In a case of this kind the absence of pancreatic juice from the intestine would be manifested by deficient lipolysis; this finding would not, however, decide positively in favor of such a diagnosis, for it would be equally possible for a carcinoma of the common duct to occlude the exit of the pancreatic duct secondarily. From the standpoint of treatment this question is an insignificant one.

Examination with the Röntgen rays may give some information in regard to tumors that are so situated that they cannot be palpated. This method will show the exact location and the size of the tumor.

Treatment.—Treatment of a malignant tumor, as a rule, can only be palliative. In exceptional cases surgeons have succeeded in extirpating a growth that was situated favorably for operative interference and in removing all diseased tissue so completely that there has been no recurrence.

I must refer to the monographs of Langenbuch and von Madelung for the description of the different cases that are on record, the methods of operating, etc.

Hochenegg and von Heidenhain have extirpated a *carcinomatous gall-bladder* together with a piece of carcinomatous liver tissue for cancer of this viscus. P. Bruns removed a *carcinomatous nodule* from the liver and reports that the wound healed rapidly; the nodule had been removed for diagnostic purposes. Lücke probably was the first to remove a large cancer nodule from the liver; during this operation he also removed a cancerous lymph-gland and cured his case. Very few successful operations of this kind have been performed since this occasion. Several surgeons have removed adenomata with success (Keen, Fr. Schmidt, v. Bergmann, Grube, Triconi); all the cases published were not malignant.

Sklifosowski removed a pedunculated sarcomatous fibromyoma; v. Bardeleben, a sarcoma of the abdominal wall that had grown into the liver; Israel (angiosarcoma) and d'Urso have published similar cases.

We know from the experiments of Ponfick, and from clinical observation in destructive lesions of the liver, that life can be carried on even though large pieces of the liver are removed, and that a process of regeneration and of hyperplasia soon replaces the loss. We may hope, therefore, that with a perfection of surgical technique it will soon be possible to extirpate larger tumors of the liver, such as solitary carcinomata and sarcomata, and in this way to cure many cases. [Kümmell* extirpated successfully a hazelnut-sized sarcoma of the liver, situated near the gall-bladder. He also removed a large wedge-shaped piece of liver tissue with the growth, then closing the wound.—ED.] The most popular method so far has been to excise the tumor by a wedge-shaped incision and to suture the edges of the wound to the abdominal wall. The tumor has also been first attached extraperitoneally and extirpated in the course of a second operation. As sepsis seems to occur more readily if the tumor is situated extraperitoneally, it is best to close the wound after resection, possibly with the aid of the mesentery, and then to replace the parts.

It is, however, not always possible to operate, and treatment must be directed toward making the patient as comfortable as possible. If pain is very severe, warm or cold compresses should be applied; if peritoneal irritation appears, counterirritants in the form of liniments, tincture of iodin, etc., or narcotics must be employed. For the sleeplessness chloral,

* Aerztlich. Verein in Hamburg, Oct. 16, 1894.

sulphonal, etc., can be given; the appetite can be stimulated by hydrochloric acid, tincture of cinchona, pepsin, etc. These remedies will at the same time aid digestion. The administration of alkaline waters, usually indicated in affections of the liver, should be avoided (Karlsbad, Ems, Faching, Vichy) and constipation should be treated by vegetable laxatives, such as rhubarb, senna, aloes, etc., rather than with sulphates.

Very much will depend on a rational regulation of the diet and the mode of life. In addition to warm bathing and rest, particularly in icterus, the patient should be kept on a diet that does not tax the digestive organs too much. Milk is the best food in this respect, together with easily digestible amylaceous foods, as soups, gruels, etc. Large quantities of milk should be avoided, because they may cause the formation of large lumps of casein in the stomach and hinder digestion in this way. The milk may be improved by the addition of cream, or may be given as koumiss, buttermilk, or sour milk. Patients, as a rule, have a disgust for meat, and it does not agree very well with them. In case of great decomposition of the intestinal contents milk again is the best remedy, as it seems to check the putrefaction of proteid material. The preparations of peptone and meat extracts are not so suitable. They may, however, be given in small quantities together with such preparations as somatose, eucasin, etc., as they stimulate the patient, and, owing to their ready assimilability, aid in maintaining his strength. Fats are usually not well tolerated. Food should be administered in small doses and frequently; *i. e.*, about every three hours.

LITERATURE.

Achard: "Verhandlungen der anatomischen Gesellschaft in Paris,' April 10, 1896 (Fever in Carcinoma).

Ahlenstiel: "Die Lebergeschwülste und ihre Behandlung," "Archiv für klin. Chirurgie," Bd. LII, p. 902.

Arnold: "Zwei Fälle von primärem Angiosarkom der Leber," "Ziegler's Beiträge," 1890, Bd. VIII, p. 123.

Benner: "Ein Fall von Gallenstauungscirrhose mit primärem Adenocarcinom im Ductus choledochus," Dissertation, Halle, 1892.

Birch-Hirschfeld: "Lehrbuch der pathologischen Anatomie," Bd. II, p. 617.

Bohnstedt: "Die Differentialdiagnose zwischen dem durch Gallensteine und dem durch Tumor bedingten Verschluss des Ductus choledochus," Dissertation, Halle, 1893.

Bramwell and Leith: "Enormous Primary Sarcoma of the Liver," "Edinburgh Med. Journal," October, 1896, p. 331.

Brissaud: "Adénome et cancer hépat.," "Archives générales de médecine," 1885, tome CLVI, p. 129.

Brodowski: "Ein ungeheures Myosarkom des Magens, nebst sec. Myosarkom der Leber," "Virchow's Archiv," Bd. LXVII, p. 227.

Brunswig: "Ein Fall von primärem Krebs der Gallenblase," Dissertation, Kiel, 1893.

Budd: "Krankheiten der Leber," German translation by Henoch, Berlin, 1846, p. 341.

Deetjen: "Ein Fall von primärem Krebs des Ductus choledochus," Dissertation, Kiel, 1894.

Eberth: "Untersuchungen über die normale und pathologische Leber, Adenom der Leber," "Virchow's Archiv," Bd. XLIII, p. 1.

Ewald: "Ein Fall von Carcinom der Gallenblase," "Berliner klin. Wochenschr.," 1897, p. 411.

Feickert: "Beitrag zur Genese des metastatischen Lebercarcinoms," Dissertation, Würzburg, 1892.

Frerichs: "Klinik der Leberkrankheiten," Bd. II, pp. 271 and 454, 1861.

Gilbert et Claude: "Cancer des voies bil. par effract. dans le cancer prim. du foie," "Archives générales de médecine," 1895, tome CLXXV, p. 513.

Grawitz: "Klinische Beobachtungen über den Krebs der Gallenblase," "Charité-Annalen," Bd. xxi, p. 157.

Griesinger: "Das Adenoid der Leber," "Archiv der Heilkunde," 1864, Bd. v, p. 385.

Hanot et Gilbert: "Etudes sur les maladies du foie," Paris, 1888 (complete bibliography of liver tumors).

Hanot: "Note sur le modification de l'appétit dans le cancer du foie," "Archives générales de médecine," October, 1893.

—"Verhandlungen der anatomischen Gesellschaft in Paris," Mar. 27, 1896 (fever in cancer).

Hansemann: "Ueber den primären Krebs der Leber," "Berliner klin. Wochenschr.," 1890, No. 16.

Harris: "Ueber die Entwickelung des primären Leberkrebses," "Virchow's Archiv," 1885, Bd. c, p. 139.

Hartmann: "Ein Fall von primärem Gallenblasenkrebs," Dissertation, Kiel, 1896.

Held: "Der primäre Krebs der Gallenblase,"...Dissertation, Erlangen, 1892.

Hölker: "Ueber carcinomatose Lebercirrhose," Dissertation, Freiburg i. Br., 1898.

Howald: "Die primären Carcinome des Ductus hepaticus und choledochus," Dissertation, Bern, 1890.

Index-Catalogue of the Library of the Surgeon-General's Office, vol. viii, p. 285 et seq. (literature).

v. Kahlden: "Ueber das primäre Sarkom der Leber," "Ziegler's Beiträge zur pathologischen Anatomie," 1897, Bd. xxi, p. 264.

Kelsch et Kiener: "Contribution à l'histoire de l'adénome du foie," "Archives de physiologie normale et pathologique," 1876, p. 622.

Kelynack: "Edinburgh Med. Journal," February, 1897.

Kuznezow and Pensky: (resection of the liver) "Centralblatt für Chirurgie," 1894, p. 978.

Langenbuch: "Chirurgie der Leber und Gallenblase," 2. Theil, p. 32.

Laveran: "Observ. d'épithel. à cellules cylindr. prim. du foie," "Archives de physiologie normale et pathologique," 1880, p. 601..

Leichtenstern: "Klinik des Leberkrebses," "Ziemssen's Handbuch der speciellen Pathologie und Therapie," Bd. viii, 1. Abtheilung, p. 315.

Litten: "Ueber einen Fall von infiltrirtem Leberkrebs," "Virchow's Archiv," 1880, Bd. lxxx, p. 269.

Madelung: "Chirurgische Behandlung der Leberkrankheiten" in Penzoldt und Stintzing's "Handbuch der speciellen Therapie," Bd. iv, Abtheilung vib, p. 198.

Marckwald: "Das multiple Adenom der Leber," "Virchow's Archiv," 1896, Bd. cxliv, p. 29.

Murchison: "Diseases of the Liver."

Naunyn: "Ueber die Entwickelung des Leberkrebses," "Archiv für Anatomie und Physiologie," 1866, p. 717.

Nölke: "Ein Fall von primärem Leberkrebs," Dissertation, Kiel, 1894.

Oberwarth: "Ein Fall von primärem Gallenblasenkrebs," Dissertation, Kiel, 1897.

Ohloff: "Ueber Epithelmetaplasie und Krebsbildung an der Schleimhaut von Gallenblase und Trachea," Dissertation, Greifswald, 1891.

Perls: "Histologie des Lebercarcinoms," "Virchow's Archiv," 1872, Bd. lvi, p. 448.

Rindfleisch: "Mikroskopische Studien über das Leberadenoid," "Archiv der Heilkunde," 1864, Bd. v, p. 395.

De Ruyter: "Congenitale Geschw. der Leber," "Archiv für klin. Chirurgie," 1890, Bd. xl, p. 95.

Rohwedder: "Der primäre Leberkrebs und sein Verhalten zur Lebercirrhose," Dissertation, Kiel, 1888.

Schmidt: "Ein Fall von primärem Gallenblasenkrebs," Dissertation, Kiel, 1891.

Schrader: "Noch ein Fall von Exstirpation einer Lebergeschwulst," "Deutsche med. Wochenschr.," 1897, p. 173.

Schreiber: "Ueber das Vorkommen von primären Carcinomen in den Gallenwegen," "Berliner klin. Wochenschr.," 1877, No. 31.

Schüppel: "Pathologische Anatomie des Leberkrebses," "Ziemssen's Handbuch," Bd. viii, i, 1, p. 284.

Siegenbeck van Heukelom: "Das Adenocarcinom der Leber mit Cirrhose," Ziegler's "Beiträge zur pathologischen Anatomie," Bd. xvi, p. 341.

Seigert: "Zur Aetiologie der primären Carcinome der Gallenblase," "Virchow's Archiv," 1893, Bd. cxxxii, p. 353.

Siegrist: "Klinische Untersuchungen über Leberkrebs," Dissertation, Zürich, 1887.

Simmonds: "Knotige Hyperplasie und Adenom der Leber," "Deutsches Archiv für klin. Medicin," Bd. xxxiv, p. 385

Sjöquist: "Nord. med. Arkiv," 1892.

Skorna: "Ein Fall von Carcinoma hepatis idiopathic," Dissertation, Berlin, 1895.

Thorel: "Die Cirrhosis hepatis carcinomatosa," Zeigler's "Beiträge zur pathologischen Antomie," Bd. xviii, p. 498.

Tiedemann: "Zur Casuistik des primären Gallenblasenkrebses," Dissertation, Kiel, 1891.

"Traité de médecine" (Charcot, Bouchard, Brissaud), tome iii, p. 962.

d'Urso: "Endothelioma prim. del. fegato," "Centralblatt für Chirurgie," 1897, No. 13.

Wagner, E.: "Zur Structur des Leberkrebses," "Archiv der Heilkunde," 1861, Bd. ii, p. 209.

—"Zwei Fälle von Neubildung von Lebersubstanz im Lig. suspensor. hepat.," ibidem, p. 471.

—"Drüsengeschwulst der Leber," ibidem, p. 473.

—"Primärer Krebs der Gallenblase," ibidem, 1863, Bd. iv, p. 184.

Waldeyer: "Die Entwickelung der Carcinome," "Virchow's Archiv," 1872, Bd. lv, p. 111.

Waring: "Diseases of the Liver," Edinburgh and London, 1897, p. 182.

Weber: "Ueber ein Plattenepitheliom der Gallenblase," Dissertation, Würzburg, 1891.

Weigert: "Ueber primäres Lebercarcinom," "Virchow's Archiv," 1876, Bd. lxvii, p. 500.

Willigk: "Beitrag zur Pathogenese des Leberkrebses," "Virchow's Archiv," 1869, Bd. xlviii, p. 524.

—"Beitrag zur Histogenese des Leberadenoms," ibidem, 1870, Bd. li, p. 208.

Windrath: "Ueber Sarkombildungen der Leber," Dissertation, Freiburg, 1885.

Zenker, H.: "Der primäre Krebs der Gallenblase," Dissertation, Erlangen, 1889.

Zinsser: "Beitrag zur Aetiologie dse Krebses," Dissertation, Kiel, 1895.

LEUKEMIC AND LYMPHOMATOUS TUMORS OF THE LIVER.

The lesions of the liver seen in leukemia and in pseudo-leukemia are related to the lesions seen in tumor formation. This is, however, not the place to discuss the course of these diseases nor their treatment. We will therefore limit our discussion to a description of the lesions caused by these conditions and found in connection with other diseases of the liver.

Leukemia is to-day divided into two forms, the acute and the chronic. There are transition stages between the two, though etiologically we are as yet unable to differentiate them. Pathologic germs have so far not been found, although many features of the disease, as the fever, the distribution of the lesions throughout the body, their starting-point in the fauces, etc., point to a parasitic origin. [Boinet* has reported several cases of leukemia that point to an infectious etiology. In two of these cases there was a general glandular enlargement, and in one case bacteria were obtained from the glands.—Ed.] The acute form is variously described; A. Fränkel states that it has a duration of from two and one-half to sixteen weeks; others state that it lasts much longer. According to Fränkel, the changes in the blood consist chiefly in an increase of the mononuclear leucocytes, and constitute a lymphemia or a lymphocythemia; others claim that the principal abnormalities consist in the appearance of marrow-cells and of polynuclear elements.

In the acute forms, at all events, there is an abundant new-formation of leucocytes and a flooding of the blood with young cells resembling lymphocytes.

In the chronic forms there is also an abundant formation of white

* *Wien. med. Woch.*, Nov. 3, 1900.

blood-corpuscles; in this case the older forms, the polynuclear and the eosinophilic cells, are more numerous. Different authors (H. F. Müller, Hindenberg) have shown that in the liver capillaries a proliferation of leucocytes, with the formation of mitoses, occurs; this is usually explained from the fact that in these channels the blood and its elements are, comparatively speaking, at rest, and that in this way the development of cell division is favored. In addition to the elements named, the so-called myeloplaques, giant-cells, are found; their origin is obscure.

The pathologic-anatomic finding in the liver is usually that of general enlargement of the organ. The surface is usually smooth, and occasionally the peritoneal covering is roughened from infiltration with leucocytes. The outline of the organ is not changed; its consistency is dependent upon the degree of infiltration and its weight may be as much as 7 kg. On transverse section a lobulated configuration is seen; between the lobules are wide, swollen bands that correspond to the periportal tissues; in other cases grayish-white, soft nodules are seen that contain leukemic lymphomata. These white spots are sometimes very well developed, and form white plates on the surface of the organ, from which white bands penetrate the interior of the organ; these processes may also start from the portal branches, shooting out from them into the liver tissue and forming a system of arborescent ramifications through its substance.

The portal lymph-glands are frequently enlarged. At the same time characteristic changes in the spleen, the bone-marrow, and the lymphatic apparatus are seen.

Microscopically, the most characteristic feature is the accumulation of leucocytes in the periportal connective tissues, extending from there between the columns of liver-cells into the acini. Round cells fill the capillaries within the liver and distend them. This process is first seen in the periphery near the branches of the portal vein and gradually advances toward the center of the acinus. Some investigators claim that the cell-columns are hyperplastic; liver-cells are seen that are larger than normal. If the infiltration with leucocytes occurs in this manner and reaches a considerable degree, the liver-cells become compressed, narrowed, and undergo atrophic changes. In addition, venous stasis occurs in the center of the acini, and as a result there is atrophy of this area. The hepatic cells, as a rule, contain a large quantity of iron pigment and present the picture of siderosis; this is due to the great disintegration of red blood-corpuscles that takes place toward the end. Simultaneously may be seen, in many chronic cases, round areas of leucocytes between the liver-cells, the so-called **leukemic lymphomata**. They consist of a fine network of delicate connective-tissue fibers, inclosing numerous leucocytes of various forms. In the acute cases this is not so prominent a feature. These nodules, in contradistinction to tubercles and other small tumors, show neither a tendency to necrosis nor to suppurative degeneration. The bile-passages are, as a rule, not involved, so that icterus usually does not appear. Similar accumulations of leucocytes are also seen in typhoid fever.

In **pseudoleukemia** the liver shows similar changes. Here, however, the portal lymph-glands show a greater tendency to enlargement, and, as a result, icterus from stasis and compression of the portal vein are more frequent. The whitish-yellow lymphomata are also larger than in leukemia; they may be as large as nuts, and appear with particular frequency in Glisson's capsule. From this point they send out processes into the acini that show a drumstick swelling at their distal extremity. They are also seen underneath the peritoneum. [Crowder * records a case of generalized tuberculous lymphadenitis simulating the clinical and anatomic picture of pseudoleukemia. The postmortem examination showed general glandular hyperplasia, and the appearance of lymphoid nodules in the liver, spleen, and lung. The latter, on microscopic examination, however, were seen to be tubercular foci. There seems to be no doubt that many of the so-called cases of pseudoleukemia are tuberculous.—Ed.] Sometimes cirrhotic changes may be seen in the intra-acinous connective tissue, causing the surface of the organ to become very rough. If the intra-acinous connective tissue contracts, the liver is diminished in size, and the symptoms of ordinary cirrhosis may appear —namely, ascites, etc. At the same time the hepatic cells are often infiltrated with fat. Some authors (Klein) believe that cirrhosis develops at the same time as the pseudoleukemic process, and that both diseases can be attributed to a common cause. .

Symptoms.—The liver is enlarged in more than one-half of all cases of **leukemia,** and, as a rule, a tumor of the spleen will be felt at the same time; the latter is only rarely absent in acute leukemia.

If the liver is very much enlarged, certain subjective symptoms appear, as a feeling of pressure, less frequently pain in the right hypochondrium, and a feeling of fulness even after the ingestion of small amounts of food. Schultz attributes the pain in the sternum, so frequently observed in leukemia, to the pressure of the enlarged liver. The organ can be easily palpated, its consistency is increased, it may even be extremely hard in severe cases. It is smooth, not very sensitive to pressure, the margin is not indentated, and is fairly sharp. In cases of great infiltration the liver may extend as far down as Poupart's ligament, or may be in contact on the left with the enlarged spleen. In other words, it may almost fill the abdominal cavity and cause the abdomen, and particularly the right hypochondriac region, to bulge. Icterus is hardly ever present. Ascites is not seen in the beginning; only toward the end of the disease may a slight exudate be poured into the abdominal cavity.

The liver shows similar changes in pseudoleukemia. Here, however, icterus is more frequently seen as a result of compression of the common duct by glands near the portal orifice. The surface of the organ is not so smooth, and the margin is indented owing to cirrhotic changes in the liver and the formation of lymphomata in the capsule.

In leukemia the general symptoms of the disease are also seen. Thus, in addition to the lesions of the liver there are swelling of the spleen and of the lymph-glands, muscular weakness, leukemic retinitis, edema, and hemorrhages, the latter principally toward the end of the course of the chronic form, and in the beginning of the acute form. There may also be ulcerations in the mouth, the pharynx, and the intestinal canal, besides a characteristic increase in the leucocytes, both relative and absolute. In the urine large quantities of uric acid and xanthin bodies are found; this is particularly the case if a rapid disintegration of leucocytes occur, as, for instance, in bacterial disease, miliary tuberculosis, septicopyemia, etc. At such times there may seem to be an improvement or a cure of the disease. Even the tumors of the spleen and the liver may appear to decrease.

* *Wien. klin. Woch.,* Dec. 6, 1900.

In pseudoleukemia also there is an increase in the uric acid and the xanthin bodies; also of nucleo-histon.

The diagnosis of leukemic liver must be made from the characteristic changes in the blood, and from the swelling of the spleen and lymph-glands. The pseudoleukemic form is recognized by the appearance of numerous lymphomatá, a tumor of the spleen, and the course of the fever (chronic recurrent type); [also by the absence of the blood-picture typical of true leukemia.—ED.]. The tumor of the liver itself is not character-istic, and may be caused by fatty liver, amyloid liver, or congestion of the liver from stasis.

· The **prognosis** of leukemia is unfavorable; less unfavorable in pseudo-leukemia only in those cases that are not very cachectic.

The **treatment** of these diseases consists principally in the adminis-tration of iron and arsenic, and in the regulation of the mode of life.

LITERATURE.

OLDER LITERATURE TO 1892.

Hoffmann: "Lehrbuch der Constitutionskrankheiten," Stuttgart, 1893.
v. Limbeck: "Grundriss einer klin. Pathologie des Blutes," Jena, 1892.
Mosler: "Ziemssen's Handbuch der speciellen Pathologie und Therapie," Bd. VIII, 2. Halfte, p. 155.
Rieder: "Beitrag zur Kenntniss der Leukocyten," Leipzig, 1892.

NEWER WORKS.

Askanazy: "Ueber acute Leukämie und ihre Beziehung zu geschwür Processen im Verdauungscanal," "Virchow's Archiv," 1894, Bd. CXXXVII, p. 1.
Dausac: "Leucocythémie suraiguë," "Gazette hebdomad.," p. 116.
Ebstein: "Beitrage zur Lehre von traumatischer Leukamie," "Deutsche med. Wochenschr.," 1894, p. 589.
Fränkel, A.: "Ueber acute Leukämie," ibidem, 1895, p. 639.
Hindenburg: "Zur Kenntniss der Organveränderungen bei Leukämie," "Deutsches Archiv für klin. Medicin," 1895, Bd. LIV, p. 209.
Hintze: "Ein Beitrag zur Lehre von der acuten Leukämie," ibidem, 1894, Bd. LIII, 377.
Lannois et Regaud: "Coexist.de la leucocythémie et d'un cancer epithél.," "Archives de méd.-expér.," 1895, tome VII, p. 254.
Klein, St.: "Ein Fall von Pseudoleukamie nebst Lebercirrhose," "Berliner klin. Wochenschr.," 1890, p. 712.
Schultze: "Ueber Leukämie," "Deutsches Archiv für klin. Medicin," 1894, Bd. LII, p. 464.
Zielenziger: "Ein leukämisches Lymphom der Leber," Dissertation, Würzburg, 1892.

PARASITES OF THE LIVER.

(Hoppe-Seyler.)

(A) COCCIDIA.

Coccidia (psorospermia) are very frequently found in the liver of animals, particularly of rabbits. In man they are not found frequently, although some investigators claim that carcinoma and other malignant tumors are caused by these parasites.

In a few cases coccidium oviforme has been found in man. Gubler reports a case in a man who suffered from loss of appetite, pain in the right hypochondriac region, cachexia, and anemia. The liver was enlarged and there was a nodular tumor in the region of the gall-bladder. Icterus was not present. Later there was fever, bile-colored vomit, prostration, dyspnea, and death followed. On autopsy numerous tumors were found in the liver, some of them as large as a hen's egg, and resembling medullary carcinomata. In addition, there was a cyst from 12 to 15 cm. in diameter containing slimy·masses mixed with blood. The tumors were soft, gray in the center, and translucent near the periphery. A creamy substance could be scraped from their surface, in which epithelial cells from the bile-ducts, liver-cells that had undergone fatty degeneration, fat-droplets, etc., could be seen, and, in addition, certain cells that were four times as large as the largest liver-cell, egg-shaped, had a double outline, and were finely granular. These bodies were also found on the intact portions of the liver surface. Gubler considers them to be the eggs of distoma, while Davaine and Leuckart look upon them as examples of coccidium oviforme infection. Dressler, Sattler, Perls, and Silcock have also described instances of coccidium infection in human livers. They produced either cysts or cheesy degeneration. Sattler found them in dilated bile-passages.

It is reported that coccidium perforans is also sometimes seen in the liver of man. Exact research with reference to this parasite has never been undertaken.

Braun: "Die thierischen Parasiten des Menschen," 2. Aufl., Würzburg, 1895, p. 77.
Davaine: "Traité des entozoaires," 2. Aufl., Paris, 1877, p. 268.
Gubler: "Gazette médicale de Paris," 1858, p. 657.
Leuckart: "Die menschlichen Parasiten," 2. Aufl., I, Abth. 1, 1879, p. 281.
Schneidemühl: "Die Protozoen als Krankheitserreger," Leipzig, 1878, p. 36.

(B) ECHINOCOCCUS CYSTICUS (HYDATIDOSUS).

The most important animal parasite found in the liver of man and capable of causing pathologic changes in this organ is the echinococcus. We will not attempt to describe the natural history of this organism in this place. In another volume of this series exhaustive attention has been paid to the subject ("Animal Parasites," by F. Mosler and E. Peiper); also in a monograph by Neisser; and in the works of Siebold, Küchenmeister, Leuckart, Davaine, and others. Echinococcus cysticus has of late been discussed separately from echinococcus multilocularis or alveolaris; for while these two conditions are intimately related, they still show essential differences in their pathologic nature, their symptomatology, and their geographic distribution.

Etiology.—According to the studies of Siebold, Küchenmeister, Leuckart, and others, echinococcus disease develops from eggs deposited in the intestinal tract of the dog, the wolf, or the jackal, less often in other animals. The parasite that lays these eggs is Tænia echinococcus, a small tapeworm 1.5 millimeters in length. From the intestinal tracts of these animals the eggs are carried to the stomach and the intestine of man; here a greater proportion, probably the majority, perish. Occasionally, however, the shell is digested and the embryo penetrates the intestinal wall, enters the portal vein, and in this manner penetrates the liver; here it becomes lodged, and is converted into an echinococcus cyst. At the same time, though less frequently, embryos enter the lymph-channels and the greater circulation. The method by which these embryos enter the intestinal wall is unknown. Some investigators (Neisser) assume that the organism is perfectly passive,—for instance, like a particle of silver,—and is simply passed through small spaces in the intestinal wall; others believe that it penetrates the wall owing to its motility. Leuckart, at all events, in his animal experiments, has found embryos within the roots of the portal vein, thus readily explaining why this parasite is found so frequently in the liver. Some authors have formulated the hypothesis that echinococcus enters the liver through the bile-ducts in the same manner as many other parasites. If this were the case, they should also be found in the pancreas, where echinococcus growths are exceedingly rare. The bile-current impedes the advance of the echinococcus, which is very sensitive to the action of this fluid. This is shown by the fact that the organism dies or becomes impaired in vitality if bile enters the echinococcus cyst. No anatomical connection can be found between bile-passages and recent echinococcus cysts; the latter develop in the interlobular connective-tissue structure of the liver. Naunyn * has also demonstrated a frequent connection between the smaller cysts and the vessel-walls.

It is said that trauma of the liver or of other organs favors the development of echinococcus (Boncour, Danlos, Duvernoy, Kirmisson, Sokolow, von Bramann, and others). A positive conclusion seems hardly justified in view of the scanty observations that are on record. It is possible, however, that an embryo might find a suitable nidus for its development in a portion of the liver that has been altered by trauma.

The echinococcus soon becomes converted into a nodule resembling a tubercle, and develops very slowly. Around its thick cuticle a capsule is formed from the hepatic connective tissue containing numerous wide bile-passages and blood-vessels, which provide nourishment for the parasite. Nutritive material particularly suitable for the parasite penetrates the cuticle; noxious substances, on the other hand, seem to be withheld.

As a rule, tiny scolices soon develop in the wall, and from these endogenous cysts, or secondary hydatids. In man the exogenous formation of daughter-cysts is rare. In sheep, however, this is frequently seen, and buds appear on the outer wall of the cyst. These daughter-cysts, the exact formation of which we may not discuss in this place, are sometimes sterile. Frequently they too contain scolices and tertiary hydatids, and granddaughter-cysts may be developed from them. As a rule, from twenty-five to fifty daughter-cysts are seen in one cyst. Some echinococci are altogether sterile; that is, they form no scolices, but only growths on the inner surface of the cyst-wall that may contain some calcium and fat. These so-called acephalo-cysts grow very large, and consequently produce more serious pathologic changes.

Sometimes several years pass before echinococcus disease causes symptoms. · This is due to the fact that the organism develops so slowly that the changes in the liver proceed imperceptibly; symptoms appear as soon as pressure is exerted on surrounding organs, or if some trauma injures the cyst, such as a blow or a fall, infection with pus organism, or perforation. We can thus readily understand that the disease is frequently not recognized during life and only discovered at autopsy or in the course of an operation. As a great many of these parasitic growths, therefore, are never recognized for the reason that the individuals are not examined postmortem, it is a difficult matter to give reliable statistics on the frequency of their occurrence.

There can be no doubt that the disease is frequent is Iceland, although older statements, that from one-seventh to one-sixth of the population are afflicted, seem to be exaggerated. Twenty-eight per cent. of the dogs seem to have the tenia. In Australia the disease is frequent wherever sheep culture is carried on. In Germany, certain parts of Mecklenburg and Pomerania are particularly afflicted.† According to

---

* Naunyn, *Archiv für Anatomie u. Physiologie*, 1863, p. 921.

† Madelung, "Beiträge mecklenb. Aerzte z. Lehre von der Echinococcus-krankheit," Stuttgart, 1885. Mosler, *Deutsche med. Woch.*, 1886, Nos. 7 and 8.

Peiper, 68.58 % of the cattle, 51.02 % of the sheep, and 4.93 % of the hogs are afflicted with echinococcus disease in the neighborhood of Greifswald. In other European countries, France, England, etc., echinococcus is quite frequently encountered, also iർ Algiers and Egypt. In Asia and Africa the disease seems to be rare. [W. J. Buchanan * states that hydatid disease seldom or never occurs in the natives of India. He reports as a medical rarity a case occurring in a native of Bhagalpur.— Ed.] The etiology is important for the diagnosis of echinococcus, because intimate contact with dogs (keeping them in the same room, allowing them to lick up the food from the plates, etc.) and extensive sheep culture create favorable circumstances for infection with this disease. It is said, for instance, that in Iceland one-third of the sheep are afflicted with echinococcus. [Kokall † considers at length the occurrence of echinococcus disease in Brünn, as indicated by the hospital statistics. Between 1881 and 1895 there were treated 104,366 cases of all kinds, and in 10 of these (0.009 %) a diagnosis of echinococcus was ventured. Many more were found at the autopsy table; 6943 autopsies were performed, and 24 cases of echinococcus (0.34 %) were discovered. In men it occurred 9 times, in women 15; in the liver 19 times, in the lower lobe of the right lung twice, once in the spleen, once in the muscles of the lower limbs, and once beneath the diaphragm. In only two cases was the cyst multilocular.—Ed.]

It is a peculiar fact that echinococcus disease seems to attack the female sex oftener than the male, though no adequate explanation for this phenomenon has been offered. Among 255 cases reported by Finsen, 191 were women. Neisser in his statistics saw a proportion of 148 men as against 210 women.

Pathologic Anatomy.—The echinococcus is found more frequently in the liver than in any other organ; in fact, nearly one-half of the cyst parasites attack this organ. Other parts of the body may also be attacked at the same time. If multiple echinococcus infection is present, the liver is almost always infected.

As a rule, only one echinococcus cyst is found in the liver. There may, however, be two or three, sometimes more; occasionally as many as twelve have been discovered.

The echinococcus cysticus is inclosed in a solid wall, the cuticle. On transverse section this membrane is seen to be striated in a characteristic manner, and, according to Lücke,‡ to consist of chitin; on boiling with sulphuric acid it yields dextrose. The clear contents contain no albumin, have a specific gravity of 1009 to 1015, frequently contain succinic acid (Heintze, Boedeker), inosite, dextrose (Cl. Bernard, Lücke), and occasionally leucin, tyrosin, etc. The chief mineral constituent is sodium chlorid.

Certain poisonous substances are also found in the fluid that cause collapse if injected into animals (Humphrey); these are probably ptomains (toxalbumins?), according to Moursson and Schlagdenhauffen. Brieger succeeded in isolating a body that was rapidly fatal for mice in small doses.§

The whole bladder is surrounded by a connective-tissue capsule

* *Lancet*, July 7, 1900.
† *Wien. klin. Woch.*, 1901, No. 4.
‡ Lücke, *Virchow's Archiv*, Bd. xix, S. 179.
§ Langenbuch, "Chirurgie der Leber," Bd. i, S. 109.

that is formed from the liver tissue by atrophy of parenchymatous cells. Nothing therefore remains but connective tissue, blood-vessels, and bile-channels. The latter do not seem to proliferate; at the same time certain inflammatory processes are present.

Cysts may appear in any part of the organ. They are chiefly found in the right lobe because the right branch of the portal vein is wider and is straighter, consequently the embryos enter it more readily than the left branch.

The form of the liver is altered according to the location of the echinococcus cyst. If the cyst develops centrally,—for instance, in the interior of the right lobe,—it may grow very large without producing any change in the outline of the liver; it will simply lead to a general enlargement of the organ, so that during life, and even postmortem, the presence of echinococcus cannot be even suspected without incising the organ. If the development of the cyst proceeds very rapidly, it may reach the surface and form a prominent hemispheric tumor, or may convert the whole lobe into a large round cyst. If this happens, the liver tissue is pushed aside and may be converted into a thin shell around the cyst.

If the cysts develop near the surface, they protrude at a much earlier stage of the disease, and become noticeable in this way. They usually have a broad base, though they may be connected with the organ by a narrow pedicle; they may, however, be connected with the liver simply by a more or less long stem.

If the tumor originates from the convex surface of the liver, it enlarges upward and may dislocate the diaphragm, the mediastinum, or the right lung. It may happen that the cyst reaches even the first rib, and compresses the right lung into an airless lobe. Under these circumstances the lung may be compressed either toward the spinal column or laterally toward the chest-wall, depending upon the direction of growth of the echinococcus, either along the anterior chest-wall or into the mediastinum. The heart, at the same time, may be pushed toward the left into the axillary region. In large cysts the right lobe of the liver is pushed downward so far that the horizontal diameter of the liver becomes vertical; the right lobe is beneath and the left lobe above.

Echinococcus cysts of the concave, lower surface of the liver enlarge toward the abdomen, and may occupy a large part of the abdomen, extending as far as the crest of the ilium or even into the pelvis. If they are situated very superficially, they may be found reaching down into the pelvis, and attached to the liver by a long pedicle, so that during life they appear as tumors of the abdominal organs. They may also be found in the region of the spleen, and may even penetrate this organ. If the cyst develops downward, the liver occupies a more horizontal position, is compressed, and may become atrophic. Large cysts usually cause the right hypochondrium to bulge; if the part of the liver that is situated in the epigastrium is involved, round protuberances may be seen in this region. The development of the cyst into the thorax causes compression of the lung. Growth into the abdomen does not cause compression of neighboring organs like the stomach or intestine, because there is room for them to move. Compression of the larger bile-passages, combined with icterus from stasis, is rare (Finsen saw it only 7 times among 167 cases, Neisser 20 times in 388 cases). Compression of the vena cava and of the portal vein is also rare.

We have already mentioned the fact that the liver tissue is compressed by the cyst. It becomes atrophic, and covers the echinococcus in a thin layer only. At the same time, compensatory hypertrophy of other portions of the liver may occur (Ponfick, Dürig, Flöck, Holle-feldt, Reinecke).

If one lobe is so completely filled by a cyst that it becomes converted into a shriveled-up mass as soon as the fluid is evacuated, a considerable enlargement of the other lobe will be seen, and microscopically an enlargement of the liver-cells with abundant mitoses. In may happen, therefore, that the weight of the organ, even after evacuation and contraction of the cyst, may be greater than normal. The remnants of the liver tissue that are still present in the place of the cyst often show hypertrophic change, in addition to a proliferation of connective tissue, so that nodular protuberances are formed (Reinecke).

Rarely gangrene of the liver may occur in the region of the echino-coccus. On the other hand, if pressure is exercised on the liver by a pregnant uterus, or if certain disturbances of the circulation or of nutri-tion supervene, changes are seen in the fibrous capsule, consisting in fibrous degeneration, changes in the vessels, etc.

In cases of this kind a cheesy mass is formed where the capsule and the cuticle are in contact. Owing to this surrounding area of nonvascular tissue, the nutrition of the echinococcus is impaired, the fluid becomes cloudy and gelatinous, later milky and purulent; at the same time the cyst contracts, the contents thicken, and finally a mortar-like mass is found containing large quantities of carbonate and phosphate of calcium, and cholesterin; all that testifies to the former presence of scolices is the resistant hooklets. The puriform mass that is some-times found in these cysts contains no pus-corpuscles; it is frequently malodorous, and is acid in reaction. The daughter-cysts, as a rule, also perish. They contract and undergo the same changes as the mother-cysts; it rarely happens that they perforate the latter and continue to develop independently. Another change that these cysts can undergo is purulent degeneration following some injury or wound. It may develop in the absence of such traumata in case bacteria—as, for instance, streptococci (Riedel)—enter the liver, penetrate the cuticle, and lodge in the interior of the cyst. Suppuration occurs especially if a communication is formed between the bile-ducts and the echino-coccus cyst. The bile kills the parasite; and bacteria, frequently found in the bile-ducts, develop in the cyst, and in this manner form an abscess of the liver. In such a cavity contracted hydatids, dead scolices, fat, and bilirubin are found. Sometimes nothing is found but the hooks. In the bile-tinged fluid leucocytes in all stages of fatty degeneration, fat-globules, etc., are found.

Sometimes, as a result of trauma or of punctures made for diagnostic purposes, abscesses develop in the neighborhood of the cyst, and, again, cause the death of the parasite.

The tendency of echinococcus cysts to perforate into other organs is clinically of even greater importance.

Perforation occurs relatively frequently into the right half of the thorax; the diaphragm becomes atrophic from the pressure of the tumor, and is finally perforated, either gradually or following some sudden concussion. The pleura may be perforated at the same time. Finally, the cyst bursts, and its contents are poured into the right pleura. The fluid may then penetrate the lungs and destroy them, or produce an abscess, and in this way enter the right bronchus. As a result of the communication between the pleural cavity and the lung or the bronchus, air may enter the latter and lead to pyopneumothorax.

In many cases the base of the lung becomes adherent to the diaphragm, so that the cyst opens directly into the lung, and lies, as a result, in a cavity which it forms by dislocation of the lung tissues. If perforation occurs, the fluid, containing hydatids, is suddenly poured into the bronchi, and may so overflood them as to lead to suffocation. As a rule, the material is expectorated. A large cavity is then present, filled with air and a fluid that soon becomes purulent; such a cavity may be called a pneumocyst. It may also happen that the lung becomes adherent to the diaphragm, and that the cyst ruptures directly before it has penetrated the pulmonary tissue; this frequently leads to the formation of abscesses. As a rule, however, a fistulous passage is formed leading from the echinococcus sac, through the infiltrated lung tissue, into the bronchi. If under these circumstances a communication exists with the bile-passages, a biliary fistula may be developed. Report has also been made of the occurrence of a pleural exudate, in a patient in whom an echinococcus cyst was adherent to the diaphragm and perforated the lung without becoming mixed with the exudate (Trousseau).

Perforation into the pericardium is rare. Sometimes, however, even this sac becomes filled with cystic contents (Wunderlich).

In many cases echinococcus cysts evacuate their contents into the intestine. It may happen that rupture takes place into a large bile channel, and that the contracting hydatids with the fluid contents may enter the duodenum through the common duct. If this happens, stasis of bile and dilatation of the bile-ducts occurs, and as a result inflammatory organisms or gangrenous material may enter the echinococcus cavity, causing suppuration and putrescence. Cysts may develop on the concave surface of the liver, and become adherent to the stomach or intestine as a result of adhesive peritonitis. Through such an adhesion perforation may occur, and the contents of the cyst may be poured into the intestinal tract. If the opening is small, it may close, the cyst walls contract, and cure take place. Neisser observed this occurrence 37 times in 43 cases. On the other hand, intestinal contents may make their way into the cyst cavity and cause gangrene with all its consequences.

Echinococcus growths of the liver may also penetrate the urinary passages. This occurs as the result of the formation of adhesions with the pelvis or the right kidney, perforation occurring with evacuation of the cystic contents through the urethra; or a deep-seated pedunculated cyst may become adherent to the urinary bladder and perforate into it.

If perforation occurs suddenly into the free peritoneal cavity, a serious diffuse peritonitis may be caused, provided the contents of the cyst are infectious or purulent. If the fluid is sterile, irritation of the peritoneum is the result; even here, however, daughter-cysts may develop in the peritoneum (Volkmann, Krause,* and others), as is proved by the experimental work of Lebedeff and Andrejew, who transplanted echinococcus cysts into the abdominal cavity of rabbits. They state that the hydatids continue to grow and form endogenous daughter-cysts. Peiper, however, performed similar experiments with fresh material on rabbits, dogs, and sheep, and could not discover any development in the abdominal cavity.

* F. Krause, "Sammlung klin. Vorträge," No. 325.

If perforation occurs into a sacculated cavity, which is itself the outcome of a previous circumscribed peritonitis, the sequelæ are not so serious, and the fluid may be evacuated through the skin or into some other organ. This occurs usually, if the cavity is situated near the diaphragm, into the pleura and the lungs; or if it is near the intestinal tract, into the intestine.

Cases have also been noted of perforation into the portal vein, followed by pylephlebitis and the formation of an abscess of the liver.

If perforation occurs into a hepatic vein, embolism of the pulmonary artery or of its branches may develop, and be followed by general pyemia. Evacuation into the lower vena cava has been known to lead to complete occlusion of the pulmonary artery and to rapid death. A branch of the hepatic artery has been found eroded, the accident leading to the pouring of blood into the echinococcus cavity, and to the death of the parasite.

Perforation may also take place through the abdominal wall, just as in the case of an abscess of the liver. At first adhesions form with the abdominal wall, then suppuration occurs, and perforation of the different layers of the abdominal parietes is the final result. In rare instances a long fistulous passage is formed that penetrates between the different layers of the abdominal muscles.

Symptoms.—If the cyst remains small and develops in the interior of the liver it causes no symptoms, or only such slight ones that its presence is not suspected. Cysts as large as a fist may remain altogether latent. This is explained by the slow method of growth of the parasite, the slight inflammatory reaction that it produces, the yielding character of the liver tissue, and the vicarious hypertrophy assumed by contiguous parts of the parenchyma. It has also been stated that certain urinary abnormalities can be found in echinococcus disease (Potherat); this assertion has, however, not yet been verified. It is further claimed that the absorption of certain toxic substances from the cyst may lead to urticaria (Dieulafoy, Debove,[*] Achard [†]), to certain digestive disorders, to a repulsion for meat and fatty foods that may be so severe as to cause vomiting, or to diarrheas immediately after or during eating (Bouilly). It cannot, however, be proved that these symptoms are primarily due to this cause, and the same may be said of the psychoses that are occasionally observed in the course of echinococcus disease (Nasse [‡]). Of all the symptoms enumerated, urticaria appears to be the only one that we are at all justified in attributing to intoxication with certain ingredients of the cystic contents, since this symptom has been seen after bursting of the veins of the cyst-wall (Davaine), in perforation of the cyst into the abdomen, and following evacuation of the fluid into the latter cavity or into the vena cava, or the hepatic vein. The remaining symptoms can probably be explained by the mechanical pressure exercised by the tumor on the gastro-intestinal organs at a time when it is still so small that it cannot be detected by physical examination. They certainly are not characteristic.

At the same time, a feeling of fulness and heaviness is often complained of in the hypochondriac region; pain on pressure or motion, on the other hand, is comparatively rare.

It is owing to the vague character of these symptoms that echino-

[*] Debove, *Gaz. hebdomadaire*, 1888, No. 11.
[†] Achard, *Arch. gen. de. med.*, Oct., Nov., 1888, T. CLXII, p. 410.
[‡] Nasse, *Allgem. Zeitschr. f. Psychiatrie*, 1863.

coccus disease so often remains unrecognized. According to Frerichs, 11 cases out of 23 that were found at the autopsy were not discovered during life; according to Bocker, 13 out of 22; and Neisser, 31 out of 47.

The appearance of a palpable tumor in the liver region or the appearance of symptoms of dislocations of other organs leads to the discovery of the disease. Sometimes the tumor is discovered by chance without having caused any disturbances. Such tumors as are situated on the anterior surface of the organ in the epigastric region are, of course, discovered early in the course of the disease. Those that are located underneath the costal arch or on the upper or the lower surface of the organ may remain unrecognized for a long time. If they continue to develop, they may attain a great size before they are discovered.

If the tumor develops within the organ, a general enlargement of the liver into the abdominal cavity may be observed, and the impression may be created that the swelling is due to some other cause.

If the tumor develops in the epigastrium,—*e. g.*, in the left lobe,—a flat or hemispheric protuberance is felt that remains quite hard as long as the normal tension of the sac is maintained. If several cysts are present, several protuberances will be felt. If the tumor develops on the right side of the liver, the ribs of the right side are pushed out; if the tumor is situated in a corresponding position in the left lobe, the ribs of the left side may be pushed out, or the spleen may be compressed. At the same time, the tumor continues to grow downward, particularly if it is situated on the lower aspect of the organ, in the same manner as other cysts that are similarly located. A cyst of this character may extend as far as the pelvis or the crest of the ilium, so that the lower border cannot be palpated. Under these circumstances diagnostic errors may occur and the growth be taken for an ovarian cyst, etc.

Echinococcus cysts that are accessible to direct palpation feel hard on account of the tension of their walls, and do not, as a rule, fluctuate. Sometimes a characteristic vibration, the hydatid thrill, may be felt on percussion; the percussion sound over the tumor is dull.

The hydatid thrill was first described by Blatin *; its diagnostic value emphasized by Briancon, Piorry, and von Tarral; and its origin studied experimentally by Davaine and others. Cruveilhier and others attribute it to the collisions between the daughter-cysts, and deduce the presence of secondary cysts from the presence of the thrill. Occasionally, however, the symptom is noticed in sterile cysts, and experiments with rubber sacs showed that daughter-sacs played no rôle whatever. Küster † formulated the theory that the thrill denoted the presence of a second cyst in the vicinity of the first one in those cases where daughter-cysts were absent; this view, however, is also erroneous. In order to elicit the phenomenon, the wall of the cyst must be in a state of tension and the fluid contents of the cyst must be under high pressure. These conditions are fulfilled in such cysts as those of the ovary, the mesentery, etc., in hydronephrosis, in simple ascites, and in cystosarcoma of the liver (Landau), and the thrill has been discovered in all these conditions. Some authors claim to have felt it only exceptionally in cases of echinococcus. Létienne in two cases was enabled to elicit the thrill only after aspirating a small portion of the fluid; in other words, after reducing the pressure a little. It appears, therefore, that too high tension causes rigidity of the membrane and a cessation of the vibrations, so that the phenomenon disappears.

The thrill can be elicited in various ways. Frerichs advises compressing the swelling lightly with the two fingers of the left hand and

---

* Quoted by Davaine, loc. cit.
† Küster, *Deutsche med. Woch.*, 1880, No. 1.

PLATE VI.

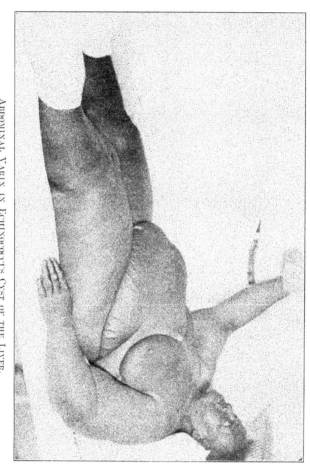

ABDOMINAL VARIX IN ECHINOCOCCUS CYST OF THE LIVER.

tapping quickly with the right; Tarral advises leaving the finger in contact with the pleximeter for some little time after the percussing.

Davaine allows three fingers of the left hand to rest on the cyst and percusses the middle one only; the other fingers feel the tremor. Desprès places one finger on the tumor and taps it quickly, withdrawing the percussing finger as rapidly as possib e.

Piorry has described the sensation as being similar to the feel of a repeater watch that is tapped while held in the hand; he has also compared it to the vibrations felt in gelatin. According to Davaine, a similar sensation is experienced by tapping the seat of a sofa that is upholstered with springs.

Löbel * describes a crackling sound elicited on palpation of a case of a large echinococcus cyst with atrophy of the surrounding tissues; he attributed the sound to peritonitic friction. On autopsy no peritonitic involvement was found, though the peculiar sound could be heard over the cyst even after death.

Cysts arising from the lower surface of the liver extend into the abdominal cavity. The liver protrudes as a hemispheric swelling that may occupy the whole right side of the abdominal cavity or its entire space. As a result, pressure is exerted on neighboring organs, so that constipation and diarrhea, and, in rare cases, even occlusion of the intestine and ileus, are seen (Reichold). If the cyst is connected with the liver by a bridge of connective tissue, the impression may be created that the tumor does not originate in that organ. There is dulness on percussion above, then a loud tympanitic sound, and further down again dulness over the cyst. The pedicle may be so long that the cyst is situated in the pelvis and simulates a tumor of that region. Compression of the common duct, of the vena cava, and of the portal vein may be caused by a cyst situated at the lower surface of the liver.

Following pressure upon the portal vein ascites is sometimes observed, rendering it difficult to outline the tumor. There may also be a tumor of the spleen and a dilatation of the venous collaterals. The vena cava inferior may be compressed to such a degree that its walls are in contact, and the vessel may be completely obliterated. This is followed by serious interference with the circulation in the lower parts of the body, particularly of the legs, with edema, venous dilatation, etc. Icterus is rare, as the common duct is not often completely compressed; albuminuria may be present, but depends almost exclusively on the amount of pressure exerted upon the kidney. Its degree may fluctuate with the position of the patient.

Echinococcus cystic involvement of the upper part of the liver enlarges toward the thorax; it causes the diaphragm to bulge, and may even produce atrophy of the latter muscle. The upper percussion boundary of the liver, therefore, is often curved convexly upward, particularly in the axillary line. This is never seen in pleuritis, and is a feature in the differential diagnosis; in pleural effusion the upper line of dulness descends from behind forward, and is concave upward. If the cyst develops near the spinal column, there will be a similar conformation, and the diagnosis may become very difficult. In general, the cyst causes more protrusion of the ribs and less lengthening of the thorax than pleuritis.

Pressure on the diaphragm causes pain and a dry cough, later dyspnea, particularly after exertion. This is due to a decrease in the size of the thorax, cyanosis, palpitation, etc. If the tumor grows still larger, there will be compression of the right lung, and atelectasis may follow.

* "Bericht des k. k. Rudolfspitales in Wien," 1869.

In such cases the left lung and the heart are also affected; the lung is compressed and the heart pushed to the left into the axillary region; in a case of this kind described by Frerichs, death occurred suddenly from asphyxia.

More frequently even than these purely mechanical injuries to the thoracic organs, caused by the pressure of a gradually enlarging cyst, is an inflammation of the pleura diaphragmatica, which usually results in adhesion between the two layers, and less frequently in exudation. If the cyst perforates the atrophied diaphragm and the adherent lung under these conditions, there will be hemoptysis, percussion dulness, and a reduction in the intensity of the breath-sounds over this area. The upper boundary of the dulness will be convex. The thorax will protrude over the cyst. It rarely happens that trauma, a fall or a blow, will cause the cyst to penetrate the pleural cavity after rupturing the diaphragm, which is already atrophic from pressure. In a case of this character the same symptoms will be observed as in perforation into the lung. As a rule, the sac will rupture and the cystic contents empty into the pleural cavity.

Suppuration of the cyst is seen most frequently in cases in which a communication is established with the biliary passages, so that bile containing bacteria enters the cyst cavity. The tenia is killed by the bile, but the bacteria continue to vegetate, and eventually may produce suppuration and gangrene. The process may in this way lead to the formation of an abscess. In the event of suppuration in some other part of the body, especially if it is located in the portal area, or in general pyemia, or, finally, after puncture of the cyst, suppuration often occurs. The pathologic picture under these circumstances is that of hepatic abscess. There is remittent fever, a chill, disturbance of the general health, localized pain radiating from the affected portion of the liver toward the shoulder. Although in ordinary echinococcus cyst peritoneal inflammation is not frequent, in case of suppuration perihepatitis is often seen. The pus may perforate into neighboring organs as in other forms of abscess, and may in this way lead to very dangerous lesions. Suppuration of an echinococcus cyst, as a rule, leads sooner or later to death, and usually with the symptom-complex of a general pyemia.

Rupture of echinococcus cysts and the **evacuation of their contents** into other organs of the body are very important events from a symptomatologic point of view.

If rupture occurs within the liver substance into the bile-passages, the parasite is, as already stated, usually killed by the action of the bile, and suppuration of the cystic contents takes place. Often the cyst is simply evacuated and undergoes contraction. If the biliary passage is small, the fluid will be poured from the cyst into the intestine *via* the bile-duct, and the daughter-cysts will remain behind because they cannot pass through the narrow channel. Sometimes these continue to vegetate; as a rule, however, they also disappear. If communication is established with a large passage, such as the main branch of the hepatic or the cystic duct, or with one of these canals themselves, the hydatids may pass into the intestine without causing any symptoms, and the cyst will collapse. Occasionally these structures, which are shriveled up and appear like raisins, can be found in the stools, together with shreds of membrane. Charcellay reports certain tubular, pseudomembranous casts of bile-channels in the stools. The hydatids may also lodge in the bile-passages, or may become impacted in the narrow opening of the common duct into the duodenum, and, like gall-stones, cause icterus from stasis, acholic stools, and catarrhal and purulent cholangitis. Attacks of colic may be produced; if repeated series of daughter-cysts attempt to pass, there may be repeated attacks of colic (Westerdyk).* In this way the picture of cholelithiasis may be simulated. Sometimes rupture takes place into the gall-bladder, and the latter is filled with fluid from the echinococcus cyst. This is then passed by the natural route, or an abnormal passageway is created into the duodenum. [A case was recently observed at autopsy at the Pennsylvania Hospital in which the entire left lobe of the liver had been replaced by an enormous echinococcus cyst, full of semi-purulent fluid containing hundreds of secondary cysts. The gall-bladder was intact, and was also full of tiny cysts full of scolices and hooklets. The cystic duct contained a few, and the common duct many intact cysts. The symptoms had been those of hepatic abscess, and at no time was there any evidence of stoppage of the bile-ducts. Death occurred from pyemia.—ED.]

Frequently a bile-passage will rupture, and yet the cystic contents be poured out by some other way, *i. e.*, into the intestine, the peritoneal cavity, the lungs, etc. In cases of this kind the bile-tinged color of the fluid, particularly of the hydatids, will indicate such an occurrence. Or the bile may be evacuated in its totality through this abnormal channel, and be expectorated, or passed in the stools, or it may be poured into the pleural or the peritoneal cavity.

Particularly those cysts that are situated on the under surface of the liver perforate into the stomach and the intestine, and in the same manner as abscesses of the liver that are similarly situated. As a rule, adhesions form first.

If perforation occurs into the stomach, an abundant quantity of a watery fluid containing hydatids is vomited; a part or all of the fluid may enter the intestine and be passed in the stools. Sometimes the perforation is preceded by pain in the stomach region as a result of peritonitis. If the opening is large, the symptoms are very acute; if it is small, the contents of the cyst may be evacuated so slowly as to cause only very slight symptoms.

If perforation occurs into the intestine, the accident is usually preceded, as above, by signs of circumscribed peritonitis; then the tumor suddenly collapses, there is a watery stool, occasionally mixed with blood, and numerous hydatids are passed. If the opening is large, serious symptoms appear, because the contents of the intestine enter the cystic cavity and cause gangrenous inflammation. If the opening is small, this does not occur so easily. The perforation is closed and some adhesions between the liver and the intestine may persist. Later peristalsis may cause a separation of these adhesions, so that a cavity remains in the liver, and contain fecal matter. This cavity is in no way connected with the intestine (F. Krause); we have, however, a fecal abscess with all its dreaded consequences.

Perforation into the peritoneal cavity occurs quite frequently. As echinococcus cysts do not show as great a tendency to the formation of adhesions as abscesses, just so the contents of the cyst are frequently poured into the free abdominal cavity. This is particularly liable to happen after trauma, contusions, a fall, etc. Following the evacuation

* Westerdyk, *Berlin. klin. Woch.*, 1877, No. 43.

of the fluid, shock becomes apparent and may lead to the death of the patient (Achard).* There will be seen a rapid pulse, costal breathing, violent abdominal pain, and the patient will be anxious and complain of a feeling as though something had given way in the belly. He feels that he is sick unto death, he may faint and lie perfectly still; his face is drawn and pale. Many recover; urticaria may then appear from the absorption of the toxins of the fluid, and nothing may remain but a freely movable fluid in the abdomen. The peritoneum seems to learn to tolerate this fluid, and it can either be removed by aspiration or may be spontaneously absorbed; it may perhaps even perforate into the urinary passages and be evacuated in this way. In rare cases daughter-cysts have been known to develop in the abdominal cavity (Volkmann, Krause). If the cystic contents are mingled with bile, the bacteria contained in the latter may cause peritonitis; this must be treated by operative measures, and may occasionally be relieved in this way. If purulent cysts burst into the peritoneal cavity, death results from suppurative peritonitis.

If the cyst bursts into some preformed peritoneal pocket, the prognosis is more favorable, as these cases are more accessible for operative interference. The fluid in these cases is not so freely movable, and will be discovered localized in a small painful area of the abdomen. The general symptoms are less pronounced, and there is less interference with the action of the heart. The peritoneal fluid can be evacuated through the skin or into the intestine without causing any very severe disturbances.

Perforation of echinococcus cyst of the liver into the urinary passages is rare. If it occurs, it usually leads, because of occlusion of the urethra with retention of urine, to renal colic and hydronephrosis. Numerous daughter-cysts colored by bile are passed in the urine and reveal their origin from the liver. If a rupture into the bile-passages occurs at the same time, bile may enter the urinary passages from the fistula.

If the echinococcus penetrates the thorax from the upper surface of the liver, the diaphragm may be torn, as previously mentioned, so that the cyst enters the pleural cavity, ruptures, and evacuates its contents. Perforation into the thoracic cavity may occur in still another manner; the echinococcus fluid may be poured into a cavity formed of peritoneal adhesions, and a subphrenic accumulation of fluid be formed, which, secondarily, perforates the diaphragm. The presence of fluid in the pleural cavity causes the ordinary symptoms of serous pleurisy and hydrothorax; namely, an increase of the diameter of the thorax on one side, obliteration of the intercostal spaces, retraction on respiration, dulness on percussion, reduction of the breathing-sounds and of the fremitus. The lung is compressed upward and backward against the spinal column, unless it is anchored anteriorly by adhesions. Bronchial breathing is heard over the lung; the heart is dislocated toward the left. On aspiration a fluid is obtained that may perhaps contain some albumin, or none at all. Scolices and shreds of membrane are usually found. If the exudate is pleuritic, the fluid will contain albumin.

Rupture of the cyst is accompanied by the feeling of a sudden tear in the chest; there is oppression, dyspnea, and a feeling of anxiety. The pulse is rapid and weak, and death may occur rapidly with all the symptoms of collapse and asphyxia. In other cases suppuration occurs, and

* Achard, *Archiv gen. de méd.*, 1888, p. 410.

empyema is formed, which may either perforate the skin or the lung, unless opened early by thoracentesis. Sometimes circumscribed pneumonia develops, with fever, sudden cough, and the expectoration of large quantities of purulent fluid containing hydatids. Complete evacuation of the fluid and a cure of the disease may be brought about in this manner; or, on the other hand, the lung tissue may undergo purulent degeneration and form an abscess. The latter usually causes death. Perforation of the lungs allows the entrance of air into the pleural cavity, and may cause pyopneumothorax. In some cases a pleuritic exudate may be present before the cyst ruptures the diaphragm, so that when the rupture occurs both fluids may be mixed. In other cases adhesions exist between the lung and the diaphragm, and the contents of the cyst may penetrate the lung without coming in contact with the pleural exudate (Trousseau).

If the cyst as a whole enters the lung without bursting, pneumonic symptoms appear; later, weakness of the breath-sounds and dulness. Finally, the sac ruptures and its contents are poured into the lungs and bronchi; this causes a sudden flooding of these parts. It may be impossible for the patient to get rid of the fluid and the hydatids quick enough; consequently he becomes asphyxiated, and drowns (as it were) in the cystic fluid. If the evacuation occurs slowly and in small quantities, a cure of the disease may be brought about. If a cystic cavity is present in the lung, a large space will remain with bronchial breathing, resonant and metallic sounds, etc. Cavities of this kind, or the remnants of abscess-cavities, gradually contract and heal. Sometimes it is necessary to open them from without, to drain them, and in this manner to produce cicatrization.

The sputum may remain purulent for a long time, or may contain bile if bile-passages have ruptured at the same time.

Perforation from the left lobe into the pericardium is rare; a few cases are on record (Wunderlich). The pericardial sac becomes rapidly distended with fluid, and the patient dies in a very short time from heart-failure.

If a communication is established between the portal vein and the echinococcus cyst, the branches of the portal vein become obstructed, and multiple abscesses are formed. Occasionally a branch of the portal vein will be punctured during exploratory aspiration. Toxic material may enter the blood in this manner and produce symptoms of poisoning, —namely, urticaria (Bouchard),—or such severe symptoms of intoxication that death may occur (Bryant).

If the lower vena cava is perforated, fluid and hydatids reach the right heart, and are forced into the pulmonary artery and occlude it. The patients die rapidly with symptoms of dyspnea and pulmonary edema, similar to those seen in embolism of the pulmonary artery following the lodgment of marantic thrombi. If perforation occurs into the hepatic vein, embolism of branches of the pulmonary artery, hemorrhagic infarcts, suppuration in the lungs, and general empyema result. Entrance of the cystic fluid into the veins is usually manifested by toxic symptoms, as, for instance, reddening of the face, pain, loss of consciousness, vomiting, spasms, or sudden stoppage of the heart.

Erosion of a branch of the hepatic artery—for instance, by trauma—may cause a large quantity of blood to enter the echinococcus cyst, and in this manner the parasites are killed.

Perforation of the echinococcus through the abdominal wall probably

51

only occurs in cases of suppuration, and the same symptoms are produced as in perforating abscess of the liver; namely, circumscribed peritonitis, inflammatory swelling of the abdominal wall, later fluctuation, thinning of the skin, bursting of the integument, and evacuation of the contents of the cyst through the fistula. [Posselt * has published a detailed discussion of echinococcus of the liver, chiefly in relation to the symptoms and diagnosis. He considers the most important sign to be the enlargement and alteration in the form of the liver. Enlargement is usually confined to the right lobe. The liver is hard, and pain and tenderness are elicited if the cyst is near the surface. Pain is, however, not a constant feature. There is usually marked jaundice, and frequently ascites. Often there is free sweating. The patient is usually constipated, and occasionally may show blood in the stools. It is noteworthy that the bodily weight seldom decreases to any marked extent, an important point in the diagnosis of this condition from carcinoma and hypertrophic cirrhosis, in both of which cachexia and loss of weight are extreme. Cachexia in echinococcus disease is a late phenomenon. There is usually no fever, and no enlargement of the spleen. Polyuria is frequently seen, due (according to Posselt)to functional hypertrophy of the kidneys. He has found the disease to be common in Bavaria, Austria, Switzerland, and Würtemburg, and rare elsewhere over the globe. Renon † describes a case of multilocular echinococcus of the pleura and right lung in a man of thirty-six. He considers this the first case of the disease in man to occur in France.—ED.]

Prognosis.—Echinococcus cyst of the liver may persist for a long time without causing any symptoms or disturbances, and even large cysts may fail to affect the general health of the patient. Their presence may be manifested by slight symptoms of dislocation of other organs. At the same time, the presence of the parasite is always dangerous, and such accidents as rupture into neighboring organs, inflammatory processes, suppuration, gangrene, etc., must always be feared. An echinococcus cyst may exist in an active condition for twenty years and more. A fall, a contusion, or a concussion is dangerous, and may lead to the rupture of the cyst. Spontaneous cures are rare; they may be brought about by the death of the parasite, or by cheesy degeneration or calcification of the cyst tissues. A natural cure by evacuation of the contents into the intestine and bronchi, etc., is quite frequently seen. In the majority of cases, however, the skill of the surgeon must be employed to remove the disease.

Suppuration and gangrenous degeneration of the echinococcus, as well as rupture into the blood-vessels (the vena cava, etc.), the peritoneum, etc., are dangerous.

Cyr has formulated the following statistics: Death occurred in 90 % of cases from rupture into the peritoneum, in 80 % into the pleura, in 70 % into the bile-passages, in 57 % into the bronchi, in 40 % into the stomach, in 15 % into the intestine, and in 3 % through the abdominal wall.

If suppuration occurs, the prognosis is probably the same as in a virulent abscess.

The prognosis, therefore, of echinococcus of the liver will only be favorable in the absence of fever and suppuration or of all symptoms

* *Deutsch. Arch. f. klin. Med.,* Aug. 18, 1899.
† *Compt. rend. de la Soc. de Biol.,* Feb. 17, 1900.

that point to a threatening perforation; or if the cyst is favorably situated for operation, as, for instance, on the anterior surface of the liver. Thanks to the perfected technique and the methods of aseptic surgery, sub-phrenic echinococcus is now accessible for operation. As long as the cyst is intact, the prognosis is favorable.

Diagnosis.—A small cyst can be recognized only if it is situated on the anterior surface of the liver immediately underneath the abdominal wall, and only if it is prominent. A cyst may be very large and still evade detection if it develops in the anterior of the liver, and only causes a general enlargement of the organ. Subjective symptoms may be completely absent or misleading. It has happened that tumors as large as a child's head have been present, but have passed unnoticed by the patient.

The anamnesis is important, and it is well to determine whether the patient comes from a region that is noted for echinococcus disease, also whether the patient has associated much with dogs, etc. It is well also to examine for tenia the stools of the animals that the patient has been in contact with; if necessary, after the administration of a vermifuge.

The following points will speak in favor of echinococcus as against other tumors of the liver, abscesses, etc.: Absence of pain or the presence of very slight pain, a tense elastic tumor (hydatid thrill) with a round, smooth surface, the absence of fever and of inflammatory symptoms in the neighborhood of the tumor (peritoneum), only slight disturbances of the general health, and a slow growth of the swelling.

If the echinococcus develops on the anterior surface of the liver, the diagnosis can frequently be made from the above symptoms. Very frequently, however, the condition is confounded with other cysts of the liver or with a chronic abscess that is unattended by inflammatory symptoms; in such cases the diagnosis is not made until an operation is performed. Other forms of cysts resemble the echinococcus cyst in shape only rarely, and if they are present, the two conditions cannot be distinguished.

Chronic abscess of the liver is usually found in subjects who have lived in the tropics; it does not present so tense a resistance to the hand in the afebrile stage as do echinococcus cysts. Other abscesses are char-acterized by fever and severe disturbances of the general health; they can only be confounded with an echinococcus cyst that has undergone purulent degeneration. Malignant tumors are frequently tense and elastic, but are generally nodular and painful; they cause greater cachexia, and develop more rapidly. In addition, primary tumors can frequently be found in other regions of the body.

The Röntgen rays frequently aid in determining the gradual enlarge-ment of the liver by echinococcus, and the procedure promises to be of value in the diagnosis, particularly in distinguishing subphrenic cysts.

Exploratory puncture is of great diagnostic value. Récamier was the first to execute this procedure in echinococcus disease, and Cru-veilhier recommended it after him. The operation is performed in the same manner as in abscess of the liver. It is well, however, to select a thin cannula in order to make the hole in the cyst-wall as small as possible; this is necessary on account of the tension of the cyst-wall, that may readily cause a rupture and an evacuation of the cystic con-tents into the peritoneal cavity. The puncture should be made diagonally through the cyst-wall, preferably with the apparatus of Dieulafoy or

Potain, rather than with a Pravaz needle. The cannula can be closed with wax or with a cock, and left in place for a little while; an inflammatory exudate is formed around the puncture, closing it still more effectually and preventing the entrance of cystic fluid into the abdomen. If the echinococcus cyst is healthy, a clear fluid is obtained in which no albumin will be found; there will be a few shreds of membrane, scolices, and hooklets. Cysts of a different character are usually filled with a fluid containing albumin, mucus, bile, etc. In abscesses, pus is found, and if the abscess is in reality an echinococcus cyst that has undergone suppuration, shreds of membrane, scolices, hooks, etc., will also be found.

The puncture may be followed by disagreeable or even dangerous results, because the wound may gape, if the walls of the cyst are fragile or rupture (Segond), and allow the escape of cystic fluid. This is particularly dangerous in purulent or gangrenous echinococcus cysts; such an accident is frequently followed by peritonitis, just as in abscess of the liver. If the cystic contents are not degenerated, intoxication of the whole organ may occur from the toxic products of the parasite.

The most frequent symptom of this intoxication is urticaria (Monneret, Rendu, Ladureau, Harley, Murchison, Dieulafoy, Finsen, v. Volkmann). In subsequent punctures this symptom does not seem to appear, possibly because the first one confers immunity. Severe poisoning has also been observed, attacks of fainting, dyspnea, nausea, vomiting, hiccup, rapidity and weakness of the pulse, signs of collapse, in some cases even death. Jenkins, Martineau, and Bryant observed death in such cases. Achard reports 8 cases of death. Fever, arthritic pains (suppuration of joints, Verneuil), diarrhea, and insomnia have all been seen.

The danger of localization and the multiple development of daughter-cysts in the abdominal cavity need not be feared, although Langenbuch, basing his statement on the experiments of Volkmann and others, calls attention to this complication. As a rule, these cases are due to the rupture of large cysts.

Sometimes puncture is performed in vain, as when the cannula becomes occluded by hydatids or by calcareous material from the wall of the cyst.

Puncture is hardly ever dangerous, though everything should be in readiness to perform a laparotomy and to remove the cyst by surgical procedures.

Sometimes the gall-bladder may be distended by stasis of bile or by hydrops, and lead to confusion. Here the position and outline of the tumor, a history of cholelithiasis, or symptoms of this condition, and the character of the aspirated fluid will decide. The contents of such a swelling are bile-tinged, or, if not, at least mucoid and albuminous. In very rare cases, it is true, a large quantity of a watery, clear, colorless fluid has been aspirated from a hydropic gall-bladder (one liter, Tuffier).

If the cyst is present on the lower surface of the liver, and the portal vein is compressed so as to cause ascites, the position of the liver may be altered by the transudate; it may become retroverted and lead to confusion with cirrhosis. Other general enlargements of the liver, as fatty liver, amyloid degeneration, etc., are simulated by echinococcus only in those cases where the parasite develops in the interior of the organ.

Cysts of the pancreas resemble those of the liver, and, owing to the close proximity of the two organs, must sometimes be differentiated. If the stomach is distended with air, the pancreatic cyst will be found behind this organ and will be clearly distinguished from the margin of the liver, which moves up and down over the cyst on inspiration. Cysts of the mesentery and of the ovary are more readily distinguished. If the former are very large, so that the liver is pushed up into the thorax, the diagnosis may be rendered difficult. Even simple meteorism has been taken for echinococcus cyst (Simpson), also cold abscesses of the abdominal wall on the right side (Trélat, Langenbuch).

If hydronephrosis of the right kidney exists, a round, tense, elastic tumor is present, which pushes the liver forward. The protrusion of the lumbar region, even in the knee-chest position, the motility of the tumor, the fact that it is situated behind the colon, will decide in favor of hydronephrosis. Exploratory puncture or catheterization of the ureter may give important information.

If echinococcus cysts are situated immediately in front of the abdominal aorta, the growth may pulsate, but in this case the pulsations are not expansile, but antero-posterior. Occasionally a cyst has been mistaken for an **aneurysm** (Neisser, Hayden).

Cysts of the spleen may be mistaken for echinococcus of the left lobe of the liver. A cyst situated in the left lobe may force its way into the spleen, or, on the other hand, a cyst of the spleen may be so close to the left lobe of the liver that it is impossible to distinguish the two organs. The diagnosis will in such cases have to be reserved for exploratory laparotomy.

The diagnosis of a subphrenic echinococcus cyst is particularly difficult. There will be dulness in the lower half of the right side of the thorax; this portion of the chest is expanded, breath-sounds are weak or absent, and there is pectoral fremitus, so that the diagnosis of a pleural exudate or of a subphrenic abscess may seem warranted. The general outline of the percussion dulness, the more circumscribed protrusion of the lower ribs, the absence of fever and of a history of inflammatory symptoms in the lungs or the pleura, above all, the results of exploratory puncture, must decide against a serous exudate in the thoracic cavity, and the entire absence of inflammatory symptoms in the abdomen will decide against subphrenic abscess. If the echinococcus cyst is situated beneath the diaphragm and is gangrenous, it cannot be distinguished from pyopneumothorax subphrenicus. The treatment of both conditions is the same, so that it is not essential to make a clear differential diagnosis.

If an echinococcus perforates into the pleural cavity, the symptoms will be so violent and so sudden (there will be collapse and a general intoxication) that even without examination of the fluid a pleurisy with exudation can be excluded.

It is said that echinococcus involvement of the pleura can be differentiated from a subphrenic echinococcus cyst by the fact that the former forces the diaphragm and the liver downward, and on inspiration the liver moves downward. In echinococcus of the liver, on the other hand, the diaphragm is forced upward, becomes paralyzed and atrophic, and for all these reasons the lower margin of the liver is not found so low as in echinococcus of the pleura; finally, on inspiration the liver moves upward.

It is sometimes difficult to decide whether the echinococcus cyst has developed primarily in the lower lobe of the right lung, or whether it was primary in the liver, later penetrating the lung.

The diagnosis of the rupture of an echinococcus into the different organs can be made from the symptomatology outlined above.

Prophylaxis.—In order to prevent echinococcus disease, all measures should be employed that will prevent infection of human beings by the eggs of the tenia. The following rules should be observed in regions where the parasite is common:

I. The number of dogs should be decreased as far as possible (by means of a dog tax), and those that have no masters should be caught and confiscated.

II. There should be a careful meat inspection for echinococcus, and all infected meat should be rendered harmless. Above all, it is important that no such meat should be fed raw to dogs.

III. People should be warned against very intimate contact with dogs, against petting and fondling them. This is particularly necessary in the case of children. After handling a dog the hands should be washed as soon as possible.

IV. In order to remove tenia the dogs should undergo a tapeworm cure about once a year, and the following prescription is useful: Flores kooso, 2.0 to 15.0 gm.; extr. filic. mar., 1.0 to 4.0 gm.; areca nut, 0.5 to 2.0 gm. of the scraped or pulverized nut on an empty stomach, followed, possibly, by 10 to 30 gm. of castor oil in two or three hours, etc.

V. All vegetables should be thoroughly cleaned, particularly if they are eaten raw, as is salad, for instance.

Treatment.—The attempt has frequently been made to treat echinococcus with drugs. Formerly emetics were given with the purpose of causing a rupture of the sac and the evacuation of the cyst into the intestine, the peritoneum, etc. This procedure, of course, is so dangerous and so uncertain that it is altogether to be condemned.

For a time ordinary salt, sometimes in combination with other salts, was recommended both for internal and external use, in the shape of compresses and baths. This treatment was based on an observation by Laennec, who saw that animals suffering from this disease were cured if they were put to pasture on a salty soil, and a few cases have been described (Laennec, Oppolzer, Bamberger) in which a decrease of the cyst was brought about by this treatment. As a rule, however, the method is fruitless.

Anthelmintics, as turpentine, Dippel's oil, and kamala, have been administered internally. Hjaltelin recommended tincture of kamala, 30 to 40 drops, three times a day; and Bird claims to have seen a quicker cure of the echinococcus after puncture and evacuation of the cyst when kamala was used in combination with bromid of potash. These remedies are probably useless, and the same can be said of inunctions of mercury ointment, or the internal administration of calomel.

Iodid of potash was popular for a long time, and has been given in these cases in considerable doses (Havkis, Wilkes, and others). Budd advises the administration of iodid of potash, together with inunctions with an iodin salve. Frerichs examined the cystic contents for iodin after this treatment, but failed to find it. Other investigators, as Mosler and Peiper, succeeded in demonstrating its presence.

In any event the results of internal medication are very uncertain, and the condition of the patient frequently calls for a prompt removal of the parasite. In the days before antisepsis the fear of operation was justified in echinococcus disease, because even a simple puncture sometimes led to suppuration. At the present time, however, it is possible to terminate the disease rapidly and safely by surgical inter-ference.

This is not the place to discuss the different methods that have been recommended. A detailed description will be found in the work of Langenbuch. The following brief description is largely based on this work.

For the general practitioner **puncture** is the most important pro-cedure.

Electro-puncture is no longer employed, although the method was used with some success in Iceland, particularly by Durham and Fagge. Two steel needles are inserted into the cyst and connected with the nega-tive pole of a battery, the other electrode terminating in a moist sponge applied to the skin. Hydrogen develops in the cyst and forces the fluid through the puncture into the abdomen. Even repeated sittings may not succeed in destroying the parasite, and unless asepsis is rigorously carried out suppuration may occur.

The **dangers of puncture** have already been discussed in our section upon exploratory puncture. If, later on, symptoms appear that can be referred to the peritoneum or to other organs, the cyst should be thoroughly removed by laparotomy.

Evacuation of the cystic contents by puncture is an old procedure. Hippoc-rates and his pupils have described the difficulties incident to this operation owing to occlusion of the cannula by hydatids.

As the cyst usually collapses after the evacuation of the fluid, and the disease is thereby cured (Hulke, Borgherini, Mosler, and Peiper), the idea suggested itself to remove only a small quantity of fluid with a fine cannula (Hulke, Savory). This, however, is rarely successful. Sibson attaches a tube to the cannula and allows it to remain in place so as to remove as much as possible of the contents.

In general, trocars of medium caliber should be employed and as much of the contents evacuated at one time as possible. In this way echinococcus disease has frequently been cured, sometimes after one puncture, in other cases after repeated attempts. During this manipula-tion, particularly if it is not carried out with aseptic precautions, purulent infection may occur; and it is indeed possible that in such instances the death of the parasite has been brought about by the entrance of bacteria (Kussmaul, Wright, Brodbury, Fuller, and others). Another danger is rupture of the bile-passages and blood-vessels in the walls of the cyst. This may cause the entrance of bile and blood into the cavity, and the death of the scolices; or, again, the membrane may become separated from the connective-tissue capsule, and in this way the death of the para-site be brought about by interference with its nutrition.

Harley reports 34 cases of cure out of 77 cases in which puncture was per-formed; Murchison, 80 cures in 103 cases. The latter advised allowing the fluid to flow into the abdominal cavity, and claims that it is absorbed there. Such a procedure, of course, is fraught with danger, owing to the possibility of intoxi-cation and infection.

Puncture and aspiration: As the entrance of air into the cyst is to be dreaded, and as, formerly, suppurative processes were attributed to the presence of air, the older operators began to devise methods of remov-ing the cystic contents, and at the same time of aspirating the air. Budd was the first to advise the employment of a suction apparatus. Dieulafoy and Potain both invented apparatus of this kind and recommended this method of treating echinococcus cysts. A great many cases have been treated in this manner. The walls of the cysts, it is true, are frequently hard and inelastic, and under these circumstances it is impossible to remove all the fluid and to cause the collapse of the cyst. In case the cyst is sterile a cure may be obtained; but if it is not sterile, or if the parasite has not been killed by suppuration or by the entrance of bile, the fluid will collect again, and it may be necessary to repeat aspiration many times. There are cases on record in which this operation was performed as often as 300 times. After aspiration a tympanitic sound will often be heard over the cyst as a result of the dilution of the gases contained in the cavity. Pain, nausea, vomiting, and urticaria have all been observed after evacuation. Sudden death is reported in a few cases (Guyot, Martineau, Moissenet). According to Braine, the mortality from the operation is as high as 15 %.

As simple aspiration has not led to the desired goal in cases in which the cyst has not been sterile, the attempt has been made to destroy the parasite by the injection of certain substances into the cyst.

As early as 1851 Boinet injected tincture of iodin, and his example was followed by Velpeau, Richard, Weber, Aran, Demarquay, and Chassaignac, Schroetter, and others. A few successes are on record, but the operation was again uncertain, was very painful, and in one or two cases was followed by the death of the patient, so that it was soon abandoned.

Filix mas (Pavy), ox-gall (Dolbeau and Voisin, Landouzy, and others), and alcohol (Richet) have all been employed for the same purpose, and have all been abandoned.

Injections of solutions of corrosive sublimate and thorough irrigation of the cyst have been more successful, and promise good results as soon as the technique is further perfected.

Mesnard probably was the first to inject a solution of this substance into a cyst; this was followed by an increase of the suppuration; he injected more sublimate and thoroughly flushed the cavity with the drug; this, finally, led to a cure of the case. The strength of the sublimate solution was one pro mille, and injection was followed by irrigation with alcohol.

Sennet and Baccelli removed a small quantity of the cystic fluid (2.5 to 30 (?) gm.) and injected the same quantity or a slightly smaller quantity of sublimate solution (1 to 2 pro mille) and obtained good results. Dujardin-Beaumetz and Blumer proceeded in the same way, and report the contraction of an echinococcus cyst after one injection, and the cure after two injections of 20 to 30 gm. of a one pro mille sublimate solution. Cimbali saw death occur after this operation; the case, however, was hardly a suitable one. Kétly saw fever following the injection that persisted for 20 days; at the end of this time, however, the cyst had disappeared. After another period the fluid again accumulated. Sublimate was again injected and the cyst disappeared again; he does not state whether the disease was finally cured. Chauffard and Widal state that 36 c.c. of a one pro mille solution of sublimate are sufficient to sterilize an echinococcus cavity of 2 liters; according to other statements, the cyst should contain as much as 1 or 2 cgm. of sublimate.

Debove advises as complete an evacuation of the contents as possible, and the injection of 100 c.c. of a one pro mille solution of sublimate; this is to be removed by aspiration after ten minutes. Terillon removed 450 c.c. of fluid, injected 100 c.c. of sublimate of the above strength, and left it in the cavity; the case was cured.

Langenbuch states that among 16 cases that were treated with injections of sublimate 14 recovered, 1 died, and 1 showed no improvement.

A 5 % solution of copper sulphate has also been employed for this purpose (Debove). Chauffard succeeded in causing the disappearance of a cyst by the injection of 150 c.c. of a 0.5 % solution of β-naphthol.

In many cases puncture and drainage have been employed, as in abscess of the liver.

Owen Rees, and later Boinet and Verneuil, operated as follows: A thick trocar was inserted and allowed to remain in place for several days, until it became loose; a little fluid then oozed out. The walls of the parietal peritoneum were adherent by this time. A drainage-tube or a double catheter can be inserted, or the opening can be dilated with laminaria, sponge tents, etc.; and in this manner the evacuation of shreds of membrane and of hydatids is made possible. As suppuration and gangrene may readily occur during this operation, abundant drainage should be provided and care should be taken that the cavity is frequently irrigated with antiseptic solutions. Jónassen, Harley, and others have treated many cases by this method. If the skin is thoroughly disinfected and the trocar is sterile, the operation promises good results. While the cannula is in place, opium should be administered. The sac should be frequently flushed and thorough drainage secured, so that the danger of suppuration and of gangrene is minimized. Gradual and complete collapse of the cavity will occur; a biliary fistula may persist for a long time afterward in case some of the bile-passages rupture into the cyst-cavity.

This method is particularly adapted for the general practitioner. Reclus states that the mortality is 28 %, but this is due to the fact that in many cases rigid antisepsis has not been observed.

In order to obliterate the cyst and to prevent oozing of its contents into the peritoneal cavity, several methods have been employed; among these were the insertion of a small cannula and allowing it to remain in place until adhesions had formed, application of cauterizing pastes, etc. At the present time the leaves of the parietal peritoneum are sutured together prior to making the large opening that is considered necessary and expedient.

Simon inserted two thin trocars two to three centimeters apart and allowed them to remain in place for two weeks. As soon as it could be assumed that adhesions had formed with the peritoneum (reduced mobility of the needles on respiration, oozing of pus or fluid, etc.) an incision was made between the two needles. Boinet inserted a curved trocar and pushed it through the cyst in such a manner that it protruded again; this he left in place for some time, and then made his incision. Bégin and Trousseau inserted several needles, Hirschberg as many as five, in order to cause the formation of adhesions. As this method can produce suppuration if it is not carried out with all aseptic precautions, and as, on the other hand, it fails to cause the formation of adhesions if it is carried out altogether aseptically, it is not a useful procedure and has been discarded.

In the seventeenth century Mayley and Dodard attempted to bring about adhesions between the surfaces of the peritoneum by the application of certain pastes that were at first applied to the skin and later to the deeper tissues.

Recamier in particular was responsible for this method. He used caustic potash; Demarquay employed "Vienna paste," or chlorid of zinc. Finsen has cured many cases in Iceland by applying caustics to the incision through the skin every three days; in this manner he has worked his way down to the cyst. The latter finally ruptures and is evacuated spontaneously; sometimes the cyst-wall is incised. Many modifications of this method have been reported. Sometimes an incision has been made down to the peritoneum and caustic paste applied to the latter. In this way it has been found possible to open the cyst within a few days. Graves simply packed the wound, thus bringing about adhesions between the folds of the peritoneum.

If this operation is well performed it is free from danger, and a wide gaping wound is produced through which the cystic contents can be thoroughly evacuated. The method is, however, painful and tedious (two weeks to six months).

In place of the foregoing appeared the method originally recommended by Recamier and Bégin, consisting in a broad incision through the abdominal walls and the peritoneum (about 10 cm.) and the use of tampons, which are left in the wound for a week or so. The incision is then completed. Without rigid asepsis this method meets with poor success, but with aseptic precautions Volkmann found it very valuable. According to the statistics of Langenbuch, some 48 cases have been cured by this method of double incision.

Of late years the single incision has been more universally employed; by this operation the echinococcus sac can be opened, the cavity emptied, and the parasite permanently removed at one stroke.

Lindemann reports several successful operations of this kind; before him Schmidt chronicled several failures. The former operator opens the peritoneum, incises the cyst, and attaches the margins of the incision to the abdominal walls. Sanger sutured the cyst before incising. Landau and others first evacuated the cyst by puncture and aspiration, or through a thick trocar. Other modifications have been described, but need not be discussed here.

The method of operating by one incision has given good results and has been responsible for the death of the patient in rare cases only. It is performed as follows:

A large incision is carried through to the peritoneum; if the wound does not gape sufficiently, a portion of the abdominal wall is resected. The peritoneum is then incised and the wall of the cyst sutured to the abdominal wall. The fluid is now aspirated, the sac opened, the margins of the wound inverted, and sutured to the abdominal wall, and the cavity flushed with water sterilized by boiling. If the walls of the cyst are soft and fragile, if the cyst contains pus, or if the patient is very restless, it is probably better to perform the operations by two incisions. The cyst-wall is in this event attached to the abdominal wall by stitches, the wound is tamponed for several days, and a second incision into the cyst, followed by evacuation of its contents, is performed at the expiration of this time.

If the cyst is already adherent to the abdominal wall, it is sometimes possible to operate by a single incision, to evacuate the fluid, and to cure the disease. In cases of echinococcus cyst that have not undergone purulent degeneration it is rare, however, for adhesions to form, and dangerous to assume that they are present. It has happened that such an error of diagnosis has been made and the peritoneal cavity inadvertently opened. Rare cases are also reported in which the cysts contained pus, which burrowed through to the lumbar region. The cyst was opened here by a single incision, the pus evacuated, and the case cured.

After opening the cyst an attempt should be made to remove the membrane as completely as possible. Sometimes the cysts are found to be pedunculated, and in such cases it is an easy matter to ablate the whole growth. In other cases the cyst has been enucleated with its capsule (Pozzi, Beckhaus). In the case of some of the larger cysts it has been found necessary to resect a part of the cyst-wall in order to bring about a cure. [Deve * states as the result of his experience: (1) that hydatid cysts can develop from daughter-cysts and scolices; (2) that cysts of the subperitoneal cellular tissue may give rise to various echinococcus growths (cysts, daughter-cysts, proligerous cysts, and scolices), which may in this way enter the peritoneal space. He suggests, therefore,

* *Gaz. hebdom. de Méd. et de Chir.*, Feb. 7, 1901.

that there is a necessity of protecting the tissues from the vesicles and from the invisible scolices, by injecting some teniacide before opening the mother-cyst, and thus destroying the sources of new infection.—ED.]

If the contents of the cyst are purulent, the same rules apply as in abscess. The operation is usually more difficult than in abscess because adhesions are not always formed, and because it is necessary to remove daughter-cysts, shreds of membrane, etc. Moreover, the walls of the cysts are usually rigid, so that the cavity does not collapse so readily. On the other hand, the prognosis is more favorable because the cavity is walled in by a dense membrane that is usually in an accessible location; pyemia does not result as often as after abscess.

The treatment of cysts that are situated in the upper portion of the liver underneath the diaphragm is more difficult. Occasionally they become accessible from the abdominal cavity after forcing the liver downward (Landau), or after resection of the anterior portions of the eighth to the eleventh costal cartilages (Lannelongue). If this can be done, a single incision will cure the disease; in other cases it becomes necessary to open the pleural cavity and to reach the cyst by resection of the ribs, and by incision of the diaphragm.

Roser was the first to suggest this method, and Israel and Volkmann carried it out. Sometimes the operation was performed at one time. The leaves of the pleura were sutured together and incised at once; or the pleura was entered (Israel), tampons were put in place for several days, the diaphragm was then incised, and after a few days the cyst was opened. Subphrenic cysts have also been treated by simple puncture and by injections of sublimate without an operation. Cysts that enter the pleural cavity are treated as above, *i. e.*, resection of ribs, suturing the cyst-wall to the pleura, incision of the cyst, and evacuation. If such a cyst ruptures into the pleural cavity, thoracentesis with resection of ribs is all that is needed.

Cysts that penetrate the lungs are best reached *via* the pleura, even if they pour their contents into the bronchi. Again the cyst-wall should be attached to the pleura and the cyst opened and drained. Pus-cavities in the lungs or gangrene must be treated by pneumotomy.

Cysts that rupture into the peritoneum may be treated by simple puncture and evacuation of the fluid; or the latter may even be spontaneously absorbed.

The fluid has also been removed by incision (Roux and others); Langenbuch advises flushing the abdominal cavity with a 0.7 % solution of common salt followed by one liter of sublimate solution of the strength of 1 : 5000 to 1 : 20,000; he then removes all traces of the sublimate by renewed washing with salt solution.

Rushton-Parker saw general peritonitis and the formation of a purulent exudate follow puncture; all this happened within twenty-four hours. He immediately opened the abdominal cavity, drained thoroughly, and the case recovered.

[Von Bokay * has reported an echinococcus cyst of the pleura in a boy five years of age. This case and three others of echinococcus disease of the liver, all in children, were treated by Baccelli's method (aspiration, and injection of bichlorid of mercury). Shrinkage of the cyst soon followed, and none of the cases showed a relapse.—ED.]

Perforation into the stomach and the intestine is only recognized in purulent or gangrenous cysts; the only treatment consists in laparotomy and evacuation of the cystic contents.

* Jacobi, Festschrift; *Phila. Med. Jour.*, May 26, 1900.

LITERATURE.

Achard: "De l'intoxication hydatique," "Archives générales de médecine," 1888, tome CLXII, p. 410.

Baccelli: "Berliner klin. Wochenschr.," 1894, p. 302.

Blümer: "Correspondenzblatt für Schweizer Aerzte," 1894, p. 216.

Bókay: "Der Werth des Bacelli'schen Verfahrens bei Leberechinococcus des Kindes," "Archiv für Kinderheilkunde," 1897, Bd. XXIII, p. 310.

Braune: "Beitrag zur Casuistik über den Echinococcus der Bauchhöhle und ihrer Organe," Dissertation, Marburg, 1897.

Budd: "Krankheiten der Leber," pp. 90 and 425.

Cobbold: "Parasites," p. 112, London, 1879.

Davaine: "Traité des entozoaires," Paris, 1860 and 1877.

Delbet: "Sur un traitement des kystes hydatiques de l'abdomen," "Gazette hebdomad.," 1896, No. 15.

Dürig: "Ueber vicariirende Hypertrophie der Leber bei Leberechinococcus," "Münchener med. Abhandlungen," 1. Reihe, 13. Heft.

Frerichs: "Lehrbuch der Leberkrankheiten," Bd. II, p. 218.

Heller: "Ziemssen's Handbuch der speciellen Pathologie und Therapie," Bd. VIII, 1. Abtheilung, p. 429.

Huber: "Bibliographie der klinischen Helminthologie," Heft 1, "Echinococcus cystic," 1877–1890.

Humphrey: "The Lancet," 1887, vol. I, p. 120.

Index-Catalogue of the Library of the Surgeon-General's Office, vol. VIII, 1887, p. 264 (literature).

Kahn: "La régénér. du foie dans les états pathologiques," Thèse de Paris, 1897.

Kétly: "Berliner klin. Wochenschr.," 1897, p. 1082.

Krause, F.: "Ueber den cystischen Leberechinococcus," "Sammlung klin. Vorträge," 1888, No. 325.

Küchenmeister: "Die in und an dem Körper des lebenden Menschen vorkommenden Parasiten," p. 169, Leipzig, 1855.

Lebedeff and Andrejew: "Transplantation von Echinococcusblasen vom Menschen auf Kaninchen," "Virchow's Archiv," 1889, Bd. CXVIII, p. 522.

Langenbuch: "Chirurgie der Leber," 1. Theil, 1894, p. 36 (literature).

Létienne: in "Manuel de médecine," tome VI, p. 210, Paris, 1895.

Leuckart: "Die menschlichen Parasiten," 1. Auflage, 1863, Bd. I, p. 328, 2. Auflage, 1879, bis 1886, Bd. I, Abtheilung 1.

Madelung: "Chirurgische Behandlung der Leberkrankheiten," "Penzoldt und Stintzing's specielle Therapie," Abtheilung VI b, p. 178.

Mosler and Peiper: "Thierische Parasiten." This work, vol. VI, including the latest bibliography.

Mourson and Schlagdenhauffen: "Comptes-rendus de l'académie des sciences," 1882, tome XCV, p. 791.

Murchison: "Diseases of the Liver."

Neisser: "Die Echinococcenkrankheit," Berlin, 1877 (literature).

Peiper: "Zur Symptomatologie der thierischen Parasiten," "Deutsche med. Wochenschr.," 1897, p. 765.

Reichold: "Fall von Ileus, bedingt durch Echinococcen der Leber," "Münchener med. Wochenschr.," 1897, p. 17.

Reinecke: "Compensatorische Leberhypertrophie bei Syphilis und bei Echinococcus der Leber," "Ziegler's Beiträge zur pathologischen Anatomie," Bd. XXIII, p. 238.

v. Siebold: "Ueber die Band- und Blasenwürmer," Leipzig, 1854.

Terrier: "Kyste hydatique d. foie," "Gazette hebdomad.," 1896, No. 13.

Waring: "Diseases of the Liver," p. 125.

Westerdyk: "Berliner klin. Wochenschr.," 1877, No. 43.

(C) ECHINOCOCCUS ALVEOLARIS (MULTILOCULARIS).

This form of echinococcus differs so essentially from the more frequent cystic form in regard to its pathologic anatomy, its geographic distribution, and, above all, its clinical manifestations, that it may be described as a clinical entity.

Ruysch (in 1721) was the first to observe such a case, and after him Buhl and Luschka reported similar growths in the liver. They considered them to be alveolar, colloid, or gelatinous forms of cancer. Zeller found the hooks and scolices, and Virchow first recognized the parasitic origin of the tumor, and gave it the name "multilocular ulcerative echinococcus-tumor." Although the symptoms produced are different, and although the geographic distribution and the form and structure vary considerably, yet this form of echinococcus was until recently considered to be identical with the form described above. The differences observed were attributed to the location of the swelling and to other anatomic conditions. Küchenmeister, it is true, had already assumed that there were several forms of echinococcus, and Vogler had called attention to certain differences in the form of the hooklets; but all this was denied by Leuckart and others, particularly after Klemm claimed to have produced typical echinococcus disease in a dog that he fed with multilocular echinococcus; unfortunately the animal was not examined for tenia before the administration of the multilocular echinococcus. Feeding experiments by Mangold also showed the presence of tenia; these, as in the case of Vogler, had longer and less curved hooks and longer roots with a knob-shaped protuberance. Fully developed specimens, moreover, had a ball-shaped accumulation of eggs that were never seen in the last links of tenia of echinococcus cysticus. Mangold also succeeded in inoculating a hog with these tenia and in producing typical young multilocular echinococci in the liver. Müller compared and corroborated these morphologic differences (compare also v. Bider).

An argument in favor of the difference between the two is found in the fact that metastases from the two varieties are different and growths similar to the primary form always being produced.

It is also remarkable that in certain regions only echinococcus alveolaris is seen, and that in other regions, again, where there is much echinococcus cysticus disease (Iceland, Mecklenburg, Pomerania), the former is rarely or never seen.

Among a number of regions in which the alveolar form is prevalent are: Southern Germany, Austria, Switzerland, and southeastern Russia.* The cases seen in other countries are usually in people that come from one of these four countries.

Vierordt has named the following German districts as prolific in echinococcus alveolaris infection; Southern Bavaria, southern Würtemberg (Black Forest and the Danube counties), Switzerland, and the German Tyrol (Posselt). Within these regions certain localities seem to be particularly exposed: Munich, the vicinity of Memmingen, the lower valley of the Inn and its surroundings, and the entrance to the Fuster Valley. Here several cases are often found in the same hamlet or even in the same family. Both of Morin's cases, for example, came from Villeret (in the Jura), and two cases from the little village of Oberzell. The disease is so frequent that the people are struck by its occurrence and have given it special names, as "Gilm" or "black jaundice," in the Tyrol. In these localities echinococcus alveolaris is by far the most frequent form of the two; also in the Tyrol the proportion of the cystic to the alveolar form is as 11 to 26, and it is worthy of note that nearly all the cases of the first category come from Wälsch Tyrol (Posselt).

The disease is found especially in the **middle years of life,** between twenty-seven and fifty; more rarely cases are also seen in younger or in older subjects. There is no appreciable influence exerted by the sex; or,

* Tokarenco, Dissertation, St. Petersburg, 1895.

if so, it is more apparent than real. It would appear that men are infected a little more frequently than women, about as 3:2 (Vierordt).

The origin, the mode of entrance, and the entire pathogenesis of the echinococcus alveolaris are still comparatively obscure, and many experiments will be required before these matters are thoroughly understood. No positive statement can as yet be made as to whether cattle-raising, which is so extensively carried on in the regions named, has anything to do with the disease.

In cattle this form of echinococcus has often been observed (Huber, Bollinger, Perroncito, Harms, and others), but no reliable statistics exist. It would appear that the disease is frequently confounded with tuberculosis (Müller).

People of the lower classes, peasants and other country folks, are most frequently affected (in Tyrol, Posselt). It is probable that the occupation of these people, and their uncleanliness, have something to do with this fact.

Pathologic Anatomy.—An alveolar echinococcus is distinguished from the cystic form by the following peculiarity: The cystic variety, as we have seen, often develops daughter-cysts within the cavity of the primary growth; the former variety, on the other hand, does not possess this power, but forms exogenous cysts, one cyst seeming to bud from the other. The mechanism is, in fact, a process of budding, either within the cuticle of the parasite (Morin, Leuckart), or in some portion that has become separated from the main body (Klebs, Leuckart, Prougeansky). Other distinguishing features are its greater tendency to perish from slight causes, and the formation of cysts containing no hooks and no scolices. The parasite irritates the liver tissues and causes an abundant proliferation of connective tissue. The center of the growth disintegrates readily and large cavities filled with debris are formed. The parasite, moreover, has a marked tendency to advance into healthy tissue in a manner that may be compared to the growth of a neoplasm. It involves bile-passages, blood-vessels, such as the portal vein, the vena cava, and the hepatic vein, also lymph-channels, and may even extend to neighboring organs, as the diaphragm. Metastases may form in the lungs, the lymph-glands, etc., in the same manner as in carcinoma or sarcoma.

The original seat of the echinococcus is obscure. Virchow and Klebs believed that it first became localized in the lymph-vessels; Friedreich, Schroeder van der Kolk, and Morin claimed the same for the bile-passages, Leuckart for the blood-vessels, and Heschl for the acini of the liver. The question is a difficult one to decide in the absence of animal experiments; in well-developed cases numerous organs are usually involved, so that it is difficult to find out which one was first affected. The opinion of Leuckart is the only one that we can accept in the light of our present knowledge; namely, that the parasite may infect any of these organs.

The macroscopic picture of the growth varies, of course, according to its age and its location. The outline of the liver need not necessarily be changed if the tumor develops in the interior of the organs; on transverse section a great development of the echinococcus will often be seen, even though its presence was hardly suspected. Sometimes small or large nodular protuberances are seen on the surface of the liver, or little bodies that are clearly defined as cysts; as a rule, they are found in the right lobe. Occasionally cicatricial contraction will be noticed. The consistency of the liver is increased, and the organ may be as hard as stone, owing partly to fibrous and partly to calcified connective tissue. In rare instances a softening of the echinococcus occurs so that fluctuation is noticed. The margin of the tumor, however, remains hard even if the center fluctuates. The liver often reaches a very high degree of enlargement; in small and young tumors the enlargement may not be so considerable. Griesinger reports a case in which the sac was as large as two adult heads, and Posselt describes a case from which over 7 liters of fluid were evacuated during an operation. At the same time there may be vicarious hypertrophy of the liver; in another case of Posselt the left lobe of the liver was 35 cm. long, 20 cm. broad, and 10 cm. thick.

The color of the tumors is different from that of the liver tissue; they are easily distinguished on transverse section. The tumor mass is whitish or bile-tinged, whereas the parenchyma is darker and occasionally also bile-tinged. Several tumors are often seen at the same time. On cutting, the tumor tissue gives a grating sound, and, owing to the cicatricial and the calcareous character of the tissue, it is often a matter of considerable difficulty to distinguish between the growths. The transverse sections appear as a vacuolated, alveolar structure similar to brown bread, cheese, honeycomb, or a sponge.

These peculiarities have probably earned for this parasite the name of alveolar echinococcus, and the name is better than the one more generally employed of multilocular echinococcus. For several echinococci of either form would constitute a multilocular cyst, whereas a single one of the alveolar form is indeed alveolar in the arrangement, and different in this respect from the cystic form.

The alveoli differ greatly in size; they may be punctiform or as large as peas. Between the single cysts bands of connective tissue are seen that may be broad or narrow. Occasionally the alveoli are not spherical, but are distorted into different shapes, owing to the pressure of the connective tissue and to the confluence of several cysts. In this manner the periphery of such an accumulation of cysts may appear gyrated and contain numerous varicose passages and cavities. The contents consist of a gelatinous, translucent, yellowish mass, that may become thickened, dry, grayish-yellow, cheesy, or mortar-like, from the admixture of calcium salts. The formation of cavities as a result of necrosis and degeneration is a conspicuous characteristic of the older cysts. These older cysts may develop to enormous sizes, as we have seen; they may fluctuate distinctly, and reach as far as the periphery of the organ. The walls have ridges containing blood-vessels. Several large cavities from different tumors may now coalesce. In such cases the walls are covered by bile-tinged or brick-red masses of bilirubin or remnants of blood. The contents of these old cysts consist of a puriform, creamy, brownish, viscid, and occasionally a bile-tinged mass containing chalk concretions, crystals of cholesterin, remnants of membrane, precipitates of bile-pigments, and crystals of hematoidin. In one case a sequestrum of liver tissue weighing 17 gm. was found floating in the cystic fluid (Kränzle). Albumin, bile-pigment, bile-acids, and fat are found. The cyst is not encapsulated so completely as in the cystic form of the disease and not so distinctly separated from the liver tissue. The connective tissue of the periphery is thicker and contains ridges, but liver tissue is mixed with it, and, on the other hand, the connective tissue sends processes into the parenchyma of the organ. In the latter new echinococcus alveoli are found. At the same time, cirrhotic changes are occasionally seen in other parts of the liver.

The bile-passages are often involved, either by compression or by inclosure in the tumor mass, both accidents leading to a closure of their lumen.   Thus the common duct may become occluded by an echinococcus that develops near the porta hepatis and all the bile be excluded from the intestine.   The cystic and the hepatic ducts may be occluded in the same way.   This will lead to stasis of bile in the gall-bladder or to dilatation of the smaller bile-passages, and as a result we will have hydrops of the gall-bladder or of the smaller bile-passages.   Concretions may develop as a result of stasis.   The tumor grows into the walls of the gall-bladder, into the cystic and the hepatic ducts and their branches, and leads to similar lesions.   Occasionally, when the tumor begins to soften, larger bile-ducts become eroded and in this manner communicate with the central cyst-cavity.   The latter becomes filled with bile, or the contents of the cyst may be poured into the bile-passages or into the gall-bladder.

If the portal vein becomes occluded or compressed, stasis in the region supplied by this vessel supervenes, and is followed by a swelling of the spleen and occasionally by ascites.   The vena cava has been found flattened and obliterated by the pressure exercised by the tumor.   Following this there was edema of the lower extremities, dilatation of the abdominal veins, etc.   Posselt describes a case in which a communication was established between the vena cava and the cyst-cavity, and in which death occurred from hemorrhage.

The lymph-channels are quite frequently involved, and appear in the region of the tumor as rosaries, the single beads of which consist of small echinococcus cysts.   Sometimes they form thick strands that run toward the porta hepatis and the abdominal aorta, or form a network of threads from 2 to 3 mm. thick.   The portal lymph-glands are frequently swollen, and contain echinococcus cysts.

Metastases are often found in the lungs.   These may be in a state of cheesy degeneration, particularly if they are situated in the lower lobes.   Sometimes occlusion of the branches of the pulmonary artery takes place.   Bosch and Morin have reported eruptions upon the diaphragmatic pleura, in the mediastinal glands, and even the formation of large alveolar echinococcus tumors containing scolices in the latter.   Metastases have even been found in the endocardium of the right side of the heart in a case in which the lower vena cava was embedded in tumor masses (Buhl).   Large strands and single cysts may often be found in the peritoneum.

Among other symptoms that may be traced to the complete obstruction of bile-passages are hemorrhages, fatty degeneration of the heart-muscles, the kidneys, etc.   Tubercular foci have also frequently been found at autopsy; these, of course, have nothing to do with the disease.

Histologic examination of alveolar echinococcus cysts reveals strands of connective tissue and a fibrous meshwork consisting of coarse fibers of elastic strands, which may be tinged with bile, and contain amorphous pigment, fat-globules, chalk concretions, etc.   These different accidental admixtures are seen chiefly in the vicinity of the central cavity.   Within this reticulum the alveoli are seen surrounded by a structureless, wavy membrane which gives the impression that the cysts are held in close contact by pressure, or suggests that the latter have attempted to grow and have been prevented from doing so by the connective tissue.   In the interior the granular layer of parenchyma will be found. The whole tumor, if still young, is translucent, colloid, and can be readily enucleated from its capsule of connective tissue as a round gelatinous lump. In some cases hooks and scolices will be found; in others they have been searched for in vain; in other cases they have been found in the lymph-gland metastases, but not in the primary tumor. As the tumor grows older the originally clear contents become cloudy from the admixture of fat-globules, pigment-granules, crystals of hematoidin, and fatty acids. In large cysts a network of stellate bodies will be seen in the parenchymatous layer; these bulge at the crossing-points, but have very thin connecting processes (Virchow). Here and there they are broader and contain granules and calcareous bodies that show a laminated structure. The chemical properties of the sac-wall are the same as those of the cuticular layer of the cystic echino-coccus, and consist essentially of chitin. Within the dry, cheesy, mortar-like paste that is found in older cysts, numerous chalk-granules, cholesterin, shreds of echinococcus membrane, etc., are found. Calcified scolices may also be found. The purulent mass often found in cysts consists largely of cholesterin needles, pieces of cuticular membrane, chalk concretions, granules of bile-pigment, crystals of hematoidin and of cholesterin, scolices and an amorphous detritus containing no pus-corpuscles. In the paren-chyma of the liver hyperplastic processes are occasionally seen if the echinococcus grows very large. There may also be fatty degeneration of the hepatic cells and proliferation of the interstitial connective tissue in the vicinity of the tumor.

Symptoms.—Echinococcus alveolaris develops so gradually that the condition often causes no symptoms and may be discovered only at the postmortem.

The first symptoms usually are, however, a feeling of pressure and distention, pain in the hypochondriac and epigastric regions, disturbances of appetite, nausea, and vomiting. Fever is sometimes present, but may be absent. If the tumor develops in the neighborhood of the large biliary passage, icterus may be the first symptom. Constipation and diarrhea may be complained of. The patient grows weak and emaciates. The liver is enlarged, its margin protrudes below the costal arch, and the hepatic dulness reaches further upward than is normal. The motility of the diaphragm is impaired above the tumor. The consistency of the liver is usually increased. If the tumor is not hidden beneath the ribs of the diaphragm, a hard nodular mass will be felt that can be distinctly outlined and distinguished from other organs. Occasionally it can be felt at the margin of the liver, and is then lost beneath the costal arch. The liver is, as a rule, freely movable unless adhesions anchor it. The organ may also be diffusely enlarged and hardened, so that it feels like a cirrhotic liver. In the portions involved by the tumor the margin is hard and nodular; it may also be hard and rounded in other parts, owing to compensatory hyper-trophy of the liver. Later, the center of the tumor may soften and fluctuate while, at the same time, the tumor decreases in size and the symptoms of oppression decrease. Generally, the tumor is not painful to pressure; if the disease is, however, complicated by perihepatitis, it may become sensi-tive, and even the pressure of the clothing may distress the patient; there may also be pain when slight pressure is exercised during palpa-tion. The liver continues to increase in size. Very large tumors may result, which extend laterally as far as the ilium and to Poupart's liga-ment, and toward the middle line as far as the umbilicus. Sometimes

52

they contain several liters of fluid. It is probable that such a cavity can evacuate its contents through the bile-passages, but no positive evidence of the passage of the fluid contents of one of these cysts *via* the rectum has so far been reported. [W. Althaus,* Clayton,† and others have recently described cases in which large echinococcus cysts compressed and finally discharged their contents through the biliary passages. In Clayton's case daughter-cysts were discovered in the bowel movements.—ED.] Buhl observed a case in which bile-tinged masses mixed with chitinous membrane were expectorated, but no fistulous channel was discovered postmortem. Sometimes it is possible, in cases in which the cystic or the common duct is compressed, to palpate the gall-bladder as a fluctuating tumor at the side of the echinococcus cyst.

Icterus from stasis is an important symptom. As a rule, icterus develops early; in certain cases, however, it may be a late symptom or may not appear at all, notwithstanding a rapid development of the cyst (Posselt). The intensity of the icterus generally remains constant. If the tumor undergoes softening, however, and in this manner relieves the pressure on the ducts; or if the intensity of the catarrh of the bile-passages is reduced, the icterus may grow less decided. For the same reasons it is occasionally noticed that acholic stools alternate with those which again temporarily contain urobilin (case of Erismann). In many cases icterus is due to partial occlusion of one of the larger ducts within the liver so that an abundant quantity of bile enters the intestine; in other cases, again, there is total retention of bile from compression of the common duct. [L. Ferralesco ‡ reports a case in which a large cyst compressed and totally occluded the main biliary passages.—ED.] In these cases the highest degrees of icterus may be seen, blackish-green color of the skin, itching, furunculosis and ulceration, and large quantities of bile-pigment may be noted in the urine. The latter, in such cases, may also contain urobilin, and as a result of the irritation of the kidneys, albumin and nucleo-albumin, and, owing to the decomposition of the intestinal contents in the absence of bile, indoxyl. Sometimes there is polyuria, and the urine has a low specific gravity, so that the patients complain of thirst. Hepatargy (cholemia) may appear; there may be a tendency to hemorrhage, epistaxis, bleeding from the mouth, the gums, from carious teeth, from the alveoli after extraction of teeth, hematemesis, passage of bloody stools, hematuria (from hemorrhage into the bladder), and hemoptysis. Any small wound of the skin may be followed by severe bleeding (razor-cuts, leech-bites, scratches, etc.). Petechiæ appear and intracerebral hemorrhages have been reported. The number of blood-corpuscles is reduced, but the blood is not otherwise affected by the disease.

The hemorrhages must be attributed to the retention of bile. A few cases, however, have been reported in which there was no icterus of long duration, and in which, nevertheless, severe hemorrhages appeared, as in a case described by Bauer, in which there was degeneration of the liver parenchyma and incipient acute atrophy of the liver. In some cases xanthopsia and hemeralopia are seen.

In the majority of cases severe icterus causes death. It may, however, occur that an echinococcus cyst grows steadily until it assumes

* *Münch. med. Woch.*, 1900, No. 33.
† *Lancet*, Sept. 15, 1900.
‡ *Gaz. degli Osped.*, July 19, 1900.

enormous dimensions without causing icterus. In cases of this kind the disease usually runs a more protracted course with the formation of large cavities in the liver and softening of the parenchyma.

Griesinger reports a case in which a remittent form of icterus existed for six years. As a rule, the time is shorter and the average case lasts for several months, although cases lasting over a year are by no means rare. Much will depend upon the completeness of the occlusion of the ducts, and as to whether some bile enters the intestine or none at all.

Narrowing or occlusion of the portal vein by the tumor is manifested by ascites and other symptoms of stasis. Ascites may be so intense as to interfere with respiration, causing dyspnea and cyanosis, and calling for puncture. The fluid is serous and bile-tinged. The splenic tumor that is occasionally seen must be attributed to stasis more than to the effect of toxic or infectious agencies.

The lower vena cava may be occluded and may even become totally obliterated (Buhl, Carrière); if this occurs, a collateral circulation is established from the inguinal through the epigastric veins to the axilla (vena axillaris) and to the sternum (vena mammaria interna); besides, there is usually edema of the lower extremities. In one case reported by Posselt the echinococcus cyst degenerated, perforated into the vena cava, and produced a fatal hemorrhage.

There is nothing characteristic about the fever which sometimes is seen; the temperature usually fluctuates irregularly and may depend on the presence of complications.

Intestinal disturbances are frequently seen, as meteorism, and diarrheas that undermine the strength of the patient. The appetite and general power of assimilation may remain good for a long time; in fact, there may be polyphagia. As a result the patient is able to attend to his affairs for a considerable period; later the appetite is lost, there is deficient power to assimilate the food, etc., the general strength is reduced, and nutrition becomes altogether inadequate.

Hypostatic processes and infarcts are seen in the lungs, and the disease may be complicated by tuberculosis of these organs. In rare instances an echinococcus cyst has been known to rupture into the lung (Predtetschenski).

The heart is not directly affected though occasionally it may be dislocated. The pulse is slowed as a result of the icterus.

Death occurs from collapse; toward the end there is edema and general loss of strength. The fatal issue is accelerated by obstinate hemorrhages, diarrhea, lack of assimilation, and deficient nourishment. It is possible that certain toxic substances play a rôle, as in the case of other parasites.

The disease usually lasts for several years. No definite length of time can be given, because the process remains latent and is unrecognized for a long time. Cases in which the tumor develops in a marked manner from the beginning in the vicinity of the large bile-ducts, and in which, as a result, icterus appears early, are more rapidly fatal than those in which the bile-ducts are involved at a later stage of the disease.

Prognosis.—Almost all of the cases of echinococcus alveolaris that are on record have terminated fatally. It is, however, to be hoped that, with a better knowledge of the pathologic picture and of the frequency of its occurrence, we shall soon be able to recognize the disease in an earlier stage and to extirpate the tumor completely, together with some of the surrounding liver tissue, and in this way cure the trouble. In cases in which the tumor is situated near the margin of the liver this will be particularly easy. If, on the other hand, the tumor is very large when it is discovered, or if it develops in the interior of the organ, at the porta, or in some inaccessible part of the liver, such measures will be inapplicable.

Diagnosis.—The diagnosis of alveolar echinococcus is by no means easy. In many cases it is altogether impossible to state positively that we are dealing with such a condition.

The course of the disease is similar to that of carcinoma of the liver, and more closely similar to this disease than to cystic echinococcus. The nodular tumor, the symptoms of stasis, the cachexia, and the biliary stasis may be very misleading. As a rule, it is true, the patient is young, and evidence of primary tumors in the stomach or the intestine is absent; these growths are, as we know, the chief source of cancer of the liver. The geographic location is of paramount importance, and many diagnoses of echinococcus have been made rather upon a geographic than a clinical basis. [L. Renon * reports a case of multilocular echino-coccus of the pleura and right lung in a man of thirty-six years. He claims that is the first case of the disease in man in France.—Ed.] In short, if the patient comes from a region in which a case of alveolar echinococcus has been previously found, the diagnosis is made in favor of this disease rather than of cancer. The course, too, is more pro-tracted than that of cancer, the latter rarely existing longer than a year; whereas echinococcus may easily last for a longer time. The patient, moreover, is able to attend to his affairs for a longer time and is not incapacitated by pain; he does not become reduced in strength until icterus appears in a severe form. The nodules of echinococcus are usually as hard as stone, whereas cancer nodules are softer. Tumor of the spleen is a frequent complication of echinococcus, and is rare in cancer; the same applies to the fever. If cancer tumors begin to soften, a feeling of fluctuation may sometimes be imparted, though indistinct; in echinococcus there may be such widespread disintegration that fluctua-tion is very distinct, and, in addition, a tympanitic sound may be heard over the cavities on percussion (Griesinger).

The following features, therefore, must be considered in the differen-tial diagnosis between echinococcus alveolaris and carcinoma of the liver: the age of the patient, the location from which he comes, the duration of the disease, disturbances of the stomach and intestine, the presence or absence of a splenic tumor, and fever.

The differential diagnosis from malignant adenoma may also be difficult. This lesion is, however, rare. It is characterized by nodular tumors, icterus, tumor of the spleen, and resembles echinococcus in the duration of the disease. Leichtenstern has reported a case that was very similar to echinococcus in its whole clinical course.

Exploratory puncture does not furnish very important information. Sometimes analysis of the aspirated fluid is of no value at all. It is impossible in many cases to find hooklets and scolices, and they should hardly be expected. Occasionally shreds of membrane are found, and crystals of hematoidin, fat, fatty-acid needles, cholesterin, pigment-granules, chalk concretions, red blood-corpuscles, occasionally also a few pus-corpuscles and isolated liver-cells. Chemical analysis will reveal

* *Deutsch. med. Woch.*, April 26, 1900.

the presence of albumin, bile-pigment (fat often in abundance), and salts. Hüfner analyzed the fluid from a growth of this kind and found: Urea, 0.014 %; chlorid of sodium, 0.003 %; chlorid of potassium, 0.712 %; albumin, 0.2 %; fat, cholesterin, and bile-pigment, altogether 0.1 %. Phosphoric acid, magnesia, and calcium were absent. The absence of the latter was noteworthy because in other cases large quantities of calcium have been found in the fluid.

It is probable that the cystic contents vary in different cases according to the presence or absence of communications with bile-passages, blood-vessels, or lymph-channels. The fluid always contains albumin, in contradistinction to the fluid in the other form of echinococcus. Exploratory puncture seems to be well borne in all cases and not to cause symptoms of peritonitic irritation.

Of late years exploratory laparotomy has been performed in a number of cases. A small portion of the tumor was excised and examined microscopically; after the diagnosis was made in this way, the cavity was opened and the tumor excised.

The disease may be taken for hypertrophic cirrhosis of the liver if the tumor develops in the interior of the liver or on its lower surface. In this condition, however, icterus is not so severe and the enlargement of the liver and the splenic tumor appear earlier. In contradistinction to syphilis of the liver, the liver in echinococcus alveolaris is harder, larger, and less indentated.

It is distinguished from the cystic form by its nodular surface (even in the stage of softening), by the greater frequency of icterus and splenic tumor, and by examination of the fluid contents.

Abscess of the liver and amyloid degeneration need hardly be considered. Gall-stones are readily differentiated by colic, the passage of concretions, etc.

Treatment.—Until very recently we were powerless to treat echinococcus alveolaris even if the condition was recognized early and the growth was small. Within late years, however, the attempt has been made to eradicate the condition by operative treatment. Terillon removed a piece of the liver that contained several cysts (probably cystic echinococci). Bruns cured a woman by excising an alveolar echinococcus from the liver.

The cyst-cavities have also been punctured, but without good results; the method of the double incision has also been tried; the cavity has been scraped and cauterized. Brunner claims to have cured a case in this manner by operating through the pleural cavity. In other cases success has not been chronicled because it was impossible to remove all of the diseased and infected tissue; thus, the parasite began to grow again from the periphery. Bobrow has recorded such an experience. Predtetschenski opened a swelling which he took for an abscess of the lung, and the case seemed to get well. Later the patient died from pneumonia and nephritis, and in the scar tissue of the lung were found echinococcus cicatrices. Large cavities may develop so near to important blood-vessels that fatal hemorrhage into the wound may occur. Nicoladoni (quoted by Posselt) reports a case of this kind in which the bleeding occurred from the vena cava.

It might be a useful procedure to attempt the destruction of the parasite by injections of sublimate in the same manner as described in the treatment of echinococcus cysticus.

LITERATURE.

Bider: "Echinococcus multilocularis des Gehirns, nebst Notiz über das Vorkommen von Echinococcen in Basel," "Virchow's Archiv," Bd. cxli, p. 190.

Bobrow: "Alveoläre Echinococcen der Leber," "Die Chirurgie," 1897, Heft 1 (Russian); "Centralblatt für Chirurgie," 1897, p. 1115.

Brunner: "Ein Beitrag zur Behandlung des Echinococcus alveolaris hepatis," "Münchener med. Wochenschr.," 1891, No. 29.

Bruns, P.: Leberresection bei multiloculärem Echinococcus," Bruns' "Beiträge zur klin. Chirurgie," Bd. xvii.

Buhl: "Zeitschr. für rationelle Medicin," 1854, Bd. iv, p. 356.

—Ibid., 1857, Bd. viii, p. 115.

Friedreich: "Beiträge zur Pathologie der Leber und Milz," "Virchow's Archiv," 1865, Bd. xxxiii, p. 16.

Griesinger: "Zur klin. Geschichte des vielfächerigen Echinococcus," "Archiv der Heilkunde," 1860, Bd. i, p. 547.

Huber: "Zur Diagnose des Echinococcus multilocularis," "Deutsches Archiv für klin. Medicin," 1865, Bd. i, p. 539.

—"Ein Fall von Echinococcus multilocularis der Gallenblase," ibidem, Bd. xlviii, p. 432.

Klemm: "Zur Kenntniss des Echinococcus alveolaris der Leber," Dissertation, München, 1883.

Leuckart: Loc. cit.

Löwenstein: "Multiloculärer Echinococcus," Dissertation, Erlangen, 1889.

Luschka: "Gallertkrebs der Leber," "Virchow's Archiv," 1852, Bd. iv, p. 400.

—"Zur Frage der Echinococcenkrankheit der menschlichen Leber," ibidem, 1856, Bd. x, p. 206.

Mangold: "Ueber den multiloculären Echinococcus und seine Taenie," Dissertation, Tübingen, 1892; and "Berliner klin. Wochenschr.," 1892, pp. 21 and 50.

Morin: "Deux cas de tumeurs à échinocoques multiloc.," Dissertation, Bern, 1876.

Mosler and Peiper: "Thierische Parasiten," Bd. vi, Nothnagel's Encyclopedia.

Müller: "Beitrag zur Kenntniss der Taenia echinococcus," "Münchener med. Wochenschr.," 1893, p. 241.

Nahm: "Ueber den multiloculären Echinococcus der Leber," ibidem, 1887, p. 674.

Peiper: in "Ergebnisse der allgemeinen Pathologie und pathologischen Anatomie," 1896, p. 40.

Predtetschenski: "Ein aus vielkammerigem Echinococcus entstandener, in die rechte Lunge durchgebrochener Leberabscess," "Med. Rundschau" (Russian), 1895, No. 10, from "Virchow-Hirsch's Jahresbericht," 1895.

Posselt: "Der Echinococcus multilocularis in Tirol," "Deutsches Archiv für klin. Medicin," 1897, Bd. lix, p. 1.

Prougeansky, M.: "Ueber die multilolcuäre ulcerirende Echinococcusgeschwulst in der Leber," Dissertation, Zürich, 1873.

Reiniger: "Multiloculärer Echinococcus, Dissertation, Tübingen, 1890.

Schiess: "Zur Lehre von der multiloculären ulcerirenden Echinococcusgeschwulst der Leber," "Virchow's Archiv," 1858, Bd. xiv, p. 371.

Schwarz: "Ein Fall von Echinococcus multilocularis hepatis," "Deutsches Archiv für klin. Medicin," Bd. li, p. 616.

Tokarenko: "Ueber Echinococcus multilocularis hominis," Dissertation, St. Petersburg, 1895, from "Virchow-Hirsch's Jahresbericht," 1895.

Tochmarke: "Ein Beitrag zur Histologie des Echinococcus multilocularis," Dissertation, Freiburg, 1891.

Virchow: "Verhandlungen der physikalisch-med. Gesellschaft zu Würzburg," 1856, Bd. vi, p. 84.

Vierordt, H.: "Ueber den multiloculären Echinococcus" (a monograph with complete references to cases and the literature). Freiburg, 1886.

—"Der multiloculäre Echinococcus der Leber," "Berliner Klinik," Heft 28.

Vogler: "Correspondenzblatt für Schweizer Aerzte," 1885, pp. 191 and 587.

Waldstein: "Ein Fall von multiloculärem Echinococcus der Leber," "Virchow's Archiv," 1881, Bd. lxxxiii, p. 41.

(D) ASCARIS LUMBRICOIDES (SPULWÜRMER).

Ascarides enter the bile-passages from the duodenum, developing first in the intestine from eggs that are introduced per os. They do not seem to develop within the bile-passages, though it is possible that sometimes they enter the ducts when they are still young, and continue to grow there. As they seem to have the power of crawling through wire loops and glass rings (pearls), it is possible that a fully developed parasite may push its conical head through the orifice of the common duct and gradually work its way into the gall-bladder, or the hepatic duct and its branches. Many clinical and anatomic observations speak in favor of this possibility. It is not correct, of course, to assume that ascarides enter the gall-bladder and the bile-passages during life in every case in which these parasites are found in the bile-channels at the autopsy; nor are we justified in basing our interpretation of the disease to which the case has succumbed, upon the presence of ascarides in this abnormal location. In very many cases they have probably entered the ducts postmortem.

All cases of hepatic disease, icterus, swelling of the liver, etc., that seem to recover after the passage of ascarides in the stools must be carefully analyzed before any rôle in the causation of the condition is attributed to the parasites. A duodenal catarrh, for instance, due to the presence of ascarides, may cause the icterus, etc.; or, again, the treatment may have caused the evacuation of the ascarides, although the latter had nothing whatever to do with the production of the lesions that were being treated. In certain cases, however, icterus has been seen to disappear at the same time with the passage of an ascaris per rectum that was bile-stained at one extremity only. In a case of this kind we are probably justified in assuming that there has been a causal connection between the presence of the ascaris and the icterus.

When these parasites enter the bile-passages, they may irritate the mucous membrane, may occlude the ducts, or may carry intestinal bacteria into the liver. The ascarides as foreign bodies cause stasis of bile, and the bacteria find thus a suitable nidus for their development in the dilated channels, filled with bile, and can penetrate the mucous membrane more easily because it is in a state of inflammation. In this way they may penetrate the liver parenchyma, and cause single or multiple abscesses.

Pathologic Anatomy.—Often no changes will be found in the liver and the bile-passages, so that the conclusion seems justified that the parasites enter the latter after the death of the patient. Only such anatomic changes can be utilized as point directly to the action of ascarides during life; such as stasis of bile in the liver, the gall-bladder, and the bile-passages; distention of these channels with thickened bile in cases in which the common duct is occluded by the parasite; and distention of the gall-bladder if the worm is situated in the cystic duct. Often there is cholangitis in the locality in which the parasite is found; also ulceration of the mucosa, formation of cavities originating from the bile-channels and filled with pus, eggs, or ascarides. Further, abscesses of the liver may be present containing a macerated worm, or metastatic foci in different places of the parenchyma, and originating from suppurative cholangitis, which in its turn owes its origin to an ascaris. Finally, the formation of a gall-stone around an ascaris has been observed.

Broussais, Wierus, Lieutaud, Buonaparte, Treille, and others have reported cases in which the worm occluded the common duct but had only entered the channel half-way, so that one-half was found protruding into the intestine. In the cases reported by Lobstein numerous ascarides occluded the common duct. An ascaris has been seen in the interior of a gall-stone that was impacted in the orifice of the ductus choledochus. Davaine quotes a case in which a large number of worms were found in the bile-ducts, and had made pockets in the walls of the passages extending for a varying distance into the liver tissue. Bourgeois reports a similar case. Laennec saw a case in which a communication existed between the common duct and the stomach and in which ascarides were present in the gall-bladder and in the bile-passages. The walls of the bile-passages were reddened, thickened, eroded, or destroyed, and cavities were formed in the liver, as large as almonds and filled with worms. Laennec attributes such a destructive action on the part of ascarides to suction performed with their mouths. Davaine believes that suppurative processes have a causal connection. Tonnelé describes a case in which pus was found around an ascaris, and in which there were several abscess-cavities in its immediate vicinity. Pellizari determined that two abscesses, found on the surface of the liver (in a shoemaker), contained ascarides and were in reality dilated bile-passages; after the worms were removed they were found to communicate with the hepatic duct and to contain pus-corpuscles, ascaris eggs, and bile-duct epithelia. Forget found an ascaris in the common duct and one in the hepatic duct; in addition, he found a cavity as large as a walnut filled with pus, which represented a dilated bile-passage and contained a dead worm in a state of maceration and decay. Further, there were found ten abscesses varying in size from a pea to a chestnut. The walls of these cavities were covered by a thick pseudomembrane and were surrounded by a hyperemic liver tissue. In a case of Lebert numerous worms were found in the bile-passages, and a number of small abscess-cavities varying in size from a pea to an apple, all through the liver tissue. The abscesses did not communicate with the portal vein; some of them, however, communicated with bile-passages and some of them contained macerated ascarides. One of the abscesses had perforated the diaphragm and had entered the lung, so that pneumothorax was present at the same time. Lobstein also describes multiple abscesses of the liver, one of which penetrated the lung; he attributes all the lesions to the presence of ascarides. These worm-abscesses may also perforate the skin, such an occurrence having been seen and reported by Kirkland. Kartulis found 80 ascarides, some of them alive, in a liver filled with small pus-cavities. Of late, Hoehler has furnished a description of multiple abscesses of the liver, caused by an ascaris which was found in one of the pus-cavities. Röderer and Wagler describe a case in which an ascaris was found within an echinococcus cyst; it appears doubtful, however, whether this worm entered the cyst during the life of the patient.

In all the cases described the worms were situated with their heads toward the liver and their tails toward the intestine. Only in the gall-bladder does it appear that they can turn around and crawl out again. Some of the worms were adults, some of them (particularly in the abscesses) young ones. Occasionally a large number of ascarides will be found together; Vinay, for instance, saw 20 lying together near the orifice of the common duct. It is probably owing to the protected and hidden location of the orifice of the common duct that invasion of the liver by ascarides does not occur more frequently.

The symptoms of ascarides are so indefinite and so little characteristic that a diagnosis of invasion of the bile-passages or the liver by these parasites can hardly be made. If the common duct is occluded (Broussais, Lieutaud, Buonaparte), the liver and the gall-bladder swell, and there will be intense icterus, and discoloration of the feces. The patients complain of fever and of violent pain in the liver region. Sometimes icterus does not appear because the worms crawl through the duct too rapidly to cause stasis of bile; in such cases the temperature is usually high, there is pain in the liver region, the organ will swell, there is lack of appetite, vomiting, diarrhea or constipation, and ultimately the symptoms of cholangitis and of abscess of the liver appear. The patient usually dies in a short time. In the case of children, there may be convulsions, coma, great weakness, and serious disturbances of the heart-action before death terminates the scene. If the worms penetrate the lung, symptoms of pneumonia or of pulmonary abscess develop; pneumothorax is also occasionally seen. In Kirkland's case the abscess broke through the skin at the level of the last false rib on the right side, and the worm was evacuated with the pus. As the fistula continued to secrete bile for a long time thereafter, it is probable that a connection existed with a bile-duct or with the gall-bladder.

We must be very skeptical as to all reports of cures of ascarides infection of the liver. It is true that many cases have been described in which certain liver symptoms disappeared after the passage of ascarides, but in these cases a simple duodenal catarrh may have been caused by the parasites, and cured as soon as the worms were removed.

The following case reported by Mallins can hardly be interpreted to signify anything else than the presence of ascarides in the common duct: An officer complained for three months of icterus and there was complete absence of bile from the intestine; at this time an ascaris was passed, one-half of which was bile-tinged; as soon as the worm was removed, icterus disappeared, bile appeared in the intestine, and the case was cured.

It is possible that cases of this kind occur more frequently, but we must not forget that the worm, if it has once succeeded in engaging its head in the common duct, will certainly have a tendency to progress, and will try to penetrate the liver as it penetrates other organs and cavities. It will not, naturally, show a tendency to work its way back into the duodenum. Only in the gall-bladder might the worm possibly turn around, and, finding no other exit, slip back into the intestine through the cystic and the common duct.

In general the prognosis is unfavorable if the worm penetrates branches of the hepatic duct, and cholangitis, abscess, etc., seem to be the inevitable consequences of this occurrence.

The only internal therapy that can be employed must be directed to that portion of the worm that is still dangling in the intestine. Laxatives, as castor oil, etc., and santonin should be given in order to induce the parasite to leave the choledochus. If the worm has entered the gall-bladder or if it has crawled into the common duct so that no part of its tail-end protrudes into the intestine, surgical measures are the only ones that promise any relief. A laparotomy will have to be performed, the affected parts exposed, and examined for worms; the bile-passages should then be opened and the parasites removed in the same manner as gall-stones.

Davaine: Loc. cit., p. 156.
Hoehler: "Ein Fall von Leberabscessen, verursacht durch einen Spulwurm," Dissertation, Greifswald, 1895.
Kartulis: "Ueber einen Fall von Auswanderung einer grossen Zahl von Ascariden in die Gallengänge und die Leber," "Centralblatt für Bakteriologie und Parasitenkunde," Bd. i.
Langenbuch: Loc. cit., p. 167.
Leuckart: Loc. cit., Bd. ii, p. 236.
Schüppel: "Krankheiten der Gallenwege," in "Ziemssen's Handbuch," 1880, p. 171.

Anguillula (Leptodera) stercoralis, also called *Rhabdonema strongyloides,* is a parasite that is found in the intestine in Cochin China diarrhea. It is usually present in large numbers, and occasionally enters the bile-passages and the gall-bladder without causing any symptoms during life that indicate its presence. Its pathologic significance is not very great.

Cobbold: Loc. cit., p. 234.
Davaine: Loc. cit., 2. Aufl., p. 966.

(E) DISTOMATA.

Distomata of the Bile-passages. Distomum s. Distoma hepaticum, lanceolatum, sinense, conjunctum, crassum, felineum.

In the bile-passages and in the gall-bladder liver flukes (German, *Leberegel;* French, *douve*) are occasionally found; not so frequently, however, as in sheep, cattle, and other animals. The disturbances seen in man are not so serious as those seen in sheep; of the latter a great number perish every year from this disease with the symptoms of severe cachexia, anemia, and hydrops. These cases are, as a rule, due to Distoma lanceolatum and hepaticum, both of which are usually present at the same time in the same animal.

These flukes vegetate in the bile-passages of the animals and produce dilatation of the bile-ducts, cholangitis, and pericholangitis. The dilated bile-passages are found incrusted with chalk; the connective tissue around the ducts then becomes inflamed, interstitial hepatitis develops, followed by contraction and, later, ascites. General edema and anemia are then seen. In cattle the disease runs a less severe course.

Distoma hepaticum is a leaf-shaped trematode about 25 to 30 mm. long, and when fully developed 8 to 12 mm. broad. The anterior portion of the body is only 4 or 5 mm. long; here are seen two suckers, and longitudinal and circular muscle-fibers. This part of the body is covered with rows of chitinous scales turned posteriorly.

The worm enters the bile-ducts in the following manner: The wedge-shaped head and the first millimeters of the body enter the common duct as the result of attachment of the suckers when the body is fully extended. The muscles of the body then contract and cause the worm to become thicker, and in this way to dilate the passage. Finally the sucker situated on the abdominal side is pulled in and attached to the mucosa. At the same time, the scales of chitin become wedged against the walls of the duct, and a position is thus occupied that offers resistance enough to allow the parasite to push its way further into the duct. The flat posterior end of the worm is usually rolled up and wrinkled so that the parasite resembles a faded leaf; owing to its brown color, it may easily be overlooked.

Distoma lanceolatum appears very similar; it is narrower and shorter, however—*i. e.,* 8 to 9 mm. long and 2 to 2.4 mm. broad; its surface is smooth.

The eggs of Distoma hepaticum are 0.13 to 0.14 mm. long and 0.075 to 0.09 mm. broad; they have a flattened anterior pole covered with a lid-like structure, and a pointed posterior pole. The eggs of Distoma lanceolatum are smaller, 0.045 mm. long and 0.03 mm. broad, have a thicker shell, and a more flattened knob-shaped extremity.

The eggs of distoma are passed out of the bile-passages together with the bile, enter the intestine and are evacuated with the stools; in this manner they may infect the pasture. As soon as the embryo (in the flagellated stage) comes in contact with water its covering separates, it is liberated, and enters the body of certain water-snails, particularly Limnæus minutus. It enters the respiratory cavity of the latter, forming a sporocyst; later these develop caudate cerceria. These are either eaten by the sheep with the grass on which they are lying, or the body of the snail is injured and the parasite liberated in this way; in the latter instance the worms become attached to water plants, grass, etc., to which they are glued with a gummy substance.

They are eaten by different animals with grass, or are swallowed with the water of pools and ditches. After entering the stomach and intestine, they penetrate the bile-ducts or may reach the liver by way of the portal vein.

Infection probably occurs in the lower animals and in man in a similar manner. An argument in favor of this view is the fact that this form of parasite is usually found in human subjects who have been known to quench their thirst by drinking well- or ditch-water, or who have eaten water-cress, etc.

This, for example, was the case in a patient of Kirchner (quoted by Leuckart), a shepherdess who had been in the habit of drinking the water of a swampy meadow, and of eating the water-cress that grew there. In Bastroem's case the patient was a laborer, working near the Main-Danube canal. Baelz reports that in Japan, particularly in the neighborhood of Okayama, distoma is frequently found in human subjects. This is a swampy region that has been reclaimed from the sea; similar conditions exist in Katayama. He distinguishes two species of liver-flukes, Distoma hepaticum endemicum s. perniciosum and Distoma hepaticum innocuum. Leuckart, however, has shown that the two are identical and are both members of the family, Distoma sinense s. spathulatum. The peasants in the region named used the dirty water of the ditches for washing their kitchen utensils, etc., and in this manner, it is said, some 20 % are afflicted.

In tropical regions distoma infection is frequently seen and is due, in all probability, to the use of dirty water. Bierner, McConnell, Carter, McGregor, Chester, and others have reported cases that seem to demonstrate this fact. The parasite was named by Cobbold Distoma sinense, and by Leuckart Distoma spathulatum; it was first found by McConnell in a Chinese, who died of a severe affection of the liver. Blanchard has found many of these worms in the livers of soldiers in Anam. Jjima found the parasite in cats in Japan.

The worm is 10 to 13 mm. long and 2 to 3 mm. broad. Its cuticle is smooth, and its eggs are from 0.028 to 0.03 mm. long and from 0.016 to 0.017 mm. broad, brown to black in color, with a thin shell and a small lid at the narrower end. There is occasionally a knob at the dull extremity.

Another kind of fluke has been found in the bile-passage of Mohammedans in Calcutta (McConnell), and in the livers of Indian dogs (Lewis and Cunningham), called Distoma conjunctum and resembling Distoma sinense. This worm is distinguished from the other species by certain fine processes and by the presence of hairs on the cuticle. It is possible that certain forms of severe cirrhosis of the liver that have been described by Ghose and Mackenzie in India are due to distoma infection.

In isolated cases Distoma crassum, a worm 4 to 6 mm. long and 1.7 to 2 mm. broad, has been known to cause serious disturbances in man. This organism was first described by Busk in the duodenum of a Lascar; in this case it was not found in the bile-passages nor in the gall-bladder (Budd). Cobbold and Johnson also found it in a missionary and his wife and child. It appears that the last-named three had become infected during a sojourn in China (Ningpo), possibly from eating oysters.

Winogradoff saw a form of distoma in Siberia which he called Distoma Sibericum. Braun claims that this form is identical with that seen in Europe in cats, and called Distoma felineum Rivolta.

Pathologic Anatomy.—Sometimes distomata produce only very slight disturbances. They have often been found first at the autopsy, or they are discovered in the stools, and in the absence of symptoms (Pallas, Fortassin, Wyss, Virchow, and others). On the other hand, fatal and severe diseases have been known to follow their entrance into the bile-ducts. Wherever they lodge, inflammation and dilatation of bile-passages occur, so that cavities are often formed as large as a walnut and resembling cysts. In cases in which the distoma is present in large numbers, as in the Japanese form, the bile-passages are uniformly dilated and may contain hundreds of worms. The walls of the ducts are usually thickened and the liver tissue in their vicinity atrophic (*vide* the Siberian form), or cirrhotic changes may occur and be followed by ascites (Winogradoff). If the cysts are very superficially situated, they may burst and cause death from bleeding into the peritoneum (Chester). Or the distoma may lodge in one of the main stems of the bile-ducts and cause ulceration by the combined action of the suction it exercises and as a result of the pressure of the chitin scales on the membrane lining the duct, particularly if violent contractions occur. Bostroem has shown that in cases of this kind the walls of the bile-passages become thickened; there is atypical proliferation of the epithelium, and hypertrophy of the musculature; the parasite may completely occlude the lumen of the duct, causing retention and absorption of bile.

In the vicinity of the worm there was in this case newly formed connective tissue which led to occlusion of the cystic duct and to hydrops of the gall-bladder. In the contents of the latter distomata were found, a proof that the worms were there before the cystic duct became occluded. Thus the conclusion seems justified that the parasites were the direct cause of the occlusion of the channel. In the case reported by Biermer, there was cicatricial occlusion of the hepatic duct at its point of division, and below the scar a distoma was found. In this instance the bile-passages were filled with a clear, slimy substance. Distoma hepaticum may also be found in the gall-bladder (Partridge). Duval claims to have found several large distomata in the portal vein and in the hepatic branches of this vessel. Miura reports numerous nodules in the peritoneum containing distoma eggs; these seemed to be connected with lymph-channels. They were found in a Japanese who had died of beri-beri, and in whom during life no symptoms attributable to involvement of the liver were observed. In distomiasis the spleen is usually enlarged.

Symptoms.—The pathologic picture is usually quite indefinite, and often there are no important symptoms to be observed. In other cases (Baelz, Biermer, Bostroem, Kirchner, and others) there are pronounced symptoms which point more or less definitely to the liver as the chief seat of the trouble.

There may be pain in the region of the stomach and the liver, loss of appetite (or, on the other hand, bulimia—Baelz), thirst (Sagarra), and constipation, all of these being initial symptoms. Later, there will be a feeling of pressure in the epigastric and the hypochondriac regions as a result of the swelling of the liver. Then vomiting and diarrhea, with the passage of bloody masses, weakness, and lassitude; on the other hand, the general health may remain good for many years (Baelz). In cases in which the hepatic duct becomes occluded (Biermer, Bostroem), icterus develops; in all other cases it is absent, or present in a mild form and of varying intensity. The liver usually enlarges, becomes hard, smooth, and rarely nodular. The gall-bladder may also appear to be enlarged. A tumor of the spleen is, as a rule, present. In the serious cases that end fatally there is cachexia and anemia, due in all probability to hemorrhages from the mucous membranes caused by the parasites. The worms seem to thrive on the bloody masses with which the bile-passages are lined. In some cases the disease is cured; this may even occur after the evacuation of bloody, slimy stools containing large numbers of the worms (Mehlis, Prunac, Wilson, and others). Distoma sinense in particular seems to produce a pathologic picture that resembles the same infection in animals, including enlargement of the liver, fluctuating icterus, an exhausting bloody diarrhea, ascites, edema, and cardiac weakness. Cases reported by J. P. Frank and Kirchner demonstrate that the European species of distoma can also produce a similar picture.

Distomiasis in Siberia resembles the course of cirrhosis of the liver (Winogradoff); in the event that the parasites are evacuated, it is asserted that the disease can be cured.

The discovery of the eggs is diagnostically important. They are passed with the feces and may be found there on microscopic examination, as has been shown by Bostroem, Perroncito, and Baelz.

Prophylaxis consists in the avoidance of unboiled water for drinking purposes, especially such as comes from pools or ditches, and in abstinence from the use of raw water-cress, particularly in regions where distomiasis is frequent.

Treatment consists essentially in the administration of laxatives and of anthelminthics. Prunac gave extractum filicis maris, and Sagarra castor oil, and both witnessed the passage of distomata as the result of the exhibition of these remedies. Bitter-waters and alkaline-saline waters (Karlsbad, etc.) may also be useful.

If the parasite occludes the hepatic duct, operative interference should be considered in order to remove the worm and to reestablish the flow of bile.

LITERATURE.

Aschoff: "Ein Fall von Distomum lanceol. in der menschlichen Leber," "Virchow's Archiv," Bd. cxxx, p. 493.
Braun: "Die thierischen Parasiten," Würzburg, 1895, p. 119.
Budd: Loc cit., p. 444.
Baelz: "Ueber einige neue Parasiten des Menschen," "Berliner klin. Wochenschr.," 1883, p. 234.
Blanchard: "Note sur quelques vers parasit. de l'homme," "Comptes-rendus de la société de biologie," tome vii, Paris, 1891.
Bostroem: "Ueber Distomum hepatic. beim Menschen," "Deutsches Archiv für klin. Medicin," 1883, Bd. xxxiii, p. 557.
Braun: "Ueber ein für den Menschen neues Distomum aus der Leber," "Centralblatt für Bakteriologie und Parasitenkunde," 1894, p. 602.
Chester: "British med. Journal," October 16, 1886.
Cobbold: "Parasites," p. 14, London, 1879.
Davaine: "Traité des entozoaires," 2. éd., Paris, 1877.
Frank, J. P.: "De curandis hominum morbis," vol. v, Liber vi, pars iii, p. 113. Florentiae, 1832.
Ghose-Mackenzie: "The Lancet," 1895, February 2, p. 321.
Humble: "A Case of Dist. Hep. in Man," "British Med. Journal," July 16, 1881.
Küchenmeister: "Die Parasiten," Abtheilung 1, p. 179, Leipzig, 1855.
Leuckart: "Die menschlichen Parasiten," 1879-1886, 2, Aufl., Bd. i, pp. 94 and 355.
Miura: "Fibröse Tuberkel, verursacht durch Parasiteneier," "Virchow's Archiv," Bd. cxvi, p. 310.
Mosler and Peiper: "Thierische Parasiten," Nothnagel's Encyclopedia, Bd. vi, p. 169.
Prunac: "De la douve ou dist. hép. chez l'homme;" "Gazette des hôpitaux," 1878, p. 1147.
Sagarra: "Un caso de dist. hep. en el hombre," "Rev. de med. y chir.," 1890, vol. xiv, p. 505; nach "Centralblatt für Bakteriologie und Parasitenkunde," 1891.
Scheube: "Krankheiten der warmen Länder," Jena, 1896, p. 261.

Distomata Inhabiting the Portal Vein. Distoma Hæmatobium (Bilharzia sanguinis).—This fluke is found in the portal vein, and may cause marked lesions of the liver. These have been observed with particular frequency in Egypt where the parasite is common.

For the morphology and the habits of life compare Loos and the text-books of Leuckart, Davaine, Cobbold, etc. The male is 12 to 14 mm. long and 1 mm. broad. The larger and also thinner female is often found (16 to 18 mm. long, 0.13 mm. broad, within the canalis gynækophorus. The eggs are 0.12 mm. long and 0.04 mm. broad and have a tiny prickle at one end; occasionally the latter is seen on one side.

The worm enters the intestine with contaminated drinking-water which contains the embryo. Thence it makes its way into the portal vein. [A new appearance (*Bilharzia hæmatobia*) has been met with in the larvæ of the bilharzia by Lazarus-Barlow and Douglas,* and commented upon in a recent preliminary note. It would appear that in the case of certain larvæ, while still living, there occurs a formation of spherical bodies, "with double contour and provided with long cilia." The spheres exhibit an intense vibratile movement of protoplasmic granules. The cilia also have been observed in active motion, though usually motionless. The spheres are able to carry on an independent existence. Many authors have described non-ciliated spheres, though none have called attention to the ciliated forms.—ED.] The pathologic process is usually more pronounced in the kidneys and the bladder, and the patient usually succumbs to lesions of these organs. Eggs are often deposited in the liver and cause inflammatory processes. Even when there is no deposition of eggs circulatory disturbances may be produced. The greater the number of parasites present in the portal vein, the more violent the signs of inflammation. Kartulis, among 22 cases of Bilharzia liver, found hypertrophic cirrhosis 12 times, atrophic cirrhosis twice, fatty degeneration twice; in one case there was an abscess following dysentery. In all other respects the microscopic appearance of the organ was normal. The liver is, as a rule, enlarged, hyperemic, and shows proliferation of the connective tissue in the neighborhood of the portal capillaries, round-cell infiltration, and dilatation of the bile-capillaries. The eggs are found in the capillaries or free in the tissues in the periphery of the acini, usually surrounded by round-cells. Sometimes the central portions of the acini will be found degenerated, and the walls of the capillaries thickened, even in the absence of eggs. It is possible that these disturbances are due to the lesion of the kidneys and of the urinary passages. It may also be true that metabolic products of the parasite present in the portal vein are carried to the liver and exercise their toxic effect on the capillaries and the surrounding tissues.

It appears that the parasites can leave the liver by way of the bile-passages. Gautrelet, for instance, found eggs of Bilharzia in a gall-stone that was passed with the symptoms of colic (following a course of Vichy water) by a patient of Willemins, twenty years after a two-year sojourn in Egypt. The eggs were also found in the liver tissue; they were impregnated with bile-pigment and incrusted with carbonate of lime.

In many cases of Distoma hæmatobium no hepatic symptoms are apparent since cirrhotic changes are absent or only mild. Occasionally the patient complains of indefinite pains in the liver region. In

* *British Med. Jour.*, Jan. 3, 1903.

more pronounced and well-developed cases the organ is enlarged, and presents the picture of hypertrophic cirrhosis. Icterus and ascites are rare. Atrophy of the liver has been reported by Kartulis in cases in which there were very many parasites. If concretions form in the bile-passages around the eggs, the symptoms of cholelithiasis may appear.

The diagnosis is based on the presence of characteristic lesions in the urinary organs, hematuria, the passage of eggs in the urine, and of the liver symptoms described.

Treatment is limited to care of the diseased urinary passages, to the administration of a nourishing and strengthening diet, and to the exhibition of iron, etc. If possible, a change of climate should be obtained.

LITERATURE.

Lehrbücher von Cobbold, Davaine, Leuckart, Mosler, und Peiper.

Chaker, Mahomed: "Etude sur l'hématurie d'Egypte," Thèse de Paris, 1890.

Kartulis: "Ueber das Vorkommen der Eier vom Distomum haematobium in den Unterleibsorganen," "Virchow's Archiv," 1895, Bd. xcix, p. 139.

—"Ueber verschiedene Leberkrankheiten in Aegypten," "Verhandlung des viii. Congresses für Hygiene und Demographie in Budapest," 1896, p. 650.

Loos: "Zur Anatomie und Histologie der Bilharzia heamatobia," "Archiv für mikroskopische Anatomie," 1895, Bd. xlvi, p. 1.

(F) PENTASTOMUM DENTICULATUM AND CONSTRICTUM.

Pentastomum denticulatum is the larva of Pentastomum (lingua-tula) tænioides, a parasite found in the nasal cavities, the frontal sinus, the ethmoidal sinus, and in the larynx of the dog, the wolf, and, less frequently, of the horse, the mule, and the sheep. Occasionally it enters the liver of man. The eggs of the parasite are swallowed and the embryos are liberated in the stomach; infection of human beings usually occurs from dogs, the embryos penetrating the liver after perforating the walls of the intestinal tract. They are found with particular frequency in the left lobe of the liver because they can get there by the shortest route after perforating the stomach wall (Zenker). Here the parasite becomes encysted and forms a larva, having numerous prickly processes and rings of chitin, also claws in the region of its cephalo-thorax. In general these animals, despite their formidable appearance, produce very slight disturbances. This may be due to the fact that they produce no toxic products, and also because they leave the intestinal tract as very small embryos and consequently cannot act as carriers of bacteria.

Laudon reports the case of a man who complained of pain in the liver, icterus, and gastric disturbances, epistaxis, and pain in the left nasal cavity for many years; finally he passed a female Pentastomum tænioides. It is a difficult matter to establish a causal connection between the liver affection and the presence of the parasite in this case.

Pentastomata are frequently first found during autopsies. Zenker found the worm 9 times in 168 autopsies performed in Dresden; Heschl 5 times in 20; Wagner once in 10. According to Sievers, they were found in the Pathologic Institute of Kiel 22 times in 3066 autopsies; 17 times in the liver.

Pentastomum constrictum is more dangerous (Linguatula constricta). Pruner found this parasite in the liver of a negro in Cairo (identified

as Pentastomum constrictum by Bilharz and v. Siebold, from its difference
from Pentastomum denticulatum—larger and more prickly). Bilharz
in many cases found it in the liver and the lungs of negroes, and Aitken
mentions two cases of encysted Pentastomum constrictum in the liver
and the lungs. It would appear that this parasite can produce peritonitic irritation, but does not cause any symptoms that point directly
to the liver.

Bilharz und v. Siebold: "Zeitschr. für wissenschaftliche Zoologie," Bd. iv, p. 63.
Cobbold: Loc. cit., p. 259.
Laudon: "Berliner klinische Wochenschr.," 1878, No. 49.
Pruner: "Krankheiten des Orients," 1847, p. 245.
Sievers: "Schmarotzerstatistik," Dissertation, Kiel, 1887.
Zenker: "Zeitschr. für rationelle Medicin," 1854, Bd. v, p. 224.

PARENCHYMATOUS CHANGES AND DEGENERATIONS.

(A) HYPERTROPHY OF THE LIVER.

(Hoppe-Seyler.)

Just as all lesions of the liver that lead to a decrease in the size of
the organ are termed atrophic, so all processes that cause an increase
are called hypertrophic. A great variety of such pathologic processes
may be responsible for an increase in the volume of the organ, as, for
instance, proliferation of interstitial tissues, the development of neoplasms, the deposit of fat, of amyloid, etc., also an increased vascularity
and, finally, the liver-cells themselves may enlarge or proliferate. Only
that increase in the volume of the liver which is due to an increase in the
size and number of the cells is properly called hypertrophy, or hyperplasia, and only this form of enlargement will be discussed in this section.
The words hypertrophy and hyperplasia are employed interchangeably,
and no distinct difference between the two can be formulated from an
anatomic point of view. In general, hypertrophy means enlargement
of the volume of individual hepatic cells, hyperplasia an increase in the
number of these cells. In all processes of this kind, however, that occur
in the liver the two conditions are found coexisting.

We distinguish further between circumscribed and general hypertrophy. The former may be a vicarious or a compensatory enlargement
of certain parts of the liver, to take the place of other parts that have
been destroyed or have become functionally inactive. Again, the enlargement of the liver may be due to a benign, and frequently to a congenital tumor. The so-called vicarious hypertrophy corresponds to
those processes that Ponfick and others have noted in animals after the
experimental extirpation of large portions of the liver (compare page
408). There occurs in this way a substitution for the missing tissue, so
to speak; the acini enlarge, and there is an abundant new-formation
of liver-cells, bile-passages, etc. The same thing occurs in echinococcus
disease, abscess, or destruction of the liver tissue by trauma, syphilis,
etc.

Heller has noted a case in which the right lobe of the liver was almost
completely destroyed by a cystic echinoccocus, and in which the left
lobe enlarged until its size was as great as that of the right one. Dürig,
Reinecke, and others report similar cases. Sometimes the lobus Spigelii

and quadratus also become hypertrophic. The echinococcus alveolaris quite often causes hypertrophic enlargement of those portions of the liver that are not involved by the primary disease, and particularly of the left lobe (Posselt and others). Heller saw a vicarious hypertrophy of the left lobe following (probably) traumatic destruction of the greater portion of the right one. Virchow, in a case of tertiary syphilis, in which a large portion of the liver was destroyed, saw enlargement of the acini as well as of the individual cells of the portion of the organ that remained intact. Reinecke made the same observation. The nodular form of hyperplasia often seen after cirrhosis of the liver is well known; this, too, is a compensatory process, intended to replace destroyed cells. Nodules of this kind may be as large as an apple though, as a rule, they are no larger than a pinhead or a pea. Kretz describes several larger tumors of the liver of this character, in which a distinct enlargement of the acini and an increase in the volume of the cells were seen. Sometimes structures of this character form transition stages to malignant adenomata, and to certain forms of carcinomata of the liver (Schuppel). Kelsch and Kiener have described similar processes in the liver following malaria.

In certain cases of partial hypertrophy there are benign tumors, often congenital, which probably belong to the class of malformations. Rokitansky, Hoffman, Klob, Mahomed, Simmonds, and Beneke have described tumors of this kind in which the acinous structure was indistinct, and which did not seem to participate in the functions of the liver. However, they were not involved in the diseases of the latter organ. Occasionally these growths are separated from the parenchyma by a connective-tissue capsule; in other cases they are not distinguishable from their surroundings. They have been discussed at length in the section on tumors (compare page 766).

General hypertrophy and hyperplasia of the liver is seen in very vigorous people that are addicted to the abuse of alcohol. In cases of this kind the organ is usually very vascular and contains much secretion in the bile-passages; the acini are not enlarged, but are more numerous than normal. No changes are seen in the cells of the liver.

The margin of the organ is rounded, and the liver is more solid than normal. In diabetes mellitus, also, the liver may present a similar appearance to the naked eye. On microscopic examination it will be found that the liver cells are filled with glycogen. As a result they are distended and rounded; their protoplasm is shiny and slightly granular. On the addition of a solution of iodid of potash in iodin the cell-contents are colored red. As the amount of glycogen in the liver-cells varies in different cases of diabetes, this change may be absent, and, in fact, is absent in the majority of cases, particularly if they are examined in the later stages of the disease. Under different circumstances the liver may be atrophic, flaccid, or tough, and the cells may be angular, not enlarged, and in a state of fatty degeneration.

In the case of people who make their residence in the tropics the liver is frequently found to be enlarged very soon after their arrival; and as soon as they remove from the tropics a reduction in the size of the organ may take place (Heymann). This enlargement has been termed hypertrophy in cases in which no abscesses, etc., developed, and where all inflammatory symptoms were absent. It seems probable, however, that changes of this character are to a large extent due to inflammatory processes, hyperemia of the organ, etc., and are due to the absorption of

53

toxic substances from the intestine, the blood, etc. With respect to this point we would refer to the sections on hyperemia and hepatitis (compare page 614 and page 626).

In **leukemia** and **pseudoleukemia** there is a general enlargement of the liver and an increase in the size of the majority of the liver-cells. Infiltration of the connective tissue, however, and distention of the capillaries with leukocytes, as well as the formation of lymphomata, all play their part in the process, and it is therefore more practical to discuss this form of hypertrophy in a separate paragraph in the section on tumors.

The **symptom-complex** of simple hypertrophy eventually consists in the presence of a hepatic tumor, which may cause a feeling of pressure to the patient, but otherwise gives no evidence of its existence.

In **circumscribed hypertrophy or hyperplasia** round tumors may occasionally be felt, of medium consistency; this is especially true if they happen to be situated in a portion of the surface that is accessible to palpation, or upon the margin of the liver. They may easily be confused with malignant tumors, though the absence of cachexia and metastases, the fact that the tumors develop slowly or do not grow at all, that they show no tendency to degeneration, etc., and finally exploratory incision, will prevent such an error in the diagnosis. Congenital tumors of this nature are very rare. In nodular hyperplasia the signs of cirrhosis are usually quite pronounced, and sometimes the vicarious enlargement of a lobe to replace the diseased or absent portions of the organ can be determined both by percussion and palpation.

General hypertrophy is manifested by an enlargement of the organ that can easily be determined by palpation or percussion. Often the liver is more resistant than normal. Symptoms of stasis in the portal system and in the bile-passages are altogether absent. Sometimes it may be possible to discover an increased production of bile, with an increased quantity of urobilin in the urine and in the stools.

There is no need of any special **therapy** in simple hypertrophy, either of a local or a general kind. The removal of hyperplastic hepatic tumors of the liver is of no avail, and the treatment of diabetes is not modified in any way by the presence of an enlarged liver.

(For nodular hyperplasia, hypertrophic hepatic enlargements, see Tumors, p. 783.)
Dürig: "Ueber vicariirende Hypertrophie," "Munchener med. Abhandlungen,"
    I, Reihe, 13. Heft.
Frerichs: "Klinik der Leberkrankheiten," Bd. II, p. 201.
Heller: "Mangelhafte Entwickelung des rechten Leberlappens," "Virchow's Archiv,"
    1876, Bd. LI, p. 355.
—Ziemssen's "Handbuch der speciellen Pathologie und Therapie," Bd. VIII,
    1. Halfte, 1. Abtheilung, p. 431.
Heymann: "Ueber Krankheiten in den Tropenlaändern," "Verhandlungen der
    physikalischmed. Gesellschaft in Würzburg," 1855, Bd. V, p. 40.
Klebs: "Handbuch der pathologischen Anatomie," 1869, Bd. I, 1. Abtheilung,
    p. 370.
Ponfick: "Experimentelle Beiträge zur Pathologie der Leber," "Virchow's Archiv,"
    1895, Supplement zu Bd. CXXXVIII, p. 81.
Posselt: "Der multiloculare Echinococcus in Tirol," "Deutsches Archiv für klin.
    Medicin," 1897, Bd. LIX, p. 1.
Reinecke: "Compensatorische Leberhypertrophie," Ziegler's "Beiträge zur patho-
    logischen Anatomie," Bd. XXIII, p. 238.
Rindfleisch: "Lehrbuch der pathologischen Gewebelehre," p. 411.
Thierfelder: "Ziemssen's Handbuch," 1878, Bd. VIII, 1. Hälfte, 1, Abtheilung, p. 377.
Virchow: "Ueber die Natur der constitutionellen syphilitischen Affection," "Vir-
    chow's Archiv," 1858, Bd. XV, p. 281.

(B) FATTY LIVER.

(Hoppe–Seyler.)

We include in the term fatty liver all processes in the organ that are characterized by an increased presence of fat. Under normal conditions the amount of fat present in the liver varies, and is dependent upon the character of the food. An abundant ingestion of fat increases the fat in the liver a few hours after eating, so that the peripheral cells of the acini contain more fat-globules at this time than several hours later. With regard to the physiology of this process we would refer to our introductory discussion on page 414. Under certain pathologic conditions we sometimes see a constant presence of 40 % of fat in the liver, instead of the normal 3 % to 5 %.

An abnormally large quantity of fat can usually be discovered in the liver from the naked-eye appearance. Such an appearance may, however, be the result of an increased imbibition of the parencyhma of the liver with fat, in the absence of any pathologic fatty change in the protoplasm of the hepatic cells; or, again, the accumulation of fat in the liver-cells may be present at the same time with lesions of the cell-contents, as, for instance, degeneration of the protoplasm and of the nucleus, necrobiosis, and fatty degeneration of the parenchyma. Clinically these two forms of fatty liver should be distinctly separated. If the parenchyma of the liver is affected, and is involved in a degenerative process, and can no longer functionate normally, the disturbances will be considerable. If, on the other hand, the parenchyma is not degenerated and merely contains a little more fat than normally, general symptoms will seldom be observed, because the functionating power of the organ remains intact. For this reason fatty degeneration is chemically to be differentiated from fatty infiltration. It has been shown, however, that these two conditions may be present in combination, and that there may be an imbibition of fat (as in simple infiltration) in addition to a degeneration of the liver-cells with a disappearance of their protoplasm and replacement of the latter by fat. Also that as soon as the liver-cells become infiltrated with fat to such a degree that the function of the cells is damaged, a degeneration of protoplasm will occur that resembles closely the primary degeneration described above.

Formerly the difference between fatty infiltration and fatty degeneration was considered to be the following: It was believed in the first place, that in fatty infiltration the fat was derived from the food, or from the fat deposits throughout the body, whereas in degeneration it was formed from the dying protoplasm and the proteid constituents of the cell itself. These views were founded chiefly upon the teaching of Voit, who stated that the fat of the body, provided it was not introduced with the food, was chiefly formed from albumin; Liebig, on the other hand, believed that it was derived from the carbohydrates. This view was the dominant one for many years, notwithstanding the objections formulated by F. Hoppe-Seyler. After Pflüger, however, in a series of carefully executed metabolic experiments, had reasserted the correctness of Liebig's view, considerable discussion arose, and to-day the proteid of the protoplasm is no longer considered to be the source of fat in fatty degeneration, and it is believed that this fat comes from the subcutaneous adipose tissue, etc. The experiments of Lebedeff and Rosenfeld lend strong support to this theory.

The latter was able to demonstrate that even in the form of hepatic degeneration produced by phosphorus, the large quantity of fat found in the liver-cell is carried there mainly from the other fat deposits of the body. Thus in dogs fed with mutton fat until the greater part of their fat consisted of the latter, and then starved and later poisoned with phosphorus, the liver-cells were found distended with fat, and this fat was mutton fat.

Lebedeff even before this time had called attention to the fact that the fat of the liver and of the adipose layers was always the same, and that after feeding linseed oil to a dog that had been poisoned with phosphorus, foreign fat was found in the liver, and that consequently the fat of the liver could not have been formed from proteid but must have come from the adipose layer of the body.

It was also shown that in the case of chickens, starved until there was no more fat present in their bodies, fatty liver did not occur after phosphorus-poisoning. In such cases the fat had plainly not been formed from the proteid of the liver-cells.

It would be too radical, however, to disclaim the possibility of the formation of fat from cellular proteid under certain pathologic conditions. That this can occur is indicated by the fact that carbohydrate is readily formed from proteid, and, as we know, fat can be formed from carbohydrate. The presence in certain cells of lecithin also signifies a fat-forming process within these cells (Heffter).

Previous analyses had already shown that in phosphorus liver the amount of fat present did not correspond to the amount of proteid lost (v. Starck and others); and that for this reason the greater part of the fat found in the liver must be derived from the fatty parts of the body. Thus in addition to a degeneration, an infiltration had to be assumed.

Infiltration of the liver-cells with fat is also found in degeneration of their protoplasm, such as is seen in phosphorus-poisoning. Degeneration of the protoplasm can, of course, be determined by the increased nitrogen excretion in the urine.

For all these reasons it is impossible to draw a sharp distinction between fatty infiltration and fatty degeneration of the liver.

The appearance of fat and the disappearance of the cellular elements of the liver parenchyma is probably analogous to the formation of fat in contraction of certain organs, as the kidneys, the pancreas, and the muscles.

All that we can really say is that a pathologic accumulation of fat may occur in the liver without degeneration and without functional impairment of the cells; and, again, that it may equally well occur with serious alterations of the cell protoplasm. Clinical symptoms are slight or altogether absent in the event of the function of the liver-cells remaining intact, even though the fat deposit may be great. Distinct symptoms appear, however, if the protoplasm and nucleus of the cell itself are affected. We may say, therefore, that in fatty liver the fat itself plays no essential rôle in the causation of the clinical pathologic picture, notwithstanding the fact that it is the most conspicuous feature, both macroscopically and microscopically. The chief point is the condition of the cell-contents.

Etiology.—A marked deposit of fat in the liver may be the result of anomalies in the mode of life, in the general constitution of the patient, and in the quality and quantity of the food.

If a diet rich in fat and carbohydrates is taken for a long time, the quantity of fat in the liver-cells increases as well as in all parts of the body. The liver in this case acts as a reservoir; for this reason the livers of children who drink very much milk, and of adults who eat large quantities of fatty and carbohydrate food, contain very much fat.

In fattening animals food containing an excess of carbohydrate is given (*e. g.,* maize or noodles in geese), and a fatty liver is produced in this manner. Also when the yolk is absorbed, the chick embryo shows an accumulation of fat in the liver which disappears later on. If dogs are fed with large quantities of fat, fatty liver is developed (Magendie, Frerichs).

The tendency to such an accumulation of fat is encouraged by lack of exercise, of bodily and mental activity, by life in small, warm rooms, because under these circumstances metabolism is not active, and oxidation processes are less thorough. Under these circumstances the carbohydrates are not completely decomposed into carbonic acid and water, and instead, owing to deficient oxygenation, fat is formed from them. For this reason fatty liver is seen in people who do not exercise very much, who shirk mental effort, and like to sit still in warm rooms. In prisoners, or in people who have to remain in bed for a long time (rest-cure), in paralyzed people, etc., an enormous deposit of fat may occur. Animals that are to be fattened are kept in narrow, warm stables for the same reason.

It still appears to be questionable whether the acute fatty degeneration of the new-born can be attributed to anomalies in the supply of nourishment. A similar condition is seen in lambs and hogs (Fürstenberg, Roloff), developing during fetal life. It is attributed to deficient exercise and to a deficient ingestion of salt by the mother, followed by an excessive production of fat, and consequently by an abnormal quantity of fat in the blood. The milk of these animals also contains more fat than normal. Birch-Hirschfeld attributes the condition in men partly to umbilical infection, which naturally would first involve the liver. In other words, he considers the condition as an infectious form of fatty liver. Infections of the body that start from other points—for instance, the intestinal tract—must also be prominently considered.

In obesity proper there seems to be on the part of the tissues a particular tendency to the formation of fat that has never been explained. Such phrases as reduced vitality, deficient oxidation-powers of the cells, etc., have been employed, without offering anything new in the way of an explanation. Obesity and fatty liver undoubtedly occur in many families. The condition is particularly frequent in the middle years of life, and is seen more frequently in women than in men, and particularly in the former after the menopause. The same result is brought about by castration, and disturbances of the thyroid gland are also said to favor a deposit of fat. That all these unexplained processes play a rôle in the formation of fat is certain; yet people are seen who indulge in a diet containing abundant fats and carbohydrates, who do not exercise the body or the mind, and whose digestive organs are perfectly normal, and who, nevertheless, do not grow fat; whereas, on the other hand, certain people, although they eat very little, grow very corpulent.

That there must be some hereditary, racial peculiarity is indicated by experience in cattle-raising also (English hogs, certain forms of cattle, etc.).

It has been claimed that in obese subjects there is a deficient secretion of bile, and as a result a decreased elimination of fat by these channels from the liver, so that ultimately there is an accumulation of fat. This view, however, is purely hypothetic, since we are as yet unable to measure the quantity and the composition of the bile secreted by the liver during life.

The process of oxidation in the tissues is, of course, seriously diminished if there is a deficient supply of oxygen, such as may be due to a lack of hemoglobin in the blood. For this reason an abnormal deposit of fat, particularly in the liver, readily occurs in anemia (chlorosis, leukemia, pernicious anemia). Moreover, a large proportion of obese people, particularly women, are anemic. If blood is repeatedly withdrawn from animals, the fattening process is aided; this procedure corresponds to the processes that take place in certain intoxications that lead to fatty liver. The fatty liver of consumptives has been attributed to lack of oxygen following a decrease in the breathing-space of the lungs. In other diseases of the lungs, however, as in emphysema, pneumonia, contraction of the lungs from pleurisy, etc., fatty liver is not found, so that we must assume that in the former disease other factors are concerned. Disturbances of the circulation, as in congestion of the liver and in tumor-formation, frequently lead to a fatty degeneration of the liver-cells. Thus fatty change of the peripheral portions of the acini is seen in venous stasis, forming the well-known picture of nutmeg liver. The red center of the acini is clearly distinguished from its yellowish periphery. In carcinomata and other tumors a zone of fatty tissue surrounds the growth.

Intoxications of varying kind play a very important rôle in fatty degeneration of the liver. The action of such a poison may consist in a direct effect upon the protoplasm of the cell, causing degeneration and a replacement of the destroyed protoplasm by fat; or the effect of the poison may be exercised upon the blood, causing a destruction of hemoglobin, and consequently a reduction in the oxygen-carrying function of the blood. Here we see the same conditions as in anemia (*vide* above). Our knowledge in regard to these different factors is too slight to allow us in any given instance to determine which effect of the poison has produced the changes in the liver.

Phosphorus-poisoning is probably the most important of this class, and has been made the subject of the most careful investigation. Von Hauff was the first to call attention to the hepatic changes in phosphorus-poisoning. His experiments, however, and those of others, as Köhler and Renz, combined with numerous clinical observations, do not enable us to say in what manner phosphorus-poisoning acts upon the parenchymatous cells of the liver. There can be no doubt that oxidative processes are reduced, that hydrolytic processes (particularly in nitrogen-metabolism) are increased, that the syntheses, which occur with the elimination or the formation of water, are hindered. No changes can be demonstrated in the red blood-corpuscles; in fact, they may be increased in the beginning (Taussig, v. Jaksch). In intoxications that do not end fatally within the first few days the amount of hemoglobin is gradually reduced.

Lack of oxygen as a result of destruction of hemoglobin can, therefore, not be regarded as the cause of this anomaly of metabolism. The disturbance of the heart and circulation may, however, be made responsible. In phosphorus-poisoning the amount of oxygen consumed and of carbon dioxid given off are both decreased (Bauer and others), the amount of carbon dioxid in the blood being also reduced (H. Meyer). On the other hand, in cases lasting over a long period, which do not terminate fatally within the first few hours or days, an increased excretion of nitrogen is discovered that must be due to an increased disintegration of proteids

(Storch, Bauer, and others). The urea is often increased. In many cases ending fatally the ammonia-excretion is enormously increased (Englien, Münzer), and there is a corresponding relative decrease in the output of urea. This is due to a disintegration of cells, and to the formation of acid products (lactic acid—Schultzen and Riess, Araki, and others) that require alkali for their neutralization. Münzer's experiments demonstrate that the increased excretion of ammonia is due to an increased formation of acid, and is not a manifestation of the disturbance of the urea-forming function of the liver. This investigator determined that the administration of alkalies decreased the excretion of ammonia, but that in rabbits, which do not possess the power of forming ammonia in acid intoxication, no such increase occurred after phosphorus-poisoning. It may be assumed, therefore, that acid intoxication plays a certain rôle in such cases, and manifests itself by a decrease of the alkalescence of the blood, Occasionally tyrosin or leucin appears, and indicates a disintegration of proteid combined with an insufficient oxygenation of catabolic products (A. Fränkel, Beaumann, and others). Peptone (Schultzen and Riess, Robitschek, and others) or a body similar to it (Harnack) may appear in the urine. These products are, however, only rarely found. As a result of the breaking-up of lecithin, usually after the first stage of the poisoning is over (twenty-four hours), there may be an increase in the excretion of phosphates (Münzer). Nuclein catabolism does not seem to play any rôle in this increased excretion of phosphoric acid, as is determined by the absence of an increase in the uric-acid excretion. Sugar has also occasionally been found in the urine (Bollinger, Huber, Araki).

At first there is a decided fatty infiltration of the liver-cells, beginning a few days after the intoxication with phosphorus, and rapidly leading to a distention of the liver-cells with fat. This may be so intense that nothing can be seen of the nucleus or the protoplasm; these structures, however, remain well preserved, and reappear when the fat is removed. At the same time there is a decrease in the quantity of lecithin present in the liver (Heffter), so that we may assume that a portion of the fat.is formed from this substance. This fact is in harmony with the increased excretion of phosphates already noted. At the expiration of a few days signs of disintegration of the parenchyma appear, manifested by the above-mentioned disturbances of metabolism. In poorly nourished individuals and in such as have only a slight adipose fatty covering, fatty degeneration of the liver develops in phosphorus-poisoning from the very beginning; thus a picture of acute atrophy may be created which ordinarily would not appear before the second week. If death does not occur, as usual, by the end of the first week, atrophy of the liver may take place later on, and, as a rule, in the first half of the second week (Hedderich). The quantity of fat decreases, the liver-cells perish, and a symptom-complex develops similar to that observed in acute yellow atrophy (compare page 641).

Arsenic and **antimony poisoning** may lead to similar fatty degeneration of the liver, as may also intoxication by **copper, mercury,** and **aluminium.** Certain mineral acids, as hydrochloric, sulphuric, and nitric, may also cause moderate degrees of fatty liver. Other substances that may cause the condition are carbon monoxid, petroleum, chloroform, iodoform, ethyl-bromid, nitrous oxid, carbolic acid, phloridzin, ricin, abrin, chronic morphin-poisoning, poisoning with fungi (mushrooms), certain meat-, fish-, and mussel-poisons, spoiled maize (pellagra), etc. In addition to the direct effect on the liver-cells, many of these substances destroy hemoglobin and diminish oxygenation, a process that is often manifested by an increased excretion of lactic acid. Thus in poisoning with many substances that lead to the destruction of hemoglobin fatty degeneration of the parenchyma may be seen. It may be noted, finally, that extensive burns may be responsible for these changes in the liver in the same way.

Fatty degeneration of the liver is especially frequently seen in drunkards. **Chronic alcoholism** leads to deficient oxidation of both the carbohydrates and fats, in that alcohol reduces oxygenation by using up a large proportion of the oxygen for its own combustion. This has been determined from the decrease in the power of assimilation of oxygen, and in the excretion of carbonic acid. As a result there is a great accumulation of fat in all parts of the body, and also in the liver. This condition may be combined with the cirrhotic changes so often produced by alcohol, and thus the picture of cirrhotic fatty liver may be created (Sabourin, Garel, Merklen). Fatty liver is found in the majority of drunkards who die in delirium tremens (Frerichs, Murchison, and others). Pupier, Magnan, Strassmann, Sabourin, and others have succeeded in causing fatty degeneration of the liver experimentally by the administration of small doses of alcohol over a long period of time. Affanassiew and v. Kahlden administered ethyl-alcohol (the first-mentioned author mixed it with amyl-alcohol) during a long period, and observed a consequent infiltration of the stellate and hepatic cells. They did not, however, succeed in producing cirrhosis of the liver, and other authors (Siegenbeck van Heukelom) also failed in this attempt. [*Vide* Cirrhosis for a qualification of this statement by subsequent experimental results.—ED.]

Ungar, Strassmann, and Ostertag have noted fatty degeneration of the liver following prolonged administration of **chloroform,** though it does not appear from their examinations of the tissues whether the cell parenchyma became fatty or whether there was simply a fatty infiltration. A. Fränkel, on the other hand, observed well-developed necrosis of the liver-cells after narcosis of long duration. Certain of the cells were in a state of fatty degeneration.

From a clinical standpoint phosphorus- and alcohol-poisoning furnish the most interesting toxic forms of fatty liver; all the more rare forms of poisoning present conditions in which the general disease-picture is so severe that fatty degeneration of the liver is comparatively of no importance, and is often completely overlooked.

Infectious diseases may also produce fatty liver. Fatty degeneration of the liver-cells occurs chiefly owing to the presence of toxic substances that are produced by bacteria, and act in a similar manner to mineral or vegetable poisons, damaging the protoplasm and perverting nitrogen metabolism. We see fatty liver in septicopyemic diseases, particularly if they are of long duration; for instance, in puerperal fever, osteomyelitis, severe cases of syphilis, prolonged suppuration, etc. The liver in such cases often has fatty degeneration that can be detected with the naked eye; the organ is large, soft, frequently fragile, and of a distinct yellowish color. Charrin and others have succeeded in producing fatty degeneration of the liver in animals by injecting cultures of Bacillus pyocyaneus. In many cases there is so much hyperemia in the infectious form of fatty liver that the fat cannot be recognized with the naked eye, and only microscopic examination reveals its presence. Fatty degeneration is also seen in smallpox, in severe cases of diphtheria and scarlatina, and occasionally in typhoid, cholera, pneumonia, and eclampsia, though it is not clinically significant. In diphtheria it is probably exclusively due to the actions of toxins.

Certain diseases of the digestive tract may also lead to fatty degenerations of the liver; as, for instance, chronic dysentery, and in children catarrhs of the gastrointestinal tract. [A thorough study of the changes in the liver in gastroenteritis of infancy has been published by Lesle and Merklen.* They found no specific changes, and in the main an epithelial degeneration or sclerosis or simple congestion, according to the duration of the disease. Glycosuria they found sometimes to occur in the chronic but not in the acute forms, and ascribed its occurrence to faulty hepatic action.—ED.] It is possible that the fatty liver frequently seen in rachitic children also belongs in this category.

In infectious diseases inflammatory processes are frequently though not always seen, coexistent with degenerative changes. This feature distinguishes such a fatty liver from that seen after pure intoxications, the characteristics of which we have described in another place in the section on hepatitis as well as those of fatty degeneration of the liver parenchyma in acute yellow atrophy and in pernicious icterus.

Finally, it should be observed that fatty liver is often seen in **phthisis.** In cases of this kind fat is frequently found in the blood, and may be present in such abundance as to give the serum a milky appearance. We are justified, therefore, in assuming that the fat found in the liver is deposited there from the adipose tissues of the body which are in a state of rapid dissolution. For this reason fatty liver is more frequently seen in tuberculous women than in men, since the former have, as a rule, larger fat deposits. When fatty liver is found in men, it is usually observed that the subject has been well nourished previously. Certain toxic substances that are formed in tuberculous foci, particularly in the presence of a mixed infection or in autointoxications, and other toxic principles formed in the intestine, may also play a rôle. Drugs, especially such as are destructive to the hemoglobin; certain narcotics which are frequently administered in large quantities; and, finally the overabundance and the fatty character of the food usually given to phthisical subjects (cod-liver oil, alcohol); may all be concerned in the process.

Fatty liver often develops in subjects suffering from **carcinoma** or other malignant tumors. Here the condition is probably due to a rapid loss of the adipose layer and the transportation of this fat to the liver. The reason for this occurrence we understand all too imperfectly. To what extent the rapidly appearing anemia, or how far the toxic products that are formed in the neoplasm or as the result of micro-organismal action, play a rôle, it is difficult to state.

The etiology and pathogenesis of fatty liver are still obscure. We know too little of the processes that occur in a cell during fatty degeneration; moreover, the causes of fatty infiltration have been so imperfectly studied, owing to the complicated processes in the liver, in which degeneration and infiltration are so closely related and so often coexistent, that it is difficult even to speculate as to the probable sequence of events in the hepatic cells. [Freeman† has made an extensive study of fatty liver, and finds that it occurs with considerable frequency in infants and children. The general condition of the child, as measured by the body fat

* *Revue Mens. des Med. de l'Enf.*, Feb. 1, 1901.
† *Archives of Pediatrics*, Feb., 1900.

seemed to have no relation to the fat deposit in the liver. He also found that fatty liver occurs rarely in the following wasting diseases: Marasmus, malnutrition, rachitis, syphilis, unless an acute disease be superimposed. In tuberculosis he finds it not more frequent than in other diseases. Most often it was found to be associated with acute infectious diseases and gastro-intestinal disorders.—Ed.]

Pathologic Anatomy.—A fatty liver in which there is simple infiltration is usually increased in all diameters, and may weigh as much as 4 kg. It has a low specific gravity, however, and will readily float in water. In a normal liver there is from 1.8 % to 5 % of fat, and 72 % to 78 % of water; in fatty infiltration there is from 19 % to 43 % of fat and only 62 % to 43 % of water (Perls). In phosphorus liver there is from 17 % to 32 % of fat, and only 66 % to 57 % of water (Perls, v. Höslin, Lebedeff, v. Starck).

The margin of the organ is usually rounded, and its surface is smooth and shiny except in those cases in which cirrhotic processes such as are due to alcoholism (cirrhotic fatty liver) cause retraction of tissue and granular protuberances. The liver is usually of a yellow color, and sometimes the small veins may be seen arranged in little stars through the surface. The outlines of the acini are clear, but often not as distinct as in the normal organ. The consistency is usually increased, at least in the dead; this may, however, be due to a solidification of the fat following postmortem cooling. A fatty liver that is warmed to the body-temperature is usually much softer and the imprint of the fingers can be clearly seen on its surface. In the dead the vascularity also appears to be less than is actually the case. Although during life the cells are distended with fat, and as a result the blood-vessels are somewhat narrowed, still this distention is not so great as it appears in the dead organ; thus it may be said that stasis seldom occurs in the portal area as a result of uncomplicated fatty liver. On transverse section the yellow color and the slight vascularity are conspicuous features. The blade of the knife is covered with grayish-white fat; the acini usually protrude somewhat over the cut surface. If, at the same time, there is stasis as a result of deficient heart action or of some obstruction in the lesser circulation, the middle of each acinus will be reddish, and the multicolored picture of nutmeg liver will be presented.

In cases in which there are present fats with a melting-point higher than the ordinary, as the glycerids of stearin and palmitin, the liver appears more translucent and whitish, like wax, or somewhat yellowish in color. It is less dense if more oleic acid is present (Rokitansky).

Icterus is absent in that form of simple fatty infiltration which is found in obese, in phthisical, in cachectic, and in anemic persons. It has been stated that the bile is scanty in these cases, and that, when the process is severe, it contains no pigment; the foregoing is true probably in exceptional cases only, in which other pathologic processes are actively present in the liver at the same time.

The **microscope** reveals an enormous number of large and small fat-globules in the acini; these may be so numerous that nothing is seen of the cells. This appearance is particularly striking in the periphery of the acini. If the fat is extracted, it will then be found that the protoplasm and the nuclei of the cells are well preserved, and that both can be demonstrated with the ordinary stains.

Occasionally fatty infiltration appears in the form of small fat nodules near the edge of the acini. This is often seen in phthisis (Sabourin.)

A similar picture is seen in cases of marked fatty degeneration of the liver following intoxications, for instance, during the first week of phosphorus-poisoning. The contour of the organ remains the same, but the abundant deposit of fat is shown in the color and in the greasy coating on the section knife. In cases of this kind icterus usually appears after a few days, so that the surface as well as the transverse section of the organ appear saffron yellow.

In experimental phosphorus-poisoning the fat is seen in the liver-cells, and also in Kupffer's stellate cells. At the same time, degeneration of nuclei and vacuolization of protoplasm are frequently noted (Ziegler and Obolenski, and others). Sometimes focal necrosis is seen. In arsenic-poisoning very similar changes are seen in the parenchyma, though of not quite so pronounced a type (Ziegler and Obolenski, Wolkow, and others).

Here and there small hemorrhagic foci are observed in the liver tissue. In the biliary pasages and in the gall-bladder there is a pale, slimy bile. In the first stages of poisoning, when icterus is absent the bile in the passages contain more bile-pigment than normal owing to irritation of the liver-cells. Icterus is probably due both to an occlusion of the small bile-passages, and to injury of the cell protoplasm, so that the bile constituents are no longer excluded from the blood (see page 426).

In cases of intoxication that terminate fatally within a few hours fatty degeneration is absent. If the intoxication is not so severe, however, and if death fails to occur within the first few days, atrophy is sometimes seen as early as the second week; the liver then decreases in size and grows soft and flabby, and small reddish areas are seen in a yellowish matrix. In the reddish portions the liver parenchyma is found to have disappeared.

On microscopic examination of an ordinary case of phosphorus intoxication the liver-cells will be distended with fat, whereas the majority show no changes of their protoplasm or their nuclei. In the bile-passages will be seen a scanty amount of slimy, colorless bile. In cases that persist for a long time, necrosis of the liver-cells is observed in the center of the acini, so that nothing remains but fat-globules, granules, and detritus, all of which are bile-tinged.

In cases of this kind the similarity to acute yellow atrophy is so great that some authors have identified the two conditions. A careful histologic examination, however, reveals the distinct differences (compare page 633).

Mannkopf and others have described an interstitial proliferation of connective tissue between the acini combined with round-cell infiltration. This condition is not found in many cases of acute phosphorus-poisoning, though if the intoxication is carried on with small doses and over a long time (Wegner, in rabbits) these changes are indeed seen (Weyl, Aufrecht, Ackermann, and others).

Other authors, again, have failed to find such interstitial changes under the same conditions (Krönig, Dinckler, Ziegler and Obolenski).

In pregnant women the effect of acute phosphorus-poisoning is manifested in the liver of the fetus, which may be found in a condition of fatty degeneration (Friedländer, Miura).

Alcoholic fatty liver differs in no way from that seen in obesity, cachexia, etc. Here, too, proliferation of the interstitial tissues is occasionally seen, particularly around the branches of the portal vein (Sabourin and others). The liver is large and hard, and the contractions on its surface and on transverse section result in distinct cicatricial indentations where the intra-acinous tissues existed. These cases probably consist of fatty liver complicated by cirrhosis; possibly both conditions originate at the same time. They are seen particularly in subjects that are obese. In the ordinary form of alcoholic cirrhosis of the liver such a picture is rare; in the atrophic form of cirrhosis there is a slight fatty degeneration of the liver-cells, but here we are dealing with nutritive disturbances caused by the contraction of connective tissue and by compression of blood-vessels. In the cirrhotic hypertrophic form of fatty liver the fat may come in part from the fatty layers of the body. Tuberculosis is frequently seen in combination with cirrhotic fatty liver (compare pages 730, 732).

As in the case of phthisical subjects, the blood-serum of alcoholics is frequently chylous owing to the abundant quantity of fat suspended in it.

The livers of persons who have died from prolonged **chloroform-narcosis** show, besides an extensive fatty degeneration of the cells, a cellular necrosis (E. Fränkel).

As the poisons reach the liver from the hepatic artery or the portal vein, the first changes of the parenchyma are usually seen in the periphery of the acini; even later on the lesions are all most pronounced in this location.

In many intoxications, and particularly those that are produced by blood-poisons, there is an alteration of the protoplasm together with the formation of fat in the cell; in other words, a fatty degeneration. This may be very slight and be noted at the autopsy merely as an accidental finding of no great import. The chief lesions are usually found in the heart or the kidneys, and have more significance with respect to the course of the disease than the fatty degeneration of the liver.

In **infectious fatty degeneration** of the liver, distinct symptoms of inflammation are often observed that are more appropriately discussed under Hepatitis than in this condition. Only in **septicopyemic forms of hepatic disease** do we witness such an enormous accumulation of fat as in the forms discussed above. Here, too, the liver may be yellow and soft, and very much enlarged. **Gastro-enteritis** in children frequently leads to fatty degeneration of the liver, starting, as a rule, from the periphery of the acini, and only producing a local injury to the cells. as manifested by deficient staining properties of their nuclei. In rare cases there is fatty degeneration, and the cells are completely involved; the process in such case is not only that of degeneration, but of infiltration as well (Thiemich). We may assume that certain metabolic bacterial products exert a toxic action, although the bacteria themselves still are present in the liver-tissue. If certain pathogenic micro-organisms (streptococci, staphylococci, etc.) make their way into the liver, there will be found localized areas of fatty degeneration resulting from necrosis and fatty degeneration of the parenchyma, in addition to round-cell infiltration. Such lesions may precede abscesses of the liver. Circumscribed fatty infiltration is, however, rare (Sabourin). Other changes in the liver parenchyma seen, at the same time with fatty degeneration, in cholera and typhoid, we will not discuss in this connection. In certain cases of fatty degeneration due to infection the condition cannot be recognized owing to the marked hyperemia, and can only be discovered microscopically.

Symptoms.—In ordinary fatty liver, such as occurs in obesity, anemia, cachexia, phthisis, etc., also, as a rule, in alcoholism, the organ is soft, and often extends well into the abdomen, though its outline can be determined better by percussion than by palpation owing to the softness of the tissue. Especially in obese people are the outlines of the organ very difficult to determine, and it may be impossible to palpate the margin.

In carcinoma and phthisis where the adipose layers and the muscles are reduced, the enlarged liver may be seen as a prominent tumor, and can usually be readily palpated. In such cases, also, the soft character of the liver is conspicuous, and the feeling is created that the organ might be indented by the pressure of the fingers. Amyloid liver appears of the same general form as fatty liver; it is, however, if anything, harder than normal, and can thus be readily differentiated. The surface of simple fatty liver is smooth, the margin is rounded, and the general contour unchanged, despite the enlargement.

If the fatty layer disappears, small fat-nodules frequently remain in the subcutaneous tissue, and may simulate small nodular protuberances on the surface of the liver. This occurs particularly often in cachexia. If the patient is instructed to breathe deeply, it will be found that these nodules do not move with the liver, and alter their position only slightly.

Percussion dulness extends further down into the abdomen than normally; as a rule, its area is not increased upward. The liver is not painful to pressure, and the patient does not complain of spontaneous pain; frequently there are no subjective symptoms whatever. Occasionally the patient will complain of a feeling of pressure and fulness in the right side or in the epigastric region. In uncomplicated fatty liver symptoms of portal stasis are absent. Ascites and splenic tumor are never seen as the result of simple fatty degeneration of the liver. If such symptoms are present, they indicate a complicating cirrhosis. There may also be present carcinomatous and tuberculous lesions of the peritoneum or the spleen may be enlarged from some previous disease, or may be another symptom of the primary disease (as, for instance, leukemia) which is the cause of the fatty liver. It is possible that in severe degrees of fatty liver there may be, after all, a slight hindrance to the flow of portal blood as manifested by chronic catarrh of the intestinal tract. There may also be gastric disturbances, lack of appetite, a tendency to meteorism, flatulence, constipation, slimy stools that occasionally become diarrheic, and hemorrhoids, all symptoms attributable to the congestive catarrh. These symptoms can, of course, also be explained by the improper mode of living that is so frequently seen in obese subjects who live an easy life.

Icterus is not a symptom of fatty liver, owing to the fact that the fat cannot compress the bile-passages and lead to icterus from stasis; also because there are no disturbances of the cell protoplasm to favor the entrance of bile-products into the blood. The production of bile may be so slight in many cases that very little enters the intestine. This is particularly true in cases of deficient feeding, or in cases of reduced digestive and assimilative powers, as, for instance, in carcinoma, phthisis, anemia, etc. In diseases of this character the secretion of bile will be diminished, and consequently the production of bile-pigment; so that an analysis of the urine may even reveal a decrease of urobilin. If there is marked disintegration of blood-pigment, or if there are hemorrhages in the internal organs, the quantity of urobilin will appear to be increased; but later, even under these circumstances, it may be decreased. If the biliary secretion is deficient, the stools assume a whitish-gray color and a clay-like consistency; in other words, they become acholic.

The appearance of the patient and the condition of the other organs will naturally depend upon the primary disease; thus, the fatty covering and the large limbs of obese people and of alcoholics are in distinct contrast to the excessive emaciation and the loss of muscle-tissue as seen in phthisis, carcinoma, etc. In the first category, the vascularity of the skin and the mucous membranes is increased, and there is frequently some disturbance of the action of the heart, so that cyanosis appears; whereas in the latter form of diseases the skin is pale and yellowish-white. There are no characteristic lesions of the skin, as claimed by Addison and others. The latter is fatty and oily in some cases of obesity and alcoholism; in cachexia, however, it is very fragile and dry, shows a tendency to desquamate, and is a true pityriasis tabescentium. Occasionally edema and anasarca are seen; they are due to some primary disease, and are not, as has been claimed by some, the result of fatty liver. Anemia and cachexia are frequently found at the same time, in the same subject.

The changes in the liver exert scarcely any influence upon the course and the outcome of the disease. Disturbances in other organs, particularly in the heart, are much more important. The patient may die after weeks or months or years, as might be expected from the primary disease; or he may succumb to heart failure following myocarditis, or fatty degeneration of the heart muscle, or to some intercurrent disease, to marasmus, severe anemia, apoplexy, kidney lesions, etc.

Toxic fatty liver, as, for instance, that of phosphorus-poisoning, has an important bearing with reference to the subsequent course of the disease. Here, too, however, the degeneration of the heart muscle is the chief cause of death. In the first stage, that lasts only twenty-four hours, no hepatic symptoms are noticed. The chief symptoms of this stage are gastro-intestinal; there is vomiting of masses containing phosphorus, pain in the epigastric region, etc. Death may occur if large quantities of poison are introduced in a readily absorbable form; such cases are, however, rare. On the other hand, if the poison is ingested in a form that is only slightly soluble, or not soluble at all, or in case vomiting occurs, or lavage is instituted, the disease may be cured without having caused any other symptoms than the gastric disturbances described. The patient usually feels better before entering upon the second stage. This period of comparative well-being lasts two or three days, so that the impression is created that the case is cured. During this time there are usually a slight loss of appetite, pain in the region of the stomach, and constipation. On the third or the fourth day of the disease, rarely sooner, sometimes a few days later, icterus of the skin and mucous membranes appears, combined with other symptoms of absorption of bile-constituents in the blood; i. e., the presence of bile-pigment in the urine, decoloration of the feces, and sometimes urticaria. The icterus increases rapidly in intensity, more rarely it creates only a slight yellowish discoloration of the skin. At this time a feeling of tension and pain appears in the liver region, the organ may be enlarged, sensitive to pressure, and feel tougher. The surface remains smooth. The enlargement is usually uniform, and is rarely seen in one lobe only. In the course of the following days the volume of the organ continues to increase.

In rare cases there is not only no enlargement, but a gradual decrease in the size of the organ. (For definite instances see Hedderich.)

Other symptoms are painful vomiting, and frequently of bloody masses. The pulse is at first slow, and later, shortly before death, is very rapid, and at the same time small and weak. The heart is dilated, the sounds not clear, and there are blowing murmurs at the orifices. Bloody diarrhea and hemorrhages into the skin and the mucous membranes may be seen, and occasionally there is rise of temperature. Just before death the temperature may either become subnormal or may be very much elevated. Death usually occurs at the end of the first week, and frequently sooner, occasionally during the second week. In many cases a decrease in the size of the liver is noted before death as a result of the disintegration of the liver substance. This is seen particularly in cases that live into the second week. (Compare Hedderich.) The mental faculties remain clear until the end. Death either occurs rapidly in collapse; or there may be delirium, coma, or convulsions, as in other forms of typical hepatic intoxication (cholemia).

If the disease persists for more than a week, the case may recover, the icterus decrease, and the liver regain its normal size. Even if a certain amount of atrophy has occurred regeneration seems possible, and the organ gradually grows, the appetite returns (in fact, the patient may be very hungry), and the case recovers. Convalescence is usually very protracted, and may extend over many weeks.

West describes the case of a woman who recovered from phosphorus-poisoning but who, several weeks after recovery, suddenly developed icterus and a swelling of the liver, and died six days later. He attributes this to the disintegration of the liver-cells following the intoxication. It is possible that there is a connection only in the sense that the liver was already diseased, and that an intercurrent infection destroyed the patient. As the bile-passages frequently contain bacteria, especially if the secretion of bile is deficient, it is possible that many cases of atrophy of the liver and degeneration of the parenchyma are caused by the action of these germs. Experimental investigations in this respect are not extant. [*Vide* Experimental Procedures, under *Alcoholic Cirrhosis.*—Ed.]

There are marked changes in the quantity and the composition of the urine. Bile-pigment and bile-acids are present, and, in severe cases, lactic acid, peptone [albumoses.—Ed.] and, rarely, tyrosin. Urobilin is often present in abundance; it may then disappear, but reappears during convalescence (Riva, Lanz). The excretion of nitrogen and of phosphoric acid and the marked amount of ammonia have already been discussed. The excretion of chlorin is decreased as a result of the small ingestion of food. Sometimes, in the earlier stages, or, in certain cases, toward the end of the disease, albumin may appear in small quantities; also casts or bile-tinged kidney epithelium in a state of fatty degeneration. There may also be blood-corpuscles, crystals of hematoidin, etc., in the sediment. Sugar is rarely excreted. The quantity of urine is decreased as the disease progresses, and may even lead to complete anuria shortly before death. Re-establishment of the flow of urine is a good prognostic sign. During convalescence there may be great diuresis.

Alcoholic fatty liver corresponds to the picture described under ordinary infiltration.

If fatty liver and cirrhosis are combined, the condition is manifested by the increased resistance of the organ on palpation. The latter is enlarged, and its surface is smooth, as in simple fatty infiltration. If the cirrhotic process assumes such a degree that the circulation is interfered with in the intra-acinous connective tissue, symptoms of stasis of the portal system appear, such as tumor of the spleen, ascites, congestive catarrhs, and collateral venous enlargements. The consistency of the liver is increased, and the surface may appear nodular as a result of the contraction of connective tissue and a protrusion of the parenchyma between the cicatricial depressions. The increased quantity of fat in the superficial layers and ascites may render the recognition of these surface peculiarities difficult. The course of the disease corresponds to that of alcoholic cirrhosis (see pages 700, 732). In many other forms of intoxication fatty degeneration of the liver may be produced, and in the same manner as by phosphorus and alcohol, though not in the same degree, and yet no clinical hepatic symptoms may appear. If the organ were carefully examined, it would probably be found enlarged, but as other symptoms about the heart, the kidneys, also the intestines, and the central nervous system, are convincing, and much more prominent, fatty degeneration of the liver is frequently overlooked.

The same statement may be made with regard to infectious diseases, in which the hepatic involvement plays a secondary rôle. If there is actual inflammation of the organ, there may result an abscess of the liver, necrosis, or acute atrophy. The symptoms that may appear under these circumstances correspond to those already described as belonging to these conditions.

Diagnosis.—If the organ is only slightly enlarged, it is impossible to diagnose fatty liver, and for this reason slight degrees of this condition are not discoverable.

Pronounced cases of fatty liver, as in obesity, alcoholism, phthisis, etc., are easily recognized. The condition is to be differentiated from amyloid liver by the softness of the fatty organ; from hyperemia also by the softness and by the absence of pain. Leukemic and pseudoleukemic tumors are harder. The smooth surface and normal contour, the absence of indentations of the margin, the absence of symptoms of stasis of the portal system, are all characteristic. The existence of some primary disease that would be likely to cause fatty liver is also important.

If cirrhosis is combined with fatty liver, as in alcoholics, the organ is enlarged, and more dense than is the ordinary fatty liver, but not as resistant as that of hypertrophic cirrhosis. There may be irregularities on the margin and the surface, and occasionally symptoms of stasis in the portal system.

The differential diagnosis of phosphorus liver, from parenchymatous hepatitis, also from acute yellow atrophy, will be discussed in the appropriate sections.

Prognosis.—The prognosis is dependent upon the primary disease.

Treatment.—The treatment will also depend upon the primary cause. In obesity it is necessary to withdraw fats and carbohydrates and to decrease the formation of fat by other measures. Alcoholic beverages should be forbidden, and metabolism stimulated by exercise in the open air, by gymnastics, etc. We cannot, however, enter into the details of these measures, and refer to the discussion of the treatment in the article on "Obesity."

In the case of fatty liver in phthisical subjects it will be well to limit the ingestion of large quantities of fat, cod liver oil, etc. In cachexia there is no satisfactory therapy. With regard to the treatment of fatty degeneration following intoxication with phosphorus, etc., and resulting from infectious disease, we must refer to the works on poisoning, and infectious diseases, and to the sections on inflammation and atrophy of the liver.

LITERATURE.

Afanassiew: "Zur Pathologie des acuten und chronischen Alkoholismus," Ziegler's "Beiträge zur pathologischen Anatomie," 1890, Bd. viii, p. 443.

Araki: "Beitrag zur Kenntniss der Einwirkung von Phosphor und von arseniger Saure auf den thierischen Organismus," "Zeitschr. fur physiologische Chemie," Bd. xvii, p. 311.

Ackermann: "Virchow's Archiv," 1889, Bd. cxv, p. 216 (phosphorus).

Aufrecht: "Experimentelle Lebercirrhose nach Phosphor," "Deutsches Archiv für klin. Medicin," 1887, Bd. lviii, p. 302.

Badt: "Kritische und klin. Beiträge zur Lehre vom Stoffwechsel bei Phosphorvergiftung," Dissertation, Berlin, 1891.

Birch-Hirschfeld: "Gerhardt's Lehrbuch der Kinderkrankheiten," Bd. iv, 2. Abtheilung, p. 772.

Böhm, Naunyn, and Böck: "Handbuch der Intoxicationen," "Ziemssen's Handbuch," Bd. xv, Leipzig, 1876.

Budd: "Krankheiten der Leber," deutsch von Henoch, 1846, p. 248.

Cohnheim: "Vorlesungen über allgemeine Pathologie," Bd. i, p. 536, Berlin, 1880.

Ehrle: "Charakteristik der acuten Phosphorvergiftung des Menschen," Tübingen, 1861.

Ewald: Artikel: "Fettleber," in Eulenburg's "Realencyklopädie."

Fränkel, E.: "Ueber Chloroformnachwirkung beim Menschen," "Virchow's Archiv," 1892, Bd. cxxix, p. 254.

Frerichs: "Klinik der Leberkrankheiten," 1858, Bd. i, p. 285.

Friedländer: "Ueber Phosphorvergiftung bei Hochschwangeren," Dissertation, Königsberg, 1892.

Fürstenberg: "Virchow's Archiv," 1864, Bd. xxix, p. 152.

Garel: "Cirrhose hypertrophique graisseuse du foie," "Revue de médecine,' 1881, p. 1004.

Harnack: "Berliner klin. Wochenschr.," 1893, p. 1138.

Hecker: "Ueber einen Fall von acuter Fettdegeneration bei einem Neugeborenen," "Archiv für Gynäkologie," Bd. x, p. 537.

Hedderich: "Ueber Leberatrophie," "Münchener med. Wochenschr.," 1895, p. 93.

v. Höslin: "Deutsches Archiv für klin. Medicin," 1883, Bd. xxxiii, p. 600.

v. Jaksch: "Die Vergiftungen," Nothnagel's "Specielle Pathologie und Therapie," Bd. i.

—"Beitrag zur Kenntniss der acuten Phosphorvergiftung," "Deutsche med. Wochenschr.," 1893, p. 10.

v. Kahlden: "Experimentelle Untersuchungen über die Wirkung des Alkohols auf Leber und Nieren," Ziegler's "Beiträge zur pathologischen Anatomie," 1891, Bd. ix, p. 349.

Krönig: "Die Genese der chronischen interstitiellen Phosphorhepatitis," "Virchow's Archiv," 1887, Bd. cx, p. 502.

Lafitte: "L'intoxication alcoolique expérimentale," Thèse de Paris, 1892.

Lanz: "Berliner klin. Wochenschr.," 1895, p. 879 (phosphorus).

Leyden: "Deutsche med. Wochenschr.," 1894, p. 475 (phosphorus).

—and Munk: "Die acute Phosphorvergiftung," Berlin, 1865.

Lebedeff: "Woraus bildet sich Fett in Fällen der acuten Fettbildung?", "Pflüger's Archiv," 1883, Bd. xxxi, p. 15.

Leo: "Fettbildung und Fetttransport bei Phosphorintoxication," "Zeitschr. für physiologische Chemie," Bd. ix, p. 469.

Liebermeister: "Ueber Leberentzündung und Leberdegeneration," "Deutsche med. Wochenschr.," 1892, p. 1181.

Litten: "Ueber die Einwirkung erhöhter Temperatur auf die Organe," "Virchow's Archiv," Bd. lxx, p. 10.

Magnan: "Archives de physiologie," 1873, p. 115 (alcohol).

Merklen: "Sur deux cas de cirrhose hypertrophique graisseuse avec ictère," "Revue de médecine," 1882, p. 997.

Meyer, H.: "Arch. für experimentelle Pathologie u. Pharmakologie," Bd. xiv, p. 313.

Münzer: "Der Stoffwechsel des Menschen bei acuter Phosphorvergiftung," "Deutsches Archiv für klin. Medicin," Bd. lii, p. 199.

Ostertag: "Die tödtliche Nachwirkung des Chloroforms," "Virchow's Archiv," 1889, Bd. cxviii, p. 250.

Perls: "Zur Unterscheidung von Fettinfiltration and fettiger Degeneration," "Centralblatt für die med. Wissenschaft," 1873, p. 801.

Pilliet: Sitzungsbericht der Pariser anatomischen Gelleschaft vom 26. Januar und 22. December, 1894.

Platen: "Virchow's *Archiv*," Bd. LXXIV, p. 286 (phosphorus).

Pupier: "Comptes-rendus de l'académie des sciences," 1872, 17, May (alcohol).

Renz: "Toxikologische Versuche über Phosphor," Dissertation, Tübingen, 1861.

Riess: Article "Phosphorvergiftung," in Eulenburg's "Realencyklopädie."

v. Recklinghausen: "Handbuch der allgemeinen Pathologie des Kreislaufes und der Ernährung," "Deutsche Chirurgie," Lieferung 2 und 3, p. 377.

Robitschek: "Deutsche med. Wochenschr.," 1893, p. 569 (phosphorus).

Roloff: "Die Fettdegeneration bei jungen Schweinen," "Virchow's Archiv," Bd. XXXIII, p. 553.

Rosenfeld: "Gibt es eine fettige Degeneration?" "XV. Congress für innere Medicin," 1897.

—"Die Fettleber bei Phlorizindiabetes," "Zeitschr. für klin. Medicin," Bd. XXVIII, p. 256.

Rothhammer: "Ueber einen Fall von acuter Phosphorvergiftung," Dissertation, Würzburg, 1890.

Sabourin: "Cirrhose hypertrophique graisseuse," "Archives de physiologie," 1881, p. 584.

Scheider: "Einige experimentelle Beiträge zur Phosphorvergiftung," Dissertation, Würzburg, 1895.

Schultzen und Riess: "Ueber acute Phosphorvergiftung und acute Leberatrophie," "Charité-Annalen," 1869, Bd. XV.

Schüppel: "Fettleber," in "Ziemssen's Handbuch," Bd. VIII, 1. Hälfte, 1. Abtheilung, p. 389.

Stadelmann: "Der Icterus," 1891, p. 176.

v. Starck: "Beitrag zur Pathologie der Phosphorvergiftung," "Deutsches Archiv fur klin. Medicin," 1884, Bd. XXXV, p. 481.

Storch: "Den acute Phosphorforgiftning," Dissertation, Copenhagen, 1865.

Strassmann: "Vierteljahresschr. für gerichtliche Medicin," 1888 (alcohol); "Virchow's Archiv," Bd. CXV, p. 1 (chloroform).

Straus and Blocq: "Archives de physiologie," 1887, 2. sémestre, p. 409 (alcohol).

Thiemich: "Ueber Leberdegeneration bei Gastroenteritis," Ziegler's "Beiträge zu pathologischen Anatomie," Bd. XX, p. 179.

Thiercelin and Joyle: "Sitzungbericht der Pariser anatomischen Gesellschaft," June 1, 1894.

Ungar: "Vierteljahresschr. für gerichtliche Medicin," Bd XLVII, p. 98 (chloroform).

Wagner, E.: "Zur Kenntniss der Phosphorvergiftung," "Archiv der Heilkunde," 1862, Bd. III, p. 359.

West: "Phosphorus-poisoning," "The Lancet," 1893, February 4, p. 245.

Wolkow: "Ueber das Verhalten der degenerativen und progressiven Vorgänge in der Leber bei Arsenikvergiftung," "Virchow's Archiv," Bd. CXXVII.

Ziegler and Obolenski: "Experimentelle Untersuchung über die Wirkung des Arseniks und Phosphors auf Leber und Nieren," Ziegler's "Beiträge zur pathologischen Anatomie," Bd. II, p. 291.

(C) CHRONIC ATROPHY.

(Hoppe-Seyler.)

By the term atrophy are characterized all hepatic conditions that are accompanied by a decrease in the size of the liver.

If only a portion of the liver is reduced in size, we speak of **circumscribed atrophy**; this may be due to a congenital anomaly of development or to some pressure effect exercised by neighboring organs that have become enlarged; *e. g.*, a dilated intestine (Frerichs), pleuritic and peritonitic exudates, hypertrophy of the heart, and tumors of neighboring parts. Other compressing factors may be lacing, corsets, straps, or deformities of the thorax (kyphosis and scoliosis). Circumscribed atrophy is also seen in the vicinity of tumors of the liver (echinococcus, carcinoma, etc.), or after occlusion of certain branches of the portal vein; also in cirrhotic and syphilitic processes that lead to a contraction of the interstitial connective tissue; in amyloid degeneration, congestion of the liver, etc. Occlusion of the bile-passages (Brissaud and Sabourin) may be congenital (Lomer), and may lead to atrophy. In all the conditions enumerated there will be seen contraction of the liver, characterized either by a simple reduction in the size of the cells, or by their destruction by fatty degeneration and necrosis. All these changes have been discussed under the headings of the different diseases of the liver or in the section on the abnormalities of the form of the liver (corset liver, congenital anomalies, etc.). In many of these lesions compensatory processes will be seen in other portions of the organ.

General atrophy is, as a rule, the effect of diffuse processes in the organ. A general reduction in the size of the organ may be seen after certain degenerative processes following icterus, phosphorus-, arsenic-, antimony-, or chloroform-poisoning, or following general cirrhosis, diffuse perihepatitis with thickening of the capsule, and occlusion of the portal vein or some of its branches. Frerichs has called particular attention to the simple atrophy of the columns of liver-cells that follows the obliteration of capillaries, or thickening of Glisson's capsule around branches of the portal vein. In the different sections that treat of these various lesions atrophy will be or has been discussed.

There is left only one form of general chronic atrophy, that which is seen after inanition, marasmus senilis, cachexia, etc., and is characterized by a wide-spread decrease in the size of the hepatic cells, involving the whole organ, and without any disintegration of the protoplasm and without any changes in the interstitial connective tissue. We will limit ourselves, in this section, to a discussion of this simple chronic atrophy of the liver.

If nutrition is deficient, or if too little food is taken, the volume of the liver will decrease; if the inverse conditions obtain, the organ will enlarge. This dependence upon the food is particularly pronounced in animals, and depends essentially on fluctuations in the size of the cells. In the case of well-nourished animals the latter will be seen to be large, rounded, and with distinct nuclei; in starving animals they will be found small, angular, granular, and with small indistinct nuclei. If nutrition is poor, the amount of glycogen, too, will be diminished, or may be completely absent, causing a reduction in the size of the cell. In inanition the liver also loses water, and later some albumin. In this manner the volume of the liver may be reduced two-thirds.

The same statement may be made as to human beings if nutrition is poor or if assimilation from the intestine is deficient; no degenerative or necrotic changes are seen in the cells during this process. Such deficient nutrition may be the result of poverty, or may be due to certain disturbances of the nervous system that cause the patient to refuse nourishment (psychoses, anorexia, coma, etc.), or may be due, finally, to certain lesions that prevent deglutition, such as paralysis, stenosis of the esophagus and cardia, ulcers of the pharynx and larynx (tuberculous, etc.). Severe vomiting, stenosis of the pylorus, strictures of the intestine, may all be at times responsible for the deficient ingestion of food. All chronic disturbances of nutrition following certain gastro-intestinal lesions must be ranked with these agencies: for example, catarrhs following ulcers and tumors, both of the stomach and intestine and of the large glands of digestion. Long-drawn-out febrile diseases may bring about the same result, as phthisis, malignant neoplasms, syphilis, chronic nephritis, anemia, diabetes, etc. These will all lead to disturbances of metabolism, deficient assimilation of food and an abundant destruction of body tissue; ultimately they lead to atrophy of the liver. In senile marasmus this condition is also seen; the liver, as well as the heart, the spleen, the musculature, etc., shows signs of brown atrophy when old age comes on.

Pathologic Anatomy.—Chronic atrophy does not, as a rule, develop uniformly throughout the organ, but is usually more pronounced at the sharp margin than in the interior.

The volume and the size of the liver are greatly reduced, and may be only one-third of normal. The organ is more flaccid, darker, and drier. It is a little more solid owing to the disappearance of soft parenchymatous tissue, and the simultaneous preservation of the more dense hard connective tissue. The transverse section is non-vascular: it is brownish in color, and shows a great reduction in the number of acini. The lower margin of the liver may be translucent and tough owing to the complete disappearance of parenchyma.

Under the microscope the cells will be found to be small and angular, and to contain small nuclei; sometimes granules of brown pigment will also be seen. The interstitial connective tissue is intact. In these cases, where the parenchyma is completely destroyed, some connective tissue will be seen in the location of the acini consisting of collapsed capillaries, and all around it is more solid periportal tissue with well-preserved capillaries and bile-passages. The latter may even be increased in number (Ziegler).

The amount of water in the liver is reduced, and later on its albumin may also be diminished. Glycogen can be detected only in traces.

Symptoms.—The chief feature of the clinical picture is the progressive **reduction in the size of the organ.** This process is slow and gradual, and may extend over many weeks or months. As a rule, the liver cannot be palpated; the area of dulness is decreased in all directions. The dulness extends neither so far down into the abdomen, nor so far to the left as is customary. Often, especially in cases of meteorism, it may be difficult to determine any dulness whatsoever. The surface of the organ is not sensitive to pressure, and is smooth.

, At the same time other symptoms of deficient nutrition will be seen; the skin will be flaccid, the cutaneous fat will be gone, the spleen is small; atrophy and disappearance of the muscular tissue may all be noted. Occasionally there will be cachectic edema, particularly in the dependent parts of the body, the legs, the lumbar region, etc.; later there may even appear ascites, hydrothorax, etc. The ascites cannot be due to stasis in the portal system, because the portal branches in the liver are neither occluded nor compressed in simple atrophy. At the same time, there will be disturbances of appetite, and of the stools, all of which may be attributed to the primary causal condition.

There is usually little bile in the stools. They are clay-colored, owing to the fact that the atrophic cells of the liver produce little bile. The urine, for the same reason, is pale and contains little urobilin. In a man with carcinoma of the stomach, who took very little food, I found daily only 0.039 gm. of urobilin, and another time only 0.043 gm., whereas the normal amount should be from 0.09 to 0.15 gm., an average of 0.12 gm. This man was very cachectic and his liver was reduced in size.

In cases of inanition resulting from pyloric stenosis, and in disturbances of nutrition following tuberculosis, I found a minimum excretion of urobilin.*

The disease may be very protracted. Some of the digestive disturbances may be due in part to the lack of bile. The duration and the course of the illness are largely dependent upon the primary disease. The **prognosis** also is dependent upon the latter. If there is a difficulty in the way of ingestion of food that can be removed, or if the patient is suffering from some digestive disorder that can be cured, the liver will also recover and return to a normal condition.

Treatment can only be directed toward the latter object. An esophageal or pyloric stenosis may have to be cured, even by a gastric fistula; if necessary, neoplasms that affect the nutrition and the general strength of the patient will have to be removed; and disturbances of the gastric or intestinal functions must be relieved. The food should be very digestible, consisting chiefly of milk, etc. Iron, and cinchona, arsenic, etc., may be administered for the improvement of the general health, and may be useful in this capacity.

Afanassiew: "Ueber die anatomischen Veränderungen der Leber während verschiedenen Thätigkeitszustandes," "Pflüger's Archiv," Bd. xxx, p. 385.
Birch-Hirschfeld: "Lehrbuch der pathologischen Anatomie," Bd. ii, p. 613.
Brissaud and Sabourin: "Deux cas d'atrophie du lobe gauche du foie d'origine biliaire," "Archiv de physiologie," 1884, 3. Serie, tome iii, p. 345.
Frerichs: "Klinik der Leberkrankheiten," 1858, Bd. i, p. 257.
Kux: "Ueber die Veränderungen der Froschleber durch Inanition," Dissertation, Würzburg, 1886.
Lomer: "Ueber einen Fall von congenitaler partieller Obliteration der Gallengänge," "Virchow's Archiv," 1885, Bd. xcix, p. 130.
Thierfelder: "Krankheiten der Leber," "Ziemssen's Handbuch," Bd. viii, 1. Hälfte, 1. Abtheilung, p. 270.
Ziegler: "Lehrbuch der pathologischen Anatomie," Bd. ii, p. 573.

(D) AMYLOID LIVER.

(Hoppe-Seyler.)

Amyloid degeneration is probably never limited to the liver. The process may be localized in the liver, but it usually involves other parts of the body at the same time. The primary disease, moreover, rarely develops in this organ itself, but usually in some remote part of the body, later involving the liver also.

The physicians of two centuries ago were acquainted with this lesion of the liver, as it is sometimes very conspicuous; they did not, however, have a clear conception of its significance. Rokitansky was the first to describe the exact anatomic changes seen in amyloid degeneration of the liver and of other organs, and to call attention to the relation between this state and wasting diseases. He called it lardaceous liver; other investigators used the term waxy or colloid. Virchow, later, discovered the characteristic iodin-sulphuric-acid reaction and called the new substance amyloid; hence the names amyloid liver and amyloid degeneration. He believed that the amyloid substance was related to the carbohydrates; but the investigations of C. Schmidt, Friedreich, Kékulé, Kühne, Rudneff, and others, demonstrated that it contains nitrogen, and that it is related to the proteids. For a long time it was

* *Virchow's Archiv*, 1891, Bd. cxxiv, S. 30.

still believed that amyloid substance at least contained a carbohydrate body, but recent investigations by Grandis and Carbone seem to refute this.

Krawkow believed that amyloid substance was related to chitin, but this has not been proved. Oddi succeeded in obtaining chondroitin-sulphuric acid from an amyloid liver, and believed that this substance (which, according to Schmiedeberg, is a product of cartilage) was related to amyloid substance. The exact connection between the two has, however, not yet been established. There appears to be some relationship with hyaline substance, and it appears that amyloid can be formed from this substance. Rählmann states that he has observed this process in amyloid degeneration of the conjunctiva. Tschermak supports this view. Amyloid substance, according to these writers, is related to coagulated albumin. v. Recklinghausen believes that hyaline change is a precursor of the amyloid process, and the investigations of Stilling, Hansemann, and Lubarsch support this view. The latter was enabled to show by his experiments that at first there was hyaline change only in the spleen, and that later the amyloid transformation appeared. The histologic findings favor the view that proteid material is gradually converted into amyloid.

It would appear that the so-called amyloid is not a homogeneous substance. This is demonstrated by the different color reactions; sometimes it is colored by iodin but not with methyl-violet; in other cases the reverse is true. The iodin-sulphuric acid reaction is often not obtained at all, or it may be atypical; *i. e.*, give a reddish-brown or a blue or green color.

The following diseases have for a long time been recognized as the chief causes of amyloid degeneration: protracted suppuration, phthisis, neoplasms, malaria, syphilis, leukemia, and pseudoleukemia.

The ultimate cause of amyloid degeneration, however, remained obscure, and only recently have experiments thrown light on the subject. Animals were infected with bacteria, and a general chronic pathologic condition was produced, with marked emaciation, amyloid degeneration of the spleen, and of the liver, etc. Birch-Hirschfeld observed amyloid degeneration in a rabbit with a long-standing suppurative process; and Bouchard and Charrin have occasionally noted amyloid deposits in the kidneys of animals that had been injected with pyocyaneus and tubercle bacilli. Czerny produced amyloid degeneration in a dog by causing suppuration with long-continued injections of turpentine; and also found a body giving similar reactions in the pus-corpuscles. Krawkow especially, and later Davidsohn, succeeded in producing a deposit of amyloid material around the vessels of the spleen and the liver by repeated injections of staphylococcus cultures. Lubarsch obtained similar results by artificially inducing suppuration. Gouget injected proteus cultures into the vena portæ and the common duct; Candarelli injected Bacillus termo, and both obtained amyloid degeneration. Carrière saw the same procedure after injections of tubercle bacilli. Petrone believes that it is due to an impregnation of the vessel-walls with perverted blood-pigment; this would seem to explain the appearance of amyloid material after chronic suppuration of the bones and of the soft tissues, following tubercular processes, staphylococcus infection (osteomyelitis), etc. The appearance of amyloid in pulmonary phthisis may also be due to infection with staphylococci. Amyloid degeneration is seen with particular frequency after ulceration of the intestine, the trachea, and the larynx. In primary urogenital tuberculosis, and in other unmixed forms of tuberculosis, the condition is not frequently seen provided the foci remain closed off; as soon as such a focus is exposed, however, amyloid degeneration may appear. Among 48 cases of amyloid degeneration in tuberculosis, 42 were combined with some tubercular lesion of the intestine.

Suppurations of bones demand particular attention in this connection, in that they are difficult to cure and persist for a long time. Caries, psoas abscesses, necrosis of the bones, combined with suppuration, as in complicated fractures, osteomyelitis, etc., and all suppurative forms of arthritis; also chronic leg-ulcers, chronic empyema, bronchiectasis (with abundant production of pus), chronic liver abscess, purulent pyelitis, etc. A few cases are on record in which amyloid degeneration has followed gastric ulcer or chronic dysentery.

In syphilis such cases seem particularly to lead to amyloid degeneration as are complicated with suppurative lesions and ulcerative processes. In hereditary syphilis the condition is frequently seen, and it has even been claimed that an amyloid condition may be congenital (Rokitansky).

The rôle played by malarial cachexia, by gout, and by rachitis is a doubtful one. The statement has also been made that mercury-poisoning may cause amyloid degeneration; this is probably not the case.

In the presence of tumors amyloid degeneration is not so frequently seen as with suppurative conditions and tuberculosis. The slow-growing tumors predispose more actively to this condition than those that develop rapidly and lead to the death of the patient in a short time. Thus gelatinous carcinomata, scirrhus, etc., are more apt to cause amyloid degeneration of the organs than other forms. Neoplasms that are complicated by ulceration of the stomach or the uterus, for instance, seem to create a particular predisposition to amyloid degeneration. In many cases the cause of the degeneration cannot be determined; a thing that is not surprising when we remember that many bacteria (staphylococci), etc., develop in a latent manner and escape recognition.

Phthisis is the most frequent cause of amyloid degeneration. Hoffmann found it in 67.5 %; O. Weber in 40.5 %; Wagner in 56.25 %; Wicht in 50 %; then suppuration of bones and chronic suppuration (Hoffmann 7.5 %, Weber 38 %, Wagner 23 %, Wicht 22.8 %). Men seem to be more frequently afflicted than women. The age of twenty-one to thirty seems to offer the greatest susceptibility. The kidneys and the spleen are more frequently involved than the liver. If the liver is involved, the two former organs are usually also involved.

Pathologic Anatomy.—Slight degrees of amyloid degeneration can only be recognized by means of the microscopic examination. If the process is well developed, the whole organ enlarges and may weigh as much as 5 or 6 kg. The surface is smooth, the margin rounded, and occasionally sharp; the contour remains unchanged. The organ grows harder; its tissue becomes translucent and appears like yellow wax or boiled bacon; for this reason the degeneration has been called waxy or lardaceous (*"Speckleber"*). This appearance is in part due to the small amount of blood contained in the organ. If, on the other hand, there is a considerable quantity, the organ looks like raw ham. The outlines of the acini are, as a rule, indistinct; though a point in the center and a fine line at the periphery will designate the old location of each acinus. This appearance is due to the fact that the process of degeneration is less complete at the periphery and in the center. If Lugol's solution is poured over the transverse section of the liver, the latter is colored mahogany brown. Under the microscope it will be seen that changes have occurred in the intra-acinous capillaries. The endothelium is fairly well preserved; and exterior to it will be seen a thick, translucent, shiny mass that is colored brown by iodin and red with methyl-violet and similar stains. The same thick layers are seen around the capillaries in some of the experimental investigations (Krawkow, Davidsohn), with the production of artificial amyloid degeneration by the injection of cultures of staphylococci, etc. The walls of the blood-channels are thickened and between the latter the atrophied liver-cells are seen; they are either in a state of brown atrophy or of fatty degeneration, and finally seem to perish completely. The theory has been held that in cases of this kind the shiny masses consist of transformed liver-cells. From Böttelier's and others' studies it appears not impossible that amyloid degeneration occasionally occurs in the cell protoplasm. Certainly it is seldom distinctly evident, and is of comparatively slight significance as compared with the deposit of amyloid substance in the vessel-walls. This same deposit may sometimes be seen in the media of the branches of the hepatic artery, which run in the interacinous tissue. The middle zone of the acini seems to be the most affected, the center and the periphery being less involved. As a rule, the degeneration is uniform throughout the organ, circumscribed foci being rarely seen.

The bile-passages do not, as a rule, participate in the process, and present an absolutely normal appearance.

Marked amyloid changes are generally seen also in the other organs, as the spleen, the kidneys, the suprarenal capsules, and the intestine.

Symptoms.—Experimental investigation has shown that amyloid changes may take place in the liver within the course of a few weeks. Before the process assumes such dimensions as to be evident clinically, however, more time must elapse.

Slight degrees of amyloid degeneration cannot be detected, owing to the fact that neither the size nor the consistency of the organs involved is changed.

Only such involvement as is diffuse throughout the liver can be recognized with any certainty. In such cases the whole organ is enlarged and extends in the right mammillary line a hand's-breadth below the costal margin. Its margin is frequently sharp, occasionally somewhat rounded; it is indented only in cases that are complicated by cirrhosis or syphilis. The surface is usually smooth; even in cases of extreme enlargement no pain is felt. There is a marked resemblance between this form of degeneration and fatty liver, particularly in its contour and in the character of its surface and margin; amyloid liver is differentiated, however, by its extreme hardness. The organ, at the same time, is by no means as unyielding as in cirrhosis, but retains more of its elasticity. There is no sign of stasis in the portal system in spite of the marked involvement of the vessels; this is due to the fact that the amyloid change develops in the vessel-walls, and grows outward, so that it thickens the walls of the vessels without narrowing their lumen. The pressure exercised in this way upon the surrounding tissues causes atrophy of the liver-cells. At times there will be a serous exudate into the peritoneum, dependent upon the primary disease. There may be a cachectic transudation, or the effusion may occur in combination with edema in other parts of the body; it may also be due to tubercular peritonitis. Splenic tumor is often associated with amyloid liver, and is caused by the same changes that are operating in the liver; it is characterized by its extreme hardness. Albumin, casts, and renal epithelium are often found in the urine, as accompanying symptoms of amyloid kidney. Albuminuria may be absent, however, despite the existence of severe grades of amyloid change. If diarrhea now supervenes, with the passage of slimy stools, the probability of amyloid degeneration of the intestine is great.

At the same time, various processes, purulent, syphilitic, tuberculous, etc., may be present in different parts of the body, and may modify the pathologic picture; usually they play the most important part in the disease.

The function of the liver, apparently, remains intact for a long time. Marked degrees of amyloid degeneration and the disappearance of considerable parenchyma involve a decreased secretion of bile. The stools lose their color, and the urine contains little urobilin, being light in color. The excretion of urea is decreased, owing, probably, to the deficient assimilation of food that is so often observed in cachectic conditions. Icterus is absent, unless the disease is complicated by some other condition that leads to stasis of the bile.

Until recently amyloid degeneration was considered an irreparable condition. This view was based upon the great resistance offered by amyloid substance to the action of chemical and physical agencies. Of late years a number of reports have been published from which it appears that amyloid processes may recede. Thus, it has been ascertained that amyloid substance, when incorporated into the body of animals, may gradually become absorbed. Lubarsch extirpated a portion of the spleen from one of his animals four weeks before death, and found distinct amyloid change; when the animal died, amyloid material could no longer be discovered even in the vicinity of the scar. Rählmann, finally, has noted the disappearance of amyloid degeneration of the conjunctiva, after the condition had been positively diagnosed by microscopic examination of a small excised portion of the growth.

It would appear, therefore, that amyloid liver may recover, if the primary cause can be removed; *e. g.*, if a suppurative bone lesion, empyema, etc., can be cured by operative interference.

The **prognosis** is dependent upon the curability of the primary disease.

The **diagnosis** rests upon the character of the liver, already described, upon the absence of symptoms of stasis in the portal system, and upon the demonstration of amyloid degeneration in other organs. Particularly important is the presence of such a condition as suppuration, which predisposes to this form of degeneration.

Treatment.—Prophylaxis is important. Suppurative processes should be removed as early as possible, particularly if they involve bones or joints; old syphilitic lesions should be carefully treated; phthisis should be handled by nourishing the patient and regulating his mode of life, and all tubercular foci should, if possible, be removed, while secondary purulent infections must be cured.

Even after the disease has developed hope should not be given up. A rational and thorough treatment of the primary disease may often lead to a cure. The patient should receive a diet rich in proteids, and readily digestible, such as milk, easily assimilable meats, eggs, digestible cereals, etc. Arsenic, iron, and potassium iodid have been recommended. Particularly in cases resulting from malaria or syphilis are these drugs useful. Amyloid degeneration of the intestine and the kidneys should be regarded and treated according to the general principles enunciated in the appropriate volume of this series.

For the earlier literature of the subject *vide* Schüppel: "Amyloide Entartung der Leber," in Ziemssen's "Handbuch der speciellen Pathologie und Therapie," 1878, Bd. viii, 1. Hälfte, 1. Abtheilung, p. 359.
Index-Catalogue of the Library of the Surgeon-General's Office, 1887, vol. viii, p. 241.

Bouchard et Charrin: "Comptes-rendus de la société de biologie," tome XL, p. 688.

Carriere: "Archives de médecine expér.," 1897, tome IX.

Czerny: "Archiv für experimentelle Pathologie und Pharmakologie," 1893, Bd. XXXI, p. 209; "Centralblatt für allgemeine Pathologie," Bd. VII.

Davidsohn: "Ueber experimentelle Erzeugung von Amyloid," "Virchow's Archiv," 1897, Bd. CL, p. 16.

Gouget: "Archives de médecine expér.," 1897, 1. série, tome IX, p. 733.

Krawkow: "De la dégénérescence amyloide," ibidem, 1896, 1. série, tome VIII, p. 107.

Litten: "Ueber Amyloiddegeneration," "Deutsche med. Wochenschr.," 1888, No. 24.

Lubarsch: "Zur Frage der experimentellen Erzeugung von Amyloid," "Virchow's Archiv," 1897, Bd. CL, p. 471.

Oddi: "Ueber das Vorkommen von Chondroitinschwefelsäure in der Amyloid-leber," "Archiv für experimentelle Pathologie und Pharmakologie," Bd. XXXIII, p. 376.

Petrone: "Recherches sur la dégénérescence amyloide expérimentale," "Archives de médecine expér.," 1898, 1. série, tome X, p. 682.

Rahlmann: "Ueber hyaline und amyloide Degeneration der Conjunctiva des Auges," "Virchow's Archiv," Bd. LXXXVII, p. 325.

Tschermak: "Ueber die Stellung der amyloiden Substanz unter den Eiweisskör-pern," "Zeitschr. für physiologische Chemie," 1895, Bd. XX, p. 343.

Wicht, L.: "Zur Aetiologie und Statistik der amyloiden Degeneration," Dissertation, Kiel, 1889.

(E) SIDEROSIS OF THE LIVER.

(Iron-Liver.)

(Quincke.)

In the normal state the liver contains more iron than any other organ of the body. The absolute quantity is 30 to 90 mg. in 100 gm. of dried liver substance in normal animals, and 80 to 200 mg. in man (Oidtmann, Stahel, Granboom). Under certain pathologic conditions the amount of iron may markedly decrease, or, especially if iron is administered, increase.

Exact determination of the amount of iron present in the liver after incineration is possible in animals only when all the blood has been washed from the organ with normal salt solution. Zaleski, Gottlieb, and others have made such determinations. In human livers it is impossible to remove all the blood, and the results obtained are therefore not uniform. For this reason, and because pathologic changes cannot always be excluded, so-called normal figures are uncertain as far as the human liver is concerned; the figures given by Stabel are, however, probably too large (see table, pages 865, 866).

Occasionally it is possible to determine the differences in the quantity of iron present from the intensity of the reaction given with ammonium sulphid, a simpler method than that of estimation by weighing. Small pieces of the organ, particularly if they are finely cut (and consequently as free as possible from blood) and prepared for the microscope, usually appear green to the naked eye when treated with ammonium sulphid; with a little practice it is possible approximately to estimate the quantity of iron from the shade. In the dead body this reaction occasionally takes place as the result of the generation of sulphuretted hydrogen in the intestine. A green color is to be seen in portions of the surface of the liver that are in contact with the loops of intestine. Microscopic examination with a high-power lens shows that the liver-cells are normally diffusely colored; but that under certain conditions, and especially when pathologic changes are present, the peripheral portions of the lobules show more intense coloring, and that small granules of pigment, almost blackish-green in color, are situated in this location. As a rule, these granules are found, either in the main or exclusively, in the axis of the columns of the liver-cells. They are usually fine (not more than 2 μ in diameter) and are surrounded by a greenish areola. Iron can also be demonstrated microchemically in the capillaries. Here, too, it is more abundant in the periphery of the lobules, and consists of little lumps that are composed of fine and coarse granules. The color of these granules, which are 6 μ and over in diameter, is made darker by ammonium sulphid, indicating a greater amount of iron. [C. Bielfeld * has analyzed many livers with the aim of discovering free iron in the hepatic cells. He now asserts that preceding failures have been due to faulty methods. He used Schmidt's method, and arrived at the following conclusions: The average amount of iron present in a healthy liver is about 0.169 %. There is more iron in the liver of the male than the female. The amount of iron in the hepatic cells increases with age. The iron becomes less between the ages of twenty and twenty-five.— ED.] The clumps are frequently seen within the leucocytes; others, as Kupffer has recently shown, are found in the endothelium of the vessels, and some are free in the lumen (Kupffer). If the capillaries contain iron, the reaction may be obtained in Kupffer's stellate cells, in the connective tissue, and in the vessel-sheaths.

The iron reaction is not usually seen in the capillaries of the healthy human liver. In the dog there are always certain isolated cells that become dark when treated with ammonium sulphid; in the rabbit they are also found, but are not so numerous.

Chemical analysis will reveal the total quantity of iron present in the liver; microchemical reactions will indicate the distribution of iron in different tissues. The two methods supplement one another.

The intensity of the green coloration by ammonium sulphid may be utilized as a measure for the determination of the quantity of iron present. It must be remembered, however, that not all iron compounds react to ammonium sulphid, as, for instance, hemoglobin. The most important iron compound found in the normal liver is Schmiedeberg's ferratin; this is a ferri-albumin acid of a light brown color containing about 6 % of iron, soluble in weak alkalies, and colored dark by ammonium sulphid. The reaction does not occur at once, but requires several minutes; after the reagent has acted for a little time the substance becomes darker and then gradually a dark green. Even after several days no sulphid of iron is found. Ferratin may be dissolved by boiling fresh liver pulp with three or four volumes of water. The decoction is filtered, and the ferratin precipitated as a brown sediment upon the addition of a small quantity of tartaric acid. The fresh liver of a healthy animal contains from 0.15 % to 0.3 % of ferratin (Vay). The amount of ferratin seems to correspond to the general state of nutrition, so that in the majority of human livers there is only a comparatively small quantity. Vay succeeded in extracting some 60 % of the iron of the liver in the form of ferratin. Of the other iron compounds a small portion is dissolved in the fluid over the ferratin sediment; this also gives a reaction with ammonium sulphid. The remainder of the iron is insoluble in water, and is probably present in various combinations. One of these has been obtained by Żaleski by extracting the liver-cell pulp repeatedly,

* *Russian Archiv. Patolog. klin. Med. Bakt.*, March, 1901.

and subjecting it to artificial digestion; this was accomplished by dissolving the residue in ammonia solution, and precipitating by alcohol. The substance obtained was called hepatin, and is a nucleo-compound containing 0.0176 % of iron. It does not give an iron reaction with ammonium sulphid. Woltering has demonstrated the presence of a similar nucleo-proteid. The other iron-containing substances of the liver are not thoroughly understood, especially those which will be discussed below, which give an ammonium sulphid reaction, and are found in the liver after the administration of large quantities of iron, and in certain pathologic conditions. The liver, when it contains much of this substance, is colored a deep blackish-green. This tint can be recognized microscopically and macroscopically, and points distinctly to the presence of a large quantity of iron. This condition I have called **siderosis** of the liver. It may be called pathologic siderosis in contradistinction to the physiologic siderosis mentioned above. In marked degrees of siderosis the liver appears rust-colored to the naked eye, and reveals microscopically a number of brownish granules within the liver-cells and capillaries; less frequently there is present a diffuse brownish coloration of the cell protoplasm.

Kunkel first regarded the rust-colored pigment found in the lymph-glands after extravasation of blood as a "ferrioxyhydrate," and later Auscher and Lapicque looked upon the peculiar ochre-colored pigment of the siderotic liver as a special ferrioxyhydrate, $Fe_2O_3.3H_2O$. In my opinion the iron is more probably combined with certain organic substances, and this combination was destroyed by Auscher and Lapicque by boiling with sodium hydrate solutions.

While the iron reaction is obtained with particular intensity in these brownish masses, it is not seen in these alone. A large portion, and possibly the greatest part, of the substances (both in the cells and the capillaries) that give the iron reaction are not colored brown.

The iron found in the liver may come directly from iron compounds absorbed from the intestine. In a series of experiments a number of animals were all fed with a special diet, and at the same time certain of them received a certain amount of an iron salt; others that did not receive the iron were used for comparison. Kunkel, for example, administered a meat diet to two dogs, and gave one of them, in addition, the chlorid of iron. In the liver of the latter animal he found 51.2 mg. of iron, in the control animal 16.5 mg. In another series of experiments he fed young dogs with milk, and performed venesection several times. One of the dogs received liquor ferri albuminati. The liver of this animal contained 22.2 mg. of iron, that of the control animal 2.9 mg. We find, therefore, that the proportion of iron was as 1 to 7 in the liver; at the same time, it was only as 5 to 8 in the blood.

Gottlieb fed his animals with an abundant meat diet, and found that when iron was administered at the same time 46.7 mg. were found in these dogs, and only 20.2 mg. in the control animals. Samoiloff performed similar experiments on rats, and found that 100 gm. of dried substances contained 70 mg. of iron after the administration of oxid of iron, whereas the control animal furnished only 45 mg. Hall fed mice with carniferrin, and found 199 mg. of iron, and only 62 mg. in the control animal. Woltering obtained similar results.

Animals fed with iron gave a more intense ammonium sulphid reaction with the liver substances (Kunkel, Woltering, Filippi, Quincke and Hochhaus, Hall).

Délépine claims to have found an increase in the microchemic iron reaction of the liver eight to twelve hours after an ordinary meal.

If the metal is given in the form of the vegetable acid salt, subcutaneously or intravenously, the accumulation of iron is still greater. It is well known that these salts produce a fatal result in a very short time; in the case of a rabbit death can be accomplished with 25 mg. of iron pro kilo of body-weight, and in a dog with 20 to 50 mg.

Gottlieb, Jacoby, and Zaleski injected the tartrate of iron and sodium into the blood, and obtained the following figures upon analysis of the liver:

AUTHOR.	ANIMAL.	TARTRATE OF IRON AND SODIUM CORRESPONDING TO 10 MG. FE.	LIVER.		
			Examined after Last Injection:	Contains mg. Fe in 100 gm. of Dry Substance:	Contains of the Fe Introduced:
Gottlieb .	Dog.	100 to 200 mg. in divided doses.	1 to 4 days.	210 to 420 mg.	20% to 65%.
Jacoby ..	Dog.	200 mg.	1¼ hours.	105 mg.	40%.
Zaleski ..	Rabbit. Cat.	9.6 mg. 56 mg.	3 hours. 3 hours.	172 mg. (normal 99). 89 mg. (normal 43).	

Laevecke injected the citrate of iron subcutaneously into rabbits, giving a dose of 15 to 176 mg. of iron pro kilo. Microchemically the liver-cells gave a distinct iron reaction that was stronger and more persistent in the peripheral part of the lobules, and disappeared in the course of the second day. Iron was passed in the urine within half an hour, and was found in the bile from the fourth to the sixth hour in a form that gave a direct reaction. When the ureters were ligated, the iron reactions of the liver and the bile were particularly intense.

Nölke injected citrate of iron into rabbits daily or every other day for from one to five weeks. The animals bore 5 mg. of iron very well, and 10 mg. not so well. As long as the doses were kept small only a slight iron reaction was elicited from the kidney, though the metal accumulated in the liver, the spleen, and the bone-marrow. The liver showed a very intense iron reaction, particularly in the cells, and less so in the capillaries. In two animals cellular siderosis of the liver was found four months after the administration of iron; in a third animal, treated in the same manner, it had disappeared at the end of seven months.

Very **insoluble iron preparations,** such as ferric oxid and ferric hydrate, are absorbed, and may lead to siderosis of the spleen, the bone-marrow, and the liver. I have verified this personally by injecting these substances into the subcutaneous connective tissue of dogs, rabbits, and guinea-pigs. The iron is deposited chiefly in the liver-cells and to a lesser extent in the capillaries.

When **pure hemoglobin** is injected under the skin, there is an accumulation of iron in the liver. v. Starck and Schurig performed experiments of this kind in dogs and rabbits, the latter especially administering small doses frequently and for a long time. A portion of the injected hemoglobin (usually from the horse) was decomposed in the cellular tissues in such a manner that two (v. Starck) or four (Schurig) days after the injection the iron could be demonstrated directly. Another portion of the hemoglobin was absorbed as such, and entered the circulation, of the latter, a portion was excreted in the urine, but only when the quantity injected exceeded 1 gm. pro kilo of body-weight. A small quantity of hemoglobin was excreted by the bile; the rest was elaborated, and in part formed bilirubin, and in part was converted into substances that will be mentioned presently. Stadelmann and Gorodecki found that from 30 % to 40 % of the quantity injected was converted into bilirubin, and caused a pleiochromia of the bile.

Both the iron that is separated in this process, and the iron that is obtained from other decomposition of hemoglobin, is to a great extent retained in the body and can be demonstrated microchemically in the spleen, the bone-marrow, and the liver. In the latter organ the peripheral portions of the lobules show a distinct iron reaction. Schurig found that in certain instances more iron was deposited in the leucocytes of the liver capillaries, and in other exactly similar experiments more in the liver-cells: it did not appear to be clear what caused these variations. It has been shown also that pigeons, in the experiments of Laspeyres, tolerated injections of equine hemoglobin only so long as the quantity did not exceed 0.3 gm. pro kilo of body-weight. The conversion occurred a little more rapidly, and up to the third day an intense iron reaction was elicited in the splenic pulp and in the liver-capillaries; the iron was usually seen in the shape of large granules, whereas from the sixth day on it was found almost exclusively in the liver-cells in the form of fine granules.

In the minority of the experiments mentioned above the substance within the cells that reacted to iron was colored brown. Sometimes it had no color. It is not certain how much of this iron is formed in the liver, the spleen, and the bone-marrow, from hemoglobin brought there unaltered; and how much of it is carried to this organ in the form of decomposition products from the hemoglobin of the body. It is remarkable that (according to Schurig) the iron reaction could not be determined before the fourth day, whereas an increase in the formation of bilirubin (according to Stadelmann) begins within ten to twelve hours. It would appear that the iron radicle must be present in an unknown form for the first three days, and is then converted into a compound that gives the iron reaction.

The question of the origin of iron in the liver becomes still more complicated if the blood of an animal of the same species, instead of a solution of pure hemoglobin,* is injected into the blood-stream or the peritoneal cavity. It is possible that the artificial plethora causes a portion of the hemoglobin to be dissolved in the serum, and it is certain that a number of blood-corpuscles are taken up by the leucocytes and the marrow- and pulp-cells while they still contain hemoglobin. They are found in the spleen, the bone-marrow, and the liver-capillaries, and are here altered in such a manner that positive iron reactions become apparent. The capillaries of the periphery of the liver lobules contain a great many of these iron-holding leucocytes. If artificial plethora is induced by repeated injections of blood, the liver-cells themselves may contain iron.†

Moreover, if the blood of the animal is injected subcutaneously, the consequences are only slightly different. A partial exosmosis of hemoglobin occurs at once, so that results are seen similar to those observed after injections of hemoglobin. Here, too, we see siderosis of the spleen, the bone-marrow, and the liver-capillaries, and to a slight degree of the liver-cells, whereas the renal epithelia show a slightly increased iron reaction, just as in intravenous injections.

Similar conditions are sometimes seen in man when large extravasations of blood occur into the abdominal cavity or into the cellular tissues. In such cases siderosis of the liver and of other organs develops (Hindenlang).

I had the opportunity recently of observing a case that was very remarkable in this respect. A young man, previously in perfect health, suffered from a twist of the mesocecum and mesocolon, and died within six hours. Owing to the torsion of the vessels the whole duodenum was filled with bloody infarcts, and contained free blood. There was a pronounced siderosis of the liver, but a positive iron reaction was obtained only from the liver-cells. It would appear, therefore, that this condition of hepatic siderosis occurred within six hours by the absorption of hemoglobin from the wall and the lumen of the intestine.

---

* Quincke, *Deutsche Archiv. f. klin. Med.*, 1880, Bd. xxv, S. 580.
† Ibid., 1883, Bd. xxxiii, S. 22.

Siderosis of the liver and of other organs which follows poisoning with arseniated hydrogen (Naunyn and Minkowski), and with toluylene-diamin (Stadelmann, W. Hunter, Biondi), is of complicated origin, for under these conditions not only is hemoglobin present in solution in the blood, but remnants of red corpuscles which still contain hemoglobin (as in artificial plethora) circulate in the blood, and are gathered up by the colorless cells.

Other blood-poisons (compare page 496) act similarly, as, for instance, a poison found by Schaumann and Tallquist in Bothriocephalus latus. Destruction of red blood-corpuscles followed by siderosis of the spleen, liver, etc., may also be due to poisoning by carbon disulphid or carbon oxysulphid (Schwalbe, Kiener, and Engel). It appears, however, that the pigment that gives the iron reactions in this case is of a different nature, being brown-black in color, and yet seemingly originating within the blood-corpuscles.

From all these experiments and observations we must form the conclusion that the liver as well as the spleen and the bone-marrow is a depository in which iron (in a form that gives positive iron reactions) is arrested. It is immaterial whether it is introduced from without or whether it enters the blood-stream from other organs, particularly from red blood-corpuscles that have perished. It seems, therefore, that the liver performs a similar [storage.—ED.] function with regard to iron, as is the case with fats and carbohydrates. When needed, this reserve store of iron is reabsorbed and utilized.

A number of physiologic and pathologic facts corroborate this view. Gottlieb has seen the iron of the liver increase to five times the normal amount (from 30 to 170 mg.) in a dog, after a period of starvation extending over eighteen days. Guillemonat and Lapicque, it is true, found no differences after fifteen days of fasting. In certain hibernating animals an abundant quantity of iron is found in the liver-capillaries (Quincke), and, according to Krüger, the liver of the fetus of cattle contains much iron (up to 300 mg.). This is also true of new-born animals (cattle 180 mg., Krüger; dogs 390 mg., Zaleski), a condition of affairs which is probably intended to compensate for the small amount of iron present in the milk. After a few weeks the quantity of iron is reduced to the level of the adult animal.

Westphalen subjected the livers of a small number of human fetuses to microchemical examination, and found that the quantity of iron in the organ, as well as in the spleen, was greater in the earlier months of intrauterine life than at a later period.

In animals in which artificial anemia has been produced the color reaction with ammonium sulphid is less marked (Quincke, Schmiedeberg). In man, if there has been much loss of blood, so that anemia supervenes, either no iron reaction, or only a slight one, is obtained in the liver, the spleen, or the bone-marrow (Stühlen and Quincke, Stockmann). In cases of this kind we must assume that the iron has been lost from the system.

On the other hand, the liver of human beings may be found to contain much larger quantities of iron than normal. Normally large quantities are rarely found, because the absorption from the intestine is regulated by the demand. If iron has accumulated under pathologic conditions, it is usually derived from the blood, although some of it may come from other organs. This condition, therefore, might very well be called

IRON CONTAINED IN THE LIVER.

| | | Liver Substance Contains: In 100 Grams: | | | | |
		Milligrams of Iron in Fresh Substance.	Milligrams of Iron in Dried Substance.	Percentage of Iron in 100 Parts of Ash.	Author.	Remarks.
Dog.	Normal	12.8	89.1	...	Zaleski.*	The blood was washed out through the vessels with a 2.5 % solution of cane-sugar.
"	"	10.4	77.9	...	"	
"	"	7.4	42.9	...	"	
"	New-born	73.8	390.0	...	Gottlieb.	
"	Normal, abundant meat diet	...	36.8	...	"	Liver washed out with sodium chlorid solution.
"		...	36.6	...	"	
"		...	20.2	...	"	
"	Abundant meat diet, iron internally	...	46.7	...	"	
"	After eighteen days' fasting	...	169.6	...	"	
"	Eighteen days fasting {200 mg.	...	427.0	...	"	Intravenous injection of tartrate of iron and sodium.
"	and iron intraven- {145 mg.	...	330.0	...	"	
"	ously. {100 mg.	...	216.0	...	"	
"	Feeding of fat and iron {200 mg.	27.0	...	...	"	
"	intravenously. {200 mg.	36.1	...	...	"	
"	Young, 10 weeks old	16.5	...	...	Kunkel.	
"	The same, iron oxychlorate for 8 days internally	51.2	...	...	"	
"	Young, 3 months; diet containing little iron, repeated venesections	5.2	...	...	v. Hösslin.	2.7 mg. of this hemoglobin that could be extracted.
"	Normal	32.0	...	...	Vay.	
"	"	38.0	...	...	"	
"	Iron internally	...	161.0	...	Quincke.	} 11 or 9 mg. of this ferratin.
"	"	...	198.0	...	"	For 30 days 1.3 ferric sulphate.
"	"	...	116.0	...	"	Four weeks daily, 1.0 ferric lactate.
"	"	...	181.0	...	"	Three months daily, 1.0 ferric lactate.
"	Old chronic anemia	...	50.0	...	"	Three months daily, 0.5 ferric pulv. Gastric fistula, pregnancy, bleeding.

Animal	Condition	Observer			Min.–Max.	Remarks
Dog	Artificial plethora	Quincke		112.0		Transfusion, 64 %, 10 days.
"	"	"		196.0		Transfusion, 34 %, 29 days.
"	"	"		134.0		Transfusion, 41 %, 40 days.
"	"	"		339.0		Transfusion, 44 %, 40 days.
"	"	"		890.0		Seven abdominal ...ins (380 %) in 6 months.
"	"	"		1420.0		Seven abdominal ...ins (465 %) in 5½ months.
Horse	Normal	Zaleski	15.3	68.7		Blood-vessels washed out.
"	"	"	16.3	88.7		
Rabbit	"	"	5.8	30.8		
"	"	"	10.0	99.0		...te of iron and sodium injected into the blood.
Cat	9.5 mg. iron endovenously	"	15.0	172.0		Tartrate of iron and sodium injected into the blood.
"	Normal	"		43.0		
Hedgehog	56 mg. Fe endovenously	"		89.0		
"	Normal	"	89.0	1183.0		
"	"	"	77.0	724.0		
Skunk	"	"	56.0	250.0		
"	"	"	22.0	122.0		
Squirrel	"	"	80.0	357.0		Blood-vessels washed out.
Hare	"	"	6.8	47.0		
"	"	"	6.3	44.0		
Beaver	"	"	21.0	96.0		
Wash.	"	"	7.5	43.0		
Cattle	Average Figures	Krüger		280.0	Min. Max. 100–500	
"	Young fetus	"		140.0	100–180	
"	Fetus (40–50 cm. long)	"		3.00	140–700	
"	Fetus (70–80 cm. long)	"		180.0	30–290	
"	Calf, first week	"		32.0	12– 60	
"	Calf, ...th week	"		24.6	19– 29	
"	Ox, 3 years old	"		27.6	19– 34	
"	Cow, pregnant	Oidtmann		1.92		Washed liver-pulp was examined.
Man	56 years old, insane man	"	21.2	81.6		
"	Syphilis neonatorum	Zaleski	18.2	103.8		
"	Fetus of 8 months	Stahel	32.7	146		
"	Burn, 24 years			31.3		

* On washing out the liver seems to swell to a varying degree; it is possible that this explains the large variations in the proportion of iron to fresh liver substance and dried substance—this is not always the case; for instance, in the hedgehog.

Iron Contained in the Liver.—(Continued.)

		Liver Substance Contains: In 100 Grams:			Author.	Remarks.
		Milligrams of Iron in Fresh Substance.	Milligrams of Iron in Dried Substance.	Percentage of Iron in 100 Parts of Ash.		
Man.	Burn, 24 years..........	10.7	39.0	....	Graanboom.	(After Zaleski.)
"	Fracture of skull, 32 years......	....	167.0	....	Stahel.	
"	Fracture of sternum, 42 years...	....	201.0	....		
"	Men (average of 29 cases)	23.0	....	....	} Guillemonat and Lapicque.	After deduction of the iron contained in the hemoglobin. Min. Max. 4 45
"	Women (average of 21 cases) ...	8.0	....	....		0 20
"	Embolism of lung, female, 49 years.	....	70.0	....	R. Stockmann.	
"	Occlusion of intestine, male, 52 years.	....	90.0	....	"	
"	Myxedema, female, 60 years......	....	90.0	....	"	
"	Acute tuberculosis, male, 16 years....	....	70.0	....	"	
"	Chronic nephritis, male, 24 years....	....	35.0	....	"	
"	Marasmus, 67 years........	....	75.0	....	Stahel.	
"	Hemorrhage	....	44.0	....	"	
"	Diphtheria	....	41.0	....	"	
"	Nephritis-pneumonia	....	48.0	....	"	
"	Fatty degeneration of the heart with stain	....	38.0	....	R. Stockmann.	
"	Ulcus ventriculi, female, 18 years ...	....	18.0	....	"	
"	Repeated intestinal hemorrhage......	....	20.0	....	"	
"	Anemia from ankylostomiasis......	....	21.0	....	"	
"	"	....	20.0	....	"	
"	"	....	30.0	....	"	
"	"	....	50.0	....	"	
"	Anemia from uterine hemorrhage, female, 51 years......	....	Trace.	....	Graanboom.	(Preceded by loss of blood? Q.)
"	Carcinoma	4.8	23.1	....		
"	Pneumonia	26.7	99.0	....		

Sex	Condition				Author	Notes
Man.	Phthisis	25.3	114.0		Graanboom.	Purpura ad ...nal hemorrhage.
"	Nephritis	31.9	129.0		"	
"	Leukemia		102.0		Stahel.	
"	"	98.3	390.0		Graanboom.	
"	"	11.0	55.0		v. Bemmelen.	
"	Pernicious anemia, case T. A.		337.0		R. Stockmann.	(7.6) These ...give the t...l
"	" " case E. S.		1890.0		Quincke.	(2.2) ...ity of iron in the liver
"	" " case B. S.		539.0		"	(1.5) in grams.
"	" " case V., after Stühlen.		364.0		"	The figures in parentheses are ...ed on the basis that
"	"		1900.0		Rosenstein.	the liver ...hs 1600 grams
"	"		518.0		Stahel.	(7.6)
"	"	129.0	614.0		Zaleski.	(2.1)
"	"	25.0	623.0		Nolen.	(2.5) and yields 25% of dry sub-
"	"		122.0		R. Stockmann.	(2.5) stance.
"	"		230.0		"	
"	Bothriocephalus anemia		140.0		"	Frequent hemorrhoidal hemorrhages
"	"		166.0		"	
"	Chronic malaria		262.0		"	
"	Addison's ...e...		257.0		"	
"	Anemia, pancreatic hemorrhage		120.0		Hindenlang.	Cutaneous and other hemorrhages.
"	Mb. ...al. Werlhofi	390.0	160.0		Zaleski.	(5.0)
"	"	11.0	1246.0		Auscher and Lapicque.	
"	Tuberculosis with i ...ternal hemor- rhages	1060.0	37.0		Quincke.	
"	...a, 9 years, ...le				"	
"	...ll hydrocephalus, 26 years		294.0		Zaleski.	(2.6)
"	Diabetes ...ns	16.5	581.0		Auscher and Lapicque.	26.9
"	...sis of the liver with di ...tes	1130.0	3607.0			
"	Phthisis, 60 ...rs; at ...e same time cirrhosis hepatis	627.0	68.0	30.8	Marchand.	"Berliner klin Wochenschrift," 1882, p. 46.

hemosiderosis (in contradistinction to pharmacosiderosis, Naunyn). The débris, consisting of used-up red blood-corpuscles, is probably carried to the liver in the plasma, partly in the form of hemoglobin in solution; the old red blood-corpuscles are also taken up by the pulp-cells of the spleen and enter the liver-capillaries while still within them. Still another portion may lodge within the liver-capillaries, and be taken up by the lymph-corpuscles and the endothelial cells of the vessel-walls. From these cells iron may be passed on to the liver-cells either in the form of hemoglobin or of some iron compound that reacts to ammonium sulphid. [Minkowski * has described a curious affection, apparently heredi- tary, in which there was chronic icterus, urobilinuria, enlargement of the spleen, and siderosis of the kidneys. Several members of the family had congenital icterus lasting for years. Two brothers, aged forty-two and fifty years, were distinctly icteric, with enlargement of the spleen. The children of both of these brothers also had the same association. Previous generations were also said to have had the same jaundice and dark urine, and in spite of these conditions lived to an advanced age. There was no evidence of malarial poisoning, nor was there any tendency to hemorrhages. The examination of the blood, made wherever possible, showed nothing unusual. In the only case in which autopsy was performed there was neither cirrhosis of the liver nor obstruction of its ducts. Even on microscopic examination there was nothing abnormal found in the liver except an abnormal pigmenta- tion of the cells in the center of the lobes, this pigmentation not showing the reaction for iron. The pigmented kidneys, however, gave an intense iron reaction, and the ash of one kidney yielded 1 or 2 grams of iron. Minkowski looks upon the affection as unique and evidently dependent upon a hereditary defect, probably an anomalous transformation of the blood-pigment, perhaps due to primary splenic trouble.—ED.] The hemoglobin of the red blood-corpuscles may be disintegrated in different ways. We learn this from the behavior of extravasations into connective tissue, where we see both bilirubin and hemosiderin deposited, the latter giving ammonium sulphid reactions (Langhans, Quincke).

In certain pathologic conditions the amount of iron present in the liver is very frequently increased, as may be demonstrated both by chemical analysis and by macroscopic and microscopic reactions.

Frequently only the liver-cells show an increased iron reaction (I will designate these cases as A), while in other, rarer instances the liver-capillaries alone give the reaction (B). Occasionally iron reactions are present in both the cells and the capillaries (C).

A most conspicuous increase of iron is found in pernicious anemia (A, C). This may be so considerable that the rusty color of the liver is evident to the naked eye. Sometimes as much as 1800 mg. of iron are found (*vide* table), and the total quantity in the liver may amount to 7 gm. of the metal. Similar conditions are found in bothrioceph- alus anemia (Stockmann). [*Vide* editorial note with reference to anemic hemolysis.—ED.] Siderosis of the liver is further found in many acute and chronic conditions, in acute enteritis of children (A, Peters), in typhoid and other acute febrile diseases (A, Quincke), in phthisis (A, C), in leukemia (A, Quincke, Stockmann), diabetes (A, C,

* " Verhandlungen des Cong. f. innere Medicin," 1900, p. 316.

Quincke), congested liver (Peters), chronic diarrhea (A, and atrophy, C, Quincke, Peters), in malaria (A, Kelsch and Kiener), in granular atrophy of the kidneys (A), in artificial plethora (A, C, Quincke), and also after large subcutaneous extravasation of blood (A, C, Quincke), in massive cellular hemorrhages (Hindenlang, Auscher, Lapicque), in cirrhosis of the liver (Hanot and Chauffard, Gilbert, Kretz, and others). The largest quantity I have ever found was in a case of diabetes mellitus (3600 mg., total quantity 27 gm.).

The origin of hepatic siderosis is in certain of these cases fairly clear. In cases of tissue-waste a large number of red blood-corpuscles are destroyed, as in hunger and in hibernation; iron is at such times deposited in the liver for future use. The same principle applies in the case of blood extravasations (including congested liver), and of artificial subcutaneous injections of blood into the circulatory stream or the peritoneal cavity. In leukemia the red blood-corpuscles perish, while the white ones enormously increase in number. The manner of destruction is not always the same; sometimes the solution and diffusion of hemoglobin in the plasma are more in evidence (hemolysis); in other cases there is partial destruction of the erythrocytes (rhestocythemia), their fragments being taken up by the leucocytes in the various organs. Of the blood-poisons that have been subjected to experimental tests, some act in one, some in another manner, this fact accounting for the various pictures presented by poisoning with different toxins. The variations depend altogether upon the blood-dissolving or blood-corpuscle-destroying properties of the different substances. In certain cases, as in the acute enteritis of children, and in the above-mentioned case of volvulus of the intestine, the hemoglobin seems to be dissolved with great rapidity. The fact that in some instances the liver-cells alone become siderotic, and in others only the capillaries, can only be explained on the basis of differences in the action of the various toxins, which are as yet unintelligible to us. Thus, we have observed that in experimental injections of hemoglobin at one time the capillaries, at another time the cells, show the greater deposits of iron. Other factors must cooperate in the process of hemolytic siderosis, possibly differences in the excretion of iron from the colon (or the bile?); we assume this from our knowledge of the fact that the condition of siderosis is neither proportionate to the amount of iron that is consumed nor constant, even though the pathologic process remains the same.

Several investigators have assumed (and Kretz recently) that a functional weakness of the liver-cells favors the deposit of iron. Such a weakness is not a necessary condition, however, inasmuch as experiments by Quincke, Nölke, and Schurig have demonstrated that the deposit may occur in healthy animals. In pernicious anemia we must assume that a particularly active destruction of red blood-corpuscles, hemophthisis, occurs. In the beginning there is probably a compensatory replacement of the erythrocytes as a result primarily of an increased activity of the bone-marrow; and the iron required is probably obtained by increased absorption. This excess is, however, immediately destroyed, and iron accumulates more and more in the liver. Owing to excessive overwork, the blood-forming powers of the bone-marrow decrease, and progressive anemia results in the same manner as in repeated losses of blood, with the difference, however, that in the case of such an internal hemorrhage the iron is deposited in the liver and the spleen. The clinical picture and the microscopic blood-findings may be the same in either case.

[Auschütz * considers especially the etiology of cases of cirrhosis with pigmentation. He finds that they do not occur with the atrophic cirrhosis of Laennec, but mainly with hypertrophic cirrhosis. Fletcher † also notes 8 cases of hypertrophic cirrhosis of the liver, of which one presented a remarkable grade of bronzing of the skin. The clinical symptoms are known as the condition *diabète bronzé*, and are quite similar in all cases. The liver showed at autopsy the features of a pigmentary cirrhosis. It is enlarged, and the cells and connective tissue contain a yellow, ochre-colored pigment, containing iron. The pigment may also be found in the muscle-fibers of the heart and in the lymphglands.—ED.]

In a certain number of cases of diabetes conditions similar to those observed in pernicious anemia seem to obtain. I have frequently seen siderosis (chiefly cellular) of the liver in cases of **diabetes**. There was not so much iron as in the other conditions, and here and there siderosis was completely absent. In cases of **acute enteritis** in children, and in cases of **chronic diarrhea,** we must assume that ptomains are formed in the intestine that act as blood-poisons. In **malaria,** the finely granular dark-brown, iron-free pigment, which is formed in the red blood-corpuscles, accumulates in the liver-capillaries. The iron-containing portion, which is split off, is dissolved in the blood-plasma and reaches the liver-cells in this way. In contracted kidney deposits of iron are often seen in the liver and the spleen. In typhoid and phthisis a pronounced siderosis of the liver may occasionally be present.

Only a few diseases lead to the deposit of large quantities of iron in the liver. This is seen particularly in diseases that are complicated by the destruction of large numbers of red blood-corpuscles. It will depend upon the intensity of the disease whether or not siderosis occurs, and the condition may be seen in certain stages of the disease and be absent in others.

Siderosis of the liver is in this respect similar to fatty liver. The accumulated material is held in the liver for future use; and occasionally the amount is so large that it can no longer be regarded as reserve material, but must, in part at least, be considered as permanently placed out of circulation. This applies more to the case of iron than to fat. It is possible, too, that a large quantity of iron is deposited in a form that is indifferent and not readily acted upon by ordinary agents.

Siderosis of the liver was first described by me in 1877. Mild degrees are frequently seen, if they are only looked for (discoloration of the adjacent intestine, and the ammonium sulphid reaction). In very pronounced cases the liver is rust-colored; but, as I have repeatedly emphasized, not only the brown parts of the protoplasm, but the colorless ones may give an iron reaction. There can be no doubt but that there is a great variety of possible iron compounds; this is clearly demonstrated by the differences that are seen in the ammonium sulphid reaction, both in regard to the rapidity with which the color change appears and the shade of the color. The nature of these various iron combinations is not well understood. Ferratin appears to be the most important one found in normal livers, though even it probably participates only to a slight extent, and possibly not at all, in the development of pathologic siderosis.

* *Deutsch. Arch. f. klin. Med.*, Bd. LXII, 1899, p. 411.
† *Jour. Am. Med. Assoc.*, Sept. 28, 1901, p. 815.

Little attention has been paid to siderosis of the liver, owing to the fact that no anatomic changes are seen other than an excessive deposit of iron and an enlargement of the organ. Clinical symptoms are not caused by the condition. The deposit of iron may, of course, occur in a liver that is already pathologically altered, just as a deposit of fat may occur under these conditions. As livers of this kind have been examined more frequently than normal ones, many investigators have called attention to the excess of iron and the rusty color in various lesions of the organ; in fact, French authors have formulated a distinct clinical entity which they call pigment cirrhosis, and claim that the deposit of iron is etiologically related to the proliferation of connective tissue. I have already called attention to this idea (see page 739), and have demonstrated that it is false. In pernicious anemia the liver may be very siderotic and still show no changes whatever in its connective-tissue structures. If such changes are present, they are, as a rule, due to some other factor. In experimental siderosis (Schurig, injections of hemoglobin, and Nölke, injections of citrate of iron) no connective-tissue changes were noted.

I have already mentioned the fact that siderosis may be seen in malaria-liver, when malaria pigment is deposited in the capillaries. Peters found an abundant quantity of iron that gave the iron reactions in the capillaries of amyloid livers; I have found it in acute fatty degeneration with icterus.* I have frequently examined livers in cases of icterus from stasis of long duration, but (maybe by chance) have never discovered the iron reaction. There seems to be no connection between stasis of bile and siderosis. Délépine, in a case in which one of the smaller ducts was occluded, could elicit an intense iron reaction in the immediate vicinity of the area of stasis, in the cells, and in the capillaries.

Symptoms.—Although the diseases that lead to siderosis are important for the very reason that they withdraw iron from other parts of the body, no symptoms are caused by the deposit of large quantities of iron in the liver *per se*. It might be assumed that icterus, when it is seen in pernicious anemia, is an icterus polycholicus, and is due to the increased disintegration of red blood-corpuscles, and is in this manner related to siderosis of the liver. In view of the fact, however, that icterus may be due to so many different causes, this symptom can hardly be utilized in making the diagnosis.

The size and the consistency of a siderotic liver are not increased. We are unable, therefore, to diagnose the condition. That the condition is present may be suspected, however, when some of the diseases that can cause it, as diabetes, pernicious anemia, etc., are present. Stühlen has shown that pernicious anemia and that form of severe anemia that is caused by great loss of blood differ chiefly in that in the latter condition less iron is contained in the affected organs. It might be of value from this point of view to recognize the existence of siderosis of the liver during the life of the patient. It might even be useful to attempt exploratory puncture of the liver during life in order to examine the aspirated material for iron.

The treatment of the primary disease should prevent or hinder the formation of hepatic siderosis. In cases in which the primary cause is known, as in certain forms of anemia, in absorption of intestinal ptomains, etc., the diet may be regulated, the bowels may be thoroughly evacuated and disinfected, and such drugs as calomel, bismuth subnitrate, tannin,

* v. Starck, *Deutsch. Archiv f. klin. Med.*, 1884, Bd. xxxv, p. 484.

salol, naphthol, benzonaphthol, yeast, etc., administered for this purpose.

According to the animal experiments of Nölke with citrate of iron, artificial siderosis can recede, the iron stored in the liver probably being eliminated through the intestine and the kidneys. It is probable, therefore, that pathologic siderosis of the liver, as seen in human beings, can also be cured. It is possible that the elimination of iron can be stimulated by the administration of an abundant quantity of water, by vegetable acids, and by the salts of these acids (sodium citrate, bitartrate of potassium) and by natural acid fruits.

The liver, it appears, possesses the power to store other metals in the same manner as iron; statements to this effect have been made in regard to lead, copper, bismuth, arsenic and antimony. In cases of poisoning with these metals they have been looked for in the liver and have been found there. As a rule, the quantity discovered in the liver is very small, and in the case of arsenic and antimony other changes in the organ will be found. There are not many careful quantitative records extant in regard to the exact amount of these metals found in the liver; the majority of the statements refer to lead-poisoning, but it does not appear that the liver, as in the case of iron, is capable of storing so much more of the metal than any of the other organs.[*]

(F) PIGMENTATION OF THE LIVER.

(Quincke.)

Substances are quite frequently found in the liver that influence the color of the organ, and are usually in such cases present in the liver-cells; they are more often granular than diffuse in character. The following substances may be mentioned:

1. **Normal liver pigment,** consisting of yellowish-brown granules found in a small number of cells, either near the periphery or near the center of the lobules. This pigment is not constantly found, and is present especially in old people, and in cases of atrophy of the liver. The intensity of the color and its shade are variable, and the chemical nature of the coloring substance is not accurately known. Probably there are several substances which owe their origin to more or less pathologic processes not yet thoroughly comprehended. One of these is possibly hemofuscin (see below).

2. **Bile-pigment,** usually bilirubin, more rarely biliverdin. Normally these are found only in the bile-passages; in cases of occlusion (and sometimes in the absence of this condition) the biliary pigments may stain the liver-cells, as well as the interstitial tissue, yellow. The greatest intensity is noted in the cells near the center of the lobules, and in the large and small granules within the cells. When the color is less intense, there is a slighter, more diffuse staining of the whole protoplasm. Necrotic foci are stained very intensely; the latter are often observed in this condition following the experimental production of biliary stasis in rabbits and guinea-pigs (Steinhaus and others), or following similar experiments in dogs (Pick and others) (compare page 429).

With the microscope it is usually possible to recognize bile-staining from its peculiar yellowish tint. On the addition of nitric acid Gmelin's color reaction is characteristic in the different tissues. It must not be forgotten, however, that if the tissue is hardened with alcohol, the bile-

[*] *Vide* Kobert, "Intoxicationen," p. 140.

pigment is in great measure dissolved; whereas if the organ is hardened in sublimate or formalin it is much better preserved.

3. **Rust-colored iron pigment.** I have discussed this pigment in the preceding section. It is found principally or exclusively in the periphery of the lobules, and may be present in the liver-cells as a diffuse or a granular stain. Sometimes it is seen in the other tissues, and usually in the form of coarse granules or collections of granules. This is particularly the case within the capillaries, in which the leucocytes and epithelial cells inclose the iron granules. They may also be seen in the large cells that come from the spleen. In rare instances they may be found within the leucocytes in the lumen of the veins, a fact from which we must assume that they are present occasionally in the free blood-stream. Granules are also found that give the iron reaction in Kupffer's stellate cells, in the vessel-sheaths, and in the interstitial connective tissues. Some of the colorless constituents of the protoplasm also give the iron reaction; these substances, as well as the iron compound, are probably combinations of iron with organic bodies, the iron being present as the ferri-compound. According to Auscher and Lapicque, they are a colloidal ferri oxyhydrate, Fe_2O_2, $3H_3O$ (? Q.). The brown pigment is usually found in conditions in which large quantities of blood are destroyed, either by extravasation or within the blood-stream, so that its hemoglobin or its iron compounds are in solution; damaged blood-corpuscles themselves may be carried, as such, to the liver.

4. **Brown pigment** is seen in venous hyperemia, chiefly in the center of the lobules and within the liver-cells (Perls); sometimes it responds to iron reactions, and may be identical with the pigment last considered. Sometimes it is not changed by the action of ammonium sulphid. It is probably derived from the red blood-corpuscles that make their exit through the stomata of the distended capillaries, and are altered in the interstitial tissues, as is the case in other extravasations.

In a case of aneurysm of the hepatic artery that ruptured into the bile-passages I found isolated red blood-corpuscles in some of the acini within the liver-cells. Their form and color were not markedly changed The hemoglobin had in part been converted into a brown pigment that gave a reaction with ammonium sulphid. In this instance the pressure of the blood had forced a few of the red blood-corpuscles through the bile-capillaries directly into the liver-cells.

5. **Malaria pigment.** The finely granular dark brown or black pigment that is formed by the plasmodium malariæ in the circulating red blood-corpuscles, and which is later found floating free in the blood-plasma, is arrested in the most various capillary areas, particularly in the spleen, the liver, and the bone-marrow. This process is analogous to the arrest of injected cinnabar. In the liver this pigment is never found in the granular cells themselves, but exclusively in the capillaries near the periphery of the lobules, and in the connective tissue of the blood-vessels. Jacobson has also observed it in the lumen of the hepatic veins. This brown-black malarial pigment is distinguished from the brown iron pigment of the liver by its color and by the uniform size of its granules. It does not give iron reactions, is insoluble in concentrated acids, but disappears in potash solutions and in solutions of chlorid of calcium (Neumann). Ammonium sulphid converts it into a reddish-brown or orange-colored pigment, which ultimately becomes colorless. This can be seen in microscopic preparations (Kelsch and Kiener).

6. **The pigment** of **melanotic sarcomata.** This pigment colors thick

masses of the tumor black, though microscopically it is yellowish-brown. It forms granules of various sizes within the sarcoma cells, and remains behind as a granular mass after the cells have perished. A portion of these granules may be carried off by the blood-current, and lodge in the liver, the spleen, and bone-marrow, just as do malaria pigment and cinnabar. In contradistinction to malaria pigment, sarcoma melanin appears to be particularly soluble in the blood-plasma (possibly after undergoing some modification). Within the liver this pigment is found exclusively in the capillaries and the interstitial connective tissue; never in the liver-cells. Sometimes it is present in such enormous quantities that the liver appears characteristically colored to the naked eye (compare Nölke and Hensen, case from the clinic in Kiel).

The pigment deposit changes the color and the markings of the liver. If bilirubin is present, the general shade of the liver will be bile-yellow or -green; if iron pigment is present, it will be rust-colored; if malaria pigment is present, chocolate-colored. The outlines of the lobules are usually more distinct because the ˙pigment is not evenly distributed; thus the bile-pigment and pigments formed by stasis are found near the center, malaria and iron-pigments near the periphery of the lobules. Occasionally several pigments are present at the same time, as, for instance, bile-pigment, together with malaria pigment, or pigment from stasis; malaria with iron pigment. If the vascularity of the organ is not uniform and the deposit of fat varies in different parts, and if, finally, there is a development of interlobular connective tissue, the picture may be very interesting.

In view of their various origin the significance of the different liver pigments varies. These differences are not sufficiently appreciated. We must not forget that the color of the organ is only one of the many external symptoms, and may be the same when caused by different substances. The damage caused in the liver by pigment deposits is apparently also various. When the deposit is bilirubin, it is greater than if it consists simply of iron (whether owing to the bilirubin or to other bile-constituents?). The deposit of pigment in the capillaries, as seen, for instance, in malaria or in melanotic sarcoma and siderosis, constitutes a mechanical obstruction to the blood-stream, interferes with the nutrition of the liver-cells, and hinders the circulatory stream in the portal system. Of much greater importance is it to determine whether, in addition to the deposit of pigment, the parenchyma has suffered injury, or whether changes have occurred in the interstitial connective tissue, as is the case especially in malaria and chronic stasis of bile.

Many clinicians include in the term "pigment liver" only the pigmented malaria liver, the so-called "melanemic" liver. This is not only a one-sided view, but an incorrect and confusing one, because rust-colored pigment is frequently found side by side with the brown malaria pigment. And yet the former is found in altogether different diseases, as, for instance, in pernicious anemia and diabetes. Many, if not all, of these forms of pigment are related to hemoglobin. In the case of bilirubin, malaria brown, and of the rust-colored iron pigment, this relationship has been established. In addition to the pigmentation of the liver, other organs are also found to be stained, so that in an attempt to explain the pathogenesis of this condition the liver should not be considered alone. Experiments have been directed with a view to explaining the conversion of the blood-pigment in extravasations, in artificial plethora, and following the ingestion of hemoglobin, and appear likely to throw some light upon this question.

Hemoglobin may be disintegrated in several ways so that different substances are generated: (1) *Bilirubin*, which is formed in blood-extravasations as well as in the liver (Langhans, Quincke). (2) *Malaria brown*, which is formed within circulating red corpuscles, and enters the plasma as soon as the latter disintegrate. Neither pigment contains iron; the iron is separated, dissolved, and is in part carried to a distance from the focus of pigmentation. (3) *Yellow and brown pigments* of different shades. These have been found particularly in spontaneous blood-extravasations, and after the injection of blood into the subcutaneous cellular tissues (Langhans, Quincke); also in the lungs (M. B. Schmidt). These pigments frequently appear as granules, particularly within the leucocytes or fixed connective-tissue cells. Sometimes they seem to be formed directly from red blood-corpuscles, and in other instances hemoglobin in solution is taken up by the cells and stored as a granular material (M. B. Schmidt, Schurig). In certain stages these granules give a reaction with ammonium sulphid; one which may, however, also be obtained with certain colorless granules, with the colorless protoplasm found at the point of extravasation, and with splenic cells, marrow-cells, liver-cells, leucocytes, and the connective-tissue cells of the liver. Some of the masses that give iron reactions are rust-colored. Neumann has grouped all these derivatives of red blood-corpuscles that give iron reactions under the name of hemosiderin. If the point of extravasation is examined, it will be found that the iron reaction does not appear for several days, and that later it then decreases in intensity (M. B. Schmidt); so that in the beginning very many, and later an increasing number of brown and yellowish granules are found that do not give the iron reaction. M. B. Schmidt also found that the iron reaction decreased in intensity some nine weeks after the injection of blood into the lungs. It is probable that by this time the iron is dissolved from the golden yellow and reddish-brown granules that are seen. During the period of transition —that is, during the time in which iron-containing masses appear and disappear— the intensity of the iron reaction is slight in the protoplasm granules, and may vary in shade from a very light-green to black-green. It appears, therefore, that a considerable number of substances are formed in blood-extravasations, and that these differ not only in color, but in the intensity of the iron reaction. The same observation can be made in the case of the pigmentary substances found in the spleen, the bone-marrow, and the liver, and of the colorless ones that are present and give an iron reaction in these organs.*

Recklinghausen's hemofuscin belongs to this group; it does not respond to the iron reactions, but is found together with iron-containing brown pigments in many organs, thus presenting the condition that Recklinghausen has called hemochromatosis.†

v. Recklinghausen found iron pigment only in the glands and stellate cells of the liver, in the connective-tissue cells of the synovial membranes of the joints, in serous and subserous tissues, in superficial cartilage cells, in lymph-glands, and vessel-sheaths; but not in the glandular cells of the salivary glands, the gastric and intestinal glands, the mucus- and sweat-glands, nor in the small muscle-fibers of the intestine, the blood, or the lymph-vessels. All the latter tissues contained hemofuscin. Other observers (Quincke, Hintze, Buss) have seen the iron reaction, in addition to hemofuscin, in the heart-muscle, the glandular cells of the pancreas, of the salivary glands, of the hypophysis, the prostate, the thyroid, the epithelium of the choroid plexus, and, to a slight degree, in the small muscle-fibers of the vessels. Hintze calls attention to the fact that pigment granules sometimes give a weak iron reaction, and that here, as in the extravasations, transition stages are seen between the two pigments; for this reason Recklinghausen's strict distinction between hemosiderin and hemofuscin cannot be maintained. I am personally very much in doubt whether the last-named substance is a distinct substance of itself, or whether it is a collective name for a variety of substances. While local staining with hemofuscin may be due to extravasation of blood, we are not justified in always attributing general hemochromatosis to the hemorrhagic diathesis, as does v. Reckling-

---

* The pigment granules of the liver stain well with methyl-violet, though not all with equal intensity, and form a dark blue color. The iron-bearing leucocytes are of a dull grayish-blue, and the splenic granules (pigment) garnet-red (Quincke).

† Hemofuscin is very stable, alcohol, ether, chloroform, and strong acids exerting no influence or change upon it (Buss).

hausen. The latter condition probably originates from a long-continued process of destruction of red blood-corpuscles, during which the derivatives of hemoglobin, whether they contain iron or not (whether they are pigments or chromogens), are dissolved in the circulation, and thus reach the cells of the various organs, where they are precipitated as a finely granular deposit. In slight degrees of this hemolysis the deposit of the colorless iron as well as of the brown pigment occurs only in the liver, later in the spleen and bone-marrow; in the more severe degrees, hemosiderin or hemofuscin may be found in the other tissues.

The deposit of iron and of pigment usually occurs simultaneously, but not necessarily so, and the deposits of the two substances do not follow a parallel. The degree of hemolysis can, therefore, only be determined by estimating the quantity of both pigments.

The deposit of pigment in the liver is a very conspicuous symptom. It is impossible, however, to estimate its significance correctly without determining the nature of the pigment, and without studying all changes that occur in the body as well as those that take place in the liver.

What we have already said with regard to the diagnosis of siderosis applies also to the diagnosis of pigment deposits during life, and to the significance of the accompanying changes in the size and the consistency of the liver.

LITERATURE.

Deposits of Iron and Pigment in the Liver.

Auscher and Lapicque: "Accumulation d'hydrate ferrique dans l'organisme animal," "Archives de physiologie," 1896, tome VIII, p. 399.

Biondi, C.: "Experimentelle Untersuchungen über die Ablagerung von eisenhaltigem Pigment in den Organen infolge von Hämatolyse," Ziegler's "Beiträge zur pathologischen Anatomie," 1895, Bd. XVIII, p. 174.

Buss, W.: "Ein Fall von Diabetes mellitus, etc., mit allgemeinerHämachromatose," Dissertation, Göttingen, 1894.

Délépine: "On the Normal Storage of Iron in the Liver," "The Practitioner," 1890, vol. XLV, No. 2.

de Filippi: "Experimentaluntersuchungen über das Ferratin," "Beiträge zur pathologischen Anatomie," 1894, Bd. XVI, p. 46.

Frerichs: "Leberkrankheiten," Bd. I, p. 324, Tafel 9, 10, 11.

Glaeveke, L.: "Ueber die Ausscheidung und Vertheilung des Eisens im Thierkörper nach Einspritzung von Eisensalzen," Dissertation, Kiel, 1883; und "Archiv für experimentelle Pathologie," 1883, Bd. XVII, p. 466.

Gottlieb: "Ueber die Ausscheidungsverhaltnisse des Eisens," "Zeitschr. für physiologische Chemie," 1891, Bd. XV, p. 371.

Guillemonat: "Recherches anatomo-patholog. et expérimentales sur la teneur en fer du foie et de la rate," Thèse de Paris, 1896.

— and Lapicque: "Teneur en fer du foie et de la rate chez l'homme," "Archives de physiologie," 1896, tome VIII, p. 841.

Hall, W. S.: "Ueber die Resorption des Carneferrins," "Archiv für Anatomie und Physiologie," Physiologische Abtheilung, 1894, p. 455.

— "Ueber das Verhalten des Eisens im thierischen Organismus," "Archiv für Anatomie und Physiologie," Physiologische Abtheilung, 1896, p. 49.

Hindenlang, O.: "Pigmentinfiltration von Leber, Lymphdrusen," etc., "Virchow's Archiv," 1880, Bd. LXXIX, p. 492.

Hintze, K.: "Ueber Hämachromatose," "Virchow's Archiv," 1896, Bd. CXXXIX, p. 459.

Hochhaus and Quincke: "Ueber Eisenresorption," etc., "Archiv für experimentelle Pathologie," 1896, Bd. XXXVII, p. 159.

Hunter, W.: "The Pathology of Pernicious Anemia," "The Lancet," 1888, II, pp. 555, 608.

Jacobi: "Ueber das Schicksal der in das Blut gelangten Eisensalze," "Archiv für experimentelle Pathologie," 1891, Bd. XVIII, p. 257.

Jacobson, O.: "Malaria und Diabetes," Dissertation, Kiel, 1896.

Kelsch and Kiener: "Maladies des pays chauds," Paris, 1889, pp. 414, 550; table III, figure 4; table v, figure 2.

Kiener and Engel: "Sur les altérations d'ordre hématique produites par le sulfure de carbone," "Comptes-rendus de l'académie des sciences," 1886.
Kretz: "Hämosiderinpigmentirung der Leber und Lebercirrhose," "Beiträge zur klin. Medicin und Chirurgie," No. 15, Wien, 1896.
Krüger: "Ueber den Eisengehalt der Leber und Milzzellen in verschied enen Lebensaltern," "Zeitschr. für Biologie," 1890, Bd. xxvii, p. 439.
Kunkel: "Zur Frage der Eisenresorption," "Pflüger's Archiv," 1891, Bd. l.
— "Blutbildung aus anorganischem Eisen," "Pfluger's Archiv," 1895, Bd. lxi.
Langhans: "Virchow's Archiv," Bd. xl.
Naunyn: "Siderosis der Leber bei Diabetes," Nothnagel's "Specielle Pathologie und Therapie," vol. vii, 6, p. 240.
Neumann: "Beitrag zur Kenntniss der pathologischen Pigmente," "Virchow's Archiv," Bd. cxi.
— "Notizen zur Pathologie des Blutes," "Virchow's Archiv," 1889, Bd. cxvi, p. 318.
Peters, E.: "Ueber Siderosis," Dissertation, Kiel, 1881; und "Deutsches Archiv für klin. Medicin," 1882, Bd. xxxii, p. 182.
Quincke, H.: "Ueber perniciöse Anämie," Volkmann's "Sammlung klin. Vorträge," 1876, No. 100.
— "Ueber Siderosis," Festschrift, Bern, 1877.
— "Ueber Wärmeregulation beim Murmelthier," "Archiv für experimentelle Pathologie," 1881, Bd. xv, p. 20.
— "Zur Physiologie und Pathologie des Blutes" "Deutsches Archiv für klin. Medicin," 1880, Bd. xxv, xxvii; 1883, Bd. xxxiii.
— "Bildung von Gallenfarbstoff in Blutextravasaten," "Virchow's Archiv," 1884, Bd. xcv, p. 125.
— "Ueber Eisentherapie," Volkmann's "Sammlung klinischer Vorträge," Neue Folge, 1895, No. 129, pp. 5 to 13.
v. Recklinghausen: "Ueber Hämachromatose," "Bericht der Naturforscher-Versammlung zu Heidelberg," 1889, p. 324.
Samoiloff: "Beitrag zur Kenntniss des Verhaltens des Eisens im thierischen Organismus," "Arbeiten des pharmaceutischen Instituts zu Dorpat," 1893, p. 1.
Schaumann and Tallqvist: "Ueber die Blutkörper auflösende Eigenschaft des breiten Bandwurms," "Deutsche med. Wochenschr.," 1898, No. 20.
Schüppel, O.: "Ziemssen's Handbuch," Bd. viii, 1, p. 420.
Schurig: "Ueber die Schicksale des Hamoglobins im Organismus," "Archiv für experimentelle Pathologie," 1898, Bd. xli, p. 29.
Schwalbe, C.: "Die experimentelle Melanämie durch Schwefelkohlenstoff und Kohlenoxysulfid," "Virchow's Archiv," 1886, Bd. cv, p. 486.
Stadelmann and Gorodecki: "Ueber die Folgen subcutaner und intraperitonealer Hämoglobininjectionen," "Archiv für experimentelle Pathologie," Bd. xxvii, p. 93.
Stahel, H.: "Der Eisengehalt in Leber und Milz nach verschiedenen Krankheiten," "Virchow's Archiv," 1881, Bd. lxxxv, p. 26.
v. Starck: "Ueber Hämoglobininjectionen," "Münchener med. Wochenschr.," 1898, Nos. 3 und 4.
Stockmann, R.: "Remarks on the Analysis of Iron in the Liver," etc., "British Medical Journal," May 2, 1896.
Stühlen, A.: "Ueber den Eisengehalt verschiedener Organe bei anämischen Zuständen," "Deutsches Archiv für klin. Medicin," 1895, Bd. liv, p. 248.
Vay, Fr.: "Ueber den Ferratin- und Eisengehalt der Leber," "Zeitschr. für physiologische Chemie," 1895, Bd. xx, p. 377.
Westphalen: "Ueber den mikrochemischen Nachweis von Eisen im fötalen Organismus," etc., "Archiv für Gynäkologie," Bd. liii.
Woltering: "Ueber die Resorbirbarkeit der Eisensalze," "Zeitschr. für physiologische Chemie," 1895, Bd. xxi, p. 186.
Zaleski: "Zur Pathologie der Zuckerharnruhr und zur Eisenfrage," "Virchow's Archiv," 1886, Bd. civ, p. 92.
— "Eisengehalt der Leber," "Zeitschr. für physiologische Chemie," 1886, Bd. x, p. 6.
— "Zur Frage über die Ausscheidung des Eisens aus dem Thierkörper," "Archiv für experimentelle Pathologie," 1887, Bd. xxiii, p. 317.
— "Das Eisen der Organe bei Morbus maculosus Werlhofii," Ebendaselbst, Bd. xxiii, p. 77.

FUNCTIONAL DISTURBANCES OF THE LIVER.

(Quincke.)

In view of the numerous functions performed by the liver, the combinations of these different functions must vary greatly even under physiologic conditions. In the light of the conditions that influence these functions, moreover, how great must these variations be? The amount of food taken, the character of the diet, rest and exercise, are probably the main conditions. In addition, the different ingredients of the food, alkalies, acids, ammonia salts, spices, alcohol, etc., must all be considered; also an increase or a decrease in the biliary secretion. Any one of the functions may be excessive or may be reduced, may be stimulated or depressed.

We may assume that deviations from the normal in the different liver functions occur under the following conditions: (1) After anomalies of gastric and intestinal digestion. Anomalies of this kind will influence biliary secretion and internal metabolism. (2) General metabolic anomalies, overfeeding, plethora, diabetes, obesity, gout, as well as anemia and cachexia, for instance, after carcinomatosis, may any or all produce qualitative and quantitative changes of the liver function. (3) All febrile and many infectious diseases. (4) Psychic and other nervous influences.

In the last three groups the functional disturbance may be of hepatic origin, but may be also in part due to deviations from normal metabolic processes in other organs, owing to which the liver is secondarily influenced. As usual it is difficult to draw a strict distinction between physiologic variations and pathologic disturbances. Functional disturbances usually precede anatomic changes, and play a definite rôle in the etiology of many diseases of the liver that have been discussed above. They must be considered in the prophylaxis, the treatment, and the after-treatment of these conditions. There are always transitions from purely functional disturbances of the liver to congestive hyperemia, hypertrophy, and fatty degeneration; in considering these anomalies the purely functional disturbances of the early stages of the condition have also been considered.

In the treatment of gastrointestinal diseases, as well as in that of diseases of metabolism, functional disturbances of the liver will have to be considered with reference to therapeutic principles.

We will only refer to these functional disturbances of the liver and to their significance. As a matter of fact, we have little to aid us in their recognition, aside from slight changes in the composition of the urine and the stools. Formerly, and even to-day, in the English and French literature, certain symptoms have been directly attributed to disturbances of the hepatic function. Among these are a yellowish, sallow complexion, a feeling of pressure and fulness in the epigastric and right hypochondriac regions, a thick yellow coating of the tongue, a bitter taste, bilious vomiting, flatulency and heart-burn, irregularities of the stool, the passage of very light-colored or very dark feces, and of dark urine which forms a large sediment. In addition, there may be headache after eating, psychic irritability, etc.

None of these symptoms, however, demonstrates conclusively that the liver is involved, although it is true that they are also observed in many diseases of the liver, and also in many other pathologic conditions that may and do lead to involvement of the liver. It is confusing, however, to teach old theories or old hypotheses that have been constructed on a false basis, and it is not proper to look for functional disturbances of the liver in every case in which there are digestive disorders. On the other hand, of course, we cannot insist on a purely anatomic classification of diseases. It is just as erroneous to recognize nothing else than a catarrh of the stomach and intestine, and to discard all the older diagnoses of gastricism, weak stomach, dyspepsia, and diarrhea, as to look for functional disturbance of the liver in every case of catarrh. It is probable that catarrhal conditions are present in many cases, but we are not as yet able to recognize them in every instance.

Murchison: "Functional Derangement of the Liver," London, 1874.
Cayley, in Davidson: "Diseases of Warm Climates," 1893, p. 637. *Vide* also sections, General Etiology, p. 451; Hyperemia, p. 607; and Fatty Liver, p. 835.

NEURALGIA OF THE LIVER.

(Nervous Liver Colic.)

(Quincke.)

The term neuralgia of the liver is applied to the occurrence of violent spasmodic pain in the region of the liver which cannot be explained on anatomic grounds. The pain resembles gall-stone colic, is as violent, and may last from half an hour to several hours, or even several days.

The patient is prostrated by the pain, very much excited, restless, pale, and collapsed; the pulse is small and irregular, but may either be accelerated or retarded. The pain starts in the right hypochondriac region, and may either remain localized strictly in the region of the liver (Fürbringer) or may radiate like the typical colic. It is usually increased by pressure on the liver. In the case reported by Talma pressure over the region of the gall-bladder only was painful. Sometimes other pressure-points are also painful—the ovary, the kidneys, the uterus, the celiac plexus. During the spasm of pain vomiting often occurs, though never chills or a rise of temperature. Icterus and enlargement of the liver, which are often present in cholelithiasis, are also absent in hepatic neuralgia. When they are reported as appearing in isolated cases, suspicion is always aroused that the case was not purely of nervous origin.

The attacks of pain are frequently periodic, and may occur shortly before menstruation (Frerichs), during menstruation (Pariser), every night, every six weeks, or every three months (Fürbringer). Cyr observed a cycle of attacks occurring twice a day on the first, second, third, eighth, and fourteenth days, first and sixth months. The cause of the attack is usually not discovered; in other instances menstruation, psychic excitement, social excesses, or, in some people, the abuse of alcohol, strong spices, mustard, pepper, vinegar (Beau), or tea (Cussak) can be made responsible.

In the intervals between the attacks there is usually, though not always, an absence of pain.

Frequency of Occurrence.—Nervous hepatic colic is found exclusively in hysterical, nervous, and usually anemic individuals, consequently most often in women, and particularly in young girls. In cases of this kind other symptoms of a nervous character are usually present, as intercostal neuralgia, or facial neuralgia, and these may alternate with the liver colic, or may later take its place entirely. The patellar reflex is frequently exaggerated. Spasms of different kinds may appear independently, or together with attacks of liver colic.

Nature of the Disease.—The pathogenesis of these pains is as obscure as in other forms of neuralgia. They have been attributed to irritation of the hepatic plexus originating in the abdominal sympathetic and following the course of the hepatic artery; they have also been ascribed to spasms of the bile-passages. This would be analogous to muscular spasm of other hollow organs. This view is strengthened by certain peculiarities we know to exist in gall-stone colic. If this explanation is the correct one, the appearance of a slight icterus, or a partial obstruction to the flow of bile, or a transitory enlargement of the liver, might still be considered symptoms of purely nervous colic. The connection of the attacks with the ingestion of certain substances may indicate an idiosyncrasy, with analogies in the cardialgia following ingestion of lemons, asthma after ipecac, urticaria after crabs.

Vasomotor disturbances, spasm of the vessel-walls, particularly of the hepatic artery, must also be considered, and are analogous pictures to that of migraine. It may also be true that sensory, motor, or vaso-motor nerves may be involved, as in other organs.

Diagnosis.—While the existence of nervous colic of the liver is un-questionably established as a fact, the diagnosis of this condition must be very carefully made, and particularly when we remember the manifold appearances that an attack of gall-stone colic may present. Several authors (Beau, Cyr) have apparently not drawn a sufficiently sharp distinction, so that for a time the symptom-complex of nervous colic was either forgotten or its existence denied.

The differential points between gall-stone colic and this condition may be enumerated as follows: the disposition of the patient; the above-mentioned primary causes of the attacks; the absence of icterus, of swell-ing of the liver, and of concretions in the stools; the periodicity and limitation of the pain to the liver region. As we have stated above, none of these symptoms is absolutely diagnostic (a nervous woman may be afflicted with gall-stones, etc.). If several of these factors, however, are present together, the disease is probably a nervous one. Sometimes the diagnosis will have to be deferred until treatment has been instituted for cholelithiasis, without effecting any result. As the pain in gall-stones is only partially nervous and to a great extent inflammatory in character, the absence of all inflammatory symptoms in a given case may be of value (a palpable or percussible tumor, and the persistence of pain in the gall-bladder in the interval between the attacks).

Treatment.—The treatment of neuralgia of the liver should be di-rected with a view to improvement of the general health, and an ameliora-tion of the general nervous condition. The mode of life and the occupa-tion should be regulated, and bodily exercise and the diet supervised. It is necessary to particularize, especially in warning against the different factors that may cause an attack. Thorough regulation of the intestinal functions is invaluable; massage of the hepatic region and of the abdomen is sometimes useful. In treating the attacks the selection and dosage of narcotics must be governed by the general condition of the nervous system. In gall-stones an operation is indicated; in neuralgia of the liver it should of course be avoided, and the diagnosis is particularly important in view of rendering a decision in regard to the necessity of operative interference. In doubtful cases an operation has been performed, but the possible nervous origin of the colic should be remembered, so that if the operation reveals negative conditions it can be stopped in time.

LITERATURE.

Beau, J. H. L.: "Archives générales de médecine," 1851, tome xxv, p. 397.
Cyr, J.: "Sur la périodicité de certains symptomes hépatiques," "Archives générales de médecine," 1883, I, p. 539.
— "Causes d'erreur dans le diagnostic de l'affection calculeuse du foie," "Archives générales de médecine," 1890, I, p. 165.
Frerichs: Loc. cit., II, p. 526.
Fürbringer: "Zur Kenntniss der Pseudogallensteine und sogenannten Leberkolik," "Verhandlungen des Congresses für innere Medicin," 1892, p. 313; 1891, p. 55.
Naunyn: "Klinik der Cholelithiasis," p. 86.
Pariser, C.: "Beitrag zur Kenntniss der nervösen Leberkolik (Neuralgia hepatis)," "Deutsche med. Wochenschr.," 1893, p. 741.
Talma, S.: "Zur Kenntniss des Leidens des Bauchsympathicus. Leberschmerz," "Deutsches Archiv für klin. Medicin," 1892, Bd. xlix, p. 233.

DISEASES OF THE VESSELS OF THE LIVER.

DISEASES OF THE PORTAL VEIN.

(Quincke.)

THE portal vein has an important rôle in the genesis of many diseases of the liver in so far as it carries many noxious agencies to the organ; among the latter portions of the ingesta, products of intestinal decomposition, and also bacteria. This probably explains why so many diseases of the parenchyma of the liver begin in the periphery of the acini, where the branches of the portal vein dissolve into capillaries. It also explains why so many diffuse diseases of the liver begin in small circumscribed foci in the interlobular spaces. In so far as other diseases than those of the liver are caused by the absorption of poisonous products from the intestinal tract, the portal vein really serves as the entrance gate for all these toxic substances, so that Stahl's old proverb, "*Vena portarum porta malorum*," is justified, even though originally it was based upon theoretic speculation.

Although the portal vein is the main channel for the entrance of disease-producing agencies, it is itself comparatively seldom affected, at least to any marked extent. It is possible that certain functional disturbances occur, and escape recognition owing to the protected position and the difficulty of observing lesions of this vessel; and that such disturbances are of greater significance with respect to diseases of the abdomen than we know. Certain facts seem, indeed, to indicate this as true.

The portal vein and its branches are devoid of valves, but contain a strong internal circular musculature, as well as external longitudinal muscle-fibers. In the long and short intestinal veins there are valves, and the circular musculature is predominant. The latter fibers decrease in number as the veins converge to form the portal vein, and ultimately disappear altogether in the ramifications of the portal vein within the liver, so that the latter vessels only have a longitudinal musculature (Koeppe). The muscles of the wall of the portal vein are supplied by the splanchnic nerve. After ligation of the lower thoracic aorta in a dog, so that the amount of blood present in the portal system was reduced, P. F. Mall has observed a narrowing of the portal vein and a complete disappearance of its lumen if the splanchnic nerve was irritated.

Kronecker determined the amount of blood in the portal vessels of the intestinal canal in rabbits (colorimetrically). If the aorta was occluded and the intestine massaged gently, and then the portal vein ligated, only 1 to 2 cm. of blood were found. If, on the other hand, the portal vein was ligated first and the aorta not closed until the animals had begun to grow weak, the vessels of the intestine contained from 14 to 24 cm. of blood; that is, ten times as much. About the same amount of blood remained in the liver after ligation of the portal vein.

These experiments, and the well-known changes in the vascularity of the whole intestinal blood-vessel system during hunger and during digestion, demonstrated that both the capacity and the lumen of the total portal system are subject to great variations. To what degree this change actually occurs and what rôle it plays in the causation of abdominal disturbances of a nervous character, and what significance it has in certain diseases of the liver, we do not know. It would be a very interesting and important matter to determine this point. The experiments of Asp and others demonstrate that irritation of the splanchnic nerves causes a rise of arterial pressure, but this can only in part be attributed to an increased filling of the arteries following the emptying of the portal system; in part they must be explained by an increase of the general tone of the arteries from reflex irritation of the splanchnics.

Experiments carried on by the Ludwig school (F. Hofmann, Tappeiner, and others) show that rabbits die a few hours after ligation of the portal vein. At first this was explained by assuming a plethora of the portal system; the theory was formulated that the animal bled to death into the portal vein. This was not tenable, however, because Hofmann found only 30 % and Tappeiner only 10 % of the total blood in the roots of the portal vein. Kronecker added the amount of blood present in the liver, but even with this the amount of blood withdrawn from the general circulation is not sufficient to explain death after ligation of the portal vein. Possibly there is a paresis of the general arterial tree from reflex irritation; or an intoxication following the obstruction of the circulation and the resulting interference with the nutrition of the parts.

I refer to the experiments of Nencki and his associates on page 406 to demonstrate how complicated and obscure the results of any change in the portal blood may be. These experiments consisted in allowing the portal blood to flow into the lower vena cava.

In the light of our present knowledge we can group the diseases of the portal vein as follows: First, disturbances of the blood-stream following occlusion and narrowing of the stem of the portal vein or of its branches; second, inflammation of the walls of the portal vein.

OCCLUSION AND NARROWING OF THE PORTAL VEIN.

This condition may be caused by:

1. Diseases of the wall of the portal vein. Acute and chronic inflammations of the vessel-wall, or the extension of a neoplasm by continuity, alter the endothelium and cause the formation of a wall-thrombus which may narrow or even occlude the lumen of the vessel. It may develop rapidly or slowly, or it may dissolve away, or it may become thoroughly organized. If the latter process takes place, the occlusion of the vessel may become permanent (pylephlebitis adhæsiva). This disease of the venous wall is analogous to arteriosclerosis, but not as frequent as the latter; the investigations of Sack and Wehnert demonstrate that it is not as rare, however, as is generally believed. The resulting thrombi and vessel-occlusions in other venous areas do not

produce any serious consequences when there are free anastomotic channels. It is a different matter in the case of the portal vein, in which chronic phlebitis seems to be the chief cause of occlusion of the vessel (see statistics of Borrmann of cases quoted by Gintrac, Balfour and Stewart, Raikem, Morhead). This endophlebitic thrombosis may begin in the main trunk of the portal vein itself or may originate in the splenic or mesenteric veins. Occasionally the phlebitis is of syphilitic origin.

2. **Compression from without.** This may be brought about by tumors, particularly carcinomata, starting from the stomach, the pancreas, the mesentery, the retroperitoneal glands, or the liver itself. It may also be due to enlarged portal lymph-glands lying in close proximity to the vessel. These glands are frequently involved in cases of neoplastic growth in their neighborhood (carcinoma or tuberculosis). Gall-stones, too, may compress the vessel, if situated in the hepatic or the common duct (Key and Bruzelius). Cicatricial inflammation in the neighborhood of the portal vein accomplishes the same result; this condition is frequently caused by syphilis, and starts in the liver with gumma formation. The syphilitic process may involve the wall of the vein itself. Chronic peritonitis may also cause the formation of compressing adhesions, particularly in tuberculosis of the peritoneum (Achard), duodenal ulcers (Frerichs), or infarction of the spleen (Osler). Sometimes these circumscribed inflammations of the peritoneum are caused by concretions situated in the gall-bladder or the large bile-ducts. The very nature of these lesions renders it probable that, in addition to pressure upon the venous wall, alterations should occur in its structure, and in this way cause the complications of thrombosis.

These lesions are generally seen in that part of the portal vein that is outside of the liver; less frequently in one of its main branches, or its roots, the mesenteric and the splenic vein.

3. **Slowing of the blood-current,** as in the case of other veins, aids in the formation of thrombosis. As narrowing of the lumen may cause a slowing of the blood-stream, it constitutes of itself a cause of thrombosis. Cirrhosis of the liver also causes slowing of the blood, which in this case is due to a narrowing of the capillary area (possibly this is the cause in Case 2 of Nonne). A general lack of circulatory power rarely is the cause of the above-named lesions in the portal area, though it is well known that in the veins of the lower extremity such a weakness may lead to marantic thrombosis (Auréol; Case 1 of Nonne is very questionable). It is possible that the portal vein is so often exempt because it is never at rest, there being a constant variation in the swiftness of the current and in the fulness and position of the vessel, owing to the continual peristaltic action of the intestine.

4. **Changes in the contents** of the portal vein. It appears that the parasite which lives in the portal system, Distoma hæmatobium (see page 830), possesses very little coagulative power. At the same time, the parasites occasionally occlude one or the other branch of the portal vein by mechanical obstruction followed by coagulation. Inflammatory lesions situated in the portal area may pour their products into the portal vein, and in this way increase the coagulability of the blood; such an increase in the coagulability is apparently present in pyemia and other severe diseases. We do not understand the exact cause of this condition, and it is quite possible that it forms the basis of some obscure cases of portal thrombosis whose etiology is unknown.

Experiments by Wooldridge are worthy of mention. This investigator succeeded in causing coagulation of the blood by the endovenous injection of a peculiar proteid body, obtained from the thymus. In rabbits such an injection caused death at once; in dogs, however, coagulation seemed only to occur in the portal system; if the occlusion is complete, death will of course occur. If smaller quantities are injected, a partial coagulation is the result, followed by certain lesions of the liver which will be discussed presently.

5. It need hardly be stated that in many cases of thrombotic occlusion of the portal vein the cause remains unknown (see above).

Anatomy.—Narrowing of the portal vein may vary from one of a slight degree causing no symptoms to complete occlusion. Compression is frequently associated with the formation of thrombi. The thrombi show the well-known changes in color, consistency, laminated structure, etc. Unfortunately their character does not admit of our drawing any conclusions with regard to their age, this fact rendering the pathogenetic interpretation of the individual case extraordinarily difficult. If the thrombus becomes organized, and particularly if there is plastic inflammation of the vessel-wall, complete organic occlusion of the vein may result. On the other hand, the clinical course of some cases, as well as analogous findings in other veins, indicates that an occlusion may retrogress, and that reabsorption and contraction of the thrombotic material may occur.

Softening of the thrombus is observed with particular frequency in inflammation of the roots of the portal vein. The contents of the latter may themselves form a thrombus, or small particles of a softened thrombus may be carried on into the liver, and cause embolic occlusion of large or small branches of the portal vein within the organ. Even if the thrombus does not undergo softening, certain mechanical influences may cause a transportation of coagulates from the splenic veins (Frerichs) or the hemorrhoidal veins (Köhler) to the liver.. If a carcinoma perforates the wall of the portal vein, numerous carcinoma nodules may be formed in the liver. In other cases degeneration of the carcinoma does not occur, growth taking place within the lumen of the vessel, and ultimately filling it; then following on into its ramifications, and in this manner producing very peculiar pictures.

Whenever thrombosis is present, there is a tendency for it to extend within the vessel. This, as a rule, occurs more readily, and to a greater extent, from the roots and the stem than backward from the branches into the stem.

Any or all of the changes described, however, may be found either in the main portion of the vessel or in its roots or branches.

Other processes are frequently seen in the liver associated with occlusion of the portal vein. Among them may be a proliferation of the connective tissue, either circumscribed (cicatrix) or diffuse (in the form of Laennec's cirrhosis). There may also be atrophy of the liver tissue; this also may be diffuse, or limited to one lobe, if individual branches of the portal vein are alone occluded. In the latter event the atrophic changes are often severe. The changes in the liver may either be a result of the occlusion of the portal vein, and may be directly due to disturbances of nutrition; or extensive narrowing of the liver-capillaries may occur as a result of the cirrhotic process, leading to secondary narrowing or thrombosis of the large afferent vessel. Both interpretations have been advocated, and it is probable that in certain cases the first and in others the second theory is the correct one.

The following statistics have recently been collected by Borrmann and v. Bermant. Cases in which the liver has undergone simple atrophy as a result of occlusion of the portal vein have been described by Gintrac (three cases), Bertog (two cases), Leyden and Waldenstrom; others with cirrhotic atrophy by Gintrac (two cases), Botkin and Carson. If only single branches of the portal vein are occluded, focal lesions may develop, which resemble the *hemorrhagic infarcts* of other organs, in that the current within the hepatic veins runs backward, so to speak, causing hyperemia in the affected area. The foci are wedge-shaped or oval, and usually extend to the surface of the organ; they vary in size from that of a hazelnut to a whole lobe. In the beginning they are distinguished from their surroundings by their dark red to brown color, and are outlined clearly by a distinct jagged line. Generally they are soft (Koehler-Orth, two cases; Rattone, Dreschfeld). Later these areas are depressed as a result of the decrease in size of the liver-cells. They grow pale and undergo cicatrization (Rattone). In one case, reported by Bermant, the whole right lobe had disappeared, and in its place was seen a cicatricial mass about as large as a hen's egg.

Oré, and later Solowieff, caused experimental narrowing of the portal vein, and produced contraction of the liver, a decrease in the size of the hepatic cells, as well as an increase of the connective tissue. If the occlusion of the portal vein was brought about suddenly, death occurred in from four to twenty-two hours. The liver was found engorged with blood, its cells enlarged and cloudy. In some of the branches of the portal vein coagula were found, and the surrounding liver tissue was seen to be infiltrated with leucocytes.

Other observations seem to show that occlusion of the portal vein is not followed by these results. Asp, for instance, experimented on dogs, and found that after ligation of the portal vein the secretion of bile was decreased but not stopped; so that it appeared that the amount of blood carried into the liver through the hepatic artery was sufficient to maintain the secretion of bile. Cohnheim saw nothing but hyperemia of the center of the acini in a case of diabetes with chronic thrombosis of the portal vein. This hyperemia was limited to the areas of the liver supplied by the obstructed portal branches. Cohnheim and Litten attempted to produce artificial embolization in the liver and succeeded in obtaining only a natural injection. They found that the hepatic artery supplies the vessels of the bile-ducts, the walls of the portal vein, and the hepatic veins, as well as the connective tissue of Glisson's capsule; that the veins gathered from these capillaries pour their contents into the interlobular branches of the portal vein; and that there is only a slight communication between the arterial capillaries and the capillaries of the portal vein. This finding was opposed to that of Chronchzewsky, who claims that the periphery of the lobules is supplied by the portal vein, the center by the hepatic artery. When arterial blood was excluded from the whole liver or from a lobe by ligation of the hepatic artery, or of one of its main branches, necrosis of the liver and of the lobe occurred This was an indirect process following the death of the wall of the portal vessels and the disturbance of circulation that naturally resulted therefrom. (These experiments cannot be carried on in the dog owing to certain anastomotic connections, but they are possible in rabbits.) After necrosis of the lobe had occurred the animals survived for two or three days; in necrosis of the whole liver, for twenty hours. Cohnheim and Litten did not succeed in observing any consequences of ligation of a lobar branch of the portal vein. Litten, it is true, states in a subsequent publication that he observed the following changes in the liver after he had produced embolic foci by the injection of chromate of lead. The cells lost their nuclei, and here and there atrophy of the lobules could be seen. Notwithstanding the embolic occlusion of small portal branches within the liver, and a deficient filling of the capillaries in these areas, changes in the liver-cells themselves could not be seen. Rattone ligated the hepatic artery, and produced embolization of branches of the portal vein. He noted the development of foci in the liver, which at the expiration of four hours appeared pale, and after seven hours red, and resembled hemorrhagic infarcts. No liver structure could be recognized in these areas. Rattone, therefore, from his injection experiments assumes that the hepatic artery also supplies the capillaries of the periphery of the lobules.

There can be no doubt, therefore, that occlusion of the portal vein or of one of its main branches is of great significance to the entire liver or to a single lobe, and we see that atrophy may result, leading even to complete destruction of the glandular tissue. The connective tissue in the affected area seems to be increased. This is, however, probably a relative increase, while as a matter of fact it merely does not disappear as rapidly as the parenchymatous structures; in other cases, possibly, there may have been some proliferation before the vessel lesion occurred. Cohnheim's apparently contradictory observations cannot invalidate the positive results obtained by him. The obstruction of circulation which he produced was not of sufficiently long duration, and was too circumscribed. Occlusion of small branches of the portal vein that supply only a few lobules will allow capillary anastomoses, so that the nutrition of the parts may be maintained. If large branches are occluded, however, this process is insufficient. It may also be true that defective nutrition is withstood for a certain length of time, but ultimately slowly leads to atrophy, with a simple reduction in the size and the number of the hepatic cells.

It is possible that the case of E. Wagner mentioned on page 639 is one of atrophy following disease of the portal vein, though the author rejects this interpretation.

Connective-tissue proliferation will be more readily produced in an organ that is not sufficiently nourished than in a healthy one. The direct cause of this proliferation may be some one of the many noxious agencies that are carried to the liver from the intestine. It will depend on the character of the anatomic changes whether occlusion of the vessel occurs rapidly or slowly, and whether collateral branches shall assume the nutrition of the affected areas or not. It is not yet determined to what extent the capillary areas of the hepatic artery communicate with those of the portal vein, and to what extent, therefore, arterial blood can, under certain circumstances, take the place of portal blood.

Heidenhain mentions certain earlier cases reported by Abernethy and Lawrence in which collateral passages were formed.

In one case mentioned by Cohn the arterial stem had become dilated, so that a sufficient amount of blood was carried to the liver by the hepatic artery, maintaining the nutrition of the gland, and, to a certain extent, the secretion of bile.

It is also possible that in certain cases of occlusion of the portal vein itself Sappey's so-called "accessory portal branches," which empty into the right main branch of the portal vein, carry blood to the liver.

If a large branch of the portal vein becomes suddenly occluded, hemorrhagic infarction may be the result. At the same time, it seems that in the liver, as in other organs, the backward current from the veins which is necessary to produce a hemorrhagic infarct occurs only under certain conditions. One of these is the simultaneous occlusion of the hepatic artery (Dreschfeld, Koehler). Necrosis and cicatricial formation may undoubtedly occur without the existence of a hemorrhagic infarct. The case reported by Bermant demonstrated that occlusion of one of the main branches of the portal vein is sufficient to cause complete atrophy of the glandular tissue; in this case the branch of the hepatic artery leading to the area was patent.

Above the occlusion or stenosis the portal vein is often dilated, or the vessels may be dilated and there may be hyperemia in the area of the portal roots, so that the spleen is enlarged and even indurated. Further, there may be parenchymatous or surface hemorrhages in the mucous membrane of the stomach and intestine, or even hemorrhagic infarction of the intestine. The latter lesions occur particularly in cases in which the occlusion occurs rapidly. The thrombosis extends backward into the mesenteric veins.

Symptoms.—Thrombotic narrowing of the portal vein may lead to acute symptoms, which are either superadded to those of some prior disease (cirrhosis of the liver, chronic peritonitis, tumors of the abdomen), or may appear suddenly, while the patient is apparently in perfect health, owing to the fact that the disease of the vessel-wall has remained latent up to then. The most important symptom is the sudden appearance or the rapid increase of symptoms of stasis in the area of the portal roots. The disease is sometimes ushered in and characterized by the appearance of sudden epigastric pain followed by vomiting and diarrhea, and the passage of blood from the mouth and bowel. Ascites and swelling of the spleen may develop in the course of a few days. The former condition causes distention of the abdomen, edema of the lower extremities, and a dilatation of the cutaneous veins of the abdomen. Sometimes a venous network and edema are seen to surround the umbilicus. If the ascites increases too rapidly, puncture may be necessary. The fluid, however, reaccumulates with great rapidity. If in spite of the ascites it is possible to examine the liver, and if the organ was not previously diseased, it may sometimes be determined that the liver decreases in size as the disease progresses.

Icterus is sometimes present, and may be due to an obstruction of the flow of bile owing to compression of the bile-ducts by the thrombotic and inflamed vein, or to pressure from without, together with that exerted by the vein.

In isolated cases icterus may be due to more remote causes. Frerichs has formulated a hypothesis according to which narrowing of the portal vein causes a fall of blood-pressure in the hepatic branches, favoring a diffusion of bile into the blood-vessels. Theoretically, this is possible; it is doubtful, however, whether as a practical thing these circumstances can lead to icterus, and the hypothesis is rendered still less probable by the rare occurrence of jaundice when narrowing of the portal vein is known to be present.

We have no means of estimating the decrease in the biliary secretion that probably occurs. Possibly the reduction in the degree of icterus seen in the later stages of the disease can be attributed to this factor. If hemorrhages occur into the intestine, secondary arterial thrombosis, hemorrhagic infarcts of the intestinal wall, and peritonitis may occur. The pathologic picture then assumes the features of acute peritonitis, or of occlusion of the intestine (case reports, Boucin).

In some instances the symptoms of narrowing of the portal vein which set in so acutely gradually subside, only to reappear at a later period. These changes are probably due to variations in the size of the thrombus which are caused by partial resolution and contraction, followed again by new deposits.

In other cases of narrowing of the portal vein the symptoms of stasis develop slowly and progressively, so that the disease resembles cirrhosis. A differentiation may be particularly difficult, since both conditions may lead to a reduction in the size of the liver, and also because such a reduction need not necessarily occur in cirrhosis. The only symptoms that are fairly characteristic of occlusion of the portal vein, in contradistinction to cirrhosis, are the magnitude and the obstinacy of the gastrointestinal hemorrhages, and the rapid formation of ascites.

We must remember, however, that ascites may be absent even in complete occlusion of the portal vein. This is the case in the event of abundant and repeated hemorrhages, when there is no increase of the pressure in the portal area (Jastrowitz, Borrmann); or when collateral branches develop and carry the blood into the systemic veins. The same vessels are concerned in the latter process as in cirrhosis of the liver. As compared with other veins, these vessels are not so abundant, nor can they be so readily dilated. The principal system, the hemorrhoidal plexus, communicates, on the one hand, with the portal vein through the superior hemorrhoidal vein, and, on the other, with the vesical plexus through the middle and external hemorrhoidal vein; the latter communicates with the hypogastric vein. Another anastomotic connection is the rudimentary umbilical vein, and its branch the paraumbilical vein, which pass along the ligamentum teres and communicate with the vessels of the abdominal wall. There is an anastomosis between the coronary vein of the stomach, and the esophageal and diaphragmatic veins of the gastroepiploic vein, and between the mesenteric vein and the renal veins; also, though not constantly, there is an anastomosis of the lumbar and renal veins. Finally, there are the so-called accessory branches of the portal vein (Sappey), which run from the porta hepatis through the suspensory ligament to the diaphragmatic and epigastric veins.

The digestive functions, even aside from the effect of the hemorrhages, are disturbed. There is loss of appetite, deficient assimilation, and either retention of feces, or a watery diarrhea that often relieves the engorgement of the portal system.

Owing to the slight absorption of fluid and to the transudation into the peritoneal cavity, the urine is decreased, and it is stated, particularly by French authors, that it occasionally contains sugar, as in cirrhosis (*glycosurie alimentaire*). This is due to the fact that a part of the sugar ingested is carried past the liver by the collateral veins (see page 706). The occlusion of a branch of the portal vein, even if it leads to complete atrophy of the portion of the gland supplied, may not cause any symptoms, because the remaining portions of the liver may hypertrophy and may vicariously assume the functions of that which is destroyed (Bermant).

The condition may last for a few days or a few years. If there is profuse hemorrhage and rapid disintegration, the disease will be of short duration; the more rapidly occlusion occurs, the more rapidly will the disease progress. Occlusion of the portal vein never occurs as rapidly in human subjects as in experiments on animals; the clinical course of the disease is likewise never so rapid.

It appears that moderate degrees of narrowing, developing slowly, can be well borne for some time, even though they ultimately lead to complete occlusion of the vessel. Strümpell mentions a case that lasted for six years and in which fifteen punctures were performed; Leyden and Alexander report similar cases. A large number of instances are on record in which the course of the disease showed variations; these occupy an intermediate position.

The following case reported by Dreschfeld is a very peculiar one: There was pylephlebitis portalis in a man of forty-eight, which led to the formation of hemorrhagic infarcts. The disease lasted for five weeks, and was characterized by the appearance of icterus, fever, chills, ascites, diarrhea, and vomiting of blood. I assume that syphilis of the portal vein and of the portal cellular tissue was the cause of the trouble (Q.).

The prognosis of portal narrowing is always unfavorable, although it is not absolutely bad. Cases that are due to the presence of syphilitic gummata or to pylephlebitis syphilitica may be cured; it is also possible that such cases as are due to intestinal ulceration, cholelithiasis, or inflammatory compression may be relieved by treating the primary disease.

Treatment is, as a rule, palliative and directed toward removing some of the consequences of portal narrowing; it is similar to the treatment of cirrhosis of the liver in this respect; it is possible to relieve the engorgement of the portal system by well-selected laxatives and purges; ascites can be relieved by puncture. It is well, however, to postpone the latter operation as long as possible, because in this disease the ascitic fluid has a great tendency to return within a short time.

In syphilitic cases a course of iodin, and especially of mercury, should be instituted, and an amelioration or a cure of the disease be attempted in this way, so long as gummata or gummatous inflammations of the walls of the vein are present. If the occlusion of the portal vein is due to an organized cicatricial mass, treatment will, of course, be altogether in vain.

INFLAMMATION OF THE PORTAL VEIN.

Pylephlebitis.

1. **Chronic Pylephlebitis.**—The wall of the portal vein, as of any other vein of the body, may undergo a degeneration similar to that of arteriosclerosis in the arteries; it is characterized by a thickening of the intima with impairment of its elasticity and degeneration and calcification of the media. Phlebosclerosis of this character frequently develops from unknown causes; it may be the starting-point of thrombotic occlusion of the portal vein, as described in the preceding section. Chronic inflammatory thickening of the walls of the portal vein has also been found in cases in which some inflammatory process, caused by the presence of gall-stones, has extended into adjacent tissues, or in which the inner surface of the vessel is irritated by the Distomum hæmatobium. This parasite is frequently found within the portal vein and in large numbers (see page 829). Syphilis may also cause changes in the walls of the portal vein, consisting in circumscribed gummatous inflammation. In the new-born, syphilis frequently causes stenosis of the umbilical vein from endophlebitis (Oedmannsson, Winckel); or there may be pylephlebitis and thickening of Glisson's capsule around the larger branches of the portal vein within the liver that leads to narrowing of the lumen of the portal vein, of the branches of the hepatic artery, and of the bile-ducts (Schüppel). Weigert has described tuberculosis of the walls of the portal vein.

All these diseases of the portal vein lead to a decreased elasticity and to an impairment of the vasoconstrictor and dilator powers. They frequently cause the formation of solid mural thrombi, which may become organized or enlarged, and either reduce the lumen of the vessel or bring about complete occlusion (pylephlebitis adhæsiva). We have already discussed the symptoms of this chronic form of inflammatory stenosis.

2. **Acute Pylephlebitis.** — (*Pylephlebitis Suppurativa, Ulcerosa.*) Acute inflammation of the main trunk of the portal vein may, in rare cases, be caused by the presence of some sharp foreign body that penetrates the wall of the intestine, and, entering adjacent tissues, reaches the portal vein (fish-bones, Lambron, Winge; wire, von Jau). The inflammation may extend to the stem of the portal vein from an en-

capsulated purulent exudate (Schönlein), or from a lymph-gland that has undergone purulent degeneration.

More frequently the inflammation starts from the roots of the portal vein, or from suppurative foci, or from ulcers in the intestinal tract. Typhlitis and diseases of the appendix are particularly important in this respect. Further, the different forms of ulceration of the colon (dysentery, typhoid, tuberculosis), diseases of the rectum and of its vicinity, as hemorrhoids, carcinoma, fistula, mechanical injuries inflicted during the administration of an enema, and during operations in this region. Pylephlebitis may also start from the venous plexuses of the bladder and the uterus. Ott describes a case of this kind occurring during the puerperium. Gastric ulcers are rarely the starting-point of pylephlebitis, notwithstanding their situation (Bristowe, West, Sonsino). This is probably due to the fact that they rarely suppurate. Frerichs (II, page 394) and others have seen pylephlebitis start from an abscess of the spleen, Leudet from a glandular abscess of the mesentery, Chvostek from a purulent pancreatitis. In the new-born infection of the portal vein sometimes starts from the umbilical vein after it is cut. Focal diseases of the liver may extend by direct continuity to neighboring branches of the portal vein and cause inflammation, for instance, abscess, or ulceration of the bile-passages as a result of concretions.

Anatomy. —The suppurative processes that cause inflammation of the portal vein are probably without exception of bacterial origin. They extend to the outer surface of the wall of the vein, usually first involving a small intestinal or mesenteric vein. The vessel-wall becomes thickened, injected, and infiltrated with cells; finally, some small area in the intima is perforated, or thrombotic occlusion of the vessel occurs, followed by bacterial disintegration of the thrombus. By continuity, or by diffusion of bacterial products, the thrombus may extend centrally up the lumen of the vein, and in this manner reach the stem of the portal vein. Or, on the other hand, fragments of the softened thrombus may become loosened, and may be carried centrally until they lodge at some point in the portal vein, or in some intrahepatic branch of this vessel. Wherever these embolic masses lodge, they form the starting-point of new thrombi and new suppurative processes. The latter do not involve the thrombus alone, but extend to the inflamed and thickened vessel-wall, and further into the surrounding tissues. In this manner it may happen that the roots, the stem, and the branches of the portal vein are filled over large areas with pus; that their walls are thickened and infiltrated with pus, and may become ulcerated or even perforated. These portions of the vessel are separated from others that still carry blood by a solid thrombus that is attached to the vessel-wall. In the case of smaller veins this occlusion near the primary disease focus may lead to organization and to definite occlusion. Cases of this kind are never recognized. In the majority of cases this protective wall will only partly and incompletely fulfil its mission, so that coagulation proceeds from this point; the puriform softening, with loosening of embolic fragments, continues. If fluid pus enters the blood, the inflammatory material is more finely distributed, becomes lodged in the capillaries of the liver, and in this manner causes the formation of numerous small abscesses; larger emboli, on the other hand, usually cause the formation of a solitary abscess. According to the character of the primary focus, the secondary ones will be purulent or gangrenous.

Acute pylephlebitis beginning in the branches or the stem of the portal vein rarely shows a tendency to form thrombi in a direction opposed to the blood-stream.

Symptoms.—As long as the inflammation is limited to the wall of the vein, no other symptoms except those caused by the primary disease are noticed. As soon as the thrombus forms, or as soon as it begins to soften, symptoms appear. Mechanical disturbances following occlusion of the vessel are not important in acute pylephlebitis, and may be altogether absent. The general symptoms of pyemia are particularly conspicuous—namely, an irregular fever with high excursions, chills, sweats, collapse, and temperature remissions below normal. As in other forms of pylephlebitis, these general symptoms do not appear for some time after the inflammation of the vessel has occurred. This rule also applies when symptoms are present of softening of the thrombus, and in secondary suppuration in the liver.

Occasionally local symptoms in the abdomen designate the origin of the pyemia; thus there may be pain in the region of the cecum or the spleen. If this was present before the other symptoms appeared, it may become exacerbated as soon as pylephlebitis occurs, probably as the result of slight peritonitis. The spleen is usually enlarged as a result of inflammation, as in any case of pyemia; occasionally there is hyperemia from stasis, particularly if the portal vein is extensively occluded. There may also be parenchymatous swelling of the liver, with enlargement of the organ; or, in cases that last long, there may be abscesses. These may either be numerous and small, so as to cause a uniform enlargement of the organ, or single large abscesses and cause a circumscribed swelling.

Icterus is not constantly found in pylephlebitis. If it is present, its intensity varies, and its pathogenesis varies in different cases. Sometimes it is due to pyemia; at others it is due to stasis from compression, or from inflammatory swelling of the bile-channel walls. There is generally some disturbance of digestion, lack of appetite, vomiting, or diarrhea. If these symptoms are not caused by the primary disease, they may be considered the results of pyemia, or of the interference with the blood-current in the portal area, or of peritonitis. The latter complication frequently develops from an extension of the inflammation by direct continuity from the portal vein. Peritonitis is localized in the beginning, but may become general as the disease progresses.

Owing to the rapidity with which the disease begins and develops, the purely mechanical results of disturbances of the portal blood-stream are rarely seen, as, for instance, ascites, and dilatation of the veins in the umbilical region. Toward the end of the disease there may be bloody evacuations as a result of infarction of certain portions of the intestine. The urine is scanty and may contain albumin or indoxyl.

Course.—It is probably impossible to determine the true beginning of the inflammation of the vein during life. The first symptoms that we notice are those of the general infection, which may develop either spontaneously, or be consecutive to the primary local disease of the cecum, etc. In many instances the primary disease seems to be cured, and symptoms of pyemia fail to develop for several weeks, lasting usually from two to six weeks; less frequently for several months.

Diagnosis.—The pathologic picture of purulent pylephlebitis corresponds, on the one hand, with that of pyemia; on the other, with that of abscess of the liver. As a rule, only the diagnosis of pyemia can be found from the objective symptoms; its origin, however, remains obscure, or can only be guessed at from the history. In other instances the primary focus is still demonstrable, or can be determined, on careful examination, by such symptoms as local pain, etc.

It is impossible to formulate a clear distinction between abscess of the liver and this condition, either diagnostically or pathogenetically, owing to the fact that every metastatic abscess of the liver is caused by a perforating inflammation of a small vein. It is due to this that we see transitions from simple hectic pus-fever to most pronounced pyemia. The source of the latter is, however, always anatomically demonstrable in the region of the portal vein. Secondary pus foci are rarely found in the greater circulation, because the liver forms a protecting wall against the transportation of pus.

Local hepatic symptoms are less frequently seen in the very acute cases than in the slow chronic variety.

The prognosis of pylephlebitis, when once distinctly diagnosed, must usually be a fatal one. At the same time, it is possible that an acute nongangrenous inflammation of the stem of the portal vein might be relieved, in case the primary focus of inflammation should subside and the thrombus be reabsorbed. It is even possible that purulent embolic phlebitis of a branch of the portal vein might be cured in the same manner as dysenteric abscess of the liver (a condition genetically related to this condition), provided the primary focus—as, for instance, an inflammation in the region of the vermiform appendix—is treated surgically and in good time.

Treatment.—From a prophylactic point of view the correct treatment of all diseases that may lead to pylephlebitis is important, as, for instance, the early opening of pus foci in the region of the vermiform appendix, and of periproctic abscesses, the careful treatment of hemorrhoidal phlebitis, strict asepsis of the umbilicus in the new-born and in all operations of the rectum. It is certain that many cases of phlebitis have of late been prevented by these precautionary measures.

Even when pyemia is already pronounced these precautions should not be neglected. If the primary focus can be removed, and the secondary abscesses in the liver incised and evacuated, some cases may be cured, as in other instances of pyemia. Treatment, of course, can only be palliative and symptomatic; drugs belonging to the class of roborants, excitants, and narcotics should be used. I think that the old-fashioned decoction of Peruvian bark is more useful in these cases than quinin, antipyrin, and similar febrifuges.

Among other pathologic changes of the portal vein may be mentioned:

Dilatation of the stem of the portal vein has been noted above an old stenosis that has not completely obliterated the vessel (Virchow *); in this case the wall was thickened, and the involved area resembled an arterial aneurysm. The portal vein may be dilated to its roots, and the vessel may be tortuous. Cirrhosis may also cause dilatation of the vessel from stasis. Sometimes this condition will lead to collateral dilatation of the esophageal veins, and the formation of sub-

* Virchow, *Verhandl. der phys.-med. Gesellsch. zu Würzburg*, Bd. vii, p. 21. Extracted by Schüppel, loc. cit., p. 781.

mucous varices. The latter may burst and cause fatal hemorrhages (see pages 707, 708).

Varicose dilatation of the submucous veins of the intestine (Rokitansky,[*] Thierfelder,[†] Neelsen,[‡] and Köster [§]). These were as large as grains of wheat or peas, or even cherries, and sometimes resembled mulberries, owing to the tortuous character of the veins. Sometimes they were gathered in bunches of dozens or hundreds, and usually were limited to certain portions of the intestine, either the colon, the jejunum, or the upper part of the ileum, and, in one case, the whole intestine (here they were smaller). Köster reports two cases of subserous varices in small areas of the colon, and in the pyloric end of the stomach. Gee describes varicose veins of the gastric mucosa as thick as a goosequill, and some of them thrombosed.[||] There was no obstruction of the blood-stream in any of these cases, so that it is probable that they were formed by local disease of the walls. Neelsen believes that the lesions were due to atrophy from inactivity of the musculature of the veins following some disturbance in its innervation. These varices caused no clinical symptoms, but occasionally produced hemorrhages.

Rupture of the portal vein,[**] either of its stem or of one of its main roots, may occur spontaneously, and, of course also as the result of trauma. It is probable that in such cases there is some circumscribed lesion of the wall. Frerichs in one case (a drunkard) saw fatty degeneration of the wall; Vesal in another case perforation of the vessel by an abscess of its wall. Perforation occurred either into the abdominal cavity or between the layers of the mesentery, sometimes immediately after a meal. Sometimes the patient has complained of a sensation as if something had torn in the upper region of the abdomen. If perforation occurs into the peritoneal cavity, death follows rapidly from internal hemorrhage. If rupture occurs between the layers of the peritoneum, the patient may survive for two days.

For parasites of the portal vein see page 829; for carcinoma, see page 777. Either condition may result in the occlusion of the blood-stream and cause various disturbances.

A remarkable anomaly has been reported by Abernethy [††] occurring in a child, the portal vein entering the lower vena cava in the neighborhood of the right renal vein. Aside from the fact that the stem of the portal vein is absent, this anastomosis corresponds to Jacobson's vein in birds, and to the so-called von Eck fistula that Pawlow, Nencki, and their associates created experimentally.

LITERATURE.

Achard: "Archives de physiologie," 1884, tome xvi, p. 484. (Compression durch tuberculöse Peritonitis.)
Alexander: "Berliner klin. Wochenschr.," 1866, No. 4.
Asp: "Zur Anatomie und Physiologie der Leber," "Arbeiten aus dem physiologischen Institut zu Leipzig," 1873, Bd. viii, p. 136; "Bericht der sächsischen Gesellschaft der Wissenschaften."

* Rokitansky, "Lehrb. der patholog. Anatomie," 1844, i, p. 672.
† Thierfelder, *Archiv der Heilkunde*, 1873, p. 83.
‡ Neelsen, *Berlin. klin. Woch.*, 1879, p. 449, 470.
§ Köster, *Berlin. klin. Woch.*, 1879, p. 634.
|| "Bartholomew's Hosp. Rep.," 1871. Jahresbericht i, p. 189.
** Frerichs, ii, p. 382.
†† Abernethy, Philosoph. Transactions, 1793, i. p. 61. Quoted by Heidenhain; Hermann's "Lehrbuch der Physiologie," v, 1, p. 237.

Auriol, L.: "Contribution à l'étude de la thrombose cachectique de la veine porte," Thèse de Paris, 1883.

Bermant: "Ueber Pfortaderverschluss und Leberschwund," Dissertation, Königsberg, 1887. (Literature.)

v. Birch-Hirschfeld: "Beitrag zur pathologischen Anatomie der hereditären Syphilis Neugeborener," "Archiv der Heilkunde," 1875, Bd. xvi, p. 166.

Borrmann: "Beitrag zur Thrombose des Pfortaderstammes," "Deutsches Archiv für klin. Medicin," 1897, Bd. lix, p. 283. (Literature.)

Botkin: "Fall von Pfortaderthrombose," "Virchow's Archiv," 1864, Bd. xxx.

Boucey, H. O.: "Des lésions intestinales consécutives a la thrombose de la veine porte ou de cas branches d'origine," Thèse de Paris, 1894.

Budd: "Diseases of the Liver," 1845, p. 136.

Chauffard: in Charcot's "Traité de Médecine," tome iii, p. 816.

Chvostek: "Krankheiten der Pfortader und der Lebervenen," "Wiener Klinik," 1882, Heft 3. (Literature.)

Cohn, B.: "Klinik der embolischen Gefässkrankheiten," p. 490, Berlin, 1860.

Cohnheim and Litten: "Ueber Circulationsstörungen in der Leber," "Virchow's Archiv," 1876, Bd. lxvii, p. 153.

Couturier: "De la glycosurie dans les cas d'obstruction totale ou partielle de la veine porte," Thèse de Paris, 1875.

Dreschfeld: "Ueber eine seltene Form von Hepatitis interstitialis mit hämorrhagischen Infarcten," "Verhandlungen des X. Internationalen Congresses," 1891, Abth. v, p. 184.

Ewald: in Eulenburg's "Realencyklopädie," Bd. xvi, p. 286.

Frerichs: "Leberkrankheiten," ii, p. 363. (Casuistik.)

Gintrac: "Journal de médecine de Bordeaux," 1856, Jan.-Mar.; "Journal de l'anatomie et de la physiologie," 1864, i, p. 562.

Goodridge: "The Lancet," June, 1887. (Injury to the portal vein, due to cicatricial bands.)

Jastrowitz: "Deutsche med. Wochenschr.," 1883, No. 47. (Thrombose aus luetischer Ursache.)

Koehler, B.: "Ueber die Veränderungen der Leber infolge des Verschlusses von Pfortaderästen," "Arbeiten aus dem pathologischen Institut in Göttingen," Berlin, 1893.

Koeppe, H.: "Muskeln und Klappen in den Wurzeln der Pfortader," "Archiv für Anatomie und Physiologie," 1890, Supplement, p. 168.

Kronecker: "Ueber den Tonus des Pfortadersystems," "Bericht über die Versammlung deutscher Naturforscher und Aertze," 1889, p. 311.

Lambron: "Observations d'inflammations: 1. de la veine porte, 2. des veines sus-hépatiques," "Archives générales de médecine," p. 129, June, 1842.

Leyden: "Fälle von Pfortaderthrombose," "Berliner klin. Wochenschr.," 1866, No. 13.

Mall, F.: "Archiv für Anatomie und Physiologie," Physiologische Abtheilung, 1892; 1890, Supplement, p. 57.

Nonne, M.: "Zur Aetiologie der Pfortaderthrombose," "Deutsches Archiv für klin. Medicin," 1885, Bd. xxxvii, p. 241.

Oré: "Journal de l'anatomie et de la physiologie," 1864, tome i, p. 565.

Osler: "Case of Obliteration of the Portal Vein," "Journal of Anatomy," p. 208, January, 1882; Jahresbericht, ii, p. 178.

Ott, A.: "Zur Casuistik der Pylephlebitis," "Prager med. Wochenschr.," 1883, No. 14.

Pippow, R.: "Ueber die Obturation der Pfortader," Dissertation, Berlin, 1888.

Quincke: "Krankheiten der Gefässe," in Ziemssen's "Handbuch der speciellen Pathologie," 2. Auflage, 1879, Bd. vi, p. 574.

Sack: "Ueber Phlebosklerose," "Virchow's Archiv," Bd. cxii.

Schiff, M.: "Ueber das Verhaltniss der Lebercirculation zur Gallenbildung," "Schweizer Zeitschr. für Heilkunde," 1862, i, 1.

Schüppel: in "Ziemssen's Handbuch," Bd. viii, Anhang, p. 269.

— "Ueber Peripylephlebitis syphilitica der Neugeborenen," "Archiv der Heilkunde," 1870, Bd. ii, p. 74.

Solowieff: "Veränderungen der Leber unter dem Einflusse künstlicher Verstopfung der Pfortader," "Virchow's Archiv," 1875, Bd. lxii, p. 195.

Sonsino: "Lo sperimentale," 1888, Ottobre. (Pylephlebitis following gastric ulcer.)

Stahl, G. E.: "De vena portae, porta malorum hypochondriaco-splenetico-sulfocativo-hysterico-colico-hamorrhoidariorum," Halae, 1698.

Strümpell: "Lehrbuch der speciellen Pathologie," 5. Auflage, ɪ, p. 783.
Tappeiner: "Ueber den Zustand des Blutstroms nach Unterbindung der Pfortader,"
    "Arbeiten aus der physiologischen Anstalt zu Leipzig," 1872, Bd. vɪɪ, p. 11.
West: "Pylephlebitis suppurativa durch Magengeschwür," "Transactions of the
    Pathological Society," 1890; Jahresbericht, ɪɪ, p. 261.
Winge: "Pylephlebitis durch Fischgräte," "Norsk. Magazin f. Lägeridensk.," 1880;
    Jahresbericht, ɪɪ, p. 197.
Wooldridge: "On Hemorrhagic Infarction of the Liver," "Transactions of the
    Pathological Society of London," 1888, vol. xxxɪx, p. 421.

DISEASES OF THE HEPATIC ARTERY.

Aside from aneurysms of the hepatic artery, which are comparatively rare, we know very little of the pathology of this vessel. We have already discussed the peculiarities of the blood-stream within the liver (see page 615), and especially in cases in which the portal vein is diseased (see page 885). The latter vessel and its capillaries may be termed a functional system, whereas the hepatic artery furnishes blood for the nutrition of the connective-tissue structures, the walls of the blood-vessels and the bile-passages. Wherever there is new formation of connective-tissue the capillaries of the hepatic artery are implicated. This is particularly the case in cirrhosis (Frerichs). The hepatic artery also sends vessels into neoplasms, so that in large carcinomata there may be dilatation of the main stem of this vessel (Frerichs).

As we have demonstrated above, the capillary blood of the hepatic artery may act vicariously for the portal blood in case the latter vessel is obstructed. This can only occur in an imperfect degree, and if large areas of the portal system are occluded the compensation is altogether inadequate. In cases of this character, also, Cohn has seen a dilatation of the stem of the artery. Spontaneous disease, sclerosis of the hepatic artery and its branches, is rare in comparison with its frequency in other vessels. Duplaix claims that the thickening of the smallest arteries is an important factor in the development of interstitial connective-tissue proliferation (see page 688).

If the main stem of the hepatic artery or one of its main branches is occluded in rabbits, necrosis of the connective tissue will follow, and as a consequence, indirectly, of the whole liver or of one lobe. In dogs, however, this does not occur, owing to the existence of so many arterial anastomoses (Cohnheim and Litten). It is not known what occurs in occlusion of the main stem of the hepatic artery in man (after excluding anastomosis with right coronary arteries of the stomach and the gastro-duodenal artery), because only one such case is on record (Ledien), and here the occlusion by an aneurysm developed so slowly that there was plenty of time for the formation of anastomoses.

If a branch of the artery is occluded within the liver, in the course of animal experiments, no circulatory disturbances are evident owing to the numerous anastomotic connections that are formed.

We know nothing of the results of embolic occlusion of the hepatic artery in man, though it is probable that such embolic occlusion may lead, for instance, to verrucose endocarditis. If in cases of this kind we see no local involvement of the liver, nor any cicatrices of the organ as in the case of the spleen, we can only assume that in man the collateral circulation is sufficient to compensate such a lesion. If there are infectious arterial emboli, general pyemia and abscess of the liver will result.

ANEURYSM OF THE HEPATIC ARTERY.

Aneurysm of the hepatic artery is not frequent. Mester, up to 1895, found 20 cases in the literature, 11 of which were studied clinically. In 16 cases the aneurysm started from the main stem or from one of the two main branches (in the case of Standhartner there were aneurysms of both branches), once from the cystic artery (Chiari); in 4 cases the aneurysm was situated outside of the liver. The extrahepatic aneurysmal sacs may become as large as a goose-egg or a child's head; the intrahepatic sacs remain small, and are never larger than a hazelnut. They are usually true aneurysms, their walls being formed by the layers of the artery. These aneurysms may perforate into the bile-passages, the gallbladder, the duodenum, into the stomach, through an abscess to the lower surface of the liver, into the peritoneal cavity. Generally, there are several hemorrhages. Ledieu, in one instance, found an aneurysmal sac that had healed spontaneously by coagulation.

Etiology.—In one case a traumatic origin was established, the lesion following a kick in the abdomen by a horse (Mester); in another case (Borchers) traumatic origin was probable. In the case of M. B. Schmidt and Chiari the aneurysm resulted from injury to the wall of the artery from without by a gall-stone. In Irvine's case the hepatic artery was eroded by an abscess of the liver, in the same manner as occurs in pulmonary cavities. In the case of Uhlich the wall of the artery was sclerotic.

In the majority of the cases the cause of the aneurysm is obscure. Of recent years syphilis has been recognized as an important etiologic factor, and a history of syphilis has probably not been elicited in all the cases in which it actually played a rôle. Here and there the existence of some infectious disease, as typhoid, pneumonia, osteomyelitis, is mentioned as preceding the formation of aneurysm; it is doubtful, however, whether such a history is of any significance. The majority of the cases have been under forty years of age.

Symptoms.—If any symptoms indeed are recognized during life, the three following are the most important—namely, pain, hemorrhage, and icterus.

Pain, when present, is localized in the epigastric or the right hypochondriac region, and once it was noted, in an aneurysm of the left branch, in the left hypochondriac region (Irvine). The origin of the pain in extrahepatic aneurysm is probably pressure on the hepatic plexus which surrounds the vessel; in intrahepatic aneurysm, local distention of the capsule of the liver, adhesive inflammation in the vicinity of the aneurysm; and in perforation of the vessel, distention of the bile-passages by the blood that is poured into them. In the latter instance the pain may be spasmodic, as in gall-stone colic, and may be accompanied by other symptoms of this condition.

Hemorrhage, as in other forms of aneurysm, is the most frequent cause of death. Sometimes the first hemorrhage is copious and at once fatal, the blood pouring into the abdominal cavity or into the intestines; in other instances several (sometimes a dozen) hemorrhages occur with intermissions, so that anemia from hemorrhage occurs. The patient in the intermissions may recover from the effects of the bleeding. The latter form of hemorrhage is seen particularly in cases in which the aneurysm perforates the bile-passages, for as soon as the latter become distended with blood the pressure becomes so great that the bleeding ceases; thrombotic occlusion of the tear in the aneurysm may thus occur.

The blood may enter the intestinal tract through the bile-ducts, or if the perforation occurs in some other place by another channel, but always in the first portion of the intestine. The greater portion of the blood is, therefore, passed in the stools, and only in rare cases does a portion of it enter the stomach so as to be vomited. As a rule, the quantity of blood poured out is large, so that the presence of blood can be readily detected in the intestinal evacuations. In one case observed by the author the blood coagulated in the intestine and formed casts of the folds of Kerkring, proving that the hemorrhage had occurred in the uppermost portion of the small intestine.

Icterus is present in the majority of cases, either because of direct aneurysmal pressure or owing to changes produced by the tissues causing an obstruction to the flow of bile. The icterus may be intermittent, as in the cases of the author and of Lebert and Mester, and be due to the temporary distention of the bile-passages with blood. If icterus is combined with paroxysmal pain, the picture of hepatic colic may be simulated. In the author's case most of the attacks were accompanied by a rise of temperature, and sometimes by a chill. In the same manner as the concretion is passed in the stools after an ordinary attack of colic, blood is passed within the next twenty-four hours. It is probable that the latter flushes the larger passages of bile so thoroughly that the second portion of blood is coagulated. In cases of this kind the attack of colic, of course, will be very severe, and it may even occur that casts of the bile-passages are found in the stool.

Enlargement of the liver is rarely observed; this, as we know, is variable also in stasis of bile. In a case reported by Stokes the left lobe was pressed against the abdominal wall by the aneurysm, so that an enlargement of this portion of the organ seemed to be present. In a few cases there has been an enlargement of the gall-bladder, due, as in the case of Niewerth, to hemorrhage into this viscus.

A pulsating tumor, as yet, has never been felt; but it is quite probable that such a lesion occurs, although it cannot be determined. In a few instances a systolic murmur has been heard (Rovighi).

Course.—Some cases run a very acute course, and lead to the death of the patient from hemorrhage into the stomach, the intestine, or the peritoneal cavity. Others run a longer course; Mester's statistics give as the average duration four and a half months. Pain is the first symptom to appear, and is soon followed by repeated hemorrhages, with icterus; this picture is characterized by remissions, and lasts for several months. The patient usually recovers during the intervals, and death finally results from exhaustion or some complication.

Diagnosis.—A diagnosis cannot be made in cases that end suddenly with hemorrhage. In others there is repeated hemorrhage into the bile-passages, and the diagnosis can then be made from the combination of symptoms of duodenal hemorrhage and biliary colic. If a great deal of blood is passed in the stools and there is only occasional vomiting of blood, the former possibility can be suspected. As a matter of fact, the diagnosis of duodenal ulcer is frequently made. If casts of Kerkring's folds are found, the intestinal hemorrhage can most certainly be located in the small intestine.

It is possible that the duodenal ulcer may be complicated by icterus,

57

because there may be cicatricial contraction in its vicinity with torsion and occlusion of a bile-duct. Such a complication will, however, never produce paroxysmal icterus, or attacks of colic. Aneurysms of the hepatic artery have been seen, associated with cholelithiasis, and the latter disease may also be complicated by hemorrhages * (from ulcers, fistulas, or chronic icterus). The large quantity of blood that is poured into the intestine is of some significance in the diagnosis of aneurysm.

Treatment.—Internal treatment of an aneurysm of the hepatic artery promises very little. Syphilis rarely plays a rôle, so that the treatment of this taint will lead to no results. If the diagnosis can be made, operative interference is justifiable. As a preliminary step it will be necessary to determine how well human beings tolerate ligation of the hepatic artery.

In three cases operative treatment has been attempted, although for other indications; namely, in two cases reported by Mester and Sauerteig for ulcerative internal hemorrhage, in one case reported by Niewerth for threatened Ileus. In all of these cases such severe hemorrhage occurred during the operation that it could not be finished.

Marion describes erosion of the hepatic artery by a carcinoma of bile-duct. Fatal hemorrhage rapidly ensued; the blood was poured into a cavity near the gall-bladder and through a duct that communicated with the duodenum into the intestine.

LITERATURE.

Duplaix: "Contribution à l'étude de la sclérose," "Archives générales de médecine," 1885, I, p. 166.
Frerichs: Loc. cit., p. 353; Atlas II, Tafel III, IV, V.
Langenbuch: Loc. cit., II, p. 67.
Marion: "De la mort par hémorrhagie dans la lithiase biliaire," "Mercr. médical," 1894, No. 51; Jahresbericht, II, p. 223.
Quincke: "Krankheiten der Gefässe," in Ziemssen's "Handbuch der speciellen Pathologie," Bd. VI, p. 547, 422.
Schüppel: Loc. cit., p. 325.

ANEURYSMS.

Borchers: Dissertation, Kiel, 1878.
Chiari: "Aneurysma der Arteria cystica," "Prager med. Wochenschr.," 1883, No. 4.
Hansson, A.: "Hygiea," 1897, I, p. 417; "Centralblatt fur die Grenzgebiete der Medicin und Chirurgie," I, p. 299.
Irvine: "Transactions of the Pathological Society," London, 1878.
Lebert: "Anat. pathologique," tome II, p. 322.
Ledien: "Journal de Bordeaux," 1856; "Schmidt's Jahrbücher," Bd. XCIII, p. 56. (Verschluss durch Aneurysma.)
Mester, B.: "Zeitschr. für klin. Medicin," 1895, Bd. XXVIII, p. 92.
Niewerth, A.: Dissertation, Kiel, 1894.
Quincke, H.: "Berliner klin. Wochenschr.," 1871, p. 349.
Rovighi: "Riv. clin. die Bologna," 1886, No. 52.
Sauerteig: Dissertation, Jena, 1893.
Schmidt, M. B.: (Aneurysma durch Gallensteine.) "Deutsches Archiv für klin. Medicin," 1894, Bd. LII, p. 536.
Wallmann: "Virchow's Archiv," Bd. XIV.

DISEASES OF THE HEPATIC VEINS.

Dilatation of the hepatic veins is frequently seen, particularly in diseases of the heart and the lungs that lead to an engorgement and an insufficiency of the right side of the heart. Dilatation of all the finer branches and the capillaries is observed in the center of the lobules, and

* Arndt, E., Dissertation, Strassburg, 1893.

is usually combined with thickening of the vessel-wall. The consequences and the symptoms of this condition coincide with those of hyperemia of the liver from stasis (see page 608).

NARROWING AND OCCLUSION OF HEPATIC VEINS.

Narrowing and occlusion are found less frequently than dilatation of one or several of the branches of the hepatic veins. This condition may be due to:

1. **Compression** by tumors or cicatrices, particularly gummata that develop within the liver and extrahepatic tumors, as, for instance, lymph-glands. The latter usually compress the vena cava at the same time.

2. **Disease of the vessel-wall.** These are rarely primary, and usually originate in the adjacent liver tissues and extend to the thin vessel-wall by direct continuity. There may be a new-formation, or, more frequently, chronic inflammation, with a development of connective tissue starting from the capsule of the liver (Frerichs, Hainski) or from interstitial hepatitis (Brissaud and Sabourin *). Many of the latter forms develop from the central veins of the lobules. This has been particularly emphasized by French authors. Some of the larger veins of the liver may also be narrowed in interstitial hepatitis, and if the hepatitis is of syphilitic origin, the proliferative changes seem to involve the walls of the veins, or they may even start from these walls (as in the case of the portal vein). Whenever perihepatitis involves the liver veins, the right pleura and the pericardium are usually the seat of chronic adhesive inflammation.

3. **Thrombosis.** This is often a complication of the above-mentioned diseases of the vessel-wall; the subsequent changes of the thrombus are determined by the character of the disease; *i. e.*, whether there is new-formation of connective tissue, purulent degeneration, or carcinomatous development. Marantic thrombi rarely originate in the liver veins, probably because the right heart is so near this organ that the current of blood is maintained; the cardiac action is, moreover, aided by the constant movement of the diaphragm. In a case of hyperemia from stasis I was enabled to diagnose thrombosis of the hepatic veins during life and to corroborate my diagnosis postmortem. It is possible that in this disease thrombosis is more frequent than we suspect (see below). It may occur secondarily after occlusion of the stem or branches of the portal vein, followed by a general obstruction of the blood-current in the liver.

Schüppel reports a case in which the coagulability of the blood seemed to be increased, a factor which appears to play a certain rôle in the formation of the thrombus.

4. **Embolic occlusion** is quite frequently seen in the area of the liver veins when the blood-stream is reversed (Heller). It will depend on the nature of the embolus whether simple occlusion, suppuration, or tumor-formation occurs.

The forces that cause a reversal of the blood-current are gravity, contraction of the right heart, particularly of the auricle, coughing and other violent expiratory efforts.

Cohn and Arnold noted simple coagulates within the liver veins that were propelled there from the heart, and originated in the spermatic veins. The last-named author also saw an embolus at the bifurcation of one of the hepatic veins. Heller

* *Archiv. de physiologie*, 1884, p. 444.

found small tumor particles that came from the lower vena cava; and Bonome saw tumor fragments that were carried through the heart-blood into the hepatic veins.

Frerichs, Heller, Arnold, and others, have attempted to study the conditions obtaining in these lesions by animal experiments. It was found that mercury, oil, and air did not form suitable emboli because their specific gravity differed from that of the blood. The majority of their experiments were performed by injecting wheat-grits into the veins of different parts of the body. If sufficiently large quantities were injected, the pulmonary blood-vessels were occluded over large areas, so that respiration was seriously interfered with and the action of the right heart was impaired. In cases of this character emboli may be carried backward as far as the crural and cerebral veins, and into the liver as far as the central veins of the acini and their surrounding capillaries (Arnold). If less was injected, the granules were surrounded with a thin layer of fibrin and moved along in the peripheral layers of the blood-column, hugging the walls of the blood-vessels. These particles were hardly moved by the fluctuations of the blood-current caused by the respiratory movements; they were propelled, however, by the more sudden waves that started from the heart (Arnold and Ribbert). These heart-waves propelled them against the blood-current either in stages or in jerks. Some of them entered the central blood-current and were carried along in the direction of the blood-current; others, again, became lodged in the narrow venous branches. We may consider the movements of the heart, therefore, as the principal force that causes recurrent embolisms. It is probable that violent expiratory efforts play a certain rôle within the area of the upper vena cava and the lower extremities, but with respect to the hepatic veins and the abdominal cavity they seem to be of no significance. This is due to the fact that these portions of the body are exposed to the same pressure as the thorax, so that only in exceptional cases can material be forced from the vessels of the thorax into those of the abdominal cavity. Factors, on the other hand, that hinder normal respiration may aid in the formation of embolism of the hepatic veins by causing distention and increased activity of the right heart.

Anatomy.—Occlusion of isolated central lobular veins causes a reversal of the capillary blood-stream in these lobules, but owing to the abundant capillary anastomoses this occurrence is not followed by any serious lesions. The same principle probably applies to the smaller branches of the hepatic veins. The anastomoses here are, however, not so abundant as in the case of the portal branches, and occlusion of large venous branches is followed by hyperemia and congestion in their roots. If this condition develops slowly, atrophy of the columns of liver-cells occurs as a result of pressure, and the hepatic cells may disappear completely. If the occlusion occurs more rapidly, there will be complete stasis of blood in the distended capillaries, and hemorrhagic infarcts with bloody infiltration, coagulation, necrosis of glandular tissue, and formation of connective-tissue cicatrices take place. The first stages of these venous infarctions have never been studied anatomically. It is probable that their outline is not so regular as that of portal vein infarcts, because the hepatic veins are less regularly distributed.

Cicatrices formed by occlusion of hepatic veins may be of various shapes, and follow the course of the branches of the hepatic vein; they are seen with particular frequency in the region of the posterior margin of the liver, sometimes in the interior of the organ. Occasionally they enable the investigator to recognize venous walls that have become glued together, or a thrombus in the lumen of the vessel and in different stages of organic metamorphosis. Heller and Lange saw an annular arrangement of the thrombus, which was pierced by a narrow canal; this lesion was the result of chronic endophlebitis.

Owing to venous congestion the liver is enormously enlarged during life. At the autopsy, however, the organ will be found normal, or even smaller than normal. On transverse section it will appear like a congested liver, *i. e.*, flaccid and slightly nodular (both on the surface and transverse section), as a result of the above-mentioned irregular development of cicatricial tissue. It is possible that some of the strands and layers of connective tissue that have been described in congested liver by Liebermeister are due to thrombi of the hepatic veins. The capsule of the liver is usually thickened in the region of the cicatrized veins, particularly at the posterior margin of the liver. Adhesions may exist with neighboring organs, and the thickening may involve large portions of the surface of the liver. In addition, as in ordinary congested liver, there may be wide-spread inflammatory thickening of the peritoneum, and, here and there, the formation of cicatrices, as, for instance, in the covering of the spleen or in the peritoneal layers of the pelvis.

In a case reported by Barth (occlusion of a vein by a gumma) stasis and enlargement were seen only in the left lobe; the right lobe was no larger than an adult fist, and atrophic, probably as a result of infarction. In a case reported by Hainski a number of small nodular hyperplasias (compensatory?), which varied in size from a pin-head to a pea, were disseminated throughout the liver.

Eppinger reports a case in which the liver cicatrix extended to the wall of the vena cava, and occluded this vessel. In one of my own cases this scar extended into the vena cava and caused the formation of a mural thrombus.

The anatomic picture resembles that of ordinary congested liver; it simply constitutes a more advanced stage of this disease.

When thrombosis and occlusion of the hepatic veins is found, in combination with diffuse or cicatricial interstitial hepatitis, the symptoms of stasis are not so pronounced. Moreover, the rôle played by the occlusion of the hepatic veins in the causation of the liver lesions is not always a certain one.

When carcinomatous nodules of the gland penetrate the hepatic veins, the blood-current is only slightly interfered with. The carcinoma in such cases shows a tendency to proliferate along the vessel, and throughout its lumen, and in this manner material is furnished for the formation of carcinomatous metastases in the lungs. It would appear that emboli are not often formed from simple thrombi of the hepatic veins.

When the total lumen of the hepatic veins is diminished, the trunk of the portal vein is usually dilated, and its walls thickened. If the former is completely occluded, thrombi may form in the portal vein.

The spleen is large and indurated as a result of the stasis. Its covering is frequently fibrous. The gastric mucosa shows ridges and wart-like thickening (Maschka).

Symptoms.—Occlusion of single branches of the hepatic veins is not recognized during life. The resulting circumscribed swelling of the hepatic tissue remains unrecognized, as a rule, because of its situation at the posterior margin of the organ. It is possible that this condition is responsible for the exacerbations and the attacks of pain in congested liver and in interstitial, particularly syphilitic hepatitis. In extensive involvement and occlusion of the hepatic veins, engorgement and enlargement of the liver result. The organ can be readily palpated over large areas, and is hard; its shape, however, is not changed. Occasionally its margin is perhaps more rounded, and, if the disease is acute, palpation is painful. The symptoms of occlusion of the blood-stream in the liver are those of atrophic cirrhosis and occlusion of the portal vein—namely, ascites and enlargement of the spleen. As in thrombosis of the portal vein, ascites seems to recur more rapidly after puncture than in cirrhosis, because obstruction of the blood-stream is more complete. In two cases observed by me there was from 3.5 % to 5 % of albumin in the ascitic fluid; this is a very large proportion. In another instance the fluid was milky. If ascites is present, palpation of the liver naturally becomes difficult; as a rule, however, the organ, as in simple stasis, is not much enlarged. Occasionally the enlargement of the liver diminishes, either because the blood-stream is re-established in certain areas of the organ, or because a portion of the liver parenchyma undergoes atrophic changes.

Icterus is never seen in thrombosis of the hepatic veins.

The spleen is often very much enlarged, so that it can be readily palpated. As a rule, it is hard, and sensitive to pressure.

As in other cases of ascites, there is a partial suppression of urine, and there may be edema of the lower extremities. Both are the result of pressure on the kidneys and the lower vena cava.

I have personally studied three cases of occlusion of the hepatic veins. The first case has been described by Lange, and occurred in a working-woman of thirty-nine. Nine months after the birth of a healthy child the abdomen began to enlarge. While the case was under clinical observation the liver was found enlarged and resistant; its surface in the beginning smooth, and later nodular. There was much ascites (circumference 119 cm.). Aspiration was performed four times in eight weeks. The fluid was cloudy (in later aspirations still more so), and deposited a thin, whitish, creamy layer consisting of small granules that seemed to be albuminoid in character, but from which fat could be extracted by ether (quantity 7000 to 14,000 c.c.; pressure up to 47 cm.). It was impossible to decide during life whether this was a case of carcinoma of the liver and the peritoneum, or of syphilis of the liver. Death occurred half a year after the beginning of her symptoms.

The second case was that of a merchant, forty-one years old, who was a sufferer from chronic heart lesion. (On section myocarditis and pericarditis were found.) Four years before the death of the patient a sudden exacerbation of his symptoms appeared; there was rapid enlargement of the abdomen, so that puncture had to be performed three times. I saw the patient with his physician, Dr. A. Bockendahl, and I could palpate the liver very well, notwithstanding the great amount of ascitic fluid. The organ was large and hard (formerly had been still larger), the spleen was enlarged, occasionally painful, and the lower part of the body edematous. Digitalis, which up to this time had helped the case, became inefficient. I suspected the presence of thrombosis of hepatic veins, possibly complicated by exudative peritonitis, particularly because stasis in the upper part of the body was slight as compared to that in the abdomen. The treatment seemed to corroborate this diagnosis, for after the exhibition of senna, diuresis and diarrhea occurred and the edema disappeared. Later on, it was found, similar conditions could always be remedied by the same treatment. The volume of the liver decreased, although the organ was never reduced to its normal size. The patient was able to attend to his office-work for many years, and finally died from an embolism of the brain.

The third patient was a working-woman of thirty-two. Two weeks after delivery her abdomen began to enlarge, though there were no other symptoms. Three months later a diagnosis of peritoneal tuberculosis was made, and a laparotomy performed. The peritoneum was found normal. Ascites returned, and had to be aspirated five times in the three months that elapsed between the operation and the death of the patient. The circumference of the abdomen was 125 cm. The liver was examined four months after the beginning of the disease, and was found to be palpable and hard, but only slightly enlarged; its surface was somewhat uneven. Following later punctures, the organ was found to be smaller, less hard, somewhat nodular, and lobulated. The spleen was enlarged and palpable. Death occurred after six months. During life a diagnosis of syphilis of the liver had been made.

The last two cases have been described in a dissertation by Thran.

Course.—The anatomic beginning of narrowing of the hepatic veins cannot be recognized clinically. As in the case of other obstructions of the hepatic blood-current, a diagnosis is possible only after the lesion has reached a certain grade, and caused ascites. It appears that in persistent occlusion the disease lasts only from three to six months. The dominant symptom is ascites, so that tuberculosis, or carcinomatosis of the peritoneum, or hepatic ascites, is usually diagnosed.

My second case demonstrates the fact that the obstruction of the blood-stream and the enlargement of the liver, as well as the ascites, may diminish. This occurrence may be due to the development of collateral channels in cases in which the occlusion occurs gradually. The blood is carried through the coronary and suspensory ligaments, or through adhesions between the liver and the diaphragm, or between the liver and the anterior abdominal wall.

The veins of the diaphragm and the right internal mammary vein have been found dilated (Gee).

Diagnosis.—Thrombosis of the hepatic veins has up to this time been studied chiefly from an anatomic point of view. My Case II shows that the condition can be diagnosed from the occurrence of hepatic ascites, with the simultaneous and uniform enlargement of the liver.

The enlargement of the spleen is important in the recognition of the lesion, since it seems to be particularly pronounced in this condition. Another important point would appear to be the rapid development of ascites after puncture. It is possible, also, that a large quantity of albumin and a milky clouding of the ascitic fluid, if present, is significant. The absence of microscopic tumor elements may be of value.

The enlargement of the liver may be due to other factors, as, for instance, primary carcinoma or one of the forms of cirrhosis; the history of the case and the symptoms in other organs will have to be carefully considered with this in view. Absence of icterus, which is more frequently seen in carcinoma and cirrhosis, is also important. The uniform enlargement of the liver, the absence of nodules, the rapidity with which the swelling of the liver and ascites develop, and, finally, the occasional reduction in the size of the liver in later stages of the disease, are all significant. In cases of the latter variety, flat, ridge-like irregularities of the surface of the organ may be palpated. A secondary reduction in the size of the organ is also seen in many cases of cirrhosis, but does not, as a rule, occur so rapidly. The general appearance of the organ is similar to that of hyperemia of the liver from stasis in heart lesions. Cardiac involvement, however, is rare in thrombosis of the hepatic veins. When such a lesion is present, the enlargement of the liver is more rapid, more considerable, and more persistent; and there is less fluctuation in the size of the organ than in simple hyperemia from stasis. The engorgement of the liver, moreover, is out of proportion to the symptoms of stasis in other parts of the body.

The only case in which a genetic relationship between syphilis and obliteration of the hepatic veins has been established is that of Maschka. In two of my own cases (I and III) is it quite probable that lues played a rôle, and in my other cases also the character and the multiplicity of the scars, and their relation to the vessel-walls, make it probable, from an anatomic point of view, that syphilis was concerned in their formation also. It will be well in future to remember this point, and possibly to utilize it in the diagnosis.

It is remarkable that in my Cases I and III, and in Maschka's case, the symptoms of the disease appeared several weeks or months after delivery. Future cases will decide whether this was a coincidence or not.

Prognosis. —The prognosis of occlusion of the hepatic veins is usually bad if the larger branches are involved. In rare cases, and particularly if heart lesions coexist, the condition may be cured, and some of the sequels of the lesions may be compensated.

Treatment.—When the primary cause of the disease is known, the attempt should be made to remove it. Cardiac disease should be treated with digitalis, diuretics, baths, etc.; syphilis with iodin and mercury. For reasons mentioned above, it will always be a good plan to try anti-syphilitic medication in cases of which the etiology is obscure.

Repeated aspiration of the ascitic fluid will be necessary; occasionally drastics administered over a long period are beneficial in relieving the engorgement of the portal system. By decreasing abdominal pressure such drugs exercise a beneficial effect indirectly, inasmuch as they help to re-establish the normal flow of urine.

INFLAMMATION OF THE PORTAL VEINS.

Chronic inflammation of the walls of the veins, analogous to arterio-sclerosis, is occasionally seen. There is generally some local thickening of the wall, and the inflammation is carried into the liver tissue or the interstitial connective tissues of the organ; syphilis is probably a prolific cause of this condition. Following these changes in the vessel-walls, we see thrombosis and narrowing and occlusion of the lumen (adhesive phlebitis), the results of which we have discussed in the preceding paragraph.

Acute purulent inflammation of the hepatic veins is more frequent than chronic inflammation, and, as a rule, the former condition originates in some pus focus within the liver. It may happen, therefore, that infection occurs from an abscess, in its turn produced by pylephlebitis; purulent cholangitis and a suppurating echinococcus cyst may also cause suppurative inflammation of the hepatic veins. The walls of these vessels are very thin and favor the entrance of pus into the vessel, either by permitting perforation or by favoring the formation of a purulent thrombus that later undergoes degeneration. From the hepatic veins pus emboli may be carried to other organs and produce abscesses in the lungs, or of other parts of the body.

It would appear that purulent inflammation of the hepatic veins occurs, and by no means seldom, as the result of infection from an embolus carried in a direction opposed to the blood-stream. This will explain the occurrence of secondary pyemic abscesses in the liver alone when there is a primary pus focus in another organ. Wagner, for example, mentions two cases of this kind in which infection of the liver originated in a thrombus of the jugular vein due to an operative lesion of that vessel. [Lubarsch * calls attention to emboli formed entirely of liver-cells. They are principally of traumatic origin. These emboli have been observed by others in the pulmonary and hepatic capillaries, especially after puerperal eclampsia.—Ed.]

Th. Aubert claims that many of the areolar abscesses of the liver start in the veins. He believes that the central vein of the lobules is thrombosed, undergoes puriform softening, thus leading to the destruction of the adjacent tissues. The areolæ formed are of different size, some as large as millet-seeds, others as large as peas; they may then become confluent and in this manner form cavities that are as large as a hen's egg or even larger. They are always wedge-shaped with the

* " Zur Leber von der Geschwülsten," 1899.

base near the surface of the liver. Occasionally phlebitis of the wall of the gall-bladder is the starting-point.

Suppurative phlebitis hepatica causes no recognizable symptoms, although it must invariably have existed in cases in which suppuration in the portal area leads to general pyemia. We can be certain of its presence when abscesses of the lung follow abscesses of the liver.

The diagnosis of embolization against the blood-stream may also be made if an abscess of the liver develops from a pus focus situated in the periphery of the body; *e. g.*, in the region of the neck. It is hardly probable, however, that an hepatic abscess of this nature can develop and attain such large dimensions that it can be clinically recognized without, at the same time, leading to the formation of secondary abscesses in other organs.

LITERATURE.

Aubert, Th.: "Etudes sur les abscès aréolaires du foie," Thèse de Paris, 1891.
Barth, H.: "France médicale," 1882, citirt bei Barthelémy, "Archives générales de médecine," 1884, tome I, p. 527. (Verschluss durch Gumma.)
Budd: Loc. cit., p. 146.
Chvostek: "Krankheiten der Pfortader und der Lebervenen," "Wiener Klinik," 1882, Heft 3.
Cohn: Loc. cit., p. 484.
Eppinger: "Prager med. Wochenschr.," 1876, No. 39, 40.
Frerichs: Loc. cit., II, pp. 92 and 408.
Gee: "Complete Obliteration of the Mouth of the Hepatic Veins," "Bartholomew's Hospital Reports," 1870, VII; Jahresbericht, I, 159.
Hainski, O.: "Ein Fall von Lebervenenobliteration," Dissertation, Gottingen, 1884.
Lambron: "Archives générales de médecine," June, 1842, p. 129.
Lange, W.: "Ein Fall von Lebervenenobliteration," Dissertation, Kiel, 1886. (Literaturangaben.)
v Maschka: "Vierteljahresschr. für gerichtliche Medicin," Bd. XLIII.
Quincke: Loc. cit., p. 568.
Rosenblatt: Dissertation, Würzburg, 1867.
Schuppel: Loc. cit., p. 323.
Thran: Dissertation, Kiel, 1899.

RECURRENT EMBOLISM.

Arnold, J.: "Rückläufige Thrombose." (Literature.) "Virchow's Archiv," Bd. CXXIV, p. 385.
Bonome: "Archivo per le scienze mediche," 1889, vol. XIII.
Diemer, L.: "Ueber Pulsation der Vena cava inferior," Dissertation, Bonn, 1876.
Heller, A.: "Zur Lehre von den metastatischen Processen der Leber," "Deutsches Archiv für klin. Medicin," 1870, Bd. VII, p. 127.
Ribbert: "Ueber den rücklaufigen Transport im Venensystem," "Centralblatt für allgemeine Pathologie," 1897, p. 433.
Scheven: Dissertation, Rostock, 1894.
Wagner, E.: "Allgemeine Pathologie." 6. Auflage, p. 263.

INDEX.

907

SAUNDERS' BOOKS

on

GYNECOLOGY

and

OBSTETRICS

W. B. SAUNDERS & COMPANY

925 WALNUT STREET   PHILADELPHIA

NEW YORK   LONDON
Fuller Building, 5th Ave. and 23d St.   9. Henrietta Street, Covent Garden

SAUNDERS' AMERICAN TEXT-BOOKS

THE phenomenal success attending the publication of the American text-books is a source of gratification alike to the Editors and Publishers. The advent of each successive volume has been signalized by the most flattering comment from both the Profession and the Press. In the short period that has elapsed since the issue of the first volume of the series, over **138,000 copies** of the various text-books have found their way into the hands of students and into the libraries of physicians; and the American Text-Books have been adopted and recommended as text-books and books of reference in **155 leading Medical Schools and Universities** of the United States and Canada.

A Complete Catalogue of our Publications will be Sent upon Request

Penrose's
Diseases of Women

Fourth Revised Edition

A Text-Book of Diseases of Women. By CHARLES B. PENROSE, M. D., PH. D., formerly Professor of Gynecology in the University of Pennsylvania; Surgeon to the Gynecean Hospital, Philadelphia. Octavo volume of 539 pages, with 221 fine original illustrations. Cloth, $3.75 net.

FOUR EDITIONS IN AS MANY YEARS

Regularly every year a new edition of this excellent text-book is called for, and it appears to be in as great favor with physicians as with students. Indeed, this book has taken its place as the ideal work for the general practitioner. The author presents the best teaching of modern gynecology, untrammeled by antiquated ideas and methods. In every case the most modern and progressive technique is adopted, and the main points are made clear by excellent illustrations. The new edition has been carefully revised, much new matter has been added, and a number of new original illustrations have been introduced. In its revised form this volume continues to be an admirable exposition of the present status of gynecologic practice.

PERSONAL AND PRESS OPINIONS

Howard A. Kelly, M. D.,
Professor of Gynecology and Obstetrics, Johns Hopkins University, Baltimore.
" I shall value very highly the copy of Penrose's ' Diseases of Women ' received. I have already recommended it to my class as THE BEST book "

E. E. Montgomery, M. D.,
Professor of Gynecology, Jefferson Medical College, Philadelphia
" The copy of ' A Text-Book of Diseases of Women ' by Penrose, received to-day. I have looked over it and admire it very much. I have no doubt it will have a large sale, as it justly merits "

Bristol Medico-Chirurgical Journal
" This is an excellent work which goes straight to the mark. . . . The book may be taken as a trustworthy exposition of modern gynecology."

American
Text-Book of Gynecology

Second Edition, Thoroughly Revised

American Text-Book of Gynecology: MEDICAL AND SURGICAL. By 10 of the leading Gynecologists of America. Edited by J. M. BALDY, M. D., Professor of Gynecology in the Philadelphia Polyclinic. Handsome imperial octavo volume of 718 pages, with 341 illustrations in the text, and 38 colored and half-tone plates. Cloth, $6.00 net; Sheep or Half Morocco, $7.00 net.

MEDICAL AND SURGICAL

This volume is thoroughly practical in its teachings, and is intended to be a working text-book for physicians and students. Many of the most important subjects are considered from an entirely new standpoint, and are grouped together in a manner somewhat foreign to the accepted custom. In the revised edition of this book much new material has been added and some of the old eliminated or modified. More than forty of the old illustrations have been replaced by new ones. The portions devoted to plastic work have been so greatly improved as to be practically new. Hysterectomy, both abdominal and vaginal, has been rewritten, and all the descriptions of operative procedures have been carefully revised and fully illustrated.

OPINIONS OF THE MEDICAL PRESS

The Lancet, London

" Contains a large amount of information upon special points in the technique of gynecological operations which is not to be found in the ordinary text-book of gynecology."

British Medical Journal

" The nature of the text may be judged from its authorship; the distinguished authorities who have compiled this publication have done their work well. This addition to medical literature deserves favorable comment."

Boston Medical and Surgical Journal

" The most complete exponent of gynecology which we have. No subject seems to have been neglected . . . and the gynecologist and surgeon, and the general practitioner who has any desire to practise diseases of women, will find it of practical value. In the matter of illustrations and plates the book surpasses anything we have seen."

GET
THE BEST

American

THE NEW
STANDARD

Illustrated Dictionary

Second Edition, Revised

The American Illustrated Medical Dictionary. A new and complete dictionary of the terms used in Medicine, Surgery, Dentistry, Pharmacy, Chemistry, and kindred branches; with over 100 new and elaborate tables and many handsome illustrations. By W. A. NEWMAN DORLAND, M. D., Editor of "The American Pocket Medical Dictionary." Large octavo, nearly 800 pages, bound in full flexible leather. Price, $4.50 net; with thumb index, $5.00 net.

Gives a Maximum Amount of Matter in a Minimum Space, and at the Lowest Possible Cost

TWO LARGE EDITIONS IN LESS THAN EIGHT MONTHS

The immediate success of this work is due to the special features that distinguish it from other books of its kind. It gives a maximum of matter in a minimum space and at the lowest possible cost. Though it is practically unabridged, yet by the use of thin bible paper and flexible morocco binding it is only 1⅝ inches thick. The result is a truly luxurious specimen of book-making. In this new edition the book has been thoroughly revised, and upward of one hundred important new terms that have appeared in recent medical literature have been added, thus bringing the book absolutely up to date. The book contains hundreds of terms not to be found in any other dictionary, over 100 original tables, and many handsome illustrations, including 24 colored plates.

PERSONAL OPINIONS

Howard A. Kelly, M. D.,

Professor of Gynecology, Johns Hopkins University, Baltimore.

"Dr. Dorland's dictionary is admirable. It is so well gotten up and of such convenient size. No errors have been found in my use of it."

Roswell Park, M. D.,

Professor of Principles and Practice of Surgery and of Clinical Surgery, University of Buffalo.

"I must acknowledge my astonishment at seeing how much he has condensed within relatively small space. I find nothing to criticize, very much to commend, and was interested in finding some of the new words which are not in other recent dictionaries."

Garrigues'
Diseases of Women

Third Edition, Thoroughly Revised

A Text-Book of Diseases of Women. By HENRY J. GARRIGUES, A. M., M. D., Gynecologist to St. Mark's Hospital and to the German Dispensary, New York City. Handsome octavo, 756 pages, with 367 engravings and colored plates. Cloth, $4.50 net; Sheep or Half Morocco, $5.50 net.

INCLUDING EMBRYOLOGY AND ANATOMY OF THE GENITALIA

The first two editions of this work met with a most appreciative reception by the medical profession both in this country and abroad. In this edition the entire work has been carefully and thoroughly revised, and considerable new matter added, bringing the work precisely down to date. Many new illustrations have been introduced, thus greatly increasing the value of the book both as a text-book and book of reference. In fact, the illustrations form a complete atlas of the embryology and anatomy of the female genitalia, besides portraying most accurately numerous pathologic conditions and the various steps in the gynecologic operations detailed. The work is, throughout, practical, theoretical discussions being carefully avoided.

PERSONAL AND PRESS OPINIONS

Thas. A. Reamy, M. D.
Professor of Clinical Gynecology, Medical College of Ohio.

"One of the best text-books for students and practitioners which has been published in the English language; it is condensed, clear, and comprehensive. The profound learning and great clinical experience of the distinguished author find expression in this book in a most attractive and instructive form."

Bache Emmet, M. D.
Professor of Gynecology in the New York Post-Graduate Medical School.

"I think that the profession at large owes you gratitude for having given to the medical world so valuable a treatise. I shall certainly put it forward to my classes as one of the best guides with which I am familiar, not only with which to study, but for constant consultations."

American Journal of the Medical Sciences

"It reflects the large experience of the author, both as a clinician and a teacher, and comprehends much not ordinarily found in text-books on gynecology. The book is one of the most complete treatises on gynecology that we have, dealing broadly with all phases of the subject."

Hirst's
Text-Book of Obstetrics

Third Edition, Thoroughly Revised and Enlarged

A Text-Book of Obstetrics. By BARTON COOKE HIRST, M. D., Professor of Obstetrics in the University of Pennsylvania. Handsome octavo, 873 pages, with 704 illustrations, 36 of them in colors. Cloth, $5.00 net; Sheep or Half Morocco, $6.00 net.

MANY BEAUTIFUL ILLUSTRATIONS, 36 IN COLORS

Immediately on its publication this work took its place as the leading text-book on the subject. Both in this country and in England it is recognized as the most satisfactorily written and clearly illustrated work on obstetrics in the language. The illustrations form one of the features of the book. These are numerous and are works of art, most of them being original. In this edition the book has been thoroughly revised. New matter has been added to almost every chapter, notably those treating of Diagnosis of Pregnancy, the Pathology of Pregnancy, the Pathology of Labor, and Obstetric Operations. More than fifty new illustrations, including three colored plates, have been introduced.

OPINIONS OF THE MEDICAL PRESS

British Medical Journal

"The popularity of American text-books in this country is one of the features of recent years. The popularity is probably chiefly due to the great superiority of their illustrations over those of the English text-books. The illustrations in Dr. Hirst's volume are far more numerous and far better executed, and therefore more instructive, than those commonly found in the works of writers on obstetrics in our own country."

Bulletin of Johns Hopkins Hospital

"The work is an admirable one in every sense of the word, concisely but comprehensively written."

The Medical Record, New York

"The illustrations are numerous and are works of art, many of them appearing for the first time. The author's style, though condensed, is singularly clear, so that it is never necessary to re-read a sentence in order to grasp the meaning. As a true model of what a modern text-book on obstetrics should be, we feel justified in affirming that Dr. Hirst's book is without a rival."

The American Text-Book of Obstetrics

Second Edition, Thoroughly Revised and Enlarged

The American Text-Book of Obstetrics. In two volumes. Edited by RICHARD C. NORRIS, M. D.; Art Editor, Robert L. Dickinson, M. D. Two handsome imperial octavo volumes of about 600 pages each; nearly 900 illustrations, including 49 colored and half-tone plates. Per volume: Cloth, $3.50 net; Sheep or Half Morocco, $4.00 net.

JUST ISSUED—IN TWO VOLUMES

Since the appearance of the first edition of this work many important advances have been made in the science and art of obstetrics. The results of bacteriologic and of chemicobiologic research as applied to the pathology of midwifery; the wider range of the surgery of pregnancy, labor, and of the puerperal period, embrace new problems in obstetrics. In this new edition, therefore, a thorough and critical revision was required, some of the chapters being entirely rewritten, and others brought up to date by careful scrutiny. A number of new illustrations have been added, and some that appeared in the first edition have been replaced by others of greater excellence. By reason of these extensive additions the new edition has been presented in two volumes, in order to facilitate ease in handling. The price, however, remains unchanged.

PERSONAL AND PRESS OPINIONS

Alex. J. C. Skene, M. D.,
Late Professor of Gynecology, Long Island College Hospital, Brooklyn.

" Permit me to say that ' The American Text-Book of Obstetrics ' is the most magnificent medical work that I have ever seen. I congratulate you and thank you for this superb work, which alone is sufficient to place you first in the ranks of medical publishers."

Matthew D. Mann, M. D.,
Professor of Obstetrics and Gynecology in the University of Buffalo.

" I like it exceedingly and have recommended the first volume as a text-book for our sophomore class. It is certainly a most excellent work. I know of none better."

American Journal of the Medical Sciences

" As an authority, as a book of reference, as a ' working book ' for the student or practitioner, we commend it because we believe there is no better."

Dorland's
Modern Obstetric*s*

Modern Obstetrics: General and Operative. By W. A. NEWMAN DORLAND, A. M., M. D., Assistant Demonstrator of Obstetrics, University of Pennsylvania; Associate in Gynecology in the Philadelphia Polyclinic. Handsome octavo volume of 797 pages, with 201 illustrations. Cloth, $4.00 net.

Second Edition, Revised and Greatly Enlarged

In this edition the book has been entirely rewritten and very greatly enlarged. Among the new subjects introduced are the surgical treatment of puerperal sepsis, infant mortality, placental transmission of diseases, serum-therapy of puerperal sepsis, etc. By new illustrations the text has been elucidated, and the subject presented in a most instructive and acceptable form.

Journal of the American Medical Association
" This work deserves commendation, and that it has received what it deserves at the hands of the profession is attested by the fact that a second edition is called for within such a short time. Especially deserving of praise is the chapter on puerperal sepsis."

Davis' Obstetric and
Gynecologic Nursing

Obstetric and Gynecologic Nursing. By EDWARD P. DAVIS, A. M., M. D., Professor of Obstetrics in the Jefferson Medical College and Philadelphia Polyclinic; Obstetrician and Gynecologist, Philadelphia Hospital. 12mo of 400 pages, illustrated. Buckram, $1.75 net.

This volume is designed for the obstetric and gynecologic nurse. Obstetric nursing demands some knowledge of natural pregnancy and of the signs of accidents and diseases which may occur during pregnancy. It also requires knowledge and experience in the care of the patient and child. Gynecologic nursing is really a branch of surgical nursing, and as such requires special instruction and training. This volume presents this informatiou in the most con-venient form.

The Lancet, London
" Not only nurses, but even newly qualified medical men, would learn a great deal by a perusal of this book. It is written in a clear and pleasant style, and is a work we can recommend."

Schäffer and Edgar's
Labor and Operative Obstetrics

Atlas and Epitome of Labor and Operative Obstetrics. By DR. O. SCHÄFFER, of Heidelberg. *From the Fifth Revised and Enlarged German Edition.* Edited, with additions, by J. CLIFTON EDGAR, M. D., Professor of Obstetrics and Clinical Midwifery, Cornell University Medical School, New York. With 14 lithographic plates in colors, 139 other illustrations, and 111 pages of text. Cloth, $2.00 net. *In Saunders' Hand-Atlas Series.*

This book presents the act of parturition and the various obstetric operations in a series of easily understood illustrations, accompanied by a text treating the subject from a practical standpoint. The author has added many accurate representations of manipulations and conditions never before clearly illustrated.

American Medicine

"The method of presenting obstetric operations is admirable. The drawings, representing original work, have the commendable merit of illustrating instead of confusing. It would be difficult to find one hundred pages in better form or containing more practical points for students or practitioners."

Schäffer and Edgar's
Obstetric Diagnosis and Treatment

Atlas and Epitome of Obstetric Diagnosis and Treatment. By DR. O. SCHÄFFER, of Heidelberg. *From the Second Revised German Edition.* Edited, with additions, by J. CLIFTON EDGAR, M. D., Professor of Obstetrics and Clinical Midwifery, Cornell University Medical School, N. Y. With 122 colored figures on 56 plates, 38 text-cuts, and 315 pages of text. Cloth, $3.00 net. *In Saunders' Hand-Atlas Series.*

This book treats particularly of obstetric operations, and, besides the wealth of beautiful lithographic illustrations, contains an extensive text of great value. This text deals with the practical, clinical side of the subject. The symptomatology and diagnosis are discussed with all necessary fullness, and the indications for treatment are definite and complete.

New York Medical Journal

"The illustrations are admirably executed, as they are in all of these atlases, and the text can safely be commended, not only as elucidatory of the plates, but as expounding the scientific midwifery of to-day."

Galbraith's
Four Epochs of Woman's Life

The Four Epochs of Woman's Life: A STUDY IN HYGIENE. By ANNA M. GALBRAITH, M. D., author of "Hygiene and Physical Culture for Women"; Fellow of the New York Academy of Medicine, etc. With an Introductory Note by JOHN H. MUSSER, M. D., Professor of Clinical Medicine, University of Pennsylvania. 12mo volume of 200 pages. Cloth, $1.25 net.

MAIDENHOOD, MARRIAGE, MATERNITY, MENOPAUSE

In this instructive work are stated, in a modest, pleasing, and conclusive manner, those truths of which every woman should have a thorough knowledge. Written, as it is, for the laity, the subject is discussed in language readily grasped even by those most unfamiliar with medical subjects.

Birmingham Medical Review, England
" We do not as a rule care for medical books written for the instruction of the public. But we must admit that the advice in Dr. Galbraith's work is in the main wise and wholesome."

American Year-Book

Saunders' American Year-Book of Medicine and Surgery. A Yearly Digest of Scientific Progress and Authoritative Opinion in all Branches of Medicine and Surgery, drawn from journals, monographs, and text-books of the leading American and foreign authors and investigators. Arranged, with critical editorial comments, by eminent American specialists, under the editorial charge of GEORGE M. GOULD, A.M., M. D. In two volumes : Vol. I.—*General Medicine*, octavo, 715 pages, illustrated ; Vol. II.—*General Surgery*, octavo, 684 pages, illustrated. Per vol.: Cloth, $3.00 net ; Half Morocco, $3.75 net. *Sold by Subscription.*

EQUIVALENT TO A POST-GRADUATE COURSE

The contents of these volumes is much more than a compilation of data. The extracts are carefully edited and commented upon by eminent specialists, the reader thus obtaining also the invaluable annotations and criticisms of the editors, all leaders in their several specialties. The Year-Book is amply illustrated.

The Lancet, London
" It is much more than a mere compilation of abstracts, for, as each section is entrusted to experienced and able contributors, the reader has the advantage of certain critical commentaries and expositions . . . proceeding from writers fully qualified to perform these tasks."

Schäffer and Norris' Gynecology

Atlas and Epitome of Gynecology. By Dr. O. Schäffer, of Heidelberg. *From the Second Revised and Enlarged German Edition.* Edited, with additions, by Richard C. Norris, A. M., M. D., Gynecologist to Methodist Episcopal and Philadelphia Hospitals. With 207 colored figures on 90 plates, 65 text-cuts, and 308 pages of text. Cloth, $3.50 net. *In Saunders' Hand-Atlas Series.*

The value of this atlas to the medical student and to the general practitioner will be found not only in the concise explanatory text, but especially in the illustrations. The large number of colored plates, reproducing the appearance of fresh specimens, give an accurate mental picture and a knowledge of the changes induced by disease of the pelvic organs that cannot be obtained from mere description.

American Journal of the Medical Sciences
" Of the illustrations it is difficult to speak in too high terms of approval. They are so clear and true to nature that the accompanying explanations are almost superfluous. ' We commend it most earnestly."

Hirst's Diseases of Women

A Text-Book of Diseases of Women. By Barton Cooke Hirst, M. D., Professor of Obstetrics in the University of Pennsylvania. Handsome octavo volume of about 800 pages, magnificently illustrated. *In Preparation.*

This new work of Dr. Hirst's will be on the same lines as his Text-Book of Obstetrics. The wealth of illustrations will be entirely original from photographs and water-colors made especially for this work.

Webster's Obstetrics

A Text-Book of Obstetrics. By J. Clarence Webster, M. D., F. R. C. P. E., Professor of Obstetrics and Gynecology, Rush Medical College, in affiliation with the University of Chicago, etc. Handsome octavo volume of 900 pages, finely illustrated. *In Preparation.*

This is an entirely new work by an eminent teacher of wide experience. The book will be thoroughly practical and the text magnificently illustrated.

American Pocket Dictionary   Third Revised Edition

THE AMERICAN POCKET MEDICAL DICTIONARY. Edited by W. A. NEWMAN DORLAND, A.M., M. D., Assistant Obstetrician to the Hospital of the University of Pennsylvania; Fellow of the American Academy of Medicine. Over 500 pages. Full leather, limp, with gold edges. $1.00 net; with patent thumb index, $1.25 net.

James W. Holland, M. D.,
Professor of Medical Chemistry and Toxicology, and Dean, Jefferson Medical College, Philadelphia.
" I am struck at once with admiration at the compact size and attractive exterior. I can recommend it to our students without reserve "

Long's Syllabus of Gynecology

A SYLLABUS OF GYNECOLOGY, arranged in conformity with "American Text-Book of Gynecology." By J. W. LONG, M. D., Emeritus Professor of Diseases of Women and Children, Medical College of Virginia, etc. Cloth, interleaved, $1.00 net.

Brooklyn Medical Journal
" The book is certainly an admirable *résumé* of what every gynecological student and practitioner should know, and will prove of value. "

Cragin's Gynecology.   Fifth Revised Edition

ESSENTIALS OF GYNECOLOGY. By EDWIN B. CRAGIN, M. D., Professor of Obstetrics, College of Physicians and Surgeons, New York. Crown octavo, 200 pages, 62 illustrations. Cloth, $1.00 net. *In Saunders' Question-Compend Series.*

The Medical Record, New York
" A handy volume and a distinct improvement on students' compends in general. No author who was not himself a practical gynecologist could have consulted the student's needs so thoroughly as Dr. Cragin has done."

Boisliniere's Obstetric Accidents, Emergencies, and Operations

OBSTETRIC ACCIDENTS, EMERGENCIES, AND OPERATIONS. By the late L. CH. BOISLINIERE, M. D., Emeritus Professor of Obstetrics, St. Louis Medical College ; Consulting Physician, St. Louis Female Hospital. 381 pages, illustrated. Cloth, $2.00 net.

British Medical Journal
" It is clearly and concisely written, and is evidently the work of a teacher and practitioner of large experience. Its merit lies in the judgment which comes from experience."

Ashton's Obstetrics.   Fifth Edition, Revised and Enlarged

ESSENTIALS OF OBSTETRICS. By W. EASTERLY ASHTON, M. D., Professor of Gynecology in the Medico-Chirurgical College, Philadelphia. Crown octavo, 252 pages, 75 illustrations. Cloth, $1.00 net. *In Saunders' Question-Compend Series.*

Southern Practitioner
" An excellent little volume containing correct and practical knowledge. An admirable compend, and the best condensation we have seen "

Lightning Source UK Ltd.
Milton Keynes UK
UKHW020627011218
333024UK00012B/2028/P